# THE WHO WORLD MENTAL HEALTH SURVEYS: GLOBAL PERSPECTIVES ON THE EPIDEMIOLOGY OF MENTAL DISORDERS

The effect of mental illness on a global level is profound, with an impact on communities worldwide from a social, cultural, and economic perspective. Although most psychiatry and psychology texts provide some statistical analyses of mental health disorders and their treatment, the epidemiology of mental illness is still poorly understood. This book reports results from the World Health Organization (WHO) World Mental Health (WMH) Survey Initiative, the largest coordinated series of cross-national psychiatric epidemiological surveys ever undertaken. Results from discrete surveys of seventeen different countries on four continents are reported here for comparison and cross-referencing. Many of the countries included in the WMH surveys had never before collected data on the prevalence or correlates of mental disorders in their country, and others had information on mental disorders only from small regional studies prior to the WMH survey. These surveys provide valuable information for physicians and health policy planners and provide greater clarity on the global impact of mental illness and its undertreatment.

Dr. Ronald C. Kessler is a professor in the Department of Health Care Policy at Harvard Medical School.

Dr. T. Bedirhan Üstün works in the Classification, Assessment, Surveys, and Terminology Division of the Department of Health Financing and Stewardship at the World Health Organization, Geneva, Switzerland.

# The WHO World Mental Health Surveys: Global Perspectives on the Epidemiology of Mental Disorders

Edited by

**Ronald C. Kessler**
Harvard Medical School

**T. Bedirhan Üstün**
World Health Organization

*Published in collaboration with the World Health Organization, Geneva, Switzerland*

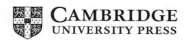

CAMBRIDGE
UNIVERSITY PRESS

CAMBRIDGE UNIVERSITY PRESS
Cambridge, New York, Melbourne, Madrid, Cape Town, Singapore, São Paulo, Delhi

Cambridge University Press
32 Avenue of the Americas, New York, NY 10013-2473, USA

www.cambridge.org
Information on this title: www.cambridge.org/9780521884198

First published 2008

Printed in the United States of America

*A catalog record for this publication is available from the British Library.*

*Library of Congress Cataloging in Publication Data*

The WHO World Mental Health Surveys : global perspectives on the epidemiology of mental disorders /
edited by Ronald C. Kessler, T. Bedirhan Üstün.
   p. ; cm.
Includes bibliographical references and index.
ISBN 978-0-521-88419-8 (hardback)
1. World Mental Health Survey Initiative.   2. Mental health – Statistics.   3. Mental health
surveys.   4. Psychiatric epidemiology.   I. Kessler, Ronald C.   II. Üstün, T. B.
III. World Health Organization.
[DNLM: 1. Mental Disorders – epidemiology.   2. Health Surveys. WM 140 W927 2008]
RA790.5.W15   2008
362.2′0422–dc22        2008007732

ISBN   978-0-521-88419-8 hardback

---

---

# Contents

# Acknowledgments

The World Health Organization (WHO) World Mental Health (WMH) Survey Initiative had its beginnings in the late 1990s in the work of an earlier WHO research consortium (Kessler 1999). That earlier consortium was created to facilitate cross-national comparisons of the results obtained in community epidemiological surveys in which the WHO Composite International Diagnostic Interview (CIDI) (Robins et al. 1988) was used to estimate the prevalence and correlates of ICD-10 and DSM-III-R disorders. The members of that earlier consortium were frustrated by the lack of consistency in the measurement of the many nondiagnostic variables in early CIDI surveys that are of interest to researchers who carry out surveys of this type, such as measures of risk factors, social consequences, and treatment. As new researchers began contacting the consortium for advice in planning future CIDI surveys, we saw the opportunity to correct the problem of incomparability by bringing together these new researchers in order to coordinate the measurement of nondiagnostic variables in future CIDI surveys. Our hope at that time was that we might be able to coordinate such surveys from a half-dozen countries for purposes of rigorous cross-national comparison. We never anticipated that the new consortium would end up including the current complement of interviews with nearly 200,000 respondents in close to 30 countries, nor that our efforts to include nondiagnostic measures would result in the complete revision of the CIDI that has subsequently occurred (Kessler & Üstün, 2004).

This first volume in the series of volumes that will report key WMH results presents an overview of the Initiative and descriptive data on patterns and correlates of prevalence and treatment in the first 17 countries that completed their WMH surveys. Future volumes will investigate more targeted issues and will expand the number of countries included as the data from these countries come on line. The results in the current volume will be updated for new WMH countries as the data from these countries become available. Our web site (www.hcp.med.harvard.edu/wmh) will provide details on access to these new results. The web site also lists the many journal articles and reports prepared by WMH collaborators to present country-specific, regional, and worldwide WMH results in a wide variety of topic areas. These postings are updated on an ongoing basis to provide current information on all available WMH reports.

We want to thank many people for making the WMH Survey Initiative possible. To begin at the beginning, we thank Darrel Regier for his vision and Lee Robins for her implementation in creating the first fully structured research diagnostic interview capable of being used by trained lay interviewers to make accurate diagnoses of mental disorders in general population samples. The instrument they developed, the Diagnostic Interview Schedule (DIS) (Robins et al. 1981), was used in the landmark Epidemiologic Catchment Area (ECA) surveys in the United States. The widespread dissemination of ECA results (Robins & Regier 1991) led to a new generation of psychiatric epidemiological studies being carried out in many countries around the world (Cross-National Collaborative Group 1992; Weissman et al. 1993; Weissman et al. 1994) and these, in turn, led to the development of the CIDI.

The Institute for Social Research (ISR) at the University of Michigan helped us early in the development of WMH in supporting and hosting several collaborator meetings. Steve Heeringa and Beth-Ellen Pennell from ISR, in addition, have been key collaborators from the beginning of WMH as Co-Directors of the WMH Data Collection Coordinating Centre. Pennell spent a year in Geneva at WHO to help jump-start the training and quality control monitoring phases of the centralized data collection process. She and Heeringa and their staff have subsequently been the driving force behind the WMH data collection effort. We cannot thank them enough for their past and continued collaboration.

Norman Sartorius, the Director of the Department of Mental Health at WHO at the time the CIDI was developed, worked with Drs. Robins and Regier to expand the DIS to include ICD-10 criteria and in this way created the first version of the CIDI. Dr. Sartorius also worked to promote use of the CIDI once it became available, leading to the creation of the first WHO CIDI Consortium and indirectly to the WMH Survey Initiative. All WMH collaborators are very grateful to him, as we are to Drs. Robins and Regier, for their vision and their foundational work. Later Directors of the Department of Mental Health at WHO, including Jorge Alberto Costa e Silva and Benedetto Saraceno, along with WHO Executive Directors Tim Evans, Julio Frenk, Chris Murray, and Yasuhiro Suzuki, also supported our work in carrying out systematic cross-national comparative studies. Their help is gratefully acknowledged.

We would also like to thank the Pan American Health Organization (PAHO) for their assistance in helping us expand the WMH Survey Initiative into the countries of their region. We are especially grateful to José Miguel Caldas de Almeida, the past Chief of the Mental Health and Specialized Programs Unit at PAHO. His support was invaluable to us in promoting WMH and encouraging a number of countries in this part of the Americas to carry out WMH surveys. We are also grateful for the support of Itzhak Levav and Claudio Miranda during their tenures at PAHO, as well as for the support of Jorge Rodriguez, the present Unit Chief of the PAHO Mental Health, Substance Abuse and Rehabilitation Unit.

Bob Rose, during his tenure as Director of the Health Program at the John D. and Catherine T. MacArthur Foundation, supported the early developmental phases of WMH work. We are very grateful to Dr. Rose and the MacArthur Foundation for affording us the opportunity to hold international planning meetings and for supporting the work of the WMH Data Collection Coordinating Centre. We also want to thank the Pfizer Foundation, which provided additional core WMH support during the critical early phases of the Initiative. The Pfizer Foundation also funded the initial WMH surveys in China, as well as early Initiative planning meetings. They continue to support WMH in numerous ways that are essential to our success.

An important development in the early days of the WMH Survey Initiative was the simultaneous funding of surveys in six Western European countries in a public-private collaboration between the European Commission and SmithKlineBeecham, with subsequent continued support of this project by GlaxoSmithKline. We were fortunate to have very helpful and enthusiastic project officers, Marc Ratcliffe and Bruce Wang, who helped launch this project under the leadership of Jordi Alonso, providing us with a critical mass that sustained us during the early years of WMH. We thank them for this vital support.

The U.S. National Institute of Mental Health (NIMH) has also provided us with valuable support for a number of important WMH activities, including funding for surveys in three countries (South Africa, Ukraine, USA), for centralized data analysis, for our most recent annual WMH collaborator meetings, and for meetings to translate and adapt the CIDI into Spanish. We would like to thank our project officers, Karen Bourdon, Lisa Colpe, and Mercedes Rubio for all their help in these undertakings. We also thank Juan Ramos, who during his tenure at NIMH was instrumental in helping us expand our initiative into the PAHO countries, and the late Ken Lutterman, who during his tenure at NIMH was instrumental in helping us expand the WMH into South Africa.

Centralized WMH analyses have also been supported by a number of other funders whose assistance we would like to acknowledge here. In addition to NIMH (R01 MH070884, R13-MH066849, R01-MH069864), the John D. and Catherine T. MacArthur Foundation, and the

Pfizer Foundation, these include AstraZeneca International, Bristol-Myers Squibb, Eli Lilly and Company Foundation, the Fogarty International Center (FIRCA R03-TW006481), GlaxoSmith-Kline, the U.S. National Institute of Drug Abuse (NIDA; R01 DA016558), Ortho-McNeil Pharmaceuticals, and the Pan American Health Organization.

Finally, we want to thank our support staff for their tireless work in helping us assemble this first WMH series volume. We are especially grateful to Alison Hoffnagle for her efforts in coordinating the preparation and processing of all the chapters in this volume. We also thank Julie Berenzweig, Eric Bourke, Jerry Garcia, Keri Godin, Emily Phares, Nancy Sampson, Todd Strauss, Laurel Valchuis, Elaine Veracruz, and Lisa Wittenberg for all their hard work on this volume to bring it to completion.

The author alone is responsible for the views expressed in this publication, and they do not necessarily represent the decisions, policy, or views of the World Health Organization.

## REFERENCES

Cross-National Collaborative Group. (1992). The changing rate of major depression. Cross-national comparisons. *Journal of the American Medical Association*, 268, 3098–105.

Kessler, R. C. (1999). The World Health Organization International Consortium in Psychiatric Epidemiology (ICPE): Initial work and future directions – The NAPE lecture 1998. *Acta Psychiatrica Scandinavia*, 99, 2–9.

Kessler, R. C. & Üstün, T. B. (2004). The World Mental Health (WMH) Survey Initiative Version of the World Health Organization (WHO) Composite International Diagnostic Interview (CIDI). *The International Journal of Methods in Psychiatric Research*, 13, 93–121.

Robins, L. N., Helzer, J. E., Croughan, J. L. & Ratcliff, K. S. (1981). National Institute of Mental Health Diagnostic Interview Schedule: Its history, characteristics and validity. *Archives of General Psychiatry*, 38, 381–9.

Robins, L. N. & Regier, D. A., eds. (1991). *Psychiatric Disorders in America: The Epidemiologic Catchment Area Study*. New York: Free Press.

Robins, L. N., Wing, J., Wittchen, H. U., Helzer, J. E., Babor, T. F., Burke, J., Farmer, A., Jablenski, A., Pickens, R., Regier, D. A., Sartorius, N. & Towle, L. H. (1988). The Composite International Diagnostic Interview. An epidemiologic Instrument suitable for use in conjunction with different diagnostic systems and in different cultures. *Archives of General Psychiatry*, 45, 1069–77.

Weissman, M. M., Bland, R. C., Canino, G. J., Greenwald, S., Hwu, H. G., Lee, C. K., Newman, S. C., Oakley-Browne, M. A., Rubio-Stipec, M. & Wickramaratne, P. J. (1994). The cross national epidemiology of obsessive compulsive disorder. The Cross National Collaborative Group. *Journal of Clinical Psychiatry*, 55 Suppl. 5–10.

Weissman, M. M., Bland, R., Joyce, P. R., Newman, S., Wells, J. E. & Wittchen, H. U. (1993). Sex differences in rates of depression: Cross-national perspectives. *Journal of Affective Disorders*, 29, 77–84.

# Contributors

Olusola Adeyemi, MBBS, FWACP
Federal Psychiatric Hospital, Kaduna, Nigeria

Sergio Aguilar-Gaxiola, MD, PhD
Center for Reducing Health Disparities,
   University of California, Davis School of
   Medicine, Sacramento, CA, USA

Josué Almansa, BSc
Institut Municipal d'Investigació Mèdica
   (IMIM-Hospital del Mar), Barcelona,
   Spain

Jordi Alonso, MD, PhD
Institut Municipal d'Investigació Mèdica
   (IMIM-Hospital del Mar), Barcelona, Spain;
   CIBER en Epidemiología y Salud Pública
   (CIBERESP), Barcelona, Spain

Matthias C. Angermeyer, MD
Center for Public Mental Health, Gösing am
   Wagram, Austria

James C. Anthony, MSc, PhD
Department of Epidemiology, School of
   Medicine, Michigan State University, East
   Lansing, MI, USA

Saena Arbabzadeh-Bouchez, MD
Hôpital Fernand Widal, Paris, France

Jaume Autonell, MD
Sant Joan de Déu-SSM. Fundació Sant Joan de
   Déu, Barcelona, Spain

Corina Benjet, PhD
Ramón de la Fuente National Institute of
   Psychiatry, Mexico City, Mexico

Patricia A. Berglund, MBA
Institute for Social Research, University of
   Michigan, Ann Arbor, MI, USA

Ipek Bilgen, MA
University of Nebraska–Lincoln, NE, USA

Jerónimo Blanco, BS
Ramón de la Fuente National Institute of
   Psychiatry, Mexico City, Mexico

Anke Bonnewyn, MA
Department of Neurosciences and Psychiatry,
   University Hospital Gasthuisberg, Leuven,
   Belgium

Guilherme Borges, ScD
Department of Epidemiology, National Institute
   of Psychiatry, Mexico City, Mexico

Ashley Bowers, MS
Institute for Social Research, University of
   Michigan, Ann Arbor, MI, USA

Joshua Breslau, PhD
Center for Reducing Health Disparities,
   University of California–Davis School of
   Medicine, Sacramento, CA, USA

Evelyn J. Bromet, PhD
State University of New York, Stony Brook, NY,
   USA

Ronny Bruffaerts, PhD
Department of Neurosciences and Psychiatry,
   University Hospital Gasthuisberg, Leuven,
   Belgium

Traolach S. Brugha, PhD, MRCPsych
Department of Health Sciences, University of
   Leicester, United Kingdom

Martine Buist-Bouwman, PhD
Netherlands Institute of Mental Health and
   Addiction, Utrecht, Netherlands; University
   Medical Center Gronigen, University of
   Gronigen, Netherlands

Huibert Burger, MD, PhD
University Medical Center Groningen,
   University of Groningen,
   Netherlands

**Stephanie Chardoul, BA**
Institute for Social Research, University of
    Michigan, Ann Arbor, MI, USA

**Somnath Chatterji, MD**
Global Programme on Evidence for Health
    Policy, World Health Organization, Geneva,
    Switzerland

**Wai-Tat Chiu, MA**
Department of Health Care Policy, Harvard
    Medical School, Boston, MA, USA

**Miquel Codony, MD, MPH**
Institut Municipal d'Investigació Mèdica
    (IMIM-Hospital del Mar), Barcelona,
    Spain

**Giovanni de Girolamo, MD**
Health Care Research Agency, Emilia-Romagna
    Region, Bologna, Italy

**Ron de Graaf, PhD**
Netherlands Institute of Mental Health and
    Addiction, Utrecht, Netherlands

**Sara Delmonte, MD**
Psychiatric University Clinic, University of
    Modena and Reggio Emilia, Modena, Italy

**Olga Demler, MA, MS**
Department of Biostatistics, Boston University,
    MA, USA

**Koen Demyttenaere, MD, PhD**
Department of Neurosciences and Psychiatry,
    University Hospital Gasthuisberg, Leuven,
    Belgium

**Hani Dimassi, PhD**
Institute for Development Research Advocacy
    and Applied Care (IDRAAC), Beirut,
    Lebanon; School of Pharmacy, Lebanese
    American University, Byblos, Lebanon

**Karl Dinkelmann, BA**
Institute for Social Research, University
    of Michigan, Ann Arbor, MI, USA

**Antonia Domingo, MD, PhD**
Institut Municipal d'Investigació Mèdica
    (IMIM-Hospital del Mar), Barcelona,
    Spain

**Patricia Duque, TS**
Colegio Mayor de Cundinamarca University,
    Bogota, Colombia

**Michael Ekpo, MBBS, FWACP**
Federal Psychiatric Hospital, Calabar,
    Nigeria

**Nonyenim Enyidah, MBBS, FWACP**
Psychiatric Hospital, Port Harcourt,
    Nigeria

**John A. Fayyad, MD**
Institute for Development, Research, Advocacy
    and Applied Care (IDRAAC), the
    Department of Psychiatry and Clinical
    Psychology at the Balamand University
    Faculty of Medicine and St George Hospital
    University Medical Center, Beirut, Lebanon

**Ana Fernández, BA**
Sant Joan de Déu-SSM, Fundació Sant Joan de
    Déu, Barcelona, Spain

**Clara Fleiz, BA**
Ramón de la Fuente National Institute of
    Psychiatry, Mexico City, Mexico

**Silvia Florescu, PhD**
National School of Public Health and Health
    Services Management, Bucharest, Romania

**Toshiaki A. Furukawa, MD**
Department of Psychiatry and
    Cognitive–Behavioral Medicine, Nagoya City
    University Graduate School of Medical
    Sciences, Japan

**Alexandra Garzón, TS**
Colegio Mayor de Cundinamarca University,
    Bogota, Colombia

**Isabelle Gasquet, MD, PhD**
INSERM U669, Hôpital Cochin, Paris, France

**Nancy Gebler, MA**
Institute for Social Research, University of
    Michigan, Ann Arbor, MI, USA

**Antonella Gigantesco, PsyD**
National Centre for Epidemiology, Health
    Promotion and Surveillance, National
    Institute of Health, Rome, Italy

**Meyer Glantz, PhD**
National Institute on Drug Abuse, Bethesda, MD, USA

**Semyon F. Gluzman, MD**
Ukrainian Psychiatric Association, Kiev, Ukraine

**Michael J. Gruber, MS**
Harvard Medical School, Department of Health Care Policy, Boston, MA, USA

**Oye Gureje, DSc, FRCPsych**
Department of Psychiatry, University College Hospital, Ibadan, Nigeria

**Zinoviy Gutkovich, MD**
St. Luke's–Roosevelt Hospital Center, New York, NY, USA

**Margaret E. Guyer, PhD**
Massachusetts Mental Health Center, Boston, MA, USA

**Janet Harkness, PhD**
University of Nebraska–Lincoln, NE, USA; ZUMA, Mannheim, Germany

**Josep Maria Haro, MD, PhD**
Sant Joan de Déu-SSM, Fundació Sant Joan de Déu, Barcelona, Spain

**Yukihiro Hata, MD**
Department of Psychiatry, Field of Social and Behavioral Medicine, Kagoshima University Graduate School of Medical and Dental Sciences, Japan

**Johan M. Havenaar, MD, PhD**
Free University of Amsterdam, Netherlands

**Yanling He, MD**
Shanghai Mental Health Center, P. R. China

**Steven G. Heeringa, PhD**
Institute for Social Research, University of Michigan, Ann Arbor, MI, USA

**Allen A. Herman, MD, PhD**
Medical University of Southern Africa, Pretoria, South Africa

**Yueqin Huang, MD, MPH, PhD**
Institute of Mental Health, Peking University, Beijing, P. R. China

**Frost Hubbard, MA**
Institute for Social Research, University of Michigan, Ann Arbor, MI, USA

**Irving Hwang, MA**
Harvard Medical School, Department of Health Care Policy, Boston, MA, USA

**Noboru Iwata, PhD**
Department of Clinical Psychology, Hiroshima International University, Japan

**Robert Jin, MA**
Harvard Medical School, Department of Health Care Policy, Boston, MA, USA

**Aimee N. Karam, MD**
Institute for Development, Research, Advocacy and Applied Care (IDRAAC), the Department of Psychiatry and Clinical Psychology at the Balamand University Faculty of Medicine and St George Hospital University Medical Center, Beirut, Lebanon

**Elie G. Karam, MD**
Institute for Development, Research, Advocacy and Applied Care (IDRAAC), the Department of Psychiatry and Clinical Psychology at the Balamand University Faculty of Medicine and St George Hospital University Medical Center, Beirut, Lebanon

**Norito Kawakami, MD**
Department of Mental Health, Tokyo University Graduate School of Medicine, Japan

**Ronald C. Kessler, PhD**
Department of Health Care Policy, Harvard Medical School, Boston, MA, USA

**Takehiko Kikkawa, MD**
Department of Human Well-Being, Chubu Gakuin University, Gifu, Japan

**Masayo Kobayashi, MD**
Department of Public Health, Jichi Medical School, Minamikawachi, Japan

**Stanislav Kostyuchenko, MD**
Ukrainian Psychiatric Association, Kiev, Ukraine

**Vivianne Kovess-Masfety, MD, PhD**
MGEN Foundation for Public Health, Paris, France

**Michael C. Lane, MS**
Department of Health Care Policy, Harvard
   Medical School, Boston, MA, USA

**Carmen Lara, MD**
Autonomous University of Puebla, Mexico;
   Ramón de la Fuente National Institute of
   Psychiatry, Mexico City, Mexico

**Sing Lee, MB, BS**
Department of Psychiatry, University of Hong
   Kong, P. R. China

**Jean-Pierre Lépine, MD**
Hôpital Lariboisière Fernand Widal, Assistance
   Publique Hôpitaux de Paris, France

**Yaacov Lerner, MD**
Falk Institute for Mental Health Studies,
   Jerusalem, Israel

**Itzhak Levav, MD**
French Research Center of Jerusalem, Israel

**Daphna Levinson, PhD**
Department of Research and Planning, Mental
   Health Services, Ministry of Health,
   Jerusalem, Israel

**Zhaorui Liu, MD, MPH**
Institute of Mental Health, Peking University,
   Beijing, P. R. China

**Montserrat Martínez, BSc**
Institut Municipal d'Investigació Mèdica
   (IMIM-Hospital del Mar), Barcelona,
   Spain

**Fausto Mazzi, MD**
Universita degli Studi dio Modena e Regio,
   Emilia, Italy

**Maria Elena Medina-Mora, PhD**
Ramón de la Fuente National Institute of
   Psychiatry, Mexico City, Mexico

**Kathleen Ries Merikangas, PhD**
Division of Service and Intervention Research,
   National Institute of Mental Health,
   Bethesda, MD, USA

**Yuko Miyake, PhD**
National Institute of Mental Health,
   National Center of Neurology and Psychiatry,
   Tokyo, Japan

**Zeina N. Mneimneh, MPH**
Institute for Development, Research, Advocacy
   and Applied Care (IDRAAC), Lebanon,
   Beirut; University of Michigan, Institute for
   Social Research, Ann Arbor, MI, USA

**Hashim Moomal, MD**
University of the Witwatersrand, Johannesburg,
   South Africa

**Pierluigi Morosini, MD**
National Centre for Epidemiology, Health
   Promotion and Surveillance, National
   Institute of Health, Rome, Italy

**Yoichi Naganuma, PSW, MSc**
National Institute of Mental Health, National
   Center of Neurology and Psychiatry, Tokyo,
   Japan

**Yosikazu Nakamura, MD, MPH, FFPH**
Department of Public Health, Jichi Medical
   School, Minamikawachi, Japan

**Hideyuki Nakane, MD**
Division of Neuropsychiatry, Department of
   Translational Medical Sciences, Nagasaki
   University Graduate School of Biomedical
   Sciences, Japan

**Yoshibumi Nakane, MD**
Division of Human Sociology, Nagasaki
   International University Graduate School,
   Japan

**Soumana C. Nasser, PharmD**
Institute for Development Research Advocacy
   and Applied Care (IDRAAC), Beirut,
   Lebanon; School of Pharmacy, Lebanese
   American University, Byblos, Lebanon

**Laurence Negre-Pages, PhD**
Toulouse University Hospital, Pharmacology
   Unit, Toulouse, France; LN Pharma,
   Toulouse, France

**Matthew Nock, PhD**
Department of Psychology, Harvard University,
   Cambridge, MA, USA

**Mark A. Oakley-Browne, PhD**
Department of Rural and Indigenous Health,
   School of Rural Health, Faculty of Medicine,
   Nursing and Health Sciences, Monash
   University, Victoria, Australia

**Susana Ochoa, PhD**
Sant Joan de Déu-SSM, Fundació Sant Joan de
    Déu, Barcelona, Spain

**Mark Olfson, MD, MPH**
Department of Psychiatry, Columbia University,
    New York, NY, USA

**Yutaka Ono, MD**
Health Center, Keio University, Yokohama, Japan

**Johan Ormel, PhD**
Netherlands Institute of Mental Health and
    Addiction, Utrecht, Netherlands

**Volodymyr I. Paniotto, PhD**
Kiev International Institute of Sociology and
    National University of Kyiv-Mohyla
    Academy, Kiev, Ukraine

**Beth-Ellen Pennell, MA**
Institute for Social Research, University of
    Michigan, Ann Arbor, MI, USA

**Maria Petukhova, PhD**
Harvard Medical School, Department of Health
    Care Policy, Boston, MA, USA

**Harold A. Pincus, MD**
Department of Psychiatry, Columbia University,
    New York, NY, USA

**Alejandra Pinto-Meza, PhD**
Sant Joan de Déu-SSM, Fundació Sant Joan de
    Déu, Barcelona, Spain

**Jacob Polakiewicz**
Department of Research and Planning, Mental
    Health Services, Ministry of Health,
    Jerusalem, Israel

**José Posada-Villa, MD**
Medico Psiquiatra, U. Javerina, Centro Medico
    de la Sabana, Bogota, Colombia

**Blanca Reneses, MD**
Hospital Clinico San Carlos, Department of
    Psychiatry, Madrid, Spain

**Marcela Rodríguez, MD**
Colegio Mayor de Cundinamarca University,
    Bogota, Colombia

**G. Estela Rojas, BA**
Ramón de la Fuente National Institute of
    Psychiatry, Mexico City, Mexico

**Ayelet Ruscio, PhD**
University of Pennsylvania, Philadelphia, PA,
    USA

**Mariana M. Salamoun, BA, BS**
Institute for Development, Research,
    Advocacy and Applied Care (IDRAAC),
    Beirut, Lebanon

**Nancy A. Sampson, BA**
Harvard Medical School, Department of Health
    Care Policy, Boston, MA, USA

**Kathleen Saunders, JD**
Group Health Cooperative Center for Health
    Studies, Seattle, WA, USA

**Joseph E. Schwartz, PhD**
State University of New York, Stony Brook, NY,
    USA

**Kate M. Scott, PhD**
Department of Psychological Medicine,
    Wellington School of Medicine and Health
    Sciences, University of Otago, Wellington,
    New Zealand

**Soraya Seedat, MD**
MRC Research Unit on Anxiety and Stress
    Disorders, Cape Town, South Africa

**Yucun Shen, MD, PhD**
Institute of Mental Health, Peking University,
    Beijing, P. R. China

**Dan J. Stein, MD, PhD**
Department of Psychiatry, University of Cape
    Town, South Africa

**Hisateru Tachimori, PhD**
National Institute of Mental Health, National
    Center of Neurology and Psychiatry, Tokyo,
    Japan

**Tadashi Takeshima, MD**
National Institute of Mental Health,
    National Center of Neurology and Psychiatry,
    Tokyo, Japan

**Margreet ten Have, PhD**
Netherlands Institute of Mental Health and
    Addiction, Utrecht, Netherlands

**Nathan L. Tintle, PhD**
Hope College, Holland, MI, USA

**Toma Tomov, MA, PhD**
Alexandrovska Hospital, Department of
    Psychiatry, Sofia, Bulgaria

**Juan Vicente Torres, BSc**
Sant Joan de Déu-SSM, Fundació Sant Joan de
    Déu, Barcelona, Spain

**Cheuk Him Adley Tsang, BSocSci**
Hong Kong Mood Disorder Center, The Chinese
    University of Hong Kong, Hong Kong Special
    Administrative Region, P. R. China

**Hidenori Uda, MD**
Director General of the Health, Social Welfare,
    and Environmental Department, Osumi
    Regional Promotion Bureau, Kagoshima
    Prefecture, Japan

**Owoidoho Udofia, MBBS, FMCPsych**
Department of Psychiatry, University of
    Calabar, Nigeria

**T. Bedirhan Üstün, MD**
Department of Classifications and Terminology
    (CAT), World Health Organization, Geneva,
    Switzerland

**Richard Uwakwe, MBBS, FMCPsych**
Faculty of Medicine, College of Health Sciences,
    Nnamdi Azikiwe University, Awka, Nnewi,
    Nigeria

**Maria Carmen Viana, MD, PhD**
Escola de Medicina da Santa Casa de
    Misericórdia de Vitória, Departamento de
    Clínica Médica, Disciplina de Psiquiatria,
    Vitoria, Brasil

**Gemma Vilagut Saiz, BSc**
Institut Municipal d'Investigació Mèdica
    (IMIM-Hospital del Mar), Barcelona, Spain;
    CIBER en Epidemiología y Salud Pública
    (CIBERESP), Barcelona, Spain

**Ana Villar, PhD**
University of Nebraska–Lincoln, NE, USA

**Jorge Villatoro, MA**
Ramón de la Fuente National Institute of
    Psychiatry, Mexico City, Mexico

**Michael R. Von Korff, ScD**
Group Health Cooperative, Center for Health
    Studies, Seattle, WA, USA

**Abba Wakil, MBBS, FWACP**
Federal Psychiatric Hospital, Maiduguri,
    Nigeria

**Ellen E. Walters, MS**
Department of Health Care Policy, Harvard
    Medical School, Boston, MA, USA

**Philip S. Wang, MD, PhD**
Division of Service and Intervention Research,
    National Institute of Mental Health,
    Bethesda, MD, USA

**Makoto Watanabe, MD, PhD**
Department of Public Health, Jichi Medical
    School, Minamikawachi, Japan

**Charles P. M. Webb, PhD**
State University of New York, Stony Brook, NY,
    USA

**J. Elisabeth Wells, PhD**
Department of Public Health and General
    Practice, Christchurch School of Medicine
    and Health Sciences, University of Otago,
    Christchurch, New Zealand

**Kenneth B. Wells, MD, MPH**
University of California, Los Angeles, CA,
    USA

**David Williams, PhD, MPH**
Harvard School of Public Health, Boston, MA,
    USA

**Victoria Zakhozha, MA**
Kiev International Institute of Sociology and
    National University of Kyiv-Mohyla
    Academy, Kiev, Ukraine

**Joaquín Zambrano, BS**
Ramón de la Fuente National Institute of
    Psychiatry, Mexico City, Mexico

**Alan M. Zaslavsky, PhD**
Department of Health Care Policy, Harvard
    Medical School, Boston, MA, USA

**Mingyuan Zhang, MD**
Shanghai Mental Health Center, P. R.
    China

**Nelly Zilber, ès Sc**
Falk Institute for Mental Health Studies, French
    Research Center of Jerusalem, Israel

PART ONE

# Methods

# I Introduction

RONALD C. KESSLER AND T. BEDIRHAN ÜSTÜN

## ACKNOWLEDGMENTS

The authors appreciate the helpful comments of the World Mental Health (WMH) Survey Initiative regional coordinators on an earlier draft of this chapter, including Sergio Aguilar-Gaxiola, Jordi Alonso, and Sing Lee.

Preparation of this chapter was supported by U.S. Public Health Service grants (K05MH00507, R01DA016558), the National Institute of Mental Health (R01MH070884), the Fogarty International Center (FIRCA R03TW006481), and by the unrestricted educational grants for core support of the WMH Survey Initiative from the John D. and Catherine T. MacArthur Foundation (R13MH066849), the Pfizer Foundation (R01MH069864), the Pan American Health Organization, Eli Lilly and Company Foundation, Ortho-McNeil Pharmaceutical, GlaxoSmithKline, and Bristol-Myers Squibb. Professor Kessler has received no additional relevant support in the past two years. Professor Üstün received support from the John D. and Catherine T. MacArthur Foundation.

## I. INTRODUCTION

As medical expenses continue to escalate, it becomes increasingly clear that no society can assume the health-care needs of all its constituents. Fiscal triage rules are needed, whether explicit or implicit, to rationalize the distribution of costly resources (Bobadilla et al. 1994). Evidence of large mismatches between current and optimal health-care allocations suggests that such rules may reap substantial benefits by considering evidence regarding a comparative disease burden and treatment cost–effectiveness (Gold et al. 1996).

Mental disorders are perhaps the largest class of diseases for which evidence exists of a substantial discordance between societal burden and health-care expenditures. The World Health Organization (WHO) Global Burden of Disease (GBD) Study estimated in the mid-1990s that commonly occurring mental disorders such as major depression, bipolar disorder, schizophrenia, and substance abuse are among the highest-ranked diseases in the world in terms of disease-specific disability (Murray & Lopez 1996). Safe, effective, and comparatively inexpensive treatments for most of these disorders were available at that time (e.g., Leonard 1996; Bradley et al. 2005; Haby et al. 2006). Yet the proportion of total health-care dollars devoted to the treatment of mental disorders was then, and continues to be, disproportionately low in the vast majority of countries (Ormel et al. 2008).

Concern about this disparity between mental health service demand and supply led the WHO to launch the World Mental Health (WMH) Survey Initiative in an effort to focus the attention of health policy makers on the problems of unmet needs. A key assumption on which the WMH was based is that government public policy makers continue to neglect mental disorders, at least partially because they discount the GBD because its results were based largely on expert ratings of comparative illness impact rather than on empirical evidence (Cohen 2000; Sanderson & Andrews 2001). The WHO had hoped that policy makers could be motivated to address the problem of unmet treatment needs if evidence of such needs were more concrete and better publicized. The approach taken by the WMH is to conduct rigorous general population surveys in nationally representative samples in many countries throughout the world, to generate reputable data from those surveys on the prevalence and societal costs of mental disorders in comparison to common physical disorders, and then to develop data on unmet mental health treatment needs and to speculate on potentially modifiable barriers to recovery.

The current volume is the first in a series that will report key WMH findings. Our focus in this first volume is on WMH study design (Part One), initial results concerning the prevalence, severity, course, and basic sociodemographic correlates of mental disorders and their treatment within each of the first 17 WMH surveys (Part Two), and cross-national comparison of these results (Part Three). A brief overview of these results is presented here in Chapter 1. It should be noted that the seventeen countries included in this report represent only slightly more than half of those participating in the WMH Survey Initiative. Those that are not represented joined the initiative after the initial enrollment period and are still in the process of either finishing data collection or finalizing data cleaning and coding. A complete list of participating WMH countries and collaborators can be found in Table 1.1. Rather than postpone publication of the first volume of WMH data because of the delayed entry of some countries, we decided to proceed by posting parallel information for other participating countries on the WMH Web site, at http://www.hcp.med.harvard.edu/wmh, as soon as they become available.

## 2. THE PSYCHIATRIC EPIDEMIOLOGICAL TRADITION OF THE WMH SURVEYS

Although the need for nationally representative data on patterns and predictors of mental disorders was recognized by mental health policy planners throughout the world many years before the WMH Survey Initiative, it was extremely difficult to implement such surveys prior to the early 1980s. This difficulty was due to a lack of sophisticated measures available to assess mental disorders; previously, researchers were limited to either simple screening scales that yielded only true prevalence figures (Langner 1962) or expensive clinician-administered diagnostic interviews that required a cadre of experienced clinicians

who could be carefully trained and monitored (Endicott & Spitzer 1978). Although surveys of the latter type were feasible in small areas in developed countries where there was ready access to many skilled clinicians (Weissman, Myers & Harding 1978), such surveys were not feasible in most parts of the world.

The options available for psychiatric epidemiological surveys improved in the early 1980s with the development of the Diagnostic Interview Schedule (DIS) (Robins et al. 1981), the first fully structured diagnostic interview of mental disorders designed for use by trained lay interviewers rather than clinicians. The development of the DIS was facilitated by the publication of the third edition of the Diagnostic and Statistic Manual of Mental Disorders (DSM-III), which was the first diagnostic system to specify diagnostic criteria for mental disorders in a sufficiently concrete way such that these criteria could be operationalized with fully structured diagnostic interviews. Recognizing this potential, the U.S. National Institute of Mental Health launched a program of epidemiological research known as the Epidemiologic Catchment Area (ECA) Program, subsequent to the publication of the DSM-III, which funded the development of the DIS and implemented large-scale DIS surveys in a number of mental health catchment areas in five U.S. metropolitan areas (Robins & Regier 1991).

The ECA results were widely disseminated, leading to the subsequent adoption of the ECA methodology and instrumentation in similar surveys around the world (Horwath & Weissman 2000). Both the ECA surveys and the later ECA-influenced surveys documented a high prevalence of mental disorders and widespread unmet need for treatment of these disorders (Canino et al. 1987; Bland, Orn & Newman 1988; Hwu, Yeh & Cheng 1989; Lépine et al. 1989; Wells et al. 1989; Lee et al. 1990; Wittchen et al. 1992). However, as the DIS operationalized only DSM-III diagnostic criteria and International Classification of Diseases (ICD-10) criteria were used in many countries, the WHO recognized the need to develop an instrument comparable to the DIS that used ICD criteria. An initiative to develop such an instrument was launched by the WHO

**Table 1.1.** The 27 WMH Initiative participating countries: Survey information

| Country | Status | Sample size |
| --- | --- | --- |
| **WHO: Regional Office for the Americas (AMRO)** | | |
| Brazil | Completed[b] | 5037 |
| Colombia | Completed[a] | 4426 |
| Mexico | Completed[a] | 5782 |
| Peru | Spring 2008 | 3912 |
| United States | Completed[a] | 9282 |
| **WHO: Regional Office for Africa (AFRO)** | | |
| Nigeria | Completed[a] | 6752 |
| South Africa | Completed[a] | 4351 |
| **WHO: Regional Office for the Eastern Mediterranean (EMRO)** | | |
| Iraq | Completed[b] | 4332 |
| Lebanon | Completed[a] | 2857 |
| **WHO: Regional Office for Europe (EURO)** | | |
| Belgium | Completed[a] | 2419 |
| Bulgaria | Completed[b] | 5318 |
| France | Completed[a] | 2894 |
| Germany | Completed[a] | 3555 |
| Israel | Completed[a] | 4859 |
| Italy | Completed[a] | 4712 |
| Netherlands | Completed[a] | 2372 |
| Northern Ireland | Winter 2007 | 3097 |
| Portugal | Winter 2008 | 10,000 (estimated) |
| Romania | Completed[b] | 2357 |
| Spain | Completed[a] | 5473 |
| Turkey | Completed[b] | 5115 |
| Ukraine | Completed[a] | 4725 |
| **WHO: Regional Office for the Western Pacific (WPRO)** | | |
| Australia | Spring 2008 | 10,000 (estimated) |
| Japan | Completed[a] | 2436 |
| New Zealand | Completed[a] | 12,992 |
| People's Republic of China | | |
| Beijing | Completed[a] | 2633 |
| Guangzhou | Spring 2008 | 7000 (estimated) |
| Shenzhen | Spring 2008 | 7134 |
| Shanghai | Completed[a] | 2568 |
| **WHO: Regional Office for South-East Asia (SEAR)** | | |
| India | Completed[b] | 2992 |

[a] Included in the current volume.

[b] Although these surveys were recently completed, we are still in the process of data cleaning. As a result, they could not be included in the current volume, but their results will be posted on the WMH web site (http://www.hcp.med.harvard.edu/wmh/) as they become available.

in the mid-1980s with support from the U.S. Department of Health and Human Services. This initiative used the DIS as the foundation for an expansion to include ICD criteria and to create culturally valid translations of the instrument in many different languages. The instrument was known as the WHO Composite International Diagnostic Interview (CIDI) (Robins et al. 1988).

The first large-scale national survey to administer the CIDI was the U.S. National Comorbidity Survey (NCS) (Kessler et al. 1994). The NCS was carried out in the early 1990s. The NCS, unlike the earlier ECA surveys, was nationally representative, making it possible to draw much more powerful inferences than from ECA surveys about prevalence, correlates, and patterns of mental disorder treatment in the United States. Like the ECA, the NCS also documented high prevalence of mental disorders and substantial unmet treatment need. The NCS also documented that much of the U.S. treatment that was provided failed to meet even the most minimal published criteria for treatment adequacy (Wang, Demler & Kessler 2002).

As was the ECA, the NCS was followed by a number of replications in other parts of the world. These replications were greater in number than after the ECA, though, because the CIDI, unlike the DIS, was developed by the WHO, included ICD criteria, was translated into many languages, and was supported by a firm foundation of international reliability and validity studies. The WHO created a cross-national research consortium that united the investigators who carried out the many replications of the NCS to collaborate in systematic cross-national comparisons (Kessler 1999). High prevalence, early age of onset, substantial persistence, and high comorbidity were all documented consistently in these comparative analyses (WHO International Consortium in Psychiatric Epidemiology 2000).

Perhaps the most concerning issue raised by the ECA, NCS, and most other surveys prior to the WMH surveys was that the number of people estimated to meet criteria for a mental disorder in any given year in most countries' surveys was much higher than the number of people who could realistically access medical care. Commentators suggested that such observations might be overstated when some untreated cases almost certainly had mild or self-limiting disorders that did not need treatment (Narrow et al. 2002). However, in the absence of information about disorder severity, it was impossible to specify biases of this sort. The ECA and NCS were unable to provide definitive data on this issue, as the main concern of the surveys was to make categorical assessments of specific DSM disorders, not to evaluate severity. Nonetheless, post

hoc analyses were able to provide some indirect information about severity. These analyses strongly suggested that a substantial proportion of DSM cases in the general population of most countries were mild (Narrow et al. 2002; Bijl et al. 2003).

As these results regarding disorder severity were based on post hoc analyses using indirect measures of severity, it soon became clear that future CIDI surveys needed to invest more heavily in the assessment of severity. To this end, the WHO consortium that coordinated CIDI surveys developed a revised version of the CIDI in the late 1990s in the hope that future CIDI surveys would collect more fine-grained data on severity (Kessler & Üstün 2004; see also Chapter 4). Shortly after this new version of the CIDI was finalized, the WHO established the WMH Survey Consortium to encourage countries around the world to implement CIDI surveys using this new version of the instrument.

Generous support from a number of funding agencies made it possible for WMH to pay centrally for core infrastructure development. This allowed participating countries to carry out high-quality, large-scale mental health epidemiological needs assessment surveys at a much lower cost than if they had attempted to launch such surveys on their own. Even putting aside cost, local investigators in many of the participating countries would not have been able to replicate this infrastructure regardless of cost because they lacked the personnel with the required expertise, which means that WMH made it possible to begin a tradition of community mental health needs assessment in these countries.

## 3. WMH METHODS

Chapters 2 through 6 in Part One present an overview of WMH methods. A WMH innovation compared to the surveys that were carried out in the wake of the ECA and the NCS was that the WMH surveys were conducted in coordinated fashion rather than assembled for post hoc comparative analysis. Sample design, interviewer training, and field quality control were all coordinated by the worldwide WMH Data

Collection Coordination Centre, directed by Steven Heeringa and Beth-Ellen Pennell from the University of Michigan's Survey Research Center at the Institute for Social Research. The activities of the WMH Data Collection Coordination Centre guaranteed consistency in survey implementation by developing and training collaborators in each country to use consistent procedures and by carrying out audits to confirm that the procedures were being implemented. The WMH Data Collection Coordination Centre also interacted on an ongoing basis with country collaborators throughout the data collection period. For example, internal consistency checks of survey responses were carried out centrally by analysts at the center using special consistency-checking software. The results of these checks were provided to interviewer supervisors in the participating countries to assist in quality-control monitoring of interviewers and data-entry specialists. The first two chapters in Part One describe these activities. The first substantive chapter, by Heeringa (Chapter 2), describes WMH sampling and design procedures. Chapter 3, by Pennell, describes WMH field quality-control procedures.

The following three chapters in Part One present information on the expanded version of the CIDI that was used in the WMH surveys. A broad overview of the many methodological issues considered and the preliminary studies needed to develop this new version of the CIDI is first presented by Kessler and Üstün (Chapter 4). Pennell and Harkness (Chapter 5) then discuss the complexities involved in translating the instrument into the many languages used in the WMH surveys. Finally, Haro and colleagues (Chapter 5) present the results of the WMH CIDI clinical reappraisal studies, in which diagnoses based on the CIDI were compared to independent clinical diagnoses based on blinded reinterviews conducted in subsamples of the WMH samples using semistructured research diagnostic interviews implemented by trained clinical interviewers. As shown in that chapter, good concordance was found between diagnoses based on the CIDI and those based on independent clinical assessments.

Once surveys were completed, all WMH data were sent to the WMH Data Analysis Coordination Centre at the Department of Health Care Policy, Harvard Medical School, for centralized cleaning in collaboration with the individual countries. Once cleaning was completed, centralized coding and analysis were carried out at the WMH Data Analysis Coordination Centre. Cleaned and coded data sets and the results of preliminary analyses were then returned to the participating countries for more in-depth analysis, the initial results of which are reported in Part Two of this volume. Subsequent within-country data analyses were then carried out both centrally at the WMH Data Analysis Coordination Centre and by collaborators in the individual countries. Cross-national WMH work groups were created to analyze particular aspects of the data. More than a dozen such work groups are currently active, investigating cross-national patterns and correlates of particular disorders, such as posttraumatic stress disorder and major depression; delving into the determinants of such well-known associations as the higher prevalence of anxiety and mood disorders among women than men; and studying modifiable barriers to seeking professional treatment. Each of these work groups interacts on an ongoing basis with the senior statisticians and analysts at the WMH Data Analysis Coordination Centre at Harvard Medical School to discuss statistical methods and interpretation of results, to share computer programs, and to troubleshoot various problems that arise in the course of data analysis. Peer consultation in the work groups is used to review drafts of papers prior to submission for publication and to provide mentorship for less experienced investigators.

This broadly collaborative process has effectively helped a number of countries that would not otherwise have been able to carry out and analyze the results of WMH surveys independently because of either lack of expertise or resources. In this way, WMH is expanding the infrastructure for psychiatric epidemiological research and training a new generation of psychiatric epidemiologists in countries that lack strong epidemiological grounding. This cadre of trained researchers will be of great value to health-care policy planners as evidence-based methods are introduced into health policy planning in the coming years.

The WMH is also leveraging the resources available in participating countries to avoid duplication of efforts and to share joint work in instrument development, training, creation of data-entry and data-cleaning software, creation of statistical analysis protocols, and preparation of state-of-the-art literature reviews. On the basis of these rich cross-national collaborations, the WMH consortium is now expanding its work to include expanded methodological studies under the direction of the WMH Data Collection Coordination Centre, genetic-epidemiological and clinical epidemiological studies, and community interventions. Although none of these new developments is discussed in the current volume, they will be the focus of a future volume in this series.

## 4. BRIDGING THE GAP BETWEEN CLINICAL AND EPIDEMIOLOGICAL STUDIES

Before turning to a discussion of Part Two, we want to comment on the importance of the efforts made by the WMH collaborators to close the traditional divide between psychiatric epidemiology and clinical practice that has limited the value of psychiatric epidemiological studies. Many of the WMH surveys include a clinical reappraisal component in which a probability sample of survey respondents is interviewed by clinical interviewers who are blind to the results of the CIDI interviews. Our original hope was that these clinical interviews would be carried out in all WMH countries, but it proved impossible to do this. The clinical interviewers are carefully trained in the use of a gold-standard, semistructured research diagnostic interview that is the basis for their clinical assessments. We consider this clinical reappraisal phase of the surveys central to the overall WMH undertaking because it helps build a heretofore-missing bridge between community epidemiological research and clinical practice.

Another part of this bridge-building activity involves the assessment of clinical severity. As

noted previously, much of the impetus for the expansion of the CIDI and the subsequent initiation of the WMH Survey Initiative came from evidence in earlier DIS and CIDI surveys that very high proportions of the populations in many countries meet criteria for some mental disorder. It is critical to advance beyond this sort of simple "head counting" to distinguish among disorders on the basis of severity. The WMH surveys have accomplished this by embedding fully structured versions of standard clinical severity measures into the assessments of specific disorders. For example, the Quick Inventory of Depressive Symptoms Self-Report (QIDS-SR) (Rush et al. 2003) is used to assess the severity of 12-month major depressive episodes, the Young Mania Rating Scale (Young et al. 1978) to assess the severity of 12-month manic episodes, and the Panic Disorder Severity Scale (Shear et al. 2001) to assess the severity of 12-month panic disorder. As with the clinical reappraisal studies, this use of standard clinical severity scales is designed to create a crosswalk between epidemiological studies and clinical research and practice.

The WMH surveys also include much more information about role impairments and disability than did previous psychiatric epidemiological surveys. As with the assessment of clinical severity, the assessment of role impairment was expanded in the WMH surveys to help establish the clinical significance of community diagnoses to clinicians and mental health policy advocates. Importantly, these assessments of role impairment are also carried out in the WMH surveys for a selected group of chronic physical conditions in an effort to provide comparative information about the burdens of mental disorders.

## 5. PREVALENCE AND TREATMENT OF MENTAL DISORDERS IN THE WMH SURVEYS

The chapters in Part Two of this volume present parallel descriptive data for each of the first 17 WMH surveys on lifetime prevalence, age of onset, persistence, and severity of the core diagnoses in the WMH surveys, along with data on patterns and correlates of treatment. The core diagnoses include a wide range of anxiety disorders (e.g., panic disorder, phobia, generalized anxiety disorder, posttraumatic stress disorder), mood disorders (major depressive disorder, dysthymic disorder, bipolar disorder), impulse-control disorders (attention deficit/hyperactivity disorder, oppositional-defiant disorder, conduct disorder, intermittent explosive disorder), and substance disorders (alcohol and illegal drug abuse and dependence). Other disorders were also assessed in subsets of the WMH surveys or as exploratory disorders in subsamples in individual surveys, but results regarding these other disorders are not presented in this first volume. Our main focus in these initial analyses is on basic description that can be used for purposes of mental health policy planning. We present data on the proportion of people in the population of each participating country who meet criteria for each core disorder at some time during their lives, the typical age of onset of each disorder, the typical course of the disorder, and the distribution of disorder severity. We also study the proportion of people with individual disorders in each country who ever receive treatment for the disorder, the typical length of time between onset of the disorder and first contact with the treatment system, and patterns of treatment in the 12 months before interview. Basic sociodemographic correlates of all these outcomes are also examined.

The chapters in Part Two make clear that a substantial proportion of the population in each participating country meets criteria for one or more of the core WMH mental disorders at some time during their lives, that age of onset is often quite early, that many of these disorders are persistent, and that a substantial proportion of these persistent disorders are seriously impairing. Sociodemographic correlates and patterns of treatment are variable, but there is a consistent pattern across countries for substantial delays between first onset of most mental disorders and first contact with the treatment system. A consistent pattern also can be seen in the data for relatively low rates of treatment in a given year and for much of this treatment's failure to meet even minimal standards of treatment adequacy. Sectors of treatment (e.g., specialty mental health treatment as compared to treatment in the general medical system or in the human services

system) vary widely as a function of the size and structure of the mental health care delivery system in the participating country. Variations in these broad patterns can be seen in each country, as detailed in the separate chapters, with associated variation in policy implications that are discussed in the chapters.

## 6. CROSS-NATIONAL COMPARISONS

The chapters in Part Three present systematic cross-national comparisons of the results, focusing more on consistencies than on the country-specific patterns documented in Part Two. Broad conclusions and policy implications are discussed, dealing with the possible public health implications of expanding programs for timely intervention with early-onset disorders, programs for secondary prevention of comorbid conditions, and quality-improvement programs designed to address the pervasive cross-national problem of low treatment quality. These recommendations are placed in the context of a broad perspective on the wide variation in the existing systems for organizing and financing the delivery of mental health services across the WMH countries.

## 7. THE IMPORTANCE OF DESCRIPTIVE PSYCHIATRIC EPIDEMIOLOGY

The results presented in this first WMH volume are largely descriptive rather than analytical (i.e., they do not search for causes of mental disorders). Descriptive data of this sort are much more important in psychiatric epidemiology than in other branches of epidemiology because psychiatric epidemiology has traditionally been hampered by difficulties in conceptualizing and measuring disorders. Indeed, the descriptive data presented here are in most cases the first representative data on the prevalence, correlates, and treatment of mental disorders ever available to the mental health policy planners in the participating countries.

As we continue with more in-depth WMH analysis, we will go beyond description to consider modifiable risk factors for disorders and barriers to treatment. The more in-depth

analyses will address the ultimate goals of epidemiology: to understand and control disease by
investigating empirical associations among variation in exposure to pathogens external to the
individual, variation in the resistance of individuals exposed to the pathogens, and variation
in resistance resources in the environments of
exposed individuals. Although these investigations should initially be carried out by examining natural variations of the sort assessed in
the WMH surveys, it is important subsequently
to move beyond this initial step by focusing
on hypotheses that can be tested in naturalistic quasi-experimental situations with matching
or statistical controls used to approximate the
conditions of an experiment.

If the hypotheses withstand these preliminary
tests, they then need to be evaluated in interventions aimed at preventing the onset or at altering
the course of the disorders. These evaluations
cannot be carried out with the WMH data, but
data of the sort collected in the WMH surveys
create a critically important empirical foundation for later studies of this sort. This means
that the WMH surveys should be viewed as a
necessary step in the evolution of epidemiological research on mental disorders, as these data
provide a firm empirical foundation for further analytic and experimental epidemiological
research. The WMH surveys also can be used to
provide provisional tests of a number of hypotheses about psychosocial risk factors for the onset
and course of mental disorders as well as about
barriers to seeking treatment. As multipurpose
data collection efforts rather than focused investigations of single disorders, the WMH surveys
lend themselves to a great many descriptive and
analytic purposes that will be elaborated on in
later volumes in this series.

## 8. THE COST–BENEFIT RATIO OF LARGE-SCALE PSYCHIATRIC EPIDEMIOLOGICAL RESEARCH

An important issue to address in considering the
value of the WMH Survey Initiative is whether a
massive undertaking of this sort is cost-effective.
At least one pair of critics has argued that it is not

(Weich & Araya 2004). These critics believed that
the usefulness of the WMH could be called into
question based on its cross-sectional design and
its use of the ICD and DSM systems to classify
cases. The cross-sectional design was criticized
because it forces us to rely on potentially biased
retrospective reports to make inferences about
the dynamics of illness. The use of ICD and DSM
categories was criticized because the validity of
these categorical systems is questionable, especially in non-Western countries.

We agree with these criticisms but not with the
conclusion that the WMH is not cost-effective
because of them. The problem with this conclusion is that it is based on an inaccurate assessment of the counterbalancing advantages of the
WMH. The two main advantages in the critics'
view were (1) that the WMH surveys would generate prevalence estimates of mental disorders
that could be used by policy planners and (2) that
the WMH surveys would generate estimates of
the societal burden of mental disorders. The first
of these two presumed advantages was criticized
on the grounds that categorical models of mental disorder lack validity, and the second presumed advantage was criticized on the grounds
that the methods used to estimate the global burden of disease in previous WHO studies have
been severely criticized (Musgrove 2003).

These criticisms can be summarily dismissed.
The criticism of strict adherence to invalid categorical systems is misplaced because the WMH
questions were designed explicitly to allow for the
assessment of subthreshold cases in an effort to
explore the validity of the diagnostic boundaries
currently specified in the ICD and DSM systems.
The criticism of using controversial methods to
estimate disease burden is misplaced because the
main criticism of these methods has been that
they rely on imputation rather than empirical
analysis. The WMH surveys are carrying out pre-
cisely the kind of empirical analysis called for
by the critics of previous disease-burden estimates. The criticism that the WMH data are
based on cross-sectional surveys that use retrospective questions to reconstruct information
about course of illness is being addressed in a
number of planned prospective studies that are

using the cross-sectional WMH surveys as baselines.

The WMH investigators recognize that the initiative has inevitable limitations. We want to be as aware of these limitations as we can be, to address them to the extent that we can within the constraints of the WMH design, and to use the WMH as a stepping stone to launch future studies that resolve the limitations that cannot be addressed adequately within the constraints of the WMH design. We know that some limitations are imposed by the rigidity of existing diagnostic systems, that other limitations are based on the constraints of cross-sectional data collection, and that others are due to the fact that we used fully structured assessments rather than semistructured clinical assessments to make diagnoses. The WMH collaborators are well aware of all these limitations and are now actively engaged in thoughtful and subtle methodological studies that address these limitations, including nosological analyses aimed at informing future ICD and DSM revisions (e.g., Hudson et al. 2007; Kessler et al. in press).

It is noteworthy that the WMH surveys are also constrained by their focus on the household population and their exclusion of population segments likely to have high proportions of the severely mentally ill (e.g., the homeless and the institutionalized). Furthermore, systematic survey nonresponse (i.e., people with mental disorders having a higher survey refusal rate than those without disorders) and systematic nonreporting (i.e., recall failure, conscious nonreporting, or error in the diagnostic evaluation) could lead to bias in the estimates of disorder prevalence or unmet need for treatment in these surveys, particularly for lifetime events. Given what we know about the associations between true prevalence and these errors (Allgulander 1989; Eaton et al. 1992; Turner et al. 1998), it is likely that disorder prevalence is underestimated, and the prevalence estimates found in these surveys is therefore conservative. The wide range of substantive analyses currently under way with the WMH data considers these conservative biases. In addition, efforts are under way to investigate these limitations using the baseline surveys as sampling frames

for methodological follow-ups aimed at studying nonrespondents and improving the questions and procedures used to assess mental disorders in future research. Results found on these ongoing substantive and methodological analyses will be reported in a future volume in this series.

## REFERENCES

Allgulander, C. (1989). Psychoactive drug use in a general population sample, Sweden: Correlates with perceived health, psychiatric diagnoses, and mortality in an automated record-linkage study. *American Journal of Public Health*, 79, 1006–10.

Bijl, R. V., de Graaf, R., Hiripi, E., Kessler, R. C., Kohn, R., Offord, D. R., Üstün, T. B., Vicente, B., Vollebergh, W. A., Walters, E. E. & Wittchen, H.-U. (2003). The prevalence of treated and untreated mental disorders in five countries. *Health Affairs (Millwood)*, 22, 122–33.

Bland, R. C., Orn, H. & Newman, S. C. (1988). Lifetime prevalence of psychiatric disorders in Edmonton. *Acta Psychiatrica Scandinavica*, 77, 24–32.

Bobadilla, J. L., Cowley, P., Musgrove, P. & Saxenian, H. (1994). Design, content and financing of an essential national package of health services. *Bulletin of the World Health Organization*, 72, 653–62.

Bradley, R., Greene, J., Russ, E., Dutra, L. & Westen, D. (2005). A multidimensional meta-analysis of psychotherapy for PTSD. *American Journal of Psychiatry*, 162, 214–27.

Canino, G. J., Bird, H. R., Shrout, P. E., Rubio-Stipec, M., Bravo, M., Martinez, R., Sesman, M. & Guevara, L. M. (1987). The prevalence of specific psychiatric disorders in Puerto Rico. *Archives of General Psychiatry*, 44, 727–35.

Cohen, J. (2000). The Global Burden of Disease Study: A useful projection of future global health? *Journal of Public Health Medicine*, 22, 518–24.

Eaton, W. W., Anthony, J. C., Tepper, S. & Dryman, A. (1992). Psychopathology and attrition in the Epidemiologic Catchment Area Study. *American Journal of Epidemiology*, 135, 1051–9.

Endicott, J. & Spitzer, R. L. (1978). A diagnostic interview: The schedule for affective disorders and schizophrenia. *Archives of General Psychiatry*, 35, 837–44.

Gold, M. R., Siegel, J. E., Russell, L. B. & Weinstein, M. C. (1996). *Cost-Effectiveness in Health and Medicine*. Oxford: Oxford University Press.

Haby, M. M., Donnelly, M., Corry, J. & Vos, T. (2006). Cognitive behavioural therapy for depression, panic disorder and generalized anxiety disorder: A meta-regression of factors that may predict outcome. *Australian and New Zealand Journal of Psychiatry*, 40, 9–19.

Horwath, E. & Weissman, M. M. (2000). The epidemiology and cross-national presentation of obsessive-compulsive disorder. *Psychiatric Clinics of North America*, 23, 493–507.

Hudson, J. I., Hiripi, E., Pope, H. G., Jr. & Kessler, R. C. (2007). The prevalence and correlates of eating disorders in the National Comorbidity Survey Replication. *Biological Psychiatry*, 61, 348–58.

Hwu, H. G., Yeh, E. K. & Cheng, L. Y. (1989). Prevalence of psychiatric disorders in Taiwan defined by the Chinese diagnostic interview schedule. *Acta Psychiatrica Scandinavica*, 79, 136–47.

Kessler, R. C. (1999). The World Health Organization International Consortium in Psychiatric Epidemiology (ICPE): Initial work and future directions – The NAPE Lecture 1998, Nordic Association for Psychiatric Epidemiology. *Acta Psychiatrica Scandinavica*, 99, 2–9.

Kessler, R. C., Gruber, M., Hettema, J. M., Hwang, I., Sampson, N. & Yonkers, K. A. (in press). Comorbid major depression and generalized anxiety disorders in the National Comorbidity Survey follow-up. *Psychological Medicine*.

Kessler, R. C., McGonagle, K. A., Zhao, S., Nelson, C. B., Hughes, M., Eshleman, S., Wittchen, H.-U. & Kendler, K. S. (1994). Lifetime and 12-month prevalence of DSM-III-R psychiatric disorders in the United States: Results from the National Comorbidity Survey. *Archives of General Psychiatry*, 51, 8–19.

Kessler, R. C. & Üstün, T. B. (2004). The World Mental Health (WMH) Survey Initiative Version of the World Health Organization (WHO) Composite International Diagnostic Interview (CIDI). *International Journal of Methods in Psychiatric Research*, 13, 93–121.

Langner, T. S. (1962). A twenty-two item screening score of psychiatric symptoms indicating impairment. *Journal of Health and Human Behavior*, 3, 269–76.

Lee, C. K., Kwak, Y. S., Yamamoto, J., Rhee, H., Kim, Y. S., Han, J. H., Choi, J. O. & Lee, Y. H. (1990). Psychiatric epidemiology in Korea: Part I. Gender and age differences in Seoul. *Journal of Nervous and Mental Disease*, 178, 242–6.

Leonard, B. E. (1996). New approaches to the treatment of depression. *Journal of Clinical Psychiatry*, 57, 26–33.

Lépine, J. P., Lellouch, J., Lovell, A., Teherani, M., Ha, C., Verdier-Taillefer, M. G., Rambourg, N. & Lempérière, T. (1989). Anxiety and depressive disorders in a French population: Methodology and preliminary results. *Psychiatric Psychobiology*, 4, 267–74.

Murray, C. J. L. & Lopez, A. D., eds. (1996). *The Global Burden of Disease: A Comprehensive Assessment of Mortality and Disability from Diseases, Injuries, and Risk Factors in 1990 and Projected to 2020*. Cambridge, MA: Harvard University Press.

Musgrove, P. (2003). Judging health systems: Reflections on WHO's methods. *Lancet*, 361, 1817–20.

Narrow, W. E., Rae, D. S., Robins, L. N. & Regier, D. A. (2002). Revised prevalence estimates of mental disorders in the United States: Using a clinical significance criterion to reconcile 2 surveys' estimates. *Archives of General Psychiatry*, 59, 115–23.

Ormel, J., Petukhova, M., Chatterji, S., Aguilar-Gaxiola, S., Alonso, J., Angermeyer, M. C., Bromet, E. J., Burger, H., Demyttenaere, K., de Girolamo, G., Haro, J. M., Karam, E., Kawakami, N., Lépine, J. P., Medina-Mora, M. E., Posada-Villa, J., Scott, K., Üstün, T. B., Von Korff, M., Williams, D., Zhang, M. & Kessler, R. C. (2008). Disability and treatment of specific mental and physical disorders across the world: Results from the WHO World Mental Health Surveys. *British Journal of Psychiatry*, 192, 368–75.

Robins, L. N., Helzer, J. E., Croughan, J. & Ratcliff, K. S. (1981). National Institute of Mental Health Diagnostic Interview Schedule: Its history, characteristics, and validity. *Archives of General Psychiatry*, 38, 381–9.

Robins, L. N. & Regier, D. A., eds. (1991). *Psychiatric Disorders in America: The Epidemiologic Catchment Area Study*. New York: Free Press.

Robins, L. N., Wing, J., Wittchen, H.-U., Helzer, J. E., Babor, T. F., Burke, J., Farmer, A., Jablenski, A., Pickens, R., Regier, D. A., Sartorius, N. & Towle, L. H. (1988). The Composite International Diagnostic Interview: An epidemiologic instrument suitable for use in conjunction with different diagnostic systems and in different cultures. *Archives of General Psychiatry*, 45, 1069–77.

Rush, A. J., Trivedi, M. H., Ibrahim, H. M., Carmody, T. J., Arnow, B., Klein, D. N., Markowitz, J. C., Ninan, P. T., Kornstein, S., Manber, R., Thase, M. E., Kocsis, J. H. & Keller, M. B. (2003). The 16-Item Quick Inventory of Depressive Symptomatology (QIDS), clinician rating (QIDS-C), and self-report (QIDS-SR): A psychometric evaluation in patients with chronic major depression. *Biological Psychiatry*, 54, 573–83.

Sanderson, K. & Andrews, G. (2001). Mental disorders and burden of disease: How was disability estimated and is it valid? *Australian and New Zealand Journal of Psychiatry*, 35, 668–76.

Shear, M. K., Rucci, P., Williams, J., Frank, E., Grochocinski, V., Vander Bilt, J., Houck, P. & Wang, T. (2001). Reliability and validity of the Panic Disorder Severity Scale: Replication and extension. *Journal of Psychiatric Research*, 35, 293–6.

Turner, C. F., Ku, L., Rogers, S. M., Lindberg, L. D., Pleck, J. H. & Sonenstein, F. L. (1998). Adolescent sexual behavior, drug use, and violence: Increased reporting with computer survey technology. *Science*, 280, 867–73.

Wang, P. S., Demler, O. & Kessler, R. C. (2002). Adequacy of treatment for serious mental illness in the United States. *American Journal of Public Health*, 92, 92–8.

Weich, S. & Araya, R. (2004). International and regional variation in the prevalence of common mental disorders: Do we need more surveys? *British Journal of Psychiatry*, 184, 289–90.

Weissman, M. M., Myers, J. K. & Harding, P. S. (1978). Psychiatric disorders in a U.S. urban community: 1975–1976. *American Journal of Psychiatry*, 135, 459–62.

Wells, J. E., Bushnell, J. A., Hornblow, A. R., Joyce, P. R. & Oakley-Browne, M. A. (1989). Christchurch Psychiatric Epidemiology Study, part I: Methodology and lifetime prevalence for specific psychiatric disorders. *Australian and New Zealand Journal of Psychiatry*, 23, 315–26.

WHO International Consortium in Psychiatric Epidemiology (2000). Cross-national comparisons of the prevalences and correlates of mental disorders. *Bulletin of the World Health Organization*, 78, 413–26.

Wittchen, H.-U., Essau, C. A., von Zerssen, D., Krieg, C. J. & Zaudig, M. (1992). Lifetime and six-month prevalence of mental disorders in the Munich Follow-up Study. *European Archives of Psychiatry and Clinical Neuroscience*, 241, 247–58.

Young, R. C., Biggs, J. T., Ziegler, V. E. & Meyer, D. A. (1978). A rating scale for mania: Reliability, validity and sensitivity. *British Journal of Psychiatry*, 133, 429–35.

# 2  Sample Designs and Sampling Procedures

STEVEN G. HEERINGA, J. ELISABETH WELLS, FROST HUBBARD,
ZEINA N. MNEIMNEH, WAI-TAT CHIU, NANCY A. SAMPSON, AND
PATRICIA A. BERGLUND

## ACKNOWLEDGMENTS

The authors appreciate the helpful review and comments from Professor Ronald C. Kessler and Alison Hoffnagle on early versions of this chapter. Appreciation is also due to the principal investigators and supporting staff of the World Mental Health Initiative countries that completed the detailed input of information to the Survey Metadata Documentation System (SDMS). The WMH SDMS metadata archive was essential to complete the detailed tables and comparative summaries presented in this chapter.

Preparation of this chapter was supported by the U.S. National Institute of Mental Health (R01MH070884, R01MH059575), the John D. and Catherine T. MacArthur Foundation, the Pfizer Foundation, the U.S. Public Health Service (R13-MH066849, R01-MH069864, and R01-DA016558), the Fogarty International Center (FIRCA R03-TW006481), the Pan American Health Organization, Eli Lilly and Company Foundation, Ortho-McNeil Pharmaceutical, Inc., GlaxoSmithKline, and Bristol-Myers Squibb. We thank the WMH staff for assistance with instrumentation, fieldwork, and data analysis. A complete list of WMH publications can be found at http://www.hcp.med.harvard.edu/wmh/.

## I. INTRODUCTION

International scientific programs of demographic, social, epidemiological, and health-related research have entered a period of rapid new development and expansion. Much of this new global research activity involves the survey method as a source of data. Fundamental to this work is the standardization of methods for developing sample designs, survey measures, questionnaire formats, data collection procedures, and postsurvey data-processing procedures. This chapter describes just one of these issues: the standardization of the probability sample designs used in the WMH Survey Initiative.

Before turning to a discussion of WMH sample design, it should be noted that the procedures used in the WMH surveys are closely related to those originally developed for the World Fertility Survey (WFS) program. The WFS was among the first and largest efforts to coordinate a global gathering of survey data (Verma, Scott & O'Muircheartaigh 1980). The decisions made in developing sample designs for the WMH surveys drew heavily on the lessons of the WFS experience. Like the WFS and many more recent successful international programs of population research, the WMH surveys required collaborating countries to employ probability sample designs to select nationally or regionally representative samples of adults for the survey interview.

In the strictest sense, the WMH sample designs were standardized on the principles of probability sampling with less emphasis placed on the specific probability sample design features employed across the WMH country surveys. The collaborators in each WMH country were provided with a list containing a common set of requirements and performance standards that their probability sample design would be expected to meet. Unique opportunities available in individual countries were then used to develop a sampling plan that achieved the requirements and met the WMH standards. The staff of the WMH Data Collection Coordination Centre worked closely with local collaborators to develop a plan for a sample design, which was reviewed by a panel of technical experts and then revised on the basis of feedback from this panel. Once the design was finalized, day-to-day oversight of implementation was the responsibility of the local research team.

Most WMH countries developed a similar sampling plan that featured multistage area probability sampling. Several countries, though, adopted an alternative probability sampling procedure, such as the use of a national registry or combined uses of area probability methods and registry sampling, to achieve the required probability sampling of the designated target population. All these samples, though, were probability samples. No WMH survey used a convenience sample, an interviewer-managed quota sampling, or any other nonprobability method of sample selection.

The purpose of this chapter is to document the sample designs and design-based estimation procedures for the 17 WMH countries whose data contribute to this volume. In documenting the sample design and estimation procedures, the aim of this chapter is to approach the WMH surveys as a collective, examining their commonalities and differences, discussing the universally successful outcomes of all the surveys, and discussing features of the surveys that could be improved in future programs like the WMH.

## 2. THE WMH SURVEY POPULATIONS

Probability sample surveys are designed to describe a target population of elements that spans a specific geographic space during a specific window of time. In theory, the observed WMH samples of population elements were designed to be representative of a defined target population. Although the term "representative" lacks a precise definition in survey sampling, for practical purposes we can assume that it connotes that survey estimates will be unbiased (or nearly so) and that the precision of sample estimates will be sufficiently high to permit useful probability statements concerning the true population value that the survey sample is designed to estimate.

As WMH investigators set out to define the target population for their country's survey, they faced a number of questions. How would the simple definition of the target population be operationalized in the design of the sample survey? What about persons who were temporary residents, guest workers, or had legal claim to medical treatment or services? Did the government and nonprofit agencies that supported the WMH country surveys wish to focus survey resources on the de jure population or on the de facto population? What about adults in the target population who were incapable of participating in the survey because they were institutionalized or cognitively or physically impaired in ways that made it impossible for them to participate in a conventional survey? What about population elements in remote places that required disproportionate amounts of survey resources to sample and interview? From the perspective of the core, a decision was needed as to whether a requirement should be made that all these questions be answered in the same ways across all the participating countries. In the end, a decision was made to allow the definition of the target population to vary across countries within a range of options described subsequently.

The survey population is defined as the subset of the target population that is truly eligible for sampling under the survey design (Groves et al. 2004). A decision was needed as to what restrictions would apply in each participating WMH country to establish a survey population definition that would conform to the survey's scientific objectives, available sample frames, and budget limitations. Multiple dimensions were included here. One of these involved the age range of the sample. WMH was designed to focus on adults. However, the age that defines adulthood (commonly referred to as the "age of majority") varies across the participating countries (most typically either 18 or 21). In addition, some countries decided to impose an upper age limit on the sample (usually 65). Other dimensions that defined the survey population involved geographic scope limitations, language restrictions, citizenship requirements, and whether to include special populations such as persons living in military barracks and group quarters or persons who were institutionalized at the time of the survey (e.g., hospital patients, prison inmates).

Table 2.1 provides a summary of the survey populations for the 17 WMH countries that are included in this volume. Starting with the different age limits, 14 of the 17 countries had a minimum age of 18 years. The lowest minimum age was age 16 (New Zealand) and the oldest was 21 (Israel). For maximum age requirements, Colombia, China, and Mexico mandated that respondents be no older than 65 or 70. Turning to the geographic scope of the survey population, 14 of the 17 countries defined the geographic scope of their survey population as the entire country, whereas China, Nigeria, and Japan restricted their survey populations to specific regions, states/provinces, or cities. Colombia and Mexico conducted national surveys but limited the survey populations to urban places with a specified population size greater than a certain threshold (e.g., more than 2500 persons in Mexico). As Table 2.1 shows, fluency in a specific language was an eligibility criterion in 13 of the 17 surveys, whereas 5 of the 17 required respondents to be citizens of the country.

Finally, there were specific residence types or living arrangements that each country could choose to include or exclude in defining its survey population. Specifically, the participating countries could decide whether to include the following settings in the survey population: seasonal residences; hospitals; nursing homes or dependent-living facilities; jails/prisons; group quarters (e.g., rooming houses, group homes, convents); military bases; and homeless, migrant, and nomadic segments of the population. Table 2.1 lists the decisions made by each country on each of these dimensions.

## 3. SAMPLING FRAMES

Probability sampling requires a sampling frame that provides a high level of coverage for the defined survey population. The sampling frame is defined as the list or equivalent enumeration procedure that identifies all population elements and enables the sampler to assign nonzero selection probabilities to each element (Kish 1965). We carefully reviewed the available choices of sample frames with the collaborators in each WMH country before deciding on a final frame. Options could have included population registries, new or existing area probability sampling frames, postal address lists, voter registration lists, and telephone subscriber lists. The final choice of the frame for each country was determined by a number of factors, including the extent of coverage and statistical efficiency of available frame alternatives, the cost of developing and using the frame for sample selection, and the experience of the data collection organization in the use of the sample frame.

The final sampling frames for the WMH surveys were generally of three types: (1) a database of individual contact information provided in the form of national population registries, voter registration lists, postal address lists, or household telephone directories; (2) a multistage area probability sample frame (Kish 1965); or (3) a hybrid multistage frame that combined area probability methods in the initial stages and a registry or population list in the penultimate and/or final stages of sample selection. Table 2.1 identifies the sample frame type chosen by each of the participating countries. Further details on the sample selection for each country survey are summarized in Table 2.2 and are discussed subsequently.

Each of the three basic sample frame types was used in roughly one-third of the participating countries. Six countries chose to sample directly from a registry for individuals or households. Another six used a conventional multistage area probability sampling approach. The remaining five combined area probability sampling in the primary stage of sampling with the use of local registries or databases for penultimate sampling of households and/or final sampling of individuals within selected area units.

## 4. COMPLEX SAMPLE DESIGNS FOR THE WMH SURVEYS

The goal of all survey sample designs is either to minimize sampling variance and bias for a fixed

**Table 2.1.** WMH sampling frames and survey population definitions

| Region/country | Survey | Sampling frame | Geographic scope | Ages | Language restrictions | Survey population Citizens only? | Survey population Other special inclusions/exclusions and notes |
|---|---|---|---|---|---|---|---|
| **WHO: Regional Office for the Americas (AMRO)** | | | | | | | |
| Colombia | NSMH | Area probability, population registry | National, urban areas only | 18–65 | Spanish | No | Urban places representing 73% of national population; San Andres and Providence Island included. |
| Mexico | M-NCS | Area probability | National, urban places of 2500+ persons | 18–65 | Spanish | No | Urban places of 2500+ persons included (or approximately 75% of the national population). |
| United States | NCS-R | Area probability | National | 18+ | English | No | Alaska and Hawaii residents excluded. |
| **WHO: Regional Office for Africa (AFRO)** | | | | | | | |
| Nigeria | NSMHW | Area probability | Major regions | 18+ | Yoruba, Hausa, Islo, Efik | No | Seasonal residences included; regions are SW, North Central, SE, South-South and NW. |
| South Africa | SASH | Area probability | National | 18+ | Afrikaans, English, N. Sotho, Xhosa, Zulu | No | Group quarters included. |
| **WHO: Regional Office for the Eastern Mediterranean (EMRO)** | | | | | | | |
| Lebanon | LNMHS | Area probability | National | 18+ | Arabic | Yes | Minor geographic exclusion in Beirut due to political unrest. |
| **WHO: Regional Office for Europe (EURO)** | | | | | | | |
| Belgium | ESEMeD | Population registry | National | 18+ | Dutch, French | Yes | |
| France | ESEMeD | National telephone directory | National | 18+ | French | No | Telephone subscribers only; seasonal residences included. |
| Germany | ESEMeD | Area probability, population registry | National | 18+ | German | No | Nursing homes and group quarters included. |
| Israel | NHS | Population registry | National | 21+ | Arabic, Hebrew, Russian | No | |
| Italy | ESEMeD | Area probability, voter registry | National | 18+ | Italian | Yes | Oversample in Piedmont. |
| Netherlands | ESEMeD | Area probability | National | 18+ | Dutch | No | Group quarters, including military housing and seasonal residences, included. |
| Spain | ESEMeD | Area probability, voter registry | National | 18+ | Spanish | No | Oversample in Catalonia. |
| Ukraine | CMDPSD | Area probability, postal registry | National | 18+ | Russian | No | Chernobyl, Pripyat, and villages with populations of <100 persons excluded. |
| **WHO: Regional Office for the Western Pacific (WPRO)** | | | | | | | |
| Japan | WMHJ | Population registry | 4 urban areas | 20+ | Japanese | Yes | Group quarters included. |
| New Zealand | MHES | Area probability | National | 16+ | English, Pacific Islands languages | No | Offshore islands (except Waiheke) representing <0.1% of population excluded; oversample of Maori and Pacific Islands ethnic groups. |
| People's Republic of China | B-WMH, S-WMH | Population registry | Beijing, Shanghai | 18–70 | Mandarin | Yes | |

**Table 2.2.** WMH sample design, stages, selection units, and special features

| WMH country | Design stages | Stratification | Primary sampling stage — Units — Description | Primary sampling stage — Units | Additional stages of selection — Second | Third | Fourth | Special design features |
|---|---|---|---|---|---|---|---|---|
| **WHO: Regional Office for the Americas (AMRO)** | | | | | | | | |
| Colombia | 4 | Urban area size | Community: cities, towns | NA | Area segment | Household | Random adult | |
| Mexico | 4 | Geographic region, urban/rural status | Census ED | 200 | Household | Random adult | – | |
| United States | 4 | Census region, urban/rural status, demographic groups | Counties, MSAs | 62 | Area segment | Household | Random adult | 25% subsample of R spouses. |
| **WHO: Regional Office for Africa (AFRO)** | | | | | | | | |
| Nigeria | 4 | Geographic region, urban/rural status | Municipality | 40 | Census ED | Household | Random adult | Subsample of R spouses. |
| South Africa | 3 | Regions, ethnic composition of ED | Census ED | 960 | Household | Random adult | – | |
| **WHO: Regional Office for the Eastern Mediterranean (EMRO)** | | | | | | | | |
| Lebanon | 3 | Geographic region, urban rural status | Area segment (sectors) | 342 | Household | Random adult | – | Subsample of R spouses. |
| **WHO: Regional Office for Europe (EURO)** | | | | | | | | |
| Belgium | 1 | None | Adult | 10,910 | – | – | – | Subsample of R spouses. |
| France | 2 | Region, municipality size | Household | 147 | Random adult | – | – | |
| Germany | 2 | Urban status, population size | Municipality unit | 7075 | Adult (registry) | – | – | |
| Israel | 1 | Gender, age, ethnicity, geographic region | Adult (registry) | | – | – | – | |
| Italy | 3 | Geographic region, municipality size | Municipality unit | 170 | Electoral districts | Adult (registry) | – | |
| Netherlands | 2 | Region, county, urban/rural status | Household (postal list) | 5116 | Random adult | – | – | Next birthday method used for sampling adults in HHs. |
| Spain | 4 | Municipality status (autonomous) and size | Municipality unit | 88 | Census ED (tracts) | Household | Random adult | Max. 2 adults/HH, subsample of R spouses. |
| Ukraine | 3 | Region (oblast), urban/rural status | Municipalities | 193 | Postal districts | Household cluster | Adult (listing) | Random adults sampled sequentially from HH lists. |
| **WHO: Regional Office for the Western Pacific (WPRO)** | | | | | | | | |
| Japan | 1 | City, prefecture | Adult (registry) | 3224 | – | – | – | Sample is composition of 4 city/prefecture samples. |
| New Zealand | 3 | Race, ethnicity, geographic region | Census ED (mesh blocks) | 1320 | Household | Random adult | – | Oversampling for Maori and Pacific ethnicity |
| People's Republic of China | 3 | None | Neighborhood community | 50 | Household | Random adult | – | Sample is composition of Beijing, Shanghai samples. |

*Notes:* ED = enumeration district, MSA = metropolitan statistical area, NA = not available, R = respondent, and HH = household (in column 9).

total cost or to minimize total cost while meeting predetermined analysis objectives. The analysis objectives are typically formulated as fixed targets for the variance and bias components of the total survey error for key survey estimates or the parameter estimates for important population models. In the WMH and other multinational survey programs, there was no single to path to this goal. The surveys shared a set of common analysis objectives, primarily centered around estimating the population prevalence of mental health conditions, modeling the etiology of individual disorders, and studying comorbidity with other mental and physical health conditions.

Survey cost structures were highly variable from one country to another, depending on factors such as availability and accessibility of survey infrastructure (government or commercial survey organizations), availability and costs for databases and map materials required to develop sample frames, labor rates for field interviewers and team leaders, and transportation costs for getting trained interviewers to distributed samples of households. Total funding for the survey also varied widely across the participating countries. In many cases, funding restrictions not only limited the total size of the interviewed sample but also limited the scope of the survey populations or the use of costly sample design options.

The individual WMH sample designs employed the full range of probability sampling techniques that survey statisticians can use to improve sample precision and to reduce the costs of sample observation. Stratification of the samples by geographic regions and demographic characteristics of the population was employed to increase the precision of sample estimates and to control sample allocation to domains and subpopulations that were critical to analysis plans. Multistage designs that employed modest clustering of sample households in the initial stages of sampling were used to control travel time and expense to reach the selected probability samples of households. A version of the double sampling technique (Cochran 1977) was used in all but two of the participating countries to determine the subsample of initial Part 1 CIDI screening interview respondents who would complete the more intensive Part 2 CIDI diagnostic questionnaire.

Table 2.2 summarizes the general features of the complex sample designs used by each of the WMH collaborators. The variety of probability sample designs evident in this summary table reflects the differences in the essential survey conditions faced by the participating countries. With the exception of Belgium, Israel, and Japan, three studies that sampled adults directly from high-quality population registries, the great majority of WMH countries employed a multistage probability sampling method. Two countries chose a first-stage probability sample of households directly from national postal lists (the Netherlands) or telephone directories (France) and then chose a random adult respondent within the selected households. Germany used a two-stage design that involved a first-stage sampling of municipalities and a second-stage sampling of adults from population registries available within each of the selected municipalities. Italy and Ukraine used a similar design but added an intermediate second-stage sampling of electoral or postal districts before selecting eligible adults from the district registry (Italy) or an enumerated list of residents within selected districts (Ukraine).

China, Lebanon, Mexico, New Zealand, and South Africa chose efficient three-stage, area probability sample designs: a first-stage sampling of census enumeration districts or neighborhood units, followed by a second-stage sampling of households and a third-stage random selection of an eligible adult within households. Colombia, Nigeria, Spain, and the United States employed four-stage probability sample designs, beginning the sampling sequence with the selection of larger county or municipal units, progressing to the selection of area segment blocks, and then to households and a randomly selected adult within the household.

Two examples are useful as illustrations of the variation in complex sample designs used in the WMH studies. Israel provides a first example of the use of a population registry as the sampling frame. To select their sample, the Israeli WMH collaborators stratified their official population registry by ethnicity (i.e., Jewish, Arab), age, sex, and population size and urban status of the locality where the individual lived. From this stratified list frame, a stratified random sample of 7075 individuals was selected to participate in the survey. This is an efficient approach in that it avoids the within-household clustering that occurs in area probability sampling and improves on simple random sampling by building in stratification aimed at reducing random sampling errors across a number of critical population dimensions.

Lebanon provides a second example in which area probability methods were used to build the frame and select a multistage sample. Unlike the situation in Israel, where there was a well-developed population registry of individuals, only limited population data existed in Lebanon. As a result, the primary stage of sampling in Lebanon selected area segments (sectors) from a comprehensive list developed by the WMH collaborators that was stratified by region and urban status. From this list, 342 area segments were selected with probabilities proportional to size. Prior to the second stage of sampling, the Lebanese team sent trained field staff to each selected area segment to create a list of the housing units in the segment. Once this enumerative list of dwelling units was completed for each area segment, a second-stage sample was selected of housing units, with 34 to 35 such units selected from each of the 342 primary-stage area segments. Interviewers then traveled to the area segments, contacting each of the 11,765 selected housing units to attempt to obtain an interview from a randomly selected member of the household. The interviewer used an objective household-selection table method developed by Kish (1949) to select randomly one of the eligible household members to participate in the survey. In a probability subsample of households, the spouse of the selected respondent was also selected to take part in the survey. In total, 2857 adults participated in the WMH survey in Lebanon.

## 5. FINAL SAMPLE DISPOSITIONS AND RESPONSE RATES

The WMH guidelines specified a target response rate target of 65% on the basis of a precise method required to calculate the response rate (the American Association for Public Opinion Research [2000] RR4 definition). This target response rate was achieved by 12 of the participating countries, with 6 having response rates in the range of 70%–75%, 4 in the range of 75%–80%, and 2 greater than 80%. The five surveys that failed to meet the target had response rates in the range 45.9%–57.8%. Survey response rates were influenced by many factors, including government privacy rules, population resistance to survey participation, experience and norms of the chosen data collection organization, and availability of financial resources to invest in incentives or other refusal-aversion efforts.

The results on final sample dispositions and response rates reported herein are based on data the participating country research teams entered into the Survey Metadata Documentation System (SMDS) developed by the Institute for Social Research at the University of Michigan. Participating WMH sites were asked to fill in the SMDS when it became available in October 2005. For many countries, this was several years after their surveys were conducted, and consequently there are gaps in the information that was provided. In some cases, countries were not able to provide the detailed sample disposition data requested for the SDMS system, and therefore data from prior reports or papers has been used here.

To simplify the discussion of the WMH survey sample outcomes, it is useful to define a set of standard terms used to code the final dispositions of the individual sample cases. The major categories and subcategories of WMH final sample dispositions include the following: interviews (I = completed interview, P = partial interview); noninterviews (R = Refusal, NC = no contact with eligible respondent, O = other noninterviews due to illness, disability, hospitalization, etc.); screening noninterviews (UH = unknown

**Table 2.3.** WMH sample sizes, completed interviews, and response rates

| Country | Initial sample size (units) | Completed interviews | | Rates based on disposition codes for main respondent | | |
|---|---|---|---|---|---|---|
| | | Primary | Secondary | Reported overall response rate | Screening rate | Eligibility rate |
| WHO: Regional Office for the Americas (AMRO) | | | | | | |
| Colombia | – | 4544 | – | 87.7 | – | – |
| Mexico | 10,377 | 5826 | – | 76.6 | 97.4 | 87.1 |
| United States | 10,377 | 7693 | 1589 | 70.9 | 99.1 | 82.9 |
| WHO: Regional Office for Africa (AFRO) | | | | | | |
| Nigeria | 8413 | 6329 | 424 | 79.3 | 94.2 | 96.4 |
| South Africa | – | 4351 | – | 87.1 | – | – |
| WHO: Regional Office for the Eastern Mediterranean (EMRO) | | | | | | |
| Lebanon | 11,765 | 2563 | 294 | 70.0 | 99.9 | 59.2 |
| WHO: Regional Office for Europe (EURO) | | | | | | |
| Belgium | 5378 | 2594 | 213 | 50.6 | 100.0 | 95.3 |
| France | 10,910 | 2874 | 83 | 45.9 | 99.6 | 57.2 |
| Germany | 8290 | 3555 | – | 57.8 | 97.0 | 81.1 |
| Israel | 7075 | 4859 | – | 72.6 | 95.8 | 89.3 |
| Italy | 6508 | 4354 | 315 | 71.3 | 98.0 | 93.3 |
| Netherlands | 5103 | 2372 | – | 56.4 | 100.0 | 100.0 |
| Spain | 7119 | 5382 | 323 | 78.6 | 96.7 | 97.8 |
| Ukraine | 6200 | 4725 | – | 78.3 | 92.5 | 97.1 |
| WHO: Regional Office for the Western Pacific (WPRO) | | | | | | |
| Japan | 3224 | 1663 | – | 56.4 | – | – |
| New Zealand | 75,340 | 12,992 | – | 73.3 | 95.5 | 22.7 |
| PRC-Beijing | – | 2633 | – | 74.8 | – | – |
| PRC-Shanghai | – | 2568 | – | 74.6 | – | – |

*Note:* PRC = People's Republic of China.

if housing unit exists, unable to reach/locate address, UO = unknown if eligible respondent in unit/no screener completed/other); and ineligible sample (INEL = not an eligible housing unit, including businesses, vacant units, households with no eligible respondent).

The other important quantity in the calculation of the response rate is the estimated proportion of cases of unknown eligibility (UH + UO) that are eligible for the survey interview. For the WMH response rates reported here, this eligibility parameter was estimated from the eligibility rate in cases where eligibility could be established:

$$\hat{e} = \frac{(I + P + R + NC + O)}{(I + P + R + NC + O + INEL)}. \quad (1)$$

Table 2.3 summarizes the initial sample sizes and number of completed interviews for each WMH country. With the exception of Ukraine, each country attempted to interview at least one randomly selected primary adult from each eligible sample household. The Ukraine sample used a special listing procedure in which all eligible persons in sample households were first identified and a one-in-three sample of persons was designated for the survey interview. Under this procedure, the number of primary respondents from a sample household could be zero, one, or greater than one. Seven countries (Belgium, France, Italy, Lebanon, Nigeria, Spain, and the United States) also interviewed a secondary probability subsample of spouses of the selected primary respondents. This spouse subsample ranged from 3% (France) to 22% (United States) of eligible spouses of the selected primary respondents.

## 5.1. Screening and Eligibility Rates

The screening response rate for the survey sample is an indicator of the interviewers' success in contacting the sample households and conducting a short screening interview to determine the eligibility of household members. Using the disposition category acronyms defined previously, the screening response rate for each WMH survey was computed as follows:

$$(Total - UH - UO)/Total. \quad (2)$$

Table 2.3 provides the screening response rates for each country that provided detailed sample disposition data. Detailed final disposition data were not provided for China (Beijing and Shanghai sites), Japan, South Africa, or Colombia. The remaining WMH countries did provide the detailed disposition data needed to compute the screening response rates, eligibility rates, and final interview rates for the survey sample.

Screening rates were greater than 90% in all participating countries, indicating a universally high rate of success in contacting and establishing eligibility for sample households. The percentage of screened housing units that contained one or more eligible individuals (the eligibility rate) was more variable across countries. In general, sample household eligibility for the WMH survey interview ranged from 80% to 100%.

The exceptions occurred in Lebanon (59.2% eligible), France (57.2% eligible), and New Zealand (22.7% eligible). In Lebanon, many sample households were ineligible because the residents were not Lebanese citizens or the sample dwelling was a seasonal residence. The low eligibility rate for France arose because initial contact was by telephone and many sample telephone numbers were not assigned to household residences. In New Zealand the low eligibility occurred as a result of a special screening procedure used to oversample two ethnic groups. For the majority of countries where eligibility rates exceeded 80%, ineligible sample units were limited primarily to vacant and seasonal housing units, non-

residential units, or address errors in the sample frame. Depending on the country's survey population definition (see Table 2.1), additional sample units could be coded as ineligible if the occupants were incarcerated, hospitalized, out of the country during the survey period, unable to speak the languages of the survey, or did not meet the survey age criteria.

## 5.2. Interview Response Rates

The WMH Data Collection Coordination Centre staff provided guidelines, advice, and assistance to the country collaborators to ensure high response rates to the survey interview request. Emphasis was placed on interviewer and supervisor training; refusal-aversion and conversion techniques; incentives; and, more generally, careful monitoring of the data collection process during the field period. The WMH collaborators in each country were also asked to maintain detailed records of sample dispositions from the field survey so that standardized response rates could be computed according to the definition:

$$RR = \frac{I + P}{I + P + R + NC + O + \hat{e}(UH + UO)}. \quad (3)$$

Comparison of response rates across the WMH countries was complicated by the fact that the local survey data collection organizations differed in their practices related to sample disposition coding. The comparison was also complicated by the fact that we needed to account for differences in survey design features employed to achieve somewhat different country-specific analysis objectives. For example, New Zealand's survey included an extensive oversampling of ethnic groups that led to substantial screening, which complicated the calculation of the response rate by introducing uncertainty about eligibility in households that could not be screened.

Total survey nonresponse can be divided into two major components: refusals and noncontact. Groves and Couper (1998) point out that these two sources of nonresponse may have very different implications for potential bias in the unadjusted survey data. The experience with refusal rates (not shown) differed markedly across WMH countries, from a low of 1.8% in Nigeria to an exceptionally high 51.9% in France. The France design was distinct from all others in the series in that it was based on a first-stage telephone screen rather than a first-stage in-person recruitment effort. This design decision, which was recommended against by the WMH Data Collection Coordination Centre, was a requirement of the funding agency. As we had feared, it led to a very high rate of initial refusal that could not be made up for in later phases of the design, despite efforts to mount an intensive refusal-conversion effort in a probability subsample of people who initially refused. Refusal rates for the other European countries, where initial contacts were made face-to-face, ranged from 19.4% to 30.4%. Refusal was the main source of nonresponse in all these surveys. Only Belgium (19.0%) and Nigeria (14.4%) had a substantial percentage of final noncontact with eligible sample respondents.

As noted previously, an attempt was made to interview a subsample of spouses in seven of the 17 countries. In three countries where the sample disposition data permit a separate calculation by respondent type, the conditional response rates for spouse respondents were as follows: Lebanon, 78.2%; Nigeria, 86.7%; and United States, 74.4%. On the basis of the results for these three countries, it appears that once a main respondent was contacted and agreed to participate, his or her spouse was also likely (although not certain) to participate. This finding is consistent with much previous experience in surveys of a strongly positive intraclass correlation for survey response within households.

## 5.3. Factors Related to Response Rates

An extensive literature exists on survey response and its components (de Leeuw & de Heer 2002; Couper & de Leeuw 2003). Quite different factors may affect each component. For example, de Leeuw and de Heer (2002) found that whereas refusal rates differed across countries and across surveys within countries, noncontact rates were much less variable for surveys conducted in a given country. Several factors were investigated in the WMH surveys to determine whether they related in any way to the cross-national patterns of variation in response rates. No clear relationships were found with the average interview length or the type of agency that carried out the fieldwork (i.e., government agency vs. private survey firm vs. investigator-constructed field force). In addition, the minimum or maximum number of contacts employed in the survey did not show an association with the achieved response rates, though this is likely true because the number of contact attempts was expanded in the midst of the surveys in some countries in an effort to guarantee that the target response rate was achieved.

Our failure to observe significant associations between survey characteristics and response rates could be due to the fact that countries used various combinations of strategies to maximize their response rates. In addition, the survey populations in the participating countries may have had quite different attitudes toward survey participation. Previous methodological research has found that populations in Europe and other more economically developed regions of the world are more resistant than those in other parts of the world to requests to participate in surveys (de Leeuw & de Heer 2002). Table 2.3 provides evidence from the WMH surveys to support this general finding, as four of the five surveys with low response rates were in Western Europe (Belgium, France, Germany, and the Netherlands).

We also know from anecdotal evidence that complications in fieldwork occurred in all four of the Western European countries with low response rates, which might have contributed to the low response. In the case of Belgium, the survey was implemented in two parts in different languages (Dutch in the north and French in the south) by separate organizations. Complications arose in negotiating with the government for access to the sampling frame, which led to delays in fieldwork and time pressures to complete the survey on time. These issues might well have contributed to the low response rate. The special situation in France was already noted previously, where the funding agency insisted that we use telephone screening. The same agency required us to use a particular commercial survey firm to carry out this screening, which resulted in our loss of quality control. Although we were subsequently able to carry out a nonrespondent survey to weight the data for bias in response, the low response rate could not be corrected with this post hoc design enhancement.

The situation was somewhat different in Germany, where the commercial data collection agency that carried out the survey was discovered midway through the study to have failed to implement the required WMH data collection quality-control procedures. This discovery required us to exclude all interviews collected up to that time in several major parts of the German sample and to carry out new interviews in those subsamples. The delays, complex negotiations with the survey firm, and extra expense introduced by this problem could well have contributed to the low response rate in the final German survey. The situation in the Netherlands, finally, was different yet, as the survey firm we hired to carry out the survey had gone through reorganization shortly before the time our survey was fielded. We had counted on the high level of field quality control this firm had exhibited in the previous work of collaborators with the firm, but this turned out not to be the case. We responded to this problem by reducing the target sample size midway through the survey and diverting financial resources for fieldwork to increased effort in completing fewer interviews. Financial incentives for refusal conversion were also included here along with enhanced quality-control monitoring, but these efforts were not able to make up for the initial low response in the main sample replicates, which resulted in a low overall response rate.

The last WMH country to have a low response rate was Japan. Fieldwork in Japan was carefully designed and monitored, but the response rate was nonetheless low for reasons that appear to have involved two things. First, the informed consent script required by the funding agency led many respondents to refuse to participate.

Second, a high proportion of designated households were never contacted for reasons that appear to be due to the fact that the population in the metropolitan areas studied had a very high not-at-home rate, presumably for reasons involving long work hours, long commutes, and lifestyle factors. Together, these factors led to rather high rates of both initial refusal and failure to contact, which resulted in a very low response rate.

## 6. NONRESPONSE SURVEYS

Collaborators in all countries were encouraged to carry out systematic nonresponse surveys in an effort to evaluate and, to the extent possible, correct for the effects of systematic survey nonresponse. The basic design of the nonresponse survey was to select a stratified probability subsample of initial survey nonrespondents who were approached one last time and asked to participate in a brief (typically 10- to 20-minute) interview that would provide the investigators with basic information about people who were not able to participate in the full survey. Respondents were typically offered a financial incentive to participate in this brief survey. The survey was typically carried out either by telephone or face-to-face. The questions in the survey included a small number of basic sociodemographic (e.g., age, sex, education, marital status) and diagnostic stem questions for diagnoses of core mental and substance disorders. Importantly, identical questions were asked in the main survey. Comparison of responses to these questions in the main sample and the nonrespondent sample was used to make inferences about nonresponse bias, and weighting adjustments described subsequently were used to adjust the main sample for these biases.

## 7. WEIGHTING

Person-level analysis weights that incorporated sample selection, nonresponse, and poststratification factors were constructed for each WMH survey data set. In the Netherlands, Germany, France, Spain, Italy, Israel, and New Zealand, the analysis weights were developed by survey statisticians on the individual country-research teams. Analysis weights for the remaining WMH countries were prepared by the Harvard Data Analysis Coordination Centre using sample design and population control data supplied by the local project teams. The case-specific analysis weights were used in computing estimates of descriptive statistics for the survey population and for estimation of analytical statistics (e.g., regression coefficients, odds ratios) that are reported in this volume.

## 7.1. Construction of Analysis Weights

In general, the final analysis weight for each WMH survey respondent was computed as the product of the three weight components:

$$W_{final,i} = W_{sel,i} \cdot W_{nr,i} \cdot W_{psc,i}, \qquad (4)$$

where

$W_{sel,i}$ = the selection weight factor for respondent $i = 1, \ldots, n$;

$W_{nr,i}$ = the nonresponse weight adjustment factor for respondent $i = 1, \ldots, n$; and

$W_{psc,i}$ = the poststratification factor for respondent $i = 1, \ldots, n$.

The exact sequence of weight calculation steps differed slightly across WMH surveys. In some countries, a separate nonresponse adjustment step was skipped and the final weight was derived as the product of the sample selection factor and a final, all-encompassing poststratification to external population controls. This section of the chapter describes the procedures used to compute the three individual components of the analysis weight for individual WMH cases.

### 7.1.1. The Sample Selection Weight

The sample selection weight, $W_{sel} = W_{sel,hh} \times W_{sel,resp} \times W_{sel,Part\,II}$, the first component of the analysis weight, is designed to compensate for the differing sampling probabilities for selecting individuals as WMH respondents. The selection weight factor, $W_{sel}$, is generally the product of the reciprocals of three factors (1) $W_{sel,hh}$,

the reciprocal of the multistage probability of selecting the respondent's housing unit from the sample frame; (2) $W_{sel,resp}$, the reciprocal of the conditional probability of selecting the WMH respondent at random within the eligible household (Kish 1965); and (3) $W_{sel,Part\,II}$, the reciprocal of the probability that an eligible WMH survey respondent was subsampled to complete the in-depth Part 2 diagnostic section of the WMH interview. It is noteworthy in this regard that all WMH respondents completed Part 1 of the WMH interview. On the basis of the results of Part 1, the majority of the country surveys selected a stratified subsample of respondents to complete Part 2 of the interview, oversampling Part 1 respondents who met criteria for any of the mental disorders assessed in that first half of the interview.

### 7.1.2. The Nonresponse Adjustment Weight

The nonresponse adjustment weight, $W_{nr}$, could be computed to account for differential patterns of response across categories of eligible respondents for a country-specific survey. When this weight was applied, nonresponse adjustments to survey weights were based on endogenous data, that is, on data from the sample frame that was known for both sample respondents and nonrespondents. In baseline or cross-sectional surveys such as the WMH studies described here, the data available to develop nonresponse adjustments is often limited to geographic and possibly demographic information available for respondents and nonrespondents in the sample frame, such as population census data collected by the government.

In cases where nonresponse adjustment was implemented, a nonrespondent survey of the sort described in Section 6, was used to generate this weight. The nonresponse sample was first weighted to be representative of all nonrespondents using the sample selection weights (see Section 7.1.1) and then this weighted subsample was compared to the similarly weighted main sample in an effort to determine whether the two samples differed meaningfully on the variables assessed in both samples. When differences of this sort were found, either a weighting class method or a propensity modeling approach (Little & Rubin 2002) was used to develop the adjustment factors.

The weight calculations for most of the WMH survey data sets, however, did not include a separate nonresponse adjustment. Instead, an adjustment for differential nonresponse and sample noncoverage of the survey population was integrated into one consolidated adjustment in the poststratification weighting step, which is described subsequently. In such cases, the factor $W_{nr}$ can be viewed as taking a value of 1.0 in the final composite weight calculation. Readers who are interested in detailed case studies of nonresponse adjustment weighting for selected WMH data sets are referred to the work of Alonso and colleagues (2004) and Kessler and colleagues (2004).

### 7.1.3. The Poststratification Weight

The final component in the WMH individual analysis weight is a poststratification factor, $W_{ps}$. The poststratification weighting adjustment differs from the nonresponse adjustment factors in that poststratification weighting uses data that are exogenous to the survey design to calibrate the weights for survey estimation. The WMH poststratification used estimates of population values from external sources, such as a recent national census or demographic population estimation program, to standardize the sampling weights to known population distribution values, such as the distribution of the population of the cross-classified by age (in categories), sex, and education. The logic of the general procedure used in each country was to form a matrix of adjustment cells by cross-classifying age, sex, and major geographic regions (data permitting) of the survey population. Within each cell of this matrix, the poststratification weight factors were computed as the ratio of the external population count for each cell to the sum of computed sample selection weights for the WMH survey cases assigned to that cell:

$$W_{pstrat,c,i} = \frac{\hat{N}_c}{\sum_{i \in c}^{n_c} W_{sel,i} \cdot W_{nr,i}}, \qquad (5)$$

where

$W_{pstrat,c,i}$ = the poststratification factor for all cases in cell c;

$\hat{N}_c$ = WMH country population estimate for cell c;

$n_c$ = WMH country sample size in cell c;

$W_{sel,i}$ = the composite sample selection weight for case $i = 1, \ldots, n_c$;

$W_{nr,i}$ = the nonresponse adjustment for case $i = 1, \ldots, n_c$.

In some countries, it was possible to include much more information than a few sociodemographic and geographic variables because of the availability of much more detailed population data on a wide range of social and demographic variables that were also assessed in the WMH survey. In cases of this sort, data analyses were carried out to compare the WMH survey data, with other weights imposed on the data, to the population data in an effort to pinpoint any variables that were meaningfully discrepant between the two. When the number of such variables was small, a modified poststratification table of the sort described in the previous paragraph could have been carried out that constructed poststratification tables from only those variables. However, this procedure would run the risk of creating discrepancies between the weighted sample and the population on other variables that were originally nondiscrepant. To guard against this possibility, propensity score adjustment was used whenever a large number of poststratification variables was present. In this approach, logistic regression analysis was used to develop a multivariate prediction equation from the poststratification variables that discriminated between the WMH sample and the population, where a dichotomous outcome variable was used to distinguish the sample from the population in an analysis that combined both data files. This prediction equation allowed for interactions among the poststratification variables and sequentially evaluated a wide range of predictors to arrive at a final model that included core variables (i.e., age, sex, education, geography) and significant discriminating variables. Appropriately weighted predicted probabilities generated from this final equation were used to adjust the final WMH sample to approximate the multivariate distribution of the population on these variables.

## 7.2. Weighted Estimation and Inference for WMH Population Statistics

Although poststratification can potentially reduce sampling variances for survey estimates, the primary purpose of weighting was to eliminate potential sources of bias that would be present in an unweighted analysis. Those biases could arise as a result of differences in the original selection probabilities for respondents, differential nonresponse (probabilities of observation), and differential sample noncoverage for elements of the target population.

Procedures for weighted estimation of population statistics are standard features of the major statistical software systems. The weighted estimate of the population prevalence for a mental health disorder is:

$$p_w = \frac{\sum_{i=1}^{n} W_{i,final} \cdot Y_i}{\sum_{i=1}^{n} W_{i,final}}, \qquad (6)$$

where

$Y_i = 1$ if individual $i$ has the disorder of interest, 0 otherwise.

Weighted estimation of linear regression models for finite survey populations can be achieved by applying the computational algorithms originally derived for weighted least squares regression. Weighted pseudo-maximum likelihood methods are employed in estimation of logistic or other generalized linear models of regression relationships in the survey population (Skinner et al. 1989).

The pursuit of "unbiasedness" of estimates, which is at the heart of weighted analysis of the WMH survey data, may have a price in the form of increased variance of survey estimates compared to an unweighted estimate based on the same sample size. Weighting effects on standard errors arise from several factors, including the association between the distributions of the weights and the variables of interest and variance of the weight values assigned to the individual

cases. In the process of developing the final analysis weights for the WMH data sets, sensitivity analyses were conducted to determine the effect of extreme weight values on the estimated sampling errors and the potential bias of key survey estimates. If sampling variances proved highly sensitive to the most extreme weight values, the computed weights in the extreme lower and upper ranges were trimmed using methods that retained the sum of weights but distributed those weights across cases at each tail of the distribution. This trimming was typically carried out for respondents with the highest and lowest 1%–2% of weights and, in extreme cases, for those in the highest and lowest 5% of weights.

## 7.3. Influence of WMH Analysis Weights on Sample Estimation and Inference

Table 2.4 provides a simple illustration of the effect of weighted analysis on WMH survey estimates and confidence intervals for descriptive statistics. The descriptive statistic chosen for this illustration is the estimated percentage of each target population that experienced any of the DSM-IV mental disorders assessed in the surveys within the preceding 12-month period. The second column in Table 2.4 presents the unweighted estimates of the 95% confidence intervals for the population percentage in each WMH country. The third column of the table presents the same confidence interval correctly estimated using the survey weight and accounting for the complex sample design.

Note that, for most countries, there is a substantial shift in the range of values included in the 95% confidence intervals for the unweighted and weighted estimates. In large part this is because estimated prevalence is based on the CIDI Part 2 data and the weighting factor, $W_{sel,\,Part\,II}$, reflects differential sampling of respondents who reported greater numbers of symptoms in the CIDI Part 1 screening interview. In the majority of WMH countries, the unweighted estimates overrepresent persons with larger numbers of symptoms and therefore are biased for the true population prevalence. In countries such as South Africa, where all respondents completed

**Table 2.4.** The effect of weights on the precision of estimates of the 12-month prevalence of any DSM-IV disorder

| Country | 95% Confidence Interval for the estimated 12-month prevalence of any DSM-IV disorder | | Part 2(n) |
|---|---|---|---|
| | Unweighted (design biased) | Final WMH weight (design unbiased) | |
| WHO: Regional Office for the Americas (AMRO) | | | |
| Colombia | (33.0%, 37.8%) | (19.0%, 23.0%) | 2381 |
| Mexico | (26.1%, 30.5%) | (11.6%, 15.2%) | 2362 |
| United States | (40.0%, 42.8%) | (25.1%, 28.7%) | 5692 |
| WHO: Regional Office for Africa (AFRO) | | | |
| Nigeria | (8.5%, 10.9%) | (4.8%, 7.2%) | 2143 |
| South Africa | (15.2%, 18.0%) | (14.7%, 18.7%) | 4315 |
| WHO: Regional Office for the Eastern Mediterranean (EMRO) | | | |
| Lebanon | (27.4%, 35.0%) | (14.4%, 21.2%) | 1031 |
| WHO: Regional Office for Europe (EURO) | | | |
| Belgium | (18.5%, 24.5%) | (9.7%, 16.1%) | 1043 |
| France | (24.4%, 30.0%) | (15.9%, 21.1%) | 1436 |
| Germany | (16.9%, 22.5%) | (8.2%, 13.4%) | 1323 |
| Israel | (8.8%, 10.4%) | (8.9%, 10.5%) | 4859 |
| Italy | (13.5%, 16.7%) | (7.1%, 9.9%) | 1779 |
| Netherlands | (22.8%, 27.6%) | (11.6%, 15.6%) | 1094 |
| Spain | (17.0%, 19.8%) | (7.7%, 10.9%) | 2121 |
| Ukraine | (37.3%, 42.5%) | (18.8%, 24.0%) | 1720 |
| WHO: Regional Office for the Western Pacific (WPRO) | | | |
| Japan | (13.9%, 19.9%) | (5.6%, 9.2%) | 887 |
| New Zealand | (36.1%, 38.5%) | (19.5%, 21.9%) | 7435 |
| People's Republic of China | (12.0%, 16.4%) | (5.3%, 8.9%) | 1628 |

CIDI Parts 1 and 2, the differences in the weighted and unweighted confidence intervals are much smaller.

## 8. SAMPLING ERROR AND INFERENCE FROM THE WMH SURVEY DATA

The WMH surveys are based on a variety of probability sample designs – each design is adapted to the resources, experiences, and cost structures that are unique to the collaborating countries. Despite the variations in probability sample design forms, each survey aims to support robust, design-based estimation of population statistics, such as prevalence of mental health, in a chosen survey population.

The survey literature refers to designs like the ones used in the WMH surveys as "complex

designs," a loosely used term meant to denote that the sample incorporates special design features such as stratification, clustering, and differential selection probabilities (i.e., weighting), which analysts must consider in computing sampling errors, and confidence intervals for sample estimates of descriptive statistics and model parameters (Heeringa & Liu 1997). Standard programs in statistical analysis software packages assume simple random sampling (SRS) or independence of observations in computing standard errors for sample estimates. In general, the SRS assumption results in underestimation of the variances of survey estimates of descriptive statistics and model parameters. This means that the confidence intervals based on computed variances that assume independence of observations will be biased (generally too narrow) and

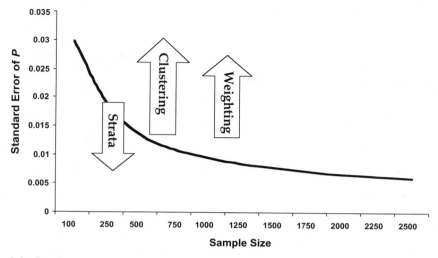

**Figure 2.1.** Complex sample design effects on standard errors of prevalence estimates. *Note:* Illustration for $P = 0.10$.

design-based inferences will be affected accordingly. This section focuses on sampling error estimation and construction of confidence intervals for WMH survey estimates of descriptive statistics such as means, proportions, ratios, and coefficients for linear and logistic regression models.

### 8.1. Sampling Error Computation Methods and Programs for the WMH Data

Over the past 50 years, advances in survey sampling theory have guided the development of a number of methods for estimating variances from complex sample data sets correctly. Several sampling error programs that implement these complex sample variance estimation methods are available to WMH data analysts. The two most common approaches (Rust 1985) are the Taylor series linearization method (and corresponding approximation to its variance) and resampling variance estimation methods, such as the balanced repeated replication (BRR) method and the jackknife repeated replication (JRR) method. The sampling error estimates presented in the substantive chapters of this volume were, for the most part, estimated in SUDAAN Version 9 (Research Triangle Institute 2004) using the Taylor series linearization method, though some

of the more complex estimates required the use of the JRR method.

### 8.2. Design Effects for WMH of Descriptive Statistics

Most practical sample designs in health-related surveys use stratification and clustering. Stratification is introduced to increase the statistical and administrative efficiency of the sample. Sample elements are selected as clusters in multistage designs to reduce travel costs and to improve interviewing efficiency. Disproportionate sampling of population elements may be used to increase the sample sizes for subpopulations of special interest, which results in the need to employ weighting in the estimation of population prevalence or other descriptive statistics. Relative to SRS, each of these complex sample design features influences the size of standard errors for survey estimates. Figure 2.1 illustrates the effects of these design features on standard errors of estimates. The curve plotted in the figure represents the SRS standard error of an estimate as a function of sample size. At any chosen sample size, the effect of sample stratification is generally a reduction in standard errors relative to SRS. Clustering of sample elements and designs that require weighting for unbiased estimation

**Table 2.5.** Design effects for estimates of the 12-month prevalence of major classes of DSM-IV disorders

| Country | Anxiety disorders | Mood disorders | Substance disorders | Any disorder | Part 2 (n) |
|---|---|---|---|---|---|
| WHO: Regional Office for the Americas (AMRO) | | | | | |
| Colombia | 2.19 | <1.0 | 1.40 | 1.44 | 2381 |
| Mexico | 1.55 | 1.32 | 1.17 | 2.40 | 2362 |
| United States | 1.80 | 1.03 | 2.49 | 2.34 | 5692 |
| WHO: Regional Office for Africa (AFRO) | | | | | |
| Nigeria | 2.82 | <1.0 | <1.0 | 2.03 | 2143 |
| South Africa | 2.01 | 2.39 | 3.03 | 2.90 | 4315 |
| WHO: Regional Office for the Eastern Mediterranean (EMRO) | | | | | |
| Lebanon | 1.37 | 1.06 | 5.14 | 2.04 | 1031 |
| WHO: Regional Office for Europe (EURO) | | | | | |
| Belgium | 2.57 | 1.26 | 1.30 | 2.38 | 1043 |
| France | 1.45 | 1.23 | 1.63 | 1.61 | 1436 |
| Germany | 2.10 | <1.0 | 1.79 | 2.32 | 1323 |
| Israel | 1.36 | 1.27 | <1.0 | 1.20 | 4859 |
| Italy | 1.04 | <1.0 | 1.78 | 1.12 | 1779 |
| Netherlands | 1.07 | 1.07 | 1.05 | <1.0 | 1094 |
| Spain | 2.75 | 1.35 | 2.84 | 1.61 | 2121 |
| Ukraine | 1.25 | 1.22 | 1.84 | 1.73 | 1720 |
| WHO: Regional Office for the Western Pacific (WPRO) | | | | | |
| Japan | 0.73 | 0.56 | 1.20 | 1.05 | 887 |
| New Zealand | 1.45 | 1.63 | 1.98 | 1.63 | 7435 |
| People's Republic of China | 1.35 | 1.21 | 1.65 | 2.00 | 1628 |
| *Average* | 1.70 | 1.08 | 1.89 | 1.81 | |

generally have larger standard errors than does an SRS sample of equal size (Kish 1965).

The combined effects of stratification, clustering, and weighting on the standard errors of estimates are termed the "design effect" ($D^2$) and are measured by the following ratio:

$$D^2 = \frac{SE(p)^2_{complex}}{SE(p)^2_{srs}} = \frac{Var(p)_{complex}}{Var(p)_{srs}}, \quad (7)$$

where,

$D^2$ = the design effect;
$Var(p)_{complex}$ = the complex sample design variance of the sample statistic $p$; and
$Var(p)_{srs}$ = the simple random sample variance of $p$.

Table 2.5 provides the estimated design effects for estimates of the prevalence of major classes of DSM-IV mental disorders for each of the WMH surveys included in this volume. The design effect

estimates are based on diagnoses from Part 2 of the WMH survey. With several exceptions, design effects for prevalence estimates are greater than 1.0, the average across countries being 1.7 for anxiety disorders, 1.1 for mood disorders, 1.9 for substance disorders, and 1.8 for any disorder. Within individual WMH country samples, the estimated design effects have a consistent trend such that

$$D^2(p_{substance}) > D^2(p_{anxiety}) > D^2(p_{mood}). \quad (8)$$

The lesser values of $D^2(p)$ for mood disorders could reflect smaller intracluster correlations in the survey populations for depression than for other disorders. The intraclass correlations for substance disorders may be greatest because of more geographic clustering of substance problems in urban areas or other localized areas of the survey population. Across WMH surveys, design effects are lower in countries that employed only limited clustering of observations in the survey sample design, such as Israel and the Netherlands. Design effects for prevalence estimates were greatest in larger countries such as the United States, Mexico, and South Africa, where distances between sample points necessitated greater primary-stage clustering of the sample selection.

An interesting observation regarding the use of Part 2 subsampling is that the design effects for disorders assessed in Part 1 do not differ greatly when they are estimated instead in the Part 2 sample. This result cannot be seen in Table 2.5, but it would be observed if we replicated the results in Table 2.5 for the specific disorders assessed in the Part 1 sample twice: once using the Part 1 weights with the full Part 1 sample and a second time using the Part 2 weights with the smaller Part 2 sample. The reason for this pattern is that 100% of respondents with any of the DSM-IV disorders assessed in Part 1 were retained in the Part 2 sample. This means that the Part 2 sample can be considered a case-control sample that undersamples persons who do not have mental disorders. As individual mental disorders are minority phenomena in each of the WMH countries, the number of cases (i.e., respondents who meet criteria for a given disorder) is much smaller than the number of controls (i.e., respondents who do not meet criteria for the disorder). In situations of this sort, standard errors of odds ratios and weighted prevalence estimates are not importantly influenced when sample sizes are as large as they are in the WMH surveys (Schlesselman 1982). This accounts for the observation that Part 2 subsampling did not adversely affect the efficiency of the design for estimating prevalence of most disorders.

## 9. SUMMARY

This chapter has reviewed the sample design characteristics, sample outcomes, and design-based estimation and inference procedures for the WMH surveys. It needs to be emphasized that each WMH survey used a probability sample design for the selection of a representative sample of its target population. Specific features of individual country's sample designs

were adapted to the sample frames available in the countries, which differed from one country to another, and were adapted to prior survey sampling experience and resources and available budget for the survey data collection.

The probability sample designs developed by the WMH country research teams in consultation with the staff of the WMH Data Analysis Coordination Centre provided a statistically sound and analytically robust framework for the collection of WMH survey data. The total error in the survey data not only is a function of the sample design and its influence over sampling variability and bias but also is affected by nonsampling errors that arise in the survey response, interviewing, measurement, and data-coding processes. These latter components of total survey error were addressed through equally rigorous attention to data collection design, interviewer training, questionnaire construction and translations, and general procedures for quality control throughout the entire survey process. These activities and their role in addressing total survey error in the WMH survey data are the topics of subsequent chapters in this first part of the volume.

## REFERENCES

Alonso, J., Angermeyer, M. C., Bernert, S., Bruffaerts, R., Brugha, T. S., Bryson, H., de Girolamo, G., de Graaf, R., Demyttenaere, K., Gasquet, I., Haro, J. M., Katz, S. J., Kessler, R. C., Kovess, V., Lépine, J. P., Ormel, J., Polidori, G., Russo, L. J., Vilagut, G., Almansa, J., Arbabzadeh-Bouchez, S., Autonell, J., Bernal, M., Buist-Bouwman, M. A., Codony, M., Domingo-Salvany, A., Ferrer, M., Joo, S. S., Martínez-Alonso, M., Matschinger, H., Mazzi, F., Morgan, Z., Morosini, P., Palacín, C., Romera, B., Taub, N. & Vollebergh, W. A. M. (2004). Sampling and methods of the European Study of the Epidemiology of Mental Disorders (ESEMeD) project. *Acta Psychiatrica Scandinavica*, 109, 8–20.

American Association for Public Opinion Research (2000). *Standard definitions: Final dispositions of case codes and outcome rates for surveys.* Ann Arbor, MI: American Association for Public Opinion Research.

Cochran, W. G. (1977). *Sampling techniques.* New York: John Wiley & Sons.

Couper, M. P. & de Leeuw, E. D. (2003). Nonresponse in cross-cultural and cross-national surveys. In *Cross-cultural survey methods*, ed. J. A.

Harkness, F. R. van de Vijver & P. P. Mohler, pp. 157–78. New York: John Wiley & Sons.

de Leeuw, E. D. & de Heer, W. (2002). Trends in household survey nonresponse: A longitudinal and international comparison. In *Survey Nonresponse*, ed. R. M. Groves, D. A. Dillman, J. L. Ettinge & R. J. A. Little, pp. 41–54. New York: John Wiley & Sons.

Groves, R. M. & Couper, M. P. (1998). *Nonresponse in household interview surveys*. New York: John Wiley & Sons.

Groves, R. M., Fowler, F. J., Couper, M. P., Lepkowski, J. M., Singer, E. & Touangeau, R. (2004). *Survey methodology*. New York: John Wiley & Sons.

Heeringa, S. G. & Liu, J. (1997). Complex sample design effects and inference for mental health survey data. *International Journal of Methods in Psychiatric Research*, 7, 56–65.

Kessler, R. C., Berglund, P., Chiu, W. T., Demler, O., Heeringa, S. G., Hiripi, E., Jin, R., Pennell, B.-E., Walters, E. E., Zaslavsky, A. & Zheng, H. (2004). The U.S. National Comorbidity Survey Replication (NCS-R): Design and field procedures. *International Journal of Methods in Psychiatric Research*, 13, 69–92.

Kish, L. (1949). A procedure for objective respondent selection within the household. *Journal of the American Statistical Association*, 44, 380–7.

Kish, L. (1965). *Survey sampling*. New York: John Wiley & Sons.

Little, R. J. A. & Rubin, D. B. (2002). *Statistical analysis with missing data*, 2d ed. New York: John Wiley & Sons.

Research Triangle Institute (2004). *SUDAAN 9.0 user's manual: Software for statistical analysis of correlated data*. Research Triangle Park, NC: Research Triangle Institute.

Rust, K. (1985). Variance estimation for complex estimators in sample surveys. *Journal of Official Statistics*, 1, 381–97.

Schlesselman, J. (1982). *Case-control studies: Design, conduct, analysis*. New York: Oxford University Press.

Skinner, C. J., Holt, D. & Smith, T. M. F. (1989). *Analysis of complex surveys*. New York: John Wiley & Sons.

Verma, V., Scott, C. & O'Muircheartaigh, C. (1980). Sample designs and sampling errors for the World Fertility Survey. *Journal of the Royal Statistical Society*, 143, 431–73.

# 3 Implementation of the World Mental Health Surveys

BETH-ELLEN PENNELL, ZEINA N. MNEIMNEH, ASHLEY BOWERS,
STEPHANIE CHARDOUL, J. ELISABETH WELLS, MARIA CARMEN VIANA,
KARL DINKELMANN, NANCY GEBLER, SILVIA FLORESCU, YANLING HE,
YUEQIN HUANG, TOMA TOMOV, AND GEMMA VILAGUT SAIZ

## ACKNOWLEDGMENTS

Preparation of this chapter was supported by the U.S. National Institute of Mental Health (R01MH070884), the John D. and Catherine T. MacArthur Foundation, the Pfizer Foundation, the U.S. Public Health Service (R13-MH066849, R01-MH069864, U01MH060220, U01MH057716-05S1, and R01 DA016558), the Fogarty International Center (FIRCA R03-TW006481), the Pan American Health Organization, Eli Lilly and Company Foundation, Ortho-McNeil Pharmaceutical, Inc., Glaxo-SmithKline, and Bristol-Myers Squibb. We thank the WMH staff for assistance with instrumentation, fieldwork, and data analysis. A complete list of WMH publications can be found at http://www.hcp.med.harvard.edu/wmh/.

## I. INTRODUCTION

Large-scale cross-national surveys have been undertaken for decades (for a concise history, see Heath, Fisher & Smith 2005), but there is surprisingly little written that addresses the practical aspects of implementing such projects. Although the necessity of cultural adaptation of survey methods is widely recognized as necessary to achieve equivalence in measurement across countries (Bulmer 1998; Jowell 1998; Kuechler 1998; Lynn 2001), few details are provided in the literature as to how to achieve this equivalence across the many phases of a project's development. In the absence of such standards of practice, many cross-national projects have been left to accept the research traditions of individual countries, which vary widely in methodological rigor. An approach at the other extreme is to implement a "one-size-fits-all" methodology that naively imposes the same procedure and protocols across all countries and cultures on the basis of the assumption that good practice in one culture will be good practice in other cultures (Harkness, Van de Vijver & Mohler 2002).

The WMH Survey Initiative sought to implement an approach between these two extremes. This was done by establishing guidelines that set minimum standards for each phase of project implementation but allowed for country-specific adaptations. For example, as noted by Heeringa and colleagues in the previous chapter, the WMH guidelines required probability sampling methods at all stages of sample selection but acknowledged that appropriate country-specific variations were not only inevitable, but also essential and appropriate. The difficulty for the staff of the WMH Data Collection Coordination Centre was determining when variations in approach were necessary and appropriate rather than simply expedient. Staying with the preceding sampling example, survey organizations in some parts of the world have a tradition of quota sampling and respondent substitution that violates the WMH requirement of probability sampling. This kind of potential conflict between local practices and best practices was found in every phase of the WMH survey implementation.

In addition to imposing quality-control constraints on the survey data collection processes in all WMH countries, we sought to achieve a level of documentation that has been lacking in many cross-national surveys (Harkness 1999; Harkness et al. 2002; Heath et al. 2005). To assist in this goal, the WMH Data Collection Coordination Centre at the University of Michigan developed a system for integrated quantitative documentation of critical design and implementation procedures. This system, known as the Survey Metadata Documentation System (SMDS), covered all aspects of the survey production processes and operated much like a Web survey. The information presented in the current chapter is based largely on the data collected in the SMDS.

This chapter details the data quality-control standards set by the WMH Data Collection Coordination Centre and the ways in which these standards were implemented in the individual countries. Study design, questionnaire development, interviewer recruitment and training, research ethics, field structure, data collection procedures and quality control, and data preparation are all discussed. Reflections on what worked, what did not work, and recommendations for future studies that face similar data collection challenges are presented at the end of this chapter. The issues involved in instrument translation and adaptation are sufficiently complex that they are discussed in a separate chapter (Chapter 5).

## 2. STUDY DESIGN

Although a total of 27 participating countries are included in the WMH collaboration, this chapter focuses on only the 17 of those countries that finished data collection and processing in time to be included in this volume. These 17 are distributed across five World Health Organization (WHO) regions: AMRO (Colombia, Mexico, United States), AFRO (Nigeria, South Africa), EMRO (Lebanon), EURO (Belgium, France, Germany, Israel, Italy, Netherlands, Spain, Ukraine), and WPRO (People's Republic of China, Japan, New Zealand). All 17 implemented probability sample designs representative of their adult populations. As noted in Chapter 1, most countries met the WMH response rate target of 65%. Sample sizes ranged from 2372 (the Netherlands) to 12,992 (New Zealand). Interviews were

conducted face-to-face using either paper-and-pencil interviews (PAPIs) or computer-assisted personal interviews (CAPIs).

Both the PAPI and the CAPI versions of the interview schedule were based on an updated version of the WHO Composite International Diagnostic Interview (CIDI) that was designed specifically for the WMH Survey Initiative. (This instrument is described in Chapter 4.) Each country was responsible for translating and adapting this interview schedule from its source language (American English) using a systematic protocol that is described in Chapter 5. Interviewer training across all the surveys was modeled on the central train-the-trainer sessions developed by the WMH Data Collection Coordination Centre at the University of Michigan. This model is described later in this chapter.

As each country was responsible for securing funding to conduct its study, fieldwork and data collection time frames varied widely. This sort of variation is typical of collaborative studies that are based on separate funding of the individual components (Jowell 1998). Most of the surveys considered in this volume were conducted between 2001 and 2002, but others were completed as late as 2007. Fieldwork duration ranged from 3 to 33 months, with about half the surveys completed in a 12-month time interval. Figure 3.1 shows the activity dates and duration of each survey.

A critical issue concerned the decision to administer interviews face-to-face rather than by telephone. Face-to-face interviewing offered a number of important advantages in implementing the WMH surveys. The CIDI is a lengthy, complex instrument and thus is well-suited to a face-to-face interaction in which the interviewer can clarify questions, probe responses, and assess respondent fatigue (Oishi 2003; Groves et al. 2004). In addition, interviewers can present visual aids (e.g., respondent booklets) to improve respondent comprehension of questions or response categories (Oishi 2003; Groves et al. 2004). Response rates are typically higher in face-to-face surveys than those surveys that use other modes of data collection (Groves & Lyberg 1988; Hox & de Leeuw 1994; Groves et al. 2004).

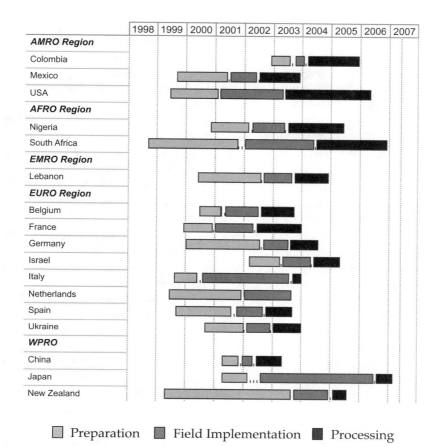

Preparation ▪ Field Implementation ▪ Processing

**Figure 3.1.** Preparation, field implementation, and processing durations for WMH Survey Initiative.

For countries that use area probability sampling, area probability frames provide more complete coverage of the household population than do frames based on telephone numbers or mailing addresses (Groves et al. 2004).

On the other hand, face-to-face interview costs can be five to ten times as high as those of telephone surveys in Western countries (Groves et al. 2004). Large field data collections require significant time for planning and implementation. The presence of an interviewer may cause respondents to change their answers to survey items to report socially appropriate or desirable responses (Groves et al. 2004). This was partially addressed in the WMH surveys by providing respondents with booklets and asking them to read the question on their own and answer with yes or no so that the actual question was not overheard by others in the household or in

close proximity. However, the impact of the interviewer's presence on respondent reporting and the effectiveness of the respondent booklet may also vary by culture and literacy levels across and within countries. Despite these limitations, face-to-face implementation was considered essential to the WMH surveys because of the complexity of the instrument.

## 3. THE INTERVIEW SCHEDULE

All participating WMH countries used the same fully structured interview, although several sections were optional and were not administered in all countries. As noted previously, the instrument is described in some detail in Chapter 4. For our present purposes, it is enough to know that the interview was designed to be administered by trained lay interviewers rather than by clinicians, and that the interview was considerably more complex than standard survey interviews. Because of this complexity, the 40-hour study-specific interviewer-training period was considerably longer than in typical surveys.

Somewhat different technical challenges of implementing and fielding surveys like the WMH surveys are raised by CAPI and PAPI implementation (Pennell et al. 2004). The advantages of CAPI include higher data quality, reduced time in the postsurvey processing phase, and potentially lower cost (Baker, Bradburn & Johnson 1995; Couper & Nicholls 1998), although the evidence on cost savings is mixed (Baker et al. 1995; Groves & Tortora 1998). In terms of gains in data quality, the amount of missing data can be reduced by automating questionnaire skip patterns (Groves et al. 2004; Kessler et al. 2004). The use of range checks (i.e., programmed checks built into the interview that determine whether entered values lie within a valid range) and consistency checks (i.e., programmed checks that compare two or more entered values that should be in agreement) allow interviewers to resolve inconsistencies in respondent reporting during the interview.

In addition, the wording of items can be customized in CAPI on the basis of previous responses in ways that are difficult to approximate in PAPI administration. Help screens and look-up features that allow interviewers to access information sources, such as a list of commonly used medications or question-level instructions, can be incorporated in computer-assisted interviewing applications more easily than in PAPI. Quality-control monitoring can be much more sophisticated in CAPI than in PAPI, as the clocks in the laptops that implement CAPI interviews can be used to time data entry (as a way to detect possible interviewer falsification), and the rapid analysis of computerized CAPI interviews can be used to detect missing values and other signs of low interview quality.

In terms of cost, for surveys with complex instruments and large data-entry requirements, the savings from direct entry of paper-and-pencil interviews using CAPI can sometimes outweigh the added costs of interviewer training and computer hardware needed for CAPI implementation (Baker et al. 1995). These cost savings can be especially large when, as for the WMH, the costs of computer programming are paid for centrally. Administration time is also somewhat shorter in CAPI interviews, as interviewers do not have to navigate complex skip patterns or perform calculations that are common in PAPI questionnaires.

There are, however, potential drawbacks and limitations associated with CAPI administration. The development of computerized specifications incorporating the features described in the previous few paragraphs requires significant time and cost commitments in the preproduction phase of the survey (House & Nicholls 1988). In the case of WMH, the development and testing of the CAPI program required more than five person-years to complete. However, as noted previously, the costs of this work were borne centrally, which meant that the incremental costs to any individual WMH country in this regard were very small.

Although CAPI resolves a number of implementation problems, a problem that is relatively specific to CAPI administration is that interviewers are more likely than in PAPI administration to lose track of where they are in the sequence of questions. This problem occurs because CAPI interviewers are able to see only one screen at a time, whereas in a paper format it is easier to gauge location in the instrument and move back and forth as needed (Groves & Mathiowetz 1984; House & Nicholls 1988; Couper 2000). An additional problem is that CAPI interviewers must be trained in the use of the computer-assisted application, which may divert attention away from training on other important interpersonal aspects of survey implementation. Although concerns have been raised that this diversion of attention might reduce the quality of interviewing, few studies have investigated this potential effect (Groves et al. 2004).

There is also the issue of the technical experience and infrastructure of the data collection organization needed to implement CAPI surveys. Although the WMH Data Collection Coordination Centre facilitated the countries' gaining access to the laptop computers needed to carry out CAPI surveys, the data collection organizations in the countries that provided the interviewers needed to have the technical expertise to accept and keep track of the completed CAPI interviews. The interviewers needed to have access to a reliable electrical power source to maintain the functioning of their laptops. The potential safety of interviewers carrying expensive computer equipment into the field also had to be considered in deciding whether to use CAPI.

In balancing these pros and cons, the majority of WMH countries opted for CAPI administration. Not surprisingly, the countries that used PAPI were almost entirely developing, whereas the developed countries used CAPI. Anticipating this divide, a centralized decision had to be made at the onset as to whether we wanted to require all WMH surveys to be implemented using the same mode. If so, this would have had to be PAPI, as CAPI implementation was logistically impossible in some countries. We decided against this requirement on the basis of the overarching perspective described at the beginning of this chapter: that optimal survey implementation allows for the best methods and procedures to vary cross-nationally.

A question can be raised as to whether the decision to allow cross-national variation in the use of CAPI versus PAPI introduced cross-national variability in survey estimates as a result of mode of data collection. It is impossible, in the absence of a controlled experiment, to answer this question definitively. We were influenced in our decision to allow both modes by the results of experimental studies of mode effects, which have generally found few significant differences in survey estimates (Baker et al. 1995; Nicholls, Baker & Martin 1997; Couper 2000), although some evidence has been found for improved reporting of sensitive items with CAPI (Baker et al. 1995). These experimental studies were all carried out in developed countries, which raises the possibility that mode effects might be greater in developing countries. However, as we knew it was not feasible to use CAPI in the developing countries that participated in WMH, we decided that the practical decision – whether to allow CAPI in developed countries even though PAPI would be

used in developing countries – should be decided in the affirmative.

Each country fielded a unique version of the WMH interview schedule. This was the result of both adaptation procedures (e.g., adding country-specific content) and because the source English version of the interview schedule was modified over time to correct errors or confusions found in earlier versions. There were four major revisions of the English source interview schedule over the course of the study, from the first version developed in 1999 to the most recent modifications made in 2007. These changes necessitated the implementation of a comprehensive set of version control procedures to allow for comparison across countries. The extent of the instrument changes was not anticipated at the beginning of the study; instead, the following procedures evolved from experience as the study progressed and countries were added to the initiative.

For the PAPI version of the instrument, a separate computerized data-entry program was developed that paralleled the CAPI version. Therefore, for both the PAPI and the CAPI instruments, it was necessary to maintain an up-to-date gold-standard English version. The process of modifying the PAPI instrument and keeping track of each country's version of the instrument began with modifications to the English source interview schedule. Modifications were reviewed by technical staff, and summary documents outlining the changes to the current version were created and posted in a secure Web-based collaborative content management system, EMC Documentum eRoom (http://software. emc.com/). As changes were made to the instruments, programming and checking were implemented in the source version.

Once all of the summary documentation and supporting material for each proposed modification were posted in eRoom, a separate e-mail was sent to each country alerting researchers of the recent changes and where to locate them in eRoom. The previous version of the English source code was sent along with the new gold-standard source code for comparison purposes. At this point, the collaborators began to update their country-specific questionnaire. A version-numbering system was established to track these changes. File comparison programs were then used to incorporate instrument changes. Two programs that were useful in this process were Windiff.exe (see http://tinyurl.com/obegs) and UltraEdit-32 (see http://www.ultraedit.com). Tracked version notes (a feature of the eRoom system), a file comparison program, and line-by-line review were used to maintain a record of changes to the instrument for study documentation purposes. The integration of the translated text is described in more detail in Chapter 5.

One key to keeping track of the many instrument corrections and modifications that were made over the course of the study was to make sure all questions across all versions kept the same question-numbering scheme. Unique country-specific items were given unique section identifiers. Such consistency in numbering greatly facilitated data analysis. Maintaining detailed records and a universal numbering scheme enabled the WMH Data Collection Coordination Centre to create two Web-based, interactive grids (for the PAPI and CAPI versions) that compared each country's version of the survey with the English gold standard. The grids compared instruments on several dimensions – whether a question was added or omitted, whether a response category changed, whether a skip sequence changed, and so on. Each grid had a drill-down function that allowed the user to start with a view of all sections across countries and then to drill down to sections of the questionnaire to view side-by-side comparison between the English gold standard and the country version. These grids have proved to be extremely useful as quick reference guides for WMH analysts as they implement cross-national comparative analyses.

## 4. PRETESTING

Pretesting the survey instrument and data collection procedures prior to main study data collection is widely recommended to maximize survey data quality (Sheatsley 1983; Converse & Presser 1986; Groves et al. 2004; Harkness,

Pennell, & Schoua-Glusberg 2004; Smith 2004). Pretests are small-scale tests of the questionnaire, sampling, and data collection procedures to be used in the main study. It is generally advised that the pretests mirror the main study in most aspects. The sample should be representative of the type(s) of respondents who will be included in the main study, although a strict probability sample is not needed.

Pretest interviews can be evaluated in a number of ways. Interviewers and respondents are often debriefed to identify potential problem areas with the instrument and survey procedures. The distributions of items are often checked for high rates of missing data and out-of-range values. The average length of the interview is estimated on the basis of the pretest interviews. Evaluation of pretest results lead to modifications to the survey instrument and data collection procedures prior to main study data collection.

Pretesting is especially important in cross-national studies (Smith 2004). A considerable challenge in such studies is that languages, social conventions, and response styles vary across cultures, making it difficult to extrapolate from the pretest experiences in any one country to those in another country (Smith 2004). Because of these complexities, we required that a separate series of pretests be carried out in each WMH country. Initial pretests focused on evaluating the translations, as discussed in Chapter 5. Once the translated instrument was finalized, each country was required to carry out a pretest of at least 40 respondents to test the questionnaire and field procedures. As substantive results were not important in this exercise, selection of respondents was left to the discretion of the country and depended on several factors. Countries that added new content modules needed to test those modules with targeted segments of the population relevant to the content. In New Zealand, for example, areas with a high concentration of Maori were selected to ensure that health services and demographic items specifically developed for the Maori population were adequately tested. The diagnostic sections of the instrument were tested in patient populations to make sure that all diagnostic sections were thoroughly tested. In addition, general population samples were used to pretest the field procedures. These were generally convenience samples, although in some cases this aspect of pretesting was carried out with quota samples (China, France, Mexico) or probability samples (China, Germany, Israel, Japan, Lebanon, New Zealand, Spain, Ukraine).

The number of pretest rounds varied from one to three, with approximately two-thirds of the countries conducting just one round of pretests and six conducting two rounds. Three pretest rounds were completed in the United States, as the U.S. version of the instrument was the basis of the source questionnaire. The WMH surveys were all based on face-to-face interviews. As a result, the pretest interviews were conducted face-to-face. In the typical case, the survey organization responsible for the main survey carried out the pretests under the supervision of WMH investigators. In five countries (Belgium, China, Mexico, New Zealand, United States), members of the WMH research team also administered some pretest interviews. Debriefing sessions with interviewers were led by field supervisors and WMH collaborators after each round of pretest interviews with a script developed by the WMH Data Collection Coordinating Centre.

The pretest debriefing sessions identified country-specific difficulties with questionnaire wording and response categories that were modified prior to the beginning of production interviewing. These sessions, along with quantitative analyses of responses, detected skip-pattern errors in the PAPI version and programming errors in the CAPI version that were corrected prior to the beginning of production interviewing. The general population component of the pretests also allowed the investigators to evaluate the adequacy of survey procedures and sample management systems. Other country-specific aims included further testing of language versions in countries that used multiple languages (e.g., South Africa), evaluating the work of interviewers, and testing the efficacy of communication strategies. The pretests also provided preliminary information on the length of the interview. Countries that used PAPI administration tended to have somewhat longer interviews than those

that used CAPI administration, although part of this difference was due to the inclusion of additional sections in a number of the PAPI surveys. This same pattern held in the production phase of the surveys (Table 3.1). There was also considerable variation in interview duration within the CAPI countries, largely due to variation in the inclusion of optional sections.

## 5. INTERVIEWER RECRUITMENT AND TRAINING

Because of the complexity of the data collection task, recruitment of qualified and capable interviewers was critical to the success of each country's survey. In some countries, the research team was responsible for interviewer recruitment and management; in other countries, the interviewing component was subcontracted to an external survey organization. During the design and planning phase of the surveys, each country worked with the WMH Data Collection Coordination Centre to decide on the structure, size, and composition of the field staff and the duration of the field period. These decisions were driven by parameters such as the sample size and location, the timing of data collection, budget constraints, and the languages in which the interviewing would occur.

### 5.1. Training the Trainers

Before starting the interviewer recruitment and training process, each country sent at least two interviewer supervisors to a train-the-trainer session presented by the WMH Data Collection Coordination Centre at the University of Michigan. These sessions lasted, on average, six days and were designed to prepare the interviewer supervisors to train and monitor interviewer performance, as well as to manage data collection and data processing in their country. Through these sessions, research teams obtained all of the information and materials necessary to train their own interviewing staff using consistent procedures. These trainers, who for almost all countries came from a pool of experienced interviewers, then trained a team of supervisors to help

**Table 3.1.** Study implementation features across WMH Survey Initiative

| | Type of organization | Mode | Length of interview (minutes) | Supervisor–interviewer ratio | Advance letter | Incentives | Response rate |
|---|---|---|---|---|---|---|---|
| **WHO: Regional Office for the Americas (AMRO)** | | | | | | | |
| Colombia | Nonprofit organization | CAPI | 104 | 1:3 | Y | Alarm clock | 87.7 |
| Mexico | Private for-profit company | CAPI | 150 | 1:6 | N | None | 76.6 |
| United States | Academic center/institute | CAPI | 123 | 1:10 | Y | Cash/check: US$50 & 100 | 70.9 |
| **WHO: Regional Office for Africa (AFRO)** | | | | | | | |
| Nigeria | Government agency; academic center/institute | PAPI | 90 | 1:4 | Y | Bath towel | 79.3 |
| South Africa | Private for-profit company | PAPI | 210 | 1:10 | N | None | 87.1 |
| **WHO: Regional Office for the Eastern Mediterranean (EMRO)** | | | | | | | |
| Lebanon | Private for-profit company | PAPI | 97 | 1:5 | N | Free psychiatric consultation | 70.0 |
| **WHO: Regional Office for Europe (EURO)** | | | | | | | |
| Belgium | Government agency | CAPI | 71 | 1:7 | Y | None | 50.6 |
| France | Private for-profit company | CAPI | 73 | – | – | Gift certificate: EUR 24 | 45.9 |
| Germany | Private for-profit company | CAPI | 75 | – | Y | None | 57.8 |
| Israel | Government agency | CAPI | 60 | 1:6 | Y | None | 72.6 |
| Italy | Private for-profit company | CAPI | 49 | 1:20 | N | Gasoline coupon: EUR 15 & 50 | 71.3 |
| Netherlands | Private for-profit company; academic center/institute | CAPI | 90 | 1:50 | Y | Gift certificate: EUR 5 & 20 | 56.4 |
| Spain | Private for-profit company | CAPI | 71 | 1:20 | Y | Gift certificate: EUR 12 & 25 | 78.6 |
| Ukraine | Academic center/institute[a] | PAPI | 98 | 1:2 | N | Cash: UAH 25 | 78.3 |
| **WHO: Regional Office for the Western Pacific (WPRO)** | | | | | | | |
| China | Academic center/institute | PAPI | 90 | 1:5 | Y | None | 74.8 (Beijing); 74.6 (Shanghai) |
| Japan | Government agency; academic center/institute | CAPI | 70–80 | 1:20 | N | None | 56.4 |
| New Zealand | Private for-profit company | CAPI | 73 | 1:5 | Y | Free family meal[b] | 73.3 |

[a] In addition to a professional organization of psychiatrists.

[b] Only for potential respondents who were reluctant to take part.

in interviewer recruitment, training, and field quality-control monitoring.

## 5.2. Selection Criteria for New Interviewers

All countries employed interviewers who traveled to the selected geographic locations, determined household eligibility, and attempted to interview the respondents in their homes. Many of the countries were required to recruit and hire new interviewers for the WMH Survey Initiative, while others were able to use existing field staff from established survey organizations. In most countries where new interviewers were recruited, recruitment was carried out in the general population. In a few countries, though, interviewers were recruited exclusively from among college students. All new interviewers were required to complete written applications, which were screened before candidates were invited to an in-person interview. The criteria assessed during the interviewer screening varied across countries, but most commonly included elements such as interviewing experience, language skills, computer or technical skills, education, location, ability to meet production goals, and capability to handle potentially emotional or stressful interactions with respondents. The personal interviews also evaluated the accuracy and clarity with which the applicants could read the survey questions. When the survey was to be conducted in multiple languages – such as in Belgium, Israel, Nigeria, and South Africa – a formal assessment of language competency was also conducted.

## 5.3. Interviewer Training

Whether the data collection was being carried out by a private research firm, an organization affiliated with a university, or a statistical agency, we repeatedly received feedback that the WMH interview schedule was one of the most complex and challenging the organization had ever administered. Although interviewers were not required to have mental health expertise to administer the CIDI, they were required to be skilled in the techniques of standardized interviewing and to understand the CIDI-specific

conventions and rules. In addition to administering the interview, interviewers needed to implement all aspects of the sampling and respondent selection procedures, to attain a high respondent cooperation rate, and to complete numerous administrative tasks.

The interviewer training consisted of two parts: general interviewing techniques and CIDI-specific training. General interviewing training (GIT) was designed to introduce interviewers to the basic components of standardized questionnaire administration, covering such topics as question reading, appropriate techniques to probe for more information, seeking clarification, providing feedback, and recording data accurately. The length of GIT sessions varied, ranging from two to three days in most countries. All sessions were conducted in person, and all interviewers were provided with a comprehensive study manual. The following elements were included in all GIT sessions: description of the data collection process; the interviewer's role in the research process; addressing respondent reluctance to participate; standardized interviewing techniques; data-recording/data-entry procedures; interviewer evaluation procedures and criteria; and administrative tasks such as sample management.

In addition, countries that used computer-assisted interviewing trained their interviewers in computer hardware and software use, including the use of CAPI questionnaire administration with the software system used in the surveys. Some countries added other country-specific topics in their GIT session, such as New Zealand's inclusion of cultural empathy to Maori and Pacific Islander households and Colombia's special training on interacting with governmental authorities and armed guerrilla and paramilitary groups. All interviewers were required to demonstrate competence with GIT concepts and procedures before moving on to study-specific training. Methods to assess interviewers included the use of a scripted interview in which the "respondent" was one of the trainers or a supervisor. Other methods included recruiting one or more respondents who were briefed for this purpose. Here, supervisors and trainers could directly observe the interviewers. Other methods included role-playing exercises and a variety of written and/or oral tests.

Following GIT, all interviewers were required to complete study-specific training. This portion of training averaged 30 hours across countries. The content was presented as a mix of lecture and round-robin practice sessions, with the following information covered: general background on the project and its importance, administration of the survey introduction and elements of informed consent, eligibility and respondent selection procedures, interviewing on sensitive topics, all aspects of the WMH interview schedule, and meeting production goals. During the train-the-trainer sessions that prepared supervisors to train the interviewers, the importance of hands-on practice was emphasized. All countries consequently incorporated this into their interviewer training. While conducting small group exercises, trainers assessed the skill level of each interviewer. Many countries held tailored "after-hours" special sessions to address areas where interviewers needed additional assistance and practice, such as in applying the respondent selection algorithms and using the laptop computer.

In addition to presenting the "mechanics" of using the CIDI, study-specific training also was designed to convey the unique challenges of the instrument. To navigate this complex interview schedule, interviewers had to remember that they were asking very personal and potentially sensitive questions. Interviewers and supervisors alike reported that it generally took several weeks of interviewing to become fully competent in the interviewing task. As a result, it was difficult to fully prepare interviewers for the range of experiences they might encounter in the training phase. Most countries followed the suggestion of the WMH Data Collection Coordination Centre to add to the training team a clinical consultant, typically a psychiatric social worker or clinical psychologist, who could provide interviewers with background information about the kinds of symptoms of emotional problems they might encounter during production interviewing. This clinical contact person (CCP) was also a resource person for both interviewers and respondents during data collection – for a respondent who might need counseling or a referral for follow-up and for an interviewer who might need to debrief after a particularly difficult interview. In most cases, the CCP was available to interviewers 24 hours a day, seven days a week. Many countries developed protocols that allowed interviewers to contact their CCP privately, without first going through a supervisor. This provided interviewers with a unique opportunity to speak freely about their own and their respondents' experiences. Allowing the interviewers to meet the CCP during training and to hear directly from this person about the types of situations they were likely to encounter was a very effective way to put the interviewers at ease and to better prepare them for the experience of administering the interview to a general population sample.

All countries required interviewers to pass a certification test before being approved for production work. Interviewers who did not pass the certification process either were terminated from the project or received retraining and another opportunity to obtain certification. During production, many countries continued their interviewer training through methods such as periodic in-person seminars, telephone conference calls, and periodic bulletins or newsletters. Interviewers were terminated from production interviewing if they were found not able to perform up to required standards. Toward the end of the data collection period, focused training sessions were provided that concentrated on addressing respondent concerns and maximizing response rates.

## 5.4. Interviewer Characteristics and Conditions of Employment

The number of interviewers working in each country ranged from 28 (Mexico) to 400 (South Africa), with an average staff size of 113. Most countries had a higher proportion of female than male interviewers, with an overall average of 67% female (from a low of 40% in Mexico to a high of 94% in Ukraine). Most interviewers had university degrees (62%), with a range from 5% in the Netherlands to 90% in the United States. The average age of interviewers across countries was 37, with a range from 24 in Lebanon to 52 in the United States. The majority of interviewers had previous interviewing experience, with an average of 68% having previous interviewing experience (from 20% in Israel and Lebanon to 100% in Belgium and Ukraine).

There was considerable variation across countries in the conditions of interviewer employment. The WMH Data Collection Coordination Centre provided overall guidelines on interviewer management, but countries were allowed to adapt these to meet the unique needs of their study and the constraints of the data collection organizations with which they worked. Perhaps the most important issue involved interviewer payment. Given the wide variation in the length of interview schedule (from less than an hour to many hours), countries were strongly encouraged to pay interviewers by the hour rather than by the interview to mitigate interviewers' incentive to take shortcuts or, in the worst case, to falsify interviews. However, the research tradition in most countries was to pay by the interview, and in some countries the employment contract with interviewers could not be changed. When this was the case, the Data Collection Coordination Centre strongly encouraged the use of interviewer bonuses and higher per-unit payments for long interviews to counteract the tendency for interviewers to rush through interviews in cases where payment was on a per-interview basis.

Approximately one-third of the countries required interviewers to work a minimum number of hours per week. In these countries, the required number of hours ranged from 16 to 56 hours per week, with the average hours worked per week being 31. Work-hour requirements varied depending on the sample type (list or area), the at-home patterns of respondents, the length of the field period, and the structure of the field staff (limited to one or several geographic areas or traveling teams of interviewers).

Many countries experienced high interviewer attrition rates as a result of the length of the data collection period and the complexity and difficulty of the interview. The interviewers who stayed with the project and successfully completed their assignments were a remarkable group. Stories from the interviewers include many instances of meeting challenges that ranged from the mundane (e.g., finding a private spot to interview the selected respondent of a large family living in close quarters) to the exceptional (e.g., hearing stories from respondents who revealed to the interviewer for the first time a rape, abuse, or other traumatic event). Interviewer safety was also a concern in some areas of every country. Steps were taken from hiding laptops for fear of robbery to working in pairs for safety and hiring escorts to minimize risk. In Colombia, the survey team at times had to negotiate with local paramilitary groups to gain access to areas under their control.

## 6. RESEARCH ETHICS

As specified in international codes and guidelines, including the Nuremberg Code and the Declaration of Helsinki, internationally accepted ethical standards and principles exist that apply to research on human subjects. However, there are cross-national differences in ethics practices, such as procedures to document respondent consent, that reflect variation in government regulations, professional codes of ethics, and cultural norms and practices. As described in this section, the WMH surveys were implemented according to widely accepted ethical standards, including review of human subject research by an independent ethics board and voluntary consent. The protocols used for obtaining informed consent, though, varied across participating countries.

Originally developed by the World Medical Association in Helsinki, Finland, in 1964, and most recently revised in 2004, the Declaration of Helsinki sets forth a series of ethical guidelines that have been adopted internationally by researchers conducting medical and social science human subject research. The principles outlined in the Declaration of Helsinki are based on principles initially established in the landmark Nuremberg Code, a set of ten principles developed in response to the atrocities committed in medical research experiments carried out under the Nazi regime. One of the basic principles listed in the declaration is the necessity of an independent ethics committee to review study protocols. The WHO also issued a set of guidelines for ethics committees that addresses a range of areas, such as the role of an ethics review board, board composition, and review procedures (WHO 2000). A human subject review board or ethics committee reviewed the study protocol for the survey in each participating country. In some countries, the WMH study was reviewed by multiple committees.

Although voluntary consent has been established as a universally accepted ethical standard, there is variability in how consent procedures are implemented across countries, depending on cultural traditions and norms regarding individual decision making and the signing of official documents. Family members and community leaders can play a key role in decision making in some cultures, whereas in others the consent decision will typically be an individual one (Bulmer 1998; Marshall 2001; Sugarman et al. 2001; Dawson & Kass 2005). In some countries, respondents may be concerned about providing a signature on a consent form because of past experience with oppressive governments that used signed documents to persecute individuals (National Bioethics Advisory Committee [NBAC] 2001). This concern appears to be particularly prevalent in African and Latin American countries (NBAC 2001). Methodological research conducted in the United States suggests that there is a small but not insignificant minority of respondents (7%–13%) who would be willing to participate in an interview but unwilling to sign a consent form (Singer 1978, 2003). The literacy level of the population and the use of technical language in the written form or oral script are also important considerations when developing culturally appropriate consent procedures (Dawson & Kass 2005).

In the WMH Survey Initiative, interviewers were required to read a statement of voluntary participation, but the WMH protocol allowed for variation across countries in how interviewers obtained respondent consent. In eight countries (France, Japan, Lebanon, the Netherlands,

New Zealand, South Africa, Spain, Ukraine), respondents were required to provide written consent that documented their understanding of the study and their willingness to participate before the start of the interview. In Lebanon and Ukraine, an interviewer could record his or her own signature to indicate respondent consent if the respondent was uncomfortable providing a signature. Oral consent was obtained in the remaining WMH surveys. In the latter countries, respondents were required to agree to participate after they were informed about the purpose of the study and the nature of the survey request before the interview could begin.

## 7. FIELD STRUCTURE AND IMPLEMENTATION

The WMH surveys were large field data collection efforts that involved the planning and implementation of data collection protocols and the close management of field staff to meet production goals and data-quality standards. Participating countries shared many of the same challenges in implementing this study and often adopted similar strategies to manage production and to maximize data quality. However, it is interesting to note differences in a number of areas of data collection implementation, including the use of computerized management systems and various techniques used to reduce nonresponse. This section addresses three main features of data collection field structure and implementation: the structure of the field operations, the implementation of data collection procedures, and field supervision.

### 7.1. Structure of Field Operations

As is detailed in Chapter 2, the majority of WMH surveys were administered to national samples. The supervisory structure of most of these surveys included a field coordinator who headed a team of field supervisors that directly oversaw the interviewers' work. The wide geographic dispersion of the sample, the long duration of the survey, and the large sample size often required several supervisory levels. In the majority of the surveys, each interviewer was assigned to a specific geographic area near his or her home. In some countries, traveling interviewing teams were also used to accommodate interviewing in households located in remote areas or to deal with security concerns. The latter approach was used in Colombia, Japan, Lebanon, Mexico, Nigeria, and Spain.

In many cases, countries received assistance from the WMH Data Collection Coordination Centre in selecting the data collection organization. The pool of organizations from which to choose varied greatly by country, as did contractual arrangements. The Data Collection Coordination Centre provided minimum specifications and a budget template for organizations to bid, but frequently these were questioned or challenged, depending on the firm's experience or the data collection traditions in the country. For example, we were repeatedly questioned about the length of the training required. Most data collection organizations simply did not have experience with such a complex project and could not understand why training would take more than a few hours or a day at most. The organizations that conducted interviewing for the WMH Survey Initiative were most commonly private, for-profit research companies. However, academic research centers or institutes, government agencies, and not-for-profit research organizations were also involved in implementing data collection for the WMH surveys (Table 3.1).

## 7.2. Field Implementation

The majority of organizations carrying out data collection for the WMH Survey Initiative used a paper-and-pencil–based case management system to deliver sample cases to interviewers, to determine study eligibility, to implement respondent selection procedures, and to record information for each contact attempt (e.g., date, time, outcome of each call attempt). However, there were some countries, including France, Israel, Italy, Japan, Mexico, the Netherlands, Spain, and the United States, that relied exclusively on a computerized case management system or implemented both computerized and paper-based components. CAPI case management systems automate activities at two or more lev-

els of field operations, including at the level of the decentralized interviewing staff in the field who complete work on laptop computers and at the level of the supervisors in the field who oversee and manage field staff and/or staff at the central office who direct field operations (Nicholls & Kindel 1993). At the interviewer level, CAPI case management systems often perform the following functions: storage of interviewing assignments, selection of cases to interview (including random sampling within the household), recording of the outcome for each contact attempt, storage of interview data, and communications functions (Nicholls & Kindel 1993; Connett 1998). CAPI case management systems support a number of supervisory or office staff activities, including assignment and reassignment of sample cases, receipt of survey data, reporting of production and cost data, and additional administrative functions. Computerized case management systems may offer a number of advantages over paper-and-pencil methods, including more timely access to cost and quality information from the field and the ability to identify and resolve problem cases more quickly (Nicholls & Kindel 1993). Countries varied in terms of their available technical expertise and experience in designing and implementing computer applications for survey interviewing and operations. The Data Collection Coordination Centre provided technical assistance to help support those countries with less experience.

As noted previously, interviews were conducted face-to-face in all participating countries. In the United States, if the respondent had privacy concerns or if the interview took two or more sessions to complete, later parts of the interview could be administered by telephone. Screening and respondent selection procedures were also typically completed in person, although screening and respondent selection in France were carried out entirely by telephone, and these steps were carried out partially by telephone in Belgium and the Netherlands. Most interviewing was conducted in the respondent's home, but in some countries, a limited number of interviews were completed in other locations. These locations included the respondent's place of employment, hostels or other group quarters, libraries, churches, meeting rooms of apartment buildings, cafés, the office of the research organization conducting the study, and the yard outside the respondent's residence.

## 7.3. Techniques for Maximizing Cooperation

Planning for and implementing techniques that minimize nonresponse are vital to the success of a field data collection effort. Two major sources of survey nonresponse are refusals (cases in which the selected respondent refuses to participate or in which another household member does so on the respondent's behalf) and noncontacts (cases in which the interviewer is unable to contact the sample household/respondent). Quite different factors may affect each component; for example, de Leeuw and de Heer (2002) found that while refusal rates differed across countries and across surveys, noncontact rates differed across countries but not across types of surveys. The survey topic was the same in all WMH surveys, although some surveys introduced the topic as health and stress, whereas others explicitly mentioned mental health. We can expect attitudes to being asked about mental health problems to have differed across countries.

As part of their conceptual framework for survey cooperation, Groves and Couper (1998) identify a set of survey design features that researchers can use to maximize cooperation. These include sending an advance notification of the survey request (typically a letter sent from the sponsoring agency that introduces the request), the use of respondent incentives, repeated attempts to contact households, and specialized interviewer training addressing respondent concerns in order to reduce non-response. Each of these was used in the WMH Survey Initiative and is discussed in turn subsequently.

As Table 3.1 shows, many countries sent an advance letter and/or study brochure or informational material as called for in the WMH Survey Initiative protocol. In addition, some countries used a media announcement that provided information about the upcoming study. In Colombia, establishing contact with local community leaders was a successful strategy to maximize the response rate, particularly in low-income areas. It was also valuable as a protective measure for interviewers working in areas controlled by militias.

Respondent incentives – typically money or gifts offered by the survey organization to encourage participation – have been shown to boost response rates in face-to-face surveys (Groves & Couper 1998; Singer et al. 1999; Groves et al. 2004). Monetary incentives appear to be more effective than gifts, and there appears to be a linear relationship between amount and response rate (Singer et al. 1999). Incentives are particularly powerful when respondents are asked to participate in a burdensome interview (Singer et al. 1999). Incentives can actually lower survey costs by reducing the amount of interviewer effort needed to gain cooperation (Groves et al. 2004). However, much of the incentives literature is based on U.S. studies, and there is clearly a need for further research on the use of incentives in cross-national studies (Lynn 2001).

As Table 3.1 shows, more than half of the WMH countries used a respondent incentive. These incentives were used either for all respondents or for a particular group of sample cases as a special measure to increase participation. Money and gift certificates were the most commonly used types of incentives. In Lebanon, all respondents were offered free psychiatric consultation after the interview, although few availed themselves of the service. A voucher for home delivery of a meal, such as a pizza, was offered to busy, reluctant respondents to make it easier for them to participate in New Zealand. In Spain, sample members who initially refused were offered EUR 25 paid upon completion of the interview. In an attempt to maximize response rates, the United States increased respondent incentives from US$50 to US$100 near the end of the field period.

As identified in the work of Groves and colleagues (2004), a second major contributor to survey nonresponse is the inability to contact sample households. According to the Groves and Couper (1998) model of contactability, the likelihood of establishing contact with a sample household is, in part, a function of the number of call attempts and the timing of the calls. Using data from large U.S. face-to-face household surveys, Groves and Couper (1998), Bates (2003), and Groves and colleagues (2004) found that weekday evenings and weekends were the most productive times to contact sample households. Purdon, Campanelli, and Sturgis (1999) reported that evenings were most productive in the U.K. Family Resources Survey. However, Groves and Couper (1998) noted that calling patterns may vary across countries. For example, in some countries where there is a strong Christian religious tradition, data collection agencies may choose to limit call attempts made on Sundays. De Leeuw and de Heer (2002) also provide evidence that differences in at-home patterns across countries may influence contactability. Although the timing of call attempts has been addressed in several studies, there has been limited research on the optimum number of attempts for face-to-face surveys. Bates (2003), for example, suggested that 14 attempts might be the optimum number for the U.S. Survey of Income and Program Participation, on the basis of analysis of call history data.

The WMH Survey Initiative protocol called for a minimum of ten call attempts to each sample household that were varied across days and time to ensure that contact would be made with nearly all sample households. Most countries followed this guideline, but several countries were able to reach the established response rate without making ten contacts. Countries adapted these requirements on the basis of known at-home patterns. Other strategies used to maximize the probability of contact included leaving brochures at the doorstep and mailing letters to households that were particularly difficult to reach. Enlisting the help of neighbors and local governments and health authorities also seemed to be a valuable strategy for contacting hard-to-reach households in some countries.

As mentioned previously, interviewer training addressed the importance of high response rates. The length, content, and frequency of trainings addressing this issue varied depending on how much effort was needed to reach the Initiative's response rate goals. For example, in the United States, where response rates for surveys continue to decline, considerable time and effort was spent on this topic in the initial interviewer training. Several workshops were also held, and weekly conference calls and periodic newsletters emphasized successful techniques and strategies for maximizing response rates.

In most participating countries, an attempt was made to convert sample members who initially refused to participate in the survey. The WMH Survey Initiative protocol required that efforts be made to reduce nonresponse through these methods. However, each country adapted the protocol on the basis of cultural appropriateness (Heath et al. 2005). For example, a supervisor made the refusal conversion attempt in Colombia. In Israel, initial refusal conversion attempts involved one to three personal visits, a persuasion letter, that is, a letter addressing the specific concerns about participation sent to households that initially refused, and a telephone call from the regional supervisor. Some countries used specially designated interviewers to address reluctant respondent concerns.

## 8. INTERVIEWER EFFECTS AND INTERVIEW PRIVACY

This section focuses on the monitoring strategies implemented in the WMH Survey Initiative to optimize data quality. As mentioned earlier, all WMH surveys used face-to-face interviewing. Although face-to-face interviewing has a number of advantages, it involves respondent-interviewer interaction that can lead to response bias (Biemer & Lyberg 2003; Groves et al. 2004), which makes it important to address the issues of interviewer effects and privacy as part of the supervision and quality-control process.

The behavior, mannerisms, appearance, and vocalization of the interviewer have long been known to have a potential effect on the respondents' answers to questions. Although most of the literature on interviewer effects is based in the United States, we can expect variation across cultures and countries. These variations could be the result of cultural factors such as the ease of building rapport between the interviewer and respondent, the respondents' expectations about the interviewer's behavior and the interviewing task, and the need for conformity (Harkness et al. 2002).

Interviewer variation occurs even when interviewers are well trained (Biemer & Lyberg 2003). Interviewer behavior may vary in the determination of household and respondent eligibility; how questions are asked, probed, and clarified; how feedback is provided; how the respondent's answer is interpreted; and how answers are recorded (Groves 1989; Fowler & Mangione 1990; Fowler 1992; Lessler & Kalsbeek 1992; Biemer & Lyberg 2003; Groves et al. 2004).

Interviewers can also induce systematic effects that bias respondents' answers as a result of their mere presence, their observable traits (which may interact with the survey topic, such as questions on race), or their level of experience (Schuman & Hatchett 1976; Kane & Macaulay 1993; Turner et al. 1998; Gfroerer, Eyerman & Chromy 2002).

A number of survey design factors have been reported to influence the magnitude of interviewer effects. These include length and complexity of the interview, mode of the interview, hiring and training methods, interviewing protocols (e.g., the level of standardization required in the interview), the interview setting (e.g., whether it allows for sufficient privacy and attentiveness), and above all, the extent of field supervision (Biemer & Lyberg 2003).

Systematic monitoring is considered the key element for supervision (Billiet & Loosveldt 1988; Fowler & Mangione 1990). In *Introduction to Survey Quality*, Biemer & Lyberg (2003) describe four key areas of performance that are usually targeted in the supervision process: detection and prevention of falsified information, compliance with the interviewing rules and guidelines set forth in the training, performance of noninterview tasks, and identification of interviewer-questionnaire interface problems. These areas could be evaluated by a number of methods including reinterview, verification, observation, audio recording, questionnaire review, analysis of performance and production measures, keystroke/trace file analysis (files that record keystrokes and movement of the interviewer through the computerized instrument), and mock interviews/tests of knowledge and practice. The WMH Survey Initiative used a combination of all of these strategies to address the key areas of performance.

The WMH guidelines required a fairly rigorous training protocol (described previously); interviewing aids such as the respondent booklet (also described previously); respondent and interviewer matching on race, ethnicity, and gender; privacy during the interview as appropriate and feasible; interview verification; interview editing; and data review (described in the section herein "Manual Editing").

In face-to-face surveys containing sensitive questions about symptoms, behaviors, and experiences, such as those asked in the CIDI, controlling the presence of others in the interview interaction is critical for data quality. This can be difficult in the best of circumstances, but it is much more difficult in some cultures and in some households. Housing arrangements, family size and structure, and the norms with regard to being interviewed in private by a stranger vary across countries and cultures (Harkness et al. 2002). These factors very much influenced interviewers' success in securing a private setting for the WMH interview. Privacy concerns were raised in countries such as China, Colombia, Lebanon, Mexico, Nigeria, South Africa, and Ukraine. In Colombia, Nigeria, Mexico, and South Africa, the challenge came in poorer communities, where the entire family lived in one room. In these cases, interviewers tried to use churches, cultural "houses," other nearby institutions, or simply a nearby outside space to conduct the interview. In Mexico, where CAPI was used, interviewers carried extra laptop batteries to enable them to conduct the interview outside the house. In Lebanon, privacy concerns were partially dealt with by matching the gender of the respondent to that of the interviewer when it would have been inappropriate for a female household member to be interviewed by a male interviewer. Race and ethnicity matching also occurred in some countries or occurred as a result of matching language.

## 9. FIELD SUPERVISION AND QUALITY CONTROL

Considering data collection costs and data quality, the optimum recommended supervisor-to-interviewer ratio is 1 for every 8 to 10 experienced interviewers (Groves 1989). Most of the WMH surveys had a supervisor-to-interviewer ratio in this range, despite the wide variation in field structure (Table 3.1). However, surveys using the PAPI mode had a higher ratio than CAPI surveys, which reflects the greater control over the data collection process offered by computerized interviewing (Williams 1986; Lavrakas 1993).

One of the main roles of a field supervisor is monitoring an interviewer's work. Supervisory observation provides a wider range of information on interviewer's performance during the interview than does any other method (Biemer & Lyberg 2003). Common observational methods for face-to-face interviewing include direct observation – when the supervisor observes the interview – or audio recording of part or all of the interview. More than half of the WMH surveys used either one or both of these methods. Those using these methods reported that they randomly recorded or observed between 5% and 10% of each interviewer's work. This is a level of observation that is generally recommended (Groves et al. 2004). Some countries combined methods. For example, in Israel, the first two interviews were observed directly and then randomly selected cases were audio recorded.

Observational methods, however, do not detect deliberate violation of interview guidelines (Biemer & Lyberg 2003). Other methods such as recontacting respondents who completed an interview become essential for this purpose. The WMH Survey Initiative required that 10% of each interviewer's work be verified. Factual questions from the beginning, middle, and end of the interview were to be verified by supervisory staff either by phone or through face-to-face visits. Although the majority of the countries implemented the required rate or more, strict consistency in implementing these guidelines across countries was impossible. The geographic dispersion of the population, the structure of the field operation, and cultural and behavioral norms, as well as funding, determined what could be accomplished.

Cases identified for verification were either randomly selected or were targeted, such as in the case of Ukraine (where carelessness or falsification was suspected in a limited number of interviews). Information gathered during verification varied by survey but included at least two of the following items: study eligibility, response to key questionnaire items, length of interview, feedback on interviewer's professionalism, use of incentives, and date and time of interview. The most common mode of recontacting respondents was by telephone (China, Belgium, Israel, Italy, Spain), followed by face-to-face visits and telephone (Colombia, Lebanon, New Zealand, Ukraine), mail only (Germany, Japan), face-to-face visits only (Nigeria), and a combination of the three modes (United States).

Inadequate interviewer training and supervision and poor quality control are the main organizational factors that contribute to interviewer falsification. However, when appropriate quality-control methods are used, interview falsification is rare and typically involves only a small percentage of interviewers (American Association for Public Opinion Research [AAPOR] 2003; Groves et al. 2004). Falsification includes fabricating all or part of the interview, miscoding the answer to a question, deliberately misreporting the disposition of a case, and deliberately interviewing a nonsampled person. Of the 17 WMH surveys discussed here, six reported confirmed falsification of data. These included surveys conducted in China, Germany, Lebanon, New Zealand, Spain, and the United States. In the majority of these surveys, few interviewers were involved. In two countries, there appears to have been widespread irregularities. In these latter countries, it appeared that as an interviewer became more familiar with the instrument, fewer positive answers were recorded on the screening questions near the beginning of the instrument. Two things should be noted: a "yes" answer to any screening question resulted in longer survey administration time, and interviewers in these countries were paid by the completed interview. In one of these countries, the data were discarded and the survey had to be repeated. In the other, the data from only one area was found to be unstable and was eliminated from the sample.

In the remaining countries, suspected falsification was dealt with by reviewing all the sample lines worked by the interviewer (e.g., China, Lebanon, Nigeria, and United States), by reviewing only completed interviews (Spain), or by a combination of both (New Zealand). Attempts to retake these interviews were the most common practice, except in Nigeria and Spain, where falsified interviews were deleted from the data set. Countries using CAPI reported that review of the audit files that record keystrokes and section timings was very helpful in detecting such falsification.

Another effective method of quality monitoring is reviewing completed interviews and other interview-related materials, such as respondent selection materials (Biemer & Lyberg 2003; AAPOR 2005). This was also recommended in the WMH Survey Initiative guidelines. This type of review is important for both modes of interviewing used in the WMH study (CAPI and PAPI), but even more so for the PAPI version, given the highly complex nature of the WMH instrument. In recognition of this, the WMH guidelines required all completed PAPI interviews to be edited.

In addition to reviewing completed questionnaires (described subsequently), reviews were also conducted to check whether the appropriate respondent was selected. Except for countries that used a population registry to select their respondents, all WMH surveys included some level of quality control on eligibility and respondent selection procedures, with the majority reviewing all completed selection procedures. In nearly all of the surveys, cases with errors were sent back to the field for follow-up.

Although the type and level of supervision methods implemented in the WMH surveys varied from one country to another, countries employed a variety of effective methods to monitor data quality, with many countries going well

beyond the minimum requirements specified in the WMH guidelines.

## 10. DATA PREPARATION

As Figure 3.1 illustrates, the majority of the WMH countries spent at least as much time processing their data as collecting it. Data-processing operations – which generally include editing, coding, data entry, cleaning, weighting, and variance estimation (Biemer & Lyberg 2003) – are costly, time consuming (Gagnon, Gough & Yeo 1994), and above all, error prone. The errors introduced by such operations vary by the type of processing activity and the data collection mode (Lyberg et al. 1997). Although keying errors in CAPI surveys have been reported as quite small, usually between 0.095% and 1.6% (Henderson & Allen 1981; Jabine, King & Petroni 1990; U.S. Bureau of the Census 1993; Dielman & Couper 1995), coding errors could reach as high as 20% for some variables (Biemer & Lyberg 2003). Thus, some processing errors are inevitable in any large-scale survey. Computer-assisted interviewing, continuous monitoring, verification protocols, and better staff training can minimize the frequency and effect of these errors (U.S. Federal Committee on Statistical Methodology 2001). As with all phases of data collection, resource constraints limit the type and level of such error-reduction techniques.

We limit our discussion here to manual editing, data entry, coding, and data editing and/or cleaning. Other processing operations such as weighting and variance estimation are discussed in Chapter 2. Manual editing is recommended by most survey method guidelines (AAPOR 2005; Biemer & Lyberg 2003; Groves et al. 2004). This becomes more critical in the case of PAPI administration (Groves & Mathiowetz 1984; Olsen 1992). During the editing process, questionnaires are usually checked for legibility, missing data, and certain reporting standards (Lyberg et al. 1997). The WMH guidelines required all completed PAPI interviews to be edited. General, as well as study-specific, detailed guidelines were provided to all WMH countries regarding the editing process and items to be reviewed. As a result of the complexity and length of the CIDI, editing a completed PAPI questionnaire was estimated to take about half of the interview administration time. All PAPI WMH surveys followed these guidelines, and all completed interviews were reviewed by some level of supervisory staff or specially trained editors. This also extended to most CAPI surveys (Colombia, Germany, Israel, Japan, Mexico, New Zealand, Spain, United States) but on a much smaller sample (United States: 5%; Germany, Israel, Japan, and Spain: 10%). Countries using CAPI were also able to monitor the quality of the data through a more timely review of basic summary statistics (e.g., prevalence rates and questionnaire/section timings by interviewer) to determine any irregularities.

For the majority of the WMH surveys (where cost and logistic feasibility allowed), questionnaires with errors in administration were sent back to the field for follow-up. In two surveys (Mexico, United States), questionnaires were sometimes sent to the field depending on the type of error and whether an interviewer was still in proximity to the household. Only in Israel and Japan were questionnaires with administration errors never sent back to the field.

The WMH countries that used the PAPI version of the interview had to enter their data manually. Given the length and complexity of the paper interview schedule, this was a fairly labor-intensive task. The task was eased somewhat through the creation of a data-entry program designed by the WMH Data Collection Coordination Centre. Modeled after the CAPI program, automatic skips, range checks, and some consistency checks were built into the program. These programs were then adapted for each country. However, countries that added new sections to the main CIDI or incorporated numerous revisions to noncore sections designed either an independent data-entry program or one that supported the WMH data-entry application.

Data-entry verification protocols used by the majority of the WMH countries evaluated keying errors on a sample of entered interviews rather than on all interviews. Such an approach, called acceptance sampling, is a commonly practiced quality-assurance scheme in the face of budget limitations (U.S. Federal Committee on Statistical Methodology 2001). Keying sampling rates in the WMH surveys ranged from 10% (Ukraine) to 20% (Lebanon), with two countries (Nigeria, South Africa) relying only on the edit checks built into the data-entry program to check the data quality. Although independent double entry was recommended in the WMH guidelines and is known to be more effective in minimizing keying errors, dependent review of the keyed entries against the completed questionnaires was also used (e.g., in Lebanon).

Establishing a diagnosis of a mental disorder on the basis of responses to the WMH interview required ascertaining that the symptoms were not due to a physical cause or to the use of medication or drugs (i.e., organic causes). To avoid any misinterpretation of the cause of symptoms, organic exclusion questions were included in every diagnostic section of the instrument. These questions were open ended and required specialized coding. A standard coding scheme and protocol was distributed to all countries and required that a mental health professional review and code these questions.

Occupation coding was also performed in almost half of the WMH surveys (China, Israel, Japan, Lebanon, the Netherlands, New Zealand, Ukraine, United States). All used the International Standard Classification of Occupations (ISCO-88) coding scheme to enable comparisons across the surveys. Coders ranged from special designated teams (e.g., editors) to field supervisory staff and research staff.

To reduce the frequency of coding errors, the WMH guidelines required 10% double coding. However, only a few countries (Israel, Lebanon, New Zealand, Nigeria, United States) verified a sample of interviews (ranging from 10% to 20%) using either dependent revision – having a supervisor review the codes already assigned (e.g., Lebanon, Nigeria) – or double coding (New Zealand). Variations and lack of adherence to the recommended guidelines are explained by the lack of resources in many countries. Because coding typically comes near the end of the survey life cycle, this is also when projects may feel budget constraints more acutely and are forced to cut back on quality-control procedures.

Bringing all the WMH survey data sets to a standard clean format required a considerable amount of time and effort. Data cleaning was carried out iteratively between the country and the WMH Data Analysis Coordination Centre at Harvard Medical School. Each country was required to provide a clean data set checked for commonly recommended items (Biemer & Lyberg 2003; Council of American Survey Research Organizations 1994), including a unique interview-identification number scheme, absence of blank or all-missing variables, variables with only one response, out-of-range responses, consistency checks (e.g., symptoms, recency, age greater than or equal to age of onset, consistent gender information) and requiring complete data on a minimum set of items such as the screening section and main stem questions in each section. Programs were then run on all data sets to ensure that these minimum standards were met. Records with errors were flagged and returned to the country for clarification. There were a few local variations on this process. About half of the countries conducted additional cleaning by reviewing illogical values or inappropriate missing data for descriptive statistics (e.g., China, France, Israel, Lebanon, Mexico, New Zealand, Nigeria, Spain, United States) or by cleaning open-ended responses (China, France, Germany, Israel, Lebanon, Nigeria, Spain, the Netherlands, Ukraine). The latter was done by translating the responses (e.g., Ukraine), by reclassifying them into precoded answers (e.g., Israel), or by checking the legibility and appropriateness of certain items such as medication names (e.g., Lebanon).

Despite efforts to monitor data quality throughout data collection, including reviewing all completed PAPI interviews, all countries reported spending significant time and resources cleaning data. This speaks to the considerable complexity of the interview schedule but also is a result of variability in quality control in the data-entry process that was subsequently detected in review of preliminary data files by the WMH Data Analysis Coordination Centre. In retrospect, it might have been more cost-effective to have spent additional resources checking the data entry, which would have necessitated fewer resources in cleaning the data after the fact.

## 11. IMPUTATION OF ITEM MISSING DATA

The WMH questionnaire was a complex survey instrument, and, as is the case in all surveys, there was a small amount of missing data for individual variables including the key demographic items that are routinely used in the analyses reported in other chapters of this volume. To prepare the core tables of survey estimates and analytical statistics for this book, the Harvard WMH Data Analysis Coordination Centre applied a hierarchical series of rules to impute missing values for selected key demographic variables: age, gender, marital status, education, and income category. Generally, hot-deck methods (Little & Rubin 2003) were used to impute missing values for these five category variables. Imputations were also performed for key substantive variables (e.g., age of onset) using hot-deck imputation. In a limited number of cases in which the rates of missing data were higher (e.g., income), regression methods were used to impute missing values.

## 12. CONCLUSIONS

Although cross-national surveys have been undertaken for decades, coordinated surveys that anticipate comparisons across nations, known as *ex ante* study designs, are a relatively new approach (Harkness et al. 2004; Heath et al. 2005). Although monocultural best practices are generally well established, we know little about how to specify and implement best practices across a wide variety of cultures and nations. The right balance between standards and local adaptations to achieve comparability is as yet not known. In the absence of guidance about this balance, the WMH Data Collection Coordination Centre attempted to adapt monocultural best practices to the circumstances and contexts of the participating countries, modifying the approach as needed, to achieve consistent cross-national goals of data quality. We also sought to document as much of the survey implementation process as feasible to be able to inform and contribute to future developments in cross-national survey methods.

We believe that several key features of the WMH Survey Initiative have contributed to its success. The core features were the existence of standards and guidelines, ongoing technical and methodological support from the WMH centres, and commitment and engagement on the part of the country collaborators and their staff. As we have detailed, guidelines were developed for all phases of the WMH Survey Initiative, from sample design through data processing. These were created with the goal of ensuring best practices across the Initiative, but with the recognition that these practices had to be adapted to local conditions. For example, with regard to the sample design specifications, the initiative set the goal of implementing a probability sample, a minimum sample size, and a minimum response rate. Countries varied in the sampling frames, stages of selection, age of majority, and response rate. The interview had core modules, but countries were free to add country-specific content. Guidelines were developed for translation and assessment, but the collaborators in each country were responsible for their implementation and quality. Training content, protocols, and length of training were specified, but countries adapted these as needed. Ethics reviews were required but were implemented according to local laws, regulations, and norms. Guidelines and recommendations were given with regard to field structure and interviewer remuneration but were constrained by local norms, contracts, geographic challenges, and the length of the field period. Quality-control steps were detailed, and in many cases countries added additional steps. The software application for data collection was provided, but the decision of whether to use CAPI or PAPI was left to the country.

Although some of these guidelines violated local research traditions, they were largely followed. This is rather remarkable, given that each country complied voluntarily. However, implementation of some aspects of these guidelines was met with more success than others. Two areas

that were difficult to realize were interviewer payment protocols and data editing and processing for quality control – the former because of entrenched organizational research traditions and limited experience with an instrument of this complexity, as well as contractual limitations, and the latter largely because of cost constraints.

Simply establishing guidelines was not sufficient. Ultimately, decisions had to be made with regard to their enforcement. Indeed, as compelling as it was to have as many countries as possible participate in the Initiative, the quality of any one country's data affected the overall initiative. Although done with great reluctance and only after all other avenues for correction were explored, in the end, data from four countries were eliminated from the final data set for failure to meet these standards. These countries are not named here because of confidentiality reasons and are no longer included in the WMH Survey Initiative. Three of the four countries had problems that were the result of an inability to resolve serious discrepancies found in the final data set. The other was the result of changing the instrument so fundamentally that it was no longer comparable to the other countries.

An important fact that distinguishes the WMH Survey Initiative from many large-scale research projects of this kind is that there was no central funding that flowed to the countries. Each country had to seek its own funding for data collection and secure the services of a data collection organization. Although technical support came from the WMH Data Collection Coordination Centre, this support was limited to providing the instrument, computer software for CAPI implementation and PAPI data entry, training, and periodic consultation with the local collaborators in each country.

It took great effort and perseverance for countries to raise the necessary funds to implement a study that could meet these guidelines. For many, this took several years. For countries with governments that changed several times over the course of the Initiative, funds sometimes had to be secured more than once. Once funding was obtained, finding an organization that would undertake the survey was yet another challenge. Several countries also had to do this more than once, when the organization they first selected could not meet the quality-control standards. Even countries that used offices of official statistics or academic research institutes encountered some level of skepticism regarding the length and complexity of the instrument, the level of training needed, and the quality control required.

Funding also drove the schedules in most countries. Countries that fielded their studies earliest were affected most acutely, as procedures and protocols were still under development while data collection preparation was well under way. A particular source of tension was the need to start translations (especially given the length of the instrument) while the instrument was still under development. This was necessary given the schedule constraints but created some significant inefficiencies.

In retrospect, there are a number of areas where we would suggest changes in approach in future initiatives of a similar kind. The first recommendation would be to ensure adequate time for the study development stage. As with any such enterprise, more planning would have made for a smoother implementation of the WMH Survey Initiative. Again, the constraints imposed by funding and schedules affected what could be accomplished. Much more core funding for infrastructure development than was available to us would be needed to implement this suggestion.

The second recommendation would be to challenge preconceived ideas of where CAPI could and could not be used. Several developing countries used CAPI with great success (e.g., Colombia); and several other countries, in retrospect, wished they had implemented the CAPI version of the instrument. The PAPI version was so long (more than 500 pages) and complex, that even with strict quality-control protocols and 100% review of completed questionnaires, errors were inevitable. If use of the CAPI instrument was not possible, then securing enough laptops to facilitate entry of completed cases on a daily basis would have made a significant difference. Here, earlier feedback to the field would have

allowed supervisors to intervene more effectively when problems were encountered.

The third recommendation would be to require more rigor than existed in many WMH surveys with respect to checking data quality. Despite many cautions about regularly reviewing data, some countries (even some using CAPI) simply did not have the means to check the data on a regular basis. Although the Initiative specified use of the same questionnaire application software, we left sample management up to each country. We provided guidelines on what data items should be tracked and specified the detail needed to determine response rates across countries. We also suggested replicate samples to control costs and response rates, but countries were largely left on their own to implement sample control procedures. If we had implemented even a rudimentary sample management system that would have allowed countries to monitor and review data on a daily or even a weekly basis, countries would have been able to detect problems much more quickly. Such a system also would have allowed the WMH coordination centres to provide a higher level of guidance. Often, when a country sought the advice of the centres, in the absence of detailed sample control information, it was difficult to diagnose the source of the problem.

The fourth recommendation would be to build in a much longer period of time for pretesting the instrument and field procedures than we did in the WMH Survey Initiative. This would be especially important in countries where the estimated prevalence of mental disorders turned out to be implausibly low. Pretesting should focus on the full range of field procedures and, in particular, should include a clinical reappraisal component that evaluates the concordance of diagnoses based on the CIDI with diagnoses based on blinded clinical reappraisal interviews.

Despite these recommendations for future improvements, some of them implying that the data quality of the WMH surveys could have been improved, the WMH Survey Initiative has to be seen as a major achievement. The Initiative successfully implemented a methodologically rigorous protocol across a wide variety of developing and developed countries. This success was due to the development and implementation of guidelines for the flexible attainment of specified data-quality goals by an extraordinary cadre of highly committed country-based collaborators who were willing to bridge the gap between the central organization and the unique conditions of local circumstances. The local expertise and epidemiological survey infrastructure created in this way will serve as a firm foundation for future expansions and refinements.

## REFERENCES

American Association for Public Opinion Research (AAPOR) (2003). Interviewer falsification in survey research: Current best methods for prevention, detection and repair of its effects. Lenexa, KS: AAPOR.

American Association for Public Opinion Research (AAPOR) (2005). AAPOR standards and best practices. Lenexa, KS: AAPOR. Available at http://www.aapor.org/bestpractices.

Baker, R. P., Bradburn, N. M. & Johnson, R. A. (1995). Computer-assisted personal interviewing: An experimental evaluation of data quality and cost. *Journal of Official Statistics*, 11, 413–31.

Bates, N. (2003). Contact histories in personal visit surveys: The Survey of Income and Program Participation (SIPP) Methods Panel. Proceedings of the Survey Methods Section of the American Statistical Association.

Biemer, P. & Lyberg, L. (2003). *Introduction to survey quality*. New York: John Wiley & Sons.

Billiet, J. & Loosveldt, G. (1988). Interviewer training and quality of responses. *Public Opinion Quarterly*, 52, 190–211.

Bulmer, M. (1998). The problem of exporting social survey research. *American Behavioral Scientist*, 42, 153–67.

Connett, W. (1998). Automated management of survey data: An overview. In *Computer-assisted survey information collection*, ed. M. P. Couper, R. P. Baker, J. Bethlehem, C. Z. F. Clark, J. Martin, W. L. Nicholls II & J. M. O'Reilly, pp. 245–62. New York: John Wiley & Sons.

Converse, J. & Presser, S. (1986). *Survey questions: Handcrafting the standardized questionnaire*, Sage Series No. 63. Thousand Oaks, CA: Sage Publications.

Council of American Survey Research Organizations (1994). *Business practices guidelines*. Port Jefferson, NY: Council of American Survey Research Organizations.

Couper, M. P. (2000). Usability evaluation of computer-assisted survey instruments. *Social Science Computer Review*, 18, 384–96.

Couper, M. P. & Nicholls, W. L., II. (1998). The history and development of computer assisted survey information collection. In *Computer-assisted survey information collection*, ed. M. P. Couper, R. P. Baker, J. Bethlehem, C. Z. F. Clark, J. Martin, W. L. Nicholls II & J. M. O'Reilly, pp. 1–22. New York: John Wiley & Sons.

Dawson, L. & Kass, N. E. (2005). View of U.S. researchers about informed consent in international collaborative research. *Social Science & Medicine*, 61, 1211–22.

de Leeuw, E. & de Heer, W. (2002). Trends in household survey nonresponse: A longitudinal and international comparison. In *Survey nonresponse*, ed. R. M. Groves, D. A. Dillman, J. L. Eltinge & R. J. A. Little, pp. 41–54. New York: John Wiley & Sons.

Dielman, L. & Couper, M. (1995). Data quality in a CAPI survey: Keying errors. *Journal of Official Statistics*, 11, 141–6.

Fowler, F. (1992). How unclear terms affect survey data. *Public Opinion Quarterly*, 56, 218–31.

Fowler, F. & Mangione, T. (1990). *Standardized survey interviewing: Minimizing interviewer-related error*. Newbury Park, CA: Sage Publications.

Gagnon, F., Gough, H. & Yeo, D. (1994). *Survey of editing practices in Statistics Canada*. Technical report for Statistics Canada.

Gfroerer, J., Eyerman. J. & Chromy, J., eds. (2002). *Redesigning an ongoing national household survey: Methodological issues*, DHHS Pub. No. SMA 03-3768. Rockville, MD: Substance Abuse and Mental Health Services Administration.

Groves, R. (1989). *Survey errors and survey costs*. New York: John Wiley & Sons.

Groves, R. M. & Couper, M. P. (1998). *Nonresponse in household interview surveys*. New York: John Wiley & Sons.

Groves, R. M., Fowler, F. J., Jr., Couper, M. P., Lepkowski, J. M., Singer, E. & Tourangeau, R. (2004). *Survey methodology*. New York: John Wiley & Sons.

Groves, R. & Lyberg, L. (1988). An overview of nonresponse issues in telephone surveys. In *Telephone survey methodology*, ed. R. M. Groves, P. P. Biemer, L. E. Lyberg, J. T. Massey, W. L. Nicholls II & J. Waksberg, pp. 191–211. New York: John Wiley & Sons.

Groves, R. M. & Mathiowetz, N. A. (1984). Computer-assisted telephone interviewing: Effect on interviewers and respondents. *Public Opinion Quarterly*, 48, 356–69.

Groves, R. M., & Tortora, R. D. (1998). Integrating CASI into existing designs and organizations: A survey of the field. In *Computer-assisted survey information collection*, ed. M. P. Couper, R. P. Baker, J. Bethlehem, C. Z. F. Clark, J. Martin, W. L. Nicholls II & J. M. O'Reilly, pp. 45–61. New York: John Wiley & Sons.

Harkness, J. (1999). In pursuit of quality: Issues for cross-national survey research. *International Journal of Social Research Methodology,* 2, 125–40.

Harkness, J. A., Pennell, B. E. & Schoua-Glusberg, A. (2004). Survey questionnaire translation and assessment. In *Methods for Testing and Evaluating Survey Questionnaires*, ed. S. Presser, J. Rothgeb, M. P. Couper, J. T. Lessler, E. Martin, J. Martin & E. Singer, pp. 453–74. Hoboken, NJ: John Wiley & Sons.

Harkness, J. A., Van de Vijver, J. R. & Mohler, P. P. (2002). *Cross-cultural survey methods*. New York: John Wiley & Sons.

Heath, A., Fisher, S. & Smith, S. (2005). The globalization of public opinion research. *Annual Review of Political Science*, 8, 297–333.

Henderson, L. & Allen, D. (1981). *NLS data entry quality control: The fourth follow-up survey.* Washington, DC: National Center for Education Statistics, Office of Educational Research and Improvement.

House, C. C. & Nicholls, W. L., II (1988). Questionnaire design for CATI: Design objectives and methods. In *Telephone survey methodology*, ed. R. M. Groves, P. P. Biemer, L. E. Lyberg, J. T. Massey, W. L. Nicholls II & J. Waksberg, pp. 421–36. New York: John Wiley & Sons.

Hox, J. & de Leeuw, E. (1994). A comparison of nonresponse in mail, telephone, and face-to-face surveys: Applying multilevel modeling to meta-analysis. *Quality and Quantity*, 28, 329–44.

Jabine, T., King, K. & Petroni, R. (1990). *Quality profile for the Survey of Income and Program Participation (SIPP)*. Washington, DC: U.S. Bureau of the Census.

Jowell, R. (1998). How comparative is comparative research? *American Behavioral Scientist*, 42, 168–77.

Kane, E. W. & McCauley, L. J. (1993). Interviewer gender and gender attitudes. *Public Opinion Quarterly*, 57, 1–28.

Kessler, R. C., Berglund, P., Chiu, W. T., Demler, O., Heeringa, S., Hiripi, E., Jin, R., Pennell, B.-E., Walters, E. E., Zaslavsky, A., and Zheng, H. (2004). The U.S. National Comorbidity Survey Replication (NCS-R): Design and field procedures. *International Journal of Methods in Psychiatric Research*, 13, 69–92.

Kuechler, M. (1998). The survey method: An indispensable tool for social science research everywhere? *American Behavioral Scientist*, 42, 178–200.

Lavrakas, P. J. (1993). *Telephone survey methods: Sampling, selection, and supervision*. Thousand Oaks, CA: Sage Publications.

Lessler, J. T. & Kalsbeek, W. D. (1992). *Nonsampling error in surveys*. New York: John Wiley & Sons.

Little, RJA & Rubin, DB (2003). Statistical analysis with missing data, 2nd Ed. New York: John Wiley & Sons.

Lyberg, L., Biemer, P., Collins, M., de Leeuw, E., Dippo, C., Schwartz, N. & Trewin D. (1997). *Survey measurement and process quality*. New York: John Wiley & Sons.

Lynn, P. (2001). Developing quality standards for cross-national survey research: Five approaches. Institute for Social and Economic Research Working Papers Nos. 2001–21.

Marshall, P. A. (2001). The relevance of culture for informed consent in U.S.-funded international health research. In *Ethical and policy issues in international research: Clinical trials in developing countries*, Vol. 2, pp. C1–C38. Bethesda, MD: National Bioethics Advisory Commission.

National Bioethics Advisory Committee (NBAC) (2001). *Ethical and policy issues in international research: Clinical trials in developing countries*, Vol. 1. Bethesda, MD: National Bioethics Advisory Committee.

Nicholls, W. L., II, Baker, R. P. & Martin, J. (1997). The effect of new data collection technologies on survey data quality. In *Survey measurement and process quality*, ed. L. Lyberg, P. Biemer, M. Collins, E. de Leeuw, C. Dippo, N. Schwarz & D. Trewin, pp. 221–48. New York: John Wiley & Sons.

Nicholls, W. L., II & Kindel, K. K. (1993). Case management and communications for computer assisted personal interviewing. *Journal of Official Statistics*, 9, 623–39.

Oishi, S. M. (2003). *The Survey Kit, 2nd ed. Volume 5: How to conduct in-person interviews for surveys* Thousand Oaks, CA: Sage Publications.

Olsen, R. (1992). The effects of computer assisted interviewing on data quality. Paper presented at the fourth Social Science Methodology Conference, Trento, Italy.

Pennell, B., Bowers, A., Carr, D., Chardoul, S., Cheung, G., Dinkelmann, K., Gebler, N., Hansen, S. E., Pennell, S. & Torres, M. (2004). The development and implementation of the National Comorbidity Survey Replication, the National Survey of American Life, and the National Latino and Asian American Survey. *International Journal of Methods in Psychiatric Research*, 13, 241–69.

Purdon, S., Campanelli, P. & Sturgis, P. (1999). Interviewers' calling strategies on face-to-face interview surveys. *Journal of Official Statistics*, 15, 199–216.

Schuman, H. & Hatchett, S. (1976). White respondents and race-of-interviewer effects. *Public Opinion Quarterly*, 39, 523–8.

Sheatsley, P. B. (1983). Questionnaire construction and item writing. In *Handbook of survey research: Quantitative studies in social relations*, ed. P. H. Rossi, J. D. Wright & A. B. Anderson, pp. 195–230. New York: Academy Press.

Singer, E. (1978). Informed consent: Consequences for response rate and response quality in social surveys. *American Sociological Review*, 43, 144–62.

Singer, E. (2003). Exploring the meaning of consent: Participation in research and beliefs about risks and benefits. *Journal of Official Statistics*, 19, 273–86.

Singer, E., Van Hoewyk, J., Gebler, N., Raghunathan, T., and McGonagle, K. (1999). The effect of incentives on response rates in interviewer-mediated surveys. *Journal of Official Statistics*, 15, 217–30.

Smith, T. W. (2004). Developing and evaluating cross-national survey instruments. In *Methods for testing and evaluating survey questionnaires*, ed. S. Presser, J. M. Rothgeb, M. P. Couper, J. T. Lessler, E. Martin, J. Martin & E. Singer, pp. 431–52. New York: John Wiley & Sons.

Sugarman, J., Popkin, B., Fortney, J. & Rivera, R. (2001). International perspectives on protecting human research subjects. In *Ethical and policy issues in international research: Clinical trials in developing countries*, Vol. 2, pp. E1–E30. Bethesda, MD: National Bioethics Advisory Commission.

Turner, C., Forsyth, B., O'Reilly, J., Cooley, P., Smith, T., Rogers, S. & Miller, H. (1998). Automated self-interviewing and the survey measurement of sensitive behaviors. In *Computer-assisted survey information collection*, ed. M. P. Couper, R. P. Baker, J. Bethlehem, C. Z. F. Clark, J. Martin, W. L. Nicholls II & J. M. O'Reilly, pp. 455–73. New York: John Wiley & Sons.

U.S. Bureau of the Census (1993). Memorandum for Thomas C. Walsh from John H. Thompson, 1990 Quality Assurance Evaluation, M. Roberts, author, October 18.

U.S. Federal Committee on Statistical Methodology (2001). Measuring and reporting sources of error in surveys. Statistical Policy Working Paper 31. Washington, DC: U.S. Office of Management and Budget.

Williams, B. J. (1986). Suggestions for the application of advanced technology in Canadian collection operations. *Journal of Official Statistics*, 2, 555–60.

World Health Organization (WHO) (2000). *Operational guidelines for ethics committees that review biomedical research*. Geneva: World Health Organization.

# 4 The World Health Organization Composite International Diagnostic Interview

RONALD C. KESSLER AND T. BEDIRHAN ÜSTÜN

## ACKNOWLEDGEMENTS

Preparation of this chapter was supported by the U.S. Public Health Service (U01MH060220, R13MH66849, 3U01MH057716-05S1), the U.S. National Institute of Mental Health (R01MH070884), the John D. and Catherine T. MacArthur Foundation, the Pfizer Foundation, the U.S. Public Health Service (R13-MH066849, R01-MH069864, and R01 DA016558), the Fogarty International Center (FIRCA R03-TW006481), the Pan American Health Organization, Eli Lilly and Company Foundation, Ortho-McNeil Pharmaceutical, Inc., Glaxo-SmithKline, and Bristol-Myers Squibb. We thank the WMH staff for assistance with instrumentation, fieldwork, and data analysis. A complete list of WMH publications can be found at http://www.hcp.med.harvard.edu/wmh/.

Portions of this chapter are based on Kessler, R. C. & Üstün, T. B. (2004). The World Mental Health (WMH) Survey Initiative Version of the World Health Organization (WHO) Composite International Diagnostic Interview (CIDI). The International Journal of Methods in Psychiatric Research, 13(2), 93–121. Copyright © 2004 John Wiley & Sons Limited. All Rights Reserved. Reproduced with permission.

The authors appreciate the helpful comments on earlier drafts by Robert Belli, Beth-Ellen Pennell, Norbert Schwarz, and Hans-Ulrich Wittchen. Portions of this chapter were previously published in Kessler and colleagues (2000) and Kessler and Üstün (2004) and are used here with the permission of the publishers, Lawrence Erlbaum Associates and John Wiley & Sons. The development of CIDI 3.0 depended on the efforts of a great many individuals. Clinical research experts who worked with us on specific diagnostic sections include the following: Jules Angst (major depression, mania), Gavin Andrews (anxiety disorders), James Anthony (substance disorders), Naomi Breslau (posttraumatic stress disorder), Emil Coccaro (intermittent explosive disorder), Ian Falloon (nonaffective psychosis), Abby Fyer (agoraphobia, specific phobia), Josep Maria Haro (family burden), Richard Heimberg (social phobia), David Katzelnick (obsessive-compulsive disorder), Martin Keller (generalized anxiety disorder), Mark Lenzenweger (personality disorders), Armand Lorenger (personality disorders), Bruce Lydiard (irritable bowel syndrome), Susan McElroy (intermittent explosive disorder), Kathleen Merikangas (major depression, mania, nicotine dependence), Dan Mroczek (nonspecific psychological distress), Tom Roth (sleep disorders), John Rush (major depression), Marc Schuckit (substance use disorders), Kathy Shear (panic disorder, separation anxiety disorder), Derrick Silove (separation anxiety disorder), Dan Stein (posttraumatic stress disorder, obsessive-compulsive disorder), Mauricio Tohen (bipolar disorder), Michael Von Korff (chronic pain disorder), Lynn Wallisch (pathological gambling), Philip Wang (services, pharmacoepidemiology), Ken Winters (pathological gambling), and Hans-Ulrich Wittchen (anxiety disorders). Survey methodology experts who worked with us on the various question-wording studies and refinements discussed in the first half of this chapter include Robert Belli, Charles Cannell, Barbel Knauper, Beth-Ellen Pennell, and Norbert Schwarz. CIDI 3.0 is built on the pioneering work of Lee Robins in developing the DIS and the original CIDI and on the work of

Hans-Ulrich Wittchen in developing a number of important CIDI innovations in his M-CIDI. Neither the original DIS nor the CIDI and its extensions would have been possible without the vision of Darrel Regier, who launched the program of research that led to the DIS and subsequently the CIDI.

## I. INTRODUCTION

This chapter presents an overview of the methodological issues involved in modifying the World Health Organization (WHO) Composite International Diagnostic Interview (CIDI) for use in the WMH surveys. The first fully structured psychiatric diagnostic interview that could be administered by trained lay interviewers was the Diagnostic Interview Schedule (DIS) (Robins et al. 1981). The DIS was developed by Lee Robins and her colleagues at Washington University, with support from the National Institute of Mental Health for use in the U.S. Epidemiologic Catchment Area (ECA) Study (Robins & Regier 1991). The ECA was a landmark community-based survey of mental disorders carried out in selected neighborhoods in five U.S. communities. The wide dissemination of ECA results in high-profile publications led to replications in other countries, as well as to the development of other structured diagnostic interviews. The most widely used of the latter is the CIDI (WHO 1990). In fact, the CIDI is an expansion of the DIS that was initially developed by Lee Robins and a group of international collaborators (Robins et al. 1988) under the auspices of WHO to address the problem that DIS diagnoses were exclusively based on the definitions and criteria of the American Psychiatric Association's (APA) *Diagnostic and Statistical Manual of Mental Disorders* (DSM). The WHO was keen to expand the DIS to generate diagnoses based on the definitions and criteria of the WHO International Classification of Disease (ICD). This was especially important for cross-national comparative research, as the ICD system is the international standard diagnostic system.

The initial CIDI development process was carried out in such a way as to encourage scientists in many different countries to carry out community epidemiological surveys. To this end, a multi-national CIDI Editorial Committee translated and field-tested the original version of CIDI in many different countries (Wittchen 1994), while WHO encouraged researchers around the world to carry out CIDI surveys beginning in 1990, when the CIDI was first made available. These efforts were successful, as more than a dozen large-scale CIDI surveys in as many countries were completed during the first half of the 1990s. The WHO created the International Consortium in Psychiatric Epidemiology (ICPE) in 1997 to bring together and compare results across these surveys (Kessler 1999). The ICPE subsequently published a number of useful descriptive studies of cross-national similarities and differences in prevalence and sociodemographic correlates of mental disorders (e.g., Aguilar-Gaxiola et al. 2000; Alegria et al. 2000; WHO International Consortium in Psychiatric Epidemiology 2000; Bijl et al. 2003). However, the work of the ICPE with this first generation of CIDI surveys was hampered by the fact that comparability across surveys was limited to the assessment of mental disorders. Measures of risk factors, consequences, patterns and correlates of treatment, and treatment adequacy were not assessed in a consistent manner across the surveys, as none of these was included in the original version of CIDI.

Recognizing the value of coordinating the measurement of these broader areas of assessment, the ICPE launched an initiative in 1997 to bring together senior scientists who were planning to carry out CIDI surveys over the following few years to coordinate measurement across surveys. Within a short period of time, research groups in more than a dozen countries joined this initiative. The WHO officially established the WHO World Mental Health (WMH) Survey Initiative to coordinate this undertaking in 1998. Since that time, the number of participating WMH countries has expanded to 28 with an anticipated combined sample size of more than 200,000 interviews. The authors of this chapter are the codirectors of both the ICPE and the WMH Survey Initiative, as well as the

**Table 4.1.** An outline of CIDI Version 3.0

| | | |
|---|---|---|
| I. | Screening and lifetime review | |
| II. | Disorders | |
| | A. Mood | Major depression, mania |
| | B. Anxiety | Panic disorder, specific phobia, agoraphobia, GAD, posttraumatic stress disorder, obsessive-compulsive disorder |
| | C. Substance abuse | Alcohol abuse, alcohol dependence, drug abuse, drug dependence, nicotine dependence |
| | D. Childhood | Attention-deficit/hyperactivity disorder, oppositional-defiant disorder, conduct disorder, separation anxiety disorder |
| | E. Other | Intermittent explosive disorder, eating disorders, premenstrual disorder, nonaffective psychoses screen, pathological gambling, neurasthenia, personality disorders screens |
| III. | Functioning and physical disorders | Suicidality, 30-day functioning, 30-day psychological distress, physical comorbidity |
| IV. | Treatment | Services, pharmacoepidemiology |
| V. | Risk factors | Personality, social networks, childhood experiences, family burden |
| VII. | Sociodemographics | Employment, finances, marriage, children, childhood demographics, adult demographics |
| VII. | Methodology | Part One–Part Two selection, interviewer observations |

principal developers of the revised version of CIDI, CIDI Version 3.0, which was created for use in the WMH surveys (Kessler & Üstün 2004).

## 2. AN OVERVIEW OF CIDI 3.0

In the course of expanding the CIDI to include broader areas of assessment, we also took the opportunity to make the diagnostic sections of the CIDI more operational. We expanded questions to break down critical criteria, including the clinical significance criteria required in the DSM-IV system. We expanded the diagnostic sections to include dimensional information along with the categorical information that existed in previous CIDI versions. We also expanded the number of disorders included in the CIDI.

The 41 sections in CIDI 3.0 are listed in Table 4.1 (for the full English source text of CIDI 3.0, see http://www.hcp.med.harvard.edu/wmhcidi/instruments_download.php). The sections listed in Table 4.1 are not in order of assessment, but rather in a conceptual order. The first section in the instrument is an introductory screening and lifetime review section, the logic of which is discussed later in this chapter. Some 22 diagnostic sections follow this intro-

ductory section. Two of these assess mood disorders; while seven, anxiety disorders; two, substance use disorders; four, childhood disorders; and seven, other disorders. Four additional sections assess functioning and physical comorbidity, two assess treatment of mental disorders, four assess risk factors, and seven assess sociodemographics. Two final sections are methodological. The first of these two includes rules for determining which respondents to select into Part 2 of the interview and which ones to terminate after Part One of the interview. The second methodological section consists of interviewer observations that are recorded after the interview has ended.

The entire CIDI takes an average of approximately two hours to administer in most general population samples. Interview time varies widely, though, depending on the number of diagnostic sections for which the respondent endorses diagnostic stem questions. As mentioned in the previous paragraph, the interview has a two-part structure that allows early termination of a representative subsample of respondents who show no evidence of lifetime psychopathology. The sampling fraction used in this subselection procedure influences average interview time. A number of CIDI sections are optional and can be administered to subsamples rather than to the entire sample. This, too, reduces average interview length.

In addition to the interview schedule, we developed an elaborate set of training materials to teach interviewers how to administer the CIDI and to teach supervisors how to monitor the quality of data collection. We developed a computer-assisted version of the interview (CAPI) that can be used with laptop computers. We also developed a direct data-entry (DDE) software system that can be used to key responses to the paper-and-pencil version of the interview (PAPI). Finally, we developed computer programs that generate diagnoses from the completed survey data using the definitions and criteria of both the ICD-10 and the DSM-IV diagnostic systems.

Use of CIDI 3.0 requires successful completion of a training program offered by an official WHO CIDI Training and Reference Centre (CIDI-TRC). Another innovation associated with the CIDI is a state-of-the art interviewer-training program that includes an intelligent 40-hour, CD-ROM self-study module in addition to a three-day, face-to-face training module that requires the trainee to travel to an authorized CIDI-TRC. The three-day, face-to-face training program is designed for individuals who have successfully completed the self-study module, as indicated by passing the self-administered tests embedded throughout the CD-ROM. Remedial training elements are embedded in the CD-ROM whenever a trainee fails a test. Trainees who successfully complete the certification process at the end of the training program are given access to all CIDI training materials for use in training interviewers and supervisors and are also given copies of the CIDI, CAPI, and DDE programs and the computerized diagnostic algorithms. Contact information for CIDI training can be obtained from the CIDI Web page (http://www.who.int/msa/cidi).

## 3. THE VALIDITY OF CIDI DIAGNOSTIC ASSESSMENTS

A number of DIS and CIDI validity studies were carried out prior to the launch of the WMH Survey Initiative. These studies aimed to determine whether the diagnoses generated by the DIS and CIDI are consistent with those obtained independently by trained clinical interviewers who administer blinded semistructured research diagnostic interviews to people who previously completed the DIS or CIDI. Wittchen (1994) reviewed these studies up through the early 1990s. Only a handful of DIS or CIDI validity studies have been published since that time (Kessler et al. 1998; Wittchen, Üstün & Kessler 1999; Brugha et al. 2001). Results of all these studies showed that diagnoses based on the DIS and on earlier versions of the CIDI are significantly related to independent clinical diagnoses, but that individual-level concordance is far from perfect. Some part of this lack of concordance is doubtlessly due to unreliability of clinical interviews. Indeed, the literature is clear in showing that test-retest reliability is higher for diagnostic classifications based on DIS-CIDI interviews than on semistructured clinical interviews. However, there is also the issue of validity, which is presumably higher in semistructured clinical interviews than in fully structured DIS-CIDI interviews. As a result of concerns about validity, we were very interested in improving the accuracy of the CIDI for use in the WMH surveys.

On the basis of previous evaluations of the CIDI by survey methodologists in preparation for the U.S. National Comorbidity Survey (NCS) (Kessler et al. 1998; Kessler, Mroczek & Belli 1999; Kessler et al. 2000), four main methodological challenges in implementing the instrument were noted and became the focus of our work revising the diagnostic sections of the CIDI for use in the WMH surveys. One is that respondents might not understand some of the CIDI questions, a number of which include multiple clauses and vaguely defined terms. A second is that some respondents might not understand the task implied by the questions, which sometimes requires careful memory search that is unlikely to be carried out unless respondents are clearly instructed to do so. A third is that respondents might not be motivated to answer accurately, especially in light of the fact that many CIDI questions deal with potentially embarrassing and stigmatizing experiences. A fourth is that respondents might not be able to answer some

CIDI questions accurately, especially those that ask about characteristics of mental disorders that are difficult to remember (e.g., age of onset, number of lifetime episodes).

A considerable amount of methodological research has been carried out by survey researchers on each of these four methodological problems (e.g., Turner & Martin 1985; Tanur 1992; Sudman, Bradburn & Schwarz 1996). This research has advanced considerably over the past two decades, as cognitive psychologists have become interested in the survey interview as a natural laboratory for studying cognitive processes (Schwarz & Sudman 1994, 1996; Sirken et al. 1999). A number of important insights have emerged from these studies about practical ways to improve the accuracy of self-reported psychiatric assessments. As we describe subsequently, we used these insights to help develop CIDI 3.0. The next four sections of this chapter provide a quick review of these insights as well as a brief discussion of the ways they were used to address each of the four methodological problems.

## 4. QUESTION COMPREHENSION

It is obvious that ambiguous questions are likely to be misconstrued. It is perhaps less obvious, though, just how ambiguous most structured survey questions are and how often respondents must read between the lines to make sense of questions. In the first systematic study of this issue, Belson (1981) debriefed a sample of survey respondents on a set of standard survey questions and found that more than 70% of respondents interpreted some questions differently from the researcher, leading Belson to conclude that subtle misinterpretations are pervasive in survey situations. Similar conclusions were subsequently reached in other survey debriefing studies (Oksenberg, Cannell & Kanton 1991). Our own debriefing studies of the CIDI found much the same result: a great many respondents misunderstood important aspects of key diagnostic questions.

How is it possible for so much misunderstanding to occur? As Oksenberg and her colleagues (1991) discovered, the answer lies partly in the fact that many terms in surveys are vaguely defined. But beyond this is the more fundamental fact that the survey interview situation is a special kind of interaction in which the standard rules of conversation – rules that help fill in the gaps in meaning that exist in most speech – do not apply. Unlike the situation in normal conversational practice, the respondent in the survey interview often only vaguely knows the person to whom he or she is talking or the purpose of the conversation (Cannell, Fowler & Marquis 1968). The person who asks the questions (i.e., the interviewer) is not the person who formulated the questions (i.e., the researcher), and the interviewer is often unable to clarify the respondent's uncertainties about the intent of the questions. Furthermore, the flow of questions in the survey interview is established prior to the beginning of the conversation, which means that normal conversational rules of give-and-take in question and answer sequences do not apply. This leads to more misreading than in normal conversations even when questions are seemingly straightforward (Clark & Schober 1992), a problem that is compounded when the topic of the interview is one that involves emotional experiences, which are in many cases difficult to describe with clarity.

Clinical interviews attempt to deal with this problem by being "interviewer-based" (Brown 1989); that is, by training the interviewer to have a deep understanding of the criteria being evaluated, by allowing the interviewer to query the respondent as much as necessary to clarify the meaning of questions, and by leaving the ultimate judgment about the rating with the interviewer rather than with the respondent. Indeed, one might say that the interview is, in some sense, administered to the interviewer rather than to the respondent in interviewer-based interviews, as the responses of interest are responses to interviewer-based questions of the following sort: "Interviewer, based on your conversation with the respondent, would you say that he definitely, probably, possibly, probably not, or definitely does not meet the requirements of Criterion A?"

Fully structured psychiatric interviews like the CIDI cannot use this interviewer-based approach because, by definition, they are designed so that interviewer judgment plays no part in the responses. These "respondent-based" interviews use totally structured questions that the respondent answers, often in a yes-no format, either after reading the questions to themselves or after having an interviewer read the questions aloud. When the criterion of interest is fairly clear, there may be little difference between interviewer-based and respondent-based interviewing. It is a good deal more difficult, though, to assess conceptually complex criteria with fully structured questions.

In an effort to investigate the problem of question misunderstanding in the CIDI as part of the pilot studies for an early CIDI survey, Kessler and colleagues (Kessler et al. 1998; Kessler et al. 1999) carried out a series of debriefing interviews with community respondents who were administered sections of the CIDI and then asked to explain what they thought the questions meant and why they answered the way they did. A great deal of misunderstanding was found. However, enormous variation across questions was also found in the frequency of misunderstanding.

Four discriminating features were found among questions that had high versus low levels of misunderstanding. First, some commonly misunderstood questions were found to be too complex for many respondents to grasp. Second, some commonly misunderstood questions were found to involve vaguely defined terms, not complex concepts. A third type of commonly misunderstood CIDI question involved questions about odd experiences that could plausibly be interpreted in more than one way, such as questions about seeing and hearing things that others do not. Many respondents were found to have a tendency to normalize these questions and to respond positively when the correct answer was actually negative. A fourth type of commonly misunderstood CIDI question, finally, involved a contextual misunderstanding; that is, a misunderstanding that derived more from the position of the question in the flow of the interview than from lack of clarity in the question.

A good example of the last of these four problems can be found in the evaluation of Criterion A in the DSM-III-R diagnosis of simple phobia, which stipulates that the fear of circumscribed stimuli must be "persistent." CIDI 1.0 operationalized this criterion by asking, "Did this strong unreasonable fear continue for months or even years?" Although seemingly not ambiguous in itself, pilot work by Kessler and colleagues (Kessler et al. 1998; Kessler et al. 1999) found that this question was misunderstood by a great many respondents because of the location of the question in the instrument. Specifically, this question followed an open-ended question that asked the respondent to give an example of a specific fear. In many cases, the respondent would respond to this open-ended question by describing the autonomic arousal symptoms that occur on exposure to the stimulus, such as feeling dizzy or having trouble breathing. When the follow-up question was administered right after this description – asking whether this fear continued for months or even years – the question was often misunderstood as asking about the duration of the arousal symptoms. The respondent would invariably answer no, the nausea or dizziness or other physiological symptoms typically lasted no more than a few hours and certainly never lasted months or years. Confusions of this sort led to substantial errors in the original version of the CIDI.

On the basis of the work of Kessler and colleagues (2000), we carried out detailed CIDI debriefing interviews with volunteer respondents in methodological studies to support the development of CIDI 3.0 in an effort to pinpoint CIDI questions with each of the above four types of comprehension problems. Misunderstandings based on complex questions were addressed by breaking down the original CIDI questions into less complex subquestions. Especially complex questions were presented in a respondent booklet (RB) that provided a visual aid to respondents as the questions were being read by the interviewer. Misunderstandings based on the vagueness of terms were addressed by introducing clarifications and examples. Misunderstandings based on normalization of questions about odd experiences were addressed by prefacing the questions with clarification that we were actually asking about odd experiences and informing respondents that it was important for us to learn how often these experiences occur. Contextual misunderstandings were resolved by reordering questions to remove the contextual effects and by adding clarifying clauses into questions where residual confusion might exist. Although the number of modifications of this sort was so large that each one cannot be reviewed here, the appendix to this chapter presents one example of each of the main types of modifications.

## 5. TASK COMPREHENSION

Respondents not only sometimes misunderstand survey questions but also sometimes misunderstand the fundamental task that they are being asked to carry out. Debriefing studies have shown that misunderstandings of the second sort are especially common with the diagnostic stem questions in the CIDI (Kessler et al. 2000). These stem questions are the first questions asked in each diagnostic section. They are used to determine whether a lifetime syndrome of a particular sort might have ever occurred. These questions provide what are, in effect, brief vignettes and ask the respondent whether he or she ever has had an experience of this sort. If a diagnostic stem question is endorsed, additional questions are asked to assess the specifics of the syndrome. If all diagnostic stem questions for a particular disorder are denied, the remaining questions about this syndrome are skipped.

Our methodological studies found that substantial confusion arises from respondent failure to understand the purpose of diagnostic stem questions. In particular, only about half of pilot respondents in the Kessler study (2000) interpreted these questions as they were intended by the authors of the CIDI; namely, as a request to engage in active memory search and to report the lifetime occurrence of episodes of the sort in the question. The other respondents interpreted the question as a request to report whether a memory of such an episode was readily accessible. These latter respondents did not believe that

they were being asked to engage in active memory search and did not do so. Not surprising, the latter respondents were much less likely than those who understood the intent of the question to remember lifetime episodes.

Why did so many respondents misinterpret the intent of these lifetime recall questions? As Marquis and Cannell (1969) discovered in their early research on standard interview practice, in general respondents are ill informed about the purposes of the research and poorly motivated to participate actively. Furthermore, cues from interviewers often reinforce the inclination of respondents to participate in a halfhearted way. For example, when an interviewer asks a question that requires considerable thought, in the absence of instructions to the contrary, the respondent is likely to assume that the interviewer is operating under normal conversational rules and, as such, is really asking for an immediate and appropriate answer. Cannell, Miller, and Oksenberg (1981) showed that this conversational artifact can be minimized by explicitly instructing respondents to answer completely and accurately and that the use of such instruction can substantially improve the quality of data obtained in surveys. On the basis of this result, we built in clarifying statements throughout CIDI 3.0 that aimed to inform respondents that accuracy was important (for an example of such a statement, see the Appendix).

## 6. MOTIVATION

One problem with emphasizing to respondents the need to work hard at a series of demanding and potentially embarrassing recall tasks is that more respondents than otherwise may refuse to engage in the task. Recognition of this problem among survey methodologists has led to the development of motivational techniques intended to increase the chances that respondents will accept the job of answering completely and accurately. Three techniques that have proved particularly useful in this regard are the use of motivational components in instructions, the use of contingent reinforcement strategies embedded in interviewer-feedback probes, and the use of respondent commitment questions.

## 6.1. Motivational Instructions

Evidence exists that the use of introductory remarks at the beginning of a survey that clarify the research aims can help motivate respondents to provide a more complete and accurate report than they would otherwise (Cannell et al. 1981). Debriefing shows that respondents are more willing to undertake laborious and possibly painful memory searches if they recognize some altruistic benefit of doing so. Even such an uncompelling rationale as, "It is important for our research that you take your time and think carefully before answering," has motivational force. This is the case even more so when instructions include statements that have universal appeal, such as, "Accuracy is important because social policy makers will be using these results to make decisions that affect the lives of all of us." On the basis of this evidence, we developed and presented a statement containing a clear rationale for administering the interview at the onset of the CIDI 3.0 interview schedule and emphasized the importance of the survey for social policy purposes (for the text, see the Appendix). In addition, in the case of especially important questions that require long-term recall to answer correctly, we included the questions in the RB along with a written instruction at the top of the RB page in capital letters urging the respondent, "Take your time and think carefully before answering."

## 6.2. Contingent Reinforcement

Consistent with research on behavioral modification of verbal productions through reinforcement (e.g., Centers 1964), several survey researchers have demonstrated that verbal reinforcers such as "thanks" and "that's useful" can significantly affect the behavior of survey respondents (Marquis & Cannell 1969). On the basis of this observation, Cannell and associates (Oksenberg, Vinokur & Cannell 1979a) devel-

oped a method for training interviewers to use systematic feedback – both positive and negative – to reinforce respondent effort in reporting. The central feature of this method is the use of structured feedback statements coordinated with the content and timing of instructions aimed at reinforcing respondent performance. It is important to recognize that it is performance that is reinforced, not the content of particular answers. For example, a difficult recall question may be prefaced with the instruction, "This next question may be difficult, so please take your time before answering." In contingent feedback instruction, interviewers issue some expression of gratitude whenever the respondent seems to consider his or her answer carefully, whether or not they remember anything. Alternatively, the interviewer might instruct the precipitous respondent: "You answered that awfully quickly. Was there anything (else), even something small?" Such invitations to reconsider would occur whenever the respondent gives an immediate answer, whether or not anything was reported.

Experiments carried out by Cannell and associates (Miller & Cannell 1977; Vinokur, Oksenberg & Cannell 1979) documented that the combined use of these contingent reinforcement probes with instructions explaining the importance of careful and accurate reporting leads to substantial improvement in recall of health-related events in general population surveys, including validated dates of medical events. Their results also importantly showed that self-enhancing response biases are reduced when these strategies are used, as indicated by both a decreased tendency to underreport potentially embarrassing conditions and behaviors (e.g., gynecologic problems, seeing an X-rated movie), and a decreased tendency to overreport self-enhancing behaviors (e.g., number of books read in the last three months, having read the editorial page of the newspaper the previous day). On the basis of these results, the Cannell contingent feedback approach was included as a fundamental part of the interviewer-training materials developed for CIDI 3.0.

## 6.3. Commitment Questions

Instructions that define the nature of interviewer expectations for respondent behavior help establish a perspective on the interview that can have motivational force. The literature on cognitive factors in surveys contains many examples of the subtle ways in which perspectives established in questions subsequently influence respondent behaviors (e.g., Loftus & Palmer 1974). This same literature shows that perspective can have motivational force when it implies a common purpose (Clark & Schober 1992). That is, if a question is posed in such a way that it implies that hard work will be invested in arriving at an answer, it is incumbent on the respondent either explicitly to demur or tacitly to accept the task of working hard as part of the common understanding between interviewer and respondent. By answering the question, the respondent, in effect, makes a commitment to honor the injunction implied in the perspective of the question. This implied commitment, in turn, creates motivation to perform this task (Marlatt 1972). On the basis of this type of thinking, Cannell and colleagues showed that it is possible to motivate respondents to accept the goal of serious and active reporting by asking an explicit commitment question as part of the interview. Experimental studies carried out by Cannell and associates (Oksenberg et al. 1979a; Oksenberg, Vinokur & Cannell 1979b; Cannell et al. 1981) showed that these commitment questions improve accuracy of recall. Thus, we added a commitment question in the screening section of CIDI 3.0 just before the administration of the lifetime diagnostic stem questions (for the text of this question, see the Appendix).

## 7. THE ABILITY TO ANSWER ACCURATELY

### 7.1. Episodic and Semantic Memories

Research on basic cognitive processes has shown that memories are organized and stored in structured sets of information packages that are commonly called "schemas" (Markus & Zajonc 1985). When the respondent has a history of many instances of the same experience that cannot be discriminated, the separate instances tend to blend together in memory to form a special kind of memory schema called a "semantic memory," a general memory for a prototypical experience (Jobe et al. 1990; Means & Loftus 1991). For example, the person may have a semantic memory of what panic attacks are like but, because he or she has had many such attacks in his lifetime, cannot specify details of any particular panic attack. In comparison, when a respondent has had only a small number of lifetime experiences of a certain sort, or when one instance stands out in memory as much different from the others, a memory can likely be recovered for that particular episode. This is called an "episodic memory."

In the case of memories of illness experiences, memory schemata tend to include not only semantic memories of prototypic symptoms but also personal theories about causes, course, and cure (Leventhal, Nerenz & Steele 1984; Skelton & Croyle 1991). Some of these theories will conceptualize the experience in illness terms, whereas others will conceptualize the experience as a moral failing, a punishment from God, or a normal reaction to stress (Gilman 1988). These interpretations can influence the extent to which different memory cues are capable of triggering the schemas.

The effects of memory schemas and the difference between semantic and episodic memories are central themes in research on autobiographical memory. In the survey context, a critical issue related to this research is whether the respondent is able to recover episodic memories in answering a particular survey question, or if the respondent is answering the question by drawing inferences of what the past must have been like on the basis of more general semantic memories. Research shows that people are more likely to recover episodic memories for experiences that are recent, distinctive, and unique, and people are more likely to rely on semantic memories for experiences that are frequent, typical, and regular (Brewer 1986; Belli 1988; Menon 1994). The implications of this fact for the design of survey questions is discussed in the next subsection.

## 7.2. Asking Questions without Knowing the Limits of Memory

When a survey question is designed to ask about a particular instance of an experience, it must be posed in such a way that the respondent knows that he or she is being asked to recover an episodic memory. Furthermore, the researcher must have some basis for assuming that an episodic memory can be recovered for this experience. If it cannot, a question that asks for such a memory implicitly invites the respondent to guess rather than to remember, which can have adverse effects on quality of reporting later in the interview (Pearson, Ross & Dawes 1992). In comparison, when a question is designed to recover a semantic memory or to use semantic memories to arrive at an answer by estimation, that should be made clear.

One difficulty with these injunctions in the case of retrospective recall questions about lifetime psychiatric disorders is uncertainty about what level of recall accuracy to expect. Therefore, as part of the CIDI pilot work in preparation for the WMH surveys, we debriefed pilot respondents with an explicit eye toward pinpointing questions that were difficult to answer on the basis of episodic memory. When questions of this sort were discovered, an attempt was made to revise the questions to reduce the memory problem by allowing explicitly for estimation (e.g., explicitly asking respondents to provide a rough estimate), by providing categorical responses that reduce the complexity of the task, or by decomposing the question into subquestions that mimic effective memory search processes. Examples of modifications to question wording that employ each of these strategies are presented in the Appendix.

## 8. THE LIFETIME REVIEW SECTION

The previous four sections of this chapter reviewed a number of strategies that we used to optimize data quality in our revisions of the CIDI by improving understanding, by enhancing respondent commitment, or by adjusting questions to recognize that some respondents are less able than others to provide completely accurate responses. We used some additional strategies to deal with two or more of these problems at once. The most important of the latter was a life review section that we included in CIDI 3.0 near the beginning of the interview in an effort both to motivate and to facilitate active memory search in answering diagnostic stem questions. This section of CIDI 3.0 starts out with an introduction that explains to respondents that the following questions might be difficult to answer because they require respondents to review their entire lives. The introduction then goes on to say that despite this difficulty it is very important for the research that these questions are answered accurately. The introduction ends with the injunction, "Please take your time and think carefully before answering," and a commitment question that asks respondents if they were willing to do this.

The diagnostic stem questions for all core diagnoses are administered directly following this commitment question. The questions are all included in the RB with the written instruction, "Take your time and think carefully before answering." Interviewers are instructed both to read the diagnostic stem questions slowly in an effort to emphasize their importance, and to use motivational probes to encourage active memory search. Our intent in developing this section was both to explain the serious and difficult nature of the task and to motivate respondents to engage in active memory search, which we hoped to stimulate by combining all the stem questions after a fairly detailed motivational introduction. We also recognized, as a result of our debriefing studies, that CIDI respondents quickly learn the logic of the stem-branch structure after a few sections and recognize that they can shorten the interview considerably by saying no to the stem questions. This problem is removed by asking all the stem questions near the beginning of the interview before the logic of the stem-branch structure becomes clear. Another important reason for including the section near the beginning of the interview is that pilot-study respondents told us in debriefing interviews that their energy flagged as the interview progressed, which made it much more difficult to carry out a serious memory search later in the interview than at the beginning.

As previously noted, Cannell and associates carried out experiments that documented powerful effects of commitment questions on the accuracy of survey responses (Oksenberg et al. 1979a, 1979b; Cannell et al. 1981). A similar experiment was carried out to evaluate the effects of using a lifetime review section in conjunction with commitment and motivational probes. A random sample of 200 community respondents was randomized either to the standard version of CIDI 1.1, or to a version that was identical except that it included the life review section at the beginning of the interview. As reported in more detail elsewhere (Kessler et al. 1998), this experiment documented that the life review section led to a significant increase in the proportion of respondents who endorsed diagnostic stem questions. For example, whereas 26.7% of respondents in the standard CIDI condition endorsed the "sad, blue, or depressed" stem question for major depression, a significantly higher 40.6% did so in the life review condition. A clinical validity study importantly documented that this increased prevalence of stem endorsement was not accompanied by a reduction in sensitivity with regard to clinical diagnoses, documenting that additional true cases were discovered by the use of the life review section and the accompanying commitment and motivation probes. These results were the basis of adopting the lifetime review section in CIDI 3.0.

## 9. SUBSTANTIVE MODIFICATIONS OF DIAGNOSTIC SECTIONS

In addition to the methodological modifications described previously, a number of important substantive modifications aimed at addressing current uncertainties about the prevalence, impairment, and appropriate diagnostic criteria for the disorders assessed in the interview were made to the diagnostic assessments in CIDI 3.0. Perhaps the most important of these uncertainties concerns diagnostic thresholds. This uncertainty arose, in no small part, as a reaction to the results of early DIS and CIDI surveys, which showed that as many as 50% of the general population in some countries was estimated to meet lifetime criteria for one or more ICD or DSM mental disorders, and that as many as 30% of the population was estimated to meet criteria for such a disorder in the past 12 months (WHO International Consortium in Psychiatric Epidemiology 2000; Bijl et al. 2003). These percentages seemed implausibly high to many critics, leading to the suggestion that the lay-administered diagnostic interviews in these surveys were upwardly biased (Brugha, Bebbington & Jenkins 1999; Wittchen et al. 1999). However, clinical calibration studies showed that the prevalence estimates in these surveys were not upwardly biased (Kessler et al. 1998; Eaton et al. 2000), leading critics to conclude that the ICD and DSM systems themselves are overly inclusive (Pincus, Zarin & First 1998; Regier et al. 1998; Üstün, Chatterji & Rehm 1998).

This conclusion was instrumental in causing an APA task force to add a clinical significance criterion to many disorders in the DSM-IV to remind readers of the basic definition of a mental disorder in the introduction of the DSM manual as requiring clinically significant distress or impairment. However, even when this additional requirement was applied post hoc to DIS and CIDI surveys carried out in the United States, the 12-month prevalence estimate of having at least one DSM disorder, equivalent to approximately 37 million adults in the United States, continued to be very high (Narrow et al. 2002). In recognition of this problem, several more restrictive definitions were subsequently proposed to narrow the number of people qualifying for treatment (National Advisory Mental Health Council 1993; Substance Abuse and Mental Health Services Administration 1993; Regier 2000; Narrow et al. 2002; Regier & Narrow 2002).

Criticisms have been raised, though, of the proposal to narrow the definition of mental disorders merely to reduce high prevalence estimates (Mechanic 2003). Indeed, some researchers have argued that the definitions in the current ICD and DSM systems should be expanded to include what would currently be considered subthreshold cases (e.g., Merikangas et al. 2003). These critics have noted that research shows many syndromes currently defined as mental disorders are extremes on continua that appear not to have meaningful thresholds (e.g., Preisig, Merikangas & Angst 2001). Exploration of the full continua rather than the currently established diagnostic thresholds, according to these critics, would yield greater power in studies of genetic and environmental risk factors (Benjamin, Ebstein & Lesch 1998). With regard to diagnostic thresholds, these critics note that research has shown subthreshold cases on some of these continua to be quite impaired (e.g., Judd et al. 1996) and to have significantly elevated risk of serious outcomes such as suicide attempts and hospitalization for emotional problems (Kessler et al. 2003c). This means that the development of early interventions to treat these subthreshold cases might prevent progression along a given severity continuum, thereby reducing the prevalence of serious cases in a cost-effective fashion (Eaton, Badawi & Melton 1995). Removal of these subthreshold cases from the ICD or DSM systems, in comparison, might result in the importance of developing interventions for these cases to be ignored, as well as a distortion occurring in the reality that mental disorders, like physical disorders, vary widely in seriousness (Spitzer 1998; Kendell 2002).

The final resolution between these competing views will doubtlessly take years to occur and will rely on emerging information about the genetics of mental disorders as well as about treatment response across the range of the symptom severity continuum. To the extent that epidemiological data will play a part, they will, at a minimum, need to include assessments of subthreshold cases, assessments of symptom severity in dimensional terms, and evaluation of the association between symptom severity and impairment. With this recognition in mind, CIDI 3.0 was designed to do all three of these things, as briefly discussed in the next three subsections.

## 9.1. Subthreshold Disorders

Our general approach in modifying diagnostic sections for CIDI 3.0 was to include as much information as possible about subthreshold cases, with the precise nature of the subthreshold assessment guided by the literature and our preliminary studies. For example, in the case of depression, even though the diagnostic criteria require dysphoria or anhedonia that persists for most of the day, we found that a great many people otherwise meet the criteria for a major depressive episode except that their symptoms persist only for about half the day or sometimes for less than half the day. We included these people in our assessment of depressive disorders but distinguished them from people whose symptoms persisted most of the day. In addition, we included people with as few as two symptoms in their worst lifetime episode of depression to capture cases of minor depression, even though larger numbers are required in the ICD and DSM systems to be considered major depressive episodes. We also included people with depressive episodes as short as three days if they reported ever having episodes of this sort most months for an entire year in a row. This is done to allow for an assessment of recurrent brief depression (Angst et al. 1990).

To take a second example, in the case of panic, we revised CIDI 3.0 to carry out a complete assessment of people who report at least one lifetime limited symptom attack or panic attack. Age of onset and the circumstances surrounding the single attack are collected as well. Parallel information is collected about the first lifetime attack among people who meet criteria for a panic disorder. Separate information is obtained from the latter people about age of onset of the transition from panic attacks to panic disorder. These subthreshold assessments were included in the instrument on the basis of the results of previous research, which has shown that only about half the people who have a single lifetime panic attack go on to develop panic disorder (Eaton et al. 1994). The information collected in CIDI 3.0 about first attacks is designed to allow information to be collected about patterns and predictors of progression from panic attacks to panic disorder. A similar distinction is made in CIDI 3.0 between specific fears and phobias, with separate dating of age of onset of the fear, of avoidance, and of impairment in daily functioning associated either with the fears or with avoidance of the feared objects.

As a final example, we included in CIDI 3.0 a complete assessment of the symptoms of generalized anxiety disorder (GAD) for respondents who reported having episodes that persist for at least one month, the original duration requirement for GAD in DSM-III, rather than requiring the six-month minimum episode duration stipulated in ICD-10 and DSM-IV. The decision by the developers of the DSM to increase the one-month minimum duration requirement for GAD in DSM-III to six months in the revision of the DSM-III (DSM-III-R) was based on the fact that the vast majority of patients with GAD in treatment samples had comorbid depression unless their GAD persisted for at least six months (Breslau & Davis 1985). However, subsequent epidemiological research showed that pure cases of GAD with shorter durations exist in the general population, athough these cases seldom come to clinical attention because seeking professional help is usually driven by comorbid disorders. Yet this does not mean that people with recurrent episodes of GAD lasting less than six months are not impaired. Indeed, the largest and most comprehensive study of this matter, carried out by Maier and colleagues (2000) in the WHO study of mental disorders in primary care, found that the one-month duration requirement is optimal for distinguishing cases of GAD from noncases in terms of role impairment. The decision to require a minimum duration of one month rather than six months in CIDI 3.0 is based on this result.

## 9.2. Symptom Persistence and Severity

The focus of the CIDI, like that of the DIS before it, has largely been on lifetime disorders, although a 12-month version of the CIDI was developed as part of the CIDI 2.0 revision. The standard lifetime version of the CIDI provides only superficial information about recent disorders by asking no more than a single question: "How recently have you had (the disorder)?" This makes it impossible to characterize the persistence of disorders over the recent past or to know whether respondents with a lifetime disorder have met full criteria during the recent past. As 12-month prevalence is of great interest for needs assessment, this superficial consideration of 12-month prevalence is a serious limitation. We addressed this problem in CIDI 3.0 by obtaining information about 12-month symptoms and persistence. In the case of panic and intermittent explosive disorder, this was done by asking about the number of attacks in the past 12 months and about the number of months during the past 12 when the respondent had at least one attack. In the case of episodic disorders, such as depression and GAD, 12-month duration was assessed by asking how many weeks out of the past 52 the respondent was in an episode.

We included similar questions in CIDI 3.0 to increase understanding of long-term course. In earlier CIDI versions, information on course was limited to two questions about age of onset and age of recency of the disorder. CIDI 3.0, in comparison, expands this assessment to ask about persistence in the interval between these two ages along the same lines used to assess 12-month persistence (e.g., with questions about lifetime number of panic and anger attacks, lifetime number of episodes of depression and GAD, typical and longest durations of episodes, and number of years in which the respondent experienced an episode of the disorder). In keeping with the prior comments on the limits of autobiographical memory, and consistent with the results of our methodological pilot studies, we recognized that respondents with complex histories of psychopathology will be unable to recover episodic memories in answering these long-term recall questions. As a result, the questions are worded in such a way as to make it clear that we are looking for semantic memories. Even with this limitation in mind, though, these data can be extremely useful in distinguishing between broad categories of people who have had only one or two, a few, or a large number of episodes over only one or two, a few, or a larger number of years.

CIDI 3.0 also includes much more extensive information about symptom severity than did earlier CIDI versions. Each diagnostic section contains explicit questions about the depth of the distress caused by the disorder along with a 12-month symptom severity scale based on a fully structured version of a standard clinical scale. For example, the quick self-report version of the Inventory of Depressive Symptomatology (Rush et al. 1996) is included in CIDI 3.0 to assess the severity of 12-month depression, and a structured version of the Panic Disorder Severity Scale (Shear et al. 1997) is included to assess the severity of 12-month panic. Our hope in embedding these clinical symptom severity scales in CIDI 3.0 was that they would help create a crosswalk between the findings in epidemiological surveys and the findings in clinical studies.

## 9.3. Internal Impairment

Related to the issue of clinical significance is the issue of impairment. Earlier CIDI versions asked only one dichotomous disorder-specific role impairment question: "Did (the disorder) ever interfere a lot with your life or activities?" No impairment questions were asked independent of disorders. This is inadequate for evaluating whether clinically significant role impairment is associated with a particular syndrome or for investigating the implications of changing diagnostic thresholds on evaluations of impairment. As a result, we substantially expanded the number of within-section questions about the impairments caused by individual disorders in CIDI 3.0. These so-called internal impairment questions ask respondents to evaluate the impairment caused by a given disorder. As described subsequently, CIDI 3.0 also includes two important sections that assess external impairment, by which we mean overall impairment in various areas of functioning without reference to the cause of the impairment. Although most of the CIDI 3.0 internal impairment questions focus on the worst lifetime impairment due to a particular

disorder, five questions are included in each diagnostic section about impairment in the past 12 months. Four of these are the Sheehan Disability Scales (Leon et al. 1997; Sheehan et al. 1996), which ask respondents to rate the impairments caused by a focal disorder during the one month in the past year when it was most severe in each of four areas of life (household duties, employment, social life, and close personal relationships) on a 0–10 scale that uses a visual analogue scale with impairment categories of none (0), mild (1–3), moderate (4–6), severe (7–9), and very severe (10). The fifth question asks respondents to estimate the total number of days out of 365 in the past 12 months when they were totally unable to work or carry out their other usual activities because of the focal disorder.

## 9.4. External Impairment

Two sections of CIDI 3.0 assess external impairment. The first is the section on 30-day functioning, which is made up of the WHO Disability Assessment Schedule (WHO-DAS) (WHO 1998; Rehm et al. 1999). The WHO-DAS assesses both the persistence (number of days in the past 30) and severity (during the days when difficulties in functioning occurred) of health-related difficulties in the respondent's functioning during the 30 days before the interview. The dimensions of functioning assessed in the WHO-DAS are keyed to the major categories in the WHO International Classification of Functioning, Disability, and Health (WHO 2001). The second section of CIDI 3.0 that assesses external impairment is the section on employment, which includes the WHO Health and Work Performance Questionnaire (HPQ) (Kessler et al. 2003a). The HPQ is an expansion of the work impairment section of the WHO-DAS that assesses the workplace costs of illness in terms of absenteeism, decrements in performance while on the job, and critical workplace incidents (e.g., work-related accidents). The HPQ was developed to provide data to employers and government health policy makers about the indirect costs of illness on the productive capacity of the labor force, based either on the results of surveys like the WMH surveys or on the results of workplace interventions designed to evaluate the effects of treatment on human capital outcomes evaluated from the employer perspective (Wang et al. 2007).

## 9.5. Why Assess Both Internal and External Impairment?

It is noteworthy that both internal (disorder specific) and external (global) assessments of impairment are important to obtain. Disorder-specific assessments are important because they can be used to make direct comparisons among different mental and physical disorders. These direct comparisons are becoming increasingly central to health-care resource allocation decisions as evidence-based medicine becomes the basis for more and more triage decisions. However, disorder-specific assessments are limited by the fact that they require respondents to make inferences about the cause of their impairments. This can be difficult, especially among the large number of people with comorbid conditions who might have a hard time sorting out which of their conditions causes various aspects of impairment.

External assessments are important to obtain because they allow the researcher to overcome the limitation of disorder-specific assessments by empirically estimating the relative effects of different disorders from prediction equations in which measures of the prevalence of these disorders and their comorbidities are included as predictors of global impairment. However, as it is not possible to make detailed assessments of all possible disorders for inclusion in such prediction equations, estimates of the impairments due to specific disorders based on analysis of such equations are necessarily imperfect. Furthermore, replication of results involving the estimated effects of a focal disorder on impairment using external comparisons requires measurement of exactly the same set of control conditions across studies. This is infeasible. As a result, the internal assessment of impairment is more feasible despite its conceptual limitations in comparison to the external assessment of impairment.

## 9.6. Ranking the Impairments of Mental and Physical Disorders

To provide comparative information on the impairments of mental and physical disorders, a checklist of chronic physical disorders was included in CIDI 3.0. Internal impairment was assessed with the five questions, described previously, for one randomly selected chronic condition per respondent. The random sampling strategy was used because comprehensive assessment of internal impairment for all possible chronic physical disorders would be too time-consuming for a one-session survey devoted to mental disorders. However, by taking care to carry out a random selection for each respondent from among all the conditions reported by that respondent, it is possible to weight the internal impairment data by the number of conditions reported to recover an equal-probability sample for each chronic condition for purposes of comparative assessment of within-disorder role impairments.

The chronic conditions checklist was modified from the list used in the National Health Interview Survey (NHIS) (National Center for Health Statistics 2003) to ask about the lifetime occurrence, age of onset, and recency of commonly occurring chronic conditions that are thought to be associated with substantial role impairment. A number of methodological studies have found that such checklists yield valid data about disorders brought to medical attention or that significantly limit activities when compared to independent medical records (Halabi et al. 1992; Heliovaara et al. 1993; Edwards et al. 1994; Gross et al. 1996; Kriegsman et al. 1996; Mackenbach, Looman & van der Meer 1996). For example, moderate to high agreement (Cohen's $\kappa$; Cohen 1960) has been found between self-reports and medical records regarding arthritis ($\kappa = 0.41$), asthma ($\kappa = 0.55$), diabetes ($\kappa = 0.82$), and high blood pressure ($\kappa = 0.73$) (Edwards et al. 1994). These are lower-bound estimates because the medical record is not a gold standard, especially for chronic conditions often not brought to medical attention (e.g., arthritis), for poorly defined conditions (e.g., back pain), and for symptom-based conditions in which the medical record merely reproduces symptoms that are based on self-report (e.g., chronic headaches).

In the case of symptom-based conditions, a number of more extensive scales are used instead of the single yes-no questions in the chronic conditions checklist. For example, we included a brief screening scale to assess migraines that reproduces physician diagnoses much more accurately than a single checklist question (Lipton et al. 2003). Other symptom-based conditions that are assessed with screening scales include chronic fatigue syndrome, irritable bowel syndrome, insomnia, and unexplained chronic pain disorder.

Comparative analyses of internal impairment could add important information to the growing body of data that physical disorders (Stewart, Greenfield & Hays 1989; Wells et al. 1989; Ormel et al. 1994; Hays et al. 1995; van den Bos 1995; Verbrugge & Patrick 1995; Penninx et al. 1996; Kempen et al. 1997; Ormel et al. 1998; Kempen et al. 2000) and mental disorders (Zeiss & Lewinsohn 1988; Wells et al. 1989; Broadhead et al. 1990; Rhode, Lewinsohn & Seeley 1990; Coryell et al. 1993; Tweed 1993; Ormel et al. 1994; Ormel et al. 1998; Bijl & Ravelli 2000) often cause substantial role impairments. Such results have led to an interest among health policy researchers in the possibility that expanded outreach and guideline-concordant treatment of impairing chronic disorders might represent an investment opportunity for employers (Kessler et al. 2001) and for governments (Murray & Lopez 1996). However, not all mental disorders have been studied in this way. The CIDI 3.0 assessment of internal impairment for each mental disorder and for one random chronic physical condition allows for such studies to be done (Druss et al. 2008).

The CIDI 3.0 assessment of external impairment has the potential to be especially important because a central limitation of the existing literature on the role impairments of chronic conditions is the lack of attention to the co-occurrence of multiple disorders in the same patient. Many people with chronic disorders suffer from more

than one disorder (Dewa & Lin 2000). Pure disorders are, in general, less impairing than co-occurring disorders in clinical samples (Ormel et al. 1994). The co-occurrence of mental disorders with chronic physical disorders is of special importance in this regard, as strong patterns of co-occurrence with mental disorders have been found for a number of commonly occurring physical disorders both in general population samples (Neeleman, Ormel & Bijl 2001) and in primary-care samples (Berardi et al. 1999).

Clinical studies have found excess impairment associated with co-occurring mental disorders among people with chronic physical disorders (Sullivan et al. 2001). As efforts increase to rationalize the allocation of health-care resources guided by the criteria of evidence-based medicine, consideration of the role played by co-occurring mental disorders in causing impairment among patients with chronic physical disorders becomes all the more important. The inclusion of the external impairment in CIDI 3.0 makes it possible to carry out such analyses in general population samples by using information about mental disorders, physical disorders, and their comorbidities to predict external impairment (Merikangas et al. 2007).

## 10. PART ONE AND PART TWO DIAGNOSES

As noted previously, CIDI 3.0 is quite a long instrument, with an average administration time of approximately two hours for the full interview. This long administration time can create practical complications, the most important being that it is often necessary to administer the interview in two sessions. To address this length problem, a case-control approach was used in the WMH surveys, whereby a subsample of respondents who completed the first half of the interview (Part 1), which included all core diagnostic assessments, and who reported having no lifetime history of disorder, were terminated at the midpoint of the interview. All respondents who met criteria for any lifetime mental disorders in the Part 1 interview, in comparison, were retained in the second half of the interview (Part 2) along with a probability subsample of noncases. The default value for the noncase probability of selection was 33%, although this was changed in some countries. A weight equal to the inverse of this sampling fraction was applied to noncase Part 2 interviews so as to correct for the undersampling of noncases. The 33% case-control subsampling fraction of noncases yielded a high ratio of controls to cases (5–10:1) for all but the most prevalent disorders. Statistical power analyses show that increasing the number of controls to cases above these levels yields very little improvement in power (Schlesselman 1982). As the main purposes of carrying out the WMH surveys was to estimate prevalence and correlates of mental disorders, this result implies that the subsampling of noncases into Part 2 retained most of the efficiency of the full sample for central analyses and substantially reduced field costs.

Several important but lengthy diagnostic sections were included in the Part 2 WMH interviews in an effort to reduce average interview length. These included the assessments of substance use disorders, post-traumatic stress disorder, obsessive-compulsive disorder, and non-affective psychosis. It should be noted that the high comorbidity of these Part 2 disorders with the disorders assessed in Part 1 means that the great majority of respondents with these disorders were selected into the Part 2 sample, leading to only a small loss of information about the Part 2 disorders by placing them in Part 2 rather than in Part 1. In addition, disorders included in CIDI 3.0 for exploratory purposes were all placed in Part 2, including eating disorders, neurasthenia, nicotine dependence, pathological gambling, premenstrual disorder, and a screen for personality disorders.

Options for additional subsampling of the assessment of these exploratory disorders within the Part 2 sample (e.g., only a random 50% of Part 2 respondents received the assessment of pathological gambling) were built into the skip logic of the CAPI version of CIDI 3.0. In addition, a series of four diagnostic sections were included in Part 2 for retrospectively reported childhood and adolescent disorders. These sections, which were modeled on those developed by

Lee Robins and colleagues (1981) for the DSM-IV version of the DIS, include assessments of attention-deficit/hyperactivity disorder, conduct disorder, oppositional-defiant disorder, and separation anxiety disorder. On the basis of concerns about retrospective reporting bias among elderly respondents, these last four sections were administered in the WMH surveys only to respondents in the age range of 18 to 44.

## II. EXPANSIONS OF OTHER CIDI SECTIONS

As noted previously, the main reason for developing CIDI 3.0 was to expand the instrument beyond its initial focus on diagnoses to include assessments of risk factors, consequences, and treatment. Fifteen sections of this sort are included in CIDI 3.0. Seven of these 15 assess sociodemographics (i.e., employment, finances, marriage, children, adult demographics for the Part 1 sample, adult demographics for the Part 2 sample, and childhood demographics). Two sections assess treatment (i.e., services and pharmacoepidemiology). The other six sections assess external impairment, chronic conditions, nonspecific psychological distress, social networks, family burden, and childhood experiences. We already commented on the external impairment and chronic conditions sections. A few comments are in order about several of the other sections.

### II.I. Sociodemographics

Basic information about sociodemographic variables – such as age, sex, race, education, marital status, and employment status – is included in all community surveys. For the most part, though, this information is cross-sectional; that is, it assesses the respondent's current status on these variables rather than his or her history. This is fine for ascribed sociodemographic characteristics (e.g., sex and race), which do not change over time, but it misses important information about the dynamics of achieved statuses, such as marital status and employment status, which change over time. This loss of information can be important if dynamic information is relevant to mental health. Given the focus of the CIDI 3.0 diagnostic sections on lifetime course, we felt that it was important to include dynamic information about achieved statuses in the interview schedule. As a result, separate sections of the interview are devoted to the respondent's history in each of the three main areas of achieved social status (i.e., employment, marriage, and childbearing).

The details of the assessments differ across the three sections, but the basic approach is the same. We began by asking about timing of initial entry into roles (e.g., ages of first dating, first marriage, first employment, first sexual intercourse, first becoming pregnant or causing a woman to become pregnant, first having an abortion, first giving birth). We then asked about role history (e.g., age at onset and duration of each marriage, age of each child, stability of employment history). Information about current role incumbency (e.g., current employment status, current marital status, number and ages of children, which children live with the respondent), which is the focus of the assessment in most surveys, was only the final part of the assessments. The exception was that Part 1 respondents who terminated before the Part 2 interview were administered only a brief sociodemographic battery that focused exclusively on current status.

The additional three sociodemographic sections – childhood demographics, adult demographics, and finances – also included much more detailed questions than most surveys about these areas. The section on childhood demographics, for example, asked about age of parents when the respondent was born, size of sibship and birth order, marital status of parents, nativity, number of generations in the country among natives, age at immigration among the foreign born, country of origins for people who were originally from another country, native tongue, education, childhood religion and religiosity, urbanicity of childhood residence, and stability of childhood residence. The section on adult demographics asked about whether parents are living or dead, age and cause of death of each deceased parent, race/ethnicity, subjective closeness of racial-ethnic identification, citizenship, religious preference, religiosity, amount

of time during adulthood when the respondent was in a jail or prison or correctional facility, amount of time homeless, amount of time institutionalized in a hospital or nursing home, and current subjective social-class position. The section on finances asked about both objective finances and subjective financial stress. With regard to objective finances, information was obtained both on income and assets. Income information was obtained for the entire household broken down by income of the respondent, the respondent's spouse, other family members, income from government-assistance programs, and other income. This disaggregation of income was very useful in analyses of social class and mental illness, where it was possible to distinguish associations that might be due to direct selection (respondent income), assortative mating (spouse income), and other sources.

## 11.2. Treatment and Pharmacoepidemiology

Treatment, like impairment, is assessed in CIDI 3.0 both internally and externally. In the internal assessment, respondents who meet criteria for a particular disorder were asked at the end of the diagnostic section whether they had ever sought professional treatment for that disorder and, if so, at what age they first sought treatment. They are also asked whether they ever obtained treatment that they considered helpful for the disorder and, if so, how many different professionals they saw before they received helpful treatment. Respondents who said that they never received helpful treatment are asked how many professionals they ever saw for the disorder. This kind of information, when coupled with information about age of onset of the disorder, can be used to study patterns and predictors of delays in initial treatment contact after first onset of a mental disorder.

Analyses of this sort in epidemiological samples consistently find pervasive delays in initial treatment contact after first onset of a mental disorder that are inversely related to age at onset, cohort, and illness severity (Kessler, Olfson & Berglund 1998; Olfson et al. 1998). It is also unclear whether patient reports of being helped would be confirmed in objective evaluations. Nonetheless, patient perceptions, even if not entirely accurate, must be considered an important dimension of treatment effectiveness that has not previously been seriously considered in psychiatric epidemiological surveys.

In the external assessment of treatment, CIDI 3.0 asks respondents about ever having treatment for problems with their emotions or mental health. A separate section contains parallel questions about seeking help for problems associated with the use of alcohol or drugs. Questions about inpatient treatment include lifetime hospitalization, age of first hospitalization, number of lifetime hospitalizations, amount of time spent in hospitals for these problems over the life course, and hospitalization in the past 12 months. Questions about outpatient treatment include treatment from each of a wide range of professionals. For each type of professional seen, information is recorded on age of first receiving treatment and age of most recent treatment. For those who received treatment in the past 12 months, information is obtained on number of visits with each type of professional, average duration of time with the professional, whether the respondent is still in treatment, and if not, whether the termination of treatment occurred because the respondent completed the course of treatment or quit. Summary questions are then asked of all respondents who were in any type of 12-month treatment about all the money spent out of pocket for treatment with all professionals over that interval of time, reasons for seeking treatment, and reasons for terminating treatment among those who did terminate. Respondents who had not received any treatment in the past 12 months are asked whether they ever felt that they might need professional help for their emotions or mental health in the past 12 months. If so, they are asked about reasons for not seeking professional help.

A separate pharmacoepidemiology section asks about the use of prescription and non-prescription medications in the past 12 months for "problems with your emotions, nerves, mental health, substance use, energy, concentration, sleep, or ability to cope with stress." An exhaustive list of prescription medications is provided as a visual aid in answering these questions. Interviewers are instructed to use motivational probes to encourage respondents to think carefully and to exhaustively list all medications taken during the recall period. Interviewers are also instructed to have respondents get their medicine bottles if they still have them to copy down information about the name of the medicine and the recommended dose. For each medicine taken, questions are then asked about number of days taken out of the past 365, dosage, and whether the medicine is taken under the supervision of a doctor. If not, information is collected about where the respondent obtains the medicine. If taken under the supervision of a doctor, a question is asked about whether the doctor is a psychiatrist, some other mental health specialist, a primary-care doctor, or some other kind of doctor. If taken under professional supervision, a question is asked about how often the respondent failed to take the medicine at the recommended dose and times. Finally, questions are asked about whether the medicine is still being taken and, if not, reasons for terminating use, including side effects.

## 11.3. Nonspecific Psychological Distress

The Part Two WMH interview included a screening scale that asked about the frequency of nonspecific psychological distress during the 30 days before the interview and in the worst month of the past year (Kessler et al. 2002). This scale was developed originally to screen for serious mental illness (SMI) in general-purpose health surveys (Kessler et al. 2003b). The scale has subsequently been adopted in a number of countries (e.g., Australia, Canada, United States) for use in ongoing government health surveys. The ten questions in the scale were selected from a large item pool aimed at sensitively measuring the first principal factor of nonspecific psychological distress, which is consistently found in community surveys of distress, in the clinically significant range of its distribution.

Validation studies of this screening scale carried out in community samples showed that the scale does an excellent job of screening for SMI (Furukawa et al. 2003; Kessler et al. 2003b). However, the sensitivity and specificity of the scale might vary across populations, making it useful to include the scale in CIDI surveys so that new calibrations can be made across many different populations. This was our main goal in including the scale in the CIDI 3.0 and in the WMH surveys. When accurate rules of this sort exist, this brief screening scale can be very useful as an inexpensive mental health needs surveillance tool in ongoing general-purpose tracking surveys. Calibration rules and software for transforming scores on this scale into individual-level predicted probabilities of SMI and other global measures of disorder based on the WMH surveys will be posted as soon as the full WMH survey series is completed.

## 11.4. Family Burden

Although the CIDI 3.0 questions on internal and external impairment do an excellent job of assessing the ways in which mental disorders affect the people who have these disorders, the effects on the families of the mentally ill are ignored. This is a major gap, as there is clear evidence that mental disorders can create enormous family burdens (Saunders 2003; Tsang et al. 2003). In an effort to correct this problem, a separate section was developed for CIDI 3.0 on family burden. Unlike all other sections of the interview, this section treats the respondent as the "family member" whose burden is being assessed rather than as the person whose mental health is being assessed. This was done as a result of concerns that respondents would be unable to provide accurate informant information on the burdens their disorders imposed on their loved ones. An additional virtue of this method is that it provides an easy way to integrate information on burden into population estimates, something that would be extremely difficult to do without enumerating networks if the respondent was treated as the focal respondent whose illness affected many different family members rather than as a representative family member who might be burdened by the illness of any number of family members.

The logic of the section requires us to begin by defining a network of first-degree relatives. This is done by asking the respondent how many living first-degree relatives he or she has, separately reporting the number of parents, siblings, children, and whether or not he or she has a spouse. The respondent is then told that there are a few questions about the health problems of these individuals. After enumerating the network in this way, the respondent is asked whether any of these individuals has any of 12 serious health problems, which include the following in the order they are asked: cancer; serious heart problems; a serious memory problem, like senility or dementia; mental retardation; a permanent physical disability, like blindness or paralysis; any other serious chronic physical illness; alcohol or drug problems; serious depression; serious anxiety; schizophrenia or psychosis; manic depression; or any other serious chronic mental illness. Note that the threshold of problems is set high (e.g., "serious depression" rather than "depression") and that open-ended questions are included about other serious chronic physical and mental illnesses at the end of the lists of explicit physical and mental disorders. The open-ended questions are put at the end so that the earlier explicit disorders can provide a context for defining the severity level we want respondents to be thinking about when responding to the open-ended questions.

Respondents who report having any first-degree relatives with any of the 12 health problems are then asked a series of questions about how these problems, taken as a whole, affect the life of the respondent. Included here are questions about the respondent helping to wash or dress the ill person, helping with practical things (e.g., paperwork, housework, local transportation, taking medications), and spending more time with the ill person(s) or giving them more emotional support than they would if the illness(es) were not present. Respondents then estimate the number of hours per week they spend doing things related to the health problems of these family members and the amount of money they spend per month because of these problems. Emotional effects of the problems on the respondent are then briefly assessed (e.g., extent of worry, anxiety, depression, and embarrassment caused by the problems). Finally, the Sheehan Disability Scales (Leon et al. 1997; Sheehan et al. 1996) are used to have the respondent rate the extent to which family members' health problems interfere with his or her functioning in the same four areas of functioning used in the assessment of internal impairment (i.e., household duties, employment, social life, and close personal relationships).

The use of the Sheehan scales makes it possible to compare the effects on functioning of the respondent's own illnesses with the illnesses of family members. More generally, by creating 48 separate variables (for each of the 12 illnesses and for each of the four types of first-degree relatives, using counts to deal with the situation in which more than one family member of a given type has a particular type of illness), regression analysis can be used to examine the relative effects of different types of illnesses on the various dimensions of family burden included in the assessment. It is also possible, using this same analysis approach, to study whether particular aspects of burden are greater for female than for male focal respondents exposed to the same profile of family illness, to examine how burden changes when the structural relationship between the focal respondent and the ill person changes (e.g., the illness of a child versus that of a parent), and to evaluate the effects of network illness comorbidity on respondent burden. As far as we are aware, none of these has up to now been the subject of systematic analysis across a wide range of illness categories considered together in a large-scale community survey, although each has long been studied in small-scale focused studies of patients and their families (e.g., Chakrabarti, Kulhara & Verma 1993; Rupp & Keith 1993). The inclusion of the family burden section in CIDI 3.0 makes it possible to carry out this systematic kind of analysis.

## 11.5. Childhood Experiences

The final section of CIDI 3.0 that we want to mention is the section on childhood experiences.

The WMH collaborators agreed early on that the WMH surveys were uniquely positioned to study the lifetime effects of traumatic life experiences, with a special emphasis on the long-term effects of childhood adversities. As a result, a fairly extensive series of questions was included in CIDI 3.0 about childhood experiences. The questions about childhood traumatic events were placed in the trauma checklist within the post-traumatic stress disorder section. The remaining questions were included in a separate section on childhood experiences. This section begins by asking whether the respondent lived with both of his or her biological parents until age 16 and, if not, to explain his or her living situation up to that age. The nature and age at each important transition obtained in response to this question are recorded for such events as death of a parent, parental divorce, adoption, and the like. Respondents who report living with both parents up to 16 years of age are then asked whether a parent was ever away from home for six months or longer due to such things as hospitalization, imprisonment, or military service. The respondent's age at and the duration of each such event are recorded. A question is then asked about whether the respondent was ever away from home for six months or longer due to such things as hospitalization, boarding school, foster care, or residential treatment. The respondent's age at and the duration of each such event are recorded.

The remainder of the section focuses on respondent reports about their mother and father or, in the absence of a mother or father during their childhood, the man and woman who served as the equivalents of mother and father. In cases when there were multiple people of this sort, information is obtained about how many there were and the ages at which these parent-surrogates lived with the respondent. Focusing on the main parent figure, respondents are asked about their biological relationship to this individual (e.g., grandfather, stepfather) as well as about the closeness and warmth of their interpersonal relationships during the years the respondent was growing up. A modified version of the Parental Bonding Instrument (Parker 1989) is used to classify parent-child relationships as either authoritarian, authoritative, overprotective, or neglectful. A modified version of the Conflict Tactics Scale (Straus et al. 1998) is used to assess the frequency and intensity of parental violence toward the respondent during the respondent's childhood. Questions are also asked about neglect and sexual abuse. Information is then obtained on parent education, employment status, occupation if they were employed, and the stability of their employment during the respondent's childhood. Finally, a modified version of the Family History Research Diagnostic Criteria Interview (Andreasen et al. 1977) is used to assess parental psychopathology during the respondent's childhood. Separate assessments are made here of parental depression, panic disorder, GAD, substance use disorder, and antisocial personality disorder.

## 12. OVERVIEW AND FUTURE DIRECTIONS

As noted in the introduction, the CIDI was originally developed by the WHO to be a tool that could help coordinate the efforts of psychiatric epidemiologists around the world to carry out community surveys in which results could be directly compared and cumulated by virtue of using the same instrument. CIDI 3.0 continues in this tradition by refining the diagnostic assessments in the original CIDI and by adding sections that examine risk factors, consequences, and treatment. Like the original CIDI, CIDI 3.0 was designed to generate diagnoses using the definitions and criteria of the most recent versions of both the ICD and DSM systems (ICD-10 and DSM-IV). In addition, like the original CIDI, CIDI 3.0 has been translated into a number of languages using the standard WHO translation and back-translation protocol. The number of CIDI 3.0 language versions is currently more than 30 and is still growing as we continue to recruit new countries into the WMH Survey Initiative.

An important CIDI 3.0 development is the establishment of an explicit protocol for modifying the instrument. In the past, reluctance on the part of the WHO CIDI Advisory Committee (WHO CIDI-AC) to work with investigators who proposed modifications led to idiosyncratic changes made by individual users in different surveys that reduced comparability across studies. The new protocol for modifying the CIDI calls for users who want to modify diagnostic questions to include both the original CIDI 3.0 questions and the proposed new questions in their modified version of the instrument and to carry out blind clinical follow-up interviews in a stratified probability sample of concordant and discordant cases to evaluate whether the new questions increase consistency of CIDI diagnoses with clinical diagnoses. In cases where the old and new questions cannot logically be included in the same instrument, a split ballot approach is stipulated in which random subsamples receive one or the other in the same study.

Stipulations for the design, instrumentation, and quality control of CIDI 3.0 clinical reappraisal studies have been established to guarantee endorsement of results by the WHO CIDI-AC. Suggestions for such methodological studies and results of these studies will be posted on the CIDI Web page (http://www.hcp.med.harvard.edu/wmhcidi/) along with author attributions. Replication of positive results in a second endorsed methodological study will lead to proposed changes being adopted in the next revision of the CIDI. A similar system of posting proposed modifications and expansions of the CIDI in ways that do not change the diagnostic questions will also be posted on the CIDI Web page to create a library of potentially useful alternative questions for future users. Included here, for example, might be expanded questions about childhood adversity, a new section on coping, or more elaborate questions about the nature of specific fears aimed at subtyping specific phobias. As with other proposed modifications and expansions of the instrument, author attributions will be included with each of these postings.

### REFERENCES

Aguilar-Gaxiola, S., Alegria, M., Andrade, L., Bijl, R. V., Caraveo-Anduaga, J. J., DeWit, D. J., Kolody, B., Kessler, R. C., Üstün, T. B., Vega, W. A. & Wittchen, H. U. (2000). The International Consortium in Psychiatric Epidemiology. In *Social psychiatry in changing times*, ed. E. Dragomirecká, A. Palcová & H. Papežová, pp. 86–95. Prague, Czech Republic: Prague Psychiatric Center.

Alegria, M., Kessler, R. C., Bijl, R., Lin, E., Heeringa, S., Takeuchi, D. T. & Kolody, B. (2000). Comparing mental health service use data across countries. In *Unmet need in mental health service delivery*, ed. G. Andrews, pp. 97–118. Cambridge, UK: Cambridge University Press.

Andreasen, N. C., Endicott, J., Spitzer, R. L. & Winokur, G. (1977). The family history method using diagnostic criteria: Reliability and validity. *Archives of General Psychiatry*, 34, 1229–35.

Angst, J., Merikangas, K., Scheidegger, P. & Wicki, W. (1990). Recurrent brief depression: A new subtype of affective disorder. *Journal of Affective Disorders (Amsterdam)*, 19, 87–98.

Belli, R. F. (1988). Color blend retrievals: Compromise memories or deliberate compromise responses? *Memory & Cognition*, 16, 314–26.

Belson, W. A. (1981). *The design and understanding of survey questions*. Aldershot, UK: Gower.

Benjamin, J., Ebstein, R. P. & Lesch, K. P. (1998). Genes for personality traits: Implications for psychopathology. *International Journal of Neuropsychopharmacology*, 1, 153–68.

Berardi, D., Berti Ceroni, G., Leggieri, G., Rucci, P., Üstün, T. B. & Ferrari, G. (1999). Mental, physical and functional status in primary care attenders. *International Journal of Psychiatry in Medicine*, 29, 133–48.

Bijl, R. V., de Graaf, R., Hiripi, E., Kessler, R. C., Kohn, R., Offord, D. R., Üstün, T. B., Vicente, B., Vollebergh, W. A., Walters, E. E. & Wittchen, H. U. (2003). The prevalence of treated and untreated mental disorders in five countries. *Health Affairs (Millwood)*, 22, 122–33.

Bijl, R. V. & Ravelli, A. (2000). Current and residual functional disability associated with psychopathology: Findings from the Netherlands mental health survey and incidence study (NEMESIS). *Psychological Medicine*, 30, 657–68.

Breslau, N. & Davis, G. C. (1985). DSM-III generalized anxiety disorder: An empirical investigation of more stringent criteria. *Psychiatry Research*, 15, 231–8.

Brewer, W. F. (1986). What is autobiographical memory? In *Autobiographical memory*, ed. D. C. Rubin, pp. 25–49. New York: Cambridge University Press.

Broadhead, W. E., Blazer, D. G., George, L. K. & Tse, C. K. (1990). Depression, disability days, and days lost from work in a prospective epidemiologic survey. *JAMA*, 264, 2524–8.

Brown, G. W. (1989). Life events and measurement. In *Life events and illness*, ed. G. W. Brown & T. O. Harris, pp. 3–45. New York: Guilford Press.

Brugha, T. S., Bebbington, P. E. & Jenkins, R. (1999). A difference that matters: Comparisons of structured and semi-structured psychiatric diagnostic interviews in the general population. *Psychological Medicine*, 29, 1013–20.

Brugha, T. S., Jenkins, R., Taub, N., Meltzer, H. & Bebbington, P. E. (2001). A general population comparison of the Composite International Diagnostic Interview (CIDI) and the Schedules for Clinical Assessment in Neuropsychiatry (SCAN). *Psychological Medicine*, 31, 1001–13.

Cannell, C. F., Fowler, F. J., Jr. & Marquis, K. H. (1968). The influence of interviewer and respondent psychological and behavioral variables on the reporting in household interviews. *Vital and Health Statistics Series 2*, *1*, 1–65.

Cannell, C. F., Miller, P. V. & Oksenberg, L. (1981). Research on interviewing techniques. In *Sociological methodology 1981*, ed. S. Leinhardt, pp. 389–487. San Francisco: Jossey-Bass Publishers.

Centers, R. (1964). A laboratory adaptation of the conversational procedure for the conditioning of verbal operants. *Journal of Abnormal and Social Psychology*, 67, 334–9.

Chakrabarti, S., Kulhara, P. & Verma, S. K. (1993). The pattern of burden in families of neurotic patients. *Social Psychiatry and Psychiatric Epidemiology*, 28, 172–7.

Clark, H. H. & Schober, M. F. (1992). Asking questions and influencing answers. In *Questions about questions: Inquiries into the cognitive bases of surveys*, ed. J. M. Tanur, pp. 15–48. New York: Russell Sage Foundation.

Cohen, J. (1960). A coefficient of agreement for nominal scales. *Educational and Psychological Measurement*, 20, 37–46.

Coryell, W., Scheftner, W., Keller, M., Endicott, J., Maser, J. & Klerman, G. L. (1993). The enduring psychosocial consequences of mania and depression. *American Journal of Psychiatry*, 150, 720–7.

Dewa, C. S. & Lin, E. (2000). Chronic physical illness, psychiatric disorder and disability in the workplace. *Social Science Medicine*, 51, 41–50.

Druss, B. G., Hwang, I., Petukhova, M., Sampson, N. A., Wang, P. S. & Kessler, R. C. (2008). Impairment in role functioning in mental and chronic medical disorders in the United States: Results from the National Comorbidity Survey Replication. *Molecular Psychiatry*, published.

Eaton, W. W., Badawi, M. & Melton, B. (1995). Prodromes and precursors: Epidemiologic data for primary prevention of disorders with slow onset. *American Journal of Psychiatry*, 152, 967–72.

Eaton, W. W., Kessler, R. C., Wittchen, H. U. & Magee, W. J. (1994). Panic and panic disorder in the United States. *American Journal of Psychiatry*, 151, 413–20.

Eaton, W. W., Neufeld, K., Chen, L. S. & Cai, G. (2000). A comparison of self-report and clinical diagnostic interviews for depression: Diagnostic interview schedule for clinical assessment in neuropsychiatry in the Baltimore epidemiologic catchment area follow-up. *Archives of General Psychiatry*, 57, 217–22.

Edwards, W. S., Winn, D. M., Kurlantzick, V., Sheridan, S., Berk, M. L., Retchin, S. & Collins, J. G. (1994). Evaluation of National Health Interview Survey Diagnostic Reporting: National Center for Health Statistics. *Vital and Health Statistics Series 2*, 120, 1–116.

Furukawa, T. A., Andrews, G., Slade, T. & Kessler, R. C. (2003). The performance of the K6 and K10 screening scales for psychological distress in the Australian National Survey of Mental Health and Well-Being. *Psychological Medicine*, 33, 357–62.

Gilman, S. (1988). *Disease and representation: Images of illness from madness to AIDS*. Ithaca, NY: Cornell University Press.

Gross, R., Bentur, N., Elhayany, A., Sherf, M. & Epstein, L. (1996). The validity of self-reports on chronic disease: Characteristics of underreporters and implications for the planning of services. *Public Health Review*, 24, 167–82.

Halabi, S., Zurayk, H., Awaida, R., Darwish, M. & Saab, B. (1992). Reliability and validity of self and proxy reporting of morbidity data: A case study from Beirut, Lebanon. *International Journal of Epidemiology*, 21, 607–12.

Hays, R. D., Wells, K. B., Sherbourne, C. D., Rogers, W. & Spritzer, K. (1995). Functioning and well-being outcomes of patients with depression compared with chronic general medical illnesses. *Archives of General Psychiatry*, 52, 11–9.

Heliovaara, M., Aromaa, A., Klaukka, T., Knekt, P., Joukamaa, M. & Impivaara, O. (1993). Reliability and validity of interview data on chronic diseases: The Mini-Finland Health Survey. *Journal of Clinical Epidemiology*, 46, 181–91.

Jobe, J. B., White, A. A., Kelley, C. L., Mingay, D. L., Sanchez, M. J. & Loftus, E. F. (1990). Recall strategies and memory for health care visits. *Milbank Quarterly*, 68, 171–89.

Judd, L. L., Paulus, M. P., Wells, K. B. & Rapaport, M. N. (1996). Socioeconomic burden of subsyndromal depressive symptoms and major depression in a sample of the general population. *American Journal of Psychiatry*, 153, 1411–7.

Kempen, G. I., Ormel, J., Brilman, E. I. & Relyveld, J. (1997). Adaptive responses among Dutch elderly: The impact of eight chronic conditions on health-related quality of life. *American Journal of Public Health*, 87, 38–44.

Kempen, G. I., Sanderman, R., Miedema, I., Mayboom-de, J. B. & Ormel, J. (2000). Functional decline after congestive heart failure and acute myocardial infarction and the impact of psychological attributes: A prospective study. *Quality of Life Research*, 9, 439–50.

Kendell, R. E. (2002). Five criteria for an improved taxonomy of mental disorders. In *Defining psychopathology in the 21st century: DSM-V and beyond*, ed. J. E. Helzer & J. J. Hudziak, pp. 3–17. Washington, DC: American Psychiatric Publishing.

Kessler, R. (1999). The World Health Organization International Consortium in Psychiatric Epidemiology (ICPE): Initial work and future directions – the NAPE lecture 1998. *Acta Psychiatrica Scandinavica*, 99, 2–9.

Kessler, R. C., Andrews, G., Colpe, L. J., Hiripi, E., Mroczek, D. K., Normand, S. L., Walters, E. E. & Zaslavsky, A. M. (2002). Short screening scales to monitor population prevalences and trends in non-specific psychological distress. *Psychological Medicine*, 32, 959–76.

Kessler, R. C., Barber, C., Beck, A., Berglund, P. A., Cleary, P. D., McKenas, D., Pronk, N., Simon, G., Stang, P., Üstün, T. B. & Wang, P. S. (2003a). The World Health Organization Health and Work Performance Questionnaire (HPQ). *Journal of Occupational and Environmental Medicine*, 45, 156–74.

Kessler, R. C., Barker, P. R., Colpe, L. J., Epstein, A., Gfroerer, J. C., Hiripi, E., Howes, M. J., Normand, S.-L. T., Manderscheid, R. W., Walters, E. E. & Zaslavsky, A. M. (2003b). Screening for serious mental illness in the general population. *Archives of General Psychiatry*, 60, 184–9.

Kessler, R. C., Greenberg, P. E., Mickelson, K. D., Meneades, L. M. & Wang, P. S. (2001). The effects of chronic medical conditions on work loss and work cutback. *Journal of Occupational and Environmental Medicine*, 43, 218–25.

Kessler R. C., Merikangas K. R., Berglund P., Eaton W. W., Koretz D., & Walters E. E. (2003c) Mild disorders should not be eliminated from the DSM-V. *Archives of General Psychiatry*, 60, 1117–22.

Kessler, R. C., Mroczek, D. K. & Belli, R. F. (1999). Retrospective adult assessment of childhood psychopathology. In *Diagnostic assessment in child and adolescent psychopathology*, ed. D. Shaffer, C. P. Lucas & J. E. Richters, pp. 256–84. New York: Guilford Press.

Kessler, R. C., Olfson, M. & Berglund, P. A. (1998). Patterns and predictors of treatment contact after first onset of psychiatric disorders. *American Journal of Psychiatry*, 155, 62–9.

Kessler, R. C. & Üstün, T. B. (2004). The World Mental Health (WMH) Survey Initiative Version of the World Health Organization (WHO) Composite International Diagnostic Interview (CIDI).

*International Journal of Methods in Psychiatric Research*, 13, 93–121.

Kessler, R. C., Wittchen, H.-U., Abelson, J. M., Mc-Gonagle, K., Schwarz, N., Kendler, K. S., Knauper, B. & Zhao, S. (1998). Methodological studies of the Composite International Diagnostic Interview (CIDI) in the U.S. National Comorbidity Survey. *International Journal of Methods in Psychiatric Research*, 7, 33–55.

Kessler, R. C., Wittchen, H. U., Abelson, J. M. & Zhao, S. (2000). Methodological issues in assessing psychiatric disorder with self-reports. In *The science of self-report: Implications for research and practice*, ed. A. A. Stone, J. S. Turrkan, C. A. Bachrach, J. B. Jobe, H. S. Kurtzman & V. S. Cain, pp. 229–55. Mahwah, NJ: Lawrence Erlbaum Associates.

Kriegsman, D. M., Penninx, B. W., van Eijk, J. T., Boeke, A. J. & Deeg, D. J. (1996). Self-reports and general practitioner information on the presence of chronic diseases in community dwelling elderly: A study on the accuracy of patients' self-reports and on determinants of inaccuracy. *Journal of Clinical Epidemiology*, 49, 1407–17.

Leon, A. C., Olfson, M., Portera, L., Farber, L. & Sheehan, D. V. (1997). Assessing psychiatric impairment in primary care with the Sheehan Disability Scale. *International Journal of Psychiatry in Medicine*, 27, 93–105.

Leventhal, H., Nerenz, D. & Steele, D. J. (1984). Illness representations and coping with health threats. In *Handbook of psychology and health*, ed. A. Baum, S. E. Taylor & J. E. Singer, pp. 219–52. Hillsdale, NJ: Lawrence Erlbaum Associates.

Lipton, R. B., Dodick, D., Sadovsky, R., Kolodner, K., Endicott, J., Hettiarachchi, J. & Harrison, W. (2003). A self-administered screener for migraine in primary care: The ID Migraine (TM) validation study. *Neurology*, 61, 375–82.

Loftus, E. F. & Palmer, J. C. (1974). Reconstruction of automobile destructions: An example of the integration between language and memory. *Journal of Verbal Language and Verbal Behavior*, 13, 585–9.

Mackenbach, J. P., Looman, C. W. & Van Der Meer, J. B. (1996). Differences in the misreporting of chronic conditions, by level of education: The effect on inequalities in prevalence rates. *American Journal of Public Health*, 86, 706–11.

Maier, W., Gansicke, M., Freyberger, H. J., Linz, M., Heun, R. & Lecrubier, Y. (2000). Generalized anxiety disorder (ICD-10) in primary care from a cross-cultural perspective: a valid diagnostic entity? *Acta Psychiatrica Scandinavica*, 101, 29–36.

Markus, H. & Zajonc, R. B. (1985). The cognitive perspective in social psychology. In *The handbook of social psychology*, ed. G. Lindzey & E. Aronson, pp. 137–230. New York: Random House.

Marlatt, G. A. (1972). Task structure and the experimental modification of verbal behavior. *Psychological Bulletin*, 78, 335–50.

Marquis, K. H. & Cannell, C. F. (1969). *A study of interviewer-respondent interaction in the urban employment*. Ann Arbor: Survey Research Center, University of Michigan.

Means, B. & Loftus, E. F. (1991). When personal history repeats itself: Decomposing memories for recurring events. *Applied Cognitive Psychology*, 5, 297–318.

Mechanic, D. (2003). Is the prevalence of mental disorders a good measure of the need for services? *Health Affairs (Millwood)*, 22, 8–20.

Menon, A. (1994). Judgements of behavioral frequencies: Memory search and retrieval strategies. In *Autobiographical memory and the validity of retrospective reports*, ed. N. Schwartz & S. Sudman, pp. 161–72. New York: Springer-Verlag.

Merikangas, K. R., Ames, M., Cui, L., Stang, P. E., Üstün, T. B., Von Korff, M. & Kessler, R. C. (2007). The impact of comorbidity of mental and physical conditions on role disability in the U.S. adult household population. *Archives of General Psychiatry*, 64, 1180–8.

Merikangas, K. R., Zhang, H., Avenevoli, S., Acharyya, S., Neuenschwander, M. & Angst, J. (2003). Longitudinal trajectories of depression and anxiety in a prospective community study: The Zurich Cohort Study. *Archives of General Psychiatry*, 60, 993–1000.

Miller, P. V. & Cannell, C. F. (1977). Communicating measurement objectives in the survey interview. In *Strategies for communication research*, ed. D. M. Hirsch, P. V. Miller & F. G. Kline, pp. 127–51. Beverly Hills, CA: Sage Publications.

Murray, C. J. L. & Lopez, A. D. (1996). *The global burden of disease: A comprehensive assessment of mortality and disability from diseases, injuries and risk factors in 1990 and projected to 2020*. Cambridge, MA: Harvard University Press.

Narrow, W. E., Rae, D. S., Robins, L. N. & Regier, D. A. (2002). Revised prevalence estimates of mental disorders in the United States: Using a clinical significance criterion to reconcile 2 surveys' estimates. *Archives of General Psychiatry*, 59, 115–23.

National Advisory Mental Health Council (1993). Health care reform for Americans with severe mental illnesses: Report of the National Advisory Mental Health Council. *American Journal of Psychiatry*, 150, 1447–65.

National Center for Health Statistics, Division of Data Services. (2003). *2003 National Health Interview Survey (NHIS)*. Hyattsville, MD: U.S. Department of Health and Human Services, Centers for Disease Control.

Neeleman, J., Ormel, J. & Bijl, R. V. (2001). The distribution of psychiatric and somatic ill-health: Associations with personality and socioeconomic status. *Psychosomatic Medicine*, 63, 239–47.

Oksenberg, L., Cannell, C. F. & Kanton, G. (1991). New strategies for pretesting survey questions. *Journal of Official Statistics*, 7, 349–65.

Oksenberg, L., Vinokur, A. & Cannell, C. F. (1979a). The effects of instructions, commitment and feedback on reporting in personal interviews. In *Experiments in interviewing techniques*, DHEW Publication No. (HRA) 78-3204, ed. C. F. Cannell, L. Oksenberg & J. M. Converse, pp. 133–99. Washington, DC: Department of Health, Education, and Welfare.

Oksenberg, L., Vinokur, A. & Cannell, C. F. (1979b). Effects of commitment to being a good respondent on interview performance. In *Experiments in interviewing techniques*, DHEW Publication No. (HRA) 78-3204, ed. C. F. Cannell, L. Oksenberg & J. M. Converse, pp. 74–108. Washington, DC: Department of Health, Education, and Welfare.

Olfson, M., Kessler, R. C., Berglund, P. A. & Lin, E. (1998). Psychiatric disorder onset and first treatment contact in the United States and Ontario. *American Journal of Psychiatry*, 155, 1415–22.

Ormel, J., Kempen, G. I., Deeg, D. J., Brilman, E. I., van Sonderen, E. & Relyveld, J. (1998). Functioning, well-being, and health perception in late middle-aged and older people: Comparing the effects of depressive symptoms and chronic medical conditions. *Journal of American Geriatrics Society*, 46, 39–48.

Ormel, J., Von Korff, N., Üstün, T. B., Pini, S., Korten, A. & Oldehinkel, T. (1994). Common mental disorders and disability across cultures: Results from the WHO collaborative study on psychological problems in general health care. *JAMA*, 272, 1741–8.

Parker, G. (1989). The Parental Bonding Instrument: Psychometric properties reviewed. *Psychiatric Development*, 7, 317–35.

Pearson, R. W., Ross, M. & Dawes, R. M. (1992). Personal recall and the limits of retrospective questions in surveys. In *Questions about questions: Inquiries into the cognitive bases of surveys*, ed. J. M. Tanur, pp. 65–94. New York: Russell Sage Foundation.

Penninx, B. W., Beekman, A. T., Ormel, J., Kriegsman, D. M., Boeke, A. J., van Eijk, J. T. & Deeg, D. J. (1996). Psychological status among elderly people with chronic diseases: Does type of disease play a part? *Journal of Psychosomatic Research*, 40, 521–34.

Pincus, H. A., Zarin, D. A. & First, M. (1998). "Clinical Significance" and DSM-IV. *Archives of General Psychiatry*, 55, 1145.

Preisig, M., Merikangas, K. R. & Angst, J. (2001). Clinical significance and comorbidity of subthreshold depression and anxiety in the community. *Acta Psychiatrica Scandinavica*, 104, 96–103.

Regier, D. A. (2000). Community diagnosis counts [commentary]. *Archives of General Psychiatry*, 57, 223–4.

Regier, D. A., Kaelber, C. T., Rae, D. S., Farmer, M. E., Knauper, B., Kessler, R. C. & Norquist, G. S. (1998). Limitations of diagnostic criteria and assessment instruments for mental disorders: Implications for research and policy. *Archives of General Psychiatry*, 55, 109–15.

Regier, D. A. & Narrow, W. E. (2002). Defining clinically significant psychopathology with epidemiologic data. In *Defining psychopathology in the 21st century: DSM-V and beyond*, ed. J. E. Helzer and J. J. Hudziak, pp. 19–30. Washington, DC: American Psychiatric Publishing.

Rehm, J., Üstün, T. B., Saxena, S., Nelson, C. B., Chatterji, S., Ivis, F. & Adlaf, E. (1999). On the development and psychometric testing of the WHO screening instrument to assess disablement in the general population. *International Journal of Methods in Psychiatric Research*, 8, 110–23.

Rhode, P., Lewinsohn, P. & Seeley, J. (1990). Are people changed by the experience of having an episode of depression? A further test of the scar hypotheses. *Journal of Abnormal Psychology*, 99, 264–71.

Robins, L. N., Helzer, J. E., Croughan, J. L. & Ratcliff, K. S. (1981). National Institute of Mental Health Diagnostic Interview Schedule: Its history, characteristics and validity. *Archives of General Psychiatry*, 38, 381–9.

Robins, L. N. & Regier, D. A., eds. (1991). *Psychiatric disorders in America: The Epidemiologic Catchment Area Study*. New York: Free Press.

Robins, L. N., Wing, J., Wittchen, H. U., Helzer, J. E., Babor, T. F., Burke, J., Farmer, A., Jablenski, A., Pickens, R., Regier, D. A., Sartorius, N. & Towle, L. H. (1988). The Composite International Diagnostic Interview: An epidemiologic instrument suitable for use in conjunction with different diagnostic systems and in different cultures. *Archives of General Psychiatry*, 45, 1069–77.

Rupp, A. & Keith, S. J. (1993). The costs of schizophrenia: Assessing the burden. *Psychiatric Clinics of North America*, 16, 413–23.

Rush, A. J., Gullion, C. M., Basco, M. R., Jarrett, R. B. & Trivedi, M. H. (1996). The Inventory of Depressive Symptomatology (IDS): Psychometric properties. *Psychological Medicine*, 26, 477–86.

Saunders, J. C. (2003). Families living with severe mental illness: A literature review. *Issues in Mental Health Nursing*, 24, 175–98.

Schlesselman, J. (1982). *Case-control studies: Design, conduct, analysis*. New York: Oxford University Press.

Schwarz, N. & Sudman, S., eds. (1994). *Autobiographical memory and the validity of retrospective reports*. New York: Springer-Verlag.

Schwarz, N. & Sudman, S., eds. (1996). *Answering questions: Methodology for determining cognitive and communicative processes in survey research*. San Francisco: Jossey-Bass Publishers.

Shear, M. K., Brown, T. A., Barlow, D. H., Money, R., Sholomskas, D. E., Woods, S. W., Gorman, J. M. & Papp, L. A. (1997). Multicenter collaborative panic disorder severity scale. *American Journal of Psychiatry*, 154, 1571–5.

Sheehan D. V., Harnett-Sheehan K. & Raj B. A. (1996) The measurement of disability. *International Clinical Psychopharmacology*, 11 Suppl 3, 89–95.

Sirken, M. G., Herrmann, D. J., Schechter, S., Schwarz, N., Tanur, J. M. & Tourangeau, R., eds. (1999). *Cognition and survey research*. New York: John Wiley & Sons.

Skelton, J. A. & Croyle, R. T., eds. (1991). *Mental representation in health and illness*. New York: Springer-Verlag.

Spitzer, R. L. (1998). Diagnosis and need for treatment are not the same. *Archives of General Psychiatry*, 55, 120.

Stewart, A., Greenfield, S. & Hays, R. D. (1989). Functional status and well-being of patients with chronic conditions. *JAMA*, 262, 907–13.

Straus, M. A., Hamby, S. L., Finkelhor, D., Moore, D. W. & Runyan, D. (1998). Identification of child maltreatment with the Parent-Child Conflict Tactics Scales: Development and psychometric data for a national sample of American parents. *Child Abuse and Neglect*, 22, 249–70.

Substance Abuse and Mental Health Services Administration (1993). Final notice establishing definitions for (1) children with a serious emotional disturbance, and (2) adults with a serious mental illness. *Federal Register*, 58, 29422–5.

Sudman, S., Bradburn, N. & Schwarz, N. (1996). *Thinking about answers: The application of cognitive processes to survey methodology*. San Francisco: Jossey-Bass Publishers.

Sullivan, M. D., LaCroix, A. Z., Russo, J. E. & Walker, E. A. (2001). Depression and self-reported physical health in patients with coronary disease: Mediating and moderating factors. *Psychosomatic Medicine*, 63, 248–56.

Tanur, J. M. (1992). *Questions about questions: Inquiries into the cognitive bases of surveys*. New York: Russell Sage Foundation.

Tsang, H. W., Tam, P. K., Chan, F. & Chang, W. M. (2003). Sources of burdens on families of individuals with mental illness. *International Journal of Rehabilitation Research*, 26, 123–30.

Turner, C. & Martin, E. (1985). *Surveying subjective phenomena*. New York: Russell Sage Foundation.

Tweed, D. L. (1993). Depression-related impairment: Estimating concurrent and lingering effects. *Psychological Medicine*, 23, 373–86.

Üstün, T. B., Chatterji, S. & Rehm, J. (1998). Limitations of diagnostic paradigm: It doesn't explain "need." *Archives of General Psychiatry*, 55, 1145–8.

van den Bos, G. A. (1995). The burden of chronic disease in terms of disability, use of health care and healthy life expectancies. *European Journal of Public Health*, 5, 29–34.

Verbrugge, L. M. & Patrick, D. L. (1995). Seven chronic conditions: Their impact on U.S. adults' activity levels and use of medical services. *American Journal of Public Health*, 85, 173–82.

Vinokur, A., Oksenberg, L. & Cannell, C. F. (1979). Effects of feedback and reinforcement on the report of health information. In *Experiments in interviewing techniques*, ed. C. F. Cannell, L. Oksenberg & J. M. Converse. Ann Arbor: Survey Research Center, University of Michigan.

Wang, P. S., Simon, G. E., Avorn, J., Azocar, F., Ludman, E. J., McCulloch, J., Petukhova, M. Z. & Kessler, R. C. (2007). Telephone screening, outreach, and care management for depressed workers and impact on clinical and work productivity outcomes: A randomized controlled trial. *JAMA*, 298, 1401–11.

Wells, K. B., Stewart, A., Hays, R. D., Burnam, M., Rogers, W., Daniels, M., Berry, S., Greenfield, S. & Ware, J. (1989). The functioning and well-being of depressed patients: Results from the Medical Outcomes Study. *JAMA*, 262, 914–9.

Wittchen, H.-U. (1994). Reliability and validity studies of the WHO Composite International Diagnostic Interview (CIDI): A critical review. *Journal of Psychiatric Research*, 28, 57–84.

Wittchen, H.-U., Üstün, T. B. & Kessler, R. C. (1999). Diagnosing mental disorders in the community: A difference that matters. *Psychological Medicine*, 29, 1021–7.

World Health Organization (WHO) (1990). *Composite International Diagnostic Interview*. Geneva: World Health Organization.

World Health Organization (WHO) (1998). *WHO Disablements Assessment Schedule II (WHO-DAS II)*. Geneva: World Health Organization.

World Health Organization (WHO) (2001). *International Classification of Functioning, Disability and Health*. Geneva: World Health Organization.

World Health Organization (WHO) International Consortium in Psychiatric Epidemiology (2000). Cross-national comparisons of the prevalences and correlates of mental disorders. *Bulletin of the World Health Organization*, 78, 413–26.

Zeiss, A. & Lewinsohn, P. (1988). Enduring deficits after remission of depression: A test of the "scar" hypotheses. *Behavior Research Therapy*, 26, 151–8.

## APPENDIX: EXAMPLES OF CIDI MODIFICATIONS

### A.1. QUESTION COMPREHENSION

#### A.1.1. Breaking Down Complex Questions into Less Complex Subquestions

A good example of a complex question is the stem question for dysphoria in the depression section. This is a very important question because failure to endorse it or a parallel question about anhedonia leads to the respondent being skipped out of further questions about depression. The question in the standard CIDI is as follows: "In your lifetime, have you ever had two weeks or longer when nearly every day you felt sad, empty, or depressed for most of the day?" This is an exceedingly complex question, as it asks about a cluster of emotions (sad, empty, or depressed) over a duration of time (two weeks or longer), which itself can have internal variation in duration both across days (nearly every day) and within days (most of the day). Debriefing studies show that most respondents miss at least one of these core components. Therefore, we decompose the question in the CIDI. We begin by asking about a shorter period of time and omit mention of between-day variation in duration: "Have you ever in your life had a period lasting several days or longer when most of the day you felt sad, empty, or depressed?" Positive responses are then followed by a duration question: "Did you ever have a period of this sort that lasted *most of the day, nearly every day*, for *two weeks* or longer?" (The underlines are an indication to interviewers to emphasize these words.) This question is then followed by a within-day duration question: "Think of times lasting two weeks or longer when these problems with your mood were more severe and frequent. During those times, did these feelings usually last less than one hour, between one and three hours, between three and five hours, or

more than five hours?" The reader might think that this last question is unnecessary, as the question before it asked about dysphoria lasting "most of the day." However, pilot studies of the CIDI showed clearly that this aspect of the question was the least likely to be heard by respondents, leading to quite a few respondents who endorsed this question reporting in a follow-up question that their low mood lasted only for an hour or two. On the basis of this result, the follow-up question about within-day duration was retained in the final CIDI. A separate follow-up question about between-day duration (i.e., whether the dysphoria lasted every day, nearly ever day, most days, half the days, or less than half the days over the two weeks) was found not to be necessary, as all pilot respondents responded "every" or "nearly every day."

#### A.1.2. Clarifying Vaguely Defined Terms

A good example of a vaguely defined term is the single standard dichotomous CIDI question about role impairment that is used in every diagnostic section of the CIDI: "Did (SYNDROME) interfere with your life and activities a lot?" This is a critical question, as it is used to operationalize the impairment component of the DSM-IV requirement that a syndrome cause clinically significant distress or impairment to qualify as a disorder. Yet both the word "interfere" and the word "a lot" are ambiguous. Furthermore, the fact that the question is dichotomous and requires an intensity qualifier to be answered positively (i.e., it is not enough for the syndrome to interfere; it must interfere a lot) creates a source of confusion. This was clearly visible in pilot studies carried out by Kessler and colleagues (2000), who found that respondents who endorsed the standard CIDI question often responded "some" or "a little" to a follow-up question that asked, "How much did it interfere with these activities – would you say a lot, some, or only a little?"

It might seem strange that a respondent who just responded yes to a question about whether there was "a lot" of interference would characterize the interference as less intense in the very next question, but the fact that this frequently occurs is testimony to the fact that survey respondents often fail to listen carefully to secondary clauses in dichotomously worded questions. Recognizing this problem, the CIDI converts the dichotomous yes-no question about a lot of interference into a dimensional question that focuses the respondent's attention on the intensity of interference by asking, "How much did (SYNDROME) interfere – not at all, a little, some, a lot, or extremely?" A small split-ballot experiment in a pilot study carried out by Kessler and colleagues (2000) found that this wording change resulted in a significantly lower proportion of respondents reporting that the interference was severe enough to be characterized as "a lot" than in the standard dichotomous CIDI question.

In addition to turning the dichotomous response scale into a polychotomous scale, the CIDI also expands the standard CIDI interference question to make sure that respondents broadly review all major areas in their life before answering. The fully modified question is: "How much did (SYNDROME) interfere with either your work, your social life, or your personal relationships – not at all, a little, some, a lot, or extremely?" To clarify the intensity level implied by the various response categories, a follow-up question is then asked in the CIDI to all respondents who report any interference: "How often were you unable to carry out your daily activities because of (SYNDROME) – often, sometimes, rarely, or never?"

### A.1.3. Clarifying Questions about Odd Experiences that Could be Normalized

The standard version of CIDI introduces the psychosis questions with the statement: "Now I want to ask you about some ideas you might have had about other people." The questioning then begins by asking about delusions rather than about hallucinations. The first question is: "Have you ever believed people were spying on you?" This is followed by questions about believing that people are spying on you and talking about you behind your back. Each time a positive response is given, the interviewer asks: "How did you know this was happening?" An open-ended response is

recorded and rated for plausibility. A great many people answer these questions positively, the vast majority of whom give plausible answers. This is not surprising, as the experiences asked about are all quite common. The first genuinely odd experience is not asked about until the fourth question in the series: "Have you ever believed that you were being secretly tested or experimented on?" This is followed by two remaining questions about delusions that could be interpreted in plausible terms: whether someone ever "plotted against you" or "tried to hurt you or poison you"; whether the respondent ever thought that "someone you never met was in love with you"; and a question about whether the respondent ever was convinced that his or her spouse or partner was being unfaithful even though they said this was not true.

These are followed by questions about more bizarre delusions, such as mind reading (e.g., "Have you ever believed that someone was reading your mind?"), thought control (e.g., "Have you ever been convinced that you were under the control of some power or force, so that your actions and thoughts were not your own?"), and being able to receive special messages through the mass media. Finally, the symptom assessment finishes with questions about visual, auditory, olfactory, and tactile hallucinations. Most of these questions are purposefully worded in a way that is designed to normalize them. For example, the auditory hallucinations question asks: "Have you more than once heard things other people couldn't hear, such as a voice?" This normalized phrasing leads to confusion, as a great many respondents in general population samples respond positively and then, in response to the follow-up question, "How do you explain hearing things other people couldn't hear?" respond by saying "I have very good hearing."

The philosophy behind this approach to assessing psychosis is that psychotics will be more willing to admit their symptoms if these symptoms are normalized. A great difficulty with this approach is that it generates an enormous number of false positives. This substantially complicates the process of screening for psychosis and introduces the strong possibility of errors in classifying false positives as cases based on misleading open-ended responses. In addition, a question can be raised as to whether true psychotics, particularly those with paranoid tendencies, will be motivated positively or negatively to respond positively to normalized questions that they might perceive as trying to trick them into reporting their clearly abnormal experiences. The philosophy behind the CIDI approach is the opposite: to make it clear to respondents that we are asking about odd experiences; to motivate reporting with an introduction that validates the experiences and points to the importance of learning more about them; and to begin the questioning with hallucinations rather than delusions to reinforce the introductory remarks about the questions being about odd behaviors.

The CIDI introduction is as follows: "The next questions are about unusual things, like seeing visions or hearing voices. We believe that these things may be quite common, but we don't know for sure because previous research has not done a good job of asking about them. So please take your time and think carefully before answering." One can see in this introduction a number of the methodological refinements discussed in the body of the chapter: clarification of the nature of the questions, validation of the experiences, motivation for honest reporting, and facilitation of serious memory search by legitimating the respondent not answering immediately in order to think. The questions themselves are worded in such a way as to avoid confusion. Compare, for example, the CIDI question about auditory hallucinations with the standard CIDI question about the same symptom: "The next question is about hearing voices that other people could not hear. I don't mean having good hearing, but rather hearing things that other people said did not exist, like strange voices coming from inside your head talking to you or about you, or voices coming out of the air when there was no one around. Did you ever hear voices in this way?"

### A.1.4. Contextual Misunderstanding

Contextual misunderstanding is a type of misunderstanding that derives from the position of the question in the flow of the interview. An example was given there about confusion in a question regarding the duration of phobic fears. The standard question order in the CIDI was modified to correct this problem. A number of similar small, but important, cases of a related sort were found and corrected in developing the CIDI. One additional example: in asking about number of lifetime manic episodes, the standard CIDI comes directly after a question about the duration of the respondent's longest lifetime manic episode. The number-of-episodes question then follows, asking about the number of "these" lifetime episodes. Debriefing shows that the word "these" in the context of this placement leads a number of respondents incorrectly to believe that the interviewer is asking about episodes that were equally as long as the longest lifetime episode, resulting in an underestimate of the number of lifetime manic episodes. A person who had, say, 30 manic episodes, only 4 of which went on as long as the longest episode, might respond 3 rather than 30 to this question about number of episodes. This problem was corrected in the CIDI by a change in question placement.

### A.2. TASK COMPREHENSION

Survey respondents are often unaware that interviewers want them to engage in active memory search in answering complex questions. Indeed, it often occurs that investigators who write survey questions without cognitive debriefing pilot studies themselves fail to appreciate the cognitive complexity involved in answering some survey question. This is all the more true for interviewers, who, in the absence of special training in the use of feedback methods aimed at stimulating thoughtful responding, will be more concerned with the accuracy of recording answers than in the accuracy of the answers being given. The CIDI includes clarifications in a number of places to make this task clear to respondents. Earlier, in Chapter 1, we discussed one of the most important places where this is done, in the life review section of the interview.

There are numerous other places in the instrument where the same principle is used to remind the respondent to think carefully. One of the most consistent of these is in the important question about age of disorder onset, which appears in each diagnostic section of the interview. The standard CIDI question asks, "How old were you the first time you (HAD THE SYNDROME)?" We know from debriefing interviews that many respondents have a very difficult time remembering their age of onset, especially for accretion disorders. Therefore, it is important both to make clear that we are looking for a serious memory search and to deal with the possibility that we may be asking for more than the respondent knows. As described in the body of Chapter 1, we deal with the first of these issues in the CIDI by asking what is known in the survey methodology literature as a "prequest," a question designed to create a clarifying context for the substantive question that follows it: "Can you remember your *exact age* the *very first time* you (HAD THE SYNDROME)?" Even though a great many respondents answer no, this question is extremely important in making the task clear to respondents. We are interested in a precise answer, which means that serious memory search is required.

It is also noteworthy that we try to be equally clear when we want estimates rather than precise information. This is important because it is not possible to motivate respondents to engage in active memory search throughout an entire long interview. Instead, we need to pick and choose the especially important questions where extra effort is thought to be needed and to be clear both to ourselves and to respondents when we are willing to settle for approximations. So, for example, questions concerning lifetime course of illness (e.g., "About how many different years in your life did you have [SYNDROME]?") explicitly ask for approximations by using the word "about." In addition, interviewers are trained both to accept approximations as answers to these questions and to probe for rough estimates if respondents say they are unable to provide exact responses. In a similar way, we use structured response categories with prespecified ranges rather than open-ended responses in cases where we ask estimation questions that will be difficult to answer, and we recognize the inability to obtain accurate fine-grained responses from most respondents.

## A.3. MOTIVATION

### A.3.1. Motivational Instructions and Commitment Questions

We developed a statement at the beginning of the life review section to emphasize the importance of careful response to encourage complete and accurate answers. As noted earlier, a commitment question is used in conjunction with the motivational instructions to make sure that the respondent is aware of and acknowledges the importance of responding carefully. The statement and commitment question are as follows: "(READ SLOWLY) The next questions are about health problems you may have had at any time in your life. It is important for the research that you think carefully before answering. Are you willing to do this?" In cases where the respondent does not answer yes to the commitment question, the interviewer is instructed to offer to reschedule the interview for a time when the respondent is more able to give serious thought to the questions. If the respondent persists in saying that he or she is unwilling to think carefully before answering, the interviewer is instructed to terminate the interview and to code the respondent as a refusal.

### A.3.2. Contingent Reinforcement

Contingent reinforcement is an interviewer feedback strategy rather than a question wording strategy. The interviewer training manual for the CIDI (which is available only to researchers who participate in the official CIDI training described earlier in this chapter) focuses considerable attention on the use of this directive feedback strategy. A variety of probes are provided to interviewers to reinforce apparent effort in providing thoughtful answers. These are very simple feedback responses, like "thanks" and "that's useful," which are administered whether the response is positive or negative, so long as effort appears to be invested in providing a thoughtful answer.

Responses that might be thought to imply a value judgment, like "good" or "excellent," are not used.

A variety of probes are also provided to give negative feedback for apparently superficial responses. Sometimes these take the form of a follow-up question to a seemingly superficial negative response (e.g., "Are you sure there was nothing?"). At other times they take the form of an injunction (e.g., "Please take your time and think carefully."). At still other times the probe can take the form of an observation followed by a request (e.g., "You answered that one awfully quickly. Could you take a minute to think hard and make sure you didn't forget anything?"). Our experience is that the long versions of the negative probes are most useful early in the interview, when respondents who give superficial answers are being trained to be more thoughtful. Periodic short positive feedback probes, with the rare use of a short negative probe at the first signs of the recurrence of superficial responding, generally are used throughout the remainder of the interview.

## A.3.3. The Ability to Answer Accurately

We use two broad strategies to deal with the realization that autobiographical memory has limits. The main one is to accept these limits and revise our questions so as to settle for less detail than we would ideally like to have. The other is to push the limits of memory by decomposing questions in ways that mimic successful memory search strategies and bound uncertainty. We already gave examples earlier in this appendix of the first of these two strategies. As illustrated in these examples, we always signal to respondents when we want approximations rather than exact responses. This is done either by building into the question an explicit reference to wanting an approximation or by providing structured response categories in rough groupings that indicate the level of approximation we are looking for in responses. Perhaps the best example of this approach is the question series described earlier in the appendix about age of disorder onset. As noted in that description, we begin

this series with the prequest: "Can you remember your *exact age* the *very first time* you (HAD THE SYNDROME)?" Respondents who answer yes are dealt with easily by asking them to report this exact age. Respondents who say no, in comparison, are asked for an estimate: "*About* how old were you the first time?"

This same question series also illustrates the use of the second strategy used to deal with the limits of autobiographical memory: decomposing questions and bounding uncertainty for respondents who vary in accuracy of recall. As information about age of onset is of great importance for a variety of substantive research questions, special effort was invested in pushing for the limits of memory among respondents who reported that they could not recall the exact age when the syndrome first began. This is done using special probes to ask respondents to go backward in time sequentially. This requires flexibility on the part of interviewers, as a good many respondents who answer no to the question about exact recall volunteer, in conjunction with that answer, that the syndrome has been going on "my whole life" or "as long as I can remember."

This kind of inexact information is useful because it implies a very early age of onset. To confirm this, though, such responses are probed for clarification of an upper bound by asking, "Was it before you first started school?" If the respondent answers yes, the question sequence ends, with a fairly narrow bounding of uncertainty in an early age range. If, however, the respondent does not answer yes to this first probe (e.g., if the respondent says "I can't really remember" or "I don't think so" or something similar), the interviewer then moves up the age range incrementally until he or she finds an interval of time at which the respondent feels secure in saying that the syndrome was definitely in existence as of that point in the life course (e.g., "Was it before you were a teenager?" If not, "Was it before you turned 20?"). Our experience in pilot studies, which has been confirmed in WMH surveys, is that most uncertainty among respondents who begin by saying that their inability to provide an exact age is due to the syndrome going on "as long as I can remember" can be bounded before the teenage years.

Among respondents who do not volunteer a comment to the effect that the syndrome has been going on "as long as I can remember" in response to the exact age question, in comparison, the interviewer begins by probing for such a response (i.e., "Did it go on as long as you can remember?"). If so, then probing proceeds as if this response was volunteered. If the respondent says that the syndrome did not go on as long as he or she can remember, in comparison, debrief-

ing studies show that recall is quite certain for a fairly specific time in the life course but not for a particular age. Therefore, the same series of probes moving up the age range is used as described in the previous paragraph, with a final request for a best estimate of the onset age once an upper-bound age range is reached. Responses that are given in ranges (e.g., "It started during my teens, but I can't remember the exact age") are recorded initially as ranges and then analyzed as the upper end of the range to provide a consistently conservative, lower-bound estimate.

# 5 Translation Procedures and Translation Assessment in the World Mental Health Survey Initiative

JANET HARKNESS, BETH-ELLEN PENNELL, ANA VILLAR, NANCY GEBLER, SERGIO AGUILAR-GAXIOLA, AND IPEK BILGEN

## ACKNOWLEDGMENTS

Preparation of this chapter was supported by the U.S. National Institute of Mental Health (R01MH070884), the John D. and Catherine T. MacArthur Foundation, the Pfizer Foundation, the U.S. Public Health Service (R13-MH066849, R01-MH069864, U01MH060220, U01MH057716-05S1, and R01 DA016558), the Fogarty International Center (FIRCA R03-TW006481), the Pan American Health Organization, Eli Lilly and Company Foundation, Ortho-McNeil Pharmaceutical, Inc., GlaxoSmithKline, and Bristol-Myers Squibb. We thank the WMH staff for assistance with instrumentation, fieldwork, and data analysis. A complete list of WMH publications can be found at http://www.hcp.med.harvard.edu/wmh/.

## I. INTRODUCTION

One of the fundamental challenges in an undertaking such as the WMH Survey Initiative is to achieve both equivalence in meaning and consistency in measurement across surveys and, within surveys that have multiple language versions, across languages. Much of the discussion that follows in this chapter is related to translation and adaptation issues. We follow the terminology used in the translation sciences, distinguishing between source and target languages. The source language is the language out of which translations are made. The target language is the language into which translations are made.

All countries that participated in the WMH Survey Initiative administered Version 3.0 of the Composite International Diagnostic Interview (CIDI) (Kessler & Üstün 2004, see also Chapter 4), a fully structured interview designed to be used by trained lay interviewers to generate diagnoses according to the definitions and criteria of both the *Diagnostic and Statistical Manual of Mental Disorders*, fourth edition (DSM-IV) and the WHO International Classification of Mental and Behavioral Disorders (ICD-10). As described in Chapter 4, the CIDI is a lengthy and highly complex interview. An added complexity is that the focus of the instrument is on symptoms of mental disorders. Such symptoms are expressed and interpreted differently in different cultures (Prince & Tcheng-Laroche 1987; Cheng 2001), which makes it necessary in some cases to use substantially different terms or even questions in different countries to assess the presence versus absence of these symptoms.

A further complexity is that cultures differ in the ways they conceptualize and express certain psychological and emotional conditions, just as they differ in the conceptualization and expression of pain, distress, cause-and-effect perceptions, and time frameworks (Rogler 1999; Andary et al. 2003; Harkness 2004). A final noteworthy complexity is that the CIDI source language, English, has a larger lexicon (i.e., stock of vocabulary) than any other known language. This can mean that distinctions made in English cannot be matched in one or more target languages. The opposite can also be true with respect to certain areas of lexical or grammatical distinctions, in which the source language may not specify enough detail necessary for translation into a given target language.

Two issues are often confused in discussions of survey translation. One is that given source-language words or phrases do not match up on a word-to-word level in a target language. This is to be expected; it is a normal part of the work of translation to resolve grammatical, structural, and lexical differences between the source and a target language. For example, the term "feeling blue" in English refers to a mood rather than to a color, so successful translation would require using whatever expressions are appropriate for the language and targeted population to convey the intended meaning of this question, referring to (approximately) the same degree of deflated mood in the relevant time frame, and not words that are associated with the color blue.

The other issue sometimes discussed is when a target language does not have a ready means to express a given concept saliently. This could occur either because the target language does not have any readily understood words to express the concept (e.g., the degree of deflated mood suggested by the English phrase "feeling blue") or because the discourse norms of the culture make it extremely difficult to ask questions about this concept. If such a problem is not noticed at the question development stage, it may become evident in the process of translation or, in the worst case, during fielding or when the data prove biased.

This chapter describes the translation guidelines that collaborators were asked to use to translate and adapt the WMH interview questions in an effort to achieve both equivalence in meaning and consistency in measurement across surveys. A rationale for these guidelines is also presented. Systematic assessments of selected translations were undertaken after the surveys were fielded. The results of these assessments are also reported here. This chapter closes with recommendations for further empirical research on the relationship between question design and question translation in cross-cultural mental health research.

## 2. WMH TRANSLATION AND ADAPTATION GUIDELINES

One of the first tasks of the then newly formed WMH Survey Initiative was to develop a comprehensive set of procedures and guidelines to follow when translating and adapting the WMH interview schedule from the American English source instrument. These guidelines were eventually used to translate the instrument into 30 different languages (Table 5.1). The guidelines were initially developed by a working group, chaired by T. B. Üstün from the WHO and including several experienced survey researchers (J. Alonso, R. Kessler, H. U. Wittchen), as a modification of long-standing WHO guidelines for translation and back-translation. These modified guidelines were later updated by the staff of the WHO Data Collection Coordination Centre under the direction of B. E. Pennell in collaboration with the WMH co–principal investigators.

The translation guidelines designated each country's principal investigator as the editor in chief for the translation process and made this individual responsible for ensuring adherence to the guidelines. This included managing the entire translation and adaptation process, which encompassed selecting and supervising the translators, convening and chairing an expert panel, overseeing the pretest and back-translation processes, and documenting the final translated version of the instrument.

Wherever possible, countries were encouraged to start with previously translated and field-tested instruments and to work from these in developing empirically justified changes. Such root documents included earlier versions of the CIDI translations, other diagnostic interviews, and official translations of the ICD-10 and DSM-IV manuals. For those parts of the instrument that covered such topics as use of services, disability, and sociodemographics, or where scales had been adapted from other studies, it was suggested that existing survey questions should also

**Table 5.1.** WMH Initiative participating countries and languages

| Country | Languages |
| --- | --- |
| **WHO: Regional Office for the Americas (AMRO)** | |
| Brazil | Portuguese |
| Colombia | Spanish |
| Mexico | Spanish |
| Peru | Spanish |
| United States | English |
| **WHO: Regional Office for Africa (AFRO)** | |
| Nigeria | Efik, Hausa, Igbo, Yoruba |
| South Africa | Afrikaans, English, Northern Sotho, Xhosa, Zulu |
| **WHO: Regional Office for the Eastern Mediterranean (EMRO)** | |
| Iraq | Arabic |
| Lebanon | Arabic |
| **WHO: Regional Office for Europe (EURO)** | |
| Belgium | Dutch, French |
| Bulgaria | Bulgarian |
| France | French |
| Germany | German |
| Israel | Arabic, Hebrew, Russian |
| Italy | Italian |
| Netherlands | Dutch |
| N Ireland | English |
| Portugal | Portuguese |
| Romania | Romanian |
| Spain | Spanish |
| Turkey | Turkish |
| Ukraine | Ukrainian, Russian |
| **WHO: Regional Office for the Western Pacific (WPRO)** | |
| Australia | English |
| Japan | Japanese |
| People's Republic of China | Mandarin |
| New Zealand | English |
| **WHO: Regional Office for South-East Asia (SEAR)** | |
| India | Assamese, Gujarati, Hindi, Kannada, Manipuri, Marathi, Tamil, Telugu |

Total countries = 27, total languages = 30

be reviewed as a potential translation resource. In the end, nearly all WMH countries used at least some previously translated materials of this sort in their translations of the WMH instrument.

All countries other than Belgium and Israel translated from the source English to the target language. Belgium has two official languages: Flemish (similar to the Netherlands' Dutch) and French. As a result, the Belgium team used the French and Dutch translations already available from France and the Netherlands as the source documents and made modest modifications as necessary. Country-specific versions of questions in these two countries were needed, for example, for sociodemographic questions such as respondent education and income, as were small adjustments in vocabulary for substantive questions related to names of medication and illnesses. The Belgian team then conducted independent back-translations for both languages. In Israel, the English source was translated into Hebrew and then the Hebrew translation was used as the source text to produce the Arabic and Russian translations. This use of a translated questionnaire as a source text for further translations is standard practice in some countries. Research on potential advantages and disadvantages of such procedures is still outstanding.

Countries were instructed that the central aim of the translation process was to achieve target language versions of the English questionnaire that were conceptually equivalent in each of the countries and/or cultures. The focus was to be on cultural equivalence rather than on literal equivalence at the level of words or entities referred to. It was emphasized that the translation should sound natural in each language (in as far as that is possible in standardized instruments) and to perform in comparable fashion across the populations and languages. As we show later in this chapter, the independent assessors found that these aims were generally achieved, but that some of the translations were at times too close to the English questionnaire's language formulation and structure to sound natural.

Countries were required to follow a six-step process in achieving these aims. These steps included: (1) forward translation; (2) expert panel review; (3) independent back-translation; (4) harmonization of vocabulary and formulation across different country versions of a shared language (if appropriate); (5) pretesting and cognitive interviewing; and (6) final revision, creation, and documentation of a final version of the translated questionnaire. These steps are described briefly in the subsequent sections.

## 2.1. Forward Translation

Countries were instructed to employ one or more translators, preferably with a background in mental health and survey interview practice, but at least familiar with the kinds of expressions used by the target population in everyday language to talk about mental health disorders and/or survey interview skills. Although the first language of the translator(s) was to be the primary language of the target culture, they were also expected to be knowledgeable in American English culture and frames of reference to produce conceptually equivalent translated versions. Most countries produced their translation in a team effort that used more than one translator. Team approaches and the reiterated process of assessment they involve have several advantages, as outlined subsequently.

The WMH guidelines for translators emphasized the importance of aiming for conceptual equivalence using natural and acceptable language. The guidelines also emphasized the importance of the questions being understood by a broad section of the targeted population, requiring questions to be as simple, clear, and concise as possible. Translators were instructed to avoid any use of jargon or technical terms that would not be understood by some segments of the population. Similarly, translators were instructed to avoid the use of colloquialisms, idioms, and vernacular terms. Finally, translators were instructed to consider issues of applicability with respect to gender, age, and race/ethnicity and to avoid any terms that might be considered offensive to segments of the population defined in terms of these variables.

## 2.2. The Expert Panel

The editor in chief in each country was asked to convene an expert panel that would include the original translator(s) in addition to bilingual experts in mental disorders and experts in survey methodology. If possible, countries were encouraged to include researchers who had participated in the development of previous officially approved CIDI versions or in the development of other instruments included in the WMH interview. Panel members were encouraged to identify and resolve any weaknesses in their country's instrument, such as inadequate expressions/concepts in the translation, as well as any discrepancies between the forward translation and any existing or comparable versions of the questionnaire (e.g., CIDI 1.0, and the other standard instruments that were used in creating the WMH instrument). The panels had an average of six members that included the full range of expertise needed to produce and assess these challenging survey translations (see Harkness 2003; Harkness, Pennell & Schoua-Glusberg 2004). The typical panel included professional translators, individuals who had previous experience in survey translation, and subject matter experts.

## 2.3. Back-translation in the WMH

The translation protocol included a requirement for back-translation of selected items in the interview. The back-translations (translations from the target language back into English) were produced by a translator not previously involved in the effort and unfamiliar with the original English-source interview schedule. The back-translator's first language was American English. As in the initial translation, emphasis in the back-translation was placed on cultural equivalence rather than on literal equivalence.

The items selected for back-translation were items either determined by the WMH translation work group or by the local WMH collaborators as potentially problematic. Discrepancies were discussed with the national editor in chief, followed by additional steps in forward translations and further expert panel review until a satisfactory version was created. Any remaining challenges, such as formulations that did not completely capture the concept addressed by the original item, were brought to the attention of the WMH translation work group chair for review and resolution.

## 2.4. Language Harmonization

The same interview language was sometimes required for different countries, the most notable example being Spanish, which was used in Spain as well as in several countries in Latin America. When a language was "shared" in this way, additional steps were undertaken during translation to harmonize the translation decisions across countries. The Spanish-language collaborators from Chile, Colombia, Mexico, Panama, Peru, Puerto Rico, Spain, and the United States, as well as representatives from AMRO and WHO, met in a series of extended meetings to document, reach consensus, and resolve the Spanish translations of terms and phrases that teams had identified as primarily used in specific countries and not easily understood across counties. The group was chaired by S. Aguilar-Gaxiola, the WMH Initiative regional coordinator for Latin America.

The result of these meetings was a Spanish translation that was harmonized where appropriate across Spanish-speaking countries but that retained country-specific translations for specific terms or idiomatic expressions in cases where that was appropriate. For example, the English term "hangover" has no equivalent that is universally understood across Spanish-speaking countries. The Spanish translation in Mexico is *cruda*, in Spain *resaca*, and in Colombia *guayabo*. Documentation of all decisions was based on a spreadsheet framework developed by the collaborators in Spain. Table 5.2 provides an example of the documentation produced as part of this process. The first column of the table lists the English item or phrase from the source questionnaire that was judged as potentially problematic, in that it might be difficult to find one term that could be used across the countries sharing the language. Entries for column A were initially identified by the Spanish harmonization committee. Column B lists the Spanish translations first proposed. Column C lists the translation that was considered "more universal," that is, more likely to be understood across the various Spanish-language groups. These were the terms that should be used wherever possible. Column D lists the translations that were deemed to be culture specific for some or all populations; that is, where no consensus could be reached as to a single universal term or phrase. Column E documents the codes for the final recommendations of the committee. Each number after the word or phrase indicates the country or countries to which the item applies. Code A indicates that all the terms proposed were to be included because no single term was found that was suitable for all the populations. Code B indicates that an item has a more restricted meaning in Spanish than in English and should be modified as indicated. Code C is used when more than one term is suggested but selection depends on the context and order of the items. Code D indicates that the English term is a colloquialism that should be modified.

## 2.5. Pretesting and Cognitive Interviewing

All countries were required to pretest their translated version(s) of the final source questionnaire on a sample of their target population(s). This was done with a combination of in-depth, face-to-face interviews and focus groups. Countries were encouraged to use experienced CIDI interviewers or members of the translation expert panel to conduct these interviews.

Each module or section was tested on people who were representative of the WMH sample for the country. In addition, countries were encouraged to include patients diagnosed with the disorder of interest, especially if the disorder was expected to have a low prevalence and the pretest samples might not yield enough cases to test the section adequately. A minimum of ten pretest respondents were required for each section, including males and females, and as wide an age range and different socioeconomic strata as feasible.

Pretest respondents were administered the questionnaire and then systematically debriefed. The debriefing included questions about how respondents had understood the questions,

**Table 5.2.** Example of harmonization step used by Spanish-speaking countries

| A | B | C | D | E |
|---|---|---|---|---|
| Término en inglés<br>*English term* | Términos propuestos en español<br>*Proposed Spanish terms* | Términos seleccionados<br>*Selected terms* | Términos alternativos según país<br>*Alternative terms in each country* | Código<br>*Code* |
| Free base | Free base | | Basuco (1, 3, 8)/pasta base (6) | A |
| Herbalists | Herbolarios, naturistas | | Naturistas (1, 2), homeópatas (1, 2), herbolarios (1), herbalistas (2), yerberos/yerbateros (3, 8) | C |
| Hot flashes | Sofocos | | Sofocos (1), sofocones (2), bochornos (5, 6), calores (8) | A |
| Ulcer in your stomach or intestine | Úlcera estomacal o intestinal | Úlcera de estómago o intestinal | | A |
| Unhappy | Desdichado(a)<br>Desgraciado(a) | Infeliz o desgraciado(a) | | C |
| Upset | Molesto | Alterado | | A |
| Using a 0–10 scale | Utilizando una escala de 0 a 10 | En una escala de 0–10 | | A |
| Usual, usually | Habitual, habitualmente | | Habitual/habitualmente (1), usual/usualmente (2) | A |
| Normally | Normalmente | Generalmente | | A |
| Vodka, gin, or whiskey | Ron, vodka, ginebra, whiskey | Ron, vodka, ginebra, whisky | pisco (6), mezcal (5), aguardiente (2), chicha (3, 8), guarapo (3), guaro (8) | C |
| Was it before you were a teenager? | ¿Fue antes de la adolescencia? | ¿Fue antes de los trece años? | | A |
| What is the day of the week? | ¿A qué día de la semana estamos? | ¿En qué día de la semana estamos? | | A |
| What is the largest number . . .? | ¿Cuál es el mayor número? | ¿Cuál es el número máximo . . .? | | A |
| What is the longest period of days, weeks, months, or years you were . . .? | ¿Cuánto duró el periodo más largo de días, semanas. . .? | ¿Cuántos días, semanas, meses o años duró el periodo más largo durante el que. . .? | | A |
| What number describes . . .? | ¿Qué cifra describe . . .? | ¿Qué número describe mejor . . .? | | A |
| What season of the year is it? | ¿En qué estación . . .? | | En qué estación (1), época (3, 8), del año estamos? | A |

*Note:* Column D shows alternative Spanish terms of the different Spanish-speaking countries/cultures to take into account cultural differences when no consensus agreement was reached about one single term. The numbers in this column indicate the following: (1) Spain, (2) Latin America, (3) Colombia, (4) Puerto Rico, (5) Mexico, (6) Chile, (7) Argentina, and (8) Panama.

whether they could repeat the question in their own words, what came to their mind when they heard a particular phrase or term, and requests for them to explain how they chose their answer. These questions were repeated for each individual item of a section. Respondents were also asked about any word or expression they did not understand or considered unacceptable or offensive. When alternative words, expressions, or questions existed for the source material, pretest respondents were asked to choose which of the alternatives matched their normal language usage better. Instrument changes based on the results of these pretests were documented in a written report.

## 2.6. Production of the Final Version and Documentation

Countries were instructed to track changes and versions of the instrument so that all the decisions and procedures could be traced through the appropriate documents. Countries were asked to archive the products of each stage in their translation process to document decisions taken at each step. These included the initial forward version, a summary of recommendations by the expert panel, the back-translation, modifications agreed to during the harmonization phase, a summary of problems found during pretesting of the questionnaire and the modifications proposed, and the final version of the questionnaire. Countries were required to pretest their final translated instrument with at least 40 respondents.

## 2.7. Adaptation

It is not uncommon that, in addition to being translated, source questions also must be modified (i.e., adapted) to meet local requirements. Examples of fairly straightforward adaptations are changes to systems of measurement (e.g., Fahrenheit and Celsius or yards and meters) to match the system used in a target country. References to currency were also changed to refer to the national currency and to reflect the appropriate levels and income distributions of the country. In the WMH surveys, a number of features required adaptation to fit the national context in

this fashion. Countries were instructed to record details of all the changes undertaken so that these could be integrated into the study documentation. Examples include questions about ethnic or racial groups or religious affiliation. In the posttraumatic stress disorder (PTSD) section, adaptations were also made to questions that asked about experience in war-torn areas and the respondent's experiences as a combatant, relief worker, peacekeeper, or civilian. The lists of countries associated with these experiences were also adapted as needed. For example, Afghanistan and Iraq were relevant to the U.S. experience. Another example is Lebanon, where countries also expanded the PTSD section to reflect more details about war experiences. These items have subsequently been used in other countries where such experiences are relevant.

In the substance use section, several questions that asked about number of drinks of alcohol consumed were adapted to better standardize volume equivalents across countries. Countries were instructed to modify the questions, if necessary, to reflect local circumstances. For example, a half-ounce glass of a potent locally used liquor, such as sake in Japan, might be the alcohol content equivalent of one ounce of whiskey in the United States. Other examples of adaptation in the substance use section include changing the lists of legal and illegal drugs and substances. References to Librium, Valium, and diazepam, for example, were changed to appropriate local terms.

In the pharmocoepidemiology section, a prescription medication was defined as one requiring a doctor's approval, a definition that is appropriate for many countries. In countries such as India, however, people can buy prescription medications without a doctor's prescription being required, either at pharmacies or on the street. In other countries, such as South Africa, prescriptions are mostly provided by nurses rather than by doctors. Countries were therefore asked to modify the source instrument definition of prescription medication to make it appropriate for their conditions. The lists of psychotropic medications were also changed, as appropriate, to reflect national variation, including the use of herbal medications and substances.

In the services section, the lists of health professionals were modified to include locally relevant examples of mental health professionals, other health professionals, religious advisers, and other healers. The places at which these advisers and professionals could be found were also modified. In the demographic sections, modifications were also made to questions about insurance options and the official languages of the country.

## 3. TECHNICAL ASPECTS

One of the challenges faced by the first WMH countries to field their surveys was that the WMH interview schedule needed to be translated while the instrument was still under development. Given the severe time constraints, the translation process was carried out in a modular fashion. The translation and adaptation instructions given to collaborators emphasized the importance of translating each module in an equally rigorous manner and the importance of maintaining continuity in the composition of the translating staff to encourage consistency across modules. Although quality-control and review steps were built into the instrument development process, the speed with which the development and translation were accomplished may have contributed to some of the issues found in the translation assessments described in Section 4.

Countries were given instructions and templates in Microsoft Word, enabling them to create

a translated document that accomplished several goals. For example, the template allowed translators to reference the English source language on screen while they entered the target translation, obviating the need to jump back and forth between files. The format also provided for two different versions of the questionnaire: one for paper administration (PAPI) and one for computer-assisted administration (CAPI). Figure 5.1 depicts the instrument development phase as it interacted with the translation and programming phases.

The development process was quite complex, with tasks being conducted simultaneously that are typically executed sequentially. As each module was developed, it was sent out for expert review and then simultaneously for translation and programming. As subsequent modules were developed, their content and format would sometimes necessitate a change in a module or modules that had already been sent out for translation and programming. It was therefore critical to maintain a robust version control system. The secure Web-based collaborative knowledge management system that was described by Pennell and colleagues in Chapter 3 facilitated communication between the central staffs at Michigan and Harvard and the participating countries. This system was also used for version control of the English source and the various country translations. The system provided each country with the most current and all previous versions of the questionnaire for easy reference. Each night,

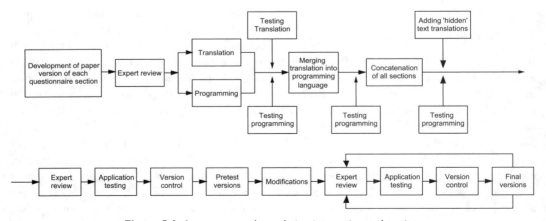

**Figure 5.1.** Instrument and translation integration and testing.

messages were automatically generated by the system to alert national collaborators of the most recent changes.

Once the programming and translations were finalized for the CAPI applications, two parallel testing activities were undertaken. One of these tested the interview (described previously), and the other tested the functionality of the computer program. Testing procedures continued as necessary until both the interview and the computer program were judged to be error free. The translations were then integrated into the programming application and the various modules merged. After this, newly produced source text on navigation and skip aids for the interviewer, as well as other interviewer and respondent instructions, were translated. The assembled instrument was then reviewed and tested again before formal pretesting began.

Countries conducted between one and four rounds of pretests with between 40 and 80 respondents. Pretest respondents were selected using a variety of methods, including random selection from the main study samples, convenience samples, samples of patients, or some combination of these. The pretests were conducted by the collaborators and their staff, members of the expert panel, staff from the data collection organization, or a combination of these staffs.

## 4. WMH GUIDELINE DEVELOPMENT

### 4.1. Overview

In the past decade or so, concepts of best practice regarding survey translation have changed noticeably, as have preferred strategies and, to some extent, the technology used. Translation guidelines published by the U.S. Census Bureau (de la Puente, Pan & Rose 2003; Pan & de la Puente 2005), by the European Social Survey (Harkness 2002, 2006), and by Eurostat for health surveys (Tafforeau et al. 2005) reflect considerable agreement on how to produce and test translated questions. This growing consensus was the foundation on which the WMH translation guidelines were developed.

The consensus view is that a team of people should develop and assess the translation, bringing together expertise in survey questionnaire design, substantive understanding of the subject, source- and target-language competence, translation training and expertise, and knowledge of the local fielding situation. Translators alone can rarely provide all of these. Coordinated team efforts have been increasingly advocated as a practical way to bring together the necessary competence and to combine translation production with translation review. It is generally agreed that different members of the team should assume different roles, with some members primarily translating and others primarily reviewing and polishing (in cooperation with the first). One person (an adjudicator) can be stipulated to make the final decisions on versions in consultation with the team. Consultants for specific aspects can be brought in as required (e.g., on adaptation issues). By monitoring team performance and output quality at an early stage in the project, adjustments can be made as needed that may both improve the product and save time and effort later.

The consensus view is that each translator should make a full draft translation whenever possible. The alternative is to have each translator do a section of the translation. The pros and cons of splitting up a translation must be carefully weighed, especially if a translation group does not have an established routine or experience working together. In contrast, when translators are providing specialized vocabulary, different translators may be required for different modules in an interview schedule. When this is the case, great care is needed to make comparisons across sections for consistency in translating phrases that are used across sections. It is generally agreed that translation and adaptation go hand in hand. It is also agreed that translated interviews should be assessed using both quantitative and qualitative procedures (for suggestions, see Harkness & Schoua-Glusberg 1998; Harkness et al. 2004; Smith 2004). Another point of agreement is that translated interview schedules should be pretested on the population for which they are intended. In terms of documentation, it is generally agreed that translators and reviewers should be required to take notes on all points of deliberation to inform the review and adjudication and to facilitate version documentation. Finally, technological support can facilitate these procedures. Templates and documentation tools are valuable in conducting review and adjudication. These tools often combine translations, source text, and note taking in one document.

## 4.2. Subsequent Changes to Guidelines

Even in the period since the WMH surveys began, perspectives and preferred strategies for instrument translation have changed. Several major translation frameworks, such as those outlined by the U.S. Census Bureau and those required to be followed by participants in the European Social Survey (ESS), now rely on team production and team review procedures as their primary quality devices within the production cycle. Research on postproduction assessment, such as the WMH assessments described subsequently, has also been under development.

The WMH guidelines have been updated to reflect these developments and have moved, for example, from employing back-translation as an assessment step to placing more emphasis on a formal implementation of a team translation protocol. As described previously, the initial WMH translation protocol featured multiple components of review, with back-translation never being the only review and assessment tool in the process. The revised WMH procedures take a more holistic view of translation production and testing, consistent with modern translation theory and the practical demands on survey translation. In contrast to back-translation, team translation efforts make review and correction of the translation an intrinsic component of the translation production process.

Back-translation was one of the earliest procedures to establish itself in survey research and, over time, became associated with quality assurance. In numerous projects, back-translation is still used to assess instrument translations after version production, and the term itself is still

frequently mentioned in reports of how studies were conducted. As noted elsewhere (Harkness & Schoua-Glusberg 1998; Harkness 2003), multiple steps can actually be involved in procedures that researchers describe as "back-translation." When projects embed a back-translation step in multiple other procedures, it is not clear what the unique contribution of back-translation might be.

The most recent WMH protocol not only checks for inappropriate changes in lexical (semantic) meaning but also focuses on issues such as whether there are changes in pragmatic meaning (meaning as shaped by context) and whether technical aspects are translated appropriately. These are just as relevant for comparable measurement across populations as considering semantic comparability (Braun & Harkness 2005). The review also assesses how well the translated questions work for a targeted population, in terms of both the level of diction appropriate for the sample population and whether design issues favor one population over another. Where possible, the review also assesses how data collected with the translated instrument compares with data collected with the original English interview schedule. This makes it possible to assess whether response patterns for what is nominally the same question differ (or do not differ) as expected across instruments and populations.

In the original WMH guidelines, final decisions on translations were made by the expert panel. The revised guidelines assign this final adjudication to a senior person or persons working in consultation with the reviewer and any other specialists needed. Adjudicator(s) should understand the research subject, know about survey design, and be proficient in the languages involved. This task often falls to the principal investigator (PI) or expert panel chair in a WMH project. In cases where the panel chair is not proficient in the languages involved, he or she is advised by a consultant or delegated adjudication authority. This situation arises most often in countries that translate into multiple languages.

The revised WMH guidelines were followed in updating the original WMH Spanish translation to the newest version of the CIDI. The WMH instrument was adopted as Version 3.0 of the CIDI in 2005 (Kessler & Üstün 2004). As such, this is now a copyrighted instrument of the WHO. Researchers wishing to use CIDI 3.0 in a language other than English are now required to update the translation using these revised guidelines for any sections they intend to use to match the English source text of the current version of the CIDI and to share their translation with the CIDI Advisory Committee so it can be used by other certified CIDI users. The current WMH translation procedures must be followed in producing any new translations.

## 5. ASSESSMENT OF WMH TRANSLATIONS

### 5.1. Introduction

In some important ways, decisions about translation quality are related to one's expectations about what a translation can and should do. The functionalist approach to translation, indeed, takes successful fulfillment of function as the key feature to determining translation quality (Hönig 1998). To measure this success, of course, one must first identify goals in a concrete fashion. At the present time, survey research still lacks a generally accepted, evidence-based framework and set of procedures for assessing the quality of translated survey instruments. Nonetheless, a number of general features can be identified that are relevant for determining survey translation quality.

Models of assessment developed in the translation sciences include a number of features that are useful to consider in the context of survey translation assessment. Several are standard features that are found in a variety of major approaches to assessment in the translation sciences (see Nord 1996; Gerzymisch-Arbogast 1997; House 1997; Hönig 1998). At the same time, these models differ from assessment required in the survey context. They are, for example, usually developed for a one-language

assessment task, not for multilingual assessments such as those undertaken in survey research. In addition, assessment models in the translation sciences are often related to meiotic correction during training or to assessment for formal grading procedures.

The assessment procedures selected for the WMH surveys take into account basic assumptions and goals that underlie the instrument design model adopted in the WMH Survey Initiative. These procedures build on earlier procedures developed in assessing the translations for two European multinational surveys, the Survey on Health, Ageing and Retirement in Europe (SHARE) and the ESS. In the SHARE surveys, a review was made of pretest translations before the study was launched to help countries recognize where revisions might be needed (Harkness 2005). Assessors were asked to comment on anything they saw as potential problems in the translations, focusing on a set of basic issues similar to those outlined subsequently. Individual countries could thus gain valuable feedback on their performance, and the central coordinator could take steps to improve translation quality.

In the ESS surveys, assessments were undertaken between rounds 2 and 3 of the biennial survey and again at the end of round 3. Feedback from the assessments was provided to participating countries to help them recognize where and how individual efforts might be improved. The assessments also gave the ESS central coordinating team a better idea of how procedures were being implemented and where modification of the ESS guidelines or instructions for country teams might be needed. In each instance, the assessments revealed problems in translations related to procedures (followed or not followed) and to inadequate briefing and/or expertise of translators or translation teams. They also highlighted certain aspects of the source instrument that might require revision.

### 5.2. Details of the Assessment Procedures

An assessment was undertaken of sections of the WMH interview in five languages and six versions: Mandarin Chinese (China), French (France), German (Germany), Spanish (Spain and Mexico) and Turkish (Turkey). The assessments were designed to gain further insight into the extent to which WMH translation procedures were successful. The primary assessors were experienced translators, most of whom had some experience in producing survey translations. A number also had experience in teaching translation and/or assessing survey translations. In addition, a second set of assessors was used who had worked in survey research or studied survey methodology at the graduate level and had native proficiency in the languages to be evaluated.

The modules chosen for assessment were the initial screening module and the depression module. The assessors were provided with the translations in a Microsoft Word template that aligned the source English text, question by question, with the translated text to be assessed. The template also provided space for comments on each question. Some of the translated versions assessed were for CAPI applications and some were for PAPI applications. These two modes differed somewhat in question content and sequence. Other differences in content are related to changes made across versions over time. In the present report, therefore, we cannot always compare assessor comments for each question across all languages.

The assessors were provided with a set of instructions on what to look for, how to code, and how to comment on translations. The instructions included a requirement to check the extent to which the translation was faithful to the semantic meaning of the source question or changed this meaning; the extent to which any special pragmatic issues were involved in the translation that did not hold for the source text; and the extent to which mistakes were found in grammatical, orthographic, typographic, and punctuation issues. Assessors were also required to rate the extent to which the translation was readily understandable or more complicated to follow than the source text, was internally consistent with respect to repeated components, had

omissions or additions, or was too close to the wording or structure of the source. Finally, assessors were instructed to comment on anything else they found relevant and to provide a general comment on the translation quality.

Much in the way team translation brings together people with different skills and expertise, the combined input from two groups of assessors with different expertise proved most useful in conducting the assessments. Because the primary assessors, the translators, could not be expected to be fully cognizant of the principles of question design and answer scale formats, they were not asked to comment on the technical measurement-related aspects of the translations. The second set of assessors was better able to comment on such aspects and had also had some exposure to translation practices in survey research. At the same time, they were not trained translators, so they were asked to focus largely on issues relevant to their expertise. Both groups were asked to report everything they noticed in terms of difference, whether or not it seemed significant. Neither group was asked to interpret what they found. In this way, we hoped to free assessors from the burden of deciding whether it was relevant to report something as a difference and to encourage more reporting to reduce the chance that something important would be overlooked. Detailed explanations and examples, culled from findings from assessment projects such as this, can be used to inform translators and assessors about issues important for survey research. These, in turn, may help future translators and assessors recognize issues that they might otherwise overlook.

Two special features of the WMH assessment remain to be mentioned. First, in most translation-assessment projects, an assessment can simply critique a target text relative to a source text, taking into account specifications provided to the translators about the goal and function of the translation. In the WMH context, the assessment was multilingual. In addition, the WMH source text changed over time; thus, there are multiple "source" texts to consider. Although all changes to the instruments were captured, matching the relevant source-language version with the fielded translated version was a challenge, especially because several of these countries fielded their studies using the oldest version of the instrument. As a result, the single source text available when assessment began does not match the source version used to produce any given translation in every respect. In addition, the PAPI version of the source interview differs somewhat in sequencing and content from the CAPI version, which again results in differences between the source texts and translations given to assessors.

## 5.3. Grammatical Mistakes

As mentioned earlier, the assessment was restricted to two modules in the WMH instrument. Both the framework for what should be covered in assessment and the guidelines to assessors on how to proceed are works in progress. Nonetheless, certain commonalities could be found across languages and assessments, and it is on these that we focus. We have separated discussion of findings into nine sections, determined partly by the kind of problem reported. Although we comment in various places about the possible relevance to translation quality of differences noted, we present more general comments on the significance of differences at the end.

We use the term "grammar" here to cover rules of structure at sentence, phrase, and word levels. Common grammar mistakes include number mismatch (e.g., plural subject with a singular verb), grammatical gender problems, and inappropriate tense or aspect usage. In many instances, the mistakes are simply grammatical infelicities. Moreover, interviewers may have automatically corrected some of these written mistakes in the process of oral delivery. Spanish, French, and German assessors point to instances in which the tense or aspect chosen subtly changed the perspective on the event or complaint referred to in the question. Mistakes related to tense and aspect may reflect the degree to which these linguistic features differ in multiple ways across languages. Their frequency within

a given module and language may also reflect cut-and-paste replacement of phrases repeated in a module, which results in the multiplication of one mistake across questions. Given that France, Germany, and Spain were three of the first countries to field the WMH study, a rushed production cycle, often an issue in survey translation, may also have played a role.

In the German depression module, the present perfect aspect (*have* you *felt* / I *have felt*) was used multiple times to refer to past events instead of imperfect forms (*did* you *feel* / I *felt*). This may have encouraged respondents to understand some of the questions as questions about their general condition or emotional state, including their present state. The source questions were about their condition at a time in the past. In the following examples, "ST" identifies source text and "TT" is an English rendering of the target text:

D26c ST: Did you gain weight without trying to within that two-week period?

TT: Have you gained weight without wanting to during this two-week period?[1]

D26d ST: How much did you gain?

TT: How much have you gained?

D26e ST: Did you lose weight without trying to?

TT: Have you lost weight without wanting to?

D26e ST: How much did you lose?

TT: How much have you lost?

Throughout this series of questions there were also references to the past time frame actually intended (i.e., the two-week period in the past). Some of the translated questions also had the appropriate imperfect verb form. Nonetheless, the time frame intended may have been unclear. It is uncertain to what extent this aspect/tense problem actually affected how respondents understood the question or even simply caused them some confusion. Nevertheless, even the

[1] Note: "that" would have been possible in German but the difference between "this" and "that" is not as pronounced in this context as in English. The difference between "without trying to" and "without wanting to" in German is, on the other hand, much the same as in English.

latter should be avoided because it adds to respondent burden.

## 5.4. Orthographic Mistakes

Most assessors noted mistakes in spelling, punctuation, or differences in underlining, bolding, and so on, between the source and the target versions. The lack of care readers often attribute to authors when confronted with such shortcomings may be less relevant for the survey context. Indeed, the fact that these questions were, in a sense, working documents for the interviewer may mean that less emphasis was placed on ensuring that these fine-tuning matters were correct. At the same time, misspelled words may impede oral presentation. In addition, bolding and underlining are intended as aids for the interviewers. Although these cannot necessarily be carried over mechanically in translation, omission of guidance provided for interviewers working with the source instrument means that interviewers working with translations have less support. Question designers, on the other hand, approved the source format on the assumption that interviewers were given certain presentational support that they did not receive when these omissions occurred.

Assessors also commented on occasional differences in the use of square brackets in CAPI versions of the instrument. These square brackets were used to enclose material used as fill inserts, so as to indicate to programmers working from this text which words or phrases were to be taken as fill material. The words to be placed inside square brackets differed from language to language. For example, in an English question such as: "When did you last visit your [mother, father, family]?" the fills are the nouns "mother," "father," and "family." In a language in which the forms of possessives match nouns, the word "your" would also be required to be inside the square brackets. Without knowing what is affected in which language, fill programming directions can go wrong.

Question D15 in the CAPI version provides an example of this: "Think of times lasting several days or longer when [these problems / this problem] with your mood [were/was] most severe and frequent. During those times, did your feelings of [sadness, discouragement or lack of interest / sadness or discouragement / sadness or lack of interest / sadness / discouragement or lack of interest / discouragement / lack of interest] usually last all day long, most of the day, about half the day, or less than half the day?" Depending on whether the respondent reported one or more problems, the reference needed to be either singular, "this problem," or plural, "these problems," and the verb accordingly had to be either "was" or "were." The source-version square bracket treatment takes this into account for English, and these bracketed elements are also necessary for Spanish. However, in Spanish, the adjectives "severe" (*grave*) and "frequent" (*frecuente*) also have singular and plural forms. These words were not in square brackets in the representation available to reviewers of the CAPI version for Spain: "Piense en los periodos de varios días o más en que [estos / este problema / estos problemas / este] problema(s) de estado de ánimo [fueron/fue] más grave(s) y frecuente(s)." This suggests that these modifications, identified as they are by parentheses, were left to the interviewers to make. In other words, programming instructions were appropriate for English but not fully so for Spanish. A more appropriate representation would have been, "Piense en los periodos de varios días o más en que [este problema / estos problemas] de estado de ánimo [fue/fueron] más [grave/graves] y [frecuente/frecuentes]."[2]

## 5.5. Mistranslations and Measurement

A wide range of features might be judged to be weaknesses, stylistic infelicities, or shortcomings in translation technique without constituting a clear-cut translation error or, indeed, contributing to survey error. Translations that change lexical meaning are described here as "mistranslations." A clear example of a mistranslation that

[2] In addition, the Spanish text refers to "problem/problems" both inside and outside of square brackets, resulting in a somewhat confusing text if this is what interviewers actually saw. These are corrected in the revised version.

affected data was found in ESS translations of an item about the conditions under which people should be allowed to immigrate to a country. The translations asked whether people allowed into the country should be "healthy." The source question, in comparison, asked whether they should be "wealthy." Recent research has shown that the effects of such mistranslations on interview interaction and on survey data are not always the same (Harkness et al. 2008). A further problem that we cannot pursue here is that respondents can produce seemingly correct answers to misunderstood (and mistranslated) questions (on misunderstood questions, see Belson 1981, 1986).

Decisions as to what counts as a mistranslation and what is simply a less successful translation are often not clear-cut. Two examples from the WMH Chinese translation illustrate this nicely. Question SC27a asks: "The next questions are about things that make some people afraid even though they know there is no real danger. Was there ever a time in your life when you had a strong fear of *any of the following things? First, bugs, snakes, dogs, or any other animals?*" In British English, "bugs" is usually taken to refer to vermin, whereas in American English, the term can refer to many kinds of insects, not necessarily just vermin. In the Chinese translation, the word "bugs" is translated as "cockroaches," an insect considered as vermin in both the United States and China. Informants suggested that cockroaches are disliked and very much avoided by some Chinese. It is not clear to what extent, if any, this might affect responses to the question.

Another example is the Chinese translation of question D17, which asked respondents, in part, "How severe was your emotional distress?" The Chinese translation was closer to, "How bad were your emotions?" Assessors agreed that the Chinese translation could be taken to refer to feelings of anger, irritability, melancholy, and other types of distress, and could thus potentially tap into something different from what the source question intended. The effect of such differences is difficult to judge. In the Spanish and French interviews, assessors noted differ-

ences in the translation of a question asking about self-worth. The source question (D26v in the CIDI) asked: "Did you feel totally worthless nearly every day?" The Spanish translation, in comparison, translates "worthless" as "useless," although a closer rendering of "worthless" would have been possible. The same term caused problems in the French translation, where worthlessness was translated as "without value" rather than by a term that implied low self-confidence or low self-assurance.

Similar shifts in focus or emphasis were found in a number of questions in the German translations. Two examples are the following:

D26r ST: Did you have a lot more trouble concentrating than is normal for you *nearly every day?*

TT: Was your *concentration considerably worse every day* than (it is) normally?

D26g ST: Did you have *a lot more trouble than usual* falling asleep, staying asleep or waking *early nearly every night* during that two-week period?

TT: During this two-week period did you have *trouble* falling asleep, trouble sleeping through *much more often than usual* or did you wake up *too early?*

It needs to be emphasized that a translation assessment is not the right tool to ascertain the degree to which changes of this sort might lead to differences in meaning in a given population in a given context. However, research indicates that respondents can sometimes be affected by changes in individual words (e.g., Schuman & Presser 1981; Fowler & Mangione 1989; Tourangeau et al. 2000). This means that changes of the sort illustrated here could be considered significant. To determine whether this is so ahead of fielding would require additional empirical research that used in-depth debriefing methods to probe for differences in perceived meaning.

## 5.6. Too-close Translation

All assessors found passages in the translations that they felt were overliteral or unnatural. Harkness, Pennell, and Schoua-Glusberg (2004) discuss the consequences of overclose translation in survey research. They suggest that if translation is overliteral, the questions will sound like translations or strangely awkward. The meanings of questions can change in such cases or respondents can fail to understand what is intended. Some issues noted by assessors appear to be related to source-text challenges, whereas others are probably the result of hurried or careless translations that were not adequately reviewed.

A number of assessors for different languages commented on overclose and unnatural sounding translations in question SC26, which asked people if they have ever been "a worrier," and question SC29, which referred to "going on a date." These concepts are familiar in many English speech communities, but they are less familiar in other cultures and languages. A concept that poses a translation challenge might induce inexperienced translators to use a word-for-word translation, such as we find in some of the translated versions of these questions. Such translations usually make little sense to respondents. At the same time, some of the close translations we found were phrases that should not have been translation challenges but occurred because of poor choices. For example, the wrong preposition was used in the German translation of "going to parties." The translation in this case was "zu Parties gehen," which reflects the English "to" instead of the German preposition *auf* (*auf Parties gehen*). Another example is the Turkish translation of SC27b, which asked about "strong fear of" various phobic situations. The translation incorrectly used a word that implied physical strength (*güçlü*). A more appropriate modifier, implying depth of the emotion, would have been *yoğun*.

## 5.7. Level of Diction

In general, assessors commented less frequently on the level of diction used than on the tendency to translate too literally. It is not clear whether this indicates that the translators used the kind of diction the assessors (who were also translators) would have used or whether it reflects that the WMH guidelines were followed. The

WMH guidelines encourage translators to use easily understandable language. This may be why, for example, the Mexican translation of the medical condition "stroke" in SC10.5e2 is *embolia*, which a Mexican assessor considered too general a term. When a different assessor checked usage frequencies for the word chosen in the WMH translation against those suggested by the Mexican assessor, *embolia* did indeed seem to be the more common word for "stroke." In contrast, a Spanish assessor identified the translation of "extremely" (*muchísimo*) in the answer scale for one particular item (D28) as colloquial and considered it successful. Standard Spanish usage, however, would caution against using this term in writing. A Turkish assessor also pointed to a few instances where she felt the words chosen were too formal, one example being the translation of "drugs" as *madde* rather than *uyuşturucu*.

## 5.8. Omissions

Some regularity can be noted in the kinds of expressions or components that are omitted and added, both within a translation and across translations. These are in part related to lexical or structural differences across languages, but they may also be related to culture-specific realizations of features of interviews. Linguists sometimes speak of the conflicting tendencies in language toward both economy and simplification and elaboration to clarify meaning (Vicentini 2003). Whereas everyday language illustrates both principles, survey instruments tend to favor elaboration and are often deliberately redundant. They repeat nouns, for example, rather than substitute pronouns. They avoid elliptical constructions in questions and repeat key phrases within a short span of text in a fashion that, in other contexts, would be unusual.

Assessors frequently noted omissions in the translations that, deliberately or not, reduced the redundancy present in the English source questions. For example, the redundant phrasing "problems with your physical health, mental health, or...," rather than the more everyday "problems with your physical or mental health, or with...." is rendered in Spanish as "problemas con su salud física, mental o . . . " (gloss: problems with your health physical, mental, or . . . ). This follows normal Spanish usage but does not, one might argue, comply with the redundancy typical of English survey language or "surveyspeak" (see Harkness 1996). It is quite possible that some languages are more resistant to creating new unusual word combinations than seems to be the case in survey language in English. It may thus not be as easy or as appropriate in Spanish to reproduce the English (often-unwritten) rules and notions of surveyspeak. The Spanish translators may also simply have aimed to produce normal discourse rather than survey discourse. Too little systematic investigation has been undertaken on this to make more than the few general observations that follow.

The first such observation involves the commonly occurring omission of discourse and text structure signals. For example, the sequencing particles "first," "second," and "third," which were used in a number of WMH questions, such as the SC27 question series, were quite often omitted in translated instruments. Although these omissions are not directly related to measurement components of the questions, they were presumably included in the original to help the respondent follow the progression of questions. It is unclear the extent to which omissions of this type influence responses.

A second observation concerns omissions of temporal references: we have already commented on grammatical problems related to tense and aspect, but translations can also differ in how they render English temporal references conveyed through time adverbials. In many instances, multiple references in the English source were reduced in translation. For example, question D14 asks, "Did you ever have a year or more in your life when just about every month you had an episode of being [sad, discouraged or uninterested / sad or discouraged / sad or uninterested / sad / discouraged or uninterested / discouraged / uninterested] each of which lasted several days or longer?" In a number of cases, the translated version of this source question omitted one of the multiple time references (typically the "lasted several days or longer" compo-

nent). This is a potential problem because multiple time references like this reflect the concern of the developers of the source question for accurate measurement and adequate priming of the respondent. However, questions of this sort break the normal conventions for written and spoken English. They also create a challenge for translation. The problem is that formulations of this sort, which just about work for English, may not work for other languages. As a result, questions that are complex and somewhat unwieldy in English can reasonably be expected to pose problems for many languages.

The best way to resolve this problem, of course, is for it to be taken into consideration at the initial question-design phase. The task of the translator would be made much easier if complex questions of this sort never appeared in the source interview schedule. When such questions appear, though, they need to be handled thoughtfully by the translator. Given that considerable differences exist across languages in the way time reference is achieved, translations of complex temporal frameworks often need to be adaptations rather than reproductions of each of the time elements mentioned in the source questions.

## 5.9. Additions and Repetitions

Reviewers also commented on additions in the translations. It is not uncommon for translated versions of interviews to add components. For instance, instructions, explanations and bridging materials, such as the phrase "the next few questions are about," are sometimes added for populations less familiar with the question-and-answer format of surveys. Occasionally, too, things are translated from the source interview that are not intended for translation and in this way are "added" to the translated interview. As it happens, assessors in the WMH assessment did not point out many additions in the material reviewed. Sometimes, an addition provided elaboration needed to clarify a concept for which only one term is used in the English source. An example of this kind occurred in the Spanish translation of the word "anxious" in question

SC20, which asked, "Have you ever in your life had an attack of fear or panic when all of a sudden you felt very frightened, anxious, or uneasy?" The Spanish translation elaborated on the source term "anxious" by adding the word *angustiado*. This example reflects the challenges inherent in translating emotions and feelings to ensure enough conceptual overlap (Wierzbicka 1992; Harkness 2004) and in dealing with differences in medical conditions in lay terms across languages (see Sartorius 1998).

Translators are trained to make sure that their translations are consistent and that they repeat in translation any phrases or terminology that are repeated in the source text. The assessors therefore pointed out when phrases repeated in the source text were not repeated in the translated texts. Inconsistency in terminology can result from having different translators work on different sections or simply from not allowing sufficient time for the proofreading and consistency-checking phases of translation revision. Consistency across languages should not be thought of as repetition at the level of words because a single word or phrase in English may be able to convey several different meanings. As a result, translations may need to differentiate and use a different translation depending on what a word or phrase is intended to convey in each case.

An interesting example occurs in the Spanish interview at D22a, which asked respondents "How old were you when *that worst episode* started?" In the Spanish version, "that worst episode" is translated as "that episode." Thus, the source follows the procedures of repetition and elaboration described earlier as typical of survey language, whereas the Spanish translation is more in line with ordinary discourse. However, the decision to translate in this way is probably dictated by structural differences between Spanish and English. These mean that the English "that worst case" can only be rendered in Spanish as either "the worst case" or "that case." Looking at the entire sequence in Spanish, the translation is probably better by not being consistent. Thus, the first translation of English "that worst episode" as "that episode" was sufficiently close to the mention of "worst episode" to be clear. In

contrast, the translation of the same phrase at a later point is further removed from mention of the identifying feature of the episode ("worst"). Not able to mimic the English exactly, the translator presumably chose the clearer phrase for the context.

## 6. ISSUES FOR SOURCE INTERVIEW DESIGN

To translate, translators first must parse the source text carefully to decide how various components contribute to the whole. This close scrutiny often leads translating teams to discover features of the source text that go unnoticed in more ordinary reading. Translators in the International Social Survey Programme (ISSP) and the ESS, for example, found a variety of problematic features in the source interview schedule. If these had been noticed at an earlier date, they could have been changed in the source text. As we suggest elsewhere, translation can be applied as a valuable tool in producing source interviews.

In the WMH assessment, assessors commented on a number of points that might usefully be reconsidered in a review of the source instrument. For example, several assessors pointed to the contradiction between question D22c and questions D22a–b, which requested that respondents "think about the worst episode" and report how old they were "when that worst episode started," and "How long did that worst episode last?" D22a presumably leads respondents to mentally identify a unique episode and D22b reinforces this. D22c, on the other hand, changes reference from the worst episode to a bad episode: "Then think of the last time you had a bad episode like this. How old were you when that last episode occurred?" The problem is that asking when the last (bad) episode occurred implies that there could be more than one such episode, and this conflicts with the superlative of "worst" in the preceding question.

Sometimes assessors raised points that are unlikely to affect measurement but are nonetheless typical of dilemmas faced by those producing other language versions. A question raised about the Spanish treatment of source question SC27f illustrates how important documentation can be in resolving small and larger details in translation. The English version of SC27f repeats the "fear" mentioned in the introduction to the question: "Sixth, fear of flying or of airplanes." The Spanish translation, in comparison, omits "fear," making the format of this question identical to that of accompanying questions in the set: "Sixth, flying or traveling on an airplane or of airplanes" ("Sexto, a volar o viajar en avión o a los aviones"). It is not clear from the documents available whether the word "fear" was deliberately repeated in the source item battery to ensure that respondents did not forget the questions are about fear or whether the inclusion of "fear" in the English item was simply a formatting oversight.

## 7. HARMONIZATION AND ADAPTATION

As described earlier, countries in Latin America met to discuss harmonization of their Spanish interviews. With the exception of a very few terms and expressions, most of the translations in these countries were identical. Occasionally, alongside a shared term, regionally favored terms were added by way of clarification. For example, in question SC20.1, the three Latin American Spanish translations used the term *enojo* as a translation of "anger," whereas the Peruvian translation also added the term *cólera*. The assumed advantage of having shared terms alongside local terms is that it might help reduce variance of interpretation.

In other cases, however, each country selected the term that would be best understood locally. Question SC29, for example, asked, "Was there ever a time in your life when you felt very afraid or uncomfortable when you had to do something in front of a group of people, like giving a speech or speaking in class?" The Latin American countries differed somewhat in their translations of the last phrase in this sentence ("like giving a speech or speaking in class"). In SC27b, which asked about fear of natural disasters, Peru added the example of "earthquakes," presumably aiming to choose a salient natural disaster for the Peruvian population. Interestingly, all four countries shared typing mistakes in D15 and D16, highlighting one of the dangers of cooperation if this also results in delegation of text production and proofreading to one unit; *interés* lacks the accent on the second "e" and, more telling, "problems" is used instead of *problemas*.

An assessor reviewing selected questions from these harmonized translations felt that the quality of translations produced seemed in general to be good. She also commented that some translation challenges were better addressed in the harmonized Latin American Spanish translations than in the European Spanish translation. We note that the Latin American countries benefited from a longer development time and the opportunity to discuss translations, as well as from Spain's earlier fielding experience. Those countries that met to discuss shared language translations in the ESS also produced translations of generally good quality. This remark is not intended to advocate harmonization. It would often not make sense to try to harmonize European Spanish with Latin American Spanish. However, the close scrutiny and discussion that harmonization efforts bring with them do seem to be beneficial in improving translations. In other words, intensive discussion of translations is useful.

We noted earlier that, in some instances, references in the English questions to culturally anchored events, behaviors, or perceptions seemed to prompt overclose translation. In other instances, the translated questions were adapted. In these cases, when the English refers to material that, although translatable would not have the intended measurement effect, the translated questions were changed. Examples are found in SC15, which asks, "How much does your health limit you now in moderate activities, such as moving a table, pushing a vacuum cleaner, bowling, or playing golf – a lot, a little, or not at all?" The term "playing golf" was adapted for Spain as "go for a long walk." The Netherlands adapted "bowling, or playing golf" into "cycling or carrying (grocery) shopping." The German interview in the same question spoke of general "sport activities," whereas the Italian translation omitted "golfing" and replaced "bowling" with the Italian ball game "bocce," even though it is by no means sure that "bocce" requires the same degree of fitness as "bowling." At the same time, the term "bowling" could itself be used to refer to very different kinds of games in the United States compared to other countries (e.g., Scotland).

A Chinese reviewer noted that an adjustment she considered necessary in D27c has not been made in Chinese. The question asked respondents whether they had ever experienced fear of "going to the dentist or doctor, getting a shot or injection, seeing blood or injury, or being in a hospital or doctor's office." The term "dentist" is probably mentioned first because many people are more afraid of dentists than of doctors. However, the assessor noted that dentists are regarded as doctors in China and that it would have been clearer for respondents if the translation had read "dentist or other doctor." In fact, the order of the Chinese translation is "doctor or dentist," so that to implement what the assessor suggested, the Chinese would have needed to follow the English order. In addition, most people in China see doctors in hospitals, so the additional reference to seeing them in a "doctor's office" was a little odd in the Chinese context. It is quite possible that these particular points do not affect measurement here. It could be dangerous, however, to generalize from individual cases. It is by no means certain that a question asking about satisfaction "with home and work" would elicit the same responses as a question asking about satisfaction "with work and home."

## 8. WHAT MATTERS AND HOW CAN WE KNOW?

Multiple differences were noted by the assessors of the five languages and six versions of the WMH interview that were assessed. Because differences are as much a part of translation as sameness, the chief interest here is the extent to which difference might contribute to survey error. The subsequent examples are intended to illustrate the difficulty encountered in trying to decide *a priori* whether a given difference contributes to survey error or detracts from the interview experience in some other sense. In many instances, further research and investigation are required. Analysis

of the data relating to some of the questions presented subsequently is planned for the coming year.

Surveys adopting a model of source questions followed by translations set out to ask the same questions to gain comparable data at the individual variable level. If the questions asked were different, the goals of the model would not have been accomplished and the questions should not have been compared. The assessments provided examples of larger and smaller differences between source and translated questions. Because analysis of the data on these questions has not yet been undertaken, for the moment we simply suggest possible directions that differences in response might take.

In the context of general survey methods research, a considerable body of research has investigated the effects of specific words, of answer scale formats, and of other design and implementation features on how respondents understand and answer questions (Schwarz et al. 1985; Schwarz et al. 1998; Tourangeau et al. 2000). This detailed consideration of words and formats stands in contrast to the world of compromise and variation across languages that we find in survey translations. If we find that questions are robust despite differences, it would be important to know what makes some questions robust and other questions less so. In addition, the effort invested in crafting source questions for comparative use is sometimes considerable. In crafting questions, the usual consensus is that small things matter (Smith 1993; Schwarz 1996). If we find that many features can be rendered differently or omitted in translation without any effect on the data, we may need to reconsider the goals of source interview drafting and the practices of survey translation. If, on the other hand, we find that small differences do matter, the same applies.

Some examples of seemingly slight differences may illustrate this point. Considered as lexemes (i.e., vocabulary items), there is a difference between "worrying a lot" and "fear." The source questions SC34 and SC35 asked whether respondents worry a lot that something will happen. The Turkish translation, in comparison, asked whether respondents fear that something will happen. In terms of intensity, there is a difference in English between being "very irritable" and being "irritable" and being "very afraid" and being "afraid." In question SC25, the source asked whether respondents were "very irritable," whereas the Turkish translation did not use a strengthening modifier ("very"). However, the Turkish word chosen for "irritable" was stronger in intensity than the English word. Thus, a proper balance was probably struck. In SC30, on the other hand, the source referred to being "afraid," whereas the Turkish translation referred to being "very afraid." This difference created an imbalance of intensity in the translation.

Question D1 asked, "During the episodes of this sort, did you ever feel discouraged about how things were going in your life?" This question was translated in Chinese as a question about whether respondents had felt discouraged and "lost faith in life." At face value, this would seem to be a more drastic response to life than suggested in the English. In similar fashion, the screening question SC11 ("During the past four weeks were you limited in the kind of work or activity you could do?") was translated in the European Spanish interview as, "During the past four weeks did you have to stop doing some of your work tasks or other activities?" The phrase "stop doing" is clearly more extreme than "being limited" in one's ability, which presumably resulted in a reduction in the number of respondents responding affirmatively to this question in Spain.

Similarly, the source text in question SC33.3 asked whether, during their adolescence, respondents often "stayed out" later than they were supposed to. The Turkish translation, however, asked whether respondents had "stayed up" longer than was expected. At face value, the consequences of staying up longer would seem to be different from staying out later, especially in terms of young people in a family context. In SC33.2, moreover, the English source asked whether respondents, as adolescents, had engaged in various types of vandalism, such as breaking into cars. The Turkish translation, in comparison, asked whether respondents had vandalized ("attacked") cars. The assessor pointing this out suggested that the words chosen would be associated with major

acts of "attacking" rather than such minor acts of vandalism as twisting mirrors or deflating tires.

## 9. OUTLOOK ON SURVEY TRANSLATION

Translation is usually one of the last procedures undertaken in producing the different versions needed to undertake multipopulation surveys. One consequence of this is that translation teams are often left to resolve any and all problems they find. Sometimes these problems may have less to do with translation in terms of language than with issues of comparability, conceptual coverage, and measurement that have gone unnoticed prior to the translation stage. We mentioned earlier that translators often engage in a closer scrutiny of texts than is necessary to understand a text that is not being translated. Perhaps this is why challenges unnoticed up to that point suddenly become apparent. One of the things to be learned from translation efforts and from assessments of translation products is that source questions might be more robust and better suited for export if some form of translation scrutiny can be built into review of draft source questions (Harkness & Van de Veer 2003).

The positive assessment of harmonized translations here suggests that translations benefit from discussion and review. Team translation efforts build discussion into the translation production process (Harkness 2002, 2006). One lesson to be learned, irrespective of the initial translation procedure used, is to make sure that the translations are discussed by a group of people who bring together the appropriate and necessary spread of expertise and knowledge.

Another lesson to be learned from the WMH assessments is that translation teams need to be trained on what quality translation involves and what steps are needed to ensure high-quality results. The overclose translations noted previously are an expression of inadequate technique and inadequate draft revision. Given the constraints that always apply in funds and time available, minor infelicities are obviously not the issue. At the same time, frequent repetition of even small infelicities may arguably affect respondent perception of the effort made to produce the interview. When respondents are requested to invest *their* time, they may unconsciously or consciously be unimpressed by the lack of effort that others have invested in producing a good translation, possibly leading to less effort being invested in responding carefully and thoughtfully.

One of the special issues faced in working on the WMH assessments was the challenge of version differences; from this, too, lessons can be learned. Occasionally, significant differences were pointed out by assessors between source English questions and translated questions. These later proved the result of differences between the source version given to assessors and that used in translation. Although all changes were recorded from version to version, the format used did not facilitate side-by-side comparisons across versions.

We still lack practical tools that allow translation efforts to match up their translations with source questions in their latest forms, to document adaptations and harmonizations, and to point, for example, to previous usage in other studies or to problems and mistakes discovered after fielding. Team translation efforts, moreover, rely on notes from the previous round of translation discussion to inform the next step. Many surveys also replicate questions already used elsewhere. It would be very useful to be able to access these questions, their available translations, the relevant documentation about adaptation, and so on, if needed. We have no doubt that such tools will be developed and will shape the future course of translation efforts in comparative research. Investigations of translation challenges and products such as those undertaken in the WMH Survey Initiative often result in better understanding of the relationship between the source question design and the translations. Our expectation is that ultimately both will benefit from the lessons to be learned.

**REFERENCES**

Andary, L., Stolk, Y. & Klimidid, S. (2003). *Assessing mental health across cultures*. Bowen Hills, Queensland: Australian Academic Press.

Belson, W. A. (1981). *The design and understanding of survey questions*. Aldershot, UK: Gower.
Belson, W. A. (1986). *Validity in survey research*. Brookvield, VT: Gower.
Braun, M. & Harkness, J. A. (2005). Text and context: Challenges to comparability in survey questions. In *ZUMA-Nachrichten Spezial No. 11. Methodological aspects in cross-national research*, ed. J. H. P. Hoffmeyer-Zlotnik & J. A. Harkness, pp. 95–107. Mannheim, Germany: ZUMA.
Cheng, A. T. A. (2001). Case definition and culture: Are people all the same? *British Journal of Psychiatry*, 179, 1–3.
de la Puente, M., Pan, Y. & Rose, D. (2003). An overview of proposed Census Bureau Guidelines for the translation of data collection instruments and supporting materials. Paper presented at the meeting of the Federal Committee on Statistical Methodology. Retrieved June 20, 2006, from http://www.fcsm.gov/03papers/delaPuente_Final.pdf.
Fowler, F. & Mangione, T. (1989). *Standardized survey interviewing: Minimizing interviewer-related error*. Newbury Park, CA: Sage Publications.
Gerzymisch-Arbogast, H. (1997). Wissenschaftliche Grundlagen für die Evaluierung von Übersetzungsleistungen. In *Translationsdidaktik: Grundfragen der Übersetzungswissenschaft*, ed. E. Fleischmann, W. Kutz, & P. A. Schmitt, pp. 573–9. Tübingen, Germany: Narr.
Harkness, J. A. (1996). The (re)presentation of self in everyday questionnaires. Paper presented at the International Sociological Association Conference on Social Science Methodology, Colchester, UK.
Harkness, J. A. (2002–2006). Round 3 ESS Translation strategies and procedures. Retrieved February 9, 2008, from (http://www.europeansocialsurvey.org/index.php?option=com_content&task=view&id=66&Itemid=112).
Harkness, J. A. (2003). Questionnaire translation. In *Cross-cultural survey methods*, ed. J. A. Harkness, F. J. R. Van de Vijver, & P. P. Mohler, pp. 35–56. Hoboken, NJ: John Wiley & Sons.
Harkness, J. A. (2004). Problems in establishing conceptually equivalent health definitions across multiple cultural groups. In *Eighth Conference on Health Survey Research Methods*, ed. S. B. Cohen & J. M. Lepkowski, pp. 85–90. Hyattsville, MD: Department of Health and Human Services.
Harkness, J. A. (2005). SHARE translation procedures and translation assessment. In *The Survey of Health, Aging, and Retirement in Europe*, ed. A. Börsh-Supan & H. Juerges, pp. 24–7. Mannheim, Germany: Mannheim Research Institute for the Economics of Ageing.
Harkness, J. A. (2008). Comparative survey research: Goals and challenges. In *International handbook*

*of survey methodology*, ed. D. Dillman, J. Hox. & E. de Leeuw, pp. 56–77. Hyattsville, VA: Erlbaum.

Harkness, J. A., Pennell, B. E. & Schoua-Glusberg, A. (2004). Survey questionnaire translation and assessment. In *Methods for testing and evaluating survey questionnaires*, ed. S. Presser, Rothgeb J., Couper M. P., Lessler J. T., Martin E., Martin J. & Singer E., pp. 453–74. Hoboken, NJ: John Wiley & Sons.

Harkness, J. A., Schoebi, N., Joye, D., Mohler, P. P., Faass, T. & Behr, D. (2008). Oral translation in telephone surveys. In *Advances in telephone survey methodology*, ed. J. M. Lepkowski, C. Tucker, J. M. Brick, E. de Leeuw, L. Japec, P. J. Lavrakas, M. W. Link & R. L. Sangster. pp. 231–49. Hoboken, NJ: John Wiley & Sons.

Harkness, J. A. & Schoua-Glusberg, A. (1998). Questionnaires in translation. In *ZUMA-Nachrichten Spezial No. 3. Cross-cultural survey equivalence*, ed. J. A. Harkness, pp. 87–126. Mannheim, Germany: ZUMA.

Harkness, J. A., Van de Vijver, F. J. R. & Johnson, T. P. (2003). Questionnaire design in comparative research. In *Cross-cultural survey methods*, ed. J. A. Harkness, F. J. R. Van de Vijver & P. P. Mohler, pp. 19–34. Hoboken, NJ: John Wiley & Sons.

Hönig, H. G. (1998). Positions, power and practice: Functionalist approaches and translation quality assessment. In *Translation and quality*, ed. C. Schäffner, pp. 6–34. Clevedon, UK: Multilingual Matters.

House, J. (1997). *Translation quality assessment.* Tübingen, Germany: Narr.

Kessler, R. C. & Üstün, T. B. (2004). The World Mental Health (WMH) Survey Initiative version of the World Health Organization (WHO) Composite International Diagnostic Interview (CIDI). *International Journal of Methods in Psychiatric Research*, 13, 93–121.

Nord, C. (1996). Text type and translation method: An objective approach to translation criticism. *The Translator*, 2, 81–8.

Pan, Y. & de la Puente, M. (2005). Census Bureau Guidelines for the translation of data collection instruments and supporting materials: Documentation on how the guideline was developed. U.S. Census Bureau Research Report Series, Survey Methodology #2005-06. Retrieved June 19, 2006, from http://www.census.gov/srd/papers/pdf/rsm2005-06.pdf.

Prince, R. & Tcheng Laroche, F. (1987). Culture-bound syndromes and international disease classifications. *Cultural Medical Psychiatry*, 11, 3–52.

Rogler, L. H. (1999). Methodological sources of cultural insensitivity in mental health research. *American Psychologist*, 54, 424–33.

Sartorius, N. (1998). SCAN translation. In *Diagnosis and clinical measurement in psychiatry: A reference manual for SCAN*, ed. J. K. Wing, N. Sartorius & T. B. Üstün, pp. 44–57. Cambridge, UK: Cambridge University Press.

Schuman, H. & Presser, S. (1981). *Questions and answers in attitude surveys: Experiments on question form, wording and context.* New York: Academic Press.

Schwarz, N. (1996). *Cognition and communication: Judgmental biases, research methods and the logic of conversation.* Mahwah, NJ: Lawrence Erlbaum Associates.

Schwarz, N., Grayson, C. E. & Knäuper, B. (1998). Formal features of rating scales and the interpretation of question meaning. *International Journal of Public Opinion Research*, 10, 177–83.

Schwarz, N., Hippler, H. J., Deutsch, B. & Strack, F. (1985). Response scales: Effects of category range on reported behavior and comparative judgments. *Public Opinion Quarterly*, 49, 388–95.

Smith, T. (1993). Little things matter: A sampler of how differences in questionnaire format can affect survey responses. *National Opinion Research Center GSS Methodological Report No. 78*. Chicago: University of Chicago.

Smith, T. W. (2004). Developing and evaluating cross-national survey instruments. In *Methods for testing and evaluating survey questionnaires*, ed. S. Presser, J. Rothgeb, M. P. Couper, J. T. Lessler, E. Martin, J. Martin & E. Singer, pp. 431–52. Hoboken, NJ: John Wiley & Sons.

Tafforeau, J., López Cobo, M., Tolonen, H., Scheidt-Nave, C. & Tinto, A. (2005). Guidelines for the development and criteria for the adoption of health survey instruments. European Commission. Retrieved June 23, 2006, from http://epp.eurostat.ec.europa.eu/cache/ITY_OFFPUB/KS-CC-05-003/EN/KS-CC-05–003-EN.pdf.

Tourangeau, R., Rips, L. J. & Rasinski, K. (2000). *The psychology of survey response.* New York: Cambridge University Press.

Vicentini, A. (2003). The economy principle in language: Notes and observations from early modern English grammars. Mots Palabras Words. Retrieved April 10, 2007, from http://www.ledonline.it/mpw/.

Wierzbicka, A. (1992). *Semantics, culture, and cognition: Universal human concepts in culture-specific configurations.* Oxford: Oxford University Press.

# 6 Concordance of the Composite International Diagnostic Interview Version 3.0 (CIDI 3.0) with Standardized Clinical Assessments in the WHO World Menvtal Health Surveys

JOSEP MARIA HARO, SAENA ARBABZADEH-BOUCHEZ, TRAOLACH S. BRUGHA, GIOVANNI DE GIROLAMO, MARGARET E. GUYER, ROBERT JIN, JEAN-PIERRE LÉPINE, FAUSTO MAZZI, BLANCA RENESES, GEMMA VILAGUT SAIZ, NANCY A. SAMPSON, AND RONALD C. KESSLER

## ACKNOWLEDGMENTS

The ESEMeD project is funded by the European Commission (Contracts QLG5-1999-01042; SANCO 2004123), the Piedmont Region (Italy), Fondo de Investigación Sanitaria, Instituto de Salud Carlos III, Spain (FIS 00/0028), Ministerio de Ciencia y Tecnología, Spain (SAF 2000-158-CE), Departament de Salut, Generalitat de Catalunya, Spain, and other local agencies, and by an unrestricted educational grant from GlaxoSmithKline. The U.S. National Comorbidity Survey Replication (NCS-R) is supported by the National Institute of Mental Health (NIMH) (U01-MH60220) with supplemental support from the National Institute of Drug Abuse (NIDA), the Substance Abuse and Mental Health Services Administration (SAMHSA), the Robert Wood Johnson Foundation (RWJF; Grant 044708), and the John W. Alden Trust. These surveys were carried out in conjunction with the World Health Organization World Mental Health (WMH) Survey Initiative. We thank the WMH staff for assistance with instrumentation, fieldwork, and data analysis. These activities were supported by the U.S. National Institute of Mental Health (R01MH070884), the John D. and Catherine T. MacArthur Foundation, the Pfizer Foundation, the U.S. Public Health Service (R13-MH066849, R01-MH069864, and R01 DA016558), the Fogarty International Center (FIRCA R03-TW006481), the Pan American Health Organization, Eli Lilly and Company Foundation, Ortho-McNeil Pharmaceutical, GlaxoSmithKline, and Bristol-Myers Squibb. A complete list of WMH publications can be found at http://www.hcp.med.harvard.edu/wmh/.

Portions of this chapter are based on Haro, J. M., Arbabzadeh-Bouchez, S., Brugha, T. S., de Girolamo, G., Guyer, M. E., Jin, R., Lepine, J. P., Mazzi, F., Reneses, B., Vilagut, G., Sampson, N. A., Kessler, R. C. (2006). Concordance of the Composite International Diagnostic Interview Version 3.0 (CIDI 3.0) with standardized clinical assessments in the WHO World Mental Health Surveys. International Journal of Methods in Psychiatric Research, 15(4), 167–80. Copyright © 2006 John Wiley & Sons Limited. All Rights Reserved. Reproduced with permission.

## I. INTRODUCTION

In Chapter 5, Harkness and colleagues reviewed the enormously complex set of issues that has to be considered in translating a source interview schedule from the source language into other target languages. Harkness and colleagues noted that it is difficult to know the extent to which each of the many complex decisions made in producing the WMH translations led to lack of comparability in responses across surveys. These authors also noted that it is difficult to study comparability of meaning even in the best of circumstances other than on the intuitive natural language level that they so well illustrated in their many examples.

In the case of survey questions designed to determine the presence of mental disorders, we have the advantage that a gold-standard assessment can be used to evaluate differential comparability across countries. This can be done at the level of the individual symptom or at the level of the diagnosis by using experienced mental health clinicians who are trained to administer research diagnostic interviews. These interviews employed semistructured probes, including conversational passages aimed at clarifying respondent meaning, to evaluate the presence of symptoms and disorders according to the definitions and criteria of an established diagnostic system. By administering these clinical reappraisal interviews to a probability subsample of WMH respondents in each of a number of different countries, it is possible to determine whether the meanings of responses to particular questions in the WMH survey are constant or variable across countries. Information about variability in meaning might then be used to adjust estimates across countries so that they correspond to a common gold-standard set of meanings, albeit with different levels of precision, in the different countries.

It was our original hope that all WMH surveys would include a systematic clinical reappraisal component that would create the kind of gold standard described in the previous paragraph that could be used to calibrate responses in all countries to a single consistent metric. This turned out to be impossible for a variety of logistical reasons. However, several WMH countries did include a clinical reappraisal phase, and others have come to see the value of doing so in the future. This chapter reviews the results of the clinical reappraisal studies of the CIDI that were carried out in conjunction with the WMH surveys in the United States and three Western European countries (France, Italy, Spain). Although additional CIDI validity studies are being carried out in other WMH countries, the ones reported here are the only ones that were completed in time for inclusion in this first volume of the WMH series.

The purpose of these clinical reappraisal studies was to determine the extent to which

diagnoses based on the CIDI are concordant with diagnoses based on blinded follow-up clinical interviews. Had the purpose been to revise the instrument as part of a pretest, we would have unblinded the clinical interviewers to respondents' answers in the CIDI and asked the clinical interviewers to probe these responses to arrive at clinically informed judgments that could be compared to the respondent reports. In this way, we could have pinpointed questions that generated responses with different meanings than those inferred by the clinical interviewers from their more probing, semistructured follow-up interviews. Revision of CIDI questions could have been based on the results of clinical interviewer debriefing sessions with respondents aimed at clarifying the confusions in meaning in the CIDI questions. However, as our purpose was to assess post hoc validity of the existing instrument, clinical interviewers were blinded to CIDI responses and asked to carry out a separate clinical reappraisal interview to arrive at independent assessments of respondent diagnoses, with the goal of assessing concordance between diagnoses based on the CIDI and diagnoses based on the gold-standard clinical interviews. The clinical interview schedule used for this purpose was the Axis I research version, nonpatient edition of the Structured Clinical Interview for DSM-IV (SCID) (First et al. 2002).

Previous clinical reappraisal studies showed that earlier versions of the CIDI, which were based on DSM-III-R criteria, generated DSM diagnoses generally consistent with those obtained in SCID clinical reappraisal interviews in community surveys (Wittchen 1994; Wittchen et al. 1995; Wittchen et al. 1996; Kessler et al. 1998). In a variety of the settings, the results of CIDI clinical reappraisal studies that generated diagnoses based on ICD-10 criteria using the Schedules for Clinical Assessment in Neuropsychiatry (SCAN) (Wing et al. 1990) as the clinical gold standard was more variable, with some studies showing the CIDI diagnoses to have poor agreement with SCAN diagnoses (Brugha et al. 2001) in a community sample and others showing agreement to be either good in a patient sample (Andrews et al. 1995) or excellent in a primary-care provider sample (Jordanova et al. 2004).

The WMH surveys are the first to administer CIDI 3.0, which operationalizes both ICD-10 and DSM-IV criteria. As noted in Chapter 4, CIDI 3.0 was developed to improve the validity of the CIDI with the benefit of insights gained from the CIDI clinical reappraisal studies cited in the previous paragraph. Methodological studies are needed to evaluate the consistency of CIDI diagnoses based on these new criteria with clinical reinterviews, as it is not legitimate to assume that the results of the earlier methodological studies hold for this new version of CIDI. The results reported in the current chapter are based on methodological studies of this sort that were carried out in probability subsamples of the four WMH samples noted previously. The data were weighted to adjust for this oversampling. Separate examinations were carried out of lifetime prevalence and 12-month prevalence.

The analysis of the clinical reappraisal data had three phases, the third of which went beyond earlier studies. The first phase considered aggregate CIDI-SCID consistency of prevalence estimates. The second phase considered CIDI-SCID consistency of individual-level diagnostic classifications. The third phase considered whether CIDI-SCID concordance would be improved significantly by developing prediction equations in which CIDI item-level data were used along with CIDI diagnostic data to predict SCID diagnoses. As discussed in more detail by Kessler and colleagues (2004a) and illustrated in a series of recent disorder-specific reports (Kessler et al. 2005; Kessler et al. 2006a; Lenzenweger et al. 2007), these predicted probabilities either can be treated as outcomes in substantive analyses or can be used as input to more complex analyses that use the method of multiple imputation (MI) (Rubin 1987) to make estimates of the prevalence and correlates of clinical diagnoses from CIDI data. Comparison with parallel estimates of the prevalence and correlates of CIDI diagnoses allows for much more fine-grained consideration of consistency with clinical diagnoses than do conventional analyses of diagnostic concordance.

## 2. THE CLINICAL REAPPRAISAL SAMPLES

The clinical reappraisal samples oversampled CIDI cases but also included noncases in each of the four WMH surveys. The methods of subsampling differed in European surveys from the U.S. survey but were based in both cases on probability procedures so that the clinical reappraisal sample could be weighted back to be representative of the total original sample. This weighting took into consideration the sample design of the original surveys, including differential probability of selection in households depending on sample size and poststratification, so that significance tests could be made using appropriate design-based methods.

The European clinical reappraisal study was based on a probability subsample of respondents who lived in targeted geographic sample areas in France, Italy, and Spain. Of the main survey respondents with any 12-month DSM-IV/CIDI diagnosis in these targeted areas, 100% were selected for participation in the clinical reappraisal study along with a random 10% subsample of other respondents in the same areas, for a sample of 428 completed clinical reappraisal interviews (87 in France, 194 in Italy, and 137 in Spain). As the focus was on consistency of assessing 12-month prevalence, the ideal design would have been one that administered reappraisal interviews within a short time of the initial interviews. However, logistical complications led to delays, with many of the reappraisal interviews carried out as much as six months after the initial WMH interviews. This means that the overlap in the recall period of 12-month prevalence estimates varied across respondents and that the number of interviews completed according to protocol (i.e., within two months of the CIDI interview) is much smaller than the total number of clinical interviews ($n = 143$). As described later in this chapter, this variation was taken into account in analysis.

The U.S. clinical reappraisal study was based on a probability subsample of all respondents in telephone households who participated in the U.S. WMH survey throughout the entire United States. The clinical reappraisal sample oversampled respondents who met DSM-IV/CIDI lifetime criteria for one or more relatively uncommon disorders (e.g., agoraphobia, panic disorder, generalized anxiety disorder, substance abuse with dependence) at a higher rate than respondents in a second sampling stratum who met criteria only for more common disorders (e.g., specific phobia, major depression, substance abuse with or without dependence), with the lowest sampling fraction for a third stratum made up of respondents who failed to meet criteria for any lifetime DSM-IV/CIDI disorder. Selection was made proportional to respondent weights in the main sample so as partially to cancel out the within-household probability of selection weight. A total of 325 clinical reappraisal interviews were completed according to protocol. In addition to the main clinical reappraisal sample, separate more focused clinical reappraisal samples were selected to validate the CIDI diagnoses of bipolar disorder (BPD) ($n = 40$) and adult attention-deficit/hyperactivity disorder (ADHD) ($n = 154$).

All the SCID clinical reappraisal interviews in the U.S. clinical reappraisal study and approximately 40% of those in the European clinical reappraisal sample were administered by telephone. The remaining clinical reappraisal interviews were administered face-to-face. Telephone administration is now widely accepted in clinical reappraisal studies on the basis of evidence of comparable validity to in-person administration (Kendler et al. 1992; Sobin et al. 1993; Rohde et al. 1997). A great advantage of telephone administration is that a centralized and closely supervised clinical interview staff can carry out the interviews throughout the entire sample area without the geographic restriction that is typically required for face-to-face clinical assessment. A disadvantage is that the small part of the population without telephones cannot be included in clinical calibration studies when interviews are done by telephone. This limitation was removed in the European study because respondents in households without telephones were interviewed face-to-face. It is a limitation of the U.S. study, though, that the roughly 5% of U.S. households without telephones were excluded from the clinical reappraisal sample.

## 3. THE CLINICAL REAPPRAISAL STUDY DESIGN

The clinical reappraisal study was designed to determine the extent to which the diagnostic classifications made on the basis of the CIDI would have been different if the surveys had been carried out entirely by carefully trained clinical interviewers using the SCID rather than by trained lay interviewers with the CIDI. As the entry questions (i.e., the diagnostic stem questions) in the CIDI and SCID are very similar, the distinction between the two types of interview hinges on two CIDI-SCID differences: differences in the ability to elicit endorsement of diagnostic stem questions based on CIDI yes-no questions versus the more flexible open-ended probing in the SCID, and differences in symptom assessments among respondents who endorse diagnostic stem questions based on fully structured CIDI questions versus the more conversational probes in the SCID. We had no doubt but that the SCID procedures were superior to the CIDI procedures in eliciting clear information about symptom characteristics. It was less clear to us, though, whether the SCID was superior to the CIDI in eliciting endorsement of diagnostic stem questions, as our previous work carrying out CIDI-SCID comparisons documented some cases in which respondents were more comfortable admitting embarrassing feelings and behaviors to lay interviewers than to clinical interviewers (Kessler et al. 1998).

A major impediment to making accurate CIDI-SCID comparisons of the sort described in the previous paragraph is that respondents are inconsistent in their reports over time. Indeed, our own previous experience and that of other researchers shows consistently that respondents in community surveys tend to report less and less as they are interviewed more and more as a result of respondent fatigue (Bromet et al. 1986). Part of this pattern is a tendency for respondents to endorse a smaller number of diagnostic stem questions in follow-up interviews than in initial interviews (Kessler et al. 1998), which leads to the biased perception that initial structured interviews overestimate prevalence more than second clinical interviews. On the basis of this observation, we modified the conventional blinded clinical reinterview design in two important ways in the WMH clinical reappraisal study. First, we unblinded the clinical interviewers to whether the respondents endorsed diagnostic stem questions in the CIDI, but not to the final CIDI diagnoses. Second, we encouraged respondents to endorse diagnostic stem questions in the clinical reappraisal interviews by reminding respondents who endorsed the CIDI stem question in their initial interview of this fact. This partial unblinding of interviewers might be seen as introducing a bias, but that turns out not to be the case because the majority of community survey respondents who endorse CIDI stem questions do not go on to meet full CIDI criteria for the associated disorder.

The stem question reminder process, in comparison, had a substantial effect on the completeness of respondent reports in clinical reinterviews. Respondents were told at the beginning of their clinical reinterview that they would be asked some of the same questions as in their earlier interview. They were also told that this was being done to test the interview and not to test their memory, so they should answer without trying to remember what they said to the previous interviewer. Respondents were then taken through the clinical interview in the usual fashion, with the exception that the sections of the clinical reinterview in which they endorsed a diagnostic stem question in the CIDI were started with the following introduction: "During the first interview, you said (presentation of the stem question endorsed in the interview). Has that happened in the past 12 months?" Reinterview respondents could still deny that they reported a diagnostic stem question in the initial interview, although this was uncommon. In cases where the respondent had not endorsed the CIDI stem question in the original interview, the SCID probing for a diagnostic stem endorsement was carried out in the conventional fashion so as to discover false negative responses in the CIDI. The clinical interviewers

also had complete flexibility to go back to a diagnostic section that was previously skipped if any information subsequently surfaced in the interview to suggest a positive response to the diagnostic stem question.

## 4. CLINICAL INTERVIEWER TRAINING AND SUPERVISION

Clinical interviewers were carefully trained by the same SCID training team in the European and U.S. studies and were closely supervised during the course of fieldwork using the same quality assurance protocol. As noted previously, the version of the SCID used was a modified version of the Axis I research version, nonpatient edition (First et al. 2002). An expanded version of the model training program created by the developers of the SCID (Gibbon et al. 1981) was used for interviewer training. This program featured (1) the use of the standard SCID training tapes and manuals, which take an average of approximately 30 hours of self-study, followed by (2) 40 hours of in-person group training by experienced SCID trainers, and (3) ongoing quality-control monitoring throughout the field period. Textual extracts from the DSM-IV manual were supplied to interviewers that described where available specific study diagnostic criteria to maximize the reliability of clinical ratings.

Quality-control monitoring included clinical supervisor review of all hard-copy-completed SCID interviews, recontact of respondents whenever the clinical supervisor believed that more information was needed to make a rating, periodic consultation with diagnostic experts who served as consultants for complex cases, consultant review of a random subsample of interview audiotapes, and biweekly interviewer–supervisor meetings to prevent drift. As training materials were all in English, the clinical interviewers in Europe had to be bilingual and were trained in what was to them a foreign language. Because of this, special care was taken to expand the second phase of training in Europe and to have the clinical supervisors in these studies specially trained by the U.S. trainers. In addition, the U.S. trainers provided ongoing telephone and e-mail consultation to clinical supervisors in the European countries throughout the field period to maintain comparability between the U.S. and European clinical reappraisal exercises.

## 5. ANALYSIS METHODS

After weighting the clinical reappraisal sample data to be representative of the main samples, we investigated whether CIDI prevalence estimates are biased in comparison to SCID prevalence estimates using McNemar $\chi^2$ tests to evaluate the statistical significance of differences in the proportions of respondents who were false positives versus false negatives. As with all our significance tests, McNemar tests were carried out using design-based estimation methods that adjusted for the effects of weighting and clustering and oversampling of CIDI cases (Kish & Frankel 1974; Wolter 1985).

Individual-level CIDI-SCID diagnostic concordance was next evaluated using two different descriptive measures, the area under the receiver operator characteristic curve (AUC) (Hanley & McNeil 1982) and Cohen's $\kappa$ (Cohen 1960). Although $\kappa$ is the most widely used measure of concordance in validity studies of psychiatric disorders, it has been criticized because it depends on prevalence and consequently is often low in situations where there appears to be high agreement between low-prevalence measures (Byrt et al. 1993; Cook 1998; Kraemer et al. 2003). An important implication is that $\kappa$ varies across populations that differ in prevalence even when the populations do not differ in sensitivity (SN) (i.e., the percentage of true cases correctly classified by the CIDI) or specificity (SP) (i.e., the percentage of true noncases correctly classified). As sensitivity and specificity are considered fundamental parameters, this means that the comparison of $\kappa$ across different populations cannot be used to evaluate the cross-population performance of a test.

Critics of $\kappa$ prefer to assess concordance with measures that are a function of SN and SP. The odds ratio (OR) meets this requirement, as $OR$ is equal to $[SN \times SP]/[(1 - SN) \times (1 - SP)]$ (Agresti 1996). However, the upper end of the OR is unbounded, making it difficult to use the OR to evaluate the extent to which CIDI diagnoses are consistent with clinical diagnoses. Yule's $Q$ has been proposed as an alternative measure to resolve this problem (Spitznagel & Helzer 1985), as $Q$ is a bounded transformation of OR $[Q = (OR - 1)/(OR + 1)]$ that ranges between $-1$ and $+1$. $Q$ can be interpreted as the difference in the probabilities of a randomly selected clinical case and a randomly selected clinical noncase that differ in their classification on the CIDI being correctly versus incorrectly classified by the CIDI. The difficulty with $Q$ is that tied pairs (i.e., clinical cases and noncases that have the same CIDI classification) are excluded, which means that $Q$ does not tell us about actual prediction accuracy.

The AUC is a measure that resolves this problem, as AUC can be interpreted as the probability that a randomly selected clinical case will score higher on the CIDI than a randomly selected noncase. Although developed to study the association between a continuous predictor and a dichotomous outcome, the AUC can be used in the special case where the predictor is a dichotomy, in which case $AUC$ equals $(SN + SP)/2$. As a result of this useful interpretation, we focus on AUC in our evaluation of CIDI-SCID diagnostic concordance. We also report SN and SP, the key components of AUC in the dichotomous case, as well as positive predictive value (PPV) (i.e., the proportion of CIDI cases that are confirmed by the SCID), negative predictive value (NPV) (i.e., the proportion of CIDI noncases that are confirmed as noncases by the SCID), and $\kappa$.

The third phase of analysis involved estimation of a series of stepwise logistic regression equations in which SCID diagnoses were treated as dichotomous outcomes and CIDI symptom variables were included along with CIDI diagnoses as predictors to determine whether CIDI symptom-level data could significantly improve the prediction of SCID diagnoses compared to predictions from CIDI diagnoses. As discussed in more detail elsewhere (Kessler et al. 2004a), significant improvement of this sort could be used to generate predicted probabilities of SCID diagnoses for each survey respondent who was not in the clinical reappraisal sample. Diagnostic imputations based on these predicted probabilities could then be used to make estimates of the prevalence and correlates of clinical diagnoses in the full sample so as to incorporate the analysis of validity into substantive investigations. For example, it would be possible in this way to carry out parallel analyses of the extent to which the correlates of predicted SCID diagnoses differ from the correlates of CIDI diagnoses.

The AUC was the descriptive statistic used to describe these improvements. As noted earlier, the AUC is typically used with a dimensional predictor and a dichotomous outcome. As a result, it is a simple matter to think of the AUC as the association between a predicted probability of a dichotomous outcome – in our case, based on prediction either from the dichotomous CIDI case classification or from a logistic regression equation containing both CIDI diagnoses and symptom measures as predictors – and the observed classifications on the outcome. This makes it possible to evaluate the extent to which AUC increases as more complex predictors are added to an equation over and above the initial CIDI dichotomous diagnostic classification.

## 6. LIFETIME AGGREGATE CONCORDANCE

Separate disorder-specific CIDI-SCID comparisons of lifetime prevalence were made in the U.S. clinical reappraisal sample for panic disorder, phobias, posttraumatic stress disorder (PTSD), major depression, bipolar disorder, and alcohol or drug abuse with or without dependence (Table 6.1) McNemar tests of CIDI versus SCID differences in estimated lifetime prevalence are insignificant for panic disorder, agoraphobia (with or without panic), specific phobia, and bipolar I–II disorder but are significant for all other disorders. As shown by the fact that PPV is consistently greater than SN, these differences are due to the CIDI lifetime prevalence estimates being conservative relative to the SCID estimates. SCID prevalence estimates are 34% greater than CIDI prevalence estimates for any anxiety disorder, 33% greater for major depression, 53%

greater for alcohol or drug abuse or dependence, and 42% greater for any of the preceding disorders.

## 7. LIFETIME INDIVIDUAL-LEVEL CONCORDANCE

Using descriptors modeled on those used for roughly comparable values of $\kappa$ (Landis & Koch 1977), individual-level CIDI-SCID lifetime prevalence concordance is moderate (AUC in the range of 0.7–0.8) for the majority of diagnoses assessed in the U.S. clinical reappraisal sample (panic disorder, any phobia, panic disorder or any phobia, any anxiety disorder, major depression, alcohol dependence, drug abuse, and any disorder; Table 6.1). Concordance is almost perfect (AUC greater than or equal to 0.9), in comparison, for bipolar disorder, substantial (AUC in the range of 0.8–0.9) for agoraphobia and alcohol abuse, and fair (AUC in the range 0.6–0.7) for the remaining disorders (specific phobia, social phobia, PTSD, drug dependence). The majority of SCID cases are detected by the CIDI (SN) for anxiety disorders (54.4%; 38.3%–62.6%), major depression (55.3%), BPD (86.8%), substance dependence (73.6%), and any disorder (62.8%). The vast majority of CIDI cases, in comparison, are confirmed by the SCID (PPV), including 74.5% (43.9%–86.1%) with anxiety disorder, 58.3%–73.7% with mood disorder, 82.0%–98.7% with substance disorder, and 84.3% with any disorder.

## 8. LIFETIME CONCORDANCE USING CIDI SYMPTOM-LEVEL DATA

Stepwise logistic regression analysis was used to select CIDI symptom questions for each diagnosis that significantly predicted the parallel SCID diagnosis after including the CIDI diagnosis in the prediction equation. Each respondent in the clinical reappraisal sample was then assigned a predicted probability of each SCID diagnosis based on the resulting logistic regression equation as a way to summarize the predictive information contained in the CIDI diagnostic and symptom data. The AUC for the predicted

**Table 6.1.** Consistency of lifetime DSM-IV CIDI and SCID diagnoses in the NCS-R clinical reappraisal sample ($n = 325$)[a]

| | McNemar $\chi^2$ test | AUC | $\kappa$ | (se) | OR | (95% CI) | SN | (se) | SP | (se) | PPV | (se) | NPV | (se) |
|---|---|---|---|---|---|---|---|---|---|---|---|---|---|---|
| **I. Anxiety disorders** | | | | | | | | | | | | | | |
| Panic disorder | 0.0 | 0.72 | 0.45 | (0.15) | 56.3* | (15.5–204.6) | 45.8 | (13.0) | 98.5 | (0.5) | 48.4 | (14.1) | 98.4 | (0.5) |
| Agoraphobia | 0.0 | 0.81 | 0.61 | (0.15) | 174.8* | (39.1–780.6) | 62.6 | (12.9) | 99.1 | (0.5) | 62.0 | (15.7) | 99.1 | (0.3) |
| Specific phobia | 0.0 | 0.67 | 0.33 | (0.07) | 6.3* | (2.7–14.6) | 45.2 | (8.7) | 88.5 | (2.3) | 43.9 | (7.6) | 89.0 | (2.8) |
| Social phobia | 5.7* | 0.65 | 0.35 | (0.07) | 8.4* | (3.9–18.2) | 36.6 | (7.0) | 93.6 | (1.4) | 53.9 | (7.6) | 87.8 | (2.6) |
| Any phobia | 7.5* | 0.71 | 0.45 | (0.06) | 9.8* | (5.0–19.4) | 51.7 | (5.7) | 90.2 | (1.9) | 68.1 | (6.0) | 82.1 | (3.0) |
| Panic or any phobia | 7.4* | 0.71 | 0.46 | (0.06) | 9.9* | (5.1–19.5) | 52.6 | (5.6) | 90.0 | (2.0) | 68.7 | (5.8) | 81.9 | (3.1) |
| Posttraumatic stress disorder | 11.4* | 0.69 | 0.49 | (0.10) | 64.9* | (14.9–281.9) | 38.3 | (11.8) | 99.1 | (0.5) | 86.1 | (7.7) | 91.3 | (3.0) |
| Any anxiety disorder | 12.1* | 0.73 | 0.48 | (0.05) | 11.6* | (6.0–22.4) | 54.4 | (5.3) | 90.7 | (1.8) | 74.5 | (5.0) | 80.0 | (3.2) |
| **II. Mood disorders** | | | | | | | | | | | | | | |
| Major depressive disorder | 7.2* | 0.75 | 0.54 | (0.06) | 18.4* | (7.9–42.9) | 55.3 | (6.8) | 93.7 | (1.9) | 73.7 | (7.0) | 86.8 | (2.7) |
| Bipolar III[b] | 0.6 | 0.93 | 0.69 | (0.3) | 582.6* | (72.6–4674) | 86.8 | (10.5) | 98.9 | (0.5) | 58.3 | (14.5) | 99.8 | (0.2) |
| **III. Substance disorders** | | | | | | | | | | | | | | |
| Alcohol abuse[c] | 7.3* | 0.81 | 0.70 | (0.06) | 93.3* | (28.0–311.3) | 64.1 | (7.4) | 98.1 | (1.0) | 88.1 | (5.6) | 92.7 | (2.0) |
| Drug abuse[c] | 8.9* | 0.76 | 0.63 | (0.08) | 111.8* | (26.3–476.3) | 53.7 | (12.7) | 99.0 | (0.5) | 88.2 | (6.0) | 93.8 | (2.7) |
| Alcohol dependence with abuse[c] | 18.5* | 0.72 | 0.56 | (0.09) | 877.0* | (105.8–7266.2) | 43.1 | (9.3) | 99.9 | (0.1) | 98.7 | (1.3) | 91.9 | (1.7) |
| Drug dependence with abuse[c] | 11.3* | 0.62 | 0.36 | (0.12) | 74.0* | (9.2–625.0) | 25.0 | (10.6) | 99.6 | (0.4) | 82.0 | (13.9) | 94.2 | (2.2) |
| Revised alcohol dependence[d] | 0.1 | 0.879 | 0.77 | (0.06) | 129.1* | (38.9–428.0) | 78.6 | (7.7) | 97.2 | (1.1) | 81.5 | (6.6) | 96.7 | (1.3) |
| Revised drug dependence[d] | 0.0 | 0.798 | 0.59 | (0.10) | 52.7* | (10.0–278.2) | 62.7 | (16.9) | 96.9 | (1.2) | 62.3 | (11.9) | 97.0 | (2.0) |
| Revised alcohol or drug dependence[d] | 2.6 | 0.856 | 0.76 | (0.06) | 113.7* | (32.8–394.8) | 73.6 | (9.1) | 97.6 | (1.1) | 86.6 | (5.5) | 94.6 | (2.3) |
| **IV Other disorders** | | | | | | | | | | | | | | |
| Adult attention-deficit/hyperactivity disorder[e] | 3.5 | 0.861 | 0.49 | (0.16) | 60.2 | (14.7–246.6) | 77.7 | (6.9) | 94.5 | (3.1) | 39.6 | (9.2) | 98.9 | (0.6) |
| **V. Any disorder[f]** | | | | | | | | | | | | | | |
| Any disorder | 21.1* | 0.76 | 0.52 | (0.05) | 13.6* | (7.3–25.4) | 62.8 | (4.4) | 89.0 | (2.1) | 84.3 | (3.2) | 71.7 | (4.3) |

* Significant at the 0.05 level, two-sided test.

[a] OR: odds ratio; AUC: area under the ROC curve; SN: sensitivity; SP: specificity; PPV: positive predictive value; NPV: negative predictive value.

[b] Results for bipolar disorder are based on a separate clinical reappraisal sample of 40 respondents (Kessler et al. 2006b).

[c] Substance abuse was diagnosed in both the CIDI and the SCID with or without dependence. The CIDI assessment of substance dependence was made only among respondents who met criteria for abuse on the basis of the finding in an earlier study that the prevalence of dependence without abuse is very uncommon (Kessler et al. 1998). However, this result has recently been called into question (Hasin & Grant 2004), leading subsequent WMH surveys to remove this restriction and to assess substance dependence even among respondents who failed to report a history of abuse.

[d] In light of the underestimation of prevalence of alcohol and drug dependence in the CIDI compared to the SCID, a revised coding scheme was used in which CIDI diagnoses of abuse were used to predict SCID diagnoses of dependence with abuse. As shown in the table, AUC increased meaningfully with this revised scoring approach.

[e] Results for adult ADHD are based on a separate clinical reappraisal sample of 154 respondents (Kessler et al. 2006a).

[f] The disorders considered here are only those included in the main clinical reappraisal sample of 325 respondents. Bipolar disorder and adult ADHD are not included.

**Table 6.2.** Area under the ROC curve (AUC) for dichotomous (DICH) DSM-IV CIDI diagnostic classifications and continuous (CONT) CIDI-based predicted probabilities in predicting lifetime DSM-IV/SCID diagnoses in the NCS-R clinical reappraisal sample ($n = 325$)

|  | DICH[a] | CONT[a] |
|---|---|---|
| **I. Anxiety disorders** | | |
| Panic disorder | 0.72 | 0.93 |
| Agoraphobia | 0.81 | 0.96 |
| Specific phobia | 0.67 | 0.84 |
| Social phobia | 0.65 | 0.74 |
| Posttraumatic stress disorder | 0.69 | 0.88 |
| **II. Mood disorders** | | |
| Major depressive disorder | 0.75 | 0.87 |
| Bipolar III[b] | 0.93 | 0.97 |
| **III. Substance disorders** | | |
| Revised alcohol dependence[c] | 0.72 | 0.99 |
| Revised drug dependence[c] | 0.62 | 0.95 |
| **IV. Other disorders** | | |
| Adult attention-deficit/ hyperactivity disorder[d] | 0.86 | 0.99 |

[a] DICH: AUC values for the dichotomous (DICH) DSM-IV CIDI diagnostic classifications; CONT: AUC values for continuous CIDI-based predicted probabilities of SCID diagnoses derived from logistic regression equations.

[b] Results for bipolar disorder are based on a separate clinical reappraisal sample of 40 respondents (Kessler et al. 2006b).

[c] In light of the underestimation of prevalence of alcohol and drug dependence in the CIDI compared to the SCID, a revised coding scheme was used in which CIDI diagnoses of abuse were used to predict SCID diagnoses of dependence with abuse. As shown in the table, AUC increased meaningfully with this revised scoring approach.

[d] Results for adult ADHD are based on a separate clinical reappraisal sample of 154 respondents (Kessler et al. 2006a).

probability is consistently greater than the AUC for the dichotomous CIDI diagnostic classification in predicting each of the SCID diagnoses (Table 6.2). This improved prediction is because the CIDI collects a substantial amount of information from respondents who endorse diagnostic stem questions but fail to meet full diagnostic criteria for DSM disorders. This information was used in the prediction equations to adjust for the consistently higher diagnostic thresholds in the CIDI than in the SCID. When the CIDI data are transformed through these equations

into predicted probabilities of SCID diagnoses, CIDI-SCID concordance changes from largely moderate (AUC in the range of 0.7–0.8) to largely substantial (AUC in the range of 0.8–0.9) or almost perfect (AUC in the range of 0.9–1.0). Bias in prevalence estimates is also removed when predicted probabilities of SCID diagnoses are used instead of dichotomous CIDI disorder classifications.

## 9. 12-MONTH AGGREGATE CONCORDANCE

Disorder-specific CIDI-SCID comparisons of 12-month prevalence were made in the European samples for most of the same disorders assessed in the United States. The one exception in the case of anxiety disorders was that generalized anxiety disorder (GAD) was assessed in the European clinical reappraisal samples but not in the U.S. clinical reappraisal sample (because the SCID includes GAD only as a current diagnosis, not a lifetime diagnosis). The two exceptions in the case of mood disorders were that dysthymic disorder was assessed in Europe but not in the United States and that BPD was assessed in the United States but not Europe. In the case of substance disorders, the European surveys assessed only alcohol abuse dependence, not illicit drug abuse dependence. Finally, the separate assessments of adult ADHD and BPD in the United States were not repeated in the European assessments.

Because of the narrower time frame of assessment in the European (12 months) than in the U.S. (lifetime) reappraisal interviews, the number of respondents with individual CIDI disorders was much smaller in the European than in U.S. reappraisal samples. As a result, CIDI-SCID 12-month diagnostic consistency was assessed by focusing on summary measures of any anxiety disorder, any mood disorder, and any overall disorder. Any alcohol disorder could not be assessed separately because of too few cases ($n = 3$). As noted in the section on the clinical reappraisal samples, logistical complications led to many of the European clinical reappraisal interviews being carried out as much as six months after the initial CIDI interviews,

**Table 6.3.** Consistency of 12-month DSM-IV-CIDI and SCID diagnoses in the ESEMeD clinical reappraisal sample with time between CIDI and SCID interviews less than 60 days ($n = 143$)

| | McNemar $\chi^2$ test | AUC | $\kappa$ (se) | OR (95% CI) | SN (se) | SP (se) | PPV (se) | NPV (se) |
|---|---|---|---|---|---|---|---|---|
| Any anxiety disorder | 6.9 | 0.88 | 0.42 (0.1) | 66.7 (18.2–244.2) | 83.7 (8.3) | 92.9 (1.7) | 31.3 (7.8) | 99.3 (0.4) |
| Any mood disorder | 0.8 | 0.83 | 0.56 (0.2) | 76.7 (21.4–274.9) | 69.1 (11.8) | 97.2 (0.9) | 49.6 (10.5) | 98.7 (0.6) |
| Any disorder | 6.0 | 0.84 | 0.49 (0.1) | 34.1 (6.6–176.8) | 77.9 (13.2) | 90.6 (2.7) | 41.5 (8.5) | 98.0 (1.5) |

* Significant at the 0.05 level, two-sided test.

*Notes:* OR: odds ratio; AUC: area under the ROC curve; SN: sensitivity; SP: specificity; PPV: positive predictive value; NPV: negative predictive value.

which resulted in the overlap in the recall period of 12-month prevalence estimates varying substantially across respondents. This variation was taken into account by carrying out the analyses separately for respondents with a time lag between CIDI and SCID interviews of less than two months, between two and four months, and more than four months. Concordance was found to increase monotonically across these three subsamples as time between the two interviews decreased. As a result, we focus here on results for the subsample with a length of time between interviews less than two months (Table 6.3). Focusing first on aggregate concordance, McNemar tests for CIDI versus SCID differences in estimated 12-month prevalence are insignificant for all four summary measures in this subsample.

## 10. 12-MONTH INDIVIDUAL-LEVEL CONCORDANCE

Individual-level CIDI-SCID concordance for 12-month prevalence is substantial (AUC in the range of 0.8–0.9) for any mood disorder, any anxiety disorder, and any overall disorder. Within-country estimates of AUC (results not shown in table but available on request) have substantial consistency for any anxiety disorder (0.83–0.94) and any mood disorder (0.83–0.84), but more variability for any disorder (0.78–0.93).

The majority of 12-month SCID cases were detected by the CIDI (SN) for any anxiety (83.7%), any mood (69.1%), and any overall disorder (77.9%). Lower proportions of CIDI cases were confirmed by the SCID (PPV) for

12-month estimates in the European clinical reappraisal surveys than for lifetime estimates in the NCS-R, including 31.3% with anxiety disorder, 49.6% with mood disorder, and 41.5% with any disorder.

## 11. 12-MONTH CONCORDANCE USING CIDI SYMPTOM-LEVEL DATA

The AUC was found to increase substantially in the case of mood disorders when CIDI symptom data were added to equations that included the dichotomous CIDI diagnosis to predict the 12-month SCID diagnosis (from 0.83 to 0.93). The AUC increased more modestly in predicting 12-month SCID anxiety disorders (from 0.88 to 0.91).

## 12. DISCUSSION

Several limitations of the WMH clinical reappraisal studies reported here should be taken into account when interpreting the results. First, most of the SCID reinterviews were carried out by telephone, while initial CIDI interviews were face-to-face. Although it has been shown that telephone interviews constitute a valid mode of clinical assessment (Kendler et al. 1992; Sobin et al. 1993; Rohde et al. 1997), we do not know what would have happened if the same mode of administration were to have been consistently employed in both cases. Second, assessment of lifetime and 12-month reliability was conducted in different countries, which makes it difficult to compare the two sets of results. Third, the investigation of

12-month concordance found strong inverse associations of CIDI-SCID concordance with time between interviews, leading us to focus on the subset of respondents in which the two interviews were carried out less than two months apart. This restriction of the sample reduced statistical power, requiring us to examine 12-month concordance only for classes of disorder rather than for individual disorders. It is conceivable that a larger sample would have shown CIDI-SCID concordance to be even greater among respondents who completed both interviews within a period of only a few days or a week. Fourth, the countries included in the study were less heterogeneous than those in the full WMH initiative. In particular, no developing countries were included in the investigation. This last limitation is being addressed in an expanded series of WMH clinical reappraisal studies that are currently under way in a diverse set of countries.

Although not a limitation, it should also be noted in interpreting the results reported here that the evaluation of clinically relevant information in epidemiological studies includes more than the simple investigation of prevalence (Brugha 2002). This is true in two ways. First, given that the population prevalence of mental disorders far outstrips available treatment resources, mental health policy decision makers have proposed several more restrictive definitions based on severity and impact that can be used to narrow the number of people qualifying for treatment (Regier 2000). Categorical measures of this sort are included in the WMH surveys (Demyttenaere et al. 2004) but were not considered in the current report. Second, dimensional measures of clinical severity are widely used in treatment studies and need to be included as well in epidemiological studies if we want to make the results of the latter relevant to clinicians (Kessler & Üstün 2004; see also Chapter 4). Fully structured versions of standard clinical severity scales are included in the WMH surveys, such as the Inventory of Depressive Symptomatology (Rush et al. 1996) and the Panic Disorder Severity Scale (Shear et al. 1997), to assess the severity of individual disorders. In addition, the WHO Disability Assessment Schedule (WHO-DAS)

(Rehm et al. 1999) is included in the WMH surveys to assess the severity of overall psychopathology. These dimensional measures were not considered in the current report.

On the basis of the additional measures described in the preceding paragraph, the assessment of clinical significance in the WMH surveys does not hinge entirely on concordance between the categorical DSM-IV diagnoses based on the CIDI and those based on the SCID. Nonetheless, information on CIDI-SCID diagnostic concordance is useful in determining whether the diagnostic thresholds and DSM-IV diagnostic criteria disorders are defined in a consistent way in the CIDI and SCID. We have seen that the CIDI diagnostic thresholds for lifetime prevalence of DSM-IV disorders are generally somewhat more conservative than those of the SCID, at least in the United States, whereas diagnostic thresholds for 12-month prevalence are generally unbiased, at least in the three Western European countries considered here. We also have seen that individual-level diagnostic concordance is generally good when we use the CIDI to make categorical diagnostic classifications and very good when we develop CIDI-based dimensional probability-of-disorder measures.

Although the word "validation" is often used to characterize the kind of investigation described in the previous two paragraphs, this is not an entirely accurate term because the SCID diagnoses cannot be taken as perfect representations of DSM diagnoses. This is true both because the test-retest reliability of the SCID is far from perfect (Segal et al. 1994), especially in community samples (Williams et al. 1992), and because some respondents in community surveys consciously hide information about their mental or substance problems from clinical interviewers (Kranzler et al. 1997). On the basis of these considerations, the estimates of CIDI-SCID concordance should be considered lower-bound estimates of CIDI validity. A good illustration can be found in the work of Booth and colleagues (1998), who compared lifetime diagnoses of major depression based on an earlier version of CIDI with diagnoses based on SCID clinical reappraisal interviews, where $\kappa$ was 0.53. However, when the CIDI was compared with more accurate Longitudinal Expert All Data (LEAD) standard diagnoses (Spitzer 1983) that used not only the SCID but also all the clinical information available to arrive at an improved estimate of clinical diagnoses, $\kappa$ increased to 0.67.

The difference in aggregate concordance between CIDI and SCID prevalence estimates is another finding that warrants comment. As noted previously, CIDI lifetime prevalence estimates are generally conservative compared to SCID estimates, but CIDI 12-month prevalence estimates are unbiased compared to SCID estimates. It is noteworthy in this regard that the CIDI first assesses lifetime prevalence of each disorder by asking the respondent to concentrate on the worst lifetime episode of the disorder. Lifetime assessment is based on that worst episode. Twelve-month prevalence is then assessed in the CIDI with a single question that asks about the last time the individual experienced an episode similar to the worse one. The 12-month SCID, in comparison, carries out a detailed assessment of all symptoms present in the past 12 months. The most plausible interpretation of the discrepancy between CIDI versus SCID lifetime and 12-month prevalence estimates based on these instrument differences is that the CIDI probably underestimates lifetime prevalence because its diagnostic thresholds are too high, while it overestimated 12-month prevalence among the lifetime cases it does not assess all required 12-month symptoms for the diagnosis. The global consequence is that 12-month CIDI prevalence estimates appear to be unbiased because the downward bias in lifetime prevalence estimates and downward bias in condition 12-month prevalence estimates among lifetime cases cancel each other out.

As mentioned earlier in the chapter and as detailed in Chapter 4, Version 3.0 of the CIDI includes a number of questions about 12-month clinical severity that were absent from earlier versions to overcome the CIDI limitations described in the preceding paragraph. These clinical questions assess disorder severity not only for respondents who meet full CIDI lifetime criteria for the disorder but also for subthreshold cases

with 12-month symptoms, allowing for correction of prevalence estimates in both time frames by decreasing diagnostic thresholds for lifetime prevalence and increasing clinical severity requirements for 12-month prevalence. A rough sense of the extent to which these recalibration exercises, which are only now beginning to be carried out in the WMH clinical reappraisal samples, might be able to improve CIDI diagnostic validity is provided by examining the increases in AUC associated with using regression-based CIDI symptom scoring rather than categorical diagnostic scoring to predict SCID diagnoses. This new work aims to refine CIDI diagnoses to correct the problem of lifetime thresholds being too high and 12-month thresholds among lifetime cases being too low.

In conclusion, the WMH clinical reappraisal studies reported here show that CIDI-SCID agreement in DSM-IV diagnoses is generally good in the surveys studied, that CIDI lifetime prevalence estimates are generally conservative relative to SCID estimates in these surveys, that CIDI 12-month prevalence estimates are generally unbiased relative to SCID estimates in these surveys, and that 12-month prevalence estimates of alcohol disorders should be interpreted with caution in these surveys as a result of a weak association with SCID diagnoses. The estimates of concordance probably underestimate true CIDI validity because SCID diagnoses, which were implicitly taken as a gold standard, are, in fact, known to be imperfect. The inclusion of subthreshold assessments and 12-month scales of clinical severity provide enough information to improve CIDI-SCID concordance on the basis of the results of currently ongoing methodological studies. An important task for the future is to extend these results to other WMH countries.

## REFERENCES

Agresti, A. (1996). *An introduction to categorical data analysis.* New York: John Wiley & Sons.

Andrews, G., Peters, L., Guzman, A. M. & Bird, K. (1995). A comparison of two structured diagnostic interviews: CIDI and SCAN. *Australian and New Zealand Journal of Psychiatry* 29, 124–32.

Booth, B. M., Kirchner, J. E., Hamilton, G., Harrell, R. & Smith, G. R. (1998). Diagnosing depression in the medically ill: Validity of a lay-administered structured diagnostic interview. *Journal of Psychiatric Research* 32, 353–60.

Bromet, E. J., Dunn, L. O., Connell, M. M., Dew, M. A. & Schulberg, H. C. (1986). Long-term reliability of diagnosing lifetime major depression in a community sample. *Archives of General Psychiatry*, 43, 435–40.

Brugha, T. S. (2002). The end of the beginning: A requiem for the categorization of mental disorder? *Psychological Medicine*, 32, 1149–54.

Brugha, T. S., Jenkins, R., Taub, N., Meltzer, H. & Bebbington, P. E. (2001). A general population comparison of the Composite International Diagnostic Interview (CIDI) and the Schedules for Clinical Assessment in Neuropsychiatry (SCAN). *Psychological Medicine*, 31, 1001–13.

Byrt, T., Bishop, J. & Carlin, J. B. (1993). Bias, prevalence and kappa. *Journal of Clinical Epidemiology*, 46, 423–9.

Cohen, J. (1960). A coefficient of agreement for nominal scales. *Educational and Psychological Measurement*, 20, 37–46.

Cook, R. J. (1998). Kappa and its dependence on marginal rates. In *The encyclopedia of biostatistics*, ed. P. Armitage & T. Colton, pp. 2166–8. New York: John Wiley & Sons.

Demyttenaere, K., Bruffaerts, R., Posada-Villa, J., Gasquet, I., Kovess, V., Lépine, J.-P., Angermeyer, M. C., Bernert, S., de Girolamo, G., Morosini, P., Polidori, G., Kikkawa, T., Kawakami, N., Ono, Y., Takeshima, T., Uda, H., Karam, E. G., Fayyad, J. A., Karam, A. N., Mneimneh, Z. N., Medina-Mora, M. E., Borges, G., Lara, C., de Graaf, R., Ormel, J., Gureje, O., Shen, Y., Huang, Y., Zhang, M., Alonso, J., Haro, J. M., Vilagut, G., Bromet, E. J., Gluzman, S., Webb, C., Kessler, R. C., Merikangas, K. R., Anthony, J. C., Von Korff, M. R., Wang, P. S., Brugha, T. S., Aguilar-Gaxiola, S., Lee, S., Heeringa, S., Pennell, B. E., Zaslavsky, A. M., Üstün, T. B. & Chatterji S. (2004). Prevalence, severity, and unmet need for treatment of mental disorders in the World Health Organization World Mental Health Surveys. *JAMA*, 291, 2581–90.

First, M. B., Spitzer, R. L., Gibbon, M. & Williams, J. B. W. (2002). *Structured clinical interview for DSM-IV Axis I disorders, research version, non-patient edition (SCID-I/NP).* New York: Biometrics Research, New York State Psychiatric Institute.

Gibbon, M., McDonald-Scott, P. & Endicott, J. (1981). Mastering the art of research interviewing: A model training procedure for diagnostic evaluation. *Archives of General Psychiatry*, 38, 1259–62.

Hanley, J. A. & McNeil, B. J. (1982). The meaning and use of the area under a receiver operating characteristic (ROC) curve. *Radiology*, 143, 29–36.

Hasin, D. S. & Grant, B. F. (2004). The co-occurrence of DSM-IV alcohol dependence: Results of the National Epidemiologic Survey on Alcohol and Related Conditions on heterogeneity that differ by population subgroup. *Archives of General Psychiatry*, 61, 891–96.

Jordanova, V., Wickramesinghe, C., Gerada, C. & Prince, M. (2004). Validation of two survey diagnostic interviews among primary care attendees: A comparison of CIS-R and CIDI with SCAN ICD-10 diagnostic categories. *Psychological Medicine*, 34, 1013–24.

Kendler, K. S., Neale, M. C., Kessler, R. C., Heath, A. C. & Eaves, L. J. (1992). A population-based twin study of major depression in women: The impact of varying definitions of illness. *Archives of General Psychiatry*, 49, 257–66.

Kessler, R. C., Abelson, J., Demler, O., Escobar, J. I., Gibbon, M., Guyer, M. E., Howes, M. J., Jin, R., Vega, W. A., Walters, E. E., Wang, P., Zaslavsky, A. & Zheng, H. (2004a). Clinical calibration of DSM-IV diagnoses in the World Mental Health (WMH) version of the World Health Organization (WHO) Composite International Diagnostic Interview (WMHCIDI). *International Journal of Methods in Psychiatric Research*, 13, 122–39.

Kessler, R. C., Adler, L., Barkley, R., Biederman, J., Conners, C. K., Demler, O., Faraone, S. V., Greenhill, L. L., Howes, M. J., Secnik, K., Spencer, T., Üstün, T. B., Walters, E. E. & Zaslavsky, A. M. (2006a). The prevalence and correlates of adult ADHD in the United States: Results from the National Comorbidity Survey Replication. *American Journal of Psychiatry*, 163, 716–23.

Kessler, R. C., Akiskal, H. S., Angst, J., Guyer, M., Hirschfeld, R. M., Merikangas, K. R., Stang, P. E. (2006b). Validity of assessment of bipolar spectrum disorders in the WHO CIDI 3.0. *Journal of Affective Disorders*, 96, 259–69.

Kessler, R. C., Birnbaum, H., Demler, O., Falloon, I. R., Gagnon, E., Guyer, M., Howes, M. J., Kendler, K. S., Shi, L., Walters, E. & Wu, E. Q. (2005). The prevalence and correlates of nonaffective psychosis in the National Comorbidity Survey Replication (NCS-R). *Biological Psychiatry*, 58, 668–76.

Kessler, R. C. & Üstün, T. B. (2004). The World Mental Health (WMH) survey initiative version of the World Health Organization (WHO) Composite International Diagnostic Interview (CIDI). *International Journal of Methods in Psychiatric Research*, 13, 93–121.

Kessler, R. C., Wittchen, H. U., Abelson, J. M., McGonagle, K. A., Schwarz, N., Kendler, K. S.,

Knäuper, B. & Zhao, S. (1998). Methodological studies of the Composite International Diagnostic Interview (CIDI) in the U.S. National Comorbidity Survey. *International Journal of Methods in Psychiatric Research*, 7, 33–55.

Kish, L. & Frankel, M. R. (1974). Inferences from complex samples. *Journal of the Royal Statistical Society*, 36, 1–37.

Kraemer, H. C., Morgan, G. A., Leech, N. L., Gliner, J. A., Vaske, J. J. & Harmon, R. J. (2003). Measures of clinical significance. *Journal of the American Academy of Child and Adolescent Psychiatry*, 42, 1524–9.

Kranzler, H. R., Tennen, H., Babor, T. F., Kadden, R. M. & Rounsaville, B. J. (1997). Validity of the longitudinal, expert, all data procedure for psychiatric diagnosis in patients with psychoactive substance use disorders. *Drug and Alcohol Dependence*, 45, 93–104.

Landis, J. R. & Koch, G. G. (1977). The measurement of observer agreement for categorical data. *Biometrics*, 33, 159–74.

Lenzenweger, M. F., Lane, M. C., Loranger, A. W. & Kessler, R. C. (2007). DSM-IV personality disorders in the National Comorbidity Survey Replication. *Biological Psychiatry*, 62, 553–64.

Regier, D. A. (2000). Community diagnosis counts. *Archives of General Psychiatry*, 57, 223–4.

Rehm, J., Üstün, T. B., Saxena, S., Nelson, C. B., Chatterji, S., Ivis, F. & Adlaf, E. (1999). On the development and psychometric testing of the WHO screening instrument to assess disablement in the general population. *International Journal of Methods in Psychiatric Research*, 8, 110–23.

Rohde, P., Lewinsohn, P. M. & Seeley, J. R. (1997). Comparability of telephone and face-to-face interviews in assessing axis I and II disorders. *American Journal of Psychiatry*, 154, 1593–8.

Rubin, D. B. (1987). *Multiple imputation for nonresponse in surveys*. New York: John Wiley & Sons.

Rush, A. J., Gullion, C. M., Basco, M. R., Jarrett, R. B. & Trivedi, M. H. (1996). The Inventory of Depressive Symptomatology (IDS): Psychometric properties. *Psychological Medicine*, 26, 477–86.

Segal, D. L., Hersen, M. & Van Hasselt, V. B. (1994). Reliability of the Structured Clinical Interview for DSM-III-R: An evaluative review. *Comprehensive Psychiatry*, 35, 316–27.

Shear, M. K., Brown, T. A., Barlow, D. H., Money, R., Sholomskas, D. E., Woods, S. W., Gorman, J. M. & Papp, L. A. (1997). Multicenter collaborative panic disorder severity scale. *American Journal of Psychiatry*, 154, 1571–5.

Sobin, C., Weissman, M. M., Goldstein, R. B., Adams, P., Wickramaratne, P. J., Warner, V. & Lisch, J. D. (1993). Diagnostic interviewing for family studies: Comparing telephone and face-to-face methods for the diagnosis of lifetime psychiatric disorders. *Psychiatric Genetics*, 3, 227–34.

Spitzer, R. L. (1983). Psychiatric diagnosis: Are clinicians still necessary? *Comprehensive Psychiatry*, 24, 399–411.

Spitznagel, E. L. & Helzer, J. E. (1985). A proposed solution to the base rate problem in the kappa statistic. *Archives of General Psychiatry*, 42, 725–8.

Williams, J. B., Gibbon, M., First, M. B., Spitzer, R. L., Davies, M., Borus, J., Howes, M. J., Kane, J., Pope, H. G., Jr., Rounsaville, B. & Wittchen, H. U. (1992). The structured clinical interview for DSM-III-R (SCID): II – Multisite test-retest reliability. *Archives of General Psychiatry*, 49, 630–6.

Wing, J. K., Babor, T., Brugha, T., Burke, J., Cooper, J. E., Giel, R., Jablenski, A., Regier, D. & Sartorius, N. (1990). SCAN: Schedules for Clinical Assessment in Neuropsychiatry. *Archives of General Psychiatry*, 47, 589–93.

Wittchen, H. U. (1994). Reliability and validity studies of the WHO-Composite International Diagnostic Interview (CIDI): A critical review. *Journal of Psychiatric Research*, 28, 57–84.

Wittchen, H. U., Kessler, R. C., Zhao, S. & Abelson, J. (1995). Reliability and clinical validity of UM-CIDI DSM-III-R generalized anxiety disorder. *Journal of Psychiatric Research*, 29, 95–110.

Wittchen, H. U., Zhao, S., Abelson, J. M., Abelson, J. L. & Kessler, R. C. (1996). Reliability and procedural validity of UM-CIDI DSM-III-R phobic disorders. *Psychological Medicine*, 26, 1169–77.

Wolter, K. (1985). *Introduction to variance estimation*. New York: Springer-Verlag.

# PART TWO

# Country-Specific Chapters

# 7 Mental Disorders in Colombia: Results from the World Mental Health Survey

JOSÉ POSADA-VILLA, MARCELA RODRÍGUEZ, PATRICIA DUQUE,
ALEXANDRA GARZÓN, SERGIO AGUILAR-GAXIOLA, AND JOSHUA BRESLAU

## ACKNOWLEDGMENTS

The Estudio Nacional de Salud Mental, Colombia 2003 (ENSM) is supported by the Ministry of Social Protection and carried out in conjunction with the World Health Organization World Mental Health (WMH) Survey Initiative. We thank the WMH staff for assistance with instrumentation, fieldwork, and data analysis. These activities were supported by the U.S. National Institute of Mental Health (R01MH070884), the John D. and Catherine T. MacArthur Foundation, the Pfizer Foundation, the U.S. Public Health Service (R13-MH066849, R01-MH069864, and R01 DA016558), the Fogarty International Center (FIRCA R03-TW006481), the Pan American Health Organization, Eli Lilly and Company Foundation, Ortho-McNeil Pharmaceutical, GlaxoSmithKline, and Bristol-Myers Squibb. A complete list of WMH publications can be found at http://www.hcp.med.harvard.edu/wmh/.

## I. INTRODUCTION

Colombia is the third most populous country in Latin America, after Brazil and Mexico, with a population of 45.6 million in 2005 (World Bank 2005). Of the population, 75% lives in urban areas, with about 35% of the population concentrated in the four largest cities, Bogotá, Cali, Medellín, and Barranquilla. The population is relatively young, with a median age of 26.3, and about 80% of the population is under the age of 45. Life expectancy at birth for the total population is 72 years (males, 68.2 years; females, 76.0 years). The majority ethnic group, comprising 86 percent of the population, includes whites of European descent and mestizos, those of mixed white and indigenous ancestry. Of the population, 10.5% is Afro-Colombian, descendants of Africans brought to Colombia as slaves, and 3.4% belong to indigenous groups. The largest majority of Colombians, 86%, are Roman Catholics.

The recent history of Colombia has been marked by persistent political and criminal violence affecting a large portion of the rural and urban populations. Armed political conflict between insurgent militant groups such as the Fuerzas Armadas Revolucionarias de Colombia (FARC) and Colombian military and paramilitary groups displaced 1.5 million people between 1995 and 2005. Political violence has also limited economic development and has fueled emigration. More than 3 million Colombians now live abroad in Europe, other countries in Latin America, in the United States, and Canada. Violence has also been fed by drug production and trafficking, in which criminal organizations such as drug cartels based in Colombia, most notably in Medellín and Cali, have been international leaders since the 1970s. The homicide rate in 2002 was one of the world's highest, at more than 60 per 100,000 people. It is also likely that the drug trade has contributed to the intransigence of political violence, with both political insurgent groups and paramilitary organizations profiting from and competing for control of drug production and distribution.

In some respects, recent economic trends suggest that conditions in Colombia are improving. The homicide rate has nearly halved in recent years. Economic growth has been sustained at around 1.5% since 2001, and the proportion of people living in extreme poverty has declined from 26% in 2002 to 15% in 2005. However, in rural areas, the prevalence of poverty remains as high as 40%, and nationwide more than 30% of the population is underemployed.

## 2. COLOMBIA'S HEALTH-CARE SYSTEM

In 2003, government spending on health accounted for 20.5% of total government expenditures and constituted 84.1% of total health expenditures. Per capita spending on health was US$150 according to 2005 figures, amounting to 5.6% of the gross domestic product. The health-care system was established in 1993 as part of structural adjustment programs with the aim to increase the role of competition among private insurers and providers in the health-care sector. The law establishing the new system, Law 100, created a hybrid public-private system that provides insurance coverage through two complementary regimes. One regime, the contributory regime (CR) covers employed workers and is funded through payroll contributions to private insurance companies selected by the covered individual. The other regime, the subsidized regime (SR), covers the poor, who are not required to make any financial contributions for health insurance coverage. The SR is funded through a combination of federal transfers to territories and a portion of payroll contribution from those enrolled in the RC.

The system established by Law 100 does not include coverage for mental health care. Consequently, treatment of even severe mental disorders is not widely available at the primary care level and treatment of less severe mental disorders is even more severely restricted. Mental health care is delivered through a mixed public and private system of psychiatric inpatient facilities (psychiatric hospitals and clinics or psychiatric units in general hospitals), outpatient facilities (outpatient services in clinics and hospitals), and rehabilitation services. The country has 3941 psychiatric beds. The professional staff in the mental health services includes licensed specialists in the field of mental health: psychiatrists

(1250), nurses (82), psychologists (4000), and larger numbers of social workers and occupational therapists. The WHO Mental Health Atlas notes that Colombia has about three psychiatrists per 100,000 persons, spends about 0.08% of it governmental health budget on mental health care, and lacks a coherent national mental health system (WHO 2005).

Despite the absence of coverage for mental health treatment, the goals of the 1993 health reform in Colombia included several that are directly related to mental health, such as promoting harmonious interpersonal relationships, increasing awareness of safe sexual practices, fostering healthy and comprehensive child development, and reducing both licit (e.g., alcohol and tobacco) and illicit (e.g., cocaine) substance use. Little information exists on these or other mental health outcomes in Colombia. The Colombia WMH survey, known as Estudio Nacional de Salud Mental (ENSM), is the first general population survey designed to estimate the prevalence of common mental disorders and to estimate the size of the population using any type of health, social, or other traditional services for the treatment of mental problems. This chapter presents descriptive data from the survey regarding the lifetime and 12-month prevalence rates of disorders and the 12-month prevalence of service use. The discussion provides the main implications of the results with reference to service provision in Colombia.

## 3. PSYCHIATRIC EPIDEMIOLOGY IN COLOMBIA

Prior to the ENSM, four other studies examined the prevalence of psychiatric disorders in national samples. The first such study, carried out in 1993, used the Zung Scale and the Self-Reporting Questionnaire (SRQ) to screen for DSM-III disorders in a national sample. This study found a lifetime prevalence of 25.1% for major depression, 9.6% for anxiety disorders, and 7.8% for alcohol abuse. A second study, carried out in 2000–2001, assessed the prevalence of depression in a national sample using a revised version of the CIDI depression module and found a past-year prevalence of 10% and the past-month prevalence of 8.5% (Gómez-Restrepo et al. 2004). The prevalence of illicit drug use and drug disorders was examined in 1987 in a third study, which was carried out in four urban areas. This study highlighted problems related to the use of *basuco* or "coca paste," in this population (Torres de Galvis and Murrelle 1990). A study of completed suicides in Bogotá in 2002, finally, found evidence suggesting increasing risk for suicide among youth between 1995 and 2000 (Sánchez et al. 2002).

Other epidemiological research in mental health in Colombia has focused on assessing the prevalence and risk factors for mental health problems among specific vulnerable groups, with a particular emphasis on displaced persons (Cáceres et al. 2002; Mogollón Pérez, Vázquez Navarrete & García Gil 2003). Puertas and colleagues used the SRQ to examine common mental disorders in a sample of urban poor in the city of Sincelejo, with a special emphasis on assessing needs among the population displaced from rural areas by political violence. Of their sample, 27% met criteria for common mental disorders, and 14% had problems with excessive alcohol consumption. The prevalence of common mental disorders was significantly higher among displaced persons (Puertas, Rios & del Valle 2006). Harpham and colleagues conducted studies of common mental disorders among the young (age 15–25) urban population in the city of Cali. These studies found high prevalence of common mental disorders, about 25%, with higher risk associated with lower education, poverty, and exposure to violence (Harpham, Grant & Rodriguez 2004; Harpham et al. 2005). Pérez-Olmos and colleagues (2005) assessed posttraumatic stress disorder (PTSD) symptoms in a sample of children age 5–14 in the department (state) of Cundinamarca. This study found high prevalence of PTSD and a strong association between PTSD symptoms and geographic proximity to political violence in the region. There has also been interest in Colombia in the mental health needs of populations that were affected by nat-

ural disasters, including an earthquake that hit the city of Armenia in 1999 (Scott et al. 2003) and a volcanic eruption that destroyed the city of Armero in 1985 (Lima et al. 1988; Lima et al. 1991).

The ENSM was designed to provide data on a broad range of psychiatric disorders and use of mental health services for the urban Colombian population. Such data are essential for informing national health policy, particularly given the lack of financial investment in mental health treatment within the framework of Colombia's national health system. Our goal in this chapter is to present findings on the lifetime and 12-month prevalence of anxiety, mood, impulse-control and substance use disorders, and use of mental health services.

## 4. METHODS

### 4.1. Study Sample

The Colombian Ministry of Social Protection conducted the ENSM as part of the WMH Survey Initiative (Posada-Villa et al. 2004; Kessler et al. 2006). A Spanish translation of the WMH version of the Composite International Diagnostic Interview (CIDI) (Kessler and Üstün 2004) was administered to a population-based sample in face-to-face interviews. Eligible respondents were aged 18–65, noninstitutionalized, ambulatory, Spanish-speaking men and women who resided in the urban areas within five regions in Colombia: (1) Bogotá, DC; (2) Atlantic (Córdoba, Sucre, Bolívar, Magdalena, Cesar, La Guajira, Atlántico; (3) Pacific (Chocó, Valle del Cauca, Cauca, Nariño); (4) Central (Caquetá, Huila, Tolima, Quindio, Risaralda, Caldas, Antioquia); and (5) Eastern (Meta, Cundinamarca, Boyaca, Santander, Norte de Santander, Arauca). The municipalities and blocks eligible for sampling were randomly selected using a stratified, multistage, clustered, probability sampling procedure. Eligible households were identified through a master sampling list owned by the Ministry of Social Protection and based on census data collected by the National Administrative

Department of Statistics (DANE). There were 4426 respondents aged 18–65 from 5526 households in 60 municipalities located in 25 departments across the country, resulting in a response rate of 87.7%. Informed consent was obtained from each respondent prior to study participation and the study was approved by a research ethics board.

## 4.2. Data Collection

All interviews were carried out using face-to-face, computer-assisted interviews by centrally trained interviewers. A detailed description of the methodology and quality-control procedures used in this study is described elsewhere (Demyttenaere et al. 2004). In terms of the interview, the standard WMH two-part interview process was used, in which all respondents completed Part 1 of the interview, and the Part 2 interview was completed by all Part 1 respondents who met lifetime criteria for any disorder in addition to a roughly 25% probability subsample of other Part 1 respondents. Noncertain Part 2 respondents were weighted by the inverse of their probability of selection into Part 2 to adjust for their undersampling. All analyses reported here used these Part 2 weights, which also included components to adjust for differential within-household probability of selection and poststratification to population distributions of sociodemographic variables.

The WMH interview was translated from English to Spanish using the standard WHO translation protocol, as described earlier in Chapter 5, which was used both in Colombia and in the Mexican National Comorbidity Survey (Medina-Mora et al. 2005). The Spanish translation was further adapted to the Spanish spoken in Colombia and pilot-tested with Colombian participants. Quality control was maintained by the WMH Data Collection Coordination Center (DCCC) at the Survey Research Center, University of Michigan. This process was conducted by checking the accuracy of data collection and specifying data cleaning and coding procedures. Data collected through the CIDI that

are used in the current report included sociodemographic variables: age (groups 18–29, 30–44, 45–54, older than 55 years), sex, marital status (married, common law, separated, divorced, widowed, single) education (none or primary school, some secondary, completed secondary, postsecondary), and family income (low, low-average, high-average, high). Income categories were defined using the standard WMH procedure of low being defined as the ratio of total family income to number of household members being less than half the samplewide median; low-average, a ratio between 0.5 and 1.0; high-average, a ratio between 1 and 3; and high, a ratio greater than 3.

## 4.3. Disorder Assessment

As in all the chapters in this volume, mental disorders were classified for purposes of this chapter according to the American Psychiatric Association (1994) DSM-IV. The disorders assessed include anxiety disorders (agoraphobia, generalized anxiety disorder, obsessive-compulsive disorder, panic disorder, posttraumatic stress disorder, social phobia, specific phobia), mood disorders (bipolar I and II disorders, dysthymia, major depressive disorder), disorders that share a problem with impulse control (oppositional-defiant disorder, conduct disorder, attention-deficit/hyperactivity disorder, intermittent explosive disorder), and substance use disorders (alcohol and drug abuse and dependence). DSM-IV organic exclusion rules were used to make the diagnoses and these were hierarchy free.

Lifetime prevalence was estimated as the proportion of respondents who ever had a given disorder up to their age at interview. The 12-month prevalence was estimated as the proportion of respondents who reported that the most recent episode of disorder included some period of the 12 months preceding the interview. The severity of 12-month disorders was classified using the standard WMH scheme into the categories "serious," "moderate," and "mild." The classification of "serious" was made if a respondent met criteria for at least one 12-month DSM-IV/CIDI disorder, was diagnosed with 12-month bipolar I, had attempted suicide in the past year, had any 12-month DSM-IV diagnosis, had substance dependence with physiological symptoms, reported at least two areas of role functioning with severe role impairment due to a mental disorder according to Sheehan Disability Scales (Leon et al. 1997), or reported overall functional impairment at a level consistent with a Global Assessment of Functioning (Endicott et al. 1976) of 50 or less. Those who were not categorized as serious were classified as moderate if they had at least one disorder and a moderate level of impairment in any Sheehan Disability Scale domain or if they had substance dependence without physiological signs. Finally, all remaining cases that met criteria for a DSM disorder were categorized as mild.

## 4.4. Treatment

Respondents were asked whether they had ever received treatment for "problems with their emotions or nerves or use of alcohol or drugs." A list of health-care services and providers was given to subjects, which included psychiatrists, general practitioners or family physicians, any other physicians, social workers, counselors, other mental health professionals, religious or spiritual advisors, or any other healer (e.g., chiropractor, herbalist). Twelve-month health services use was categorized into the following groups: psychiatrist, other mental health care (nonpsychiatrist, psychologist, social worker, or counselor in a mental health specialty setting), general medical services (primary care physician, other physician, nurse), human services (religious or spiritual advisor or social worker or counselor in any setting other than a specialty mental health setting), and complementary alternative medicine (CAM) services (other healer, e.g., a chiropractor, Internet support groups, self-help groups). Psychiatrists and other mental health care were combined into a summary category "any mental health care." Likewise, mental health care and general health care were collapsed into a broader

category "health care" and human services and CAM were combined into a "non–health-care" category.

The definition for minimally adequate treatment was the same used in earlier WMH reports based on evidence-based guidelines (Wang et al. 2005). In summary, minimally adequate treatment was defined as receiving pharmacotherapy (*two or more* months of an appropriate medication for the focal disorder plus five or more visits to any type of physician) or psychotherapy (eight or more visits with any health-care or human services professional lasting an average of *at least* 30 minutes; for substance abuse disorders, self-help visits of any duration). Appropriate medications for disorders included antidepressants for depressive disorders, mood stabilizers or antipsychotic agents for bipolar disorders, antidepressants or anxiolytic agents for anxiety disorders, and antagonists or agonists (disulfiram, naltrexone, methadone hydrochloride) for alcohol and other substance abuse disorders. In determining treatment adequacy, each 12-month disorder was considered separately.

## 5. ANALYSIS

Data were weighted to adjust for differences in probabilities of selection, differential nonresponse, residual differences between the sample and the population, and oversampling in the Part 2 sample. Prevalence estimates, patterns of service use, and standard errors were obtained using the Taylor series method implemented with the SUDAAN computer software (Research Triangle Institute, 2002). Sociodemographic predictors of lifetime disorders were examined using discrete-time survival analysis with person-years as the unit of analysis (Efron 1988). Sociodemographic variables that change over time (educational attainment, marital status) were treated as time-varying predictors in the survival analyses that are described subsequently.

Logistic regression analyses were used to identify the sociodemographic predictors of mental disorders, severity of mental illness, receiving any 12-month treatment, and the criteria for

**Table 7.1.** Demographic distribution of the sample compared to the population on poststratification variables

|          | Part 1 unweighted (%) | Part 1 weighted (%) | Part 2 unweighted (%) | Part 2 weighted (%) | Census (%) |
|----------|-----------------------|---------------------|-----------------------|---------------------|------------|
| **Age**  |                       |                     |                       |                     |            |
| 18–25    | 22.4                  | 25.2                | 24.0                  | 25.0                | 25.0       |
| 26–35    | 25.6                  | 24.6                | 25.8                  | 25.4                | 25.4       |
| 36–45    | 25.5                  | 23.2                | 24.5                  | 23.0                | 23.0       |
| 46–55    | 16.0                  | 16.2                | 15.7                  | 16.2                | 16.2       |
| 56–65    | 10.6                  | 10.9                | 9.9                   | 10.5                | 10.5       |
| **Sex**  |                       |                     |                       |                     |            |
| Male     | 38.4                  | 45.6                | 37.2                  | 45.5                | 45.5       |
| Female   | 61.6                  | 54.4                | 62.8                  | 54.5                | 54.5       |

minimal adequacy of treatment. Odds ratio (OR) estimates and their corresponding 95% confidence intervals (CIs) were adjusted for design effects. Multivariate significance tests were made with Wald $\chi^2$ tests using Taylor series design-based coefficient variance-covariance matrices. Analyses were conducted by the WMH Data Analysis Coordination Centre (DACC) at the Department of Health Care Policy, Harvard Medical School. All statistical tests were evaluated using two-tailed tests, and $p$-value less than 0.05 was considered statistically significant.

## 6. RESULTS

The unweighted sample was less likely to be young and male, compared with census data on the entire Colombian population (Table 7.1). With weighting, both the Part 1 and Part 2 samples were very close in age and sex distribution to the census data.

### 6.1. Lifetime Prevalence of Mental Disorders

The lifetime prevalence of any DSM-IV/CIDI disorder assessed in the survey was 39.1% (Table 7.2). The most common individual disorders were specific phobia (12.5%), major depressive disorder (12.0%), separation anxiety disorder (9.8%), and alcohol abuse (9.2%). Anxiety disorders were the most prevalent class of disorders (25.3%), followed by mood disorders (14.6%). Of respondents, 17.8% had two or more disorders and 8.3% had three or more.

To investigate cohort differences in risk for disorder, dummy variables defining age groups 18–34, 35–49, and 50 years or older were used to predict lifetime disorders using discrete-time survival analysis. These age groups correspond roughly to age cohorts born in 1969–1985, 1954–1968, and prior to 1954, respectively. The ORs were statistically significant in 12 of 22 comparisons, with a consistent positive association between recency of cohort and OR of onset (Table 7.2). The pattern of increasing risk across cohorts was particularly strong for four disorders, separation anxiety disorder (SAD) and/or adult separation anxiety disorder (ASA), major depressive disorder (MDD), bipolar disorder, and intermittent explosive disorder (IED), where we found a monotonic increase in risk across cohorts with significantly higher risk among both younger cohorts relative to the 50 and older cohort. The cohort effect was also consistently significant for substance use disorders. However, for substance use disorders, elevated risk was only found in the most recent cohort relative to the 50 and older cohort. The ORs comparing risk of substance use among the youngest cohort with the oldest cohort were large, ranging from 7.6 for drug abuse without dependence to 2.3 for alcohol abuse without dependence. For classes of disorder examined together, the

**Table 7.2.** Lifetime prevalence of psychiatric disorders in Colombia

| DX group | DX | n | % | (se) | OR (18–34) | LCL | UCL | OR (35–49) | LCL | UCL | OR (50+) | LCL | UCL | χ² | DF | P |
|---|---|---|---|---|---|---|---|---|---|---|---|---|---|---|---|---|
| Anxiety | Panic DX | 65 | 1.2 | (0.2) | 1.6 | 0.7 | 3.8 | 1.0 | 0.4 | 2.6 | 1.0 | 1.0 | 1.0 | 1.6 | 2 | 0.46 |
| | GAD with hierarchy | 56 | 1.3 | (0.3) | 4.1[a] | 1.4 | 12.1 | 2.6 | 1.0 | 6.7 | 1.0 | 1.0 | 1.0 | 6.6 | 2 | 0.037 |
| | Social phobia | 219 | 5.0 | (0.5) | 1.5 | 0.8 | 2.7 | 1.4 | 0.7 | 2.8 | 1.0 | 1.0 | 1.0 | 1.7 | 2 | 0.43 |
| | Specific phobia | 558 | 12.5 | (0.8) | 1.2 | 0.9 | 1.8 | 1.4[a] | 1.0 | 2.0 | 1.0 | 1.0 | 1.0 | 5.0 | 2 | 0.08 |
| | Agoraphobia without panic | 97 | 2.5 | (0.3) | 1.1 | 0.4 | 3.3 | 1.3 | 0.5 | 3.3 | 1.0 | 1.0 | 1.0 | 0.4 | 2 | 0.84 |
| | PTSD[a] | 57 | 1.8 | (0.4) | 2.5 | 0.2 | 29.0 | 0.9 | 0.1 | 7.3 | 1.0 | 1.0 | 1.0 | 4.3 | 2 | 0.12 |
| | SAD/ASA[a] | 359 | 9.8 | (0.8) | 5.4[a] | 3.1 | 9.4 | 2.0[a] | 1.1 | 3.8 | 1.0 | 1.0 | 1.0 | 64.0 | 2 | <0.001 |
| | Any anxiety[a] | 948 | 25.3 | (1.4) | 1.6[a] | 1.2 | 2.1 | 1.3 | 0.9 | 1.8 | 1.0 | 1.0 | 1.0 | 10.0 | 2 | 0.007 |
| Mood | MDD with hierarchy | 547 | 12.0 | (0.7) | 6.5[a] | 4.1 | 10.3 | 2.1[a] | 1.5 | 3.0 | 1.0 | 1.0 | 1.0 | 69.1 | 2 | <0.001 |
| | DYS with hierarchy | 40 | 0.8 | (0.2) | 1.7 | 0.4 | 6.3 | 1.9 | 0.6 | 5.8 | 1.0 | 1.0 | 1.0 | 1.4 | 2 | 0.49 |
| | Bipolar-broad | 115 | 2.6 | (0.3) | 7.3[a] | 3.3 | 16.6 | 3.6[a] | 1.7 | 7.3 | 1.0 | 1.0 | 1.0 | 24.3 | 2 | <0.001 |
| | Any mood | 666 | 14.6 | (0.7) | 6.3[a] | 4.2 | 9.3 | 2.3[a] | 1.6 | 3.1 | 1.0 | 1.0 | 1.0 | 92.7 | 2 | <0.001 |
| Impulse | ODD with hierarchy[b] | 85 | 3.1 | (0.5) | 0.9 | 0.5 | 1.7 | 1.0 | 1.0 | 1.0 | 1.0 | 1.0 | 1.0 | 0.1 | 1 | 0.82 |
| | CD[b] | 58 | 2.1 | (0.4) | 1.6 | 0.9 | 3.1 | 1.0 | 1.0 | 1.0 | 1.0 | 1.0 | 1.0 | 2.3 | 1 | 0.13 |
| | ADHD[b] | 33 | 1.2 | (0.3) | 0.5 | 0.2 | 1.0 | 1.0 | 1.0 | 1.0 | 1.0 | 1.0 | 1.0 | 3.7 | 1 | 0.05 |
| | IED with hierarchy | 206 | 4.7 | (0.4) | 4.0[a] | 2.4 | 6.7 | 1.8[a] | 1.0 | 3.1 | 1.0 | 1.0 | 1.0 | 42.3 | 2 | <0.001 |
| | Any impulse[b] | 273 | 9.6 | (0.8) | 1.4 | 0.9 | 2.0 | 1.0 | 1.0 | 1.0 | 1.0 | 1.0 | 1.0 | 2.4 | 1 | 0.12 |
| Substance | ALC abuse w/without DEP | 325 | 9.2 | (0.6) | 2.3[a] | 1.6 | 3.5 | 1.1 | 0.7 | 1.7 | 1.0 | 1.0 | 1.0 | 35.8 | 2 | <0.001 |
| | ALC DEP with abuse | 95 | 2.3 | (0.3) | 2.4[a] | 1.2 | 5.0 | 1.0 | 0.4 | 2.4 | 1.0 | 1.0 | 1.0 | 17.8 | 2 | <0.001 |
| | Drug abuse w/without DEP | 70 | 1.6 | (0.3) | 7.6[a] | 3.2 | 18.1 | 2.1 | 0.7 | 6.4 | 1.0 | 1.0 | 1.0 | 30.5 | 2 | <0.001 |
| | Drug DEP with abuse | 28 | 0.6 | (0.2) | – | – | – | – | – | – | – | – | – | – | – | – |
| | Any substance | 345 | 9.6 | (0.6) | 2.3[a] | 1.6 | 3.3 | 1.1 | 0.7 | 1.6 | 1.0 | 1.0 | 1.0 | 39.3 | 2 | <0.001 |
| All disorders | Any DX[a] | 1432 | 39.1 | (1.3) | 1.9[a] | 1.5 | 2.5 | 1.3 | 1.0 | 1.7 | 1.0 | 1.0 | 1.0 | 27.4 | 2 | <0.001 |
| | 2+ DX[a] | 729 | 17.8 | (1.0) | | | | | | | | | | | | |
| | 3+ DX[a] | 349 | 8.3 | (0.7) | | | | | | | | | | | | |

[a] Denotes Part 2 disorder.

[b] Denotes disorder in part 2 and age ≤44 years.

Notes: Part 1 sample size = 4426, Part 2 sample size = 2381, and Part 2 and ≤44 years of age = 1731.

GAD = Generalized Anxiety Disorder; PTSD = Posttraumatic Stress Disorder; SAD = Separation Anxiety Disorder; ASA = Adult Separation Anxiety; MDD = Major Depressive Disorder; DYS = Dysthymia; ODD = Oppositional Defiant Disorder; CD = Conduct Disorder; ADHD = Attention Deficit Hyperactivity Disorder; IED = Intermittent Explosive Disoder; ALC = Alcohol; DEP = Dependence.

137

**Table 7.3.** Prevalence and severity of 12-month DSM-IV disorders in Colombia

| Diagnosis | N | 12-month % | (se) | Serious % | (se) | Moderate % | (se) | Mild % | (se) |
|---|---|---|---|---|---|---|---|---|---|
| **Anxiety disorder** | | | | | | | | | |
| Panic disorder[a] | 39 | 0.7 | (0.1) | 31.5 | (8.9) | 50.6 | (9.3) | 17.9 | (7.9) |
| Generalized anxiety disorder[a] | 24 | 0.6 | (0.2) | 47.2 | (11.2) | 33.7 | (13.5) | 19.1 | (6.2) |
| Specific phobia[a] | 355 | 8.0 | (0.7) | 21.2 | (2.8) | 42.8 | (3.7) | 36.0 | (3.6) |
| Social phobia[a] | 126 | 2.8 | (0.3) | 31.5 | (5.7) | 54.1 | (6.3) | 14.4 | (3.2) |
| Agoraphobia without panic[a] | 64 | 1.5 | (0.3) | 35.8 | (6.7) | 33.7 | (9.6) | 30.5 | (11.5) |
| Posttraumatic stress disorder[b] | 24 | 0.6 | (0.2) | 44.5 | (13.0) | 22.1 | (14.5) | 33.5 | (12.0) |
| Adult separation anxiety[b] | 88 | 2.6 | (0.5) | 28.2 | (6.7) | 40.4 | (9.3) | 31.5 | (7.1) |
| Any anxiety disorder[b] | 542 | 13.5 | (0.9) | 22.3 | (2.2) | 43.6 | (3.0) | 34.1 | (2.9) |
| **Mood disorder** | | | | | | | | | |
| Major depressive disorder[a] | 245 | 5.3 | (0.4) | 33.3 | (3.9) | 52.6 | (4.1) | 14.1 | (2.3) |
| Dysthymia[a] | 29 | 0.6 | (0.2) | 32.9 | (13.5) | 59.6 | (15.0) | 7.5 | (3.3) |
| Bipolar I/II/subthreshold[a] | 65 | 1.5 | (0.2) | 54.0 | (7.1) | 31.4 | (7.3) | 14.6 | (5.4) |
| Any mood disorder[a] | 316 | 6.9 | (0.5) | 37.7 | (3.5) | 47.8 | (4.0) | 14.5 | (2.2) |
| **Impulse disorder** | | | | | | | | | |
| Oppositional-defiant disorder[c] | 13 | 0.4 | (0.2) | 29.2 | (16.7) | 11.9 | (7.0) | 58.9 | (18.3) |
| Conduct disorder[c] | 10 | 0.5 | (0.2) | 61.8 | (21.3) | 3.0 | (3.0) | 35.3 | (21.8) |
| Attention-deficit/hyperactivity disorder[c] | 11 | 0.5 | (0.2) | 14.5 | (11.4) | 25.8 | (14.5) | 59.6 | (18.0) |
| Intermittent explosive disorder[a] | 118 | 2.9 | (0.3) | 31.4 | (5.5) | 45.7 | (6.0) | 22.9 | (5.2) |
| Any impulse-control disorder[c] | 119 | 4.4 | (0.4) | 28.8 | (5.2) | 38.2 | (5.1) | 33.0 | (5.5) |
| **Substance disorder** | | | | | | | | | |
| Alcohol abuse[a] | 83 | 2.3 | (0.3) | 46.0 | (8.9) | 17.2 | (6.4) | 36.8 | (9.2) |
| Alcohol dependence[a] | 36 | 1.1 | (0.3) | 89.4 | (6.0) | 10.6 | (6.0) | 0.0 | (0.0) |
| Drug abuse[a] | 19 | 0.5 | (0.1) | 74.4 | (9.9) | 3.0 | (3.1) | 22.5 | (9.5) |
| Drug dependence[a] | 9 | 0.2 | (0.1) | 100.0 | (0.0) | 0.0 | (0.0) | 0.0 | (0.0) |
| Any substance use disorder[a] | 105 | 2.8 | (0.4) | 48.9 | (7.8) | 17.4 | (5.5) | 33.6 | (7.7) |
| **Any disorder** | | | | | | | | | |
| Any[b] | 810 | 20.1 | (1.0) | 23.7 | (2.1) | 41.4 | (2.6) | 34.9 | (2.2) |
| **Total sample** | | | | | | | | | |
| Total sample[b] | 2381 | – | – | 4.9 | (0.5) | 8.4 | (0.7) | 7.2 | (0.5) |

[a] Part 1 sample, prevalence calculated using Part 1 weights.
[b] Part 2 sample, prevalence calculated using Part 2 weights.
[c] Part 2 sample (age ≤44), prevalence and severity calculated using Part 2 weights for ages ≤44.
*Notes:* se = standard error. Severity calculated using Part 2 weights.

cohort effect was significant for mood disorders, anxiety disorders, substance disorders, and any disorder.

### 6.2. 12-month Prevalence and Severity of Mental Disorders

Of respondents, 20.1% had a mental disorder in the past 12 months, and 4.9% had a past-year disorder classified as serious (Table 7.3). The most prevalent disorders were specific phobia (8.0%), major depressive disorder (5.3%), intermittent explosive disorder (2.9%), social phobia (2.8%) and alcohol abuse (2.3%). Anxiety disorders were the most prevalent class of disorder (13.5%), followed by mood disorders (6.9%), impulse-control disorders (4.4%) and substance use disorders (2.8%). The 12-month prevalence of impulse-control disorders, assessed only in respondents under age 45, was 4.4%.

Among those who had a mental disorder, 23.7% were serious, 41.4% were moderate, and

34.9% were mild. Substance use disorders had the highest proportion of serious classifications (48.9%), whereas anxiety disorders had the lowest proportion (22.3%). The disorders that had the highest percentage of respondents who were classified as serious within each class of disorder were generalized anxiety disorder (47.2%) among anxiety disorders, bipolar I/II/subthreshold (54.0%) among mood disorders, conduct disorder (61.8%) among impulse control disorders, and drug abuse (100.0%) and alcohol dependence (89.4%) among substance use disorders.

## 6.3. Demographic Correlates of 12-month Disorders

Women were more likely to have mood or anxiety disorders, whereas men were more likely to have impulse-control disorders and substance use disorders (Table 7.4). Because of these countervailing patterns across disorders, sex is not a significant predictor of any 12-month disorder. There were no other significant demographic correlates for mood, anxiety, and impulse-control disorders. Those who were younger and not married were more likely to have substance use disorders. When the correlates were examined for severity of illness among those with a 12-month disorder, respondents who were older, from low- or low–average-income households, never married, and with postsecondary education were more likely to have a moderate or serious severity of illness.

## 6.4. Health-care Service Use and Predictors of Receiving Treatment

Of the sample, 5.5% and 14% of those with a past-year diagnosis had used mental health services in the past 12 months (Table 7.5). The prevalence of service use increased with increasing severity of illness for all sectors of care. However, even among those with severe disorders, only 27.8% received any treatment. Among those with severe disorders who received treatment, the most common source of care was the specialty mental health sector (17.5%), followed by the general medical sector (9.3%). Only 4.6% of those with

severe disorders received care in the non-health-care sector, which includes both human services and CAM.

Receipt of services in the health-care sector (combining the general medical and specialty mental health sectors) was positively associated with having high income, being separated, widowed, or divorced, and having more severe disorder (Table 7.5). The median number of 12-month visits among those receiving health-care services was 1.8 (data not shown).

## 7. DISCUSSION

The ENSM provides the first national data on the prevalence and treatment of mental disorders in urban areas of Colombia. Several findings with important implications for policy planning emerge from this study. First, psychiatric disorders are common in the general population, with about two in five people experiencing disorders in their lifetime, and one in five people experiencing disorders in the past year. On the basis of these estimates, the prevalence of psychiatric disorders in Colombia is lower than in the United States (45% lifetime and 26.2% 12-month) (Kessler et al. 2005a; Kessler et al. 2005b) and higher than Mexico (26.1% lifetime and 12.1% 12-month) (Medina-Mora et al. 2005, 2007).

Second, risk for psychiatric disorders in Colombia appears to be increasing across historical birth cohorts. A similar trend toward higher risk among more recent birth cohorts has been found in several other countries, including the United States and Mexico. Increasing risk across birth cohorts was pronounced for drug use disorders, but it was not observed for alcohol use disorders. The pattern of increasing risk across birth cohorts may also reflect age-related recall bias. Older people must recall events over a longer period of time and thus may be less likely to recall periods of poor mental health that occurred earlier in their lives. The CIDI employs several survey techniques designed to minimize recall bias by encouraging active memory searching by the respondent.

The pattern of increasing risk across birth cohorts has important implications for policy. Given the chronic nature of most psychiatric

**Table 7.4.** Correlates of 12-month psychiatric disorders in Colombia

| | Mood | | Anxiety | | Impulse control | | Substance use | | Serious disorder | | Any disorder | |
|---|---|---|---|---|---|---|---|---|---|---|---|---|
| | OR | (95% CI) | OR | (95% CI) | OR | (95% CI) | OR | (95% CI) | OR | (95% CI) | OR | (95% CI) |
| **Sex** | | | | | | | | | | | | |
| Male | 1.0 | – | 1.0 | – | 1.0 | – | 1.0 | – | 1.0 | – | 1.0 | – |
| Female | 1.5 | (1.1–2.0) | 1.5 | (1.1–2.1) | 0.6 | (0.4–1.0) | 0.1 | (0.0–0.2) | 0.8 | (0.5–1.3) | 1.1 | (0.9–1.5) |
| $\chi^2$ | | 7.2* | | 7.4* | | 4.5* | | 37.0* | | 0.8 | | 0.9 |
| **Age** | | | | | | | | | | | | |
| 18–29 | 1.3 | (0.8–2.1) | 1.2 | (0.7–2.0) | 1.7 | (0.9–3.4) | 8.5 | (1.3–53.8) | 0.5 | (0.2–1.0) | 1.7 | (1.1–2.7) |
| 30–44 | 1.0 | (0.6–1.7) | 1.2 | (0.7–2.0) | 1.0 | – | 7.3 | (1.1–46.5) | 0.7 | (0.3–1.4) | 1.5 | (1.0–2.3) |
| 45–54 | 0.8 | (0.5–1.5) | 1.2 | (0.6–2.2) | . | . | 9.8 | (1.3–75.1) | 0.6 | (0.2–1.5) | 1.2 | (0.7–2.2) |
| 55≤ | 1.0 | – | 1.0 | – | | | 1.0 | – | 1.0 | – | 1.0 | – |
| $\chi^2$ | | 2.5 | | 0.4 | | 2.6 | | 5.6 | | 4.4 | | 6.2 |
| **Income** | | | | | | | | | | | | |
| Low | 1.3 | (0.7–2.2) | 1.1 | (0.7–1.6) | 0.8 | (0.4–1.8) | 1.4 | (0.6–3.5) | 1.5 | (0.8–2.7) | 1.1 | (0.7–1.6) |
| Low average | 1.5 | (0.8–2.5) | 1.2 | (0.8–1.8) | 1.5 | (0.7–3.2) | 1.6 | (0.6–4.1) | 2.2 | (1.1–4.4) | 1.3 | (0.9–1.9) |
| High average | 1.0 | (0.6–1.8) | 1.2 | (0.7–2.0) | 0.6 | (0.3–1.4) | 0.7 | (0.3–1.9) | 1.0 | (0.5–1.9) | 1.1 | (0.7–1.8) |
| High | 1.0 | – | 1.0 | – | 1.0 | – | 1.0 | – | 1.0 | – | 1.0 | – |
| $\chi^2$ | | 4.4 | | 0.8 | | 4.6 | | 4.1 | | 14.2* | | 2.2 |
| **Marital status** | | | | | | | | | | | | |
| Married/cohabiting | 1.0 | – | 1.0 | – | 1.0 | – | 1.0 | – | 1.0 | – | 1.0 | – |
| Separated/widowed/divorced | 1.0 | (0.6–1.6) | 1.1 | (0.7–1.7) | 1.0 | (0.4–2.5) | 3.8 | (1.2–12.0) | 0.8 | (0.5–1.6) | 1.4 | (0.9–2.1) |
| Never married | 1.0 | (0.7–1.4) | 1.1 | (0.8–1.6) | 1.3 | (0.7–2.2) | 1.7 | (1.0–2.9) | 1.6 | (1.0–2.5) | 1.1 | (0.8–1.4) |
| $\chi^2$ | | 0.0 | | 0.6 | | 0.6 | | 6.2* | | 5.0 | | 1.8 |
| **Education** | | | | | | | | | | | | |
| None + primary | 0.9 | (0.5–1.7) | 1.1 | (0.7–1.9) | 1.1 | (0.4–3.1) | 1.4 | (0.6–3.0) | 0.5 | (0.3–0.9) | 1.2 | (0.8–1.9) |
| Some secondary | 1.1 | (0.6–1.9) | 1.5 | (0.9–2.5) | 1.1 | (0.5–2.5) | 1.5 | (0.7–3.1) | 0.4 | (0.2–0.6) | 1.6 | (1.1–2.4) |
| Completed secondary | 0.7 | (0.4–1.2) | 1.1 | (0.7–1.7) | 0.6 | (0.2–1.6) | 0.9 | (0.4–1.9) | 0.5 | (0.3–0.8) | 1.0 | (0.7–1.5) |
| Postsecondary | 1.0 | – | 1.0 | – | 1.0 | – | 1.0 | – | 1.0 | – | 1.0 | – |
| $\chi^2$ | | 3.9 | | 5.2 | | 3.6 | | 3.0 | | 14.2* | | 9.7 |

* $p \leq 0.05$.

**Table 7.5.** Severity and treatment of 12-month psychiatric disorders in Colombia

| Treatment | Total sample | | Any disorder | | Severe | | Moderate | | Mild | | No disorder | |
|---|---|---|---|---|---|---|---|---|---|---|---|---|
| | % | (se) | % | (se) | % | (se) | % | (se) | % | (se) | % | (se) |
| General medical | 2.3 | (0.4) | 6.0 | (1.0) | 9.3 | (2.5) | 6.1 | (1.7) | 2.7 | (0.9) | 1.4 | (0.4) |
| Mental health | 3.0 | (0.4) | 7.7 | (1.2) | 17.5 | (4.2) | 5.0 | (1.1) | 5.1 | (1.5) | 1.7 | (0.4) |
| Health care | 5.1 | (0.6) | 13.2 | (1.6) | 25.7 | (4.6) | 10.5 | (2.1) | 7.8 | (1.7) | 3.0 | (0.6) |
| Non–health-care | 0.7 | (0.2) | 1.7 | (0.8) | 4.6 | (2.7) | 0.8 | (0.5) | 0.4 | (0.4) | 0.5 | (0.2) |
| Any treatment | 5.5 | (0.6) | 14.0 | (1.6) | 27.8 | (4.8) | 10.6 | (2.1) | 8.2 | (1.7) | 3.4 | (0.6) |
| No treatment | 94.5 | (0.6) | 86.1 | (1.6) | 72.2 | (4.8) | 89.4 | (2.1) | 91.8 | (1.7) | 96.6 | (0.6) |

*Notes:* Non–health-care includes human services and CAM.

disorders, the current generation of young adults in Colombia is likely to experience a much higher burden of disease during later periods of life than has been the case for previous generations. Therefore the significance of mental health problems for health and health care across the life span is likely to increase in coming decades. Moreover, much of the burden of psychiatric disorders is shared among those with disorders, their families, and social networks. A much larger portion of the current Colombian population will directly or indirectly experience the consequences of psychiatric disorders than that of earlier periods. It is likely that this broad exposure to mental health problems will produce qualitative changes in how Colombians view mental health treatment.

Third, treatment for mental disorders is uncommon in Colombia, even among those with serious mental disorders. Nearly three-quarters of those with a severe disorder and nine-tenths of those with a moderately severe disorder received no treatment in the past year for their mental health problems. This low level of mental health treatment reflects the overall lack of mental health resources available across the country, where there are only three psychiatrists per 100,000 persons, and the low level of government investment in mental health care. The low level of mental health treatment in Colombia is at least partially a result of the lack of attention given to mental health in the planning of the current mental health system. For instance, Romero-González and colleagues compared the impact

of the 1993 health reform on access to mental health treatment with its impact on access to general medical care. This study found that access to mental health treatment decreased after the 1993 reform, as access to general medical treatment was expanding dramatically (Romero-González, González & Rosenheck 2003). Efforts to increase the availability of treatment for mental disorders across all sectors of care should be a high priority for the Colombian national health-care system. In particular, policies that address the needs of people with incomes in the lower three-quarters of the income distribution should be developed and implemented.

Several important limitations to the study need to be noted. First, the diagnosis of mental disorders was based on algorithms from survey instruments based on DSM-IV classification of disorders that are not culturally specific; therefore, this may not reflect current classifications of disorders or screening practices used in psychiatric settings in Colombia. Attempts to calibrate these diagnoses with instruments and diagnostic concepts in common use in clinical practice in Colombia would provide a better cultural contextualization of these results than is possible using the standardized instruments reported here. Such a calibration may help clinicians interpret these results with respect to their own clinical experience. Although the CIDI was previously validated in other countries (Rubio-Stipec, Bravo & Canino 1991; Rubio-Stipec, Peters & Andrews 1999), no studies of the validity of the instrument have been conducted in Colombia.

Finally, although the survey is nationally representative of people living in urban areas, it excluded people who are homeless, who live in rural or urban areas without a fixed address, who are part of Colombia's displaced populations, or who are either indigenous who speak a language other than Spanish or institutionalized people. However, given that the vast majority of the Colombian population that is included in the sampling frame for the surveys do have fixed addresses, this study provides a foundation for policy makers to use in setting new mental health agendas and developing programs.

It is important to note that the current chapter merely described the early results of our analyses of the ENSM data. Future analyses will focus on the extent to which examining how prevalence estimates and predictors vary over cohorts, over regions of the country, and in different high-risk segments of the population. Future analyses of health services use will focus on modifiable barriers to receiving treatment, more detailed patterns of service use, the adequacy of treatment in relation to published treatment guidelines, implementation of existing treatment policies, and patient satisfaction.

## REFERENCES

American Psychiatric Association (1994). *Diagnostic and statistical manual of mental disorders (DSM-IV)*, 4th ed. Washington, DC: American Psychiatric Association.

Cáceres, D. C., Izquierdo, V. F., Mantilla, L., Jara, J. & Velandia, M. (2002). Epidemiologic profile of the population displaced by the internal armed conflict of the country in a neighborhood of Cartagena, Colombia, 2000. *Biomedica*, 22 (suppl. 2), 425–44.

Demyttenaere, K., Bruffaerts, R., Posada-Villa, J., Gasquet, I., Kovess, V., Lepine, J. P., Angermeyer, M. C., Bernert, S., Girolamo, G., Morosini, P., Polidori, G., Kikkawa, T., Kawakami, N., Ono, Y., Takeshima, T., Uda, H., Karam, E. G., Fayyad, J. A., Karam, A. N., Mneimneh, Z. N., Medina-Mora, M. E., Borges, G., Lara, G., de Graaf, R., Ormel, J., Gureje, O., Shen, Y., Huang, Y., Zhang, M., Alonso, J., Haro, J. M., Vilagut, G., Bromet, E. J., Gluzman, S., Webb, C., Kessler, R. C., Merikangas, K. R., Anthony, J. C., Korff, M. R. V., Wang, P. S., Alonso, J., Brugha, T. S., Aguilar-Gaxiola, S., Lee, S.,

Heeringa, S., Pennell, B. E., Zaslavsky, A. M., Üstün, T. B. & Chatterji, S. (2004). Prevalence, severity, and unmet need for treatment of mental disorders in the World Health Organization World Mental Health Surveys. *Journal of the American Medical Association*, 291, 2581–90.

Efron, B. (1988). Logistic regression, survival analysis and the Kaplan-Meier curve. *Journal of the American Statistical Association*, 83, 414–25.

Endicott, J., Spitzer, R. L., Fleiss, J. L. & Cohen, J. (1976). The global assessment scale: A procedure for measuring overall severity of psychiatric disturbance. *Archives of General Psychiatry*, 33, 766–71.

Gómez-Restrepo, C., Bohorquez, A., Pinto Masis, D., Gil Laverde, J. F., Rondon Sepulveda, M. & Diaz-Granados, N. (2004). The prevalence of and factors associated with depression in Colombia. *Revista Panamericana de Salud Pública*, 16, 378–86.

Harpham, T., Grant, E. & Rodríguez, C. (2004). Mental health and social capital in Cali, Colombia. *Social Science and Medicine*, 58, 2267–77.

Harpham, T., Snoxell, S., Grant, E. & Rodríguez, C. (2005). Common mental disorders in a young urban population in Colombia. *British Journal of Psychiatry*, 187, 161–7.

Kessler, R. C., Berglund, P., Demler, O., Jin, R., Merikangas, K. R. & Walters, E. E. (2005a). Lifetime prevalence and age-of-onset distributions of DSM-IV disorders in the National Comorbidity Survey Replication. *Archives of General Psychiatry*, 62, 593–602.

Kessler, R. C., Chiu, W. T., Demler, O., Merikangas, K. R. & Walters, E. E. (2005b). Prevalence, severity, and comorbidity of 12-month DSM-IV disorders in the National Comorbidity Survey Replication. *Archives of General Psychiatry*, 62, 617–27.

Kessler, R. C., Haro, J. M., Heeringa, S. G., Pennell, B. E. & Üstün, T. B. (2006). The World Health Organization World Mental Health Survey Initiative. *Epidemiologia E Psichiatria Sociale*, 15, 161–6.

Kessler, R. C. & Üstün, T. B. (2004). The World Mental Health (WMH) Survey Initiative Version of the World Health Organization (WHO) Composite International Diagnostic Interview (CIDI). *International Journal of Methods in Psychiatric Research*, 13, 93–121.

Leon, A. C., Olfson, M., Portera, L., Farber, L. & Sheehan, D. V. (1997). Assessing psychiatric impairment in primary care with the Sheehan Disability Scale. *International Journal of Methods in Psychiatric Research*, 27, 93–105.

Lima, B. R., Pai, S., Santacruz, H. & Lozano, J. (1991). Psychiatric disorders among poor victims following a major disaster: Armero, Colombia. *Journal of Nervous and Mental Disease*, 179, 420–7.

Lima, B. R., Santacruz, H., Lozano, J., Luna, J. & Pai, S. (1988). Primary mental health care for the victims of the disaster in Armero, Colombia. *Acta Psiquiátrica y Psicológica de América Latina*, 34, 13–32.

Medina-Mora, M. E., Borges, G., Benjet, C., Lara, C. & Berglund, P. (2007). Psychiatric disorders in Mexico: Lifetime prevalence in a nationally representative sample. *British Journal of Psychiatry*, 190, 521–8.

Medina-Mora, M. E., Borges, G., Lara, C., Benjet, C., Blanco, J., Fleiz, C., Villatoro, J., Rojas, E. & Zambrano, J. (2005). Prevalence, service use, and demographic correlates of 12-month DSM-IV psychiatric disorders in Mexico: Results from the Mexican National Comorbidity Survey. *Psychological Medicine*, 35, 1773–83.

Mogollón Pérez, A. S., Vázquez Navarrete, M. & García Gil M., M. (2003). Health-related needs of the displaced population due to armed conflict in Bogotá. *Revista Española de Salud Pública*, 77, 257–266.

Pérez-Olmos, I., Fernández-Piñeres, P. E., & Rodado-Fuentes, S. (2005). The prevalence of war-related post-traumatic stress disorder in children from Cundinamarca, Colombia. *Revista de Salud Pública*, 7 (3), 268–280.

Posada-Villa, J., Aguilar-Gaxiola, S., Magaña, C. & Gómez, L. (2004). Prevalence of mental disorders and use of services: Preliminary results from the National Study of Mental Health, Colombia. *Revista Colombiana de Psiquiatría*, 33, 241–61.

Puertas, G., Ríos, C. & del Valle, H. (2006). The prevalence of common mental disorders in urban slums with displaced persons in Colombia. *Revista Panamericana de Salud Pública*, 20, 324–30.

Research Triangle Institute (2002). *SUDAAN: Professional software for survey data analysis 8.01.* Research Triangle Park, NC: Research Triangle Institute.

Romero-González, M., González, G. & Rosenheck, R. A. (2003). Mental health service delivery following health system reform in Colombia. *Journal of Mental Health Policy and Economics*, 6, 189–94.

Rubio-Stipec, M., Bravo, M. & Canino, G. (1991). The Composite International Diagnostic Interview (CIDI): An epidemiologic instrument suitable for using in conjunction with different diagnostic systems in different cultures. *Acta Psiquiátrica y Psicológica de América Latina*, 37, 191–204.

Rubio-Stipec, M., Peters, L. & Andrews, G. (1999). Test-retest reliability of the computerized CIDI (CIDI-Auto): Substance abuse modules. *Substance Abuse*, 20, 263–72.

Sánchez, R., Orejarena, S., Guzmán, Y. & Forero, J. (2002). Suicide in Bogotá: An increasing phenomenon in young populations. *Biomedica*, 22 (suppl. 2), 417–24.

Scott, R. L., Knoth, R. L., Beltran-Quiones, M. & Gomez, N. (2003). Assessment of psychological functioning in adolescent earthquake victims in Colombia using the MMPI-A. *Journal of Traumatic Stress*, 16, 49–57.

Torres de Galvis, Y. & Murrelle, L. (1990). Consumption of dependence-producing substances in Colombia. *Bulletin of the Pan American Health Organization*, 24, 12–21.

Wang, P. S., Lane, M., Olfson, M., Pincus, H. A., Wells, K. B. & Kessler, R. C. (2005). Twelve-month use of mental health services in the United States: Results from the National Comorbidity Survey Replication. *Archives of General Psychiatry*, 62, 629–40.

World Bank (2005). Country statistical information: Colombia. Retrieved July 16, 2007, from http://ddp-ext.worldbank.org/ext/CSIDB/getCountryStatInfoXML?id=170&format=CSIDB.

World Health Organization (WHO) (2005). *World Mental HealthAtlas*. Geneva, World Health Organization.

# 8 The Mexican National Comorbidity Survey (M-NCS): Overview and Results

MARIA ELENA MEDINA-MORA, GUILHERME BORGES, CARMEN LARA,
CORINA BENJET, CLARA FLEIZ, G. ESTELA ROJAS, JOAQUÍN ZAMBRANO,
JORGE VILLATORO, JERÓNIMO BLANCO, SERGIO AGUILAR-GAXIOLA,
AND RONALD C. KESSLER

## ACKNOWLEDGMENTS

The Mexican National Comorbidity Survey (M-NCS) is supported by The National Institute of Psychiatry Ramon de la Fuente (INPRFMDIES 4280) and by the National Council on Science and Technology (CONACyT-G30544-H), with supplemental support from the PanAmerican Health Organization (PAHO).

The MNCS is carried out in conjunction with the World Health Organization World Mental Health (WMH) Survey Initiative. We thank the WMH staff for assistance with instrumentation, fieldwork, and data analysis. These activities were supported by the U.S. National Institute of Mental Health (R01MH070884), the John D. and Catherine T. MacArthur Foundation, the Pfizer Foundation, the U.S. Public Health Service (R13-MH066849, R01-MH069864, and R01 DA016558), the Fogarty International Center (FIRCA R03-TW006481), the Pan American Health Organization, Eli Lilly and Company Foundation, Ortho-McNeil Pharmaceutical, Inc., GlaxoSmithKline, and Bristol-Myers Squibb. A complete list of WMH publications can be found at http://www.hcp.med.harvard.edu/wmh/.

## I. INTRODUCTION

The mental health of the Mexican population has improved considerably as compared to the conditions that prevailed in the first half of the past century. This improvement is due, in great part, to the new alternatives for treatment derived from advances in psycho-pharmacotherapy and successful behavioral and psychosocial treatment models. These important advances, however, are not evenly distributed, with the poor having less access to health services. Additionally, psychiatric problems, such as dementia, substance abuse and dependence, and other forms of chronic mental illnesses, have increased. This trend has resulted, in part, from the increase in life expectancy, as more people now live to the age of risk, and from the effects of globalization, which have increased access to tobacco, alcohol, and other drugs. At the same time, exposure to violence is now more prevalent, and poverty and inequity, which have resulted from continuous economic crises and the growing concentration of wealth in a small proportion of the population, have increased the vulnerability of the population and made the lives of those affected more difficult. The new treatment approaches do not reach all those in need, in part as a result of a lack of knowledge in the population as to how to discern effective treatment from the many available alternatives that have not been empirically tested or found to be effective above and beyond the placebo effect. Further, effective treatments are primarily available only in large metropolitan areas.

The Mexican health agenda has yet to solve the prevalent conditions derived from infectious diseases. Ever-increasing chronic conditions, such as mental disorders and emerging problems such as learning and behavioral difficulties, adolescent suicide, and addictions, further tax a challenged system. Improvement of the health system requires accurate data on the extent of the problem. Epidemiological studies can be very helpful in this regard by providing information on the number of people with mental disorders in a given population and the characteristics of patients with different disorders in a given context, helping match patient needs and treatment modalities, identifying variables that predict treatment outcome and determine rates of service use, and identifying pathways to care and barriers to treatment.

This chapter reports data from a national household survey undertaken in Mexico as part of the World Mental Health (WMH) Survey Initiative (Kessler et al. 2006), the Mexican National Comorbidity Survey (M-NCS). To put these data in context, we begin by describing the major social transitions that have modified the risk for mental disorders in Mexico and then provide an overview of the results from prior studies before turning to a description of the M-NCS.

## 1.1. The Social Context of Mental Disorders

Mexico is a large country, with more than 100 million inhabitants, 75% of whom live in urban areas of more than 2500 inhabitants. Important social and demographic transitions have modified the extent and characteristics of the vulnerable population. The Mexican demographic transition is characterized by an important increase in the population, which doubled in 1981 and is expected to double again in 2020, derived from the decrease in mortality (in the 1930s, life expectancy was 35 years for males and 37 for females and increased to almost 73 and 78, respectively, in 2005) and the delayed drop in birthrate that occurred only after 1980 (from 6.1 to 2.1 children per female between 1974 and 2005) (Consejo Nacional de Población 2005). The result is an increase in the absolute number of young people with insufficient educational and employment opportunities and an increase in the number of elderly people. This shift translates into an increased risk for addictions and mental health problems more characteristic of the vulnerable young population and an increased risk for dementia and other degenerative diseases more common of the older population.

Mexico is defined as a country with a high level of human development, ranking 53rd, under Argentina, Chile, Uruguay, Costa Rica, and Cuba in the Latin American and Caribbean Spanish-speaking countries (Programa de las Naciones Unidas para el Desarrollo 2006). In 2005, only 4.1% of the population lived under the poverty line (defined as earning less than US$1 per day); in 1989, the proportion was more than double, at 10.8%. Nonetheless, improvement in economic status is not evenly distributed throughout the country, with important differences related to the level of economic development. For example, in urban sites, where three-fourths of the population lives, the proportion who live under the poverty line is as low as 0.2%, but it increases to 10.5% in rural areas (defined as those with fewer than 2500 inhabitants) (Secretaría de Desarrollo Social 2005). The National Survey of Household Income and Expenditure showed that the population living in the 10% of households with the highest income concentrated 35.6% of the national income, whereas 10% of the poorest concentrated only 1.6% (Instituto Nacional de Estadística Geografía e Informática 2002). In 2002, it was estimated that 26.5% of the population did not have the required income to satisfy basic nutritional requirements or had limited access to education and health services (Secretaría de Desarrollo Social 2002). The informal economy is considerable, estimated as 50% of employment within the nonagricultural sector (Secretaría de Desarrollo Social 2005).

Economic crises have brought about new social transitions, such as the incorporation of females into the labor force, including mothers raising young children. Although females have gained an important proportion of participation in the labor market (45%), they are incorporated into more precarious occupations with less social protection; for instance, the proportion of females in the labor market increased by 91% for those in the lowest tenth percentile of income and only by 12% for the wealthier (Secretaría de Desarrollo Social 2005). The incorporation of other family members in money-raising activities means that children have joined the informal sectors of the economy, with increased risk of drug abuse and victimization (Medina-Mora, Villatoro & Fleiz 1999; Medina-Mora 2000).

The centralization of services and jobs has resulted in an increase in the size of cities; Mexico City now has 20 million inhabitants. Poor development conditions are also linked to rural-urban and international migration. In the period from 1961 to 1979, it was estimated that 30,000 persons crossed the border into the United States, growing to 440,000 between 2001 and 2004; around three-fourths of those crossing are considered illegal workers; the modifications in the border controls have resulted in a more definitive migration and the period of permanence within the United States has changed from 5.5 months to 11.2 months in the past ten years (Consejo Nacional de Población 2005). This process has modified the communities of origin of these workers in definite ways for those left behind, usually females and their children, and more recently the children left under the care of older siblings or grandparents. Females, mostly coming from rural communities with traditional gender roles, are suddenly thrust into traditionally male roles, which contributes to increased rates of stress and depression (Salgado & Díaz-Pérez 1999) and to behavioral problems in children and adolescents (Aguilera et al. 2004). These economic burdens and their impact are greater for the poor than for other segments of the population, which have more stresses and fewer resources to cope with their problems.

## 1.2. The Structure of the Health System

The health system in Mexico is coordinated by the Ministry of Health. Health services are provided by the Mexican Institute of Social Security, an organization funded by the federal and state governments; by the private sector through quotas paid per affiliated worker and by contributions deducted from salaries by workers; by the Institute of Social Security and Services for State Workers (ISSSTE); and by special organizations such as health services for workers from the oil industry, among others, such that 53 million people are protected by their affiliation to these institutions, or roughly half the Mexican population. The Ministry of Health provides services for an additional 1.3 million people. In 2004, it was estimated that 52.2 million people did not have health coverage. According to Frenk and colleagues (1999), poor families without the benefit of social security or other health coverage sources (12%) use a higher proportion of their income to pay for services, in a rate estimated at 5.2%, compared to only 2.8% among the wealthiest sector of society. By 2005, 13% of the poorest segments of the population had been affiliated with a new system known as Popular Insurance. Nine in ten persons affiliated with this system belong to the poorest sectors of society. Mental illnesses, including addictions, were recently included among the illnesses for which treatment is provided by this insurance system (Secretaría de Desarrollo Social 2005).

## 1.3. Psychiatric Eepidemiology in Mexico: Some Background

Mortality due to neuropsychiatric disorders occupies the 12th place of importance in Mexico according to the WHO analysis of the Global Burden of Disease. However, when premature death and life lived with disability (so-called disability-adjusted life years, or DALYs) are also considered, then these conditions are thought to rank in 5th place (Frenk et al. 1999), mainly because those who develop mental disorders tend to live many years with a poorer quality of life. It is important to note, though, that these rankings are based on estimates of the prevalence of neuropsychiatric disorders that might be downwardly biased.

Suicide is a growing problem in Mexico. In 2002, the mortality rate was estimated at 5.83 among males and 1.04 among females per 100,000 inhabitants, representing 6% of deaths due to external causes. According to the WHO (2000), between the years 1981 and 1983 and the years 1993 and 1995, the suicide rate increased 62%, making it one of the highest in the world.

Mexico has a long tradition of epidemiological research in substance abuse, but psychiatric epidemiology has had a later start. The first general population surveys of addictions date back to 1974 (Medina-Mora 1978). Today, four national surveys are available (Secretaría de Salud 1988, 1993, 1998, 2002), all but the last were conducted in urban areas (75% of the country's population) with an age range between 12 and 65 years (Tapia-Conyer et al. 1990; Medina-Mora, Borges & Villatoro 2000, Medina-Mora et al. 2001a, 2001b, 2004; Villatoro et al. 2004). Findings from these surveys show a high prevalence of alcohol abuse and dependence. The highest rates are found among rural males between 18 and 65 years of age, with a rate of 10.5%, followed by urban males 9.3%; rates among females are considerably lower, 0.7% among those that live in urban areas and 0.4% in rural areas. Drinking patterns are linked to elevated rates of associated problems. In other words, while there are high rates of abstention and daily drinking is not a frequent practice, drinking large quantities only on specific drinking occasions outside the home is common. Thus, emergency room entrances for trauma with positive alcohol levels are high – ranging from 23% to 35%, higher than those observed in the United States (Borges et al. 2003). Rates of death associated with liver cirrhosis are among the highest in the world, at 22 per 100,000 inhabitants. Rates of abuse/dependence among males 26 and older are similar to those reported in the National Household Survey in the United States (SAMHSA 2001) and higher than those reported in the European countries that participated in the WHO Mental Health Survey Initiative (Kessler et al. 2006).

Abuse and dependence of other drugs is considerably lower, estimated at 0.44% of the national population between 18 and 65 years of age. The main drugs of abuse are marijuana, cocaine, and inhalants. Abuse of inhalants has shown a downward trend since the 1990s (Medina-Mora & Fleiz 2003; Villatoro et al. 2004; Centros de Integración Juvenil 2005; SISVEA 2005), except among street children, for whom inhalants are the preferred drug (Medina-Mora, Villatoro & Fleiz 1999). Cocaine showed a sharp increase in the late 1980s and early 1990s but leveled off by the end of the past century and is showing a decreasing trend at the beginning of the millennium; despite this, cocaine is related to the highest treatment demand (Medina-Mora

& Fleiz 2003; Villatoro et al. 2004; Centros de Integración Juvenil 2005; SISVEA 2005). The decrease of cocaine abuse coincides with a slight increase in the abuse of amphetamine-type stimulants, mainly ecstasy and crystal methamphetamine (Centros de Integración Juvenil 2005; SISVEA 2005). Drug abuse rates in Mexico are considerably lower than those reported in national household surveys in the United States (SAMHSA 2001) and rates of dependence are considerably lower than those reported in Germany and the Netherlands (Merikangas et al. 1998).

The first epidemiological studies of mental disorders conducted in Mexico used screening instruments to detect possible mental health disorders and a psychiatric interview to confirm the diagnosis in random samples of positive and negative cases (Campillo et al. 1979; Medina-Mora et al. 1983; Ezban et al. 1984). These first studies sampled patients in general hospital settings (Caraveo et al. 1986; Gómez et al. 1990), community mental health centers (Padilla et al. 1984), and other populations such as college students (Romero & Medina-Mora 1987). Higher rates of anxiety, depression, and adaptation problems were found among the poor.

As one of the first approximations of prevalence estimates for the general population in Mexico, a subsample of the National Addictions Survey (Secretaria de Salud 1988) responded to an additional brief questionnaire. This questionnaire was designed ad hoc to provide DSM-III diagnoses. Between 15% and 18% of the population 18 to 65 years of age presented one or more of the disorders studied, excluding substance abuse disorders, with 7% reporting inability to perform daily activities as a result of their condition (Medina-Mora et al. 1993; Caraveo 1996).

A few years later, Caraveo and colleagues (1998) conducted a representative survey of Mexico City residents using a fully structured psychiatric interview (Robins et al. 1988) (a previous version of the instrument used in the present survey), which subsequently allowed for comparisons between México City residents and Mexican Americans in California (Vega et al. 1998b). In the capital city, the rates for mood disorders reached 9% of the adult population (between 18 and 65 years of age), with 7.8%

corresponding to major depressive episodes at a ratio of 2.5 females per male; dysthymia, 1.5% with a similar female-to-male ratio (2.6:1); and a lower rate of manic episodes, reaching 1.3% with a smaller difference between sexes (1.2:1). Prevalence rates for anxiety disorders were slightly lower, affecting 8.3% of the population; agoraphobia without panic (3.8%) and social phobia (2.2%) were the most common diagnoses (Caraveo, Martínez & Rivera 1998). Studies conducted in rural areas have shown lower prevalence rates (Salgado & Díaz-Pérez 1999).

These rates are significantly lower than the ones observed in the United States, where 19.5% and 25% report any mood disorder and anxiety disorder, respectively (Vega et al. 1998a). Vega and his coauthors (1998b) also reported comparatively lower rates of alcohol and drug dependence in Mexico; the difference in alcohol rates is mainly due to the low levels of use among Mexican females (Medina-Mora et al. 2004; Villatoro et al. 2004).

Other surveys have shown that poor families have higher 12-month prevalence rates of depression and anxiety disorders and that these are higher among single-parent families (Berenzon, Tiburcio & Medina-Mora 2005).

Rates of service use for mood disorders are low; data derived from a survey conducted in the capital city indicated that only 13.9% of those who qualified for the DSM-IV criteria of depression sought help (Caraveo et al. 1997). Local studies of communities of middle and low socioeconomic levels have indicated that medical doctors were the most common source of help for this population. Forty-two percent of those with an anxiety or mood disorder reported having told their problems to a general physician. Psychologists were the second (42% of females and 36% of males); psychiatrists the third source among males (32%) and religious ministers for females (26%); traditional healers were consulted by 9% of males and 11% of females (Medina-Mora et al. 1997).

Other studies that have analyzed barriers to care show that the main reasons are related to the belief that the treatment available was not effective to deal with mental problems (58% of males and 68% of females), that access was difficult

(16% of males and 22% of females) or that they had insufficient information (8% and 14%). Barriers were related to low educational attainment and family income (Medina-Mora et al. 1997). Shame associated with psychiatric conditions still prevails among the population. In the capital city, males who did not seek help reported being concerned with the opinion of their employers if they found out about their mental condition, and females reported being concerned about the opinion of family members (Caraveo et al. 1997). In rural areas the situation is worse, as there are no specialized facilities available for persons with mental problems; a visit to a psychiatrist represents a day's journey and an elevated cost. At the local level, traditional healers and other informal agents are consulted (Salgado & Díaz-Pérez 1999).

## 2. METHODS

### 2.1. Sample

A general description of the M-NCS has been presented elsewhere (Medina-Mora et al. 2005). The survey was based on a stratified, multistage clustered area probability sample of persons aged 18 to 65 years in the noninstitutionalized population living in urban areas (population 2500+) of Mexico. About 75% of the Mexican population is urban, as defined previously. Urban Mexico was stratified in six strata:

1. Self-representing metropolitan areas. Includes the three largest metropolitan areas of Mexico: Mexico City (AMCM), Guadalajara (AMG), and Monterrey (AMM).
2. Northwest. Includes the states of Baja California, Baja California Sur, Nayarit, Sinaloa, and Sonora.
3. North. Includes the states of Coahuila, Chihuahua, Durango, Nuevo León (excluding AMM), San Luis Potosí, Tamaulipas, and Zacatecas.
4. West Central. Includes the states of Aguascalientes, Jalisco (excluding AMG), Colima, Guanajuato, and Michoacán.
5. East Central. Includes the states of Guerrero, Morelos, Estado de México (excluding

counties part of AMCM), Querétaro, Hidalgo, Tlaxcala, and Puebla.

6. Southeast. Includes the states of Veracruz, Oaxaca, Tabasco, Chiapas, Campeche, Yucatán, and Quintana Roo.

Data collection took place in two phases from September 2001 through May 2002. The average length of the interview was 2.5 hours, with a range varying between 25 minutes to 9 hours in four different sessions. The response rate was 76.6% (for a total of 5826 interviews), well above the original targeted sample size of 5000) and within the range of other WMH surveys (50.6%–87.7% response rate range; Demyttenaere et al. 2004). Refusal to answer the interview once the selected person had been contacted was less than 6%, including refusal to continue the interview in a second or subsequent visit. In fact, interviewers found it challenging to limit the interviewee in their answers to questions, as they often wanted to expand upon their feelings and experiences. All respondents were administered a Part 1 interview and a selected subsample of 2362 received a supplemental number of questions on risk factors and supplemental mental disorders, Part 2. The sample receiving Part 2 consisted of all respondents who screened positive for any disorder on Part 1 plus a probability subsample of other Part 1 respondents. All interviews were conducted at the respondents' homes after a careful description of the study goals was given and informed consent was obtained. No financial incentive was given for respondents' participation. All recruitment and consent procedures were approved by the ethics committee of the National Institute of Psychiatry.

## 2.2. Measures

The instrument used to carry out the M-NCS interviews was the WMH version of the WHO Composite International Diagnostic Interview (CIDI 3.0) (Kessler & Üstün 2004, see also Chapter 4), a fully structured diagnostic interview administered by trained lay interviewers in face-to-face interviews using a laptop computer version (i.e., CAPI). Although the CIDI yields

diagnoses according to the definitions and criteria of both the ICD and the DSM systems, the results reported here, like all the others in this volume, use DSM-IV criteria (American Psychiatric Association 1994).

The Spanish-language version of CIDI that was used in the M-NCS as well as in the WMH survey in Colombia was developed using the standard WHO approach (i.e., translation, back-translation, and harmonization of modules), building upon Spanish versions of ICD-10 and DSM-IV and previous Spanish versions of the Diagnostic Interview Schedule (DIS) and CIDI. One of the first translations was performed by the team from Puerto Rico (Rubio-Stipec, Bravo & Canino 1991). The DIS (Caraveo, González & Ramos 1991) and previous versions of the CIDI in Spanish have been used in México (Caraveo, Martínez & Rivera 1998), in Spanish-speaking communities in the United States (Vega et al. 1998a; Dwight-Johnson et al. 2000), in Chile (Ruiz et al. 1996; Vicente et al. 2002), and in other Spanish-speaking countries that participated in the WMH Survey Initiative. Berumen and Associates, an established survey research firm in Mexico, conducted the fieldwork and employed a group of interviewers who received extensive CAPI training in the CIDI.

## 2.3. Disorders

We report on the lifetime and 12-month prevalence of psychiatric disorders, defined according to DSM-IV criteria and operationalized by the CIDI for diagnoses by sex. Prevalence rates according to ICD-10 have been reported elsewhere (Medina-Mora et al. 2003). All disorders used organic exclusions rules as well as hierarchy definitions to avoid double counting of disorders such as alcohol dependence and alcohol abuse or major depression and dysthymia in the same person. The disorders are grouped into the following categories:

1. Affective disorders: major depressive episode, bipolar I–II disorders, and dysthymia with hierarchy.
2. Anxiety disorders: panic disorder, agoraphobia without panic disorder, social phobia,

specific phobia, separation anxiety disorder, generalized anxiety disorder, and posttraumatic stress disorder.

**3.** Substance disorders: alcohol and drug abuse and dependence.

**4.** Impulse-control disorders (the three disorders typically manifest during childhood and adolescence): oppositional-defiant disorder, conduct disorder, and attention-deficit/hyperactivity disorder. These three disorders were assessed only in respondents in the age range of 18 to 44 because of concerns about recall bias among older respondents.

## 2.4. Disorder Severity

Twelve-month DSM-IV/CIDI cases were classified as serious, moderate, or mild (Demyttenaere et al. 2004). The criteria used here for a serious disorder was presence of a bipolar I disorder, substance dependence with a physiological dependence syndrome, a suicide attempt in conjunction with any other CIDI disorder, reporting of at least two areas of role functioning with severe role impairment due to a mental disorder as measured by the disorder-specific Sheehan Disability Scales (SDS) (Sheehan, Harnett-Sheehan & Raj 1996), or reporting of overall functioning impairment at a level consistent with a global assessment of functioning (Endicott et al. 1976) of 50 or less in conjunction with any other CIDI disorder. Respondents not classified as having a serious disorder were classified as moderate if interference was rated as at least moderate in any domain of the Sheehan Disability Scales or if the respondent had substance dependence without a physiological dependence syndrome. All other disorders were classified as mild.

## 2.5. Service Use

Information was obtained about lifetime and 12-month treatment for emotional, alcohol, or drug problems; the type and context of professional visited; and the use of self-help or support groups and hotlines. Respondents could select as many

professionals and treatment options as they used. Mental health care was divided into the following five sectors:

**1.** Psychiatrist.

**2.** Other mental health specialty: psychologists, counselors, psychotherapists, mental health nurses, or social workers in a mental health specialty setting.

**3.** General medical: family physicians, general practitioners, other medical doctors such as cardiologists or gynecologists (for women) and urologists (for men), nurses, occupational therapists, or other health care professionals.

**4.** Human services: outpatient treatment with a religious or spiritual advisor or social worker or counselor in any setting other than a specialty mental health setting; religious or spiritual advisor such as a minister, priest, or rabbi.

**5.** Complementary alternative medicine (CAM): Internet use, self-help groups, any other healer (e.g., herbalist, chiropractor, spiritualist), and other alternative therapy.

For purposes of analysis, we grouped psychiatrist and other mental health specialty together under "any mental health sector." Also, psychiatrist, mental health specialty, and general medical were grouped together under "any health care." Finally, human services and CAM professionals were grouped together under "non–health-care."

## 2.6. Analyses

The data from Part 1 and Part 2 samples were weighted to adjust for differential probabilities of selection and nonresponse. The sample receiving Part 2 was additionally weighted to adjust for differential probability of selection. Poststratification to the urban Mexican population according to the 2000 census in the target age and sex range was also made. As a result of this complex sample design and weighting, estimates of standard errors for proportions were obtained by the Taylor series linearization method using the SUDAAN software (Research Triangle Institute 2002). Logistic regression analysis (Hosmer

**Table 8.1.** Demographic distribution of the sample compared to the population on poststratification variables

| | Part 1 unweighted (n = 5826) (%) | Part 1 weighted (%) | Census (%) | Part 2 unweighted (n = 2362) (%) | Part 2 weighted (%) | Census (%) |
|---|---|---|---|---|---|---|
| **Sex** | | | | | | |
| Male | 39.4 | 47.6 | 47.7 | 36.1 | 47.7 | 47.7 |
| Female | 60.6 | 52.4 | 52.3 | 63.9 | 52.3 | 52.3 |
| **Age** | | | | | | |
| 18–24 | 21.4 | 24.5 | 24.7 | 24.3 | 25.4 | 24.7 |
| 25–29 | 14.2 | 15.5 | 15.6 | 13.6 | 15.9 | 15.6 |
| 30–34 | 14.0 | 13.6 | 13.6 | 12.2 | 12.5 | 13.6 |
| 35–39 | 13.7 | 12.3 | 12.1 | 13.1 | 11.5 | 12.1 |
| 40–44 | 11.0 | 10.1 | 9.9 | 10.3 | 10.6 | 9.9 |
| 45–49 | 8.0 | 7.7 | 7.8 | 8.3 | 7.8 | 7.8 |
| 50–54 | 6.5 | 6.3 | 6.4 | 6.9 | 6.3 | 6.4 |
| 55–59 | 4.8 | 4.7 | 4.9 | 5.6 | 4.9 | 4.9 |
| 60–65 | 6.4 | 5.3 | 5.1 | 5.7 | 5.2 | 5.1 |
| **Region** | | | | | | |
| Metropolitan | 31.5 | 28.0 | 27.6 | 32.6 | 27.6 | 27.6 |
| Northwest | 9.8 | 7.9 | 8.0 | 10.9 | 8.0 | 8.0 |
| North | 14.5 | 15.3 | 15.1 | 13.7 | 15.1 | 15.1 |
| Central West | 12.7 | 12.3 | 12.4 | 13.4 | 12.4 | 12.4 |
| Central East | 15.1 | 17.1 | 17.5 | 14.9 | 17.5 | 17.5 |
| South East | 16.4 | 19.4 | 19.3 | 14.6 | 19.3 | 19.3 |

& Lemeshow 2000) was performed to study demographic correlates of 12-month prevalence among those with a lifetime disorder. Estimates of standard errors of odds ratios (ORs) from logistic regression coefficients were also obtained by SUDAAN, and 95% confidence intervals (CI) were adjusted to design effects. Statistical significance was evaluated using two-sided design-based tests at the 0.05 level of significance. Lifetime prevalence was estimated as the proportion of respondents who ever had a given disorder up to their age at the time of the interview. Sociodemographic predictors of cohort effects on the lifetime prevalence were examined using discrete-time survival analyses with person-year as the unit of analyses (Efron 1988).

## 3. RESULTS

Table 8.1 presents the distribution of the sample, according to unweighted and weighted results.

The most relevant variable for poststratification was sex, as actual participants were more likely to be female. The age and regional distribution of actual participants were more similar to the census count. The demographic distribution of the sample after stratification and weighting (both for Part 1 and Part 2 samples) is similar to the targeted population. After weighting the data, about 52% of the sample was female and about 25% in the youngest age group (18–24 years). About 28% of the sample lived in Mexico's three main metropolitan areas.

### 3.1. Prevalence

The lifetime and 12-month prevalence of DSM-IV disorders among females and males are presented in Table 8.2. According to our summary measure, 27.4% of Mexican males and 24.9% of Mexican females respondents reported a lifetime prevalence of any disorder. Comorbidity is

**Table 8.2.** Lifetime and 12-month prevalence of DSM-IV/CIDI disorders in the M-NCS sample by gender groups

| | Lifetime | | | | 12 months | | | |
|---|---|---|---|---|---|---|---|---|
| | Male | | Female | | Male | | Female | |
| | % | (se) | % | (se) | % | (se) | % | (se) |
| **I. Anxiety disorders** | | | | | | | | |
| Panic disorder | 0.6 | (0.2) | 1.4 | (0.3) | 0.3 | (0.1) | 1.1 | (0.2) |
| Generalized anxiety disorder | 0.5 | (0.1) | 1.3 | (0.2) | 0.3 | (0.1) | 0.6 | (0.1) |
| Social phobia | 2.2 | (0.4) | 3.6 | (0.3) | 1.4 | (0.3) | 2.6 | (0.3) |
| Specific phobia | 4.2 | (0.5) | 9.6 | (0.8) | 3.0 | (0.5) | 7.2 | (0.7) |
| Agoraphobia without panic | 0.3 | (0.1) | 1.6 | (0.2) | 0.2 | (0.1) | 1.2 | (0.2) |
| Posttraumatic stress disorder[a] | 0.5 | (0.2) | 2.3 | (0.5) | 0.4 | (0.2) | 0.7 | (0.2) |
| Separation anxiety disorder[b] | 3.7 | (0.8) | 5.2 | (0.5) | 0.7 | (0.2) | 1.1 | (0.2) |
| Any anxiety disorder[c] | 10.6 | (1.1) | 17.6 | (1.4) | 5.5 | (0.8) | 11.0 | (0.9) |
| **II. Mood disorders** | | | | | | | | |
| Major depressive disorder | 4.6 | (0.6) | 9.7 | (0.6) | 2.3 | (0.4) | 4.7 | (0.4) |
| Dysthymia | 0.3 | (0.2) | 1.0 | (0.2) | 0.2 | (0.1) | 0.6 | (0.2) |
| Bipolar I–II disorders | 2.4 | (0.4) | 1.5 | (0.3) | 1.0 | (0.2) | 1.3 | (0.3) |
| Any mood disorder | 6.9 | (0.6) | 11.2 | (0.7) | 3.2 | (0.4) | 6.1 | (0.5) |
| **III. Impulse-control disorders** | | | | | | | | |
| Oppositional-defiant disorder[b] | 3.5 | (0.7) | 1.9 | (0.5) | 0.8 | (0.4) | 0.3 | (0.1) |
| Conduct disorder[b] | 2.0 | (0.6) | 0.6 | (0.2) | 0.4 | (0.3) | 0.0 | (0.0) |
| Attention-deficit/hyperactivity disorder[b] | 3.9 | (0.7) | 2.2 | (0.5) | 1.1 | (0.3) | 0.9 | (0.2) |
| Any impulse-control disorders[b] | 7.3 | (1.1) | 4.2 | (0.7) | 2.1 | (0.6) | 1.2 | (0.3) |
| **IV. Substance disorders** | | | | | | | | |
| Alcohol abuse | 14.5 | (1.1) | 1.3 | (0.3) | 4.3 | (0.7) | 0.2 | (0.2) |
| Alcohol dependence | 6.2 | (0.8) | 0.7 | (0.2) | 2.0 | (0.4) | 0.2 | (0.1) |
| Drug abuse | 2.7 | (0.3) | 0.2 | (0.1) | 0.7 | (0.2) | 0.0 | (0.0) |
| Drug dependence | 0.8 | (0.2) | 0.1 | (0.1) | 0.2 | (0.1) | 0.0 | (0.0) |
| Any substance disorders | 15.0 | (1.1) | 1.3 | (0.3) | 4.6 | (0.7) | 0.2 | (0.2) |
| **V. Any disorder** | | | | | | | | |
| Any (one or more) | 27.4 | (1.9) | 24.9 | (1.7) | 12.0 | (1.3) | 14.7 | (1.1) |
| Two or more disorders[c] | 14.1 | (1.3) | 10.1 | (0.7) | 5.3 | (0.9) | 5.0 | (0.5) |
| Three or more disorders[c] | 5.6 | (0.7) | 4.5 | (0.4) | 1.7 | (0.4) | 2.1 | (0.3) |
| **VI. Sample sizes** | | | | | | | | |
| Part 1 | 5782 | | | | | | | |
| Part 2 | 2362 | | | | | | | |
| Part 2, age ≤44 | 1736 | | | | | | | |

[a] Posttraumatic stress disorder was assessed only in the Part 2 sample.

[b] Separation anxiety disorder, oppositional-defiant disorder, conduct disorder, and attention-deficit disorder were assessed only among Part 2 respondents in the age range 18–44.

[c] These summary measures were analyzed in the full Part 2 sample. Separation anxiety disorder, oppositional-defiant disorder, conduct disorder, and attention-deficit disorder were coded as absent among respondents who were not assessed for these disorders.

not infrequent: 14.1% of males reported two or more disorders and 10.1% of females reported two or more disorders. Among males, substance use disorders, as a group, followed by anxiety disorders, were the most common disorders. As a group, anxiety disorders followed by mood disorders were the most common among females. The most prevalent single disorder in Mexico was alcohol abuse (14.5%) for males and major depression (9.7%) for females.

**Table 8.3.** Distribution of severity of DSM-IV/CIDI disorders in the M-NCS sample by group of disorders

| | Female | | | | | | Male | | | | | |
| --- | --- | --- | --- | --- | --- | --- | --- | --- | --- | --- | --- | --- |
| | Severe | | Moderate | | Mild | | Severe | | Moderate | | Mild | |
| | % | (se) | % | (se) | % | (se) | % | (se) | % | (se) | % | (se) |
| Any anxiety disorder | 20.5 | (2.2) | 41.6 | (3.9) | 37.9 | (4.0) | 25.7 | (4.7) | 34.5 | (5.7) | 39.7 | (5.3) |
| Any mood disorder | 32.8 | (3.6) | 48.4 | (4.6) | 18.8 | (3.0) | 43.8 | (6.8) | 33.9 | (4.3) | 22.3 | (6.1) |
| Any impulse-control disorders | 25.9 | (9.5) | 35.4 | (8.9) | 38.7 | (9.4) | 33.5 | (11.4) | 9.6 | (4.9) | 56.8 | (12.8) |
| Any substance disorders | – | – | – | – | – | – | 54.5 | (7.6) | 6.5 | (3.1) | 39.0 | (7.2) |
| Any disorder | 20.4 | (1.9) | 43.1 | (3.3) | 36.5 | (3.2) | 34.2 | (4.7) | 23.6 | (3.2) | 42.2 | (4.5) |

*Note:* Part 2 sample ($n = 2362$).
Assessed only for Part II sample with the age ranging from 18 to 44.

A total of 12% of Mexican males reported any 12-month disorder and a total of 14.7% of females reported so. The individual disorder with the highest 12-month prevalence was alcohol abuse for males (4.3%) and specific phobia (7.2%) for females. The most common group of disorders among males and females was anxiety disorders.

three disorders was severe for males. Mood disorders had the greatest proportion of severe cases among females (32.8%), and for males more than half of substance disorders were severe (54.5%). Anxiety disorders had the lowest distribution of severe disorders in both sexes (20.5% for females and 25.7% for males). There were too few cases of substance disorders among females for a stable estimation of the severity distribution.

## 3.2. Severity

Regarding the distribution of severity of these 12-month disorders (Table 8.3), one in every five disorders in females was severe and one in every

## 3.3. Service Use

The 12-month prevalence of any service use was 17.1% for females and 19.2% for males (Table 8.4). That is, no more than one in every

**Table 8.4.** 12-month and lifetime service usage in Mexico: Percentage treated by sectors among people with mental disorder (by sex)

| | Female | | | | | | Male | | | | | |
| --- | --- | --- | --- | --- | --- | --- | --- | --- | --- | --- | --- | --- |
| | **12-month** | | | | | | | | | | | |
| | Health care | | Non-health care | | Any | | Health care | | Non-health care | | Any | |
| | % | (se) | % | (se) | % | (se) | % | (se) | % | (se) | % | (se) |
| Any anxiety disorder | 13.9 | (2.3) | 2.5 | (1.1) | 15.3 | (2.4) | 13.8 | (4.2) | 6.5 | (3.8) | 17.8 | (5.0) |
| Any mood disorder | 17.9 | (2.2) | 4.1 | (1.4) | 21.5 | (2.7) | 25.5 | (6.2) | 7.3 | (3.8) | 29.5 | (6.3) |
| Any impulse-control disorders | 17.1 | (7.2) | 5.4 | (3.3) | 19.7 | (7.2) | 9.3 | (5.2) | 11.4 | (10.5) | 20.7 | (10.8) |
| Any substance disorders | 11.1 | (14.1) | 0.0 | (0.0) | 11.1 | (14.1) | 17.3 | (4.8) | 3.1 | (1.6) | 19.8 | (4.9) |
| Any disorder | 15.3 | (1.9) | 2.8 | (0.9) | 17.1 | (2.1) | 15.9 | (2.9) | 4.4 | (2.0) | 19.2 | (3.0) |
| | **Lifetime** | | | | | | | | | | | |
| Any anxiety disorder | 35.3 | (2.6) | 6.6 | (1.1) | 38.0 | (2.8) | 33.4 | (4.1) | 7.4 | (2.5) | 37.8 | (4.4) |
| Any mood disorder | 41.2 | (3.3) | 8.4 | (1.5) | 45.5 | (3.2) | 35.4 | (4.5) | 9.3 | (2.7) | 38.5 | (4.6) |
| Any impulse-control disorders | 43.8 | (7.7) | 10.6 | (4.0) | 48.7 | (7.3) | 26.1 | (6.3) | 7.9 | (3.8) | 31.6 | (6.7) |
| Any substance disorders | 54.2 | (14.4) | 27.8 | (10.8) | 59.8 | (13.9) | 24.4 | (3.1) | 5.1 | (1.4) | 27.1 | (3.4) |
| Any disorder | 34.7 | (2.4) | 7.1 | (1.0) | 37.5 | (2.4) | 24.6 | (2.4) | 5.1 | (1.2) | 27.2 | (2.6) |

five respondents with a psychiatric disorder in Mexico used any treatment service in the past 12 months. Mood disorder was the group that used more services for both sexes, followed by impulse-control disorders. Services were provided more frequently by the health-care sector than by the non–health-care sector. Non–health-care use was especially prevalent for impulse-control disorders in both sexes.

Lifetime treatment in Mexico was more frequent, with 37.5% of females and 27% of males using any service for treatment of a lifetime disorder. Almost 60% of any substance use disorder among females was ever treated, and almost 40% of any anxiety disorders in males was ever treated. As in 12-month treatment, most treatment is taken care of by the health-care sector. Additional analyses (Borges et al. 2008) showed that among the fraction of cases ever making treatment contacts, delays in seeking treatment were shortest for substance use disorders. Delays were longer for mood disorders and longest for anxiety disorders.

### 3.4. Cohort Effects

In previous analyses, we found that recent cohorts (18–29 years old) showed larger odds ratios in comparison with the older cohort (55+) for most groups of disorders and for "any" disorder. There was a dose-response relationship such that the younger the cohort was, the greater were the odds of having a lifetime disorder (Medina-Mora et al. 2007). We explore this association further in Tables 8.5a and 8.5b. Sex and age were associated with anxiety disorders. Among age groups, being female was consistently associated with anxiety disorders, and education was associated with anxiety disorders only for those 45–54 years old. For mood disorders, the associated variables were sex (females with higher odds), age (with the younger showing larger odds), and education (with students showing lower odds and those who did not complete high school showing larger odds). Among age groups, being female was consistently associated with mood disorders, and education was associated only for those 18–29 years old. Females

had lower odds for impulse control disorders. No other variable showed association with impulse-control disorders. Less education, being male, and being younger all had increased odds for substance use disorders, and this was consistent (although not always statistically significant) across all age groups.

### 3.5. Demographic Correlates of 12-month Psychiatric Disorder among Lifetime Cases

Prior analyses showed that age was the only variable associated with any 12-month disorder, with the younger more likely to report any disorder. Income was associated with severity, such that those with low and low-average income were more likely to report a 12-month disorder. Females were more likely to report a mood and anxiety disorder but less likely to report a substance use disorder. The younger were more likely to report an anxiety and a substance use disorder. The group of separated/widowed/divorced was more likely to report a mood and an impulse-control disorder (Medina-Mora et al. 2005). Table 8.6 shows the persistence of 12-month disorder correlates. For any disorder, females, younger age cohorts, and those with less education had greater odds of persistence. Similar correlates were found for any anxiety disorder and for mood disorders (although some variables lacked statistical significance). Among cases with a substance use disorder, females were less likely and younger respondents more likely to have a persistent disorder. It is interesting to note that, in general, for all classes of disorders, those with low income had increased odds for the persistence of disorder, but no statistically significant association was found.

### 4. DISCUSSION

The results of this survey should be interpreted in light of its limitations. The limitations common to all of the WMH surveys along with other epidemiological population surveys in general, such as sample bias, recall bias, and imperfect validity as a result of the use of nonclinical interviewers, are discussed at length in Chapters 3 and 4 of

**Table 8.5a.** Variation across cohorts in the association of sex and education with first age of onset of DSM-IV anxiety and mood disorders in the M–NCS sample

| Disorder | Education / sex / age | Total OR | Total (95% CI) | 18–29 OR | 18–29 (95% CI) | 30–44 OR | 30–44 (95% CI) | 45–54 OR | 45–54 (95% CI) | 55+ OR | 55+ (95% CI) |
|---|---|---|---|---|---|---|---|---|---|---|---|
| I. Anxiety disorders | Currently a student | 0.9 | (0.4–1.8) | 1.5 | (0.5–4.4) | 0.5 | (0.2–1.5) | 14.6* | (2.5–86.8) | 0.3 | (0.0–5.4) |
| | None/some elementary | 1.0 | (0.5–1.9) | 1.7 | (0.5–6.0) | 0.6 | (0.2–1.5) | 9.9* | (1.4–71.2) | 0.8 | (0.1–10.5) |
| | Completed elementary/some secondary | 0.9 | (0.4–1.9) | 1.3 | (0.4–4.6) | 0.5 | (0.2–1.7) | 5.7 | (0.6–52.5) | 1.9 | (0.2–20.6) |
| | Completed secondary/some high school | 0.8 | (0.4–1.7) | 1.1 | (0.3–3.9) | 0.7 | (0.3–1.9) | 1.0 | – | – | – |
| | Completed high school and more | 1.0 | – | 1.0 | – | 1.0 | – | – | – | 1.0 | – |
| | Education $\chi^2$/DF/P | 0.5 | 4/0.97 | 1.2 | 4/0.87 | 2.3 | 4/0.67 | 11.3 | 3/0.010 | 3.9 | 3/0.28 |
| | Female | 1.7* | (1.3–2.3) | 1.5* | (1.0–2.1) | 2.2* | (1.2–4.1) | 1.8 | (0.9–3.7) | 1.4 | (0.4–4.3) |
| | Male | 1.0 | – | 1.0 | – | 1.0 | – | 1.0 | – | 1.0 | – |
| | Sex $\chi^2$/DF/P | 12.6 | 1/<.001 | 4.4 | 1/0.037 | 6.2 | 1/0.013 | 2.6 | 1/0.11 | 0.3 | 1/0.57 |
| | 18–29 | 2.5* | (1.4–4.5) | – | – | – | – | – | – | – | – |
| | 30–44 | 2.2* | (1.2–4.1) | – | – | – | – | – | – | – | – |
| | 45–54 | 1.4 | (0.7–2.7) | – | – | – | – | – | – | – | – |
| | 55+ | 1.0 | – | – | – | – | – | – | – | – | – |
| | Age $\chi^2$/DF/P | 18.7 | 3/<.001 | – | – | – | – | – | – | – | – |
| | Age × Educ $\chi^2$/DF/P | – | – | – | – | – | – | – | – | 11.0 | 10/0.36 |
| | Age × Sex $\chi^2$/DF/P | – | – | – | – | – | – | – | – | 1.5 | 3/0.67 |
| II. Mood disorders | Currently a student | 0.6* | (0.4–1.0) | 0.7 | (0.3–1.4) | 0.7 | (0.3–1.7) | 0.4 | (0.1–2.5) | 1.4 | (0.1–15.3) |
| | None/some elementary | 1.1 | (0.6–1.9) | 0.7 | (0.3–1.7) | 1.0 | (0.5–1.9) | 1.7 | (0.3–9.2) | 3.8 | (0.4–39.4) |
| | Completed elementary/some secondary | 0.9 | (0.6–1.5) | 1.1 | (0.5–2.2) | 0.9 | (0.5–1.7) | 1.1 | (0.2–6.7) | 1.2 | (0.1–11.6) |
| | Completed secondary/some high school | 1.5* | (1.0–2.1) | 1.5 | (0.9–2.7) | 1.3 | (0.8–2.3) | 1.7 | (0.3–9.1) | – | – |
| | Completed high school and more | 1.0 | – | 1.0 | – | 1.0 | – | 1.0 | – | 1.0 | – |
| | Education $\chi^2$/DF/P | 28.3 | 4/<.001 | 11.7 | 4/0.020 | 3.9 | 4/0.43 | 5.6 | 4/0.24 | 2.6 | 3/0.45 |
| | Female | 1.6* | (1.2–2.2) | 1.4 | (1.0–2.0) | 1.8 | (1.0–3.1) | 2.0 | (0.7–6.0) | 4.8* | (1.6–14.4) |
| | Male | 1.0 | – | 1.0 | – | 1.0 | – | 1.0 | – | 1.0 | – |
| | Sex $\chi^2$/DF/P | 11.4 | 1/0.001 | 3.3 | 1/0.07 | 4.0 | 1/0.045 | 1.8 | 1/0.18 | 8.3 | 1/0.004 |
| | 18–29 | 5.9* | (2.5–13.8) | – | – | – | – | – | – | – | – |
| | 30–44 | 2.1 | (0.9–4.9) | – | – | – | – | – | – | – | – |
| | 45–54 | 1.5 | (0.5–4.2) | – | – | – | – | – | – | – | – |
| | 55+ | 1.0 | – | – | – | – | – | – | – | – | – |
| | Age $\chi^2$/DF/P | 90.4 | 3/<.001 | – | – | – | – | – | – | – | – |
| | Age × Educ $\chi^2$/DF/P | – | – | – | – | – | – | – | – | 17.1 | 11/0.11 |
| | Age × Sex $\chi^2$/DF/P | – | – | – | – | – | – | – | – | 5.2 | 3/0.16 |

*Note:* Models include time intervals as cohorts. Person years are restricted to 0 ≤ 29 years.

* Significant at the 0.05 level.

**Table 8.5b.** Variation across cohorts in the association of sex and education with first age of onset of DSM-IV impulse and substance disorders in the M-NCS sample

| Disorder / Education / sex / age | Total OR | Total (95% CI) | Age group 18–29 OR | 18–29 (95% CI) | 30–44 OR | 30–44 (95% CI) | 45–54 OR | 45–54 (95% CI) | 55+ OR | 55+ (95% CI) |
|---|---|---|---|---|---|---|---|---|---|---|
| **III. Impulse-control disorders** | | | | | | | | | | |
| Currently a student | 1.4 | (0.3–7.4) | 2.1 | (0.3–14.2) | 1.6 | (0.2–15.6) | – | – | – | – |
| None/some elementary | 2.2 | (0.4–11.5) | 1.3 | (0.2–8.1) | 5.7 | (0.6–49.9) | – | – | – | – |
| Completed elementary/some secondary | 1.0 | (0.2–6.0) | 0.1 | (0.0–1.6) | 6.3 | (0.5–71.6) | – | – | – | – |
| Completed secondary/some high school | 1.0 | – | 1.0 | – | 1.0 | – | – | – | – | – |
| Completed high school and more | | | | | | | | | | |
| Education $\chi^2$/DF/P | 1.5 | 3/0.69 | 6.7 | 3/0.08 | 7.2 | 3/0.07 | – | – | – | – |
| Female | 0.6* | (0.4–0.9) | 0.6 | (0.3–1.1) | 0.5* | (0.3–1.0) | – | – | – | – |
| Male | 1.0 | – | 1.0 | – | 1.0 | – | – | – | – | – |
| Sex $\chi^2$/DF/P | 5.6 | 1/0.018 | 3.1 | 1/0.08 | 4.2 | 1/0.040 | – | – | – | – |
| 18–29 | 1.6 | (1.0–2.7) | – | – | – | – | – | – | – | – |
| 30–44 | 1.0 | – | – | – | – | – | – | – | – | – |
| 45–54 | – | – | – | – | – | – | – | – | – | – |
| 55+ | – | – | – | – | – | – | – | – | – | – |
| Age $\chi^2$/DF/P | 3.4 | 1/0.07 | – | – | – | – | – | – | – | – |
| Age × Educ $\chi^2$/DF/P | – | – | – | – | – | – | – | – | 8.9 | 3/0.031 |
| Age × Sex $\chi^2$/DF/P | – | – | – | – | – | – | – | – | 0.1 | 1/0.79 |
| **IV. Substance disorders** | | | | | | | | | | |
| Currently a student | 0.2* | (0.1–0.4) | 0.2* | (0.1–0.5) | 0.2* | (0.1–0.6) | 0.4 | (0.1–1.8) | – | – |
| None/some elementary | 2.8* | (1.4–5.9) | 2.3 | (0.7–7.5) | 2.5* | (1.1–5.9) | 2.6 | (0.7–9.8) | 0.7 | (0.2–2.5) |
| Completed elementary/some secondary | 2.0* | (1.1–3.7) | 2.3 | (0.9–6.0) | 1.9 | (0.6–5.4) | 1.4 | (0.4–4.3) | 0.2* | (0.03–0.8) |
| Completed secondary/some high school | 1.9* | (1.0–3.4) | 2.1 | (0.8–5.6) | 1.6 | (0.7–4.0) | 0.7 | (0.2–2.1) | 1.0 | – |
| Completed high school and more | 1.0 | – | 1.0 | – | 1.0 | – | 1.0 | – | – | – |
| Education $\chi^2$/DF/P | 103.8 | 4/<0.001 | 53.1 | 4/<0.001 | 48.5 | 4/<0.001 | 9.3 | 4/0.05 | 5.8 | 2/0.06 |
| Female | 0.1* | (0.0–0.1) | 0.1* | (0.0–0.2) | 0.1* | (0.0–0.1) | 0.050* | (0.0–0.2) | 0.0* | (0.0–0.2) |
| Male | 1.0 | – | 1.0 | – | 1.0 | – | 1.0 | – | 1.0 | – |
| Sex $\chi^2$/DF/P | 140.3 | 1/<0.001 | 34.4 | 1/<0.001 | 60.4 | 1/<0.001 | 15.6 | 1/<0.001 | 15.7 | 1/<0.001 |
| 18–29 | 4.3* | (2.4–7.6) | – | – | – | – | – | – | – | – |
| 30–44 | 1.9* | (1.2–3.0) | – | – | – | – | – | – | – | – |
| 45–54 | 1.7 | (0.9–3.2) | – | – | – | – | – | – | – | – |
| 55+ | 1 | – | – | – | – | – | – | – | – | – |
| Age $\chi^2$/DF/P | 40.4 | 3/<0.001 | – | – | – | – | – | – | – | – |
| Age × Educ $\chi^2$/DF/P | – | – | – | – | – | – | – | – | 10.5 | 10/0.40 |
| Age × Sex $\chi^2$/DF/P | – | – | – | – | – | – | – | – | 1.4 | 3/0.72 |

*Note:* Models include time intervals as cohorts. Person years are restricted to $0 \le 29$ years.

* Significant at the 0.05 level.

**Table 8.6.** Demographic correlates of persistence of 12-month DSM-IV disorders using Part 2 weights after stratification among those with a lifetime disorder

| Risk factor | Any 12-month disorder OR | (95% CI) | Anxiety OR | (95% CI) | Mood OR | (95% CI) | Impulse control OR | (95% CI) | Substance OR | (95% CI) |
|---|---|---|---|---|---|---|---|---|---|---|
| **Sex** | | | | | | | | | | |
| Male | 1.0 | – | 1.0 | – | 1.0 | – | 1.0 | – | 1.0 | – |
| Female | 1.8 | (1.2–2.7) | 1.5 | (0.9–2.5) | 1.2 | (0.7–2.1) | 1.0 | (0.3–2.8) | 0.2 | (0.0–1.0) |
| $\chi^2$ | 9.2* | | 2.1 | | 0.4 | | 0.0 | | 4.2* | |
| **Age** | | | | | | | | | | |
| 18–29 | 2.9 | (1.6–5.1) | 1.3 | (0.5–3.2) | 2.2 | (1.1–4.4) | 1.0 | (0.3–3.5) | 43.7 | (5.7–331.7) |
| 30–44 | 1.5 | (0.8–2.7) | 0.6 | (0.2–1.6) | 1.2 | (0.6–2.4) | 1.0 | – | 12.6 | (1.7–92.0) |
| 45–54 | 1.1 | (0.6–2.0) | 0.8 | (0.3–1.9) | 1.0 | (0.4–2.3) | – | – | 3.7 | (0.4–31.7) |
| 55≤ | 1.0 | – | 1.0 | – | 1.0 | – | – | – | 1.0 | – |
| $\chi^2$ | 20.8* | | 10.2* | | 8.9* | | 0.0 | | 10.6* | |
| **Income** | | | | | | | | | | |
| Low | 1.4 | (0.8–2.6) | 1.8 | (0.9–3.7) | 1.3 | (0.6–2.7) | 2.6 | (0.4–16.3) | 1.7 | (0.6–5.4) |
| Low-average | 1.2 | (0.7–1.8) | 1.7 | (0.9–3.0) | 1.5 | (0.8–2.8) | 2.9 | (0.7–11.2) | 0.9 | (0.3–2.4) |
| High-average | 1.0 | (0.6–1.7) | 1.2 | (0.6–2.4) | 1.0 | (0.5–1.8) | 2.0 | (0.5–7.6) | 0.6 | (0.2–1.7) |
| High | 1.0 | – | 1.0 | – | 1.0 | – | 1.0 | – | 1.0 | – |
| $\chi^2$ | 1.8 | | 4.7 | | 2.6 | | 2.6 | | 6.1 | |
| **Marital status** | | | | | | | | | | |
| Married/cohabiting | 1.0 | – | 1.0 | – | 1.0 | – | 1.0 | – | 1.0 | – |
| Separated/widowed/divorced | 1.3 | (0.8–2.1) | 1.2 | (0.6–2.4) | 1.1 | (0.6–2.2) | 4.0 | (0.9–17.7) | 2.4 | (0.6–9.2) |
| Never married | 1.3 | (0.9–1.9) | 1.5 | (0.8–2.8) | 0.9 | (0.5–1.6) | 2.3 | (0.7–8.1) | 0.6 | (0.2–1.7) |
| $\chi^2$ | 2.6 | | 2.1 | | 0.5 | | 5.2 | | 3.4 | |
| **Education** | | | | | | | | | | |
| 0–5 years | 1.9 | (1.2–3.1) | 1.5 | (0.8–2.6) | 1.9 | (0.9–3.8) | 0.3 | (0.1–1.0) | 2.0 | (0.5–7.7) |
| 6–8 years | 1.7 | (1.1–2.7) | 1.7 | (0.9–3.2) | 2.0 | (1.0–3.9) | 1.3 | (0.4–4.5) | 1.2 | (0.4–3.4) |
| 9–11 years | 1.3 | (0.9–1.9) | 1.3 | (0.8–2.1) | 1.3 | (0.7–2.5) | 0.7 | (0.2–1.9) | 1.5 | (0.5–4.3) |
| 12 or more years | 1.0 | – | 1.0 | – | 1.0 | – | 1.0 | – | 1.0 | – |
| $\chi^2$ | 9.4* | | 3.4 | | 6.4 | | 6.4 | | 1.3 | |

* Significant at the 0.05 level, two-sided test.

this volume and will not be repeated here. However, there are other limitations that are specific to the M-NCS that are worthy of mention. One such limitation is the exclusion of the rural population, which represents 25% of the national population as well as the non–Spanish-speaking population, and primarily comprises indigenous people living in rural areas. Local surveys conducted among specific rural populations in Mexico have documented lower prevalence rates of mental disorders in general, with the exception of alcohol abuse and dependence, which are higher (Medina-Mora et al. 2004). Rates of service use are considerably lower in rural areas than in the urban parts of the country (Salgado & Díaz-Pérez 1999; Berenzon, Medina-Mora & Lara 2003); mental disorders often go untreated, as access to adequate service often requires a day's journey or more, representing a high cost. There is also a cultural and often linguistic gap between those needing treatment services and the caregivers. Another such limitation is the exclusion of the elderly population over the age of 65, which most likely contributes to an underestimation of certain disorders such as major depression, the incidence of which may increase in later life (Wagner, Gallo & Delva 1999).

Stigma toward mental disorders may also contribute to an underestimation of prevalence. Although in other countries the population has become more accustomed to the open discussion of mental disorders and thus is more informed, mental disorders in Mexico are less publicly visible and charged with much stigma and shame. Despite this, however, we found that participants, once they began the interview, had a great need and desire to talk to interviewers about their mental health problems, many times sharing information that they had never previously revealed to anyone.

Willingness to disclose emotional problems was presumably related to privacy, and it is important to note that privacy during interview administration was sometimes a challenge because of housing conditions in which many family members live. Although interviewers made exceptional efforts to find ways to afford the participants privacy such as conducting

interviews on the front steps, in one case on the hood of a car, and during hours when the husband was at work (this was at times requested by female participants), interviews sometimes had to be conducted in the presence of young children or extended family members.

Finally, although evidence of the reliability and validity of different versions of the CIDI has been documented in different countries (Farmer et al. 1987; Janca et al. 1992; Wacker et al. 1990), studies of the reliability and validity of the Spanish-language CIDI version used in this survey have not been conducted. Pretesting before the beginning of fieldwork with a convenience sample and a very small inpatient clinical sample suggested that participants understood the items and that the CIDI diagnoses corresponded to the clinical diagnoses of the inpatients; however, these conclusions were not based on broad-based empirical investigation. Furthermore, as Feinstein (1987) has pointed out, subjective phenomena cannot be measured against a gold standard, so criterion validity cannot truly be achieved. There have been some attempts to solve this problem, such as the proposal of Faraone and Tsuang (1994) regarding latent class analysis. Other proposals are to determine consistency (Feinstein 1987), and Kessler and colleagues (2004) proposed the use of the area under the ROC curve as a statistical index. Without a real gold standard, though, another possibility is to rely on construct validity, as defined by Feinstein (1987) as how well the instrument works. The wide usage of the Spanish-language CIDI in varying Spanish-speaking countries and communities (Caraveo, Martínez & Rivera 1998; Dwight-Johnson et al. 2000; Ruiz et al. 1996; Vega et al. 1998b; Vicente et al. 2002) and the theoretical consistency of most results should be viewed as partial evidence of validity.

Despite these limitations, the M-NCS also has strengths not often present in population surveys. One such strength was the organization of the supervision of fieldwork. Supervision was not conducted by phone or by listening to audiotapes but rather in person. Two types of supervisors traveled around the country with their teams of interviewers: logistic supervisors, primarily responsible for assuring that the proper procedures for household and participant selection were adhered to, and conceptual supervisors, who were members of the research team who sat in on face-to-face interviews throughout the entire period of fieldwork. They gave personal and immediate feedback to the interviewers on presentation, following informed consent procedures and the administration of the interview as well as circulating bulletins among all interviewers of areas to be strengthened.

The Mexican population has not yet been bombarded with being asked to participate in surveys as has occurred in many developed nations and (not considering the largest metropolitan areas where violence and crime are a concern) was very open to allowing strangers into their homes. Thus, the direct refusal rate was very low and much of the nonresponse was due to the organization of fieldwork in which interviewer teams were only in each region of the country for a short period of time.

Finally the most important contribution of this study is that it provides the first nationally representative estimates of psychiatric disorders in Mexico. The aim is to provide epidemiological data useful for guiding public health policy and planning for Mexico. Although the overall rate of any psychiatric disorder in Mexico is in the middle range as compared to the other participating countries in the WMH Survey Consortium (Demyttenaere et al. 2004), a dramatic 40% increase in lifetime risk is projected by age 65, representing one in every three Mexicans (Medina-Mora et al. 2007). This projection presents an important challenge to the health system, especially considering the low rates of service use and even lower rates of receiving minimally adequate health services.

Alcohol abuse, major depression, and specific phobia are the most prevalent mental disorders facing the Mexican adult population. Attention directed at substance use disorders is particularly important because that disorder group contains the largest proportion of severe cases. Mood disorders must also be a priority for future health policy planning because the older ages of onset and the aging of the Mexican population will contribute to an increase in the current prevalence estimate. Although substance disorders and major depression tend to be more serious, timely treatment of the very frequent but less severe earlier-onset anxiety disorders such as specific phobia may prevent the onset of other more severe disorders in the future. Schizophrenia, a very disabling mental disorder, was not evaluated in this survey, and its omission in our discussion is by no means a reflection of its unimportance as a mental health problem.

Treatment for mental health disorders in Mexico is a rarity; fewer than one in five of those with a disorder in the prior 12 months made any treatment contact. The limited service use for mental health disorders should be viewed in light of treatment availability. According to the recent World Health Report (WHO 2006), the mental health specialty team ideally should be composed of medical and nonmedical professionals: psychiatrists, general practitioners and other nonpsychiatric medical doctors, psychologists, psychiatric nurses, psychiatric social workers, occupational therapists, and other groups such as priests and traditional healers. In Mexico, by 1976, there were approximately 507 psychiatrists, mostly found in the largest cities, an alarmingly insufficient number. In the *World Mental Health Atlas* (WHO 2005), the number of psychiatrists was estimated as 2.7 per 100,000 inhabitants; of these, only 1451 psychiatrists were registered with the National Board of Psychiatrists in 2005, with a ratio of 1.5 per 100,000 inhabitants. The number of psychiatric nurses was grouped in the range of zero to one per 100,000 inhabitants in the atlas.

The largest health provider in Mexico, the Mexican Institute of Social Security, with 42,993,343 affiliates in 2004, employed only 244 psychiatrists, which clearly reflects insufficient human resources for the care of mental illnesses. The most recently created government-funded health provider, the Popular Insurance, as of 2005 had affiliated 11,404,861 persons. Although the number of mental health workers is not specified, the recent Catalogue of Universal Services (Comisión Nacional de Protección Social en Salud 2006) has included some limited aims in regard to mental health. Among 20 preventive aims, 3 are related to mental health: diagnosis and counseling for alcoholism, diagnosis and counseling for smoking in adolescents, and detection of attention-deficit/hyperactivity disorder. Ambulatory medicine includes 83 aims, only 2 of which are related to mental health. One is the diagnosis and treatment of depression including one general consultation and three subsequent follow-up consultations at two-month intervals, two specialty consultations at six months, and annual pharmacological treatment. The drugs included are fluoxetine, diazepam, clonazepam, and amitriptyline.

The other mental health–related aim is the diagnosis and treatment of psychosis, for which the same treatment scheme is proposed and includes the following medications: clozapine, risperidone, zuclopenthixol, haloperidol, lithium, diazepam, biperidene, amitriptyline, tioridazine, and trifluoperazine. Although the treatment scheme and list of medications are far from optimal, the inclusion of some minimal treatment for two mental health disorders in the Popular Insurance is a step in the right direction, considering that private insurance in Mexico explicitly excludes all mental health coverage. For example, the clause of one private health insurance states, "Exclusions applicable to all coverage (1) Mental disorders, depression, hysteria, stress, neurosis or psychosis, psychological, psychomotor, language, or learning problems whatever their manifestations" (Inburmedic & Inbursa 2005).

With one in four Mexicans having suffered a mental disorder in their lifetime and projections that one in three will do so by the age of 65, in conjunction with the abysmally low service use rates and the panorama of service availability, policy makers in public health urgently need to take action to consider mental disorders as chronic illnesses with legitimate rights to treatment as is afforded to other "nonmental" illnesses. But the challenge does not stop there; public awareness as to the existence of effective treatments and destigmatization of mental disorders is important to increase treatment demand among those affected. To meet that treatment demand, of

course, requires a greater number of mental health professionals; a redistribution and a greater allocation of resources as well as legislation is needed to ensure the availability of effective psychotherapies and medications, the modalities of which are matched to patients' needs, including culturally consonant self-perceived needs. Because these results show that the people with the lowest income have the most severe disorders, special treatment strategies to reach this vulnerable population are necessary.

Timely treatment is needed especially in the younger population, because the early onset of disorders is associated with a greater delay in treatment contact. Not receiving treatment for first-episode, early-onset depression, for example, is associated with more recurrent episodes throughout one's life (Benjet et al. 2004). As in other countries (Kessler et al. 2005; Bromet et al. 2005), psychiatric disorders have early ages of onset in Mexico. Fifty percent of the population who present a psychiatric disorder do so by the age of 21, thus affecting the population throughout a large portion of their lifetime. Early ages of onset may have far-reaching repercussions given the important developmental tasks of the first decades of life, which include, among other things, educational attainment, career choice, and selection of romantic partners.

Because the majority of people in Mexico have not sought treatment, the magnitude, severity, and largely unmet treatment needs have gone undetected or insufficiently appreciated in the public health sector. These data are available to guide in the planning and allocation of resources for the detection and treatment of mental illnesses, to prioritize specific disorders and risk groups in need of particular attention, and to form public policy regarding the availability and distribution of mental health specialty services and professionals throughout the country, as well as mechanisms of detection and referrals. The recent emergence of the new government-funded health provider for the poorest sector of society including more than 11 million people is an opportunity for government and the health ministry to translate epidemiological data such as these into action. Mexico cannot afford to lose this opportunity.

## REFERENCES

Aguilera, R. M., Salgado, N., Romero, M. & Medina-Mora, M. E. (2004). Paternal absence and international migration stressors and compensators associated with the mental health of Mexican teenagers of rural origin. *Adolescence*, 39, 711–23.

American Psychiatric Association (1994). *Diagnostic and statistical manual of mental disorders (DSM-IV)*, 4th ed. Washington, DC: American Psychiatric Association.

Benjet, C., Borges, G., Medina-Mora, M. E., Fleiz-Bautista, C. & Zambrano-Ruiz, J. (2004). Early onset depression: Prevalence, course, and treatment seeking delay. *Salud Pública de México*, 46, 417–24.

Berenzon, S., Medina-Mora, M. E. & Lara, M. A. (2003). Servicios de salud mental: Veinticinco años de investigación. *Salud Mental*, 26, 61–72.

Berenzon, S., Tiburcio, M. & Medina-Mora, M. E. (2005). Variables demográficas asociadas con la depresión: Diferencias entre hombres y mujeres que habitan en zonas urbanas de bajos ingresos. *Salud Mental*, 28, 33–40.

Borges, G., Mondragon, L., Cherpitel, C., Ye, Y. & Rosovsky, H. (2003). El consumo de bebidas alcohólicas y los servicios de urgencias: Estudios realizados por el Instituto Nacional de Psiquiatría Ramón de la Fuente. 1986–2003. *Salud Mental*, 26, 19–27.

Borges, G., Wang, P. S., Medina-Mora, M. E., Lara, C. & Chiu, W. T. (2007). Delay to first treatment of mental and substance use disorders in Mexico. *American Journal of Public Health*, 97, 1630–43.

Bromet, E. J., Gluzman, S. F., Paniotto, V. I., Webb, C. P., Tintle, N. L., Zakhozha, V., Havenaar, J. M., Gutkovich, Z., Kostyuchenko, S. & Schwartz, J. E. (2005). Epidemiology of psychiatric and alcohol disorders in Ukraine: Findings from the Ukraine World Mental Health survey. *Social Psychiatry and Psychiatric Epidemiology*, 40, 681–90.

Campillo, S. C., Medina-Mora, M. E., Martínez, L. P. & Caraveo, A. J. (1979). Cuestionario (GHQ) de detección de posibles casos psiquiátricos en una comunidad. *Cuadernos Científicos CEMESAM*, 11, 43–44.

Caraveo, A. J., Martínez, N. & Rivera, E. (1998). Un modelo para estudios epidemiológicos sobre la salud mental y la morbilidad psiquiátrica. *Salud Mental*, 21, 48–57.

Caraveo, J. (1996). La prevalencia de los trastornos psiquiátricos en la población mexicana: Estado actual y perspectivas. *Salud Mental*, 19 (suppl.), 8–13.

Caraveo, J., González, C. & Ramos, L. (1991). The concurrent validity of the DIS: Experience with psychiatric patients in México City. *Hispanic Journal of Behavioral Sciences*, 13, 63–77.

Caraveo, J., González, C., Ramos, L. & Mendoza, P. (1986). Necesidades y demandas de atención en los servicios de salud mental. *Salud Pública de México*, 28, 504–14.

Caraveo, J., Martínez, N. A., Rivera, E. & Polo, A. (1997). Prevalencia en la vida de episodios depresivos y utilización de servicios especializados. *Salud Mental*, 20, 15–23.

Centros de Integración Juvenil (2005). *Sistema de Información Epidemiológica del Consumo de Drogas (SIECD)*. Mexico City: Centros de Integración Juvenil.

Comisión Nacional de Protección Social en Salud (2006). *Seguro Popular: Catálogo universal de servicios de salud 2006*. Mexico City: Secretaría de Salud.

Consejo Nacional de Población (2005). *Migración México-Estados Unidos. Temas de Salud*, Document number 970–628-840–6. Mexico City: Consejo Nacional de Población.

Demyttenaere, K., Bruffaerts, R., Posada-Villa, J., Gasquet, I., Kovess, V., Lepine, J. P., Angermeyer, M. C., Bernert, S., de Girolamo, G., Morosini, P., Polidori, G., Kikkawa, T., Kawakami, N., Ono, Y., Takeshima, T., Uda, H., Karam, E. G., Fayyad, J. A., Karam, A. N., Mneimneh, Z. N., Medina-Mora, M. E., Borges, G., Lara, G., de Graaf, R., Ormel, J., Gureje, O., Shen, Y., Huang, Y., Zhang, M., Alonso, J., Haro, J. M., Vilagut, G., Bromet, E. J., Gluzman, S., Webb, C., Kessler, R. C., Merikangas, K. R., Anthony, J. C., Korff, M. R. V., Wang, P. S., Alonso, J., Brugha, T. S., Aguilar-Gaxiola, S., Lee, S., Heeringa, S., Pennell, B. E., Zaslavsky, A. M., Üstün, T. B. & Chatterji, S. (2004). Prevalence, severity and unmet need for treatment of mental disorders in the World Health Organization World Mental Health Surveys. *Journal of the American Medical Association*, 291, 2581–90.

Dwight-Johnson, M., Sherbourne, C. D., Liao, D. & Wells, K. B. (2000). Treatment preferences among depressed primary care patients. *Journal of General Internal Medicine*, 15, 527–34.

Efron, B. (1988). Logistic regression, survival analysis, and the Kaplan-Meier curve. *Journal of the American Statistical Association*, 83, 414–25.

Endicott, J., Spitzer, R. L., Fleiss, J. L. & Cohen, J. (1976). The global assessment scale: A procedure for measuring overall severity of psychiatric disturbance. *Archives of General Psychiatry*, 33, 766–71.

Ezban, M., Medina-Mora, M. E., Peláez, O. & Padilla, P. (1984). Sensibilidad del cuestionario general de salud de Goldberg para detectar la evolución de pacientes en tratamiento psiquiátrico. *Salud Mental*, 7, 68–71.

Faraone, S. V. & Tsuang, M. T. (1994). Measuring diagnostic accuracy in the absence of a "gold standard." *American Journal of Psychiatry*, 151, 650–7.

Farmer, A. E., Katz, R., McGuffin, P. & Bebbington, P. A. (1987). Comparison between the Present State Examination and the Composite International Diagnostic Interview. *Archives of General Psychiatry*, 44, 1064–8.

Feinstein, A. R. (1987). *Clinimetrics.* New Haven, CT: Yale University Press.

Frenk, J., Ruelas, E., Bobadilla, J. L., Zurita, B., Lozano, R., González-Block, M. A., Cruz, C., Álvarez F. & González, A. (1999). Economía y salud: Propuesta para el avance del sistema de salud en México. Mexico City: Fundación Mexicana para la Salud.

Gómez, E., Morales, F., Aretia, A. & Gutiérrez, E. (1990). Detección de alteraciones emocionales en pacientes obstétricas y ginecológicas. *Ginecología y Obstetricia de México*, 58, 112–6.

Hosmer, D. W. & Lemeshow, S. (2000). *Applied logistic regression*, 2d ed. New York: John Wiley & Sons.

Inburmedic & Inbursa (2005). *General conditions for insurance from Inburmedic & Inbursa.* Mexico City: Inburmedic & Inbursa.

Instituto Nacional de Estadística Geografía e Informática (2002). *Encuesta nacional de ingresos y gastos.* Mexico City: Instituto Nacional de Estadística Geografía e Informática.

Janca, A., Üstün, T. B., Drimmelenm, V. & Dittman, C. (1992). *ICD-10 symptoms checklist version 1.0.* Geneva: World Health Organization.

Kessler, R. C., Abelson, J., Demler, O., Escobar, J. I. Gibbon, M., Guyer, M. E., Howes, M. J., Jin, R., Vega, W. A., Walters, E. E., Wang, P., Zaslavsky, A. & Zheng, H. (2004). Clinical calibration of DSM-IV diagnoses in the World Mental Health (WMH) version of the World Health Organization (WHO) Composite International Diagnostic Interview (WMHCIDI). *International Journal of Methods in Psychiatric Research*, 13, 122–39.

Kessler, R. C., Berglund, P., Demler, O., Jin, R., Merikangas, K. R. & Walters, E. E. (2005). Lifetime prevalence and age-of-onset distributions of DSM-IV disorders in the National Comorbidity Survey Replication. *Archives of General Psychiatry*, 62, 593–602.

Kessler, R. C., Haro, J. M., Heeringa, S. G., Pennell, B.-E. & Üstün, T. B. (2006). The World Health Organization World Mental Health Survey Initiative. *Epidemiologia e Psichiatria Sociale*, 15, 161–6.

Kessler, R. C. & Üstün, T. B. (2004). The World Mental Health (WMH) Survey Initiative Version of the World Health Organization (WHO) Composite International Diagnostic Interview (CIDI). *International Journal of Methods in Psychiatric Research*, 13, 93–121.

Medina-Mora, M. E. (1978). Prevalencia del consumo de drogas en algunas ciudades de la República Mexicana: Encuesta de hogares. *Revista de Enseñanza en Investigación Psicológica*, 4, 111–5.

Medina-Mora, M. E. (2000). Abuso de sustancias. In *Estudio de Niñas, Niños y Jóvenes Trabajadores en el Distrito Federal, DIF-DF & UNICEF, Editors.* pp. 119–37. Mexico City: UNICEF.

Medina-Mora, M. E., Berenzon, S., López, E. K., Solís, L., Caballero, M. A. & González, J. (1997). Uso de los servicios de salud por los pacientes con trastornos mentales: Resultados de una encuesta en una población de escasos recursos. *Salud Mental*, 20, 32–8.

Medina-Mora, M. E, Borges G., Benjet, C., Lara, C. & Berglund, P. (2007). Psychiatric disorders in México: Lifetime prevalence in a nationally representative sample. *British Journal of Psychiatry*, 190, 521–8.

Medina-Mora, M. E., Borges, G., Lara, C., Benjet, C., Blanco, J., Fleiz, C., Villatoro, J., Rojas, E. & Zambrano, J. (2005). Prevalence, service use, and demographic correlates of 12-month DSM-IV psychiatric disorders in Mexico: Results from the Mexican National Comorbidity Survey. *Psychological Medicine*, 35, 1773–83.

Medina-Mora, M. E., Borges, G., Lara, C., Benjet, C., Blanco, J., Fleiz, C., Villatoro, J., Rojas, E., Zambrano, J., Casanova, L. & Aguilar-Gaxiola, S. (2003). Prevalencia de trastornos mentales y uso de servicios: Resultados de la Encuesta Nacional de Epidemiología Psiquiátrica en México. *Salud Mental*, 26, 1–16.

Medina-Mora, M. E., Borges, G. & Villatoro, J. (2000). The measurement of drinking patterns and consequences in Mexico. *Journal of Substance Abuse*, 12, 183–96.

Medina-Mora, M. E. & Fleiz, C. (2003). La salud mental y las adicciones: Retos, barreras y perspectivas. *Cuadernos de Nutrición*, 26, 69–76.

Medina-Mora, M. E., Natera, G., Borges, G., Cravioto, P., Fleiz, C. & Tapia, R. (2001a). Del siglo XX al tercer milenio. Las adicciones y la salud pública: Drogas, alcohol y sociedad. *Salud Mental*, 24, 3–19.

Medina-Mora, M. E., Padilla, P., Campillo, C., Mas, C., Ezban, M., Caraveo, J. & Corona, J. (1983). Factor structure of the General Health Questionnaire GHQ: A scaled version for a hospital's general practice service in Mexico. *Psychological Medicine*, 13, 355–61.

Medina-Mora, M. E., Rascón, M. L., Tapia, E. R., Mariño, M. C., Juárez, F., Villatoro, J., Caraveo, J. & Gómez, E. M. (1993). Trastornos emocionales en población urbana mexicana: Resultados de un estudio nacional. *Anales 3, Reseña de la VII Reunión de*

*Investigación, Instituto Mexicano de Psiquiatría*, 48–55.

Medina-Mora, M. E., Villatoro, J., Caraveo, J. & Colmenares, E. (2001b). Patterns of alcohol consumption and related problems in Mexico: Results from two general population surveys. In *Surveys of drinking patterns and problems in seven developing countries*, ed. A. Demers, R. Room & C. Bourgault, pp. 13–31. Geneva: World Health Organization.

Medina-Mora, M. E., Villatoro, J., Cravioto, P., Fleiz, C., Galván, F., Rojas, E., Castrejón, J. & Kuri, P. (2004). Uso y abuso de alcohol en México: Resultados de la Encuesta Nacional de Adicciones 2002. Consejo Nacional Contra las Adicciones. In *Observatorio mexicano en tabaco, alcohol y otras drogas 2003*, pp. 49–61. Mexico City: Consejo Nacional Contra las Adicciones.

Medina-Mora, M. E., Villatoro, J. & Fleiz, C. (1999). Uso indebido de sustancias. In *Estudio de niños, niñas y adolescentes entre 6 y 17 años: Trabajadores en 100 ciudades*, 7–39, UNICEF, DIF, PNUFID editors, ISBN: 970-9074-03-2, México.

Merikangas, K. R., Mehta, R., Molnar, B. E., Walters, E. E., Swendsen, J. D., Aguilar-Gaxiola, S. A., Bijl, R., Borges, G., Caraveo, A. J., Dewit, D. J., Kolody, B., Vega, A. Wittchen, H. & Kessler, R. C. (1998). Comorbidity of substance use disorders with mood and anxiety disorders: Results of the international consortium in psychiatric epidemiology. *Addictive Behaviors*, 23, 893–907.

Padilla, P., Mas, C., Ezban, M., Medina-Mora, M. E. & Peláez, O. (1984). Frecuencia de trastornos mentales en pacientes que asisten a la consulta médica general de un Centro de Salud. *Salud Mental*, 7, 72–8.

Programa de las Naciones Unidas para el Desarrollo (2006). Indicadores del desarrollo humano. In *Informe sobre desarrollo humano 2005*, pp. 141–236. Madrid: Mundi-Prensa.

Research Triangle Institute (2002). *SUDAAN: Professional software for survey data analysis 8.01*. Research Triangle Park, NC: Research Triangle Institute.

Robins, L. N., Wing, J., Wittchen, H. U., Helzer, J. E., Babor, T. F., Burke, J., Farmer, A., Jablenski, A., Pickens, R., Regier, D. A., Sartorius, N. & Towle, L. H. (1988). The Composite International Diagnostic Interview: An epidemiologic instrument suitable for use in conjunction with different diagnostic systems and in different cultures. *Archives of General Psychiatry*, 45, 1069–77.

Romero, M. & Medina-Mora, M. E. (1987). Validez de una versión del Cuestionario General de Salud, para detectar psicopatología en estudiantes universitarios. *Salud Mental*, 10, 90–7.

Rubio-Stipec, M., Bravo, M. & Canino, G. (1991). La entrevista diagnóstica Internacional compuesta (CIDI): Un instrumento epidemiológico adecuado para ser administrado conjuntamente con otros sistemas diagnósticos en diferentes culturas. *Acta Psiquiátrica y Psicológica de América Latina*, 37, 191–204.

Ruiz, A., Blanco, R., Arcos, M., Santander, J. & San Martin, A. (1996). Genetic factors study in family aggregation of schizophrenia in Santiago, Chile. *Revista Médica de Chile*, 124, 1447–52 (in Spanish).

Salgado, V. N. & Díaz-Pérez, M. J. (1999). Los trastornos afectivos en la población rural. *Salud Mental*, 22, 68–74.

SAMHSA, Office of Applied Studies (2001). *SAMHSA National Household Survey on Drug Abuse*. Rockville, MD: SAMHSA.

Secretaría de Desarrollo Social (2002). *Comité técnico para la medición de la pobreza: Medición de la pobreza, variantes metodológicas y estimación preliminar*. Mexico City: Secretaría de Desarrollo Social.

Secretaría de Desarrollo Social (2005). *Gabinete de Desarrollo Humano y Social. Los objetivos de desarrollo del milenio en México: Informe de avances 2005*. Mexico City: Secretaría de Desarrollo Social.

Secretaría de Salud, Dirección General de Epidemiología (1988). *Encuesta nacional de adicciones*. Mexico City: Secretaría de Salud.

Secretaría de Salud, Dirección General de Epidemiología (1993). *Encuesta nacional de adicciones*. Mexico City: Secretaría de Salud.

Secretaría de Salud, Dirección General de Epidemiología (1998). *Encuesta nacional de adicciones*. Mexico City: Secretaría de Salud.

Secretaría de Salud, Dirección General de Epidemiología (2002). *Encuesta nacional de adicciones*. Mexico City: Secretaría de Salud.

Sheehan, D. V., Harnett-Sheehan, K. & Raj, B. A. (1996). The measurement of disability. *International Clinical Psychopharmacology*, 11, 89–95.

SISVEA (2005). *Secretaría de Salud, Subsecretaría de Prevención y Control de Enfermedades Sistema de Vigilancia Epidemiológica en Adicciones*. Mexico City: SISVEA.

Tapia-Conyer, R., Medina-Mora, M. E., Sepúlveda, J., De la Fuente, R. & Kumate, J. (1990). La encuesta nacional de adicciones en México. *Salud Pública de México*, 32, 507–22.

Vega, W. A., Alderete, E., Kolody, B. & Aguilar-Gaxiola, S. (1998a). Illicit drug use among Mexicans and Mexican Americans in California: The effects of gender and acculturation. *Addiction*, 93, 1839–50.

Vega, W. A., Kolody, B., Aguilar-Gaxiola, S., Alderete, E., Catalano, R. & Caraveo-Anduaga, J. (1998b). Lifetime prevalence of DSM-III-R psychiatric disorders among urban and rural Mexican Americans in California. *Archives of General Psychiatry*, 55, 771–8.

Vicente, B., Rioseco, P., Saldivia, S., Kohn, R. & Torres, S. (2002). Chilean study on the prevalence of psychiatric disorders (DSM-III-R/CIDI) (ECPP). *Revista Médica de Chile*, 130, 527–36 (in Spanish).

Villatoro, J., Medina-Mora, M. E., Cravioto, P., Fleiz, C., Galván, F., Rojas, E., Castrejón, J., Kuri, P. & García, A. (2004). Uso y abuso de drogas en México: Resultados de Encuesta Nacional de adicciones 2002. In *Observatorio mexicano en tabaco, alcohol y otras drogas 2003*, pp. 71–84. Mexico City: Consejo Nacional Contra las Adicciones.

Wacker, H. R., Battegay, R., Mullejans, R. & Schlosser, C. (1990). Using the CIDI-C in the general population. In *Psychiatry: A world perspective*, ed.

C. N. Stefanis, A. D. Rabavilas & C. R. Soldatos, pp. 138–43. Amsterdam: Elsevier Science.

Wagner, F. A., Gallo, J. J. & Delva, J. (1999). Depression in late life: A hidden public health problem for Mexico? *Salud Publica de México*, 41, 189–202.

WHO International Consortium in Psychiatric Epidemiology (2000). Cross-national comparisons of the prevalences and correlates of mental disorders. *Bulletin of the World Health Organization*, 78, 413–26.

World Health Organization (WHO) (2005). *World mental health atlas*. Geneva: World Health Organization.

World Health Organization (WHO) (2006). *The world health report: Working together for health*. Geneva: World Health Organization.

# 9 The National Comorbidity Survey Replication (NCS-R): Cornerstone in Improving Mental Health and Mental Health Care in the United States

RONALD C. KESSLER, PATRICIA A. BERGLUND, WAI-TAT CHIU, OLGA
DEMLER, MEYER GLANTZ, MICHAEL A. LANE, ROBERT JIN, KATHLEEN
RIES MERIKANGAS, MATTHEW NOCK, MARK OLFSON, HAROLD A.
PINCUS, ELLEN E. WALTERS, PHILIP S. WANG, AND KENNETH B. WELLS

## ACKNOWLEDGMENTS

The National Comorbidity Survey Replication (NCS-R) is supported by the National Institute of Mental Health (NIMH) (U01-MH60220) with supplemental support from the National Institute on Drug Abuse (NIDA), the Substance Abuse and Mental Health Services Administration (SAMHSA), the Robert Wood Johnson Foundation (RWJF; Grant 044780), and the John W. Alden Trust. Collaborating NCS-R investigators include Ronald C. Kessler (principal investigator, Harvard Medical School), Kathleen Merikangas (co–principal investigator, NIMH), James Anthony (Michigan State University), William Eaton (Johns Hopkins University), Meyer Glantz (NIDA), Doreen Koretz (Harvard University), Jane McLeod (Indiana University), Mark Olfson (New York State Psychiatric Institute, College of Physicians and Surgeons of Columbia University), Harold Pincus (University of Pittsburgh), Greg Simon (Group Health Cooperative), Michael Von Korff (Group Health Cooperative), Philip Wang (Harvard Medical School), Kenneth Wells (UCLA), Elaine Wethington (Cornell University), and Hans-Ulrich Wittchen (Max Planck Institute of Psychiatry, Technical University of Dresden). The views and opinions expressed in this report are those of the authors and should not be construed to represent the views of any of the sponsoring organizations, agencies, or U.S. government. We thank Julie Berenzweig, Eric Bourke, Jerry Garcia, Keri Godin, Alison Hoffnagle, Emily Phares, Nancy Sampson, Todd Strauss, Laurel Valchuis, Elaine Veracruz, and Lisa Wittenberg for assistance with manuscript preparation. A complete list of NCS publications and the full text of all NCS-R instruments can be found at http://www.hcp.med.harvard.edu/ncs. Send correspondence to ncs@hcp.med.harvard.edu.

The NCS-R is carried out in conjunction with the World Health Organization World Mental Health (WMH) Survey Initiative. We thank the staff of the WMH Data Collection and Data Analysis Coordination Centres for assistance with instrumentation, fieldwork, and consultation on data analysis. These activities were supported by the NIMH (R01 MH070884), the John D. and Catherine T. MacArthur Foundation, the Pfizer Foundation, the U.S. Public Health Service (R13-MH066849, R01-MH069864, R01 DA016558), the Fogarty International Center (FIRCA R03-TW006481), the Pan American Health Organization, Eli Lilly and Company Foundation, Ortho-McNeil Pharmaceutical, GlaxoSmithKline, and Bristol-Myers Squibb. A complete list of WMH publications can be found at http://www.hcp.med.harvard.edu/wmh/.

Portions of this chapter are based on Kessler, R. C., Berglund, P. A., Demler, O., Jin, R., Walters, E. E. (2005). Lifetime prevalence and age of onset distributions of DSM-IV disorders in the National Comorbidity Survey Replication (NCS-R). Archives of General Psychiatry, 62(6), 593–602. 330; Wang, P. S., Berglund, P. A., Kessler,

R. C., Olfson, M., Pincus, H. A., Wells, K. B. (2005). Failure and delay in initial treatment contact after first onset of mental disorders in the National Comorbidity Survey Replication (NCS-R). Archives of General Psychiatry, 62(6), 603–613; Kessler, R. C., Chiu, W. T., Demler, O., Walters, E. E. (2005). Prevalence, severity, and comorbidity of twelve-month DSM-IV disorders in the National Comorbidity Survey Replication (NCS-R). Archives of General Psychiatry, 62(6), 617–627; and Wang, P. S., Lane, M., Kessler, R. C., Olfson, M., Pincus, H. A., Wells, K. B. (2005). Twelve-month use of mental health services in the U.S.: Results from the National Comorbidity Survey Replication (NCS-R). Archives of General Psychiatry, 62(6), 629–640. All articles copyright © 2005, American Medical Association. All rights reserved. Reproduced with permission.

## I. INTRODUCTION

A paradox exists in the United States: there is an enormous burden of mental disorders in the country and good access to high-quality care, yet the treatment of the mentally ill is often quite poor or nonexistent. This paradox exists, at least in part, because nearly one out of every five Americans lack health insurance, and the proportion is growing as a result of reductions in employer-sponsored coverage (Holahan & Cook 2005); of the uninsured, roughly three-fourths are the working poor and disproportionately racial or ethnic minority families with limited abilities to pay for mental health services (Kaiser Commission on Medicaid and the Uninsured n.d.). Even for the insured, fragmentation of U.S. mental health care occurs across disparate federal, state, and private systems and funding streams (Mark et al. 2005). Approximately two-thirds of mental health care is covered by already-strained public sectors (compared to less than half of all health care), leading to particularly strong pressures on governmental agencies to contain mental health care use and costs (Mark et al. 2005). Furthermore, even many with coverage are underinsured, perhaps explaining the widespread low intensity, poor quality, and suboptimal allocation of mental health treatments

observed previously in the United States (Kessler et al. 1997; Wang, Berglund & Kessler 2000; Wang, Demler & Kessler 2002).

As a result of this paradox, leading health-care policy groups, including the President's New Freedom Commission on Mental Health (President's New Freedom Commission on Mental Health n.d.) and the Institute of Medicine's Crossing the Quality Chasm Committee (Institute of Medicine 2006), have called for reform that would address unmet need for effective treatment, eliminate disparities in mental health and services, efficiently allocate resources, and guide future research efforts. Achieving each of these important goals requires population-based data that identify the current nature and reasons for burdens as well as potential ways to improve care and outcomes. Collecting accurate general population data on mental disorders and their treatments is a fairly recent phenomenon in the United States. The first such survey employing modern methods, the Epidemiologic Catchment Area (ECA) study, occurred in the 1980s (Robins & Regier 1991). The second, the National Comorbidity Survey (NCS), took place in the 1990s (Kessler et al. 1994). Both surveys documented high lifetime and 12-month prevalence of mental disorders as well as widespread unmet needs for services. However, the rapid pace of change in the American mental health care system has made it imperative to reexamine the burdens from mental disorders and their care. Although new forms of treatment have been introduced and promoted, their efficacy and safety have been questioned as well (Food and Drug Administration n.d.; Eisenberg et al. 1993; Eisenberg et al. 1998; Leucht et al. 1999; Kessler et al. 2001c; Olfson et al. 2002; Rosenthal et al. 2002; Schatzberg & Nemeroff 2004). Initiatives promoting awareness, detection, help seeking, and best practices for mental disorders have been launched, but little is known concerning their impacts (Agency for Health Care Policy and Research 1993; Jacobs 1995; Katon et al. 1995; Hirschfeld et al. 1997; National Committee for Quality Assurance 1997; American Psychiatric Association 1998; Lehman & Steinwachs 1998; American Psychiatric Association 2000; Wells et al. 2000;

American Psychiatric Association 2002; Katon et al. 2002; American Psychiatric Association 2004). Likewise, effects of the many delivery systems, financing, and mental health policy redesigns that have taken place are unclear (Williams 1998; Mechanic & McAlpine 1999; Sturm & Klap 1999; Williams et al. 1999; Weissman et al. 2000; Kessler et al. 2001a; Bender 2002).

To shed light on these impacts and to provide up-to-date data on the current burdens from and care of mental disorders in the United States, the National Comorbidity Survey Replication (NCS-R) was undertaken between 2001 and 2003 as part of the larger WHO World Mental Health (WMH) Survey Initiative (Kessler et al. 2006). This chapter presents basic descriptive data from the NCS-R regarding lifetime prevalence of mental disorders, delay in initial treatment seeking, 12-month prevalence of disorders, and 12-month treatment use and adequacy. Implications of these findings, including for future mental health initiatives, interventions, and policies, are discussed. We close with a review of promising future directions and potential uses for the NCS-R data and program.

## 2. METHODS

### 2.1. Sample

The NCS-R is a nationally representative household survey of respondents aged 18 and older in the coterminous United States (Kessler et al. 2004). Face-to-face interviews were carried out with 9282 respondents between February 2001 and April 2003. Like most other WMH surveys, the NCS-R used a two-part interview approach in which Part 1 of the interview, which included a core diagnostic assessment, was administered to all respondents, while Part 2 was administered to a probability subsample of Part 1 respondents. Part 2 assessed risk factors, correlates, service use, and additional disorders and was administered to all Part 1 respondents with lifetime disorders plus a probability subsample of other respondents. The overall response rate was 70.9%. The NCS-R recruitment, consent, and field procedures were approved by the Human Subjects Committees of both Harvard Medical School and the University of Michigan. A more complete discussion of the NCS-R sample design is presented elsewhere (Kessler et al. 2004).

### 2.2. Measures

#### 2.2.1. Diagnostic Assessment of Lifetime and 12-month DSM-IV Disorders

As with all WMH surveys, diagnoses were made using Version 3.0 of the WHO's Composite International Diagnostic Interview (CIDI) (Kessler & Üstün 2004), a fully structured lay-administered diagnostic interview that generates diagnoses according to the definitions and criteria of both the ICD-10 (WHO 1991) and DSM-IV (American Psychiatric Association 1994) diagnostic systems. DSM-IV criteria are used in analyses for this chapter. A detailed discussion of the instrument is presented in Chapter 4 of this volume (Kessler & Üstün 2004). The disorders considered in this chapter include the same ones as those described in the chapters on the Colombian and Mexican WMH surveys: mood disorders (major depressive episode [MDE], dysthymia [DYS], and bipolar disorder I or II [BPD] studied together for increased statistical power), anxiety disorders (panic disorder [PD], agoraphobia without panic [AG], specific phobia [SP], social phobia [SoP], generalized anxiety disorder [GAD], posttraumatic stress disorder [PTSD], and separation anxiety disorder [SAD]), substance disorders (alcohol and drug abuse and dependence [AA, DA, AD, DD, respectively]), and impulse-control disorders (intermittent explosive disorder [IED], oppositional-defiant disorder [ODD], and attention-deficit/hyperactivity disorder [ADHD]). Lifetime prevalence, age of onset, and 12-month prevalence were assessed separately for each disorder (Kessler et al. 2005a). All diagnoses are considered with organic exclusions and without diagnostic hierarchy rules. As described in Chapter 6 of this volume (see also Haro et al. 2006), a blinded clinical reappraisal study using the Structured Clinical Interview for

DSM-IV (SCID) (First et al. 2002) showed generally good concordance between DSM-IV diagnoses based on the CIDI and the SCID for anxiety, mood, and substance disorders. The CIDI diagnoses of impulse-control disorders have not been validated.

## 2.2.2. Severity of 12-month Cases

Twelve-month cases were classified by severity using a somewhat more complex classification scheme than in most other WMH surveys. Cases were classified as serious if they had any of the following: a 12-month suicide attempt with serious lethality intent; work disability or substantial limitation due to a mental or substance disorder; a positive screen for nonaffective psychosis, bipolar I or II disorder, substance dependence with serious role impairment (as defined by disorder-specific impairment questions), an impulse-control disorder with repeated serious violence, or any disorder that resulted in 30 or more days out of role in the year. Cases not defined serious were defined as moderate if they had any of the following: suicide gesture, plan, or ideation; substance dependence without serious role impairment; at least moderate work limitation due to a mental or substance disorder; or any disorder with at least moderate role impairment in two or more domains of the Sheehan Disability Scales (SDS; the SDS assessed disability in work role performance, household maintenance, social life, and intimate relationships on 0–10 visual analogue scales with verbal descriptors, and associated scale scores, of: none, 0; mild, 1–3; moderate, 4–6; severe, 7–9; and very severe, 10) (Leon et al. 1997). All other cases were classified as mild. This classification scheme is somewhat more refined than the one used in comparative analyses of all WMH surveys (Demyttenaere et al. 2004) because the NCS-R has more detailed information than the other WMH surveys. To assess the meaningfulness of these severity ratings, we compared number of days in the past 12 months that respondents were totally unable to carry out their normal daily activities because of mental or substance problems. The mean of this variable was significantly higher ($F_{2,5689} = 17.7$,

$p < 0.001$) among respondents classified as serious (88.3) than those classified as moderate (4.7) or mild (1.9).

## 2.2.3. Initial Lifetime Treatment Contact

Near the end of each CIDI diagnostic section, respondents were asked whether they had ever in their life "talked to a medical doctor or other professional" about the disorder under investigation. In asking this question, the interviewer clarified that the term "other professional" was meant to apply broadly to include "psychologists, counselors, spiritual advisors, herbalists, acupuncturists, and any other healing professionals." Respondents who reported ever talking to any of these professionals about the disorder in question were then asked how old they were the first time they did so. The response to this question was used to define age of first treatment contact.

## 2.2.4 12-month Use of Mental Health Services

All Part 2 respondents were asked whether they had ever received treatment for "problems with your emotions or nerves or your use of alcohol or drugs." Separate assessments were made for different types of professionals, support groups, self-help groups, mental health crisis hotlines (assumed to be visits with nonpsychiatrist mental health specialists), CAM therapies, and use of other treatment settings including admissions to hospitals and other facilities (each day of admission was assumed to include a visit with a psychiatrist). Follow-up questions asked about age at first and most recent contacts as well as number and duration of visits in the past 12 months.

Reports of 12-month service use were classified into the following categories: psychiatrist; nonpsychiatrist mental health specialist (psychologist or other nonpsychiatrist mental health professional in any setting, social worker or counselor in a mental health specialty setting, and use of a mental health hotline); general medical provider (primary care doctor, other general medical doctor, nurse, or any other health professional not previously mentioned); human services professional (religious or spiritual advisor, social worker or counselor in any setting other than a specialty mental health setting); and CAM professional (any other type of healer such as chiropractors, participation in an Internet support group, and participation in a self-help group). Psychiatrist and nonpsychiatrist specialist categories were combined into a broader mental health specialty (MHS) category; MHS was also combined with general medical (GM) into an even broader health care (HC) category. Human services (HS) and CAM were also combined into a non–health-care (NHC) category.

## 2.3. Minimally Adequate 12-month Treatment

As described in the chapters on the Colombian and Mexican WMH surveys, minimally adequate treatment was defined on the basis of available evidence-based guidelines (Agency for Health Care Policy and Research 1993; American Psychiatric Association 1998; Lehman & Steinwachs 1998; American Psychiatric Association 2000, 2002, 2004) using a somewhat more rigorous definition than in other WMH surveys. Treatment was considered at least minimally adequate if the patient received either pharmacotherapy (two months or longer of an appropriate medication for the focal disorder plus four visits or more to any type of medical doctor) or psychotherapy (eight visits or more with any health care or human services professional lasting an average of 30 minutes or longer). The decision to require four or more physician visits for pharmacotherapy was based on the fact that four or more visits for medication evaluation, initiation, and monitoring are generally recommended during the acute and continuation phases of treatment in available guidelines (Agency for Health Care Policy and Research 1993; American Psychiatric Association 1998; Lehman & Steinwachs 1998; American Psychiatric Association 2000, 2002, 2004).

Appropriate medications for disorders included antidepressants for depressive disorders; mood stabilizers or antipsychotics for bipo-

lar disorders; antidepressants or anxiolytics for anxiety disorders; antagonists or agonists (e.g., disulfiram, naltrexone, methodone) for alcohol and substance disorders; and any psychiatric drug for impulse-control disorders (Schatzberg & Nemeroff 2004). At least eight sessions were required for minimally adequate psychotherapy based on the fact that clinical trials demonstrating effectiveness have generally included at least eight psychotherapy visits (Agency for Health Care Policy and Research 1993; American Psychiatric Association 1998; Lehman & Steinwachs 1998; American Psychiatric Association 2000, 2002, 2004). For alcohol and substance disorders, self-help visits of any duration were counted as psychotherapy visits. Treatment adequacy was defined separately for each 12-month disorder (i.e., a respondent with comorbid disorders could be classified as receiving minimally adequate treatment for one disorder but not for another).

Respondents who began treatments shortly before the NCS-R interview may not have had time to fulfill requirements, even though they were in the early stages of adequate treatment. Furthermore, very brief treatments have been developed for certain disorders (Ost, Ferebee & Furmark 1997; Ballesteros et al. 2004). We therefore created a broader definition of minimally adequate treatment for sensitivity analyses that consisted of receiving at least two visits to an appropriate treatment sector (one visit for presumptive evaluation/diagnosis and at least one visit for treatment) or being in ongoing treatment at interview.

## 2.4. Predictor Variables

Predictor variables in analyses of lifetime data include age of onset (AOO) of the focal disorder (coded into the categories 0–12, 13–19, 20–29, and 30+ years of age), cohort (defined by age at interview in the categories 18–29, 30–44, 45–59, 60+), sex, race-ethnicity (non-Hispanic white, non-Hispanic black, Hispanic, and other), education (categorized as either current students or nonstudents with 0–11, 12, 13–15, or 16+ years of education), and marital status (categorized as either currently married/cohabitating, previously married, or never married). The last two of these predictors vary within a given individual over time. Information was obtained in the NCS-R on timing of marital histories (i.e., ages of marriage and marital dissolution), allowing for marital status to be coded for each year of each respondent's life. Information on years of education was also coded as a time-varying predictor by assuming an orderly educational history for each respondent in which eight years of education corresponds to being a student up to age 14 and other lengths of education are associated with ages consistent with this benchmark (e.g., 12 years of education is assumed to correspond to being a student up to age 18).

Variables in analyses of 12-month data included sex, race-ethnicity, cohort, education, and marital status (all categorized as described previously). In addition, family income in relation to the federal poverty line (Proctor & Dalaker 2002) (categorized as low [$\leq$ 1.5 times the poverty line], low average [1.5+ to three times], high-average [three+ to six times], and high [six+ times], urbanicity defined according to 2000 Census definitions (U.S. Census Bureau 2000) (large and smaller metropolitan areas; central cities, suburbs, and adjacent areas; and rural areas), and health insurance coverage (including private, public, or military sources) were also included.

## 2.5. Analysis Procedures

The data were weighted to adjust for differential probabilities of selection of respondents within households and differential nonresponse as well as to adjust for residual differences between the sample and the U.S. population on the cross-classification of sociodemographic variables. An additional weight was used in the Part 2 sample to adjust for differences in probability of selection into that sample. These procedures are described in more detail elsewhere (Kessler et al. 2004). Survival analysis was used to make estimated projections of cumulative lifetime probability of disorders and treatment contact from year of onset. The actuarial method (Halli & Rao 1992) implemented in SAS V8.2 (SAS Institute 2001)

was used rather than the more familiar Kaplan–Meier method (Kaplan & Meier 1958) of generating survival curves because the former has an advantage over the latter in estimating onsets within a year. The typical duration of delay in initial treatment contact was defined on the basis of these curves as the median number of years from disorder onset to first treatment contact among cases that eventually made treatment contact.

Discrete-time survival analysis (Efron 1988) with person-year as the unit of analysis was used to examine correlates of disorders and treatment contact. Models of treatment contact were estimated twice for a given disorder: once among all respondents with a history of the disorder to study the predictors of ever making a treatment contact; and then a second time among the subsample who eventually made a treatment contact to study the predictors of delay in initial contact. Basic patterns of 12-month disorders and service use were examined by computing proportions, means, and medians. Logistic regression analysis (Hosmer & Lemeshow 1989) was used to study sociodemographic predictors of having 12-month disorders, receiving any 12-month treatment in the total sample, treatment in particular sectors among those receiving any treatment, and treatment meeting criteria for minimal adequacy. Standard errors were estimated using the Taylor series method as implemented in SUDAAN (Research Triangle Institute 2002). Multivariate significance tests were made using Wald $\chi^2$ tests based on coefficient variance-covariance matrices that were adjusted for design effects using the Taylor series method. Statistical significance was evaluated using two-sided design-based tests and the 0.05 level of significance.

## 3. RESULTS

### 3.1. Lifetime Prevalence of DSM-IV Mental Disorders

Table 9.1 shows the lifetime prevalence of mental disorders in the NCS-R. The lifetime prevalence of any disorder is 46.4%; 27.7% of respondents had two or more lifetime disorders and

**Table 9.1** Lifetime prevalence of DSM-IV/CIDI disorders in the total NCS-R sample and by age

| | Total | | 18–29 | | 30–44 | | 45–59 | | 60+ | | $\chi^2_3$ |
|---|---|---|---|---|---|---|---|---|---|---|---|
| | % | (se) | % | (se) | % | (se) | % | (se) | % | (se) | |
| **I. Anxiety disorders** | | | | | | | | | | | |
| Panic disorder | 4.7 | (0.2) | 4.4 | (0.4) | 5.7 | (0.5) | 5.9 | (0.4) | 2.0 | (0.4) | 52.6* |
| Agoraphobia without panic | 1.4 | (0.1) | 1.1 | (0.2) | 1.7 | (0.3) | 1.6 | (0.3) | 1.0 | (0.3) | 4.5 |
| Specific phobia | 12.5 | (0.4) | 13.3 | (0.8) | 13.9 | (0.8) | 14.1 | (1.0) | 7.5 | (0.7) | 54.3* |
| Social phobia | 12.1 | (0.4) | 13.6 | (0.7) | 14.3 | (0.8) | 12.4 | (0.8) | 6.6 | (0.5) | 109.0* |
| Generalized anxiety disorder | 5.7 | (0.3) | 4.1 | (0.4) | 6.8 | (0.5) | 7.7 | (0.7) | 3.6 | (0.5) | 39.9* |
| Posttraumatic stress disorder[a] | 6.8 | (0.4) | 6.3 | (0.5) | 8.2 | (0.8) | 9.2 | (0.9) | 2.5 | (0.5) | 37.9* |
| Obsessive-compulsive disorder[b] | 1.6 | (0.3) | 2.0 | (0.5) | 2.3 | (0.9) | 1.3 | (0.6) | 0.7 | (0.4) | 6.8 |
| Separation anxiety disorder[c] | 5.2 | (0.4) | 5.2 | (0.6) | 5.1 | (0.6) | – | –[c] | – | –[c] | 0.0[c] |
| Any anxiety disorder[d] | 28.8 | (0.9) | 30.2 | (1.1) | 35.1 | (1.4) | 30.8 | (1.7) | 15.3 | (1.5) | 89.9* |
| **II. Mood disorders** | | | | | | | | | | | |
| Major depressive disorder | 16.6 | (0.5) | 15.4 | (0.7) | 19.8 | (0.9) | 18.8 | (1.1) | 10.6 | (0.8) | 49.9* |
| Dysthymia | 2.5 | (0.2) | 1.7 | (0.3) | 2.9 | (0.4) | 3.7 | (0.7) | 1.3 | (0.3) | 10.6* |
| Bipolar I–II disorders | 3.9 | (0.2) | 5.9 | (0.6) | 4.5 | (0.3) | 3.5 | (0.4) | 1.0 | (0.3) | 62.0* |
| Any mood disorder | 20.8 | (0.6) | 21.4 | (0.9) | 24.6 | (0.9) | 22.9 | (1.2) | 11.9 | (1.0) | 58.0* |
| **III. Impulse-control disorders** | | | | | | | | | | | |
| Oppositional-defiant disorder | 8.5 | (0.7) | 9.5 | (0.9) | 7.5 | (0.8) | – | –[c] | – | –[c] | 3.0[c] |
| Conduct disorder | 9.5 | (0.8) | 10.9 | (1.0) | 8.2 | (0.8) | – | –[c] | – | –[c] | 7.6[c,e] |
| Attention-deficit/hyperactivity disorder | 8.1 | (0.6) | 7.8 | (0.8) | 8.3 | (0.9) | – | –[c] | – | –[c] | 0.2[c] |
| Intermittent explosive disorder | 5.2 | (0.3) | 7.4 | (0.7) | 5.7 | (0.6) | 4.9 | (0.4) | 1.9 | (0.5) | 74.7* |
| Any impulse-control disorder | 24.8 | (1.1) | 26.8 | (1.7) | 23.0 | (1.3) | – | –[c] | – | –[e] | 4.0[e] |
| **IV. Substance disorders** | | | | | | | | | | | |
| Alcohol abuse | 13.2 | (0.6) | 14.3 | (1.0) | 16.3 | (1.1) | 14.0 | (1.1) | 6.2 | (0.7) | 60.2* |
| Alcohol dependence | 5.4 | (0.3) | 6.3 | (0.7) | 6.4 | (0.6) | 6.0 | (0.7) | 2.2 | (0.4) | 45.2* |
| Drug abuse | 7.9 | (0.4) | 10.9 | (0.9) | 11.9 | (1.0) | 6.5 | (0.6) | 0.3 | (0.2) | 168.7* |
| Drug dependence | 3.0 | (0.2) | 3.9 | (0.5) | 4.9 | (0.6) | 2.3 | (0.4) | 0.2 | (0.1) | 90.0* |
| Any substance disorder | 14.6 | (0.6) | 16.7 | (1.1) | 18.0 | (1.1) | 15.3 | (1.0) | 6.3 | (0.7) | 71.4* |
| **V. Any disorder** | | | | | | | | | | | |
| Any[d] | 46.4 | (1.1) | 52.4 | (1.7) | 55.0 | (1.6) | 46.5 | (1.8) | 26.1 | (1.7) | 115.4* |
| Two or more disorders[d] | 27.7 | (0.9) | 33.9 | (1.3) | 34.0 | (1.5) | 27.0 | (1.6) | 11.6 | (1.0) | 148.3* |
| Three or more disorders[d] | 17.3 | (0.7) | 22.3 | (1.2) | 22.5 | (1.1) | 15.9 | (1.3) | 5.3 | (0.7) | 140.7* |
| **VI. Sample sizes** | | | | | | | | | | | |
| Part 1 | (9282) | | (2338) | | (2886) | | (2221) | | (1837) | | |
| Part 2 | (5692) | | (1518) | | (1805) | | (1462) | | (907) | | |
| Part 2 OCD subsample | (1808) | | (493) | | (566) | | (457) | | (292) | | |

* Significant age difference at the 0.05 level.

[a] Posttraumatic stress disorder was assessed only in the Part 2 sample ($n = 5692$).

[b] Obsessive-compulsive disorder was assessed only in a random one-third of the Part 2 sample ($n = 1808$).

[c] Separation anxiety disorder, oppositional-defiant disorder, conduct disorder, and attention-deficit/hyperactivity disorder were assessed only among Part 2 respondents aged 18–44 years ($n = 3199$). These summary measures were analyzed in the full Part 2 sample ($n = 5692$). Obsessive-compulsive disorder, separation anxiety disorder, oppositional-defiant disorder, conduct disorder, and attention-deficit/hyperactivity disorder were coded as absent among respondents who were not assessed for these disorders.

[d] The $\chi^2$ test evaluates statistical significance of age-related differences in estimated prevalence. $\chi^2$ is evaluated with one degree of freedom for separation anxiety disorder, oppositional-defiant disorder, conduct disorder, attention-deficit/hyperactivity disorder, and any impulse-control disorder.

17.3% had three or more. The most prevalent class is anxiety disorders (28.8%), followed by impulse-control disorders (24.8%), mood disorders (20.8%), and substance use disorders (14.6%). The most prevalent individual lifetime disorders are major depressive disorder (MDD) (16.6%), AA (13.2%), SP (12.5%), and SoP (12.1%).

Significant differences in prevalence with age occur for almost all disorders, with generally monotonic increases found going from the youngest (18–29) to older (for the most part, 30–44) age groups, followed then by a decline in the oldest age group(s). The prevalence of disorders is always lowest in the oldest age group (60+), with the most extreme examples of this pattern of differences occurring for DA and DD, PTSD, and BPD.

### 3.2. Distributions of the Age of Onset of Mental Disorders

Table 9.2 presents the distributions of cumulative lifetime risks estimates that have been standardized and examined for fixed percentiles. Median AOOs (i.e., the 50th percentile on the AOO distribution) are earlier for anxiety disorders (age 11) and impulse-control disorders (age 11) than for substance (age 20) and mood disorders (age 30). AOO is also concentrated in a very narrow age range for most disorders, with interquartile ranges (IQRs; i.e., the number of years between the 25th and 75th percentiles of the AOO distributions) of only eight years (ages 7–15) for impulse-control disorders, nine years (ages 18–27) for substance use disorders, and 15 years (ages 6–21) for anxiety disorders, compared to 25 years (ages 18–43) for mood disorders.

### 3.3. Projected Lifetime Risk of Mental Disorders

On the basis of on the AOO distributions shown in Table 9.2, the projected lifetime risk of mental disorders as of age 75 is 9% higher than the lifetime prevalence estimates for anxiety disorders, 34% higher for mood disorders, 2% higher for impulse-control disorders, 12% higher for substance use disorders, and 9% higher for any disorder. Not surprisingly, the greatest differences between lifetime prevalence and projected lifetime risk were observed for disorders with late AOO distributions (e.g., MDD, GAD, and PTSD). The projected lifetime risk is highest for anxiety disorders (31.5%), but the order is reversed relative to lifetime prevalence estimates for impulse-control and mood disorders – with impulse-control disorders having a higher prevalence (24.8% vs. 20.8%) and mood disorders having a higher projected risk (28.0% vs. 25.4%). The lowest project risk is for substance use disorders (16.3%). Of projected new onsets of disorders, more than 80% are in people with existing disorders. This derives from the fact that the overall projected risk in the total sample is only 4.4% higher than the lifetime prevalence reported in Table 9.1 (50.8% vs. 46.4%); meanwhile, disorder-specific risk versus prevalence differences sum to 20.4%.

### 3.4. Cohort Effects in Lifetime Risk of Mental Disorders

Discrete-time survival analysis was used to predict lifetime risk of mental disorders in various age groups (i.e., 18–29, 30–44, 45–59, and 60+, corresponding roughly to cohorts born in the years 1970+, 1955–1969, 1940–1954, and earlier than 1940). As Table 9.3 shows, there were generally significant positive associations between recency of cohorts and risk of mental disorders. Drug disorders had the largest cohort effects, while phobias and childhood-onset impulse-control disorders had the smallest.

An alternative explanation for these apparent cohort effects is that lifetime risk is actually constant across cohorts but appears to vary with cohort because onsets occur earlier in more recent than in later cohorts (as might happen if there were secular changes in environmental triggers or to age-related differences in AOO recall accuracy). Another explanation might be that mortality has an increasing impact on sample selection bias as age increases. To study these possibilities, the cohort model was examined to determine whether intercohort differences

**Table 9.2.** Ages at selected percentiles on the standardized age of onset distributions of DSM-IV/CIDI disorders with projected lifetime risk at age 75

| | Projected lifetime risk at age 75 | | Ages at selected age of onset percentiles | | | | | | | |
|---|---|---|---|---|---|---|---|---|---|---|
| | % | (se) | 5 | 10 | 25 | 50 | 75 | 90 | 95 | 99 |
| I. Anxiety disorders | | | | | | | | | | |
| Panic disorder | 6.0 | (0.3) | 6 | 10 | 16 | 24 | 40 | 51 | 56 | 63 |
| Agoraphobia without panic | 1.6 | (0.2) | 6 | 7 | 13 | 20 | 33 | 48 | 51 | 54 |
| Specific phobia | 13.2 | (0.4) | 4 | 5 | 5 | 7 | 12 | 23 | 41 | 64 |
| Social phobia | 12.6 | (0.4) | 5 | 6 | 8 | 13 | 15 | 23 | 34 | 52 |
| Generalized anxiety disorder | 8.3 | (0.4) | 8 | 13 | 20 | 31 | 47 | 58 | 66 | 75 |
| Posttraumatic stress disorder[a] | 8.7 | (0.6) | 6 | 9 | 15 | 23 | 39 | 53 | 61 | 71 |
| Obsessive-compulsive disorder[b] | 1.9 | (0.3) | 10 | 11 | 14 | 19 | 30 | 48 | 54 | 54 |
| Separation anxiety disorder[c] | 5.2 | (0.4) | 5 | 5 | 6 | 7 | 10 | 13 | 14 | 17 |
| Any anxiety disorder[d] | 31.5 | (1.1) | 5 | 5 | 6 | 11 | 21 | 41 | 51 | 65 |
| II. Mood disorders | | | | | | | | | | |
| Major depressive disorder | 23.2 | (0.6) | 12 | 14 | 19 | 32 | 44 | 56 | 64 | 73 |
| Dysthymia | 3.4 | (0.3) | 7 | 11 | 17 | 31 | 43 | 51 | 57 | 73 |
| Bipolar I–II disorders | 5.1 | (0.3) | 11 | 13 | 17 | 25 | 42 | 50 | 57 | 65 |
| Any mood disorder | 28.0 | (0.8) | 11 | 13 | 18 | 30 | 43 | 54 | 63 | 73 |
| III. Impulse-control disorders | | | | | | | | | | |
| Oppositional-defiant disorder[c] | 8.5 | (0.7) | 5 | 6 | 8 | 13 | 14 | 16 | 17 | 18 |
| Conduct disorder[c] | 9.5 | (0.8) | 6 | 7 | 10 | 13 | 15 | 17 | 17 | 18 |
| Attention-deficit hyperactivity disorder[c] | 8.1 | (0.6) | 5 | 6 | 7 | 7 | 8 | 11 | 11 | 16 |
| Intermittent explosive disorder | 5.4 | (0.3) | 6 | 8 | 11 | 15 | 20 | 26 | 37 | 46 |
| Any impulse-control disorder[c] | 25.4 | (1.1) | 5 | 6 | 7 | 11 | 15 | 18 | 23 | 36 |
| IV. Substance disorders | | | | | | | | | | |
| Alcohol abuse[a] | 15.1 | (0.7) | 15 | 16 | 18 | 21 | 29 | 39 | 44 | 54 |
| Alcohol dependence[a] | 6.5 | (0.4) | 16 | 17 | 19 | 23 | 31 | 41 | 50 | 56 |
| Drug abuse[a] | 8.5 | (0.4) | 15 | 16 | 17 | 19 | 23 | 29 | 36 | 46 |
| Drug dependence[a] | 3.4 | (0.3) | 15 | 16 | 18 | 21 | 28 | 36 | 41 | 49 |
| Any substance use disorder[d] | 16.3 | (0.6) | 15 | 16 | 18 | 20 | 27 | 37 | 41 | 54 |
| V. Any disorder | | | | | | | | | | |
| Any[d] | 50.8 | (1.2) | 5 | 5 | 7 | 14 | 24 | 42 | 51 | 64 |

[a] Posttraumatic stress disorder and substance disorders were assessed only in the Part 2 sample ($n = 5692$).

[b] Obsessive-compulsive disorder was assessed only in a random one-third of the Part 2 sample ($n = 1808$).

[c] Separation anxiety disorder, oppositional-defiant disorder, conduct disorder, attention-deficit/hyperactivity disorder, and any impulse-control disorder were assessed only among Part 2 respondents aged 18–44 years ($n = 3199$).

[d] These summary measures were analyzed in the full Part 2 sample ($n = 5692$). Obsessive-compulsive disorder, separation anxiety disorder, oppositional-defiant disorder, conduct disorder, and attention-deficit/hyperactivity disorder were coded as absent among respondents who were not assessed for these disorders.

decrease significantly with increasing age. Differences were examined separately for first onsets in the age ranges 1–12, 13–19, 20–29, 30–39, 40–49, and 50–59 (as the last of these age intervals is the upper end of the age distribution of the second-oldest cohort quartile, it was impossible to study intercohort differences beyond this age).

Results in Table 9.4 show that there was no evidence of decreasing cohort effects with increasing age for anxiety or mood disorders. On the other hand, for substance use disorders there were much higher cohort effects in the teens and twenties than in either childhood or the thirties through fifties.

**Table 9.3.** Cohort (age at interview) as a predictor of lifetime risk of DSM-IV/CIDI disorders in the NCS-R[a]

| | Younger cohorts (age at interview) compared to respondents ages 60+ | | | | | | |
|---|---|---|---|---|---|---|---|
| | 18–29 | | 30–44 | | 45–59 | | |
| | OR | (95% CI) | OR | (95% CI) | OR | (95% CI) | $\chi_3^2$ |
| **I. Anxiety disorders** | | | | | | | |
| Panic disorder | 6.4* | (3.8–10.5) | 5.0* | (3.0–8.5) | 4.1* | (2.4–6.9) | 61.5** |
| Agoraphobia without panic | 2.3* | (1.2–4.6) | 2.5* | (1.2–5.1) | 2.0 | (0.9–4.1) | 7.4 |
| Specific phobia | 2.1* | (1.7–2.7) | 2.1* | (1.7–2.7) | 2.1* | (1.6–2.6) | 49.3** |
| Social phobia | 2.5* | (2.0–3.0) | 2.5* | (2.0–3.1) | 2.1* | (1.6–2.6) | 89.6** |
| Generalized anxiety disorder | 4.6* | (2.9–7.1) | 4.1* | (2.7–6.1) | 3.3* | (2.1–5.1) | 54.7** |
| Posttraumatic stress disorder[b] | 6.3* | (3.7–10.5) | 5.5* | (3.4–9.0) | 4.8* | (3.0–7.8) | 55.7** |
| Obsessive-compulsive disorder[c] | 6.3 | (1.0–37.8) | 5.0 | (0.9–28.5) | 2.5 | (0.4–14.9) | 6.0 |
| Separation anxiety disorder[d] | 1.1 | (0.8–1.5) | 1.0 | – | – | – | 0.1[f] |
| Any anxiety disorder[b,g] | 3.0* | (2.4–3.6) | 3.1* | (2.5–3.9) | 2.5* | (2.0–3.1) | 123.3** |
| **II. Mood disorders** | | | | | | | |
| Major depressive disorder | 7.3* | (5.9–9.0) | 4.5* | (3.5–5.6) | 2.7* | (2.2–3.3) | 370.7** |
| Dysthymia | 4.9* | (3.1–7.7) | 4.4* | (3.0–6.5) | 3.8* | (2.5–5.8) | 62.5** |
| Bipolar I–II disorders | 22.4* | (11.3–44.7) | 9.5* | (4.7–19.2) | 4.8* | (2.5–9.3) | 125.7** |
| Any mood disorder | 8.6* | (6.8–10.8) | 4.9* | (3.8–6.3) | 2.9* | (2.3–3.7) | 419.4** |
| **III. Impulse-control disorders** | | | | | | | |
| Oppositional-defiant disorder[d] | 1.4* | (1.1–1.8) | 1.0 | – | 1.0 | – | 6.3**[f] |
| Conduct disorder[d] | 1.4* | (1.1–1.7) | 1.0 | – | 1.0 | – | 9.4**[f] |
| Attention-deficit/hyperactivity disorder[d] | 1.5* | (1.1–2.0) | 1.0 | – | 1.0 | – | 6.1**[f] |
| Intermittent explosive disorder | 7.3* | (4.2–12.4) | 4.3* | (2.3–7.8) | 2.5* | (1.4–4.3) | 39.0** |
| Any impulse-control disorder[d] | 15.2* | (9.9–23.4)[f] | – | – | – | – | –[f] |
| **IV. Substance use disorders** | | | | | | | |
| Alcohol abuse or dependence | 4.5* | (3.4–6.1) | 3.2* | (2.5–4.2) | 2.4* | (1.8–3.3) | 133.2** |
| Alcohol dependence | 6.4* | (4.2–9.8) | 3.7* | (2.3–5.8) | 2.9* | (1.9–4.5) | 79.6** |
| Drug abuse or dependence | 61.3* | (20.4–183.6) | 49.7* | (16.6–148.2) | 24.8* | (8.2–75.4) | 99.7** |
| Drug dependence | 45.4* | (10.2–202.0) | 35.0* | (7.8–156.5) | 13.8* | (2.7–69.2) | 69.0** |
| Any substance disorder | 4.9* | (3.6–6.6) | 3.7* | (2.8–4.8) | 2.7* | (2.0–3.7) | 138.0** |
| **V. Any disorder** | | | | | | | |
| Any[e] | 4.1* | (3.5–4.9) | 3.6* | (2.9–4.3) | 2.4* | (2.0–2.8) | 280.6** |

* Significant difference compared to the 60+ year olds at the 0.05 level, two-sided test.

** Significant intercohort differences in global test.

[a] Based on discrete-time survival models with person-year as the unit of analysis.

[b] Estimated in the Part 2 sample ($n = 5692$).

[c] Estimated in a random one-third of the Part 2 sample ($n = 1868$).

[d] Estimated among respondents aged 18–44 years in the Part 2 sample ($n = 3199$).

[e] Estimated in the full Part 2 sample. Obsessive-compulsive disorder, separation anxiety disorder, oppositional-defiant disorder, conduct disorder, and attention-deficit/hyperactivity disorder were coded as absent among respondents who were not assessed for these disorders.

[f] $\chi^2$ is evaluated with one degree of freedom for separation anxiety disorder, oppositional-defiant disorder, conduct disorder, attention-deficit/hyperactivity disorder, and any impulse control disorder comparing respondents aged 18–29 to the omitted control group of respondents aged 30–44.

[g] Obsessive-compulsive disorder was coded as absent among respondents who were not assessed for this disorder.

**Table 9.4.** Variations in the effects of cohort (age at interview) in predicting lifetime risk of DSM-IV/CIDI disorders

| | Person-years | | | | | | | | | | | |
|---|---|---|---|---|---|---|---|---|---|---|---|---|
| | 1–12 | | 13–19 | | 20–29 | | 30–39 | | 40–49 | | 50–59 | |
| | OR | (95% CI) | OR | (95% CI) | OR | (95% CI) | OR | (95% CI) | OR | (95% CI) | OR | (95% CI) |
| **I. Anxiety disorders** | | | | | | | | | | | | |
| 19–29 | 2.9* | (2.4–3.6) | 3.1* | (2.2–4.4) | 3.9* | (1.8–8.4) | – | – | – | – | – | – |
| 30–44 | 3.0* | (2.3–3.9) | 3.1* | (2.1–4.5) | 4.4* | (2.1–9.0) | 5.8* | (3.4–9.9) | 2.5* | (1.1–5.8) | – | – |
| 45–59 | 2.3* | (1.9–2.9) | 2.6* | (1.8–3.8) | 3.2* | (1.5–6.7) | 2.7* | (1.3–5.5) | 3.3* | (1.8–6.2) | 4.9* | (2.7–8.9) |
| 60+ | 1.0 | – | 1.0 | – | 1.0 | – | 1.0 | – | 1.0 | – | 1.0 | – |
| | $\chi^2_3 = 135.0$** | | $\chi^2_3 = 54.4$** | | $\chi^2_3 = 18.4$** | | $\chi^2_2 = 52.5$** | | $\chi^2_2 = 15.2$** | | $\chi^2_1 = 28.4$** | |
| $\chi^2_{11} = 35.5$*** | | | | | | | | | | | | |
| **II. Mood disorders** | | | | | | | | | | | | |
| 19–29 | 8.8* | (4.8–16.0) | 8.0* | (5.5–11.6) | 9.2* | (6.1–13.9) | 9.2* | (2.3–36.0) | – | – | – | – |
| 30–44 | 6.0* | (2.9–12.3) | 4.3* | (2.8–6.6) | 4.5* | (3.0–6.8) | 6.5* | (4.1–10.3) | 5.1* | (2.9–8.9) | – | – |
| 45–59 | 3.6* | (1.9–6.9) | 2.8* | (1.9–4.2) | 2.9* | (1.8–4.5) | 2.9* | (1.9–4.3) | 3.1* | (2.0–4.9) | 3.5* | (2.3–5.5) |
| 60+ | 1.0 | – | 1.0 | – | 1.0 | – | 1.0 | – | 1.0 | – | 1.0 | – |
| | $\chi^2_3 = 68.2$** | | $\chi^2_3 = 216.7$** | | $\chi^2_3 = 133.5$** | | $\chi^2_3 = 76.5$** | | $\chi^2_2 = 35.5$** | | $\chi^2_1 = 33.0$** | |
| $\chi^2_{12} = 28.7$** | | | | | | | | | | | | |
| **III. Substance disorders** | | | | | | | | | | | | |
| 19–29 | 1.5 | (0.6–3.9) | 11.3 | (5.4–24.0) | 3.4* | (2.0–5.7) | – | – | – | – | – | – |
| 30–44 | 0.7 | (0.4–1.5) | 9.2* | (4.1–20.3) | 3.0* | (1.8–4.9) | 2.0* | (1.8–4.9) | 0.5 | (0.2–1.6) | – | – |
| 45–59 | 0.2* | (0.0–0.7) | 4.4* | (2.0–9.4) | 3.7* | (2.4–5.8) | 2.2* | (1.1–4.7) | 0.5 | (0.2–1.5) | 2.4 | (0.7–7.7) |
| 60+ | 1.0 | – | 1.0 | – | 1.0 | – | 1.0 | – | 1.0 | – | 1.0 | – |
| | $\chi^2_3 = 23.5$** | | $\chi^2_3 = 95.2$** | | $\chi^2_3 = 35.7$** | | $\chi^2_2 = 6.2$** | | $\chi^2_2 = 2.8$ | | $\chi^2_1 = 2.2$ | |
| $\chi^2_{11} = 100.8$*** | | | | | | | | | | | | |

* Significant difference compared with the before-1940 cohorts (age $\geq$ 60 years) at the 0.05 level, two-sided test in the subsample of person-years defined by the column headings.

** Significant intercohort differences in the global test in the subsample of person-years.

*** Significant interaction between cohort and person-years in the lives of respondents in the total sample.

*Notes*: Based on discrete-time survival models with person-year as the unit of analysis. Total-sample models evaluated the significance of interactions between cohort and person-year. This was not done for impulse-control disorders based on the fact that the vast majority of such disorders have onsets in a very narrow time window. Cohort by person-year interactions were significant in predicting each of the three outcomes. Based on these results, subsample models were estimated for the effects of cohort in each of the first six decades of life (including 11- to 12-year-olds with the earliest decade to distinguish teenagers from other parts of the life span). All analyses were carried out in the full Part 2 sample. In the analysis of anxiety disorders, obsessive-compulsive disorder was coded as absent among respondents who were not assessed for that disorder.

### 3.5. Sociodemographic Predictors of Lifetime Risk of Mental Disorders

Table 9.5 presents sociodemographic predictors of lifetime risk of mental disorders identified in survival analyses that adjusted for cohort. Women have significantly higher risk of anxiety and mood disorders, and men have significantly higher risk of impulse-control and substance use disorders. Non-Hispanic blacks and Hispanics have significantly lower risk of anxiety, mood, and substance use disorders (the latter only among non-Hispanic blacks) than non-Hispanic whites. Respondents with less education had higher risks of substance disorders. Three out of four disorder classes (not impulse-control disorders) were associated with marital disruption.

To examine whether the increasing prevalence of disorders in recent cohorts is concentrated in certain subgroups, interactions between sociodemographic correlates and cohort were studied (results not shown but are available on request). At least one significant interaction was found for each sociodemographic predictor (however, patterns were generally not consistent). Of note, sex differences in anxiety, mood, and impulse-control disorders did not differ across cohort, but women are more similar to men in substance disorders in recent cohorts. Significant associations between lower education or not being married and substance disorders were observed only in recent cohorts.

### 3.6. Cumulative Lifetime Probabilities of Treatment Contact

Figure 9.1 presents survival curves showing the proportion of cases with mood disorders that will eventually make treatment contact. For MDE, BPD, and DYS, these proportions are 88.1%, 90.2%, and 94.2%, respectively (with no statistically significant differences in the survival curves; $\chi_2^2 = 0.7$; $p = 0.718$). Survival curves for anxiety disorders in Figure 9.2 show that the projected proportions are more variable (ranging from 27.3% for SAD to 95.3% for PD) and statistically significant so ($\chi_5^2 = 242.4$; $p < 0.001$).

Projected proportions for impulse-control disorders shown in Figure 9.3 range from 33.9% for ODD to 51.8% for ADHD, with significant differences between curves for disorders in this class ($\chi_2^2 = 6.0$; $p = 0.050$). Projected proportions for substance disorders shown in Figure 9.4, range from 52.7% for AA to 76.9% for DD, with significant differences between curves in this class ($\chi_3^2 = 44.8$; $p < 0.001$).

### 3.7. Duration of Delays in Initial Treatment Contact

The proportion of cases that made treatment contact in the year of first onset of the disorder and the median delay among people who eventually made treatment contact after the year of first onset were estimated from survival curves and are shown in Table 9.6. Proportions of cases making treatment contact in the year of disorder onset range from highs of 37.4%–41.6% for the mood disorders to lows of 1.0%–3.4% for SP, SoP, and SAD. The median years of delay also differ greatly, from lows of 6–8 years for mood disorders to highs of 20–23 years for SP and SAD.

### 3.8. Predictors of Failure and Delay in Initial Treatment Contact

Tables 9.7–9.9 display predictors of failure to ever make a treatment contact among respondents with lifetime disorders. These are very similar to predictors of the duration of delay among respondents who eventually made treatment contact (data not shown but are available upon request). Cohort is significantly related to lifetime treatment contact in 14 of 17 comparisons (0.05 level, two-sided tests) and to delay in treatment contact among eventual patients in 17 of 17 comparisons. AOO is significantly related to treatment contact in 15 of 17 comparisons (exceptions being SAD and ADHD) and to delay among eventual patients in 17 of 17 comparisons.

Less consistency exists for sociodemographic predictors. Women have significantly higher odds of treatment contact than men for 4 (MDE, DYS, BPD, SoP) of 17 disorders. Sex differences

**Table 9.5.** Sociodemographic predictors of lifetime risk of any DSM-IV/CIDI anxiety disorder, mood disorder, impulse-control disorder, substance use disorder, and any disorder[a]

| | Anxiety[a] | | Mood[a] | | Impulse control[b] | | Substance[a] | | Any[a] | |
|---|---|---|---|---|---|---|---|---|---|---|
| | OR | (95% CI) | OR | (95% CI) | OR | (95% CI) | OR | (95% CI) | OR | (95% CI) |
| I. Sex | | | | | | | | | | |
| Female | 1.6* | (1.5–1.8) | 1.5* | (1.3–1.7) | 0.7* | (0.6–0.8) | 0.4* | (0.3–0.4) | 1.1 | (1.0–1.2) |
| Male | 1.0 | – | 1.0 | – | 1.0 | – | 1.0 | – | 1.0 | – |
| $\chi^2_1$ | 90.8* | | 44.7* | | 18.3* | | 204.6* | | 2.8 | |
| II. Race-ethnicity | | | | | | | | | | |
| Non-Hispanic white | 1.0 | – | 1.0 | – | 1.0 | – | 1.0 | – | 1.0 | – |
| Non-Hispanic black | 0.8* | (0.6–0.9) | 0.6* | (0.5–0.8) | 0.7 | (0.5–1.1) | 0.6* | (0.5–0.8) | 0.7* | (0.6–0.8) |
| Hispanic | 0.7* | (0.6–0.9) | 0.8* | (0.6–0.9) | 0.7 | (0.5–1.1) | 0.9 | (0.7–1.2) | 0.8 | (0.6–1.0) |
| Other | 1.2 | (0.9–1.5) | 1.1 | (0.8–1.4) | 1.1 | (0.7–1.7) | 1.2 | (0.8–1.9) | 1.0 | (0.8–1.3) |
| $\chi^2_3$ | 14.1* | | 28.4* | | 8.3* | | 17.7* | | 16.1* | |
| III. Education[d] | | | | | | | | | | |
| Student | 1.3 | (0.9–1.9) | 0.8 | (0.6–1.2) | 0.8 | (0.3–2.2) | 1.0 | (0.6–1.8) | 1.2 | (0.8–1.7) |
| 0–11 nonstudent | 1.1 | (0.8–1.6) | 0.9 | (0.7–1.1) | 0.9 | (0.4–2.5) | 1.9* | (1.2–3.0) | 1.1 | (0.8–1.5) |
| 12 nonstudent | 0.9 | (0.6–1.4) | 1.0 | (0.9–1.2) | 1.0 | (0.4–2.5) | 1.5 | (1.0–2.3) | 1.1 | (0.9–1.4) |
| 13–15 nonstudent | 1.1 | (0.8–1.5) | 1.2 | (0.9–1.5) | 1.1 | (0.4–3.1) | 1.4 | (0.8–2.3) | 1.1 | (0.8–1.5) |
| 16+ nonstudent | 1.0 | – | 1.0 | – | 1.0 | – | 1.0 | – | 1.0 | – |
| $\chi^2_4$ | 2.4 | | 7.0 | | 0.9 | | 39.0* | | 1.2 | |
| IV. Marital status[c] | | | | | | | | | | |
| Married/cohabitating | 1.0 | – | 1.0 | – | 1.0 | – | 1.0 | – | 1.0 | – |
| Previously married | 1.8* | (1.4–2.2) | 1.9* | (1.6–2.3) | 1.8 | (0.7–4.4) | 3.9* | (2.8–5.3) | 2.1* | (1.6–2.6) |
| Never married | 1.0 | (0.7–1.3) | 1.0 | (0.8–1.2) | 1.4 | (0.6–3.2) | 1.2 | (1.0–1.6) | 1.0 | (0.8–1.2) |
| $\chi^2_2$ | 35.8* | | 46.9* | | 1.9 | | 88.7* | | 39.3* | |
| (n) | (5692) | | (5692) | | (3199) | | (5692) | | (5692) | |

* Significant at the 0.05 level, two-sided test.

*Note:* Based on discrete-time survival models with person-years as the unit of analysis.

[a] Based on the full Part 2 sample (n = 5692). In the case of any anxiety disorder, obsessive-compulsive disorder was coded as absent among respondents who were not assessed for this disorder.

[b] Based on Part 2 respondents aged 18–44 years (n = 3199).

[c] Time-varying predictor.

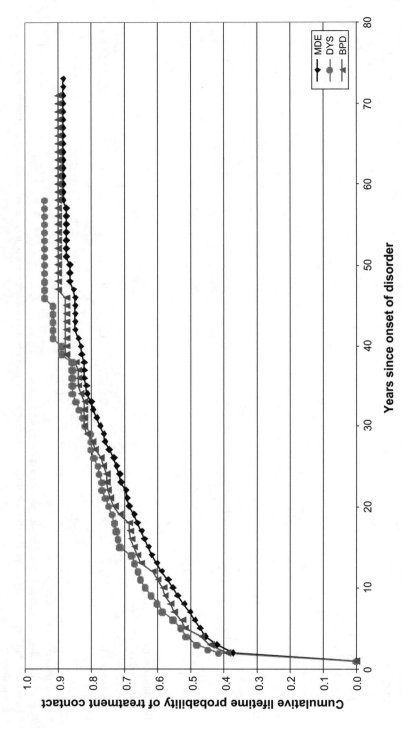

**Figure 9.1.** Cumulative lifetime probability of treatment contact for mood disorders from year of onset[*a]

* Significance of differences among curves: $\chi_2^2 = 0.7$, $p = .718$.

[a] Based on survival analysis. The projected proportions of cases that will eventually make treatment contact for each disorder are estimated to be: major depressive disorder (MDE), 88.1%; dysthymia (DYS), 94.2%; bipolar disorder (BPD) I and II, 90.2%.

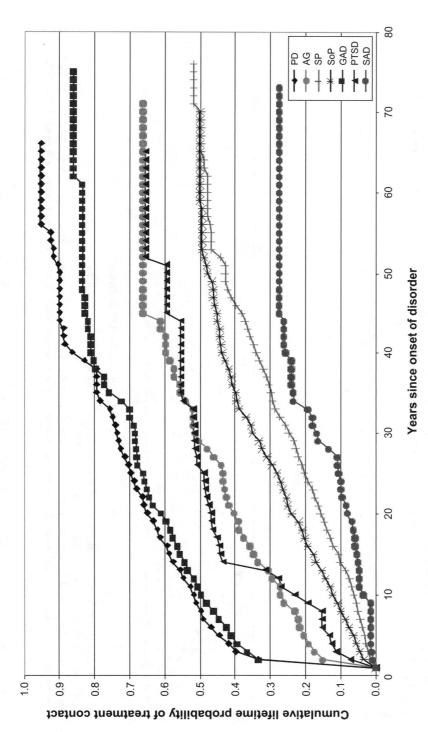

**Figure 9.2.** Cumulative lifetime probability of treatment contact for anxiety disorders from year of onset*[a]

* Significance of differences among curves: $\chi_6^2 = 242.4$, $p < 0.001$.

[a] Based on survival analysis. The projected proportions of cases that will eventually make treatment contact for each disorder are estimated to be: panic disorder (PD), 95.3%; agoraphobia without panic (AG), 66.5%; specific phobia (SP), 50.1%; social phobia (SoP), 74.0%; generalized anxiety disorder (GAD), 86.1%; posttraumatic stress disorder (PTSD), 65.3%; separation anxiety disorder (SAD), 27.3%.

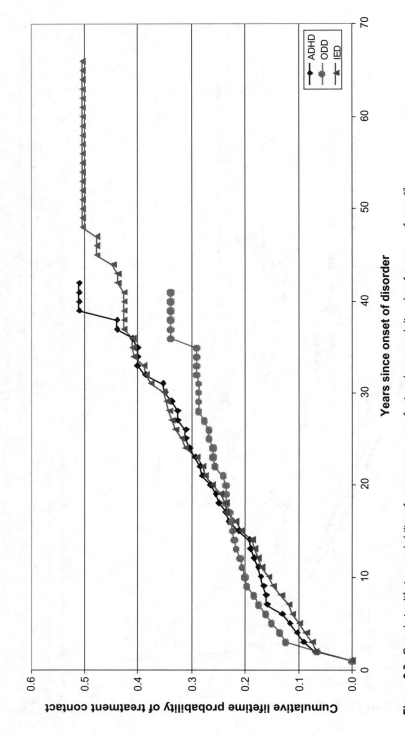

**Figure 9.3.** Cumulative lifetime probability of treatment contact for impulse-control disorders from year of onset[*a]

* Significance of differences among curves: $\chi^2_2 = 6.0$, $p < 0.050$.

[a] Based on survival analysis. The projected proportions of cases that will eventually make treatment contact for each disorder are estimated to be: attention-deficit/hyperactivity disorder (ADHD), 51.8%; oppositional defiant disorder (ODD), 33.9%; intermittent explosive disorder (IED), 50.4%.

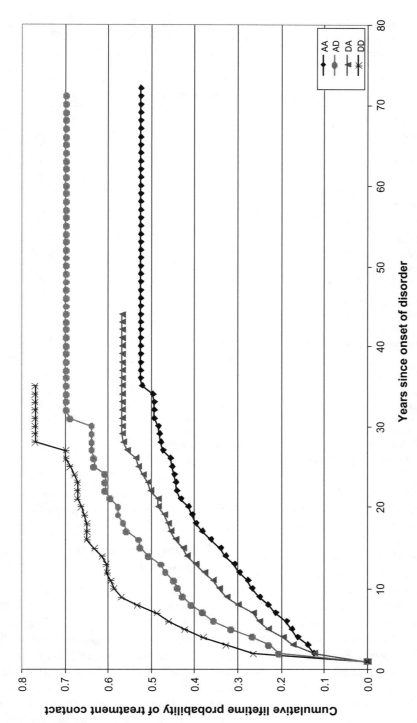

**Figure 9.4.** Cumulative lifetime probability of treatment contact for substance disorders from year of onset[*a]

* Significance of differences among curves: $\chi_2^2 = 44.8$, $p < 0.001$.

[a] Based on survival analysis. The projected proportions of cases that will eventually make treatment contact for each disorder are estimated to be: alcohol abuse (AA), 52.7%; alcohol dependence (AD), 69.8%; drug abuse (DA), 57.0%; drug dependence (DD), 76.9%.

**Table 9.6.** Proportional treatment contact in the year of disorder onset and median duration of delay among cases that subsequently made treatment contact

|  | Treatment contact made in year of onset, % | Median duration of delay (years)[a] | n[b] |
|---|---|---|---|
| I. Anxiety disorders |  |  |  |
|   Panic disorder | 33.6 | 10 | 269 |
|   Agoraphobia | 15.1 | 12 | 137 |
|   Specific phobia | 1.6 | 20 | 720 |
|   Social phobia | 3.4 | 16 | 694 |
|   Generalized anxiety disorder | 33.3 | 9 | 444 |
|   Posttraumatic stress disorder | 7.1 | 12 | 389 |
|   Separation anxiety disorder | 1.0 | 23 | 234 |
| II. Mood disorders |  |  |  |
|   Major depressive episode | 37.4 | 8 | 1092 |
|   Dysthymia | 41.6 | 7 | 229 |
|   Bipolar I–II disorder | 39.1 | 6 | 224 |
| III. Impulse-control disorders |  |  |  |
|   Attention-deficit/hyperactivity disorder | 7.0 | 13 | 253 |
|   Oppositional-defiant disorder | 6.6 | 4 | 324 |
|   Intermittent explosive disorder | 6.8 | 13 | 447 |
| IV. Substance disorders |  |  |  |
|   Alcohol abuse | 12.4 | 9 | 751 |
|   Alcohol dependence | 20.7 | 6 | 307 |
|   Drug abuse | 12.5 | 6 | 450 |
|   Drug dependence | 26.5 | 5 | 174 |

[a] Projections based on time-to-contact survival curves in Figures 9.1–9.4.
[b] Weighted number of respondents with a lifetime history of the disorder.

in delays are significant for only 1 of 17 comparisons. Differences between racial and ethnic groups are significant in 8 of 17 comparisons, with non-Hispanic whites always having higher odds of treatment than one or more minority group. For delays, 5 of 17 comparisons are significant, including some instances in which minorities have significantly shorter delays than non-Hispanic whites. In 8 of 17 comparisons of treatment contact, education is significant; the pattern of association varies depending on the disorder, with the most consistent being that students generally have higher odds of treatment than do people who have completed their education. On the other hand, 10 of 17 comparisons examining delays are significant, with college graduates generally having the shortest delays. Marital status is significant in 5 of 17 comparisons, with the unmarried more likely than married to make treatment contact; a similar relationship exists between marital status and delays, with 7 of 17 comparisons being significant.

## 3.9. Prevalence and Severity of 12-month Disorders

Table 9.10 shows the 12-month prevalence of disorders, with the most common being SP (8.7%), SoP (6.8%), and MDD (6.7%). Among classes, anxiety disorders are the most prevalent (18.1%), followed by mood disorders (9.5%), impulse-control disorders (8.9%), and substance disorders (3.8%). The 12-month prevalence of any disorder is 26.2%, with more than half of cases (14.4% of the total sample) having only one disorder and smaller proportions having two (5.8%) or more (6.0%).

Of 12-month cases, 22.3% were classified as serious, 37.3% as moderate, and 40.4% as mild. Having a serious disorder was strongly related to

**Table 9.7.** Sociodemographic predictors of lifetime treatment contact for specific DSM-IV/CIDI anxiety disorders

| | Anxiety disorders | | | | | | | | | | | | | |
| | Panic disorder | | Agoraphobia | | Social phobia | | Specific phobia | | Generalized anxiety disorder | | Posttraumatic stress disorder | | Separation anxiety disorder | |
| | OR | (95% CI) | OR | (95% CI) | OR | (95% CI) | OR | (95% CI) | OR | (95% CI) | OR | (95% CI) | OR | (95% CI) |
|---|---|---|---|---|---|---|---|---|---|---|---|---|---|---|
| **I. Cohort (age at interview)** | | | | | | | | | | | | | | |
| 18–29 | 3.3* | (1.1–9.9) | 2.5 | (0.9–6.6) | 6.3* | (3.9–10.0) | 7.5* | (3.6–15.7) | 5.4* | (2.6–11.1) | 3.9 | (0.8–18.5) | 0.9 | (0.3–2.8) |
| 30–44 | 1.9 | (0.7–5.4) | 1.3 | (0.6–3.1) | 3.5* | (2.0–6.3) | 4.1* | (2.0–8.3) | 3.0* | (1.8–5.0) | 1.7 | (0.3–8.7) | 1.3 | (0.5–3.3) |
| 45–59 | 1.2 | (0.5–3.0) | 0.5 | (0.2–1.2) | 2.3* | (1.4–3.6) | 2.4* | (1.2–4.9) | 1.9* | (1.1–3.2) | 0.9 | (0.2–5.8) | 1.0 | –[c] |
| 60+ | 1.0 | – | 1.0 | – | 1.0 | – | 1.0 | – | 1.0 | – | 1.0 | – | –[c] | –[c] |
| $\chi^2_3{}^a$ | 10.0* | | 16.8* | | 106.7* | | 57.9* | | 31.6* | | 11.5* | | 0.6 | |
| **II. Age of onset** | | | | | | | | | | | | | | |
| 0–12 | 0.0* | (0.0–0.1) | 0.1* | (0.0–0.3) | 0.1* | (0.1–0.2) | 0.3* | (0.1–0.6) | 0.0* | (0.0–0.1) | 0.1* | (0.0–0.5) | 0.8 | (0.4–1.6) |
| 13–19 | 0.1* | (0.0–0.2) | 0.1* | (0.0–0.3) | 0.2* | (0.1–0.4) | 0.4* | (0.2–0.8) | 0.1* | (0.0–0.1) | 0.2* | (0.0–0.6) | 1.0 | –[c] |
| 20–29 | 0.3* | (0.2–0.5) | 0.3* | (0.1–0.9) | 0.3* | (0.1–0.6) | 0.6 | (0.2–1.6) | 0.2* | (0.1–0.2) | 0.7 | (0.1–3.7) | –[c] | –[c] |
| 30+ | 1.0 | – | 1.0 | – | 1.0 | – | 1.0 | – | 1.0 | – | 1.0 | – | –[c] | –[c] |
| $\chi^2_3{}^b$ | 79.9* | | 22.5* | | 46.9* | | 17.4* | | 101.0* | | 20.5* | | 0.6 | |
| **III. Sex** | | | | | | | | | | | | | | |
| Female | 1.2 | (0.9–1.7) | 1.6 | (0.9–2.9) | 1.7* | (1.3–2.1) | 1.1 | (0.9–1.4) | 1.4 | (0.9–2.0) | 1.0 | (0.3–3.1) | 0.9 | (0.5–1.7) |
| Male | 1.0 | – | 1.0 | – | 1.0 | – | 1.0 | – | 1.0 | – | 1.0 | – | 1.0 | – |
| $\chi^2_1$ | 1.8 | | 2.5 | | 18.8* | | 1.0 | | 2.7 | | 0.0 | | 0.1 | |
| **IV. Race-ethnicity** | | | | | | | | | | | | | | |
| Non-Hispanic white | 1.0 | – | 1.0 | – | 1.0 | – | 1.0 | – | 1.0 | – | 1.0 | – | 1.0 | – |
| Non-Hispanic black | 0.6* | (0.4–0.9) | 0.4* | (0.2–0.8) | 0.5* | (0.4–0.8) | 0.8 | (0.5–1.2) | 0.4* | (0.2–0.6) | 0.5* | (0.2–0.9) | 0.2* | (0.0–0.9) |
| Hispanic | 0.5* | (0.3–0.8) | 0.8 | (0.3–2.0) | 0.7 | (0.4–1.2) | 0.8 | (0.5–1.3) | 0.7 | (0.3–1.5) | 2.0 | (0.7–7.8) | 0.8 | (0.3–2.3) |
| Other | 0.4* | (0.2–0.8) | 0.5 | (0.1–2.0) | 0.7 | (0.5–1.1) | 1.0 | (0.5–1.9) | 0.4 | (0.1–1.2) | 0.4 | (0.1–1.6) | 0.1* | (0.0–0.8) |
| $\chi^2_3$ | 14.4* | | 7.6* | | 12.0* | | 1.9 | | 14.2* | | 12.6* | | 18.0* | |
| **V. Education** | | | | | | | | | | | | | | |
| Student | 0.6 | (0.3–1.2) | 0.4 | (0.1–2.0) | 0.7 | (0.4–1.3) | 0.4 | (0.2–1.0) | 1.0 | (0.4–2.1) | 9.8* | (2.5–37.4) | 0.7 | (0.1–8.0) |
| 0–11 nonstudent | 0.4* | (0.2–0.8) | 1.1 | (0.4–2.8) | 1.2 | (0.7–1.9) | 0.8 | (0.6–1.2) | 0.6* | (0.3–0.9) | 2.5* | (1.1–6.1) | 0.4 | (0.2–1.2) |
| 12 nonstudent | 0.9 | (0.5–1.6) | 0.6 | (0.2–1.6) | 0.8 | (0.6–1.2) | 0.9 | (0.6–1.4) | 0.9 | (0.6–1.4) | 1.3 | (0.3–5.2) | 0.7 | (0.2–2.7) |
| 13–15 nonstudent | 0.7 | (0.4–1.2) | 1.1 | (0.4–3.0) | 0.9 | (0.6–1.2) | 0.9 | (0.6–1.4) | 0.9 | (0.6–1.5) | 1.2 | (0.2–6.7) | 0.1* | (0.0–0.3) |
| 16+ nonstudent | 1.0 | – | 1.0 | – | 1.0 | – | 1.0 | – | 1.0 | – | 1.0 | – | 1.0 | – |
| $\chi^2_4$ | 10.2* | | 6.2 | | 2.5 | | 5.1 | | 6.9 | | 14.8* | | 23.9* | |
| **VI. Marital status** | | | | | | | | | | | | | | |
| Married/cohabitating | 1.0 | – | 1.0 | – | 1.0 | – | 1.0 | – | 1.0 | – | 1.0 | – | 1.0 | – |
| Previously married | 0.8 | (0.4–1.3) | 1.2 | (0.6–2.6) | 1.7* | (1.1–2.5) | 1.2 | (0.8–1.8) | 1.2 | (0.8–1.9) | 0.9 | (0.4–1.9) | 1.1 | (0.5–2.2) |
| Never married | 0.7 | (0.4–1.1) | 1.7 | (0.8–3.6) | 1.4 | (1.0–2.0) | 1.1 | (0.8–1.7) | 1.1 | (0.8–1.5) | 0.5 | (0.1–2.8) | 2.2 | (0.6–7.1) |
| $\chi^2_2$ | 3.2 | | 2.0 | | 8.9* | | 0.8 | | 0.9 | | 0.6 | | 1.9 | |

\* Significant at the 0.05 level, two-sided test.

*Note*: Based on multivariate discrete-time survival analysis with person–year as the unit of analysis and time-varying values used for education and marital status. Referent indicated by OR of 1.0 and 95% CI.

[a] Two degrees of freedom in the separation anxiety disorder equation.

[b] One degree of freedom in the separation anxiety disorder equation.

[c] Childhood disorders only assessed in respondents up to age 44.

**Table 9.8.** Sociodemographic predictors of lifetime treatment contact for specific DSM-IV/CIDI mood and impulse-control disorders

| | Mood disorders | | | | | | Impulse-control disorders | | | | | |
| | Major depressive episode | | Dysthymia | | Bipolar disorder I or II | | Intermittent explosive disorder | | Oppositional defiant disorder | | Attention-deficit/ hyperactivity disorder | |
| | OR | (95% CI) | OR | (95% CI) | OR | (95% CI) | OR | (95% CI) | OR | (95% CI) | OR | (95% CI) |
|---|---|---|---|---|---|---|---|---|---|---|---|---|
| **I. Cohort (age at interview)** | | | | | | | | | | | | |
| 18–29 | 5.0* | (3.2–7.9) | 2.9* | (1.6–5.3) | 16.3* | (2.0–134.6) | 6.3* | (2.6–15.2) | 1.2 | (0.6–2.1) | 0.5* | (0.3–0.8) |
| 30–44 | 2.3* | (1.5–3.7) | 1.6 | (0.8–3.1) | 6.9 | (0.8–60.6) | 3.5* | (1.5–8.3) | 1.0 | – | 1.0 | – |
| 45–59 | 1.7* | (1.1–2.6) | 1.5 | (0.9–2.6) | 6.6 | (0.8–50.9) | 2.3 | (0.8–6.1) | –ᵇ | –ᵇ | –ᵇ | –ᵇ |
| 60+ | 1.0 | – | 1.0 | – | 1.0 | – | 1.0 | – | –ᵇ | –ᵇ | –ᵇ | –ᵇ |
| $\chi^2_3{}^a$ | 100.9* | | 14.4* | | 20.5* | | 35.4* | | 0.2 | | 7.4* | |
| **II. Age of onset** | | | | | | | | | | | | |
| 0–12 | 0.0* | (0.0–0.1) | 0.0* | (0.0–0.1) | 0.0* | (0.0–0.0) | 0.6 | (0.2–1.7) | 0.5* | (0.3–0.9) | 1.1 | (0.2–6.1) |
| 13–19 | 0.1* | (0.1–0.2) | 0.1* | (0.0–0.2) | 0.1* | (0.0–0.1) | 1.1 | (0.4–3.1) | 1.0 | – | 1.0 | – |
| 20–29 | 0.2* | (0.2–0.3) | 0.2* | (0.1–0.3) | 0.2* | (0.1–0.4) | 0.8 | (0.2–2.8) | –ᵇ | –ᵇ | –ᵇ | –ᵇ |
| 30+ | 1.0 | – | 1.0 | – | 1.0 | – | 1.0 | – | –ᵇ | –ᵇ | –ᵇ | –ᵇ |
| $\chi^2_3{}^a$ | 167.1* | | 96.3* | | 84.3* | | 12.9* | | 6.1* | | 0.0 | |
| **III. Sex** | | | | | | | | | | | | |
| Female | 1.5* | (1.2–1.8) | 1.6* | (1.1–2.1) | 1.5* | (1.1–2.1) | 1.4 | (1.0–1.9) | 1.6 | (1.0–2.6) | 0.8 | (0.4–1.3) |
| Male | 1.0 | – | 1.0 | – | 1.0 | – | 1.0 | – | – | – | – | – |
| $\chi^2_1$ | 10.2* | | 8.0* | | 6.0* | | 3.7 | | 3.4 | | 1.3 | |
| **IV. Race-ethnicity** | | | | | | | | | | | | |
| Non-Hispanic white | 1.0 | – | 1.0 | – | 1.0 | – | 1.0 | – | 1.0 | – | 1.0 | – |
| Non-Hispanic black | 0.5* | (0.4–0.7) | 0.5* | (0.3–0.9) | 0.3* | (0.2–0.6) | 0.8 | (0.5–1.4) | 0.2* | (0.1–0.6) | 0.8 | (0.3–1.7) |
| Hispanic | 0.5* | (0.4–0.7) | 0.9 | (0.5–1.8) | 0.4* | (0.2–0.7) | 0.9 | (0.6–1.4) | 0.7 | (0.3–1.5) | 1.0 | (0.5–2.0) |
| Other | 0.5* | (0.3–0.8) | 0.8 | (0.5–1.4) | 1.1 | (0.6–2.0) | 0.8 | (0.4–1.7) | 1.3 | (0.4–4.5) | 0.9 | (0.3–2.5) |
| $\chi^2_3$ | 63.2* | | 7.2 | | 25.5* | | 1.4 | | 8.1* | | 0.6 | |
| **V. Education** | | | | | | | | | | | | |
| Student | 1.2 | (0.8–1.8) | 1.7 | (0.8–3.6) | 0.7 | (0.2–2.2) | 1.6 | (0.8–3.5) | 7.6* | (1.6–35.3) | 0.9 | (0.2–4.1) |
| 0–11 nonstudent | 0.8 | (0.5–1.2) | 0.6 | (0.3–1.3) | 0.6 | (0.2–2.0) | 0.7 | (0.4–1.4) | 1.5 | (0.2–10.3) | 0.8 | (0.2–2.5) |
| 12 nonstudent | 0.6 | (0.4–0.8) | 0.7 | (0.4–1.3) | 0.8 | (0.3–2.0) | 0.7 | (0.4–1.1) | 1.3 | (0.2–7.5) | 0.3 | (0.1–1.0) |
| 13–15 nonstudent | 0.8 | (0.6–1.1) | 0.9 | (0.4–1.9) | 1.6 | (0.6–3.7) | 0.6* | (0.4–0.8) | 1.0 | (0.2–5.1) | 0.8 | (0.3–2.5) |
| 16+ nonstudent | 1.0 | – | 1.0 | – | 1.0 | – | 1.0 | – | 1.0 | – | 1.0 | – |
| $\chi^2_4$ | 26.9* | | 7.4 | | 7.7 | | 15.2* | | 52.0* | | 7.9 | |
| **VI. Marital status** | | | | | | | | | | | | |
| Married/cohabitating | 1.0 | – | 1.0 | – | 1.0 | – | 1.0 | – | 1.0 | – | 1.0 | – |
| Previously married | 1.3 | (0.9–1.8) | 0.9 | (0.5–1.7) | 1.8 | (1.0–3.5) | 1.6 | (0.9–2.9) | 4.6* | (1.1–18.6) | 0.8 | (0.4–1.7) |
| Never married | 1.2 | (0.9–1.6) | 1.9* | (1.2–3.1) | 1.5 | (0.8–2.6) | 1.3 | (0.8–2.1) | 1.8 | (0.4–7.6) | 0.9 | (0.4–2.4) |
| $\chi^2_2$ | 3.1 | | 8.1* | | 4.5 | | 3.8 | | 5.5 | | 0.4 | |

* Significant at the 0.05 level, two-sided test.

*Notes:* Based on multivariate discrete-time survival analysis with person-year as the unit of analysis and time-varying values used for education and marital status. Referent indicated by OR of 1.0 and 95% CI.

ᵃ One degree of freedom in the oppositional-defiant disorder and attention-deficit/hyperactivity disorder equations.

ᵇ Childhood disorders only assessed in respondents up to age 44.

**Table 9.9.** Sociodemographic predictors of lifetime treatment contact for specific DSM-IV/CIDI substance disorders

| | Substance disorders | | | | | | | |
|---|---|---|---|---|---|---|---|---|
| | Alcohol abuse | | Alcohol dependence | | Drug abuse | | Drug dependence | |
| | OR | (95% CI) | OR | (95% CI) | OR | (95% CI) | OR | (95% CI) |
| **I. Cohort (age at interview)** | | | | | | | | |
| 18–29 | 2.8* | (1.7–4.6) | 2.1 | (0.8–6.0) | 2.4 | (1.0–5.8) | 0.6 | (0.2–2.2) |
| 30–44 | 2.2* | (1.4–3.5) | 1.5 | (0.6–3.9) | 1.6 | (0.7–3.5) | 0.4 | (0.1–1.4) |
| 45–59 | 1.6* | (1.1–2.3) | 1.1 | (0.6–2.2) | 0.8 | (0.4–1.8) | 0.2* | (0.1–0.9) |
| 60+ | 1.0 | – | 1.0 | – | 1.0 | – | 1.0 | – |
| $\chi_3^2$ | 18.2* | | 4.9 | | 15.8* | | 13.5* | |
| **II. Age of onset** | | | | | | | | |
| 0–12 | 0.4* | (0.2–0.9) | 0.1* | (0.0–0.3) | 0.3* | (0.2–0.8) | 0.0* | (0.0–0.1) |
| 13–19 | 0.3* | (0.2–0.5) | 0.2* | (0.1–0.3) | 0.2* | (0.1–0.4) | 0.1* | (0.0–0.3) |
| 20–29 | 0.5* | (0.3–0.7) | 0.2* | (0.1–0.4) | 0.3* | (0.2–0.6) | 0.2* | (0.1–0.5) |
| 30+ | 1.0 | – | 1.0 | – | 1.0 | – | 1.0 | – |
| $\chi_3^2$ | 25.1* | | 34.2* | | 25.0* | | 37.6* | |
| **III. Sex** | | | | | | | | |
| Female | 1.1 | (0.8–1.4) | 0.8 | (0.5–1.2) | 1.0 | (0.8–1.5) | 1.0 | (0.7–1.5) |
| Male | 1.0 | – | 1.0 | – | 1.0 | – | 1.0 | – |
| $\chi_1^2$ | 0.1 | | 1.7 | | 0.1 | | 0.0 | |
| **IV. Race-ethnicity** | | | | | | | | |
| Non-Hispanic white | 1.0 | – | 1.0 | – | 1.0 | – | 1.0 | – |
| Non-Hispanic black | 0.9 | (0.6–1.3) | 0.4* | (0.2–0.9) | 0.7 | (0.4–1.1) | 0.6 | (0.2–1.7) |
| Hispanic | 0.9 | (0.6–1.3) | 0.8 | (0.5–1.3) | 0.8 | (0.4–1.6) | 1.1 | (0.4–2.8) |
| Other | 0.7 | (0.4–1.2) | 0.8 | (0.3–1.7) | 1.0 | (0.5–1.9) | 1.3 | (0.6–2.7) |
| $\chi_3^2$ | 3.4 | | 6.6 | | 3.0 | | 2.1 | |
| **V. Education** | | | | | | | | |
| Student | 1.2 | (0.7–1.9) | 1.1 | (0.5–2.1) | 2.0 | (1.0–3.8) | 1.5 | (0.5–4.8) |
| 0–11 nonstudent | 1.3 | (0.9–1.9) | 1.4 | (0.8–2.6) | 1.6 | (1.0–2.6) | 1.1 | (0.4–2.9) |
| 12 nonstudent | 0.8 | (0.6–1.1) | 0.8 | (0.4–1.3) | 0.8 | (0.5–1.2) | 0.7 | (0.3–1.8) |
| 13–15 nonstudent | 0.9 | (0.6–1.4) | 1.0 | (0.5–1.8) | 1.1 | (0.6–2.0) | 1.4 | (0.5–4.1) |
| 16+ nonstudent | 1.0 | – | 1.0 | – | 1.0 | – | 1.0 | – |
| $\chi_4^2$ | 18.5* | | 7.7 | | 26.9* | | 6.9 | |
| **VI. Marital status** | | | | | | | | |
| Married/cohabitating | 1.0 | – | 1.0 | – | 1.0 | – | 1.0 | – |
| Previously married | 1.4 | (1.0–1.9) | 1.0 | (0.6–1.7) | 1.7* | (1.1–2.7) | 2.5* | (1.3–4.7) |
| Never married | 1.6* | (1.1–2.2) | 1.6 | (1.0–2.5) | 1.9* | (1.3–2.9) | 2.6* | (1.2–5.5) |
| $\chi_2^2$ | 8.2* | | 3.7 | | 14.5* | | 11.2* | |

* Significant at the 0.05 level, two-sided test.

*Notes:* Based on multivariate discrete-time survival analysis with person-year as the unit of analysis and time-varying values used for education and marital status. Referent indicated by OR of 1.0 and 95% CI.

comorbidity, with 9.6% of those with one diagnosis, 25.5% with two, and 49.9% with three or more diagnoses classified as serious cases. Among disorder classes, mood disorders have the highest percentage of serious cases (45.0%) and anxiety disorders the lowest (22.8%). The anxiety disorder with the greatest proportion of serious cases is obsessive-compulsive disorder (OCD) (50.6%), while BPD has the greatest proportion of serious case (82.9%) among mood disorders, ODD the

**Table 9.10.** 12-month prevalence and severity of DSM-IV/CIDI disorders ($n = 9282$)

| | Total | | Serious | | Moderate | | Mild | |
|---|---|---|---|---|---|---|---|---|
| | % | (se) | % | (se) | % | (se) | % | (se) |
| **I. Anxiety disorders** | | | | | | | | |
| Panic disorder | 2.7 | (0.2) | 44.8 | (3.2) | 29.5 | (2.7) | 25.7 | (2.5) |
| Agoraphobia without panic | 0.8 | (0.1) | 40.6 | (7.2) | 30.7 | (6.4) | 28.7 | (8.4) |
| Specific phobia | 8.7 | (0.4) | 21.9 | (2.0) | 30.0 | (2.0) | 48.1 | (2.1) |
| Social phobia | 6.8 | (0.3) | 29.9 | (2.0) | 38.8 | (2.5) | 31.3 | (2.4) |
| Generalized anxiety disorder | 3.1 | (0.2) | 32.3 | (2.9) | 44.6 | (4.0) | 23.1 | (2.9) |
| Posttraumatic stress disorder[b] | 3.5 | (0.3) | 36.6 | (3.5) | 33.1 | (2.2) | 30.2 | (3.4) |
| Obsessive-compulsive disorder[c] | 1.0 | (0.3) | 50.6 | (12.4) | 34.8 | (14.1) | 14.6 | (5.7) |
| Separation anxiety disorder[d] | 0.9 | (0.2) | 43.3 | (9.2) | 24.8 | (7.5) | 31.9 | (12.2) |
| Any anxiety disorder[e] | 18.1 | (0.7) | 22.8 | (1.5) | 33.7 | (1.4) | 43.5 | (2.1) |
| **II. Mood disorders** | | | | | | | | |
| Major depressive disorder | 6.7 | (0.3) | 30.4 | (1.7) | 50.1 | (2.1) | 19.5 | (2.1) |
| Dysthymia | 1.5 | (0.1) | 49.7 | (3.9) | 32.1 | (4.0) | 18.2 | (3.4) |
| Bipolar I–II disorders | 2.6 | (0.2) | 82.9 | (3.2) | 17.1 | (3.2) | 0.0 | (0.0) |
| Any mood disorder | 9.5 | (0.4) | 45.0 | (1.9) | 40.0 | (1.7) | 15.0 | (1.6) |
| **III. Impulse-control disorders** | | | | | | | | |
| Oppositional-defiant disorder[d] | 1.0 | (0.2) | 49.6 | (8.0) | 40.3 | (8.7) | 10.1 | (4.8) |
| Conduct disorder[d] | 1.0 | (0.2) | 40.5 | (11.1) | 31.6 | (7.5) | 28.0 | (9.1) |
| Attention-deficit/hyperactivity disorder[d] | 4.1 | (0.3) | 41.3 | (4.3) | 35.2 | (3.5) | 23.5 | (4.5) |
| Intermittent explosive disorder | 2.6 | (0.2) | 23.8 | (3.3) | 74.4 | (3.5) | 1.7 | (0.9) |
| Any impulse-control disorder[d, f] | 8.9 | (0.5) | 32.9 | (2.9) | 52.4 | (3.0) | 14.7 | (2.3) |
| **IV. Substance disorders** | | | | | | | | |
| Alcohol abuse[b] | 3.1 | (0.3) | 28.9 | (2.6) | 39.7 | (3.7) | 31.5 | (3.3) |
| Alcohol dependence[b] | 1.3 | (0.2) | 34.3 | (4.5) | 65.7 | (4.5) | 0.0 | (0.0) |
| Drug abuse[b] | 1.4 | (0.1) | 36.6 | (5.0) | 30.4 | (5.8) | 33.0 | (6.8) |
| Drug dependence[b] | 0.4 | (0.1) | 56.5 | (8.2) | 43.5 | (8.2) | 0.0 | (0.0) |
| Any substance disorder[b] | 3.8 | (0.3) | 29.6 | (2.8) | 37.1 | (3.5) | 33.4 | (3.2) |
| **V. Any disorder** | | | | | | | | |
| Any[e] | 26.2 | (0.8) | 22.3 | (1.3) | 37.3 | (1.3) | 40.4 | (1.6) |
| One disorder[e] | 14.4 | (0.6) | 9.6 | (1.3) | 31.2 | (1.9) | 59.2 | (2.3) |
| Two disorders[e] | 5.8 | (0.3) | 25.5 | (2.1) | 46.4 | (2.6) | 28.2 | (2.0) |
| Three or more disorders[e] | 6.0 | (0.3) | 49.9 | (2.3) | 43.1 | (2.1) | 7.0 | (1.3) |

[a] Percentages in the three severity columns are repeated as proportions of all cases and sum to 100% across each row.

[b] Assessed in the Part 2 sample ($n = 5692$).

[c] Assessed in a random one-third of the Part 2 sample ($n = 1808$).

[d] Assessed in the Part 2 sample among respondents aged 18–44 years ($n = 3199$).

[e] Estimated in the Part 2 sample. No adjustment is made for the fact that one or more disorders in the category were not assessed for all Part 2 respondents.

[f] The estimated prevalence of any impulse-control disorder is larger than the sum of the individual disorders because the prevalence of intermittent explosive disorder, the only impulse-control disorder that was assessed in the total sample, is reported here for the total sample rather than for the subsample of respondents among whom the other impulse-control disorders were assessed (Part 2 respondents aged 18–44). The estimated prevalence of any impulse-control disorder, in comparison, is estimated in the latter subsample. Intermittent explosive disorder has a considerably higher estimated prevalence in this subsample than in the total sample.

highest (49.6%) among impulse-control disorders, and DD the highest (56.5%) among substance disorders.

## 3.10. Bivariate Analyses of 12-month Comorbidity

Table 9.11 shows tetrachoric correlations between hierarchy-free 12-month disorders. Nearly all are positive (98%) and statistically significant (72%). Only four correlations are negative and all involve either OCD or SAD, which are uncommon. The 12 highest correlations, each exceeding 0.60, involve well-known syndromes: BPD (MDE with mania-hypomania), double depression (MDE with dysthymia), anxious depression (MDE with GAD), comorbid mania-hypomania and ADHD, panic disorder with agoraphobia, comorbid SoP with agoraphobia, and comorbid substance disorders (both AA and AD with DA and DD).

The correlation matrix was explored with factor analysis after excluding disorders (OCD and SAD) associated with negative correlations. Eigenvalues greater than one (7.3, 2.3) were observed for two factors; the eigenvalue of the third factor was substantially smaller (0.8). As shown in Table 9.11, rigid and oblique rotations of the two-factor solution yielded similar patterns, with high factor loadings on the first factor for internalizing disorders (anxiety disorders, MDE) and on the second factor for externalizing disorders (conduct disorder, substance disorders). Factor loadings of 0.30 or higher on both factors were observed for five disorders (dysthymia, mania-hypomania, ODD, ADHD, and IED), with higher loadings on the internalizing than externalizing factor for all five.

## 3.11. Multivariate Analyses of 12-month Comorbidity

Among the $2^{19}$ or 524,288 logically possible multivariate disorder profiles that can be made from the 19 NCS-R disorders assessed, 433 were observed. As shown in Table 9.12, nearly 80% involve highly comorbid cases (three or more disorders), which account for 27.0% of all respondents with a disorder and 55.9% of all instances of these disorders. Importantly, the distribution of comorbidity is significantly different ($\chi_3^2 = 110.2$, $p < 0.001$) from the distribution we would expect to find if the multivariate structure among the disorders was due entirely to the two-way associations that are the focus of factor analysis. For this reason, confirmatory factor analysis was not used to explore comorbid profiles. Rather, nonadditive comorbid profiles were examined using latent class analysis (LCA). Because LCA assumes conditional independence within classes, AA and AD were collapsed into a single category for this analysis; DA and DD were collapsed for the same reason and MDE and DYS were collapsed because of their extremely high tetrachoric correlation.

The seven-class LCA model shown in Table 9.13 provided the best fit to the data. Prevalence of the seven classes differs greatly, from 68.5% in Class I to 0.7% in Class VII. Inverse relationships exist between prevalence and both the number of disorders (see Table 9.13, Part 3) as well as severity (see Table 9.13, Part 4); meaningful inversions between Classes IV and V exist as well. Subsets of the classes form a general hierarchy (e.g., Classes II, IV, and VI represent profiles of increasingly comorbid internalizing disorders). However, some disorders are more prevalent in the lower than in the higher classes (e.g., ODD and conduct disorder are more prevalent in Class II than Class IV, whereas PD and all three types of phobia are more prevalent in Class IV than Class VI). Such inversions provide evidence that the classes are not just points of density on the two factor analysis dimensions.

Interpretation of the seven LCA classes is assisted by examining the mean number ($\overline{x}_d$) and content of within-class disorders. Class I represents unaffected respondents ($\overline{x}_d = 0.1$); Class II represents pure ($\overline{x}_d = 1.2$) internalizing disorders; Class III represents pure ($\overline{x}_d = 1.2$) externalizing disorders; Class IV represents comorbid ($\overline{x}_d = 2.9$) internalizing disorders; Class V represents comorbid ($\overline{x}_d = 2.0$) internalizing-externalizing disorders dominated by comorbid SoP and ADHD; Class VI represents highly comorbid ($\overline{x}_d = 4.9$) MDEs; Class VII represents

**Table 9.11.** Tetrachoric correlations among hierarchy-free 12-month DSM-IV/CIDI disorders and factor loadings from a principal axis factor analysis of the correlation matrix (n = 3199)

| | PD | AG | SP | SoP | GAD | PTSD | OCD | SAD | MDE | DYS | MHE | ODD | CD | ADHD | IED | AA | AD | DA | DD |
|---|---|---|---|---|---|---|---|---|---|---|---|---|---|---|---|---|---|---|---|
| **I. Anxiety disorders** | | | | | | | | | | | | | | | | | | | |
| Panic disorder (PD) | 1.0 | | | | | | | | | | | | | | | | | | |
| Agoraphobia (AG) | 0.6* | 1.0 | | | | | | | | | | | | | | | | | |
| Specific phobia (SP) | 0.5* | 0.6* | 1.0 | | | | | | | | | | | | | | | | |
| Social phobia (SoP) | 0.5* | 0.7* | 0.5* | 1.0 | | | | | | | | | | | | | | | |
| Generalized anxiety disorder (GAD) | 0.5* | 0.4* | 0.4* | 0.5* | 1.0 | | | | | | | | | | | | | | |
| Posttraumatic stress disorder (PTSD) | 0.5* | 0.5* | 0.4* | 0.4* | 0.4* | 1.0 | | | | | | | | | | | | | |
| Obsessive-compulsive disorder (OCD)[a] | 0.4 | 0.4 | 0.2 | 0.2 | 0.3 | 0.6* | 1.0 | | | | | | | | | | | | |
| Separation anxiety disorder (SAD) | 0.4* | 0.3 | 0.3* | 0.3* | 0.4* | 0.5* | −0.8 | 1.0 | | | | | | | | | | | |
| **II. Mood disorders** | | | | | | | | | | | | | | | | | | | |
| Major depressive episode (MDE) | 0.5* | 0.5* | 0.4* | 0.5* | 0.6* | 0.5* | 0.4* | 0.4* | 1.0 | | | | | | | | | | |
| Dysthymia (DYS) | 0.5* | 0.4* | 0.4* | 0.6* | 0.6* | 0.5* | 0.4 | 0.4* | 0.9* | 1.0 | | | | | | | | | |
| Manic-hypomanic episode (MHE) | 0.5* | 0.5* | 0.4* | 0.5* | 0.5* | 0.4* | 0.4 | 0.4* | 0.6* | 0.6* | 1.0 | | | | | | | | |
| **III. Impulse-control disorders** | | | | | | | | | | | | | | | | | | | |
| Oppositional-defiant disorder (ODD) | 0.4* | 0.5* | 0.4* | 0.5* | 0.3* | 0.5* | 0.5 | 0.5* | 0.5* | 0.5* | 0.6* | 1.0 | | | | | | | |
| Conduct disorder (CD) | 0.3 | 0.2 | 0.2 | 0.3* | 0.1 | 0.3 | −0.8 | −0.1 | 0.1 | 0.3 | 0.3* | 0.5* | 1.0 | | | | | | |
| Attention-deficit hyperactivity disorder (ADHD) | 0.4* | 0.4* | 0.3* | 0.5* | 0.5* | 0.4* | 0.3 | 0.4* | 0.5* | 0.5* | 0.6* | 0.6* | 0.4* | 1.0 | | | | | |
| Intermittent explosive disorder (IED) | 0.3* | 0.4* | 0.3* | 0.3* | 0.3* | 0.2* | 0.2 | 0.3 | 0.4* | 0.4* | 0.4* | 0.4* | 0.4* | 0.4* | 1.0 | | | | |
| **IV. Substance disorders** | | | | | | | | | | | | | | | | | | | |
| Alcohol abuse (AA) | 0.3* | 0.2 | 0.1 | 0.2* | 0.2* | 0.3* | 0.3* | 0.1 | 0.2* | 0.3* | 0.4* | 0.3 | 0.4* | 0.3* | 0.4* | 1.0 | | | |
| Alcohol dependence (AD) | 0.2 | 0.3 | 0.2* | 0.3* | 0.3* | 0.3* | 0.2 | 0.1 | 0.4* | 0.4* | 0.4* | 0.4 | 0.4 | 0.3 | 0.4* | 1.0* | 1.0 | | |
| Drug abuse (DA) | 0.2 | 0.1 | 0.1 | 0.2* | 0.2* | 0.1 | 0.3 | 0.1 | 0.2* | 0.4* | 0.4* | 0.4* | 0.4 | 0.4* | 0.3* | 0.7* | 0.6* | 1.0 | |
| Drug dependence (DD) | 0.3 | 0.3 | 0.3 | 0.4* | 0.4* | 0.2 | 0.4 | −0.8* | 0.4* | 0.6* | 0.4* | 0.6* | 0.4 | 0.6* | 0.4* | 0.6* | 0.7* | 1.0* | 1.0 |
| Prevalence | 3.4 | 1.6 | 10.1 | 8.8 | 4.4 | 3.7 | 1.3 | 0.9 | 10.3 | 2.4 | 3.8 | 1.1 | 1.0 | 4.1 | 6.6 | 5.0 | 2.2 | 2.4 | 0.7 |
| Percentage comorbid | 80 | 97 | 62 | 74 | 85 | 75 | 65 | 71 | 76 | 99 | 87 | 93 | 70 | 78 | 70 | 77 | 100 | 79 | 100 |
| Factor 1[b] | 0.7 | 0.8 | 0.6 | 0.7 | 0.6 | 0.6 | – | – | 0.8 | 0.7 | 0.7 | 0.6 | 0.3 | 0.6 | 0.4 | 0.1 | 0.2 | 0.1 | 0.3 |
| Factor 2[b] | 0.1 | 0.1 | 0.0 | 0.2 | 0.2 | 0.2 | – | – | 0.2 | 0.3 | 0.3 | 0.3 | 0.5 | 0.3 | 0.4 | 0.9 | 0.9 | 0.9 | 0.9 |

* Significant at the 0.05 level, two-sided test.

*Note:* Part 2 respondents aged 18–44 years (n = 3199).

[a] Assessed in a random one-third of the Part 2 sample among respondents aged 18–44 years (n = 1025).

[b] Varimax rotation.

**Table 9.12.** Distribution of hierarchy-free 12-month DSM-IV/CIDI disorders ($n = 3199$)

| | Respondents | | Cases | | Diagnoses[a] | | Profiles[b] |
|---|---|---|---|---|---|---|---|
| | % | (se) | % | (se) | % | (se) | % |
| Disorders | | | | | | | |
| 0 | 66.4 | (0.9) | – | – | – | – | – |
| 1 | 16.9 | (0.7) | 50.3 | (1.5) | 23.2 | (1.4) | 3.9 |
| 2 | 7.6 | (0.4) | 22.7 | (1.2) | 20.9 | (1.4) | 17.1 |
| 3+ | 9.1 | (0.6) | 27.0 | (1.8) | 55.9 | (2.4) | 79.0 |

*Note:* Part 2 NCS-R respondents aged 18–44 years.

[a] The proportion of respondents with more than two diagnoses ranged from 3.8% with exactly 3 to 0.03% with 15 and averaged 4.5 diagnoses per respondent with more than 2. When the diagnosis is taken as the unit of analysis, the results in this column show that more than half of all 12-month diagnoses occurred to respondents with three or more disorders.

[b] The 19 disorders generate $2^{19}$ (524,288) logically possible multivariate disorder profiles, of which 433 are observed in the sample of Part 2 respondents aged 18–44 years.

**Table 9.13.** Conditional probabilities and distributions of hierarchy-free 12-month DSM-IV/CIDI disorders based on a seven-class latent class analysis

| | Class 1 % | Class 2 % | Class 3 % | Class 4 % | Class 5 % | Class 6 % | Class 7 % |
|---|---|---|---|---|---|---|---|
| **I. Within-class disorder prevalences** | | | | | | | |
| Panic disorder | 0.9 | 1.5 | 2.5 | 32.8 | 0.0 | 10.9 | 73.0 |
| Agoraphobia | 0.0 | 0.0 | 0.0 | 23.7 | 1.5 | 3.0 | 45.8 |
| Specific phobia | 4.8 | 15.6 | 2.0 | 53.0 | 25.4 | 36.0 | 83.9 |
| Social phobia | 2.1 | 15.9 | 3.6 | 51.3 | 40.2 | 41.0 | 88.4 |
| Generalized anxiety disorder | 0.1 | 13.2 | 3.5 | 23.2 | 0.0 | 38.6 | 50.5 |
| Posttraumatic stress disorder | 1.0 | 5.8 | 1.5 | 19.5 | 14.1 | 22.8 | 54.8 |
| Major depressive episode/dysthymia | 0.0 | 40.7 | 5.3 | 40.7 | 0.0 | 94.6 | 89.3 |
| Manic-hypomanic episode | 0.0 | 6.5 | 11.1 | 10.2 | 0.0 | 54.1 | 93.8 |
| Oppositional-defiant disorder | 0.0 | 1.1 | 1.3 | 0.7 | 15.9 | 11.7 | 39.3 |
| Conduct disorder | 0.3 | 0.3 | 3.0 | 0.0 | 15.0 | 6.7 | 11.9 |
| Attention-deficit/hyperactivity disorder | 0.9 | 5.9 | 0.0 | 7.7 | 39.0 | 56.2 | 64.0 |
| Intermittent explosive disorder | 1.4 | 12.7 | 22.1 | 14.6 | 21.8 | 40.5 | 45.1 |
| Alcohol abuse or dependence | 0.2 | 0.0 | 43.6 | 13.2 | 14.4 | 42.5 | 5.6 |
| Drug abuse or dependence | 0.0 | 0.0 | 21.5 | 0.0 | 11.9 | 31.2 | 5.2 |
| **II. Class prevalence** | 68.5 | 14.5 | 7.4 | 5.0 | 2.3 | 1.6 | 0.7 |
| **III. Within-class disorder distributions** | | | | | | | |
| 0 | 88.9 | 25.7 | 24.4 | 2.6 | 9.7 | 0.0 | 0.9 |
| 1 | 10.5 | 40.1 | 40.9 | 12.2 | 26.1 | 0.8 | 0.2 |
| 2 | 0.6 | 25.4 | 25.6 | 27.0 | 35.2 | 4.2 | 0.0 |
| 3+ | 0.0 | 8.9 | 9.1 | 58.2 | 29.0 | 95.0 | 98.8 |
| **IV. Within-class severity distributions** | | | | | | | |
| None | 86.8 | 25.1 | 23.8 | 2.6 | 9.5 | 0.0 | 0.9 |
| Mild | 7.6 | 22.7 | 28.5 | 23.2 | 30.7 | 1.3 | 0.2 |
| Moderate | 4.5 | 37.3 | 30.7 | 40.0 | 44.5 | 28.1 | 5.2 |
| Serious | 1.1 | 14.9 | 17.0 | 34.2 | 15.2 | 70.5 | 93.8 |

*Note:* Part 2 respondents aged 18–44 years ($n = 3199$).

highly comorbid ($\overline{x}_d$ = 7.5) BPD. Although classes with high comorbidity (Classes IV, VI, and VII) include only about 7% of the sample, it is worth noting that 43.6% of serious cases are in these classes.

### 3.12. Sociodemographic Correlates of 12-month Mental Disorders

Correlates of being largely unaffected by mental disorders were identified using predicted probabilities of LCA Class I membership and included being male, non-Hispanic black or Hispanic, married, having a college education, high income, and residing in a rural area (see Table 9.14). Correlates of pure internalizing disorders (Class II) include being female, married, having a high level of education, and residing in the suburbs of small metropolitan areas. Correlates of pure externalizing disorders (Class III) include being young, male, Hispanic, not low income, and residing in a rural area. Correlates of comorbid internalizing disorders (Class IV) include being female, previously married, and residing either in suburbia or in an outlying nonrural area. Correlates of comorbid internalizing-externalizing disorders (Class V) include being young, male, married, and residing in a nonrural area. Correlates of highly comorbid major depression (Class VI) include being female, non-Hispanic white or other non-Hispanic/non-black race-ethnicity, unmarried, having a low level of education, less than high income, and residing in a nonrural area. Correlates of highly comorbid BPD (Class VII) include termination of schooling with the completion of high school and residing in cities or suburbs. Sociodemographic variation is strongest and most diverse in predicting either being unaffected (Class I) or having highly comorbid major depression (Class VI). Sociodemographic variation is weakest in predicting pure internalizing disorders (Class II) and highly comorbid BPD (Class VII).

### 3.13. Probability of 12-month Service Use

In the prior year, 17.9% of respondents used mental health services, including 41.1% of those

with 12-month DSM-IV disorders and 10.1% of those without (see Table 9.15). The proportion of cases in treatment ranged from a low for IED of 29.6% to a high for DYS of 67.5%). Most of those treated receive services in HC sectors (15.3% of respondents, representing 85.5% of those in treatment); among those treated in HC sectors, most receive services in the GM sector (9.3% of respondents, representing 52.0% of those in treatment)

### 3.14. Number of Visits in the Prior Year

The median number of 12-month visits among those receiving any treatment was 2.9 and was significantly higher among those with disorders (4.5) than without (1.9; $z$ = 5.8, $p$ < 0.001) (see Table 9.16). Respondents with no disorder make up most of the population (74.6%), leading them to account for 33.2% of all visits. The median number of within-sector visits was lowest for the GM (1.6) and highest for CAM (9.2).

Mean numbers of visits are consistently much higher than the median (data not shown but are available on request). For example, among patients receiving any treatment the median was 2.9 versus a mean of 14.7. Patients with disorders made significantly more mean visits (16.9) than those without (11.6; $z$ = 3.1, $p$ = 0.001). Mean within-sector visits were lowest for GM (2.6), higher for HS (7.1), psychiatrist (7.5), nonpsychiatrist specialty (16.1), and highest for CAM (29.8). The proportion of all visits made in specific sectors was highest for nonpsychiatrist specialty (39%) and CAM (32%), lower for psychiatrist (13%), and lowest for GM (9%) and HS (9%).

The greater magnitude of means than medians implies that a relatively small number of patients receive a disproportionately high share of all visits. As shown in Table 9.17, although nearly 60% of patients seen by psychiatrists made fewer than five visits in the year, they accounted for only one-sixth of all visits to psychiatrists. On the other hand, those making 50 or more visits to psychiatrists in the year, while representing only 1.6% of all patients seen by psychiatrists, accounted for 20.2% of all psychiatrist visits. The proportion of patients who account for 50% of

**Table 9.14** Sociodemographic correlates (odds ratios) of latent class analysis class membership probabilities

| | Class 1 | | Class 2 | | Class 3 | | Class 4 | | Class 5 | | Class 6 | | Class 7 | |
|---|---|---|---|---|---|---|---|---|---|---|---|---|---|---|
| | OR | (95% CI) | OR | (95% CI) | OR | (95% CI) | OR | (95% CI) | OR | (95% CI) | OR | (95% CI) | OR | (95% CI) |
| **I. Age** | | | | | | | | | | | | | | |
| 18–29 | 0.9 | (0.7–1.1) | 0.9 | (0.7–1.0) | 1.4* | (1.2–1.6) | 0.8 | (0.7–1.0) | 1.4* | (1.2–1.7) | 1.1 | (0.8–1.4) | 1.0 | (0.9–1.1) |
| 30–44 | 1.0 | – | 1.0 | – | 1.0 | – | 1.0 | – | 1.0 | – | 1.0 | – | 1.0 | – |
| $\chi_1^2$ | 1.9 | | 2.4 | | 15.5* | | 3.1 | | 14.2* | | 0.3 | | 0.4 | |
| **II. Sex** | | | | | | | | | | | | | | |
| Female | 0.7* | (0.6–0.9) | 1.6* | (1.4–1.8) | 0.6* | (0.5–0.7) | 1.9* | (1.7–2.2) | 0.6* | (0.6–0.7) | 1.4* | (1.1–1.7) | 1.1 | (0.9–1.2) |
| Male | 1.0 | – | 1.0 | – | 1.0 | – | 1.0 | – | 1.0 | – | 1.0 | – | 1.0 | – |
| $\chi_1^2$ | 9.3* | | 52.2* | | 51.3* | | 87.0* | | 46.1* | | 9.5* | | 1.0 | |
| **III. Race-ethnicity** | | | | | | | | | | | | | | |
| Non-Hispanic white | 1.0 | | 1.0 | – | 1.0 | | 1.0 | | 1.0 | | 1.0 | | 1.0 | |
| Non-Hispanic black | 2.1* | (1.4–3.0) | 1.2 | (1.0–1.4) | 0.9 | (0.8–1.1) | 0.9 | (0.7–1.0) | 1.2 | (1.0–1.4) | 0.5* | (0.4–0.7) | 1.1 | (0.9–1.2) |
| Hispanic | 2.0* | (1.3–3.0) | 1.0 | (0.8–1.2) | 1.3* | (1.0–1.7) | 0.9 | (0.7–1.1) | 1.1 | (0.9–1.3) | 0.5* | (0.4–0.8) | 0.9 | (0.8–1.0) |
| Other | 0.9 | (0.4–1.8) | 1.0 | (0.7–1.3) | 0.8 | (0.6–1.1) | 0.9 | (0.7–1.3) | 1.4 | (0.6–2.1) | 1.1 | (0.6–2.1) | 1.2 | (0.9–1.5) |
| $\chi_3^2$ | 23.4* | | 4.4 | | 7.8* | | 3.3 | | 6.2 | | 32.7* | | 5.9 | |
| **IV. Education** | | | | | | | | | | | | | | |
| 0–11 | 0.3* | (0.2–0.5) | 0.7* | (0.5–1.0) | 1.0 | (0.7–1.3) | 1.2 | (1.0–1.6) | 1.0 | (0.7–1.3) | 2.6* | (1.7–4.0) | 1.1 | (0.9–1.4) |
| 12 | 0.5* | (0.4–0.8) | 0.8* | (0.7–0.9) | 1.0 | (0.8–1.3) | 1.0 | (0.8–1.3) | 1.0 | (0.8–1.2) | 1.6* | (1.2–2.2) | 1.2* | (1.0–1.3) |
| 13–15 | 0.6* | (0.4–0.9) | 0.9 | (0.8–1.1) | 1.0 | (0.9–1.2) | 1.2 | (1.0–1.5) | 1.0 | (0.8–1.2) | 1.4* | (1.1–1.9) | 1.0 | (0.9–1.1) |
| 16+ | 1.0 | – | 1.0 | – | 1.0 | – | 1.0 | – | 1.0 | – | 1.0 | – | 1.0 | – |
| $\chi_3^2$ | 25.2* | | 18.5* | | 0.4 | | 5.9 | | 0.2 | | 21.2* | | 7.8 | |
| **V. Marital status** | | | | | | | | | | | | | | |
| Married/cohabitating | 1.0 | | 1.0 | – | 1.0 | | 1.0 | | 1.0 | | 1.0 | | 1.0 | |
| Previously married | 0.2* | (0.1–0.4) | 0.9 | (0.7–1.1) | 0.8 | (0.6–1.2) | 1.7* | (1.2–2.3) | 0.6* | (0.5–0.9) | 3.0* | (1.9–4.8) | 1.2 | (0.9–1.6) |
| Never married | 0.6* | (0.4–0.8) | 0.8* | (0.7–0.9) | 1.2 | (1.0–1.5) | 1.1 | (0.9–1.3) | 0.7* | (0.6–0.9) | 1.5* | (1.1–2.0) | 1.0 | (0.8–1.2) |
| $\chi_2^2$ | 32.5* | | 9.1* | | 6.1* | | 8.8* | | 13.3* | | 28.0* | | 1.7 | |
| **VI. Family income[a]** | | | | | | | | | | | | | | |
| Low | 0.7 | (0.4–1.2) | 1.0 | (0.7–1.3) | 0.7* | (0.6–0.9) | 1.2 | (0.9–1.6) | 1.0 | (0.8–1.2) | 1.4 | (0.9–2.1) | 1.2 | (1.0–1.5) |
| Low average | 0.6* | (0.4–1.0) | 1.0 | (0.8–1.3) | 0.9 | (0.7–1.1) | 1.2 | (0.9–1.6) | 0.9 | (0.7–1.2) | 1.4 | (1.0–2.0) | 1.1 | (0.9–1.3) |
| High average | 0.7* | (0.5–1.0) | 1.0 | (0.8–1.2) | 1.0 | (0.8–1.3) | 1.2 | (0.9–1.5) | 1.0 | (0.8–1.3) | 1.4* | (1.0–1.8) | 1.0 | (0.9–1.1) |
| High | 1.0 | – | 1.0 | – | 1.0 | – | 1.0 | – | 1.0 | – | 1.0 | – | 1.0 | – |
| $\chi_3^2$ | 6.4 | | 0.2 | | 9.4* | | 2.7 | | 1.7 | | 7.3 | | 3.5 | |
| **VII. County urbanicity[b]** | | | | | | | | | | | | | | |
| Central city (CC) 2M+ | 0.6* | (0.4–0.8) | 1.0 | (0.8–1.3) | 0.7* | (0.6–0.9) | 1.0 | (0.8–1.3) | 1.6* | (1.3–2.0) | 2.0* | (1.4–2.8) | 1.2* | (1.1–1.4) |
| Central city (CC) <2M | 0.6* | (0.4–1.0) | 1.1 | (1.0–1.4) | 0.7* | (0.6–0.9) | 1.1 | (0.9–1.3) | 1.6* | (1.4–1.8) | 1.6* | (1.2–2.2) | 1.3* | (1.1–1.4) |
| Suburbs of CC 2M+ | 0.6* | (0.4–0.8) | 1.1 | (0.8–1.5) | 0.7* | (0.6–0.9) | 1.3* | (1.1–1.6) | 1.6* | (1.3–1.9) | 1.7* | (1.3–2.3) | 1.2* | (1.0–1.5) |
| Suburbs of CC <2M | 0.5* | (0.3–0.8) | 1.3* | (1.1–1.6) | 0.6* | (0.5–0.8) | 1.4* | (1.1–1.7) | 1.6* | (1.4–1.9) | 2.1* | (1.5–2.9) | 1.2* | (1.0–1.4) |
| Adjacent area | 0.6* | (0.4–0.8) | 1.1 | (1.0–1.4) | 0.7* | (0.6–0.8) | 1.2* | (1.0–1.5) | 1.6* | (1.2–2.0) | 1.7* | (1.3–2.1) | 1.1 | (1.0–1.3) |
| Rural area | 1.0 | – | 1.0 | – | 1.0 | – | 1.0 | – | 1.0 | – | 1.0 | – | 1.0 | – |
| $\chi_5^2$ | 19.6* | | 9.0 | | 40.2* | | 12.6* | | 74.4* | | 41.6* | | 23.0* | |

* Significant at the 0.05 level, two-sided test.

*Note:* Part 2 respondents aged 18–44 years ($n = 3199$).

[a] Family income is defined in relation to the official federal poverty line for families of the size and composition of the respondent's family (Proctor & Dalaker 2002). Low income is defined as less than or equal to 1.5 times the poverty line, low-average as 1.5+ to 3 times the poverty line, high-average as 3+ to 6 times the poverty line, and high as greater than 6 times the poverty line.

[b] Coded according to the 2000 Census definitions (U.S. Census Bureau 2000). Central cities and suburbs are defined by the Census Bureau for each consolidated metropolitan statistical area and metropolitan statistical area in the United States. Adjacent areas are defined as all area beyond the outer boundary of the suburban belt, but within 50 miles of the central business district of a central city. Rural areas include all territory more than 50 miles from the central business district of a central city.

**Table 9.15.** Prevalence of 12-month mental health service use in separate service sectors by 12-month DSM-IV/CIDI disorder

| | Health care | | | | | | | Non-health-care | | | | | | Any service use | | n[a] |
| | Mental health specialty | | | | | | | | | | | | | | | |
| | Psychiatrist | | Nonpsychiatrist[b] | | Any | | General medical[c] | | Any | | Human services[d] | | CAM[e] | | Any | | | | |
| | % | (se) | % | (se) | % | (se) | % | (se) | % | (se) | % | (se) | % | (se) | % | (se) | % | (se) | |
|---|---|---|---|---|---|---|---|---|---|---|---|---|---|---|---|---|---|---|---|
| **I. Anxiety disorders** | | | | | | | | | | | | | | | | | | | |
| Panic disorder | 21.5 | (2.5) | 24.6 | (2.8) | 34.7 | (2.6) | 43.7 | (3.3) | 59.1 | (3.3) | 10.8 | (1.9) | 8.0 | (2.0) | 17.3 | (2.3) | 65.4 | (3.3) | 251 |
| Agoraphobia without panic | – | | – | | – | | – | | 45.8 | (7.0) | – | | – | | – | | 52.6 | (7.4) | 79 |
| Specific phobia | 12.1 | (1.6) | 13.6 | (1.4) | 19.0 | (1.8) | 21.2 | (1.5) | 32.4 | (2.0) | 8.6 | (0.9) | 7.0 | (0.8) | 13.5 | (1.0) | 38.2 | (1.9) | 812 |
| Social phobia | 15.2 | (1.5) | 18.8 | (1.5) | 24.7 | (1.5) | 25.3 | (1.7) | 40.1 | (1.9) | 7.7 | (1.1) | 7.7 | (1.0) | 13.4 | (1.1) | 45.6 | (1.9) | 632 |
| Generalized anxiety disorder | 14.2 | (2.4) | 17.0 | (2.5) | 25.5 | (2.9) | 31.7 | (2.6) | 43.2 | (3.0) | 14.0 | (3.5) | 10.1 | (1.8) | 21.7 | (3.5) | 52.3 | (2.9) | 247 |
| Posttraumatic stress disorder | 22.6 | (2.4) | 26.1 | (2.3) | 34.4 | (2.9) | 31.3 | (2.5) | 49.9 | (3.3) | 10.7 | (2.4) | 12.6 | (2.0) | 19.7 | (2.4) | 57.4 | (3.3) | 203 |
| Obsessive-compulsive disorder | – | | – | | – | | – | | – | | – | | – | | – | | – | | – |
| Separation anxiety disorder | – | | – | | – | | – | | – | | – | | – | | – | | – | | – |
| Any anxiety disorder | 13.0 | (1.0) | 16.0 | (1.0) | 21.7 | (1.2) | 24.3 | (1.0) | 36.9 | (1.4) | 8.2 | (0.9) | 7.3 | (0.6) | 13.5 | (0.7) | 42.2 | (1.3) | 1036 |
| **II. Mood disorders** | | | | | | | | | | | | | | | | | | | |
| Major depressive disorder | 20.6 | (1.8) | 23.2 | (1.9) | 32.9 | (1.6) | 32.5 | (2.3) | 51.7 | (2.2) | 10.7 | (1.2) | 9.0 | (1.3) | 16.8 | (1.7) | 56.8 | (2.2) | 623 |
| Dysthymia | 27.7 | (3.7) | 23.3 | (3.2) | 36.8 | (4.1) | 39.6 | (5.1) | 61.7 | (4.5) | 13.3 | (3.2) | 7.1 | (2.3) | 17.5 | (3.9) | 67.5 | (4.1) | 135 |
| Bipolar I–II disorders | 22.5 | (2.2) | 27.1 | (2.2) | 33.8 | (2.3) | 33.1 | (3.0) | 48.8 | (2.7) | 11.7 | (2.2) | 12.2 | (2.7) | 21.6 | (3.2) | 55.5 | (3.0) | 244 |
| Any mood disorder | 21.0 | (1.3) | 24.1 | (1.5) | 32.9 | (1.3) | 32.8 | (1.8) | 50.9 | (1.8) | 11.0 | (1.2) | 9.8 | (1.3) | 18.1 | (1.6) | 56.4 | (1.8) | 884 |
| **III. Impulse-control disorders** | | | | | | | | | | | | | | | | | | | |
| Intermittent explosive disorder | 7.1 | (1.7) | 9.2 | (1.7) | 13.9 | (2.3) | 12.6 | (2.4) | 22.8 | (2.6) | 7.6 | (2.3) | 3.7 | (1.2) | 10.9 | (2.6) | 29.6 | (2.9) | 243 |
| **IV. Substance disorders** | | | | | | | | | | | | | | | | | | | |
| Alcohol abuse | 12.8 | (1.7) | 20.2 | (2.7) | 25.6 | (2.3) | 16.4 | (2.1) | 33.4 | (2.5) | 7.0 | (1.8) | 7.4 | (1.9) | 12.8 | (2.2) | 37.2 | (2.6) | 176 |
| Alcohol dependence | 19.6 | (2.9) | 28.0 | (5.8) | 35.1 | (4.4) | 19.3 | (3.7) | 43.6 | (4.9) | 8.2 | (2.8) | 14.5 | (3.3) | 19.6 | (3.9) | 48.4 | (5.4) | 76 |
| Drug abuse | 15.5 | (3.7) | 26.3 | (4.8) | 32.8 | (4.9) | 21.8 | (4.1) | 40.5 | (4.9) | 7.1 | (3.9) | 7.7 | (2.7) | 14.2 | (5.5) | 43.1 | (4.8) | 79 |
| Drug dependence | 30.4 | (10.5) | 29.4 | (8.1) | 42.9 | (10.0) | 23.9 | (7.3) | 49.8 | (9.8) | 0.0 | (0.0) | 6.0 | (3.6) | 6.0 | (3.6) | 51.5 | (9.9) | 24 |
| Any substance disorder | 13.2 | (1.5) | 21.0 | (2.9) | 26.2 | (2.5) | 18.1 | (1.7) | 34.5 | (2.6) | 7.8 | (2.1) | 7.2 | (1.7) | 13.7 | (2.6) | 38.1 | (2.7) | 219 |
| **V. Composite** | | | | | | | | | | | | | | | | | | | |
| Any disorder | 12.3 | (0.7) | 16.0 | (0.9) | 21.7 | (0.9) | 22.8 | (0.9) | 36.0 | (1.1) | 8.1 | (0.8) | 6.8 | (0.6) | 13.2 | (0.7) | 41.1 | (1.0) | 1443 |
| No disorder | 1.9 | (0.2) | 3.0 | (0.3) | 4.4 | (0.4) | 4.7 | (0.3) | 8.3 | (0.5) | 1.8 | (0.2) | 1.4 | (0.2) | 3.0 | (0.3) | 10.1 | (0.6) | 4249 |
| Total sample | 4.5 | (0.3) | 6.3 | (0.4) | 8.8 | (0.5) | 9.3 | (0.4) | 15.3 | (0.6) | 3.4 | (0.3) | 2.8 | (0.2) | 5.6 | (0.4) | 17.9 | (0.7) | 5692 |

[a] Weighted number of respondents meeting criteria for each 12-month DSM-IV/CIDI disorder.

[b] Nonpsychiatrist is defined as psychologists or other nonpsychiatrist mental health professional in any setting, social worker or counselor in a mental health specialty setting, use of a mental health hotline.

[c] General medical defined as primary care doctor, other general medical doctor, nurse, any other health professional not previously mentioned.

[d] Human services professional defined as religious or spiritual advisor, social worker, or counselor in any setting other than a specialty mental health setting.

[e] CAM defined as any other type of healer, participation in an Internet support group, or participation in a self-help group.

**Table 9.16.** Median number of visits in separate service sectors among patients treated in those sectors by 12-month DSM-IV/CIDI disorder

| | Health care | | | | | | | | | | | | | Non-health-care | | | | | | | | |
| --- | --- | --- | --- | --- | --- | --- | --- | --- | --- | --- | --- | --- | --- | --- | --- | --- | --- | --- | --- | --- | --- | --- |
| | Mental health specialty | | | | | | General medical[c] | | Any | | Human services[d] | | CAM[e] | | Any | | Any service use | |
| | Psychiatrist | | Nonpsychiatrist[b] | | Any | | | | | | | | | | | | | |
| | % | (se) | % | (se) | % | (se) | % | (se) | % | (se) | % | (se) | % | (se) | % | (se) | % | (se) |
| **I. Anxiety disorders** | | | | | | | | | | | | | | | | | | |
| Panic disorder | 5.3 | (1.0) | 8.5 | (1.7) | 10.0 | (2.3) | 1.8 | (0.1) | 3.7 | (0.7) | – | – | – | – | 4.1 | (1.1) | 4.3 | (1.0) |
| Agoraphobia without panic | – | – | – | – | – | – | – | – | 5.3 | (1.8) | – | – | – | – | – | – | 7.0 | (2.0) |
| Specific phobia | 3.6 | (0.9) | 7.2 | (2.2) | 6.1 | (1.7) | 1.5 | (0.1) | 2.9 | (0.5) | 2.0 | (0.3) | 13.3 | (3.9) | 5.1 | (1.9) | 3.9 | (0.8) |
| Social phobia | 4.3 | (1.2) | 7.7 | (1.7) | 8.6 | (1.8) | 1.7 | (0.1) | 3.4 | (0.9) | 2.4 | (0.5) | 7.4 | (2.3) | 5.2 | (1.5) | 4.6 | (1.1) |
| Generalized anxiety disorder | 4.7 | (1.7) | 14.3 | (4.4) | 7.0 | (2.1) | 1.6 | (0.2) | 3.9 | (1.2) | – | – | – | – | 3.6 | (2.4) | 4.5 | (1.8) |
| Posttraumatic stress disorder | 3.3 | (1.0) | 11.1 | (2.7) | 11.4 | (2.8) | 1.5 | (0.1) | 5.1 | (1.4) | 0.6 | (NA)[a] | 14.7 | (11.0) | 4.9 | (1.2) | 6.7 | (1.7) |
| Obsessive-compulsive disorder | – | – | – | – | – | – | – | – | – | – | – | – | – | – | – | – | – | – |
| Separation anxiety disorder | – | – | – | – | – | – | – | – | – | – | – | – | – | – | – | – | – | – |
| Any anxiety disorder | 3.8 | (0.9) | 7.6 | (1.3) | 6.4 | (1.1) | 1.7 | (0.0) | 2.8 | (0.4) | 2.1 | (0.2) | 11.2 | (2.7) | 4.4 | (1.0) | 3.8 | (0.6) |
| **II. Mood disorders** | | | | | | | | | | | | | | | | | | |
| Major depressive disorder | 3.8 | (0.9) | 9.3 | (1.3) | 7.8 | (1.6) | 1.4 | (0.1) | 3.9 | (0.8) | 2.5 | (0.7) | 9.4 | (1.9) | 7.4 | (1.5) | 5.5 | (1.0) |
| Dysthymia | 5.2 | (1.9) | 12.9 | (4.2) | 9.8 | (4.2) | 1.9 | (0.4) | 5.0 | (1.1) | – | – | – | – | – | – | 5.0 | (1.2) |
| Bipolar I or II | 4.8 | (0.9) | 7.6 | (2.1) | 11.4 | (2.7) | 1.6 | (0.3) | 5.9 | (2.1) | – | – | 16.5 | (6.9) | 6.3 | (2.8) | 9.4 | (1.8) |
| Any mood disorder | 4.2 | (0.7) | 9.0 | (1.1) | 9.4 | (1.2) | 1.5 | (0.1) | 4.5 | (0.7) | 2.7 | (0.5) | 9.8 | (3.1) | 7.1 | (1.4) | 6.0 | (0.8) |
| **III. Impulse-control disorders** | | | | | | | | | | | | | | | | | | |
| Intermittent explosive disorder | – | – | – | – | 3.5 | (2.1) | 1.4 | (0.1) | 1.9 | (0.6) | – | – | – | – | – | – | 2.4 | (0.6) |
| **IV. Substance disorders** | | | | | | | | | | | | | | | | | | |
| Alcohol abuse | – | – | 5.5 | (4.3) | 5.7 | (3.1) | 1.5 | (0.1) | 4.1 | (1.5) | – | – | – | – | 3.8 | (1.8) | 6.1 | (1.2) |
| Alcohol dependence | – | – | – | – | 5.9 | (6.2) | – | – | 4.9 | (2.1) | – | – | – | – | – | – | 6.3 | (2.6) |
| Drug abuse | – | – | – | – | 12.0 | (3.8) | – | – | 5.9 | (3.3) | – | – | – | – | – | – | 6.7 | (3.7) |
| Drug dependence | – | – | – | – | – | – | – | – | – | – | – | – | – | – | – | – | – | – |
| Any substance disorder | 3.5 | (1.1) | 10.6 | (3.7) | 8.5 | (3.1) | 1.4 | (0.1) | 5.3 | (2.3) | – | – | – | – | 3.3 | (1.5) | 6.6 | (2.0) |
| **V. Composite** | | | | | | | | | | | | | | | | | | |
| Any disorder | 3.6 | (0.7) | 7.9 | (1.2) | 7.4 | (1.0) | 1.7 | (0.0) | 3.0 | (0.3) | 2.3 | (0.2) | 9.3 | (1.5) | 3.9 | (0.6) | 4.5 | (0.4) |
| No disorder | 2.3 | (0.4) | 5.1 | (0.3) | 3.7 | (0.6) | 1.1 | (NA)[a] | 1.7 | (0.1) | 1.7 | (0.3) | 8.4 | (2.9) | 2.4 | (0.5) | 1.9 | (0.2) |
| Total sample | 3.1 | (0.4) | 6.0 | (0.6) | 5.7 | (0.4) | 1.6 | (0.0) | 2.6 | (0.1) | 2.0 | (0.2) | 9.2 | (1.2) | 3.6 | (0.2) | 2.9 | (0.2) |

*Note:* Missing cell entries indicate that the number of patients with the disorder who were treated in the sector was less than 30, in which case no estimate was made.

[a] Due to lack of sufficient variance in the distribution, standard error cannot be calculated.

[b] Nonpsychiatrist is defined as psychologist or other nonpsychiatrist mental health professional in any setting, social worker or counselor in a mental health specialty setting, use of a mental health hotline.

[c] General medical is defined as primary care doctor, other general medical doctor, nurse, any other health professional not previously mentioned.

[d] Human services professional is defined as religious or spiritual advisor, social worker, or counselor in any setting other than a specialty mental health setting.

[e] CAM is defined as any other type of healer, participation in an Internet support group, or participation in a self-help group.

**Table 9.17.** Distributions of patients by number of visits in the treatment sector and the proportions of all visits to the sector provided to patients in the various categories of individual-level visits in the Part 2 sample ($n = 5692$)

| Sector | Number of visits made by the patient in the treatment sector | | | | | | | | | | | | $n^a$ |
|---|---|---|---|---|---|---|---|---|---|---|---|---|---|
| | 1 | | 2–4 | | 5–9 | | 10–19 | | 20–49 | | 50+ | | |
| | % | (se) | % | (se) | % | (se) | % | (se) | % | (se) | % | (se) | |
| I. Psychiatrist | | | | | | | | | | | | | |
| Respondents | 18.5 | (3.6) | 40.4 | (3.3) | 17.3 | (2.2) | 16.2 | (2.5) | 6.1 | (1.5) | 1.6 | (0.7) | 258 |
| Visits | 2.5 | (0.7) | 14.8 | (2.5) | 14.1 | (2.1) | 26.4 | (4.2) | 22.1 | (4.4) | 20.2 | (7.7) | – |
| II. Nonpsychiatrist mental health specialty | | | | | | | | | | | | | |
| Respondents | 12.0 | (1.6) | 27.2 | (1.9) | 17.0 | (2.3) | 17.5 | (1.6) | 17.6 | (1.6) | 8.7 | (1.0) | 358 |
| Visits | 0.7 | (0.1) | 4.5 | (0.5) | 6.8 | (1.2) | 14.3 | (1.5) | 32.3 | (2.7) | 41.3 | (3.6) | – |
| III. General medical | | | | | | | | | | | | | |
| Respondents | 39.5 | (1.8) | 51.7 | (1.8) | 5.1 | (1.1) | 2.9 | (0.5) | 0.6 | (0.2) | 0.1 | (0.1) | 529 |
| Visits | 15.3 | (1.2) | 48.8 | (3.0) | 12.6 | (2.7) | 13.6 | (2.1) | 6.9 | (2.6) | 2.8 | (2.8) | – |
| IV. Human services | | | | | | | | | | | | | |
| Respondents | 27.6 | (3.9) | 45.9 | (4.1) | 8.2 | (1.9) | 9.3 | (1.6) | 5.6 | (1.2) | 3.4 | (1.8) | 192 |
| Visits | 3.9 | (1.1) | 17.3 | (4.1) | 6.8 | (2.1) | 16.2 | (4.4) | 22.3 | (5.5) | 33.5 | (13.9) | – |
| V. Complementary alternative medicine | | | | | | | | | | | | | |
| Respondents | 14.1 | (2.3) | 22.5 | (2.8) | 11.8 | (2.0) | 16.9 | (2.7) | 16.6 | (2.4) | 18.2 | (2.5) | 159 |
| Visits | 0.5 | (0.1) | 2.1 | (0.5) | 2.6 | (0.6) | 6.9 | (1.5) | 16.8 | (3.2) | 71.1 | (4.5) | – |

[a] Weighted number of respondents in the Part 2 sample seeking treatment in each service sector.

all visits to the sector ranged between 6.4% for the HS sector to 23.6% for the GM sector.

### 3.15. Minimally Adequate Treatment in the Prior Year

Among treated patients with disorders, only 32.7% were classified as receiving at least minimally adequate treatment in the prior year (see Table 9.18). The probability was lowest in the GM sector (12.7%) and highest in the MHS sectors (44.5% in the psychiatrist sector and 46.5% in the nonpsychiatrist specialty sector).

Using the broader definition of minimally adequate treatment (i.e., receiving at least two visits to an appropriate sector or being in ongoing treatment at the time of interview) in sensitivity analyses, the percentage of patients receiving at least minimally adequate treatment increased to 47.8% (data not shown but available on request).

The probabilities were lowest in the GM sector (33.2%), higher in HS (46.9%) and nonpsychiatrist specialty (51.1%) sectors, and highest in the psychiatrist (53.3%) sector.

### 3.16. Sociodemographic Predictors of 12-Month Treatment

As shown in Table 9.19, receiving any 12-month mental health treatment is significantly related to being younger than age 60, female, non-Hispanic white, not having low-average family income, being previously married, and not living in a rural area. Among those receiving services, treatment in one of the HC sectors is significantly related to not being in the age range of 18–29, not being non-Hispanic black, living in rural areas, and having health insurance. Among those who received HC treatment, MHS treatment is significantly related to being younger than 60 years of

**Table 9.18.** Percentage of patients who received at least minimally adequate treatment in those sectors by 12-month DSM-IV/CIDI disorder

| | Health care | | | | | | | | | | | | Non-health-care | | | | Any service use | |
| | Mental health specialty | | | | | | General medical[b] | | Any | | Human services[c] | | Self help[d] | | | |
| | Psychiatrist | | Nonpsychiatrist[a] | | Any | | | | | | | | | | | |
| | % | (se) | % | (se) | % | (se) | % | (se) | % | (se) | % | (se) | % | (se) | % | (se) |
|---|---|---|---|---|---|---|---|---|---|---|---|---|---|---|---|---|
| I. Anxiety disorders | | | | | | | | | | | | | | | | |
| Panic disorder | 58.6 | (9.0) | 48.2 | (9.0) | 55.3 | (7.7) | 20.6 | (4.7) | 41.2 | (5.3) | 19.0 | (7.8) | –e | –e | 39.8 | (5.1) |
| Agoraphobia w/o panic disorder | – | | – | | – | | – | | 42.1 | (8.1) | – | | –e | –e | 41.1 | (7.2) |
| Specific phobia | 46.2 | (6.6) | 50.6 | (5.5) | 49.9 | (5.5) | 15.7 | (3.6) | 34.4 | (4.1) | 16.3 | (4.6) | –e | –e | 33.6 | (4.0) |
| Social phobia | 51.6 | (7.5) | 53.0 | (4.2) | 55.9 | (5.4) | 14.8 | (3.8) | 38.7 | (3.9) | 20.7 | (5.4) | –e | –e | 38.2 | (3.8) |
| Generalized anxiety disorder | 51.5 | (11.5) | 69.1 | (8.9) | 60.7 | (7.7) | 20.2 | (4.2) | 43.7 | (5.6) | 24.0 | (9.0) | –e | –e | 42.5 | (5.5) |
| Posttraumatic stress disorder | 45.8 | (8.3) | 56.6 | (6.7) | 56.6 | (5.5) | 12.8 | (4.0) | 42.0 | (4.3) | 20.1 | (6.6) | –e | –e | 40.4 | (3.6) |
| Obsessive-compulsive disorder | – | | – | | – | | – | | – | | – | | –e | –e | – | |
| Separation anxiety disorder | – | | – | | – | | – | | – | | – | | –e | –e | – | |
| Any anxiety disorder | 46.1 | (6.5) | 50.5 | (4.0) | 51.5 | (4.8) | 13.4 | (1.9) | 34.3 | (3.0) | 18.9 | (2.9) | –e | –e | 33.8 | (2.8) |
| II. Mood disorders | | | | | | | | | | | | | | | | |
| Major depressive disorder | 43.2 | (7.4) | 53.2 | (3.8) | 52.0 | (5.1) | 14.9 | (2.7) | 38.0 | (3.7) | 22.0 | (5.8) | –e | –e | 37.5 | (3.1) |
| Dysthymia | 45.7 | (10.8) | 60.1 | (10.9) | 53.1 | (9.2) | 29.2 | (6.4) | 43.1 | (5.6) | – | | –e | –e | 40.7 | (5.3) |
| Bipolar I–II disorders | 47.7 | (7.2) | 49.8 | (5.8) | 53.9 | (5.9) | 9.0 | (3.5) | 38.8 | (3.9) | 20.9 | (8.9) | –e | –e | 39.2 | (4.2) |
| Any mood disorder | 44.4 | (5.8) | 52.1 | (3.1) | 52.3 | (3.8) | 14.3 | (1.9) | 38.5 | (2.4) | 21.2 | (4.7) | –e | –e | 38.3 | (2.2) |
| III. Impulse-control disorders | | | | | | | | | | | | | | | | |
| Intermittent explosive disorder | – | | – | | 36.4 | (9.5) | 7.8 | (5.1) | 26.1 | (6.5) | – | | –e | | 21.8 | (5.4) |
| IV. Substance disorders | | | | | | | | | | | | | | | | |
| Alcohol abuse | – | | 41.2 | (10.3) | 36.5 | (6.4) | 5.5 | (3.3) | 27.4 | (5.5) | – | | – | | 29.1 | (5.2) |
| Alcohol dependence | – | | – | | 39.1 | (7.8) | – | | 31.9 | (6.9) | – | | – | | 37.4 | (6.4) |
| Drug abuse | – | | – | | 28.9 | (7.7) | – | | 22.6 | (5.8) | – | | – | | 28.2 | (5.3) |
| Drug dependence | – | | – | | – | | – | | – | | – | | – | | – | |
| Any substance disorder | – | | 37.3 | (6.5) | 34.9 | (4.5) | 5.3 | (2.9) | 26.1 | (3.7) | – | | – | | 28.6 | (3.8) |
| V. Composite | | | | | | | | | | | | | | | | |
| Any mental disorder | 44.5 | (5.3) | 46.5 | (3.3) | 48.3 | (3.4) | 12.7 | (1.6) | 33.4 | (2.2) | 16.9 | (2.5) | 16.7 | (5.1) | 32.7 | (1.9) |
| (n)[f] | 177 | | 208 | | 294 | | 329 | | 504 | | 117 | | 53 | | 565 | |

*Note:* Missing cell entries indicate that the number of patients with the disorder who were treated in the sector was less than 30, in which case no estimate was made.

[a] Nonpsychiatrist defined as psychologist or other nonpsychiatrist mental health professional in any setting, social worker or counselor in a mental health specialty setting. Use of a mental health hotline removed from definition because it is not considered adequate treatment.

[b] General medical defined as primary care doctor, other general medical doctor, nurse, any other health professional not previously mentioned.

[c] Human services professional defined as religious or spiritual advisor, social worker, or counselor in any setting other than a specialty mental health setting.

[d] Standard definition of complementary and alternative medicine reduced to self-help only because only self-help is considered adequate treatment.

[e] By definition, self help is considered inadequate treatment for all disorders other than substance.

[f] Weighted number of respondents with a 12-month DSM-IV/CIDI disorder seeking treatment in each service sector.

**Table 9.19.** Demographic predictors of 12-month service use

| | Any treatment | | Health-care treatment among patients with any treatment[a] | | Mental health specialty treatment among patients with health-care treatment | |
|---|---|---|---|---|---|---|
| | OR | (95% CI) | OR | (95% CI) | OR | (95% CI) |
| I. Age | | | | | | |
| 18–29 | 1.5* | (1.1–2.1) | 0.5* | (0.2–0.9) | 4.8* | (2.4–9.4) |
| 30–44 | 2.1* | (1.6–2.7) | 0.9 | (0.5–1.7) | 3.8* | (2.5–5.7) |
| 45–59 | 1.8* | (1.4–2.5) | 1.4 | (0.6–3.3) | 2.4* | (1.6–3.6) |
| 60+ | 1.0 | – | 1.0 | – | 1.0 | – |
| $\chi^2_3$ | 40.7* | | 13.4* | | 47.0* | |
| II. Sex | | | | | | |
| Female | 1.6* | (1.4–1.8) | 1.2 | (0.8–1.8) | 0.6* | (0.5–0.8) |
| Male | 1.0 | – | 1.0 | – | 1.0 | – |
| $\chi^2_1$ | 46.8* | | 0.7 | | 12.2* | |
| III. Race-ethnicity | | | | | | |
| Non-Hispanic white | 1.0 | – | 1.0 | – | 1.0 | – |
| Non-Hispanic black | 0.5* | (0.4–0.7) | 0.4* | (0.2–0.8) | 1.3 | (0.7–2.6) |
| Hispanic | 0.6* | (0.5–0.8) | 0.8 | (0.4–1.7) | 0.9 | (0.5–1.4) |
| Other | 0.5* | (0.4–0.7) | 0.6 | (0.1–3.1) | 1.1 | (0.4–3.0) |
| $\chi^2_3$ | 31.6* | | 8.0 | | 1.6 | |
| IV. Education | | | | | | |
| 0–11 years | 1.0 | (0.7–1.3) | 1.3 | (0.7–2.6) | 0.6* | (0.3–1.0) |
| 12 years | 0.9 | (0.7–1.3) | 1.2 | (0.8–2.0) | 0.4* | (0.3–0.6) |
| 13–15 years | 1.1 | (0.8–1.4) | 1.2 | (0.8–1.8) | 0.8 | (0.5–1.1) |
| 16+ years | 1.0 | – | 1.0 | – | 1.0 | – |
| $\chi^2_3$ | 1.3 | | 1.3 | | 29.8* | |
| V. Marital status | | | | | | |
| Married/cohabitating | 1.0 | – | 1.0 | – | 1.0 | – |
| Previously married | 1.7* | (1.3–2.1) | 1.5 | (0.9–2.5) | 1.7* | (1.2–2.5) |
| Never married | 1.2 | (1.0–1.5) | 1.3 | (0.8–2.2) | 1.6* | (1.0–2.4) |
| $\chi^2_2$ | 19.0* | | 4.3 | | 12.4* | |
| VI. Family Income | | | | | | |
| Low | 1.0 | (0.7–1.4) | 1.1 | (0.7–2.0) | 0.9 | (0.5–1.5) |
| Low average | 0.7* | (0.6–0.9) | 0.8 | (0.5–1.5) | 0.8 | (0.5–1.2) |
| High average | 0.8 | (0.7–1.1) | 0.6 | (0.4–1.0) | 0.8 | (0.5–1.2) |
| High | 1.0 | – | 1.0 | – | 1.0 | – |
| $\chi^2_3$ | 15.6* | | 7.2 | | 3.0 | |
| VII. County Urbanicity | | | | | | |
| Central city (CC) 2M+ | 2.1* | (1.7–2.7) | 0.3* | (0.1–0.8) | 2.2* | (1.2–4.1) |
| Central city (CC) <2M | 2.0* | (1.5–2.6) | 0.2* | (0.1–0.4) | 1.7* | (1.0–2.9) |
| Suburbs of CC 2M+ | 2.0* | (1.6–2.6) | 0.3* | (0.1–0.5) | 2.4* | (1.3–4.3) |
| Suburbs of CC <2M | 2.2* | (1.6–3.0) | 0.3* | (0.2–0.6) | 1.4 | (0.8–2.3) |
| Adjacent area | 1.9* | (1.7–2.2) | 0.2* | (0.1–0.5) | 1.6* | (1.1–2.3) |
| Rural area | 1.0 | – | 1.0 | – | 1.0 | – |
| $\chi^2_5$ | 113.5* | | 29.6* | | 10.7 | |
| VIII. Insurance | | | | | | |
| Yes | 1.2 | (0.9–1.6) | 1.9* | (1.3–2.9) | 1.1 | (0.7–1.7) |
| No | 1.0 | – | 1.0 | – | 1.0 | – |
| $\chi^2_1$ | 1.2 | | 10.4* | | 0.1 | |
| % getting treatment | 17.9% | | 84.9% | | 57.3% | |

* Significant at the 0.05 level, two-sided test.

[a] Respondents with obsessive-compulsive disorder and the combination of any mood disorder and intermittent explosive disorder were dropped from this analysis because 100% of these subjects received health-care treatment.

age, male, college educated, not married, and not living in a rural area.

Among people who received treatment after controlling for the presence of all individual 12-month mental disorders, no significant sociodemographic correlates were found (see Table 9.20); no significant sociodemographic correlates of treatment adequacy among those receiving GM sector care were found either. Significant predictors of adequate treatment among those receiving MHS sector care include high education and living in a rural area. Significant predictors of adequate treatment in NHC sectors include being aged 18–29, male, and married.

## 4. DISCUSSION

### 4.1. Considerations in Interpreting NCS-R Findings

These results should be interpreted with the following five limitations in mind, which are consistent across the WMH surveys. First, the NCS-R excludes people who are homeless or institutionalized, who do not speak English, and who were too ill to be interviewed. As these exclusions apply only to a small proportion of the population, the results apply to the vast majority of the population. However, the excluded population segments almost certainly have a higher prevalence of mental disorders than do the segments included in the study. Another related exclusion is that the WMH CIDI did not assess all DSM-IV disorders. Therefore, some respondents in treatment not classified as not having a disorder may actually have met criteria for a DSM-IV disorder not assessed.

Second, systematic survey nonresponse (i.e., people with mental disorders having a higher survey refusal rate than those without disorders) or systematic nonreporting (i.e., recall failure, conscious nonreporting, or error in the diagnostic evaluation) could lead to bias in the estimates of disorder prevalence or unmet need for treatment, particularly for lifetime events. Given what we know about the associations between true prevalence and these errors (Cannell, Marquis & Laurent 1977; Allgulander 1989; Eaton et al.

1992; Turner et al. 1998; Kessler et al. 2004), it is likely that disorder prevalences and unmet needs for treatment have been underestimated in the NCS-R.

Third, the CIDI is a lay-administered interview. However, as is reported elsewhere (Kessler et al. 2004), a clinical reappraisal study using the SCID (First et al. 2002) found generally good individual-level concordance between the CIDI and SCID and conservative estimates of prevalence compared to the SCID.

Fourth, without corroborating data on service use, we cannot study the validity of self-reported treatment use in the NCS-R. Recent studies of the Ontario Health Survey (OHS) suggest that self-reports of mental health service use overestimate administrative treatment records, especially concerning the number or intensity of service use among respondents with more distressing disorders (Rhodes, Lin & Mustard 2002; Rhodes & Fung 2004). Unlike the OHS, the NCS-R did attempt to minimize such inaccuracies by using commitment probes (i.e., questions designed to measure a subject's commitment to the survey) and excluded the small number (<1%) of respondents who failed to endorse that they would think carefully and answer honestly. Nevertheless, potentially biased recall of mental health service use remains a limitation. To the extent that it occurred, our results are likely to underestimate unmet need for treatment, especially among those with more serious disorders.

Fifth, our definitions of minimally adequate treatment may differ from others in use and their relationships with important clinical outcomes have not been studied. In addition, respondents diagnosed shortly before interview may not have had enough time to meet our main definition. Very brief treatments have also been described for certain phobias (Ost et al. 1997) and alcohol disorders (Ballesteros et al. 2004). However, our sensitivity analyses using broader definitions (i.e., at least two visits to an appropriate sector or being in ongoing treatment at the time of interview) took these possibilities into account and still found that half of treated cases are cared for inadequately.

**Table 9.20.** Demographic predictors of treatment adequacy among people with a 12-month DSM-IV/CIDI disorder who received treatment in each service sector

| | Any treatment | | General medical | | Mental health care | | Non–health-care[a] | |
|---|---|---|---|---|---|---|---|---|
| | OR | (95% CI) | OR | (95% CI) | OR | (95% CI) | OR | (95% CI) |
| I. Age | | | | | | | | |
| 18–29 | 0.6 | (0.3–1.5) | 0.4 | (0.1–1.6) | 0.8 | (0.3–2.5) | 3.6 | (0.4–32.7) |
| 30–44 | 0.6 | (0.3–1.6) | 0.8 | (0.2–2.8) | 0.9 | (0.3–3.2) | 0.4 | (0.0–4.7) |
| 45–59 | 0.5 | (0.2–1.3) | 0.7 | (0.2–2.2) | 0.7 | (0.2–2.3) | 0.3 | (0.0–2.6) |
| 60+ | 1.0 | – | 1.0 | – | 1.0 | – | 1.0 | – |
| $\chi_3^2$ | 2.2 | | 2.6 | | 1.5 | | 15.2* | |
| II. Sex | | | | | | | | |
| Female | 1.1 | (0.7–1.7) | 0.9 | (0.4–2.0) | 1.0 | (0.7–1.7) | 0.2* | (0.1–0.7) |
| Male | 1.0 | – | 1.0 | – | 1.0 | – | 1.0 | – |
| $\chi_1^2$ | 0.1 | | 0.1 | | 0.1 | | 7.1* | |
| III. Race-ethnicity | | | | | | | | |
| Non-Hispanic white | 1.0 | – | 1.0 | – | 1.0 | – | – | – |
| Non-Hispanic black | 0.8 | (0.5–1.2) | 1.0 | (0.3–2.8) | 1.1 | (0.6–2.0) | – | – |
| Hispanic | 0.6 | (0.3–1.2) | 0.6 | (0.2–2.2) | 0.8 | (0.4–1.9) | – | – |
| Other | 1.1 | (0.3–3.6) | 0.5 | (0.1–3.2) | 0.9 | (0.3–3.5) | – | – |
| $\chi_3^2$ | 2.9 | | 1.0 | | 0.5 | | – | |
| IV. Education | | | | | | | | |
| 0–11 years | 0.7 | (0.3–1.6) | 2.1 | (0.6–7.8) | 0.3* | (0.1–0.9) | 1.3 | (0.2–8.8) |
| 12 years | 0.8 | (0.5–1.3) | 1.2 | (0.5–2.8) | 0.5* | (0.3–0.9) | 1.6 | (0.4–5.9) |
| 13–15 years | 1.2 | (0.8–1.8) | 1.3 | (0.5–3.1) | 0.8 | (0.5–1.5) | 3.2* | (1.0–9.9) |
| 16+ years | 1.0 | – | 1.0 | – | 1.0 | – | 1.0 | – |
| $\chi_3^2$ | 5.2 | | 1.5 | | 9.1 | | 6.7 | |
| V. Marital status | | | | | | | | |
| Married/cohabitating | 1.0 | – | 1.0 | – | 1.0 | – | 1.0 | – |
| Previously married | 1.2 | (0.6–2.3) | 1.4 | (0.5–3.7) | 1.3 | (0.7–2.2) | 0.5 | (0.1–2.0) |
| Never married | 1.1 | (0.5–2.6) | 1.8 | (0.7–4.4) | 1.1 | (0.5–2.4) | 0.2* | (0.0–0.7) |
| $\chi_2^2$ | 0.4 | | 1.9 | | 0.9 | | 6.3 | |
| VI. Family income | | | | | | | | |
| Low | 1.4 | (0.8–2.4) | 1.2 | (0.4–3.3) | 1.4 | (0.8–2.6) | 3.4 | (0.5–23.7) |
| Low average | 1.0 | (0.6–1.8) | 1.3 | (0.4–4.1) | 1.0 | (0.5–2.0) | 1.9 | (0.5–7.9) |
| High average | 1.6 | (0.9–2.7) | 1.7 | (0.6–5.0) | 2.0 | (1.0–4.0) | 2.0 | (0.4–9.7) |
| High | 1.0 | – | 1.0 | – | 1.0 | – | 1.0 | – |
| $\chi_3^2$ | 4.8 | | 1.2 | | 8.4 | | 1.7 | |
| VII. County Urbanicity | | | | | | | | |
| Central city (CC) 2M+ | 0.8 | (0.4–1.8) | 2.0 | (0.5–8.9) | 0.4* | (0.2–0.8) | 2.4 | (0.6–9.4) |
| Central city (CC) <2M | 0.5 | (0.2–1.2) | 0.8 | (0.2–3.5) | 0.3* | (0.1–0.6) | 1.3 | (0.3–5.3) |
| Suburbs of CC 2M+ | 0.6 | (0.3–1.5) | 0.9 | (0.2–3.5) | 0.4* | (0.2–0.9) | 0.4 | (0.1–1.7) |
| Suburbs of CC <2M | 0.5 | (0.2–1.2) | 1.0 | (0.3–3.5) | 0.3* | (0.1–0.7) | 1.0 | (0.4–2.3) |
| Adjacent area | 0.7 | (0.3–1.6) | 2.2 | (0.6–9.1) | 0.3* | (0.1–0.8) | 1.0 | – |
| Rural area | 1.0 | – | 1.0 | – | 1.0 | – | –[b] | |
| $\chi_5^2$ | 4.8 | | 10.0 | | 13.9* | | 7.9 | |
| VIII. Insurance | | | | | | | | |
| Yes | 1.2 | (0.6–2.1) | 0.6 | (0.2–1.3) | 1.0 | (0.5–2.0) | 1.4 | (0.4–4.5) |
| No | 1.0 | – | 1.0 | – | 1.0 | – | 1.0 | – |
| $\chi_5^2$ | 0.3 | | 1.7 | | 0.0 | | 0.3 | |
| % receiving adequate treatment | 31.2% | | 12.7% | | 45.4% | | 21.6% | |

* Significant at the 0.05 level, two-sided test.

[a] This model contains only respondents with a 12-month disorder treated in the human serves sector and respondents with a substance disorder who participated in a self-help group.

[b] Not included in model as a separate category due to insufficient size.

## 4.2. Lessons from the NCS-R Lifetime Prevalence Data

NCS-R estimates of the lifetime prevalence of mental disorders are broadly consistent with those found in previous community surveys in the United States (Kessler et al. 1994; Regier et al. 1998) in showing that half of the general population is afflicted by mental disorders at some time in their life. Similar to these earlier studies, anxiety and mood disorders are common classes with MDD, SP, SoP, and AA being the most prevalent individual disorders. What may be more surprising, given the paucity of prior lifetime data, is the frequency of impulse-control disorders, which have a combined lifetime prevalence that is higher than for either mood disorders or substance disorders.

In addition to their high prevalences, mental disorders examined in the NCS-R are notable for their AOOs, which are concentrated in the first two decades of life, with later-onset disorders largely occurring as temporally secondary comorbid conditions. Consistent with previous epidemiological surveys (Christie et al. 1988; WHO International Consortium in Psychiatric Epidemiology 2000), anxiety disorders have the earliest AOO and mood disorders the latest. However in spite of any between-disorder variation, it is critical to note that mental disorders are uniquely burdensome in that they typically attack the young, whereas almost all chronic physical disorders have conditional risks that increase with age, typically peaking in late middle or old age (Murray & Lopez 1996).

The cohort effect in the NCS-R, with increasing prevalence of disorders in more recent cohorts, deserves further consideration. It varies in plausible ways (e.g., largest with substance disorders, which are known independently to have increased among cohorts that went through adolescence beginning in the 1970s), sociodemographic correlates are substantively plausible (e.g., increasing similarity of women and men in substance use disorders in recent cohorts), and there was no evidence for convergence among cohorts with increasing age. These data argue for the cohort effect being due at least in part to

substantive rather than entirely to methodological factors. In addition, the NCS-R used weights from a nonresponse survey to correct for nonresponse bias (Kessler et al. 2004) as well as a special AOO probing strategy to reduce recall bias (Kessler & Üstün 2004). Nonetheless, residual effects of methodological factors are likely based on the fact that longitudinal studies show mental disorders to be associated with early mortality (Bruce & Leaf 1989) and the fact that resolved mental disorders reported in baseline interviews often are not reported in follow-up interviews (Badawi et al. 1999). To the extent that these biases are at work, the high prevalence found in the younger NCS-R cohorts might also apply to older cohorts.

Taken together, the NCS-R findings on lifetime prevalence of mental disorders plus the enormous personal and societal burdens of these disorders, suggest that greater attention be paid to public health interventions that target the childhood and adolescent years. With appropriately balanced considerations of potential risks and benefits, focus is also needed on early interventions aimed at preventing the progression of primary disorders and the onset of comorbid disorders.

## 4.3. Implications of NCS-R 12-month Findings

The NCS-R results show episodes of DSM-IV disorders to be highly prevalent during the prior year, affecting more than one-quarter of Americans. Although many cases are mild, the prevalence of moderate and serious cases is still substantial, affecting 14.0% of the population. The 5.7% with a serious disorder is remarkably close to the estimated prevalence of serious mental illness (SMI) defined by SAMHSA in the original NCS (Kessler et al. 1996). Consistent with prior studies (Bijl et al. 2003; Demyttenaere et al. 2004), anxiety disorders are the most common class of disorders, but the proportion of serious cases is lower than for other classes; mood disorders are next most common and have the highest proportion of serious cases. Impulse-control disorders, which have been neglected in previous epidemiological studies, are present in more than one-third of cases and also have a higher proportion of serious cases.

A striking finding from the NCS-R 12-month prevalence data is that more than 40% of cases in the prior year also have comorbid disorders. Patterns of bivariate comorbidity are broadly consistent with the ECA and original NCS in showing that the vast majority of disorders are positively correlated. Relative magnitudes of associations are also quite similar across the three surveys, with high rank-order correlations of odds ratios among comorbid pairs in the NCS-R versus published odds ratios (Kessler 1995) in both the NCS (0.79) and the ECA (0.57). Major internal patterns of comorbidity are also quite consistent across surveys, such as the stronger odds ratios within the mood disorders than the anxiety disorders, very high odds ratios between anxiety and mood disorders, and odds ratios between anxiety and mood disorders generally being higher than between pairs of anxiety disorders. NCS-R 12-month data on disorders also reveal that severity is strongly related to comorbidity. The sociodemographic correlates of having 12-month disorders are broadly consistent with previous surveys in finding that mental disorders are associated with a general pattern of disadvantaged social status, including being female, unmarried, and having low socioeconomic status (Canino et al. 1987; Bland, Orn & Newman 1988; Hwu, Yeh & Cheng 1989; Lépine et al. 1989; Wells et al. 1989; Lee et al. 1990; Wittchen et al. 1992; WHO International Consortium in Psychiatric Epidemiology 2000; Demyttenaere et al. 2004).

One important question raised by the high prevalence estimates in this and earlier psychiatric epidemiological surveys in the United States is whether they are scientifically implausible (Eaton et al. 1992). The generally good concordance between CIDI and SCID diagnoses and the fact that the CIDI is conservative relative to the SCID provides some reassurance that NCS-R estimates are accurate. Furthermore, NCS-R data show that even those with mild 12-month CIDI disorders have levels of impairment equivalent to those caused by clinically significant chronic

physical disorders (Allgulander 1989). Such evidence argues for the scientific plausibility of NCS-R prevalence estimates and against higher thresholds for clinical significance in future DSM criteria.

## 4.4. Unmet Needs in NCS-R Lifetime Service Use

The NCS-R lifetime data on use of mental health services reveal large and underappreciated needs for mental health treatment in the United States. First, a large number of lifetime cases never seek help. This is especially true for substance and impulse-control disorders, where nearly half of all lifetime cases failed to ever make any treatment contact. The second source of unmet need documented in the NCS-R lifetime data concerns pervasive delays in initial treatment contact. The typical delays persist for years or even decades for some disorders. This has not been a focus of previous research, as mental health services research has traditionally focused on treatment of current episodes for established cases (Joseph & Boeckh 1981; Leaf et al. 1985; Leaf, Bruce & Tischler 1986; Leaf et al. 1988; Temkin-Greener & Clark 1988; Hu et al. 1991; Padgett et al. 1994). These NCS-R findings suggest that the focus needs to be expanded to address the speed of initial help seeking because, even for disorders where eventual treatment is typical, long delays are pervasive.

There was considerable variation between disorders in the probability of eventually making treatment contacts and in typical durations of delay. The higher initial treatment contact and shorter delays for mood disorders may be because they have been targeted by educational campaigns, primary care quality improvement programs, and treatment advances (Jacobs 1995; Hirschfeld et al. 1997; Olfson et al. 2002; Pincus et al. 2003; Schatzberg & Nemeroff 2004). PD is often accompanied by prominent and dysphoric somatic symptoms, which may explain why treatment contact for it is more common and rapid than for other anxiety disorders (Katon, Von Korff & Lin 1992; Katerndahl & Realini 1995). Greater failure and delays for some anxiety disorders (e.g., phobias and SAD) could also be due to their earlier AOOs, mild impairments, and even fear of providers or treatments (Leaf et al. 1985; Leaf et al. 1988; Solomon & Gordon 1988).

Consistent with prior research (Kessler, Olfson & Berglund 1998; Olfson et al. 1998; Christiana et al. 2000; Wang et al. 2004), we found that early-onset disorders are associated with longer delays and lower probabilities of help seeking. Minors may need the help of parents or other adults, and recognition of disorders by these adults may be low unless symptoms are extreme (Morrissey-Kane & Prinz 1999; Janicke, Finney & Riley 2001). Early onset may also lead to normalization of symptoms or coping strategies (e.g., social withdrawal) that interfere with help seeking during adulthood. Child mental health services may also not be available. Sociodemographic correlates of failure and delay in making initial treatment contact (e.g., older age, male sex, being poorly educated, or racial-ethnic minority status) may reflect negative attitudes toward mental health treatments as well as financial and other barriers to care.

The shorter delays and higher proportions of cases making treatment contacts among more recent cohorts provide some grounds for optimism as well as clues for improving failure and delays in the future. This secular change could be due, at least in part, to recent programs to destigmatize and increase awareness of mental illness, screening and outreach initiatives, the introduction and direct-to-consumer promotion of new treatments, and expansion of some insurance programs (Regier et al. 1988; Bhugra 1989; Ridgely & Goldman 1989; Ross 1993; Jacobs 1995; Hirschfeld et al. 1997; Williams 1998; Kessler & Wang 1999; Leucht et al. 1999; Mechanic & McAlpine 1999; Spitzer, Kroenke & Williams 1999; Sturm 1999; Williams et al. 1999; Weissman et al. 2000; Kessler et al. 2001c; Kessler et al. 2001a; Bender 2002; Olfson et al. 2002; Rosenthal et al. 2002; Schatzberg & Nemeroff 2004). Additional large-scale public education programs (e.g., the NIMH Depression, Awareness, Recognition, and Treatment [DART] program) and expanded use of national screening

days continue to hold great promise for hastening detection and treatment (Regier et al. 1988; Jacobs 1995; Morrissey-Kane & Prinz 1999). School-based screening programs using brief self-report and/or informant scales may be needed to detect early-onset mental disorders (Connors 1994; Aseltine & DeMartino 2004). Demand management and other outreach strategies could also help reduce critical delays and failures in initial help seeking once mental disorders are identified (Velicer et al. 1995; Carleton et al. 1996). Training non–health-care professionals to recognize individuals with mental disorders and make timely referrals for health care should also be explored (Weaver 1995; Kessler et al. 2001c; Wang, Berglund & Kessler 2003). Although preclinical (Post & Weiss 1998), epidemiological (Kessler & Price 1993; Kessler et al. 1995; Forthofer et al. 1996; Kessler 1997; Kessler et al. 1997; Kessler, Walters & Forthofer 1998), and even trials (Meltzer et al. 2003) suggest that there would be benefits to reducing these delays, definitively answering how much earlier treatment improves outcomes will need to wait until long-term trials of aggressive outreach and treatment of new cases are complete (MTA Cooperative Group 1999; Beidel, Turner & Morris 2000; Dierker et al. 2001).

## 4.5. Additional Concerns Regarding 12-month Treatment of Mental Disorders

NCS-R findings on 12-month use of mental health services shed light on additional deficiencies of mental health care in the United States, including underuse of services, poor quality regimens, use of unproven modalities, and suboptimal allocation of services. On one hand, the NCS-R reveals that mental health service use remains disturbingly low, with the majority of cases not receiving any care in the prior year. Among those receiving services, many go outside of health-care sectors. For example, CAM treatments account for 32% of all mental health visits despite a paucity of data supporting their efficacy (Eisenberg et al. 1993; Weaver 1995; Eisenberg et al. 1998; Kessler et al. 2001a; Kessler et al. 2001b; Hypericum Depression Trial Study

Group 2002; Wang et al. 2003). Even those using health-care sectors fail to get sufficient visits for clinical assessments, delivery of treatments, and appropriate ongoing monitoring (SAMHSA 1996; National Committee for Quality Assurance 1997; Olfson et al. 2002). Because of these and other problems, only one-third of treatments meet minimal standards of adequacy based on evidence-based treatment guidelines (Agency for Health Care Policy and Research 1993; American Psychiatric Association 1998; Lehman & Steinwachs 1998; American Psychiatric Association 2000, 2002, 2004). A shift also appears to be occurring between sectors, with expanded use of the general medical sector for mental health services (by 17.9% of NCS-R respondents vs. 13.3% a decade earlier in the original NCS) (Kessler et al. 1999). However this trend is of concern in light of the particularly low rate of treatment adequacy in the general medical sector.

On the other hand, a considerable number of mental health services are being consumed by respondents without apparent disorders. For example, respondents without disorders make up such a large majority of the population that they account for nearly one-third of all visits. Certainly some of these are being used appropriately to treat disorders not assessed in the NCS-R, subthreshold symptoms, secondary prevention of lifetime disorders, or even primary prevention (Kessler & Price 1993). However, it remains concerning that such a high proportion of treatment resources are being potentially diverted to individuals without mental disorders when unmet needs among people with well-defined disorders are so great (Narrow et al. 2002). Another potential problem in the allocation of mental health care is suggested by the highly skewed distribution of visits, with a small proportion of patients using the majority of services. Developing and implementing a principled basis for optimally allocating treatment resources remains an enormous challenge.

The NCS-R results reveal that service use varies across disorders, with generally greater use for disorders marked by distress or impairment (e.g., PD) and lower use for externalizing disorders (e.g., substance disorders and IED), which

may be accompanied by diminished perceived needs for treatment. The sociodemographic predictors of 12-month service use confirm earlier studies in showing the greatest risks of undertreatment or ineffective treatment among vulnerable groups such as the elderly, racial-ethnic minorities, those with low education or incomes, the uninsured, and residents of rural areas (Leaf et al. 1985; Wells et al. 1986; Leaf et al. 1988; Katz et al. 1998; Rost et al. 2002; Wang et al. 2002; Fischer et al. 2003; Klap, Unroe & Unutzer 2003; McLean, Campbell & Cornish 2003).

A variety of possible interventions to improve service use are suggested by these results. Interventions to increase access and initiation of treatments could include renewed community awareness and screening programs, new means for financing mental health services, and expansion of treatment resources for underserved areas (Jacobs 1995; Hirschfeld et al. 1997; Mechanic & McAlpine 1999; Kessler et al. 2001a; Bender 2002; Rost et al. 2002). Future interventions also clearly need to focus on improving the intensity and effectiveness of care that is given to patients with mental disorders. A related challenge is understanding why non–health-care treatments such as CAM have such great appeal and whether legitimate aspects of this appeal (e.g., greater patient-centeredness) can be adopted in evidence-based treatments. Proven disease management programs that enhance treatment adequacy and adherence (Katon et al. 1995; Wells et al. 2000; Schoenbaum et al. 2001; Simon et al. 2001; Katon et al. 2002) as well as establishing performance standards hold promise for enhancing treatments and monitoring the impacts of interventions in the future (SAMHSA 1996; National Committee for Quality Assurance 1997). However, increasing uptake of such successful programs and treatment models will almost certainly require addressing existing barriers, such as competing clinical demands and distorted incentives for effectively treating mental disorders, as well as providing purchasers with metrics to help them understand what their return on investment will be for improving mental health service use in the United States (Klinkman 1997; Williams 1998; Williams et al. 1999; Frank,

Huskamp & Pincus 2003; Pincus et al. 2003; Wang, Simon & Kessler 2003).

## 5. FUTURE DIRECTIONS

This chapter has reviewed ways in which the NCS-R has been able to provide an up-to-date and detailed view of the enormous societal burdens that mental disorders impose in the United States as well as potentially fruitful ways in which unmet needs for effective mental health care can be addressed. However, the NCS-R has the potential to become an even more powerful tool in the future through its linkage with two other forms of data. First, population-based surveys such as the NCS-R can become uniquely powerful if applied longitudinally in a consistent fashion. In the industrial quality sciences, repeated application of data collection using consistent methods is an integral part of continuous cycles of improvement (Berwick 1989). Although analogous cycles of continuous quality improvement have been called for in health care, they have failed to take hold especially in the general population in part because of the lack of the requisite longitudinal data collection on which the process depends (Blumenthal 1995; Blumenthal & Kilo 1998). Examination of temporal trends between the original NCS and NCS-R have already shown lack of change in disorder prevalence (Kessler et al. 2005c) and suicidality in the United States (Kessler et al. 2005b), which suggests that efforts and changes in the past decade have not been sufficient. Such comparisons between the original NCS and NCS-R provide evidence that longitudinal application of population-based psychiatric epidemiological surveys hold great promise for identifying and reducing burdens as well as for understanding and improving poor-quality care. Repeating population-based surveys using consistent methodology can serve as the nation's quality improvement and assurance system.

A second way in which the NCS-R can become a uniquely powerful tool is when its data are pooled, supplemented, and compared with comparable data from other WMH countries. Policy makers need specific designs they can implement to achieve their goals. Some techniques employed in managed care systems (e.g., gatekeeping, increased cost sharing, utilization review, prior approval) could presumably be brought to bear on unnecessary use but not underuse – in fact, they may worsen unmet needs for treatment. The impacts of other policies, delivery system features, and means of financing that policy makers could implement are essentially unknown (Burgess et al. 2004). For these reasons, collection of detailed data on the mental health policies, delivery system features, and means of financing mental health care in different countries is a promising area for future research (Saxena, Sharan & Saraceno 2003). When merged with WMH surveys on the use and adequacy of treatments, such combined data could shed light on the impacts of policies, delivery system, and financing features and will help policy makers choose strategies that achieve their desired goals (Mezzich 2003).

## REFERENCES

Agency for Health Care Policy and Research (1993). *Depression Guideline Panel, Vol. 2: Treatment of major depression, clinical practice guideline, No 5.* Rockville, MD: U.S. Department of Health and Human Services, Public Health Service, Agency for Health Care Policy and Research.

Allgulander, C. (1989). Psychoactive drug use in a general population sample, Sweden: Correlates with perceived health, psychiatric diagnoses, and mortality in an automated record-linkage study. *American Journal of Public Health*, 79, 1006–10.

American Psychiatric Association (1994). *Diagnostic and statistical manual of mental disorders (DSM-IV)*, 4th ed. Washington, DC: American Psychiatric Association.

American Psychiatric Association (1998). *Practice guideline for treatment of patients with panic disorder*. Washington, DC: American Psychiatric Association Press.

American Psychiatric Association (2000). *Practice guideline for treatment of patients with major depressive disorder*, 2d ed. Washington, DC: American Psychiatric Association Press.

American Psychiatric Association (2002). *Practice guideline for treatment of patients with bipolar disorder*, 2d ed. Washington, DC: American Psychiatric Association Press.

American Psychiatric Association (2004). *Practice guideline for treatment of patients with schizophrenia*, 2d ed. Washington, DC: American Psychiatric Association Press.

Aseltine, R. H., Jr. & DeMartino, R. (2004). An outcome evaluation of the SOS Suicide Prevention Program. *American Journal of Public Health*, 94, 446–51.

Badawi, M. A., Eaton, W. W., Myllyluoma, J., Weimer, L. G. & Gallo, J. (1999). Psychopathology and attrition in the Baltimore ECA 15-year follow-up 1981–1996. *Social Psychiatry and Psychiatric Epidemiology*, 34, 91–8.

Ballesteros, J., Duffy, J. C., Querejeta, I., Arino, J. & Gonzalez-Pinto, A. (2004). Efficacy of brief interventions for hazardous drinkers in primary care: Systematic review and meta-analyses. *Alcoholism: Clinical and Experimental Research*, 28, 608–18.

Beidel, D. C., Turner, S. M. & Morris, T. L. (2000). Behavioral treatment of childhood social phobia. *Journal of Consulting and Clinical Psychology*, 68, 1072–80.

Bender, E. (2002). Better access to geriatric mental health care goal of new house bill. *Psychiatric News*, 2–5.

Berwick, D. M. (1989). Continuous improvement as an ideal in health care. *New England Journal of Medicine*, 320, 53–6.

Bhugra, D. (1989). Attitudes towards mental illness: A review of the literature. *Acta Psychiatrica Scandinavica*, 80, 1–12.

Bijl, R. V., de Graaf, R., Hiripi, E., Kessler, R. C., Kohn, R., Offord, D. R., Üstün, T. B., Vicente, B., Vollebergh, W. A., Walters, E. E. & Wittchen, H.-U. (2003). The prevalence of treated and untreated mental disorders in five countries. *Health Affairs (Millwood)*, 22, 122–33.

Bland, R. C., Orn, H. & Newman, S. C. (1988). Lifetime prevalence of psychiatric disorders in Edmonton. *Acta Psychiatrica Scandinavica*, 77, 24–32.

Blumenthal, D. (1995). Applying industrial quality management science to physicians' clinical decision. In *Improving clinical practice: Total quality management and the physician*, ed. D. Blumenthal & A. Scheck, pp. 25–50, San Francisco: Jossey-Bass.

Blumenthal, D. & Kilo, C. M. (1998). A report card on continuous quality improvement. *Milbank Quarterly*, 76, 625–48.

Bruce, M. L. & Leaf, P. J. (1989). Psychiatric disorders and 15-month mortality in a community sample of older adults. *American Journal of Public Health*, 79, 727–30.

Burgess, P., Pirkis, J., Buckingham, B., Burns, J., Eagar, K. & Eckstein, G. (2004). Adult mental health needs and expenditure in Australia. *Social Psychiatry and Psychiatric Epidemiology*, 39, 427–34.

Canino, G. J., Bird, H. R., Shrout, P. E., Rubio-Stipec, M., Bravo, M., Martinez, R., Sesman, M. & Guevara,

L. M. (1987). The prevalence of specific psychiatric disorders in Puerto Rico. *Archives of General Psychiatry*, 44, 727–35.

Cannell, C. F., Marquis, K. H. & Laurent, A. (1977). A summary of studies of interviewing methodology: 1959–1970. *National Center for Health Statistics. Vital Health Stat Series No. 2* (69) 1977.

Carleton, R. A., Bazzarre, T., Drake, J., Dunn, A., Fisher, E. B., Jr., Grundy, S. M., Hayman, L., Hill, M. N., Maibach, E. W., Prochaska, J., Schmid, T., Smith, S. C., Jr., Susser, M. W. & Worden, J. W. (1996). Report of the Expert Panel on Awareness and Behavior Change to the board of directors, American Heart Association. *Circulation*, 93, 1768–72.

Christiana, J. M., Gilman, S. E., Guardino, M., Kessler, R. C., Mickelson, K., Morselli, P. L. & Olfson, M. (2000). Duration between onset and time of obtaining initial treatment among people with anxiety and mood disorders: An international survey of members of mental health patient advocate groups. *Psychological Medicine*, 30, 693–703.

Christie, K. A., Burke, J. D. J., Regier, D. A., Rae, D. S., Boyd, J. H. & Locke, B. Z. (1988). Epidemiologic evidence for early onset of mental disorders and higher risk of drug-abuse in young-adults. *American Journal of Psychiatry*, 145, 971–5.

Connors, C. K. (1994). The Connors Rating Scales: Use in clinical assessment, treatment planning and research. In *Use of psychological testing for treatment planning and outcome assessment*, ed. M. Maruish, pp. 550–78, Hillsdale, NJ: Lawrence Erlbaum Associates.

Demyttenaere, K., Bruffaerts, R., Posada-Villa, J., Gasquet, I., Kovess, V., Lepine, J. P., Angermeyer, M. C., Bernert, S., de Girolamo, G., Morosini, P., Polidori, G., Kikkawa, T., Kawakami, N., Ono, Y., Takeshima, T., Uda, H., Karam, E. G., Fayyad, J. A., Karam, A. N., Mneimneh, Z. N., Medina-Mora, M. E., Borges, G., Lara, C., de Graaf, R., Ormel, J., Gureje, O., Shen, Y., Huang, Y., Zhang, M., Alonso, J., Haro, J. M., Vilagut, G., Bromet, E. J., Gluzman, S., Webb, C., Kessler, R. C., Merikangas, K. R., Anthony, J. C., Von Korff, M. R., Wang, P. S., Brugha, T. S., Aguilar-Gaxiola, S., Lee, S., Heeringa, S., Pennell, B. E., Zaslavsky, A. M., Üstün, T. B. & Chatterji, S. (2004). Prevalence, severity and unmet need for treatment of mental disorders in the World Health Organization World Mental Health surveys. *Journal of the American Medical Association*, 291, 2581–90.

Dierker, L. C., Albano, A. M., Clarke, G. N., Heimberg, R. G., Kendall, P. C., Merikangas, K. R., Lewinsohn, P. M., Offord, D. R., Kessler, R. C. & Kupfer, D. J. (2001). Screening for anxiety and depression in early adolescence. *Journal of the American Academy of Child and Adolescent Psychiatry*, 40, 929–36.

Eaton, W. W., Anthony, J. C., Tepper, S. & Dryman, A. (1992). Psychopathology and attrition in the Epidemiologic Catchment Area Study. *American Journal of Epidemiology*, 135, 1051–9.

Efron, B. (1988). Logistic regression, survival analysis, and the Kaplan-Meier curve. *Journal of the American Statistical Association*, 83, 414–25.

Eisenberg, D. M., Davis, R. B., Ettner, S. L., Appel, S., Wilkey, S. A., van Rompay, M. & Kessler, R. C. (1998). Trends in alternative medicine use in the United States, 1990–1997: Results of a follow-up national survey. *Journal of the American Medical Association*, 280, 1569–75.

Eisenberg, D. M., Kessler, R. C., Foster, C., Norlock, F. E., Calkins, D. R. & Delbanco, T. L. (1993). Unconventional medicine in the United States. Prevalence, costs, and patterns of use. *New England Journal of Medicine*, 328, 246–52.

First, M. B., Spitzer, R. L., Gibbon, M. & Williams, J. B. W. (2002). *Structured Clinical Interview for DSM-IV-TR Axis I disorders, research version, non-patient edition (SCID-I/NP)*. New York: Biometrics Research, New York State Psychiatric Institute.

Fischer, L. R., Wei, F., Solberg, L. I., Rush, W. A. & Heinrich, R. L. (2003). Treatment of elderly and other adult patients for depression in primary care. *Journal of the American Geriatric Society*, 51, 1554–62.

Food and Drug Administration (n.d.). Antidepressant use in children, adolescents, and adults. Retrieved March 22, 2004, from http://www.fda.gov/cder/drug/antidepressants/default.htm.

Forthofer, M. S., Kessler, R. C., Story, A. L. & Gotlib, I. H. (1996). The effects of psychiatric disorders on the probability and timing of first marriage. *Journal of Health and Social Behavior*, 37, 121–32.

Frank, R. G., Huskamp, H. A. & Pincus, H. A. (2003). Aligning incentives in the treatment of depression in primary care with evidence-based practice. *Psychiatric Services*, 54, 682–7.

Halli, S. S. & Rao, K. V. (1992). *Advanced techniques of population analysis*. New York: Plenum.

Haro, J. M., Arbabzadeh-Bouchez, S., Brugha, T. S., de Girolamo, G., Guyer, M. E., Jin, R., Lepine, J. P., Mazzi, F., Reneses, B., Vilagut, G., Sampson, N. A. & Kessler, R. C. (2006). Concordance of the Composite International Diagnostic Interview Version 3.0 (CIDI 3.0) with standardized clinical assessments in the WHO World Mental Health surveys. *International Journal of Methods in Psychiatric Research*, 15, 167–80.

Hirschfeld, R. M. A., Keller, M. B., Panico, S., Arons, B. S., Barlow, D., Davidoff, F., Endicott, J., Froom, J., Goldstein, M., Gorman, J. M., Marek, R. G., Maurer, T. A., Meyer, R., Phillips, K., Ross, J., Schwenk, T. L., Sharfstein, S. S., Thase, M. E. & Wyatt, R. J. (1997). The national depressive and manic-depressive association consensus statement on the undertreatment of depression. *Journal of the American Medical Association*, 277, 333–40.

Holahan, J. & Cook, A. (2005). Changes in economic conditions and health insurance coverage, 2000–2004. *Health Affairs (Millwood)*, W5-498–508.

Hosmer, D. W. & Lemeshow, S. (1989). *Applied logistic regression*. New York: John Wiley & Sons.

Hu, T. W., Snowden, L. R., Jerrell, J. M. & Nguyen, T. D. (1991). Ethnic populations in public mental health: Services choice and level of use. *American Journal of Psychiatry*, 81, 1429–34.

Hwu, H. G., Yeh, E. K. & Cheng, L. Y. (1989). Prevalence of psychiatric disorders in Taiwan defined by the Chinese diagnostic interview schedule. *Acta Psychiatrica Scandinavica*, 79, 136–47.

Hypericum Depression Trial Study Group (2002). Effect of *Hypericum perforatum* (St. John's wort) in major depressive disorder: A randomized controlled trial. *Journal of the American Medical Association*, 287, 1807–14.

Institute of Medicine (2006). *Improving the quality of health care for mental and substance-use conditions: Quality chasm series*. Washington, DC: National Academy of Sciences.

Jacobs, D. G. (1995). National depression screening day: Educating the public, reaching those in need of treatment and broadening professional understanding. *Harvard Review of Psychiatry*, 3, 156–9.

Janicke, D. M., Finney, J. W. & Riley, A. W. (2001). Children's health care use: A prospective investigation of factors related to care-seeking. *Medical Care*, 39, 990–1001.

Joseph, A. E. & Boeckh, J. L. (1981). Locational variation in mental health care utilization dependent upon diagnosis: A Canadian example. *Social Science and Medicine*, 15, 395–440.

Kaiser Commission on Medicaid and the Uninsured (n.d.). The uninsured: A primer: Key facts about Americans without health insurance. Retrieved April 20, 2006, from http://www.kff.org.

Kaplan, E. L. & Meier, P. (1958). Nonparametric estimation from incomplete observations. *Journal of the American Statistical Association*, 53, 457–81.

Katerndahl, D. A. & Realini, J. P. (1995). Where do panic attack sufferers seek care? *Journal of Family Practice*, 40, 237–43.

Katon, W. J., Roy-Byrne, P., Russo, J. & Cowley, D. (2002). Cost-effectiveness and cost offset of a collaborative care intervention for primary care patients with panic disorder. *Archives of General Psychiatry*, 59, 1098–104.

Katon, W. J., Von Korff, M. & Lin, E. (1992). Panic disorder: Relationship to high medical utilization. *American Journal of Medicine*, 92, 7S–11S.

Katon, W., Von Korff, M., Lin, E., Walker, E., Simon, G. E., Bush, T., Robinson, P. & Russo, J. (1995). Collaborative management to achieve treatment guidelines: Impact on depression in primary care. *Journal of the American Medical Association*, 273, 1026–31.

Katz, S. J., Kessler, R. C., Lin, E. & Wells, K. B. (1998). Medication management of depression in the United States and Ontario. *Journal of General Internal Medicine*, 13, 77–85.

Kessler, R. C. (1995). Epidemiology of psychiatric comorbidity. In *Textbook in psychiatric epidemiology*, ed. M. T. Tsuang, M. Tohen, & G. E. P. Zahner, pp. 179–97. New York: John Wiley & Sons.

Kessler, R. C. (1997). The prevalence of psychiatric comorbidity. In *Treatment strategies for patients with psychiatric comorbidity*, ed. S. Wetzler & W. C. Sanderson, pp. 23–48. New York: John Wiley & Sons.

Kessler, R. C., Berglund, P., Chiu, W. T., Demler, O., Heeringa, S., Hiripi, E., Jin, R., Pennell, B. E., Walters, E. E., Zaslavsky, A. & Zheng, H. (2004). The U.S. National Comorbidity Survey Replication (NCS-R): Design and field procedures. *International Journal of Methods in Psychiatric Research*, 13, 69–92.

Kessler, R. C., Berglund, P., Demler, O., Jin, R. & Walters, E. E. (2005a). Lifetime prevalence and age-of-onset distributions of DSM-IV disorders in the National Comorbidity Survey Replication. *Archives of General Psychiatry*, 62, 593–602.

Kessler, R. C., Berglund, P. A., Borges, G., Nock, M. & Wang, P. S. (2005b). Trends in suicide ideation, plans, gestures, and attempts in the United States 1990–92 to 2001–03. *Journal of the American Medical Association*, 293, 2487–95.

Kessler, R. C., Berglund, P. A., Bruce, M. L., Koch, J. R., Laska, E. M., Leaf, P. J., Manderscheid, R. W., Rosenheck, R. A., Walters, E. E. & Wang, P. S. (2001a). The prevalence and correlates of untreated serious mental illness. *Health Services Research*, 36, 987–1007.

Kessler, R. C., Berglund, P. A., Foster, C. L., Saunders, W. B., Stang, P. E. & Walters, E. E. (1997). Social consequences of psychiatric disorders, II: Teenage parenthood. *American Journal of Psychiatry*, 154, 1405–11.

Kessler, R. C., Berglund, P. A., Zhao, S., Leaf, P. J., Kouzis, A. C., Bruce, M. L., Friedman, R. M., Grosser, R. C., Kennedy, C., Kuehnel, T. G., Laska, E. M., Manderscheid, R. W., Narrow, W. E., Rosenheck, R. A., Santoni, T. W. & Schneier, M. (1996). The 12-month prevalence and correlates of serious mental illness (SMI). In *Mental health, United States, 1996*, ed. R. W. Manderscheid & M. A. Sonnenschein, pp. 59–70. Washington, DC: U.S. Government Printing Office.

Kessler, R. C., Davis, R. B., Foster, D. F., Van Rompay, M. I., Walters, E. E., Wilkey, S. A., Kaptchuk, T. J. & Eisenberg, D. M. (2001b). Long-term trends in the use of complementary and alternative medical therapies in the United States. *Annals of Internal Medicine*, 135, 262–8.

Kessler, R. C., Demler, O., Frank, R. G., Olfson, M., Pincus, H. A., Walters, E. E., Wang, P. S., Wells, K. B. & Zaslavsky, A. M. (2005c). Prevalence and treatment of mental disorders, 1990 to 2003. *New England Journal of Medicine*, 352, 2515–23.

Kessler, R. C., Foster, C. L., Saunders, W. B. & Stang, P. E. (1995). Social consequences of psychiatric disorders, I: Educational attainment. *American Journal of Psychiatry*, 152, 1026–32.

Kessler, R. C., Frank, R. G., Edlund, M., Katz, S. J., Lin, E. & Leaf, P. J. (1997). Differences in the use of psychiatric outpatient services between the United States and Ontario. *New England Journal of Medicine*, 336, 551–7.

Kessler, R. C., Haro, J. M., Heeringa, S. G., Pennell, B. E. & Üstün, T. B. (2006). The World Health Organization World Mental Health Survey Initiative. *Epidemiologia e Psichiatria Sociale*, 15, 161–6.

Kessler, R. C., McGonagle, K. A., Zhao, S., Nelson, C. B., Hughes, M., Eshleman, S., Wittchen, H.-U. & Kendler, K. S. (1994). Lifetime and 12-month prevalence of DSM-III-R psychiatric disorders in the United States. Results from the National Comorbidity Survey. *Archives of General Psychiatry*, 51, 8–19.

Kessler, R. C., Olfson, M. & Berglund, P. A. (1998). Patterns and predictors of treatment contact after first onset of psychiatric disorders. *American Journal of Psychiatry*, 155, 62–9.

Kessler, R. C. & Price, R. H. (1993). Primary prevention of secondary disorders: A proposal and agenda. *American Journal of Community Psychology*, 21, 607–33.

Kessler, R. C., Soukup, J., Davis, R. B., Foster, D. F., Wilkey, S. A., Van Rompay, M. & Eisenberg, D. M. (2001c). The use of complementary and alternative therapies to treat anxiety and depression in the United States. *American Journal of Psychiatry*, 158, 289–94.

Kessler, R. C. & Üstün, T. B. (2004). The World Mental Health (WMH) survey initiative version of the World Health Organization (WHO) Composite International Diagnostic Interview (CIDI). *International Journal of Methods in Psychiatric Research*, 13, 93–121.

Kessler, R. C., Walters, E. E. & Forthofer, M. S. (1998). The social consequences of psychiatric disorders, III: Probability of marital stability. *American Journal of Psychiatry*, 155, 1092–6.

Kessler, R. C. & Wang, P. S. (1999). Screening measures for behavioral health assessment. In *SPM handbook of health assessment tools*, ed. G. Hyner, K. Peterson, J. Travis, J. Dewey, J. Foerster, & E. Framer, pp. 33–40. Pittsburgh: Society for Prospective Medicine.

Kessler, R. C., Zhao, S., Katz, S. J., Kouzis, A. C., Frank, R. G., Edlund, M. & Leaf, P. J. (1999). Past year use of outpatient services for psychiatric problems in the National Comorbidity Survey. *American Journal of Psychiatry*, 156, 115–23.

Klap, R., Unroe, K. T. & Unutzer, J. (2003). Caring for mental illness in the United States: A focus on older adults. *American Journal of Geriatric Psychiatry*, 11, 517–24.

Klinkman, M. S. (1997). Competing demands in psychosocial care: A model for the identification and treatment of depressive disorders in primary care. *General Hospital Psychiatry*, 19, 98–111.

Leaf, P. J., Bruce, M. L. & Tischler, G. L. (1986). The differential effect of attitudes on use of mental health services. *Social Psychiatry*, 21, 187–92.

Leaf, P. J., Bruce, M. L., Tischler, G. L., Freeman, D. H., Weissman, M. M. & Myers, J. K. (1988). Factors affecting the utilization of specialty and general medical mental health services. *Medical Care*, 26, 9–26.

Leaf, P. J., Livingston, M. M., Tischler, G. L., Weissman, M. M., Holzer, C. E. & Myers, J. K. (1985). Contact with health professionals for the treatment of psychiatric and emotional problems. *Medical Care*, 23, 1322–37.

Lee, C. K., Kwak, Y. S., Yamamoto, J., Rhee, H., Kim, Y. S., Han, J. H., Choi, J. O. & Lee, Y. H. (1990). Psychiatric epidemiology in Korea: Part I. gender and age differences in Seoul. *Journal of Nervous and Mental Disease*, 178, 242–6.

Lehman, A. F. & Steinwachs, D. M. (1998). Translating research into practice: Schizophrenia patient outcomes research team (PORT) treatment recommendations. *Schizophrenia Bulletin*, 24, 1–10.

Leon, A. C., Olfson, M., Portera, L., Farber, L. & Sheehan, D. V. (1997). Assessing psychiatric impairment in primary care with the Sheehan Disability Scale. *International Journal of Psychiatry in Medicine*, 27, 93–105.

Lépine, J. P., Lellouch, J., Lovell, A., Teherani, M., Ha, C., Verdier-Taillefer, M. G., Rambourg, N. & Lempérière, T. (1989). Anxiety and depressive disorders in a French population: Methodology and preliminary results. *Psychiatric Psychobiology*, 4, 267–74.

Leucht, S., Pitschel-Walz, G., Abraham, D. & Kissling, W. (1999). Efficacy and extrapyramidal side effects of the new antipsychotics olanzapine, quetiapine, risperidone, and sertindole compared to conventional antipsychotics and placebo: A meta-analysis of randomized controlled trials. *Schizophrenia Research*, 35, 51–68.

Mark, T. L., Coffey, R. M., McKusick, D. R., Harwood, H., King, E., Bouchery, E., Genuardi, J., Vandivort, R., Buck, J. & Dilonardo, J. (2005). *National estimates of expenditures for mental health services and substance abuse treatment, 1991–2001*. SAMHSA Pub No. SMA 05-3999. Rockville, MD: SAMHSA.

McLean, C., Campbell, C. & Cornish, F. (2003). African-Caribbean interactions with mental health services in the UK: Experiences and expectations of exclusion as (re)productive of health inequalities. *Social Science and Medicine*, 56, 657–69.

Mechanic, D. & McAlpine, D. D. (1999). Mission unfulfilled: Potholes on the road to mental health parity. *Health Affairs (Millwood)*, 18, 7–21.

Meltzer, H. Y., Alphs, L., Green, A. I., Altamura, A. C., Anand, R., Bertoldi, A., Bourgeois, M., Chouinard, G., Islam, M. Z., Kane, J., Krishnan, R., Lindenmayer, J. P. & Potkin, S. (2003). Clozapine treatment for suicidality in schizophrenia: International Suicide Prevention Trial (InterSePT). *Archives of General Psychiatry*, 60, 82–91.

Mezzich, J. E. (2003). From financial analysis to policy development in mental health care: The need for broader conceptual models and partnerships. *Journal of Mental Health Policy and Economics*, 6, 149–50.

Morrissey-Kane, E. & Prinz, R. J. (1999). Engagement in child and adolescent treatment: The role of parental cognitions and attributions. *Clinical Child and Family Psychology Review*, 2, 183–98.

MTA Cooperative Group (1999). A 14-month randomized clinical trial of treatment strategies for attention-deficit/hyperactivity disorder. The MTA Cooperative Group. Multimodal Treatment Study of Children with ADHD. *Archives of General Psychiatry*, 56, 1073–86.

Murray, C. J. L. & Lopez, A. D. (1996). *Global health statistics*. Cambridge, MA: Harvard University Press.

Narrow, W. E., Rae, D. S., Robins, L. N. & Regier, D. A. (2002). Revised prevalence estimates of mental disorders in the United States: Using a clinical significance criterion to reconcile 2 surveys' estimates. *Archives of General Psychiatry*, 59, 115–23.

National Committee for Quality Assurance, ed. (1997). *HEDIS 3.0: Narrative: What's in it and why it matters*. Washington, DC: National Committee for Quality Assurance.

Olfson, M., Kessler, R. C., Berglund, P. A. & Lin, E. (1998). Psychiatric disorder onset and first treatment contact in the United States and Ontario. *American Journal of Psychiatry*, 155, 1415–22.

Olfson, M., Marcus, S. C., Druss, B., Elinson, L., Tanielian, T. & Pincus, H. A. (2002). National trends in the outpatient treatment of depression. *Journal of the American Medical Association*, 287, 203–9.

Ost, L. G., Ferebee, I. & Furmark, T. (1997). One-session group therapy of spider phobia: Direct versus indirect treatments. *Behaviour Research and Therapy*, 35, 721–32.

Padgett, D. K., Patrick, C., Burns, B. J. & Schlesinger, H. J. (1994). Ethnicity and use of outpatient mental health services in a national insured population. *American Journal of Public Health*, 84, 222–6.

Pincus, H. A., Hough, L., Houtsinger, J. K., Rollman, B. L. & Frank, R. G. (2003). Emerging models of depression care: Multi-level ('6 P') strategies. *International Journal of Methods in Psychiatric Research*, 12, 54–63.

Post, R. M. & Weiss, S. R. (1998). Sensitization and kindling phenomena in mood, anxiety, and obsessive-compulsive disorders: The role of serotonergic mechanisms in illness progression. *Biological Psychiatry*, 44, 193–206.

President's New Freedom Commission on Mental Health (n.d.). Achieving the promise: Transforming mental health care in America. Retrieved November 16, 2007 from http://www.mentalhealthcommission.gov/reports/finalreport/fullreport.htm.

Proctor, B. D. & Dalaker, J. (2002). Current population reports. In *Poverty in the United States: 2001*, pp. 60–219. Washington, DC: U.S. Government Printing Office.

Regier, D. A., Hirschfeld, R. M., Goodwin, F. K., Burke, J. D., Jr., Lazar, J. B. & Judd, L. L. (1988). The NIMH Depression Awareness, Recognition, and Treatment Program: Structure, aims, and scientific basis. *American Journal of Psychiatry*, 145, 1351–7.

Regier, D. A., Kaelber, C. T., Rae, D. S., Farmer, M. E., Knauper, B., Kessler, R. C. & Norquist, G. S. (1998). Limitations of diagnostic criteria and assessment instruments for mental disorders: Implications for research and policy. *Archives of General Psychiatry*, 55, 109–15.

Research Triangle Institute (2002). *SUDAAN: Professional software for survey data analysis*. Research Triangle Park, NC: Research Triangle Institute.

Rhodes, A. E. & Fung, K. (2004). Self-reported use of mental health services versus administrative records: Care to recall? *International Journal of Methods in Psychiatric Research*, 13, 165–75.

Rhodes, A. E., Lin, E. & Mustard, C. A. (2002). Self-reported use of mental health services versus administrative records: Should we care? *International Journal of Methods in Psychiatric Research*, 11, 125–33.

Ridgely, M. S. & Goldman, H. H. (1989). Mental health insurance. In *Handbook on mental health policy in the United States*, ed. D. A. Rochefort, pp. 341–61. Westport, CT: Greenwood Press.

Robins, L. N. & Regier, D. A., eds. (1991). *Psychiatric disorders in America: The Epidemiologic Catchment Area Study*. New York: Free Press.

Rosenthal, M. B., Berndt, E. R., Donohue, J. M., Frank, R. G. & Epstein, A. M. (2002). Promotion of prescription drugs to consumers. *New England Journal of Medicine*, 346, 498–505.

Ross, J. (1993). Social phobia: the consumer's perspective. *Journal of Clinical Psychiatry*, 54 (suppl.), 5–9.

Rost, K., Fortney, J., Fischer, E. & Smith, J. (2002). Use, quality, and outcomes of care for mental health: The rural perspective. *Medical Care Research and Review*, 59, 231–65.

SAS Institute (2001). *SAS/STAT Software: Changes and enhancements, Release 8.2*. Cary, NC: SAS Publishing.

Saxena, S., Sharan, P. & Saraceno, B. (2003). Budget and financing of mental health services: Baseline information on 89 countries from WHO's project atlas. *Journal of Mental Health Policy and Economics*, 6, 135–43.

Schatzberg, A. F. & Nemeroff, C. B. (2004). *Textbook of psychopharmacology*. Washington, DC: American Psychiatric Publishing.

Schoenbaum, M., Unutzer, J., Sherbourne, C., Duan, N., Rubenstein, L. V., Miranda, J., Meredith, L. S., Carney, M. F. & Wells, K. (2001). Cost-effectiveness of practice-initiated quality improvement for depression: results of a randomized controlled trial. *Journal of the American Medical Association*, 286, 1325–30.

Simon, G. E., Katon, W. J., VonKorff, M., Unutzer, J., Lin, E. H., Walker, E. A., Bush, T., Rutter, C. & Ludman, E. (2001). Cost-effectiveness of a collaborative care program for primary care patients with persistent depression. *American Journal of Psychiatry*, 158, 1638–44.

Solomon, P. & Gordon, B. (1988). Outpatient compliance of psychiatric emergency room patients by presenting problems. *Psychiatric Quarterly*, 59, 271–83.

Spitzer, R. L., Kroenke, K. & Williams, J. B. (1999). Validation and utility of a self-report version of PRIME-MD: The PHQ primary care study. Primary Care Evaluation of Mental Disorders. Patient Health Questionnaire. *Journal of the American Medical Association*, 282, 1737–44.

Sturm, R. (1999). Tracking changes in behavioral health services: How have carve-outs changed care? *Journal of Behavioural Health Services and Research*, 26, 360–71.

Sturm, R. & Klap, R. (1999). Use of psychiatrists, psychologists, and master's-level therapists in managed behavioral health care carve-out plans. *Psychiatric Services*, 50, 504–8.

Substance Abuse and Mental Health Services Administration (SAMHSA) (1996). *Consumer-oriented mental health report card*. Rockville, MD: Center for Mental Health Services, SAMSHA.

Temkin-Greener, H. & Clark, K. T. (1988). Ethnicity, gender, and utilization of mental health services in a Medicaid population. *Social Science and Medicine*, 26, 989–96.

Turner, C. F., Ku, L., Rogers, S. M., Lindberg, L. D., Pleck, J. H. & Sonenstein, F. L. (1998). Adolescent sexual behavior, drug use, and violence: Increased reporting with computer survey technology. *Science*, 280, 867–73.

U.S. Census Bureau (2000). *County and city databook, 2000*. Washington, DC: U.S. Government Printing Office.

Velicer, W. F., Hughes, S. L., Fava, J. L., Prochaska, J. O. & DiClemente, C. C. (1995). An empirical typology of subjects within stage of change. *Addictive Behaviors*, 20, 299–320.

Wang, P. S., Berglund, P. & Kessler, R. C. (2000). Recent care of common mental disorders in the United States: Prevalence and conformance with evidence-based recommendations. *Journal of General Internal Medicine*, 15, 284–92.

Wang, P. S., Berglund, P. A. & Kessler, R. C. (2003). Patterns and correlates of contacting clergy for mental disorders in the United States. *Health Services Research*, 38, 647–73.

Wang, P. S., Berglund, P. A., Olfson, M. & Kessler, R. C. (2004). Delays in initial treatment contact after first onset of a mental disorder. *Health Services Research*, 39, 393–415.

Wang, P. S., Demler, O. & Kessler, R. C. (2002). Adequacy of treatment for serious mental illness in the United States. *American Journal of Public Health*, 92, 92–8.

Wang, P. S., Simon, G. & Kessler, R. C. (2003). The economic burden of depression and the cost-effectiveness of treatment. *International Journal of Methods in Psychiatric Research*, 12, 22–33.

Weaver, A. J. (1995). Has there been a failure to prepare and support parish-based clergy in their role as frontline community mental health workers: A review. *Journal of Pastoral Care*, 49, 129–47.

Weissman, E., Pettigrew, K., Sotsky, S. & Regier, D. A. (2000). The cost of access to mental health services in managed care. *Psychiatric Services*, 51, 664–6.

Wells, J. E., Bushnell, J. A., Hornblow, A. R., Joyce, P. R. & Oakley-Browne, M. A. (1989). Christchurch Psychiatric Epidemiology Study, part I: Methodology and lifetime prevalence for specific psychiatric disorders. *Australian and New Zealand Journal of Psychiatry*, 23, 315–26.

Wells, K. B., Manning, W. G., Duan, N., Newhouse, J. P. & Ware, J. E., Jr. (1986). Sociodemographic factors and the use of outpatient mental health services. *Medical Care*, 24, 75–85.

Wells, K. B., Sherbourne, C., Schoenbaum, M., Duan, N., Meredith, L., Unutzer, J., Miranda, J., Carney, M. F. & Rubenstein, L. V. (2000). Impact of disseminating quality improvement programs for depression in managed primary care: A randomized controlled trial. *Journal of the American Medical Association*, 283, 212–20.

WHO International Consortium in Psychiatric Epidemiology (2000). Cross-national comparisons of the prevalences and correlates of mental disorders. *Bulletin of the World Health Organization*, 78, 413–26.

Williams, J. B. W. (1998). Competing demands: Does care for depression fit in primary care? *Journal of General Internal Medicine*, 13, 137–9.

Williams, J. W., Jr., Rost, K., Dietrich, A. J., Ciotti, M. C., Zyzanski, S. J. & Cornell, J. (1999). Primary care physicians' approach to depressive disorders: Effects of physician specialty and practice structure. *Archives of Family Medicine*, 8, 58–67.

Wittchen, H.-U., Essau, C. A., von Zerssen, D., Krieg, C. J. & Zaudig, M. (1992). Lifetime and six-month prevalence of mental disorders in the Munich Follow-up Study. *European Archives of Psychiatry and Clinical Neuroscience*, 241, 247–58.

World Health Organization (WHO) (1991). *International classification of diseases (ICD-10)*. Geneva: World Health Organization.

# 10 Mental Disorders among Adult Nigerians: Risks, Prevalence, and Treatment

OYE GUREJE, OLUSOLA ADEYEMI, NONYENIM ENYIDAH, MICHAEL EKPO,[*]
OWOIDOHO UDOFIA, RICHARD UWAKWE, AND ABBA WAKIL

## ACKNOWLEDGMENTS

We acknowledge with thanks the design and statistical advice provided by Professor E. A. Bamgboye and administrative support by Dr. Olusola Odujinrin. Funding for the NSMHW was provided by World Health Organization (WHO), Geneva and the WHO country office in Nigeria. Collaborating investigators include Dr. O. Gureje, principal investigator, along with Drs. R. Uwakwe, O. Udofia, A. Wakil, N. Enyidah, M. Ekpo, and O. Adeyemi. The NSMHW is carried out in conjunction with the WHO World Mental Health (WMH) Survey Initiative. We thank the WMH coordination staff both for their assistance with instrumentation and for their consultation on field procedures and data analysis. These activities were supported by the U.S. National Institute of Mental Health (R01MH070884), the John D. and Catherine T. MacArthur Foundation, the Pfizer Foundation, the US Public Health Service (R13-MH066849, R01-MH069864, and R01 DA016558), the Fogarty International Center (FIRCA R03-TW006481), the Pan American Health Organization, Eli Lilly and Company Foundation, Ortho-McNeil Pharmaceutical, GlaxoSmithKline, and Bristol-Myers Squibb. A complete list of WMH publications can be found at http://www.hcp.med.harvard.edu/wmh/.

## I. INTRODUCTION

The first, and to date the only, mental health policy in Nigeria was formulated and published in 1991. In formulating broad policy aims for the improvement of mental health service for the country, the authors stated explicitly the absence of reliable data on which to base much of the projections. In particular, the need was emphasized for community-based epidemiological surveys that would document the burden of mental illness in the population and identify gaps in existing service provision. The policy thus drew attention to the fact that, in spite of many years of epidemiological studies in the country, the focus of earlier studies tended to be limited. Many prior studies consisted of selected subject samples or assessed a limited range of disorders.

The emergence of fully structured diagnostic interviews that do not require highly trained clinicians for their administration has made large-scale and replicable epidemiological studies of mental disorders possible. Even with this development, such studies in developing countries are hampered by a lack of resources and are particularly rare in Africa (Gureje & Alem 2000). Large-scale surveys are expensive to mount and demand considerable survey expertise, both of which are not always available in research centers in Africa (Alem & Kebede 2003).

Effective service planning requires knowledge of the number of people affected by mental disorders. Estimates derived from studies in one country may not serve the needs of another because there is wide variation in the rates reported for both lifetime and 12-month mental disorders across studies. For example, a 12-month prevalence rate of 30% was reported for the United States, 23% Australia, and 9.6% for Western Europe, even when broadly identical ascertainment tools had been used (Andrews,

* Dr. Michael Ekpo was a coinvestigator until his death.

Henderson & Hall 2001; Kessler et al. 1994; ESEMeD/MHEDEA 2000 Investigators 2004a). Divergence of rates can be expected to be even more pronounced when demographic and socio-cultural differences are significant, as these factors are of great relevance to the occurrence of mental disorders.

Although surveys examining prevalence of disorders are important, information on met and unmet need for treatment is also required given that having a diagnosable mental disorder is not synonymous with treatment need (Spitzer 1998; Regier et al. 2000) and that the rates of met need also vary widely (Bijl et al. 2003). Evidence derived from rich industrialized countries suggests that the unmet need for treatment of mental disorders is a major problem in the community. Studies conducted in North America and Western Europe show that, although marked differences exist in the pattern and correlates of service use between countries, underuse of services by individuals with mental disorders is common (WHO International Consortium in Psychiatric Epidemiology 2000; Alonso 2002; Kessler, Olfson & Berglund 1998; Wang et al. 2005a; Oakley-Browne et al. 2006).

Information is sparse on met and unmet needs for mental health service among representative samples in communities within developing countries in general (Alegria & Kessler 2000) and virtually nonexistent in African countries specifically. The few studies from developing countries, some of them on very highly selected samples, suggest that the pattern and nature of access to service in developing countries are different from those of developed countries and that access is generally poorer (Abas & Broadhead 1997). Resources are, of course, scarce in developing countries. However, factors other than resources may also determine the receipt of care for mental disorders. Awareness that an existing impairment is due to the presence of a mental disorder and that effective intervention exists for the problem may determine whether persons with mental disorders seek care. Poor knowledge of and negative attitude toward mental illness in the community, which are often widespread in some developing countries (Gureje et al. 2005)

may prevent persons with disorders from seeking help.

This report presents data on lifetime prevalence, age of onset distributions, and projected lifetime risks of mental disorders obtained in the World Mental Health (WMH) Survey Initiative (Kessler et al. 2006) in Nigeria. We also present data on the extent and timing of initial treatment contact for mental disorders and the sociodemographic correlates of lifetime treatment.

## 2. METHOD

The surveys described in this chapter were centrally coordinated by the principal investigator in Ibadan, with site investigators based in Calabar, Kaduna, Maiduguri, Nnewi, and Port Harcourt.

### 2.1. Sample

We used a four-stage area probability sample of households to select respondents aged 18 years and older. The survey was conducted in five of the six geopolitical regions of Nigeria: South-West (Lagos, Ogun, Osun, Oyo, Ondo, and Ekiti), South-East (Abia, Anambra, Enugu, Ebonyi, and Imo), South-South (Akwa Ibom, Cross-River, and Rivers), North-Central (Kaduna, Kogi, and Kwara), and North-East (Adamawa, Bornu, Gombe, and Yobe). Collectively, these states represent about 57% of the national population. The initial plan to include states in the North-West did not succeed because of difficulties in engaging a collaborating site in the region. The surveys were conducted in four languages: Yoruba (South-West and parts of North-Central), Igbo (South-East and parts of South-South), Hausa (North-East and parts of North-Central), and Efik (parts of South-South).

Selection of local government areas (LGAs) within the states and geographically defined enumeration areas (EAs) within the LGAs constituted the first and second stages of the selection process, respectively. All selected EAs were visited by research enumerators prior to the interview phase of the survey and an enumeration and listing of all the household units contained therein were conducted. This information was fed into a computer file in the central office. In the third stage of the selection, a random selection of households was made from the computerized data file, with the probability of selection proportional to the size of the households in the EA. The final selection of respondents was made during the interview phase of the survey. Interviewers obtained a full listing of all residents in each of the randomly selected households from an informant in the household. After identifying household residents who were aged 18 years or older and were fluent in the language of the study, a probability procedure, the Kish table selection method (Kish 1965), was used to select one eligible person as the respondent. Only one such person was selected per household, except for a random 25% of households in the Yoruba-language component of the survey, in which a secondary respondent, a spouse of the primary respondent who had been interviewed, was also selected for a substudy of spouses. When the primary respondent was either unavailable following repeated calls (five repeated calls were made) or refused to participate, no replacement was made within the household.

On the basis of this selection procedure, face-to-face interviews were carried out on 6752 respondents. The overall response rate was 79.3%. However, as a result of administrative and financial difficulties, response rates varied widely: it was 95.0% for the South-East and South-South, 79.9% for the South-West and the Yoruba-speaking North-Central, and 47.0% for the North-East. The low response rate from the North-East was because more than half of the initial households could not be surveyed as a result of nonavailability of previously promised funds. The respective contributions to the overall sample were: Yoruba-speaking South-West and North-Central, 4984; Igbo-speaking South-East and Efik-speaking South-South, 1277; and North-East 491.

As a result of differences in funding sources, planning and implementation did not occur at the same time in the study sites. Thus, while fieldwork (including enumeration and interviews) was conducted in the Yoruba-speaking study areas between February and November 2002,

it was conducted in the other language groups between October 2002 and May 2003. The survey was administered in two parts. Part 1 consisted of a core of diagnoses and was administered to all respondents. Part 2 consisted of sections for the assessment of risk factors, consequences, and correlates of disorders, as well as a few non-core disorders. Part 2 was administered to respondents who met lifetime Part 1 disorders plus a probability subsample of other respondents. The total Part 2 sample was 2143. Table 10.1 shows the age and sex distribution of the sample, weighted and unweighted, compared to the national profile (WHO 2005).

Respondents were informed about the study and provided either verbal or written consent before interviews were conducted. Verbal consent was the norm because of widespread illiteracy and because some respondents seemed somewhat hesitant about the implications of appending their signature to a document. The survey was approved by the University of Ibadan/University College hospital, Ibadan Joint Ethical Review Board.

## 2.2. Measures

As with other WMH surveys, diagnostic assessment was made with Version 3.0 of the Composite International Diagnostic Interview (CIDI) (Kessler & Üstün 2004). As discussed in Chapter 4 of this volume, the CIDI is a fully structured diagnostic interview that is lay administered and can generate diagnoses according to both the ICD-10 and the DSM-IV criteria. We previously had carried out studies using earlier versions of the CIDI in Yoruba (Gureje, Obikoya & Ikuesan 1992; Gureje et al. 1995). The language versions of the CIDI used in the present survey were derived, as in the earlier Yoruba versions, from standard protocols of iterative back-translation conducted by panels of bilingual experts. The CIDI primarily ascertains lifetime disorders. For respondents with lifetime occurrence of a disorder, follow-up questions allowed for a determination of whether they had also experienced such disorders in the prior 12 months. Specifically, we considered the occurrence of anxiety

**Table 10.1.** Demographic distribution of the sample compared to the population on poststratification variables

|         | Part 1 unweighted % | Part 1 weighted % | Part 2 unweighted % | Part 2 weighted % | Census % |
|---------|---------------------|-------------------|---------------------|-------------------|----------|
| **Age** |                     |                   |                     |                   |          |
| 18–24   | 25.7                | 26.8              | 27.8                | 27.0              | 27.0     |
| 25–29   | 16.3                | 15.2              | 15.6                | 15.2              | 15.2     |
| 30–34   | 11.9                | 13.4              | 10.2                | 13.1              | 13.1     |
| 35–39   | 9.7                 | 10.3              | 8.9                 | 10.4              | 10.4     |
| 40–44   | 7.6                 | 8.0               | 8.5                 | 8.0               | 8.0      |
| 45–49   | 5.2                 | 5.9               | 6.7                 | 6.0               | 6.0      |
| 50–54   | 6.0                 | 5.8               | 4.8                 | 5.8               | 5.8      |
| 55–59   | 3.2                 | 4.5               | 3.0                 | 4.8               | 4.8      |
| 60–64   | 4.1                 | 3.8               | 5.2                 | 3.7               | 3.7      |
| 65–69   | 2.7                 | 2.7               | 2.6                 | 2.7               | 2.7      |
| 70–74   | 3.6                 | 1.8               | 3.0                 | 1.8               | 1.8      |
| 75+     | 4.0                 | 1.7               | 3.7                 | 1.7               | 1.7      |
| **Sex** |                     |                   |                     |                   |          |
| Male    | 58.5                | 49.4              | 56.2                | 49.0              | 49.0     |
| Female  | 41.5                | 50.6              | 43.8                | 51.0              | 51.0     |

disorders (panic disorder, generalized anxiety disorder, agoraphobia without panic disorder, specific phobia, social phobia, posttraumatic disorder, obsessive-compulsive disorder), mood disorders (major depressive disorder, dysthymia, bipolar disorder), and substance use disorders (alcohol and drug abuse and dependence). DSM-IV organic exclusion rules were applied to all diagnoses, as were hierarchy rules, except in the case of substance use disorders, where abuse is defined with or without dependence.

## 2.3. Severity

Ratings of severity associated with each disorder experienced in the prior 12 months were made. This was done by asking respondents to focus on the month in the past year when the symptoms of the disorder were most persistent and severe and to rate the disability associated with the disorder during that month using an expanded version of the Sheehan Disability Scales (SDS) (Sheehan, Harnnet-Sheehan & Raj 1996). Four areas of functioning (work performance, household maintenance, social life, and intimate relationship) are assessed by the SDS on a 0–10 visual analogue scale that also incorporates

verbal descriptors of none (0), mild (1–3), moderate (4–6), severe (7–9), and very severe (10). The design of the SDS, incorporating as it does both a visual and verbal dimensions for rating, is particularly useful in this setting with a large number of respondents with no formal education. Respondents with any 12-month disorder were categorized as having a severe or moderate disorder if they had a moderate or high rating on the SDS. All other respondents with 12-month disorders were rated as mild.

## 2.4. Use of Mental Health Services

### 2.4.1. Initial Lifetime Treatment Contact

For every diagnostic category that respondents were interviewed about, they were asked whether they had "talked to a medical doctor or other professional" about the disorder. The respondent was told that "other professional," included "psychologists, counselors, spiritual advisors, herbalists, acupuncturists, and any other healing professionals." Respondents who reported having ever talked to any of these professionals about the disorder in question were then asked how old they were the first time they did so. The response to this question was used to define age of first treatment contact.

### 2.4.2. 12-month Use of Services

All Part II respondents were asked whether they had ever received treatment for "problems with your emotions or nerves or your use of alcohol or drugs." Separate assessments were made for different types of professionals and for support and treatment services. When a service had been used, respondents were asked about the age at first and most recent contacts as well as number and duration of visits in the previous 12 months. Responses to these questions were used to classify service use in the 12-month period into the following categories: psychiatrist; nonpsychiatrist mental health specialist (psychologist or other nonpsychiatrist mental health professional in any setting, social worker, or mental health counselor); general medical provider (primary care doctor, other general medical doctor, nurse, and other health professional not previously mentioned); human services professional (religious or spiritual advisor, social worker or counselor in any setting other than a specialty mental health setting); and complementary-alternative medicine professional (particularly traditional healer or any other type of healer). Service providers were grouped into general medical (essentially general practitioners but also non–mental health specialists), mental health (including psychiatrists, psychologists, social workers, and psychiatric nurses), Health care (incorporating mental health, general medical, general nurses, counselors, and other trained health workers), and non–health-care (essentially alternative or traditional health workers).

### 2.4.3. Minimally Adequate Treatment

Among those in receipt of treatment, we classified some as receiving treatment that was at least minimally adequate in relation to published treatment guidelines, while others were classified as receiving treatment that failed to meet even these minimal standards of adequacy. Persons classified as receiving at least minimally adequate treatment were required to fulfill at least one of three criteria: (1) they made at least four visits in the prior 12 months to any type of provider, or (2) they made at least two visits and received any medication in the period, or (3) they were in treatment at the time of interview. It is important to note that these criteria are arbitrary and do not necessarily meet evidence-based minimum standards of care. They do, however, provide a measure to allow for an examination of the level of care that respondents were receiving.

### 2.5. Predictor Variables

Predictor variables in analyses of lifetime data include age of onset (AOO) of the focal disorder (coded into the categories early, early average, late average, and late, obtained by dividing respondents in each diagnostic group into four equal groups on the basis of the quartile, 25th, 50th, and 75th, of the AOO distribution), cohort (defined by age at interview in the categories 18–29, 30–44, 45–59, 60+), sex, education (categorized as either current students or nonstudents with 0, 1–6, 7–12, and 13+ years of education), and marital status (categorized as either currently married/cohabitating, previously married, or never married). Both marital status and educational level were coded as time-varying variables in the analysis because both vary within an individual's life.

Per capita income was calculated by dividing household income by the number of people in the household. Respondents' per capita income has been categorized by relating each respondent's income to the median per capita income of the entire sample. Thus, an income is rated low if its ratio to the median is 0.5 or less, low average if the ratio is 0.5–1.0, high average if it is 1.0–2.0, and high if it is greater than 2.0. Residence was classified as rural (less than 12,000 households), semiurban (12,000–20,000 households), and urban (more than 20,000 households).

### 2.6. Training and Quality Control

The interviews were conducted by trained interviewers, all of whom had at least a high school education. Many had been involved in field surveys and were experienced at conducting face-to-face interviews. Training sessions were conducted in Ibadan for Yoruba interviewers, in Calabar for interviewers in Igbo and Efik, and in Maiduguri for Hausa interviewers. Each training lasted at least one week and consisted of role-plays, trial interviews, and debriefing sessions. Supervisors, all of whom underwent the same level of training, monitored the day-to-day implementation of the survey.

Quality control was implemented at various levels. A supervisor was responsible for the work of four interviewers and checked every questionnaire returned by those interviewers for completeness and consistency. He or she made random field checks on at least 10% of each interviewer's prospective respondents (more at the beginning of the survey) to ensure the correct implementation of the protocol and full adherence to interview format. Special emphasis was placed on the detection of systematic errors or bias in the administration of the interview. Each supervisor made regular returns to the site co-coordinator, who was responsible for the day-to-day implementation of the project and reported to the site investigator. During the fieldwork, regular debriefing sessions were held when all interviewers and supervisors returned to the site office for review of experience and discussion of difficulties. The principal investigator also made visits to the collaborating sites during fieldwork to monitor protocol compliance and to provide technical support and clarification. Following data collection, data entry was done centrally in Ibadan. Data entry was followed by an extensive data cleaning, which was conducted in consultation with the site investigators to identify and rectify inconsistencies in dating, missing values, and so on.

## 2.7. Data Analysis

To take into account the stratified multistage sampling procedure and the associated clustering, weights were derived and applied to the rates presented in this chapter. The first weighting adjusts for the probability of selection within households and for nonresponse. Also, poststratification to the target sex and age range was made

to adjust for differences between the sample and the total Nigerian population (WHO 2005). The weight so derived, termed "Part 1 weight," was normalized to reset the sum of weights back to the original sample size of 6752.

A second weight, termed "Part 2 weight" was also derived and applied to a probability subsample that completed the long form of the interview ($n = 2143$), or Part 2. The Part 2 weight is a product of Part 1 weight as well, as the empirical probability of selection into the group with the long interview. This probability varied according to the presence or absence of selected diagnostic symptoms. Thus, all persons who endorsed a set of diagnostic symptoms in Part 1 of the interview were selected into Part 2 with certainty (i.e., probability = 1.0). All others were randomly selected into Part 2 with a constant probability of 25%. The weight was then normalized to reset the sum of weights back to the sample size of 2143.

The analysis has taken account of the complex sample design and weighting. Thus, we used the Taylor series linearization method implemented with the SUDAAN statistical package to estimate standard errors for proportions (Research Triangle Institute 2002). Demographic correlates were explored with discrete-time survival analysis using person-year as the unit of analysis (Efron 1988) in a logistic regression framework (Hosmer & Lameshow 2000). The estimates of standard errors of the odds ratio (ORs) obtained were made with the SUDAAN software system. All of the confidence intervals reported are adjusted for design effects.

## 3. RESULTS

### 3.1. Lifetime Prevalence

Specific lifetime diagnoses of one or more of the DSM-IV/CIDI disorders assessed in the survey were made in 12.0% of the sample (Table 10.2). As a group, anxiety disorders were the most prevalent (6.5%), followed by substance use disorders (3.7%). Specific phobia was the most common diagnosis, with 5.9% having a lifetime history of the disorder, followed by major depressive disorder (MDD) (3.1%) and alcohol abuse with

**Table 10.2.** Lifetime prevalence for Part 1[a] and Part 2[b] samples of DSM-IV/CIDI disorders

| DX group | N | Total % (se) | 18–34 % (se) | 35–49 % (se) | 50–64 % (se) | 65+ % (se) | $\chi^2$ | df | p-value |
|---|---|---|---|---|---|---|---|---|---|
| **Anxiety** | | | | | | | | | |
| Panic disorder | 11 | 0.2 (0.1) | 0.2 (0.1) | 0.1 (0.1) | 0.2 (0.2) | 0.2 (0.1) | 2.8 | 3 | 0.43 |
| GAD with hierarchy | 6 | 0.1 (0.0) | 0.1 (0.1) | 0.1 (0.0) | 0.2 (0.1) | 0.0 (0.0) | 5.5 | 3 | 0.15 |
| Social phobia | 10 | 0.2 (0.1) | 0.2 (0.1) | 0.3 (0.2) | 0.0 (0.0) | 0.0 (0.0) | 7.3 | 3 | 0.07 |
| Specific phobia | 355 | 5.9 (0.5) | 6.5 (0.6) | 4.7 (0.6) | 5.8 (0.8) | 5.6 (0.8) | 5.1 | 3 | 0.18 |
| Agoraphobia without panic | 18 | 0.3 (0.1) | 0.1 (0.1) | 0.6 (0.3) | 0.4 (0.1) | 0.3 (0.2) | 0.3 | 3 | 0.35 |
| PTSD* | 1 | 0.0 (0.0) | 0.0 (0.0) | 0.0 (0.0) | 0.0 (0.0) | 0.2 (0.2) | 1 | 3 | 0.79 |
| SAD/ASA* | 12 | 0.3 (0.1) | 0.2 (0.1) | 0.6 (0.3) | 0.1 (0.1) | 0.0 (0.0) | 6.9 | 3 | 0.09 |
| Any anxiety* | 169 | 6.5 (0.9) | 7.2 (1.5) | 5.6 (1.4) | 7.1 (1.3) | 2.7 (0.8) | 15.1 | 3 | 0.003 |
| **Mood** | | | | | | | | | |
| MDD with hierarchy | 229 | 3.1 (0.3) | 2.4 (0.3) | 3.6 (0.7) | 4.5 (0.5) | 4.9 (1.1) | 16.7 | 3 | 0.002 |
| DYS with hierarchy | 15 | 0.2 (0.1) | 0.1 (0.1) | 0.1 (0.1) | 0.1 (0.1) | 0.7 (0.3) | 4 | 3 | 0.27 |
| Bipolar-broad | 7 | 0.1 (0.1) | 0.2 (0.1) | 0.1 (0.1) | 0.0 (0.0) | 0.3 (0.3) | 6.7 | 3 | 0.09 |
| Any mood | 236 | 3.3 (0.3) | 2.5 (0.4) | 3.7 (0.7) | 4.5 (0.5) | 5.2 (1.1) | 13.5 | 3 | 0.007 |
| **Impulse**[d] | | | | | | | | | |
| ODD with hierarchy[c] | – | – | – | – | – | – | – | – | – |
| CD** | 4 | 0.2 (0.1) | 0.1 (0.1) | 0.7 (0.7) | – | – | 0.7 | 1 | 0.41 |
| ADHD[c] | – | – | – | – | – | – | – | – | – |
| IED with hierarchy | 14 | 0.2 (0.1) | 0.4 (0.1) | 0.0 (0.0) | 0.0 (0.0) | 0.0 (0.0) | 8 | 3 | 0.06 |
| Any impulse** | 9 | 0.3 (0.1) | 0.2 (0.1) | 0.7 (0.7) | – | – | 0.4 | 1 | 0.51 |
| **Substance** | | | | | | | | | |
| ALC abuse w/without Dep | 168 | 2.2 (0.2) | 1.5 (0.2) | 3.5 (0.6) | 2.5 (0.5) | 2.6 (0.6) | 12.6 | 3 | 0.009 |
| ALC Dep with abuse | 23 | 0.3 (0.1) | 0.1 (0.1) | 0.5 (0.1) | 0.4 (0.2) | 0.5 (0.3) | 7.8 | 3 | 0.06 |
| Drug abuse w/without Dep* | 31 | 1.0 (0.2) | 0.9 (0.3) | 1.8 (0.7) | 0.7 (0.5) | 0.2 (0.2) | 6 | 3 | 0.12 |
| Drug Dep with abuse* | 2 | 0.0 (0.0) | 0.0 (0.0) | 0.0 (0.0) | 0.0 (0.0) | 0.0 (0.0) | 2 | 3 | 0.57 |
| Any aubstance | 119 | 3.7 (0.4) | 2.3 (0.4) | 6.7 (1.4) | 5.1 (1.2) | 2.2 (0.8) | 12.7 | 3 | 0.009 |
| **All disorders** | | | | | | | | | |
| Any DX* | 440 | 12.0 (1.0) | 10.7 (1.5) | 14.2 (2.1) | 15.1 (1.8) | 8.3 (1.5) | 14.6 | 3 | 0.004 |
| 2+ DX* | 109 | 2.3 (0.3) | 1.7 (0.4) | 3.6 (1.1) | 2.3 (0.5) | 1.9 (0.6) | 2.5 | 3 | 0.47 |
| 3+ DX* | 28 | 0.6 (0.2) | 0.3 (0.1) | 1.3 (0.9) | 0.4 (0.3) | 0.5 (0.3) | 1.7 | 3 | 0.64 |

\* Denotes Part 2 disorder.
** Denotes disorder in Part 2 and age $\leq 39$ years.
[a] Part 1 sample size = 6752.
[b] Part 2 sample size = 2143.
[c] ADHD and ODD not assessed in Nigeria.
[d] Part 2 and $\leq 39$ years of age, $n = 1203$.

or without dependence (2.2%). Drug abuse (with or without dependence) was present in 1.0%. Surprisingly, very few persons fulfilled the criteria for generalized anxiety disorder and virtually none of those for posttraumatic stress disorder.

Comorbidity was relatively common: of the 12% with disorders, about 3.9% (or almost one-third) had two or more disorders. There was no apparent cohort effect in the probability of having multiple disorders.

**Table 10.3.** Disability among persons who screened positive for lifetime anxiety and trauma-related stress symptoms

| Health-related problems in prior 30 days | Screen positive to anxiety | | | Screen positive to trauma-related stress symptoms | | |
|---|---|---|---|---|---|---|
| | OR | (95% CI) | P | OR | (95% CI) | P |
| Concentration, memory, understanding, or ability to think clearly | 2.4 | (1.3–4.5) | 0.006 | 2.1 | (1.0–4.2) | 0.050 |
| Mobility | 1.2 | (0.6–2.3) | 0.65 | 2.5 | (1.3–4.8) | 0.007 |
| Self-care | 2.9 | (0.7–12.8) | 0.15 | 1.1 | (0.4–3.5) | 0.84 |
| Getting along with people, maintaining a normal usual life, participating in usual activities | 3.3 | (1.3–8.1) | 0.011 | 2.5 | (0.7–9.0) | 0.16 |

Prevalence of the major disorder groups (anxiety, mood, and substance use) varied significantly with age but the direction of variation was not the same. For anxiety, the highest estimates of 7.2% and 7.1% were obtained in the 18–34 and 35–49 age groups, respectively, and persons aged 65 years and over had the least (2.7%). The pattern for substance use disorders was slightly different: the highest rates were in the 35–49 age group, followed by the 50–64 age group, and the rates for those in the 18–34 and 65 and older groups were similar and were the lowest. The estimates for any mood disorder follow a different pattern: there was an incremental rise with age such that the lowest estimate was in the youngest age group and the highest estimate was in the oldest group.

We explored the possibility that the near absence of generalized anxiety disorder (GAD) and posttraumatic stress disorder (PTSD) was due to ascertainment bottleneck or restrictive diagnostic criteria. The screening questions for GAD enquired about being a "worrier," period in the lifetime when respondent was more nervous or anxious than most other people, or six months or more in lifetime when respondent was anxious and worried most of the time. Using these screens, 18.6% of the sample was rated positive and taken to the GAD section of the CIDI. We compared these screen positives to the rest of the sample with regard to specific features of disability in the month prior to interview,

using items from the WHO-DAS. Table 10.3 shows the results. After controlling for age, sex, and any current DSM-IV disorder, persons who screened positive were more likely to have difficulties in concentration, memory, understanding, or ability to think clearly, as well as difficulties in getting along with people, maintaining a normal social life, or participating in social activities.

The same analysis was performed for persons who reported traumatic events and responded positively to having problems like upsetting dreams, feeling emotionally distant from other people, having trouble sleeping or concentrating, and feeling jumpy or easily startled but did not receive a diagnosis of PTSD. The table shows that these respondents were more disabled than the rest of the sample with regard to concentration and mobility. In addition, compared to screen negatives, persons who screened positive to GAD questions reported more days out of role in the prior month (1.96 vs. 1.0, $t = -3.88$, $p < 0.001$). Also, persons with positive screen to PTSD reported more days out of role in the prior month than persons who did not screen positive to PTSD (2.03 vs. 1.12, $t = -2.62$, $p < 0.01$).

### 3.2. AOO Distribution and Lifetime Risks

The AOO distributions for the disorder groups are shown in Table 10.4. Small numbers precluded the presentation of figures for specific

**Table 10.4.** Ages at selected percentiles on the standardized age of onset distributions of DSM-IV disorders

| | **Ages at selected age of onset percentiles** | | | | | | | | |
|---|---|---|---|---|---|---|---|---|---|
| | **5** | **10** | **25** | **50** | **75** | **90** | **95** | **99** | **Projected risk age 75% (SE)** |
| Any anxiety disorder | 5 | 5 | 6 | 8 | 11 | 21 | 33 | 69 | 7.1 (0.9) |
| Any mood disorder | 17 | 21 | 28 | 42 | 55 | 68 | 71 | 73 | 8.9 (1.2) |
| Any substance disorder | 17 | 18 | 22 | 29 | 41 | 56 | 56 | 60 | 6.4 (1.0) |
| Any disorder | 5 | 6 | 11 | 25 | 43 | 58 | 68 | 73 | 19.5 (1.9) |

disorders. The median age of onset (represented by the 50th percentile age of onset) is 25 years for "any" disorder. Among the groups, anxiety disorder has the lowest age of onset (11 years), followed by substance use disorders (29 years), with a much higher distribution for mood disorders (42 years). The AOO for anxiety disorder is concentrated within a very narrow margin, with the difference between the 25th and 75th percentiles being only five years (6–11); for mood disorders, there is a rather wide margin of 27 years (28–55), emphasizing the relatively late age of onset distribution of mood disorders.

The projected lifetime risk at age 75 years for any anxiety disorder is 7.1%. This estimate is 9% higher than the lifetime prevalence of anxiety disorder (6.5%). The projected lifetime risk for mood disorder is 8.9%, while that of any substance use disorder is 6.4%. Thus, compared with the prevalence estimates, the lifetime risk is 73% higher for substance use disorders and about 170% higher for mood disorder. The projected lifetime risk for any disorder is 19.5%, which is 63% higher than the lifetime prevalence estimate of 12.0% for any disorder. Other than anxiety disorder, therefore, the differences between projected lifetime risks and lifetime prevalence estimates suggest that a substantial proportion of those who would develop disorders had not done so in the sample. This was particularly the case for mood disorders. Among the disorder groups, mood disorder had the highest projected risk (8.9%), even though it had the lowest lifetime prevalence estimate, further emphasizing the much later age of onset distribution of mood

disorders. The differences between the projected risks and lifetime prevalence estimates for the disorder groups add up to 8.9%, whereas the difference between the projected lifetime risk for any disorder and the lifetime prevalence estimate for any disorder (19.5% and 12.0%, respectively) is 7.5%. Thus, about 46% of projected new onsets will be among persons with no previous lifetime diagnosis.

### 3.3. Cohort Effect

Table 10.5 shows the results of discrete-time survival analysis in which the association of cohort at interview with the risk of having a disorder in each of the three main groups of disorders and the few individual disorders for which there was sufficient data was examined. Several things are observable in the table: (1) as a group, there was a significant cohort effect for anxiety disorders and for substance use disorders; (2) a cohort effect is not very apparent for mood disorders, even though the most recent cohort has a significantly higher risk than the earliest cohort; (3) among individual disorders, only drug use disorders showed the clearest cohort effect.

To examine the probability that the cohort effects observed do not reflect a true variation in lifetime risks but possibly a reporting bias, a test of intercohort effect was next conducted. Table 10.6 shows the results. Although a decreasing intercohort effect with age was seen in anxiety disorders, this was not true for either mood or substance use disorders. For mood disorders, a stronger cohort effect was observable among

**Table 10.5.** Cohort as predictor of lifetime risk of DSM-IV disorders

| | Age group | | | | $\chi^2$ | DF | P |
|---|---|---|---|---|---|---|---|
| | 18–34 | 35–49 | 50–64 | 65+ | | | |
| **Anxiety disorders** | | | | | | | |
| Panic[a] | – | – | – | – | – | – | – |
| GAD[a]** | – | – | – | – | – | – | – |
| Social phobia[a] | – | – | – | – | – | – | – |
| Specific phobia | 1.2 (0.8–1.7) | 0.8 (0.6–1.2) | 1.0 (0.7–1.6) | 1.0 (1.0–1.0) | 5.5 | 3 | 0.14 |
| Agoraphobia without panic[a] | – | – | – | – | – | – | – |
| PTSD[a] | – | – | – | – | – | – | – |
| ASA/SAD[a] | – | – | – | – | – | – | – |
| Any anxiety | 3.1* (1.4–6.9) | 2.3* (1.1–4.9) | 2.8* (1.5–5.4) | 1.0 (1.0–1.0) | 11.1 | 3 | 0.011 |
| **Mood disorders** | | | | | | | |
| MDD ** | 4.0* (1.9–8.4) | 2.0 (1.0–4.1) | 1.3 (0.7–2.3) | 1.0 (1.0–1.0) | 19.0 | 3 | <0.001 |
| DYS[a]** | – | – | – | – | – | – | – |
| Bipolar broad[a] | – | – | – | – | – | – | – |
| Any mood | 3.7* (1.8–7.6) | 1.8 (0.9–3.6) | 1.2 (0.7–2.1) | 1.0 (1.0–1.0) | 19.4 | 3 | <0.001 |
| **Substance use disorders** | | | | | | | |
| Alcohol abuse with or without dependence | 1.6 (0.8–3.1) | 1.9* (1.0–3.5) | 1.1 (0.5–2.1) | 1.0 (1.0–1.0) | 10.1 | 3 | 0.017 |
| Alcohol dependence with abuse[a] | – | – | – | – | – | – | – |
| Drug abuse with or without dependence | 6.7* (1.0–44.2) | 8.4* (1.1–65.5) | 3.4 (0.4–27.3) | 1.0 (1.0–1.0) | 4.9 | 3 | 0.18 |
| Drug dependence with abuse[a] | – | – | – | – | – | – | – |
| Any substance | 3.4* (1.1–10.1) | 4.9* (1.8–13.3) | 2.9 (1.0–8.7) | 1.0 (1.0–1.0) | 11.8 | 3 | 0.008 |
| **Any disorder** | 3.1* (1.7–5.6) | 2.8* (1.7–4.7) | 2.4* (1.5–3.8) | 1.0 (1.0–1.0) | 18.7 | 3 | <0.001 |

*Notes:* Based on discrete-time survival models with person-year as the unit of analysis. Controls are time intervals.
  * Significant at the 0.05 level.
** With hierarchy.
[a] Cell size ≤30 cases, too small to estimate.

the late-onset group than in either the early- or middle-onset group. The pattern for substance use disorders was less clear.

To explore the likelihood that the differences in the prevalence of disorders between cohorts are more applicable to some subgroups than others, we examined the interactions between socioeconomic correlates and cohort (results are not shown but are available on request). The results showed interactions between education and sex on the one hand and between education and cohort on the other. Specifically, in the cohort aged 50–64, anxiety was concentrated

among those with at least a high school education, and the same was true for substance use disorders in the cohort aged 35–49. Both anxiety and mood disorders were more likely among men in the cohort aged 65 years and older. Although there was a significant trend for men to be more likely to have substance use disorders in the cohorts aged 18–34, 35–49, and 50–64, the difference between females and males in the cohort aged 18–34 was about one-tenth of that between females and males in the other two cohorts. That is, males and females were much less different with regard to the prevalence of substance use

**Table 10.6.** Variation across life course in the association of cohort in predicting lifetime risk of DSM-IV disorders

| Disorder age group | DX | | |
|---|---|---|---|
| | Early onset OR (95% CI) | Middle onset OR (95% CI) | Late onset OR (95% CI) |
| Age at interview | Anxiety disorders | | |
| 18–34 | 39.4* (5.1–305.6) | 2.1 (0.7–6.7) | 2.0 (0.7–5.5) |
| 35–49 | 20.1* (2.2–180.9) | 2.0 (0.6–6.1) | 1.2 (0.4–4.0) |
| 50–64 | 19.4* (2.3–160.5) | 2.6* (1.0–6.7) | 1.6 (0.4–7.2) |
| 65+ | 1.0 (1.0–1.0) | 1.0 (1.0–1.0) | 1.0 (1.0–1.0) |
| $\chi^2$ | 14.7 | 4.5 | 2.5 |
| Age at interview | Mood disorders | | |
| 18–34 | 4.2 (0.8–22.6) | 1.5 (0.5–4.2) | 8.5* (1.8–40.3) |
| 35–49 | 1.6 (0.2–10.6) | 1.1 (0.4–3.3) | 2.6* (1.1–6.2) |
| 50–64 | 1.8 (0.3–10.6) | 0.4* (0.1–1.0) | 2.1* (1.1–4.2) |
| 65+ | 1.0 (1.0–1.0) | 1.0 (1.0–1.0) | 1.0 (1.0–1.0) |
| $\chi^2$ | 7.5 | 10.4 | 8.5 |
| Age at interview | Substance disorders | | |
| 18–34 | 7.4* (1.0–53.2) | 1.6 (0.2–10.5) | 1.5 (0.2–13.7) |
| 35–49 | 7.3 (0.9–61.7) | 5.1* (1.1–24.0) | 3.0 (0.8–11.7) |
| 50–64 | 4.6 (0.5–40.8) | 1.0 (0.1–7.4) | 3.0 (0.7–11.8) |
| 65+ | 1.0 (1.0–1.0) | 1.0 (1.0–1.0) | 1.0 (1.0–1.0) |
| $\chi^2$ | 4.8 | 9.4 | 3.2 |

* Significant at the 0.05 level.

*Note:* Model includes time intervals and sex as controls.

disorders in the most recent cohort than they are in earlier cohorts.

## 3.4. Sociodemographic Predictors of Lifetime Disorders

Sociodemographic predictors of lifetime disorders were few. Females had a significantly lower risk of having a substance use disorder, and younger cohorts were more likely to have anxiety disorders (Table 10.7). No clear relationship was observed between age and mood disorders. Compared to persons in the highest education category, those in the lowest education category had a significantly elevated risk for having anxiety disorders while the reverse was true for substance use disorders. No such relationship was apparent for mood disorders.

## 3.5. Lifetime Treatment Contact

Figure 10.1 shows the cumulative lifetime probabilities of treatment contacts for the three disorder groups using survival analyses. There was clear variability in the probability that persons with the disorders would seek treatment in their lifetime. Although only 0.8% of those with anxiety disorder had sought treatment in the first year of onset, 2.8% had done so among those with substance use disorders, and 6.0% of those with mood disorders (Table 10.8). The proportions that would eventually make treatment contact by 50 years were 15.2%, 19.8%, and 33.3%, respectively. The median duration of delay in seeking treatment was longest for anxiety disorders (16 years), shortest for mood disorders (6 years), and intermediate for substance use disorders (8 years). Figure 10.1 shows the cumulative lifetime percentage of treatment contact for any disorders from year of onset, and displays the relative delays in treatment contacts between the disorder groups.

Sex was not associated with the probability of making lifetime contact for any of the disorder groups (Table 10.9). Compared to the cohort

**Table 10.7.** Variation across cohorts in the association of sex and education with first age of onset of DSM-IV disorders

|  | Any anxiety | Any mood | Any substance |
|---|---|---|---|
| **Sex** | | | |
| Female | 1.0 (0.7–1.5) | 1.1 (0.8–1.7) | 0.1* (0.0–0.3) |
| Male | 1.0 (1.0–1.0) | 1.0 (1.0–1.0) | 1.0 (1.0–1.0) |
| $\chi^2$ | 0.0 | 0.4 | 15.9 |
| **Age** | | | |
| 18–34 | 4.3* (1.8–10.0) | 2.6 (0.8–8.7) | 1.9 (0.6–6.7) |
| 35–49 | 3.0* (1.4–6.7) | 1.5 (0.4–5.2) | 3.4 (1.0–11.3) |
| 50–64 | 3.2* (1.6–6.5) | 0.8 (0.2–2.5) | 1.5 (0.4–5.9) |
| 65+ | 1.0 (1.0–1.0) | 1.0 (1.0–1.0) | 1.0 (1.0–1.0) |
| $\chi^2$ | 13.4 | 8.6 | 5.1 |
| **Education** | | | |
| Student | 5.5 (0.7–43.7) | 0.7 (0.2–2.2) | 1.9 (0.3–10.3) |
| Low | 9.3* (1.2–72.6) | 0.8 (0.3–2.1) | 0.1* (0.0–0.7) |
| Low/med | 2.7 (0.3–24.2) | 0.8 (0.3–2.0) | 0.9 (0.3–2.5) |
| Med | 3.6 (0.4–34.2) | 1.7 (0.7–4.2) | 1.3 (0.5–3.6) |
| High | 1.0 (1.0–1.0) | 1.0 (1.0–1.0) | 1.0 (1.0–1.0) |
| $\chi^2$ | 17.0 | 7.9 | 12.0 |

*Note:* Models include time intervals as controls. Person-years are restricted to ≤29 years. Any impulse has a cell size ≤30 cases, too small to estimate.
* Significant at the 0.05 level.

**Table 10.8.** Proportional treatment contact in the year of disorder onset and median duration of delay among cases that subsequently made treatment contact

|  | % making treatment contact in year of onset | % making treatment contact by 50 years | Median duration of delay (years) | n |
|---|---|---|---|---|
| **I. Anxiety disorders** | | | | |
| Panic disorder | –[a] | –[a] | –[a] | –[a] |
| Generalized anxiety disorder | –[a] | –[a] | –[a] | –[a] |
| Specific phobia | 0 | 13.3 | 17 | 354 |
| Social phobia | –[a] | –[a] | –[a] | –[a] |
| Any anxiety disorders | 0.8 | 15.2 | 16 | 377 |
| **II. Mood disorders** | | | | |
| Major depressive episode | 6.6 | 28.8 | 9 | 231 |
| Dysthymia | –[a] | –[a] | –[a] | –[a] |
| Bipolar disorder (broad) | –[a] | –[a] | –[a] | –[a] |
| Any mood disorders | 6.0 | 33.3 | 6 | 237 |
| **III. Substance disorders** | | | | |
| Alcohol abuse | 3.8 | 13.3 | 8 | 168 |
| Alcohol abuse with dependence | –[a] | –[a] | –[a] | –[a] |
| Drug abuse[b] | –[a] | –[a] | –[a] | –[a] |
| Drug abuse with dependence[b] | –[a] | –[a] | –[a] | –[a] |
| Any substance disorders[b] | 2.8 | 19.8 | 8 | 119 |

[a] Disorder was omitted due to insufficient $n < 30$, but it will be included as one of the disorders in "Any" category.

[b] Assessed in the Part 2 sample.

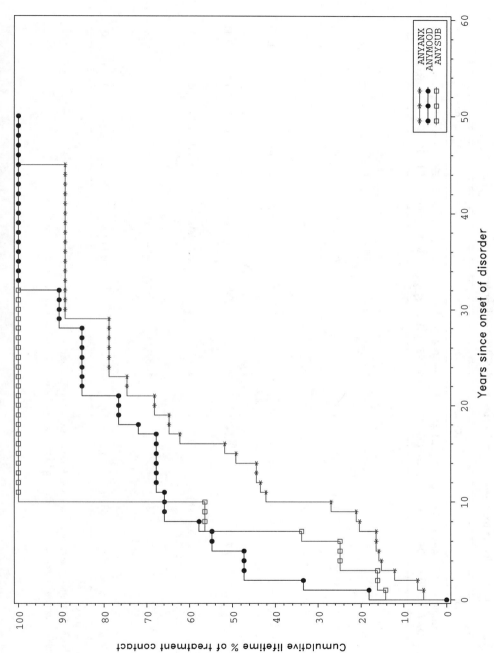

**Figure 10.1.** Cumulative lifetime % of treatment contact for any disorders from year of onset.

Table 10.9. Sociodemographic predictors of lifetime treatment contact for specific DSM-IV/CIDI disorders

| | Sex | Cohort | | | | Age of onset | | | |
| --- | --- | --- | --- | --- | --- | --- | --- | --- | --- |
| | Female OR (95% CI) | Age 18–34 OR (95% CI) | Age 35–49 OR (95% CI) | Age 50–64 OR (95% CI) | $\chi^2_{2-3}$ | Early OR (95% CI) | Early–average OR (95% CI) | Late–average OR (95% CI) | $\chi^2_3$ |
| **I. Anxiety disorders** | | | | | | | | | |
| Panic disorder | —[a]—[a] | —[a]—[a] | —[a]—[a] | —[a]—[a] | —[a] | —[a]—[a] | —[a]—[a] | —[a]—[a] | —[a] |
| Generalized anxiety disorder | —[a]—[a] | —[a]—[a] | —[a]—[a] | —[a]—[a] | —[a] | —[a]—[a] | —[a]—[a] | —[a]—[a] | —[a] |
| Specific phobia | 1.6 (0.4–5.8) | 4.2* (1.0–17.7) | 0.9 (0.2–4.7) | 1.0 – | 7.3* | 0.5 (0.2–1.4) | 0.6 (0.2–1.9) | 0.6 (0.2–2.4) | 1.8 |
| Social phobia | —[a]—[a] | —[a]—[a] | —[a]—[a] | —[a]—[a] | —[a] | —[a]—[a] | —[a]—[a] | —[a]—[a] | —[a] |
| Any anxiety disorders | 1.1 (0.4–3.3) | 0.6 (0.1–3.0) | 0.1* (0.0–0.7) | 0.3 (0.1–1.9) | 7.9* | 0.3* (0.2–0.7) | 0.6 (0.2–2.0) | 0.5 (0.2–1.5) | 10.1* |
| **II. Mood disorders** | | | | | | | | | |
| Major depressive episode | 1.3 (0.5–3.8) | 4.0 (0.3–59.2) | 0.7 (0.1–7.8) | 1.3 (0.2–8.9) | 5.5 | 1.3 (0.1–32.3) | 1.7 (0.1–43.0) | 2.6 (0.1–45.7) | 1.1 |
| Dysthymia | —[a]—[a] | —[a]—[a] | —[a]—[a] | —[a]—[a] | —[a] | —[a]—[a] | —[a]—[a] | —[a]—[a] | —[a] |
| Bipolar disorder (broad) | —[a]—[a] | —[a]—[a] | —[a]—[a] | —[a]—[a] | —[a] | —[a]—[a] | —[a]—[a] | —[a]—[a] | —[a] |
| Any mood disorders | 1.4 (0.5–3.6) | 2.7 (0.3–22.4) | 0.5 (0.1–3.7) | 1.0 – | 6.8* | 2.6 (0.2–33.6) | 1.2 (0.0–31.2) | 3.3 (0.3–41.1) | 3.0 |
| **III. Substance disorders** | | | | | | | | | |
| Alcohol abuse | —[b]—[b] | 0.9 (0.2–4.8) | 1.1 (0.3–4.2) | 1.0 – | 0.0 | 0.2 (0.0–2.4) | 0.5 (0.1–1.9) | 0.4 (0.0–8.7) | 2.2 |
| Alcohol abuse with dependence | —[a]—[a] | —[a]—[a] | —[a]—[a] | —[a]—[a] | —[a] | —[a]—[a] | —[a]—[a] | —[a]—[a] | —[a] |
| Drug abuse[c] | —[a]—[a] | —[a]—[a] | —[a]—[a] | —[a]—[a] | —[a] | —[a]—[a] | —[a]—[a] | —[a]—[a] | —[a] |
| Drug abuse with dependence[b] | —[a]—[a] | —[a]—[a] | —[a]—[a] | —[a]—[a] | —[a] | —[a]—[a] | —[a]—[a] | —[a]—[a] | —[a] |
| Any substance disorders[c] | —[b]—[b] | 4.7 (0.6–34.6) | 2.3 (0.7–7.9) | 1.0 – | 3.5 | 0.1 (0.0–1.7) | 0.5 (0.1–3.0) | 0.2 (0.0–2.8) | 3.1 |

* Significant at the 0.05 level, two-sided test.
[a] Disorder was omitted due to insufficient lifetime cases ($n < 30$) but will be included as one of the disorders in "Any" category.
[b] Sex was used as a control variable in the model except for alcohol abuse and any substance disorders (because of insufficient cases for females).
[c] Assessed in the Part 2 sample.

**Table 10.10.** 12-month prevalence and severity prevalence of DSM-IV disorders

| Diagnosis | n | 12 month<br>% (se) | Serious[b]<br>% (se) | Moderate[b]<br>% (se) | Mild[b]<br>% (se) |
|---|---|---|---|---|---|
| **Anxiety disorder** | | | | | |
| Panic disorder[a] | 9 | 0.1 (0.1) | 59.9 (19.7) | 21.9 (15.9) | 18.2 (11.8) |
| Generalized anxiety disorder[a] | 1 | 0.0 (0.0) | 100.0 (0.0) | 0.0 (0.0) | 0.0 (0.0) |
| Specific phobia[a] | 261 | 4.3 (0.3) | 3.6 (1.3) | 10.2 (2.8) | 86.2 (3.0) |
| Social phobia[a] | 9 | 0.2 (0.1) | 96.5 (4.4) | 3.5 (4.4) | 0.0 (0.0) |
| Agoraphobia without panic[a] | 9 | 0.1 (0.1) | 0.0 (0.0) | 4.5 (5.1) | 95.5 (5.1) |
| Posttraumatic stress disorder[a] | 0 | 0.0 (0.0) | – | – | – |
| Adult separation anxiety[b] | 1 | 0.0 (0.0) | 0.0 (0.0) | 0.0 (0.0) | 100.0 (0.0) |
| Any anxiety disorder[b] | 111 | 4.2 (0.5) | 10.6 (4.9) | 9.9 (2.5) | 79.5 (5.1) |
| **Mood** | | | | | |
| Major depressive disorder[a] | 75 | 1.1 (0.1) | 13.1 (4.2) | 29.8 (7.3) | 57.1 (6.6) |
| Dysthymia[a] | 7 | 0.1 (0.0) | 59.0 (17.1) | 5.1 (5.7) | 35.9 (15.9) |
| Bipolar I/II/subthreshold[a] | 2 | 0.1 (0.1) | 100.0 (0.0) | 0.0 (0.0) | 0.0 (0.0) |
| Any mood disorder[a] | 77 | 1.1 (0.2) | 16.0 (4.8) | 28.8 (7.2) | 55.2 (6.5) |
| **Impulse** | | | | | |
| Oppositional–defiant disorder[c] | – | – | – | – | – |
| Conduct disorder[c] | 0 | 0.0 (0.0) | – | – | – |
| Attention-deficit/hyperactivity disorder[c] | – | – | – | – | – |
| Intermittent explosive disorder[a] | 11 | 0.2 (0.0) | 23.4 (19.3) | 36.1 (19.6) | 40.4 (16.4) |
| Any impulse-control disorder[c] | 6 | 0.1 (0.0) | 23.4 (19.3) | 36.1 (19.6) | 40.4 (16.4) |
| **Substance** | | | | | |
| Alcohol abuse[a] | 43 | 0.6 (0.1) | 34.4 (10.5) | 5.8 (4.3) | 59.8 (10.7) |
| Alcohol dependence[a] | 15 | 0.2 (0.1) | 93.1 (6.7) | 6.9 (6.7) | 0.0 (0.0) |
| Drug abuse[b] | 9 | 0.2 (0.1) | 47.0 (22.2) | 0.0 (0.0) | 53.0 (22.2 |
| Drug dependence[b] | 0 | 0.0 (0.0) | – | – | – |
| Any substance use disorder[b] | 36 | 0.9 (0.2) | 35.7 (9.0) | 4.5 (3.3) | 59.9 (9.1) |
| **Any disorder** | | | | | |
| Any[b] | 206 | 6.0 (0.6) | 12.8 (3.7) | 12.5 (2.5) | 74.7 (4.2) |
| **Total sample** | | | | | |
| Total sample[b] | 2143 | – | 0.8 (0.2) | 0.7 (0.2) | 4.5 (0.5) |

*Note:* Severity calculated using Part 2 weights.

[a] Part 1 sample, prevalence calculated using Part 1 weights.

[b] Part 2 sample, prevalence calculated using Part 2 weights.

[c] Part 2 sample (age ≤39), prevalence and severity calculated using Part 1 weights for ages ≤39.

aged 65 years and older, younger cohorts were less likely to have made a treatment contact for anxiety disorders as a group, even though, for specific phobia, the age 18–34 cohort was more likely to have made treatment contact. AOO was also associated with the probability of making treatment contact for anxiety disorders: compared to persons with late AOO, those in the group with early AOO were least likely to have made treatment contact. There was no clear pattern in the association of cohort with the proba-

bility of making treatment contact for mood disorders and no significant association was found between sociodemographic features and treatment contact for substance use disorders.

## 3.6. 12-month Prevalence

Table 10.10 displays the 12-month prevalence disorders. The pattern is similar to the lifetime profile in that anxiety disorders were, as a group, the most common but dissimilar in that

**Table 10.11.** Demographic correlates of 12-month DSM–IV disorders using Part 2 weights after stratification

|  | Mood | Anxiety | Impulse control | Substance | Any disorder |
|---|---|---|---|---|---|
|  | OR (95% CI) | OR (95% CI) | OR (95% CI) | OR (95% CI) | OR (95% CI) |
| **Sex** |  |  |  |  |  |
| Female | 1.0 (1.0–1.0) | 1.0 (1.0–1.0) | 1.0 (1.0–1.0) | 1.0 (1.0–1.0) | 1.0 (1.0–1.0) |
| Male | 0.8 (0.4–1.8)] | 1.2 (0.6–2.2) | – | 0.0 (0.0–0.1) | 0.8 (0.5–1.3) |
| $\chi^2$ | 0.3 | 0.3 | – | 21.7* | 0.7 |
| **Age** |  |  |  |  |  |
| 18–34 | 1.1 (0.5–2.7) | 0.9 (0.4–2.1) | – | 0.4 (0.1–1.5) | 0.8 (0.5–1.6) |
| 35–49 | 0.6 (0.2–1.5) | 1.1 (0.5–2.4) | – | 0.5 (0.2–1.4) | 0.9 (0.5–1.7) |
| 50–64 | – | – | – | – | – |
| 65 ≤ | 1.0 (1.0–1.0) | 1.0 (1.0–1.0) | 1.0 (1.0–1.0) | 1.0 (1.0–1.0) | 1.0 (1.0–1.0) |
| $\chi^2$ | 2.7 | 0.2 | – | 2.5 | 0.3 |
| **Income** |  |  |  |  |  |
| Low | 0.9 (0.3–2.6) | 0.9 (0.3–2.2) | – | 0.6 (0.2–2.5) | 0.8 (0.4–1.5) |
| Low-average | 0.3 (0.1–0.9) | 1.2 (0.6–2.5) | – | 0.5 (0.2–1.7) | 0.9 (0.5–1.5) |
| High-average | 0.8 (0.4–1.8) | 0.6 (0.3–1.4) | – | 0.4 (0.1–1.4) | 0.6 (0.3–1.0) |
| High | 1.0 (1.0–1.0) | 1.0 (1.0–1.0) | 1.0 (1.0–1.0) | 1.0 (1.0–1.0) | 1.0 (1.0–1.0) |
| $\chi^2$ | 7.9* | 3.6 | – | 3.1 | 5.0 |
| **Marital status** |  |  |  |  |  |
| Married/cohabiting | 1.0 (1.0–1.0) | 1.0 (1.0–1.0) | 1.0 (1.0–1.0) | 1.0 (1.0–1.0) | 1.0 (1.0–1.0) |
| Separated/widowed/ divorced | 1.7 (0.7–4.4) | 0.9 (0.4–2.1) | – | 0.2 (0.0–1.3) | 1.0 (0.5–2.0) |
| Never married | 0.3 (0.1–1.1) | 1.5 (0.5–4.6) | – | 0.9 (0.2–3.5) | 1.1 (0.5–2.5) |
| $\chi^2$ | 4.2 | 0.6 | – | 3.1 | 0.1 |
| **Education** |  |  |  |  |  |
| No formal education | 1.2 (0.4–3.3) | 1.5 (0.5–5.0) | – | 1.1 (0.3–4.6) | 1.4 (0.6–3.6) |
| Completed secondary | 0.5 (0.2–1.3) | 1.4 (0.4–4.7) | – | 0.8 (0.2–3.3) | 1.1 (0.4–3.1) |
| Some college | 2.1 (0.9–4.5) | 1.1 (0.4–2.8) | – | 1.1 (0.4–2.8) | 1.2 (0.6–2.4) |
| Completed college | 1.0 (1.0–1.0) | 1.0 (1.0–1.0) | 1.0 (1.0–1.0) | 1.0 (1.0–1.0) | 1.0 (1.0–1.0) |
| $\chi^2$ | 15.6* | 1.0 | – | 0.4 | 0.9 |

* Significant at the 0.05 level, two-sided test.

mood disorders are now slightly more prevalent than substance use disorders. As for lifetime prevalence, the most prevalent disorder continues to be specific phobia (4.3%), and the second most prevalent remains major depressive disorder (1.1%). Both GAD and PTSD were virtually absent, as was drug dependence. Overall, the prevalence of any disorder in the prior 12 months was 6.0%.

Most cases of 12-month disorders were mild. In the entire sample, 74.7% had disorders that were rated mild, 12.5% moderate, and only 12.8% serious. However, the severity profile was variable between disorder groups and between specific disorders. Thus, although almost 80% of anxiety disorders were mild and only 10.6% were serious, the respective figures for mood disorders were 55.2% and 18.0%; for substance use disorders, they were 59.9% and 35.7%, respectively. The overall predominance of mild cases for anxiety disorders hides the variability within the disorders. The only case of GAD identified was rated serious, whereas 96.5% of those with social phobia and 59.9% of those with panic disorder were serious. Also, compared to 13.1% of serious cases of major depressive disorder, 59.0% of those with dysthymia had serious disorder. For anxiety and mood disorders, relatively uncommon

**Table 10.12.** Severity by treatment

| Treatment | Severe or moderate % (se) | Mild % (se) | None % (se) | Any % (se) |
|---|---|---|---|---|
| General medical | 11.9 (4.8) | 9.7 (2.8) | 0.5 (0.2) | 1.1 (0.2) |
| Mental health | 0.4 (0.4) | 1.9 (1.0) | 0.0 (0.0) | 0.1 (0.1) |
| Health care | 12.3 (4.8) | 10.0 (2.7) | 0.5 (0.2) | 1.1 (0.2) |
| Non–health-care | 5.3 (3.7) | 0.4 (0.4) | 0.4 (0.2) | 0.5 (0.2) |
| Any treatment | 17.7 (6.2) | 10.0 (2.7) | 1.0 (0.3) | 1.6 (0.3) |
| No treatment | 82.3 (6.2) | 90.0 (2.7) | 99.0 (0.3) | 98.4 (0.3) |

*Note:* Non–health-care includes human services and CAM.

disorders tended to be more serious than common ones, possibly reflecting a higher threshold for the detection of the former in this sample. Disorders within the substance use group also tended to have higher proportions of serious cases, reflecting the way severity was defined.

### 3.7. Sociodemographic Correlates of 12-month Disorders

Females were significantly less likely to have a substance use disorder and, compared to persons in the highest income group, those in the lower groups were less likely to have a mood disorder even though there was variability within the groups (Table 10.11). There was an overall effect of education on the probability of having mood disorders, but the pattern was not consistent. No other significant association emerged between sociodemographic factors on the one hand, and disorder groups, any disorder, or any serious disorder on the other hand.

### 3.8. Severity by Treatment

Most treatments were received from general medical practitioners (Table 10.12). Among the 1.6% of those in the entire survey who had received any treatment for mental health problems, 1.1% of them had done so from general medical settings. Only about 0.1% had received treatment from mental health specialist settings and 0.5% from complimentary alternative health providers (mainly traditional healers). The proportions of persons receiving in this sector of the health service were about the same in the seri-

ous (11.7%), moderate (12.2%) and mild (9.7%) severity categories. The pattern was variable for mental health specialist setting: 0.8% of serious, 0% of moderate, and 1.9% of mild disorders had been presented to this setting. On the other hand, the proportions presented to complementary providers followed severity gradient: more severe cases (8.9%) than moderate (1.7%) and mild (0.4%) were seen by these healers. However, traditional healers were as likely to be consulted as general practitioners for mental health problems by persons with no 12-month diagnosis. Less than 0.05% of such persons saw mental health professionals. In all, about 1.0% of those with no diagnosis in the prior 12 months had sought mental health treatment from a professional.

### 3.9. Percentage Treated by Health-care Professionals among People with Mental Health Disorders

Table 10.13 shows the percentage of persons with 12-month disorders who received any treatment during the period. Persons with mood disorders were more likely to have received treatment. Almost 21% of such persons had received some form of treatment. The proportion of persons with substance use disorders who received treatment was similar at almost 20%. Overall, 11.8% of persons with any disorder in the prior 12 months received treatment.

Most treatments were received from general medical settings and only few people had been seen by psychiatrists. Persons with substance use

**Table 10.13.** 12-month service usage in Nigeria: Percentage treated by health-care professionals among people service in mental disorder

| | Type of professional | | | | Any non-health-care | Any treatment | Unweighted n with mental disorder | Weighted n with mental disorder |
| | Psychiatrist | Any mental health-care | General medical | Any health-care | | | | |
|---|---|---|---|---|---|---|---|---|
| Any anxiety disorder[b] | 0.0 (0.0) | 0.1 (0.1) | 9.9 (3.1) | 10.0 (3.1) | 1.5 (1.0) | 11.5 (3.2) | 111 | 90 |
| Any mood disorder[a] | 3.4 (2.6) | 3.8 (2.7) | 11.7 (4.2) | 14.8 (4.8) | 8.6 (5.3) | 20.9 (6.2) | 77 | 76 |
| Any substance[b] | 6.6 (6.2) | 6.6 (6.2) | 19.8 (7.2) | 19.8 (7.2) | 0.0 (0.0) | 20.0 (7.2) | 36 | 20 |
| Any disorder[b] | 1.4 (0.8) | 1.6 (0.8) | 10.3 (2.5) | 10.7 (2.4) | 1.3 (0.7) | 11.8 (2.6) | 202 | 127 |
| No disorder[b] | 0.0 (0.0) | 0.0 (0.0) | 0.5 (0.2) | 0.5 (0.2) | 0.5 (0.2) | 1.0 (0.3) | 1941 | 2016 |
| Total Part 2 sample[b] | 0.1 (0.1) | 0.1 (0.1) | 1.1 (0.2) | 1.1 (0.2) | 0.5 (0.2) | 1.6 (0.3) | 2143 | 2143 |

*Notes*: Values are percentages with standard errors in parentheses. Disorders with unweighted *n* less than 30 do not have percentages.
[a] Denotes Part 1 weight.
[b] Denotes Part 2 weight.

disorders were more likely to be seen by psychiatrists and mental health workers. Although about 6.5% of such persons had been in the specialist mental health sector, only 3.9% of those with mood disorders had been seen in this sector. Virtually no one with an anxiety disorder was treated in the specialist mental health sector. On the other hand, persons with mood disorders were more likely to be seen by alternative health providers (mostly traditional healers) than were those with other disorders. Although 8.7% of those with mood disorders were seen by such healers, only about 1.5% of those with anxiety disorders and virtually none of those with substance use disorders were seen by alternative medical providers.

### 3.10. Sociodemographic and Disorder-type Predictors of any Treatment

Persons with disorders were predictably more likely to receive treatment than were those without a disorder. The odds varied from 5.6 for those with anxiety disorders to 16.7 for those with substance use disorders (Table 10.14). On the other hand, no sociodemographic features predicted the probability of receipt of treatment for a 12-month disorder.

### 3.11. Number of Visits in the Past Year

The numbers of cases that had received any treatment in the prior 12 months were few, both for specific disorders and for disorder groups. Thus, computation of mean or median numbers of visits for disorders or disorder groups could not be calculated. For the entire Part 2 sample, the mean number of visits among those who had received any treatment was 3.10 (standard error [se] 1.0) and the median was 1.74 (se 0.09). The mean number of visits to general practitioners was 1.86 (se 0.18) and the mean to any orthodox provider was 2.08 (se 0.23).

### 4. DISCUSSION

Community surveys of the size and scope reported here are rare in sub-Saharan Africa. Even though small-scale surveys have been conducted in Nigeria, our survey is the first known to address a broad range of mental disorders, as well as their antecedents and impact. It is the first survey of mental health problems conducted in four major Nigerian languages, with three of them spoken by more than 65% of the national population.

In considering the findings reported here, several general caveats are important to note. It is possible that the rates reported here underestimate the occurrence of mental disorders in the community for a number of reasons. First, respondents might find health assessment by lay interviewers rather novel and thus feel less inclined to disclose their symptoms. General health surveys are not novel in Nigeria. However, they are not very common either and it is very likely that most of our respondents were participating in a face-to-face assessment of their well-being by laypersons for the first time. Although it is unclear how a first encounter of such a nature might be perceived by our respondents, it is clearly plausible that some could have denied symptoms because they were unsure of whether it was safe to share them with strangers or because they doubted the utility of such disclosure to non-clinicians who had turned up at their doorsteps. Second, we have focused on categorical DSM-IV disorders and have not examined the prevalence and impact of subthreshold disorders. However, there is evidence from our previous studies that persons who did not meet the full criteria to receive a categorical diagnosis but who may have some psychological symptoms might nevertheless have associated disabilities that are similar to those with categorical diagnoses (Gureje 2000). Third, this report does not include data on non-affective psychosis because the CIDI screening questions for psychosis do not permit diagnostic assignment. Even though persons with non-affective psychosis might otherwise have been captured as cases meeting the criteria of one of the assessed disorders, some may still have been missed. Fourth, our survey was regionally, rather than nationally, representative. Even though the survey was conducted in five of the six geopolitical regions of the country, albeit to varying degrees, and our results may provide a broadly national perspective, the data on which

**Table 10.14.** 12-month service usage in Nigeria: Sociodemographic and disorder-type predictors of any treatment

| Model effect | Any treatment given<br>Any 12-month disorder<br>OR (95% CI) |
|---|---|
| **Age** | |
| 18–34 | 1.4 (0.1, 20.3) |
| 35–49 | 0.7 (0.0, 11.2) |
| 50–64 | 1.4 (0.3, 7.9) |
| 65+ | 1.0 (1.0, 1.0) |
| Overall test of effect | Wald-Chi 3 df = 1.0, $p$-value = 0.80 |
| **Any anxiety** | |
| Yes | 5.6 (1.5, 21.7) |
| No | 1.0 (1.0, 1.0) |
| Overall test of effect | Wald-Chi 1 df = 6.6, $p$-value = 0.010 |
| **Any mood** | |
| Yes | 10.1 (3.0, 33.3) |
| No | 1.0 (1.0, 1.0) |
| Overall test of effect | Wald-Chi 1 df = 14.9, $p$-value = <0.001 |
| **Any substance** | |
| Yes | 16.7 (2.5, 110.7) |
| No | 1.0 (1.0, 1.0) |
| Overall test of effect | Wald-Chi 1 df = 8.9, $p$-value = 0.003 |
| **Education** | |
| 0 years | 0.4 (0.0, 5.5) |
| 1–6 years | 1.0 (0.1, 7.0) |
| 7–12 years | 0.5 (0.1, 3.6) |
| 13+ | 1.0 (1.0, 1.0) |
| Overall test of effect | Wald-Chi 3 df = 1.2, $p$-value = 0.75 |
| **Income** | |
| Low | 3.8 (0.9, 16.8) |
| Low-average | 2.2 (0.5, 8.9) |
| High-average | 2.1 (0.5, 9.2) |
| High | 1.0 (1.0, 1.0) |
| Overall test of effect | Wald-Chi 3 df = 3.5, $p$-value = 0.32 |
| **Marital status** | |
| Never married | 0.6 (0.2, 1.9) |
| Separated/widowed/divorced | 0.5 (0.1, 3.4) |
| Married/cohabiting | 1.0 (1.0, 1.0) |
| Overall test of effect | Wald-Chi 2 df = 1.9, $p$-value = 0.39 |
| **Sex** | |
| Male | 0.4 (0.1, 1.5) |
| Female | 1.0 (1.0, 1.0) |
| Overall test of effect | Wald-Chi 1 df = 1.9, $p$-value = 0.17 |

they are based were not collected from a truly nationally representative sample. In a comparative sense, our sample was relatively more representative of Nigeria than the Epidemiological Catchment Area study (Robins & Regier 1991) was representative of the United States, but not as representative as the National Comorbidity Survey Replication was for the United States

(Kessler et al. 2005). Finally, the diagnostic groups evaluated are not exhaustive and higher rates of treatment might have occurred for persons with the unevaluated disorders such as psychotic disorders.

## 5. PREVALENCE ESTIMATES

About 1 in 8 adult Nigerians has had a mental disorder in their lifetime, and about 1 in 16 reported a disorder in the prior 12 months. Lifetime and 12-month disorders were most commonly those of anxiety disorders, followed by substance use disorders. Thus, although anxiety disorders had been experienced by 6.5% of the population, 3.7% had fulfilled the criteria for a DSM-IV substance use disorder and 3.3% a mood disorder. For 12-month disorders, anxiety disorders remained the most prevalent, and the estimate for mood disorders was marginally higher than for that of substance use disorder. The rate of 12.1% for lifetime disorders is lower than the estimate of 25.0% reported for six European countries and in the National Comorbidity Survey-Replication in the United States, both of which used identical ascertainment procedures (ESEMeD/MHEDEA 2000 Investigators 2004a; Kessler et al. 2005). However, as in other settings (Andrews et al. 2001; Kessler et al. 1994; Kessler et al. 2005), anxiety disorders were the most frequent. Impulse-control disorders were very infrequently elicited, being reported by only 0.3% of respondents. We suspect that this estimate was affected by denial. Impulse-control disorders are made on the basis of questions that might be perceived with heavy social disapproval in the Nigerian setting. It is plausible that strong denial occurred in response to these questions in the community. Substance use disorders were surprisingly relatively common: the 12-month rate of 0.6% for alcohol abuse is close to that of 0.7% for alcohol abuse reported for six European countries (ESEMeD/MHEDEA 2000 Investigators 2004a).

The variations of the estimates with age were in accord with previous literature with regard to anxiety and substance use disorders, but not so for mood disorders. Thus, the increase in rates of anxiety disorders in the younger age groups compared to the older groups and the tendency for substance use disorders to be more common in the young and middle ages are both substantially similar to findings from other community surveys. In our setting, substance use disorders, especially alcohol use disorders, tend to be most common in middle age, typically in the fourth and fifth decades of life. It would appear that the traditional restraint of young people with regard to patterns of alcohol consumption begins to wane at about that period of life. On the other hand, major depressive disorder, the main diagnosis within the mood disorder cluster, shows a rise in prevalence with age, a pattern that is different from that reported from other surveys where, characteristically, low rates are often found in the youngest and oldest age groups and the highest rates are typical of middle age.

The median AOO for any disorder was 25 years: 29 for substance use disorders and 8 for anxiety disorders. Thus, other than mood disorders, which had a median AOO of 42 years, most disorders start within the first three decades of life. Given the recurrent or chronic nature of many of the disorders, the early AOO gives a strong indication of the public health burden that mental disorders constitute. Other than anxiety disorders, for which the difference between prevalence estimate and projected lifetime risk at age 75 years was only 9%, the prevalence estimates for the other disorder groups were far less than the projected lifetime risks. This was particularly the case for mood disorders, with a difference of 170% between the two rates. These findings emphasize the relatively young age of the sample, the later AOO distribution for mood disorders, and the very conservative nature of the prevalence estimates reported. Because the majority of the survey sample had not lived through the median AOO of major depressive disorder, for example, a much higher estimate of the prevalence would be expected among samples of older respondents. This is indeed the picture that emerged in a recent community survey of 2152 elderly persons conducted in the Yoruba-speaking regions of the country (Gureje, Kola & Afolabi 2007). Using the same version of the CIDI as was used in the present survey and implemented with the same diagnostic algorithm and analytic approach, the lifetime prevalence of major depressive disorder in that survey was 26.2%. The mean AOO of the first episode was about 50 years. Both of these observations emphasize the relatively late AOO of major depressive disorder in Nigeria, and the rates reported here might underestimate the eventual extent of mental health problems in the sample (and consequently, the overall burden in the community).

There are other indications that the report here underestimates the prevalence of specific mental health disorders. Our analysis shows that persons who reported that they had lifetime history of persistent worry or anxiety and those with history of experiencing traumatic events and consequent emotional problems relating to those events but who did not receive the indicative DSM-IV diagnosis had evidence of functional role impairments in the month prior to the interview. Such impairments were not due to any other DSM-IV disorder that they might have, nor to age or sex. The results provide strong indications that a substantial proportion of those who screened positive for these disorders but who did not receive the related diagnosis continued to experience difficulties functioning in areas, which would suggest that, even though they had subthreshold syndromes, they were nevertheless in need of some form of intervention. In essence, the rates reported here may have been too conservative in their exclusion of persons with significant impairments. These observations emphasize the weakness of current assessment and diagnostic tools for mental health problems (Regier et al. 1998) and speak directly to the need for survey results to be contextualized to prevailing social and cultural attributes of the index population.

## 5.1. Cohort Effect

There is controversy about whether the phenomenon of cohort effect, in which more recent birth cohorts are reported to be at higher risk for a number of mental disorders, is real or artifi-

cial (Giuffra & Risch 1994; Kessler et al. 2005). We provide the results of the first set of analyses known to us in a sub-Saharan African sample in which cohort effect is examined. Significant cohort effect was seen for the three disorder groups of anxiety, mood, and substance use. For all three cohorts, persons in the youngest age group, 18–34 years, were at elevated risks compared to those in the oldest age group, 65 years and older. The same was true for anxiety and substance use disorders for persons in the age groups 35–49 and 50–64. An examination of intercohort variation with increasing age was conducted to determine whether the differences in lifetime risk were due to factors other than cohort effect, such as differential recall or of impact of mortality. The results provided ambiguous results: there was a significant decrease with age in intercohort differences with respect to anxiety disorders, but that was not so for mood and substance use disorders. Indeed, for mood disorders, there was a much higher cohort effect in the late-onset category than in the early-and middle-onset groups. Our results thus provide some support for the view that recent birth cohorts are at elevated risk for mood and substance use disorders. The observation with regard to anxiety disorders seems open to the possibility that reporting bias, or telescoping, rather than a true difference in lifetime risk may be the explanation. A striking feature of the pattern of lifetime risk between the cohorts is the observation that the difference between females and males in the most recent cohort in the risk for substance use disorders was much less than in earlier cohorts. This is in consonance with much of recent literature in Nigeria suggesting that substance use, in particular alcohol use, is becoming more common among females than in the past and that females are approaching males with regard to their pattern of alcohol consumption (Odejide et al. 1987).

## 5.2. Severity

Most of the 12-month disorders were mild, with just about 25% rated as moderate or serious. This finding is consistent with those of other studies that suggest that, although mental disorders are common in the community, a large proportion of people with those disorders nevertheless manage to function without considerable limitations (Bijl, Ravelli & van Zessen 1998; WHO International Consortium in Psychiatric Epidemiology 2000; Narrow et al. 2002). These findings support the contention that prevalence studies in the community require complementary assessment of severity to determine true need (Regier et al. 2000). However, we have focused on persons with specific DSM-IV diagnoses in our assessment of severity. It is often the case that persons with subthreshold disorders may suffer from associated impairment that may otherwise qualify them for a classification of having serious disorder. It is therefore essential that in determining need, such persons not be excluded.

## 5.3. Sociodemographic Predictors of Prevalence

Other than the clear association of being male with substance use disorders and the observation that females were less likely to have a lifetime disorder, there were no striking sex differences in prevalence and disorder types. In particular, the common observation of an association of being female with mood disorders, particularly with depression (Kessler 2003), was not found. In our earlier study in primary care, we also failed to find an association between being female and depression in this cultural setting (Gureje et al. 1995). However, given the small numbers of cases in these observations, there is a need for caution in drawing conclusions. Still, this observation requires further exploration as it may shed light on cultural differences between males and females in the experience of putative environmental risk factors for depression (Kessler et al. 2003). The finding that persons with lower income were less likely to have a disorder is unusual and may, at least in part, be related to a reduced willingness to report psychological symptoms. Our findings suggest a need for more studies examining the relationship between poverty and common mental disorders in developing countries (Patel & Kleinman 2003).

## 5.4. Service Use

The observations with regard to treatment delay are interesting. Although there are no previous data with which to compare our results, observations made in tertiary care settings suggest that, even among persons with psychotic disorders, considerable time often elapses between the first signs of illness and the decision to seek care. With regard to common mental disorders, about which there is even much less recognition of their medical nature in the general public, one can expect an even greater delay. The convergence of the results in this survey with those of another large-scale survey of elderly persons in the community (Gureje et al. 2007) is noteworthy. The mean duration of delay in the current survey was six years for mood disorders. This is very similar to the mean duration of five years of delay among persons with major depressive disorder in the other survey. It is instructive that both of these durations do not represent delays in getting to orthodox medical treatment, but to any treatment, including that obtained from traditional or religious healers.

We found that about 1.6% of this community sample had received any formal treatment for a mental health problem in the prior 12 months. Predictably, this is lower than what has been reported in many developed countries. For example, 13.4% of the general population of New Zealand had made a visit for a mental health reason in a 12-month period (Oakley-Browne et al. 2006); in the ESEMeD study involving six European countries (Belgium, France, Germany, Italy, Netherlands, and Spain) (ESEMeD/MHEDEA 2000 Investigators 2004b; Alonso et al. 2004), an average of 6.4% of the total sample had consulted formal health services for mental health problems in the previous 12 months. A much higher rate of 17.9% was reported in the United States (Wang et al. 2005b).

Not unexpectedly, low rates of mental health service use were also recorded among those with 12-month DSM-IV disorders. Less than 12% of such persons had received any treatment. This contrasts with a treatment rate of 41.1% for 12-month DSM-IV disorders in the U.S. National

Comorbidity Survey-Replication (Wang et al. 2005b) and 38.9% in New Zealand (Oakley-Browne et al. 2006). In our sample, even though diagnosis did make a significant difference with regard to whether respondents would have received treatment, only about 21% of persons with mood disorders, the group with the highest proportion of treated cases, actually received any treatment. We were, nevertheless, surprised that almost a similar proportion of persons with substance use disorders had received treatment. Substance use disorders are commonly regarded in Nigeria as social problems, with a greater implication of personal behavior failure than a medical problem. It is reassuring that persons with substance use disorders are seeking treatment at the level that our results suggest, especially because most of the subjects with substance use disorders who had sought treatment had done so from an orthodox treatment (general medical) setting whereas, virtually none sought treatment from complementary alternative health providers.

Despite the variation in the proportion of respondents in treatment for any mental health problem in different countries of the world, similarities exist in certain areas (Demyttenaere et al. 2004). For example, as reported by others, a small proportion of noncases also received treatment (1.0%) in this survey. This figure is on the lower side of the range of 0.3%–3.0% of noncases in developing countries receiving treatment and far indeed from the range of 2.4%–8.1% of noncases receiving treatment in developed countries (Demyttenaere et al. 2004). As previously speculated (Demyttenaere et al. 2004), the reasons might include the possibilities that the CIDI erroneously classified some true cases as being noncases, that some mental disorders were not assessed, or that some people in treatment did not meet the criteria for a DSM-IV disorder.

Most treatment was received from the general medical sector. Among those with mental health problems in the prior 12 months who received any treatment, 88% had done so from general medical providers. On the other hand, only 13% of treated cases received the treatment from the mental health specialist sector. The proportions receiving treatment from these sectors were 10.3% and 1.6%, respectively. The finding that many more individuals with any mental disorder use non–mental health specialists has been reported from diverse countries, both developing and developed. Still, the proportions of persons with 12-month disorders receiving care from specialist settings in our survey, ranging from about 0.1% for anxiety disorders to 3.9% for mood disorders, are very low when compared with findings from settings in Western Europe and North America and reflect a striking inaccessibility of that sector to patients in need. A surprising finding was the relatively low rate of use of complementary health providers by persons with mental illness. Although 48% of persons with no DSM disorders but who nevertheless received service for mental health problems did so from such providers, only 11% of those with any treated DSM disorders did so, with the proportion peaking at 41% for those with treated mood disorders. Our observation suggests that, contrary to commonly held beliefs, traditional healers provide service for only a minority of persons with mental illness. Although it can not be excluded that these providers are widely consulted for disorders not systematically assessed in this survey, such as psychotic disorders, it would appear that they draw the bulk of their clientele from persons with symptoms that may not reach usual diagnostic thresholds and from those with mood disorders. They were rarely consulted by those with anxiety disorders or those with substance use disorders. Our observation complements that made in a Chilean epidemiological survey, which suggests that, contrary to popular belief, traditional healers were rarely used for mental health problems (Gureje et al. 2005). Almost 20% of persons with substance use problems received some form of treatment, and almost all from orthodox medical settings. Indeed, the largest proportion of those in specialist treatment within any of the diagnostic groups was among those with substance use disorders. Of the treated persons with these diagnoses, 33% received treatment in the specialist mental health sector. These observations contrast with those made in the

South-West and North-Central regions of our survey, as previously published (Gureje & Lasebikan 2006), where virtually no case of substance use disorder was treated in any sector. Given that the South-West, in which the metropolis of Lagos is located, is relatively better resourced in terms of medical personnel and facilities, we suspect that this difference is not a reflection of variation within health service provision in the country but possibly differential attitude to substance use–related disorders.

In conclusion, the results of this large community survey show that mental disorders are common in the Nigerian community, even though current diagnostic categories may underestimate the extent of the burden. The disorders often start early, with anxiety disorders particularly more likely to start before or during early adolescence. Because of the young age of the population and the fact that some disorders, such as mood disorders may start in middle age, estimates of burden that are based on cross-sectional assessment of a random sample will need to be supplemented by estimates of projected lifetime risks to better reflect total community burden. Most persons with mental disorders do not receive any treatment. Those who do tend to do so from general medical rather than specialist service. There is urgent need to scale up the delivery mental health service to those in need and early detection and treatment of anxiety disorders may be a particularly important focus of preventive service.

## REFERENCES

Abas, M. A. & Broadhead, J. C. (1997). Depression and anxiety among women in an urban setting in Zimbabwe. *Psychological Medicine*, 27, 59–71.

Alegria, M. & Kessler, R. C. 2000. Comparing mental health service use data across countries. In *Unmet need for mental health service delivery*, ed. G. Andrews, pp. 97–118. Cambridge, UK: Cambridge University Press.

Alem, A. & Kebede, D. (2003). Conducting psychiatric research in the developing world: Challenges and rewards. *British Journal of Psychiatry*, 182, 185–7.

Alonso, J. (2002). The European Study of the Epidemiology of Mental Disorders (ESEMeD/MHEDEA 2000) Project: Rationale and methods. *International Journal of Methods in Psychiatric Research*, 11, 55–67.

Andrews, G., Henderson, S. & Hall, W. (2001). Prevalence, comorbidity, disability and service utilization: Overview of the Australian National Health Survey. *British Journal of Psychiatry*, 178, 145–53.

Bijl, R. V., de Graaf, R., Hiripi, E., Kessler, R. C., Kohn, R., Offord, D. R., Üstün, T. B., Vicente, B., Vollebergh, W. A., Walters, E. E. & Wittchen, H.-U. (2003). The prevalence of treated and untreated mental disorders in five countries. *Health Affairs (Millwood)*, 22, 122–33.

Bijl, R. V., Ravelli, A. & van Zessen, G. (1998). Prevalence of psychiatric disorder in the general population: Results of the Netherlands Mental Health Survey and Incidence Study (NEMESIS). *Social Psychiatry and Psychiatric Epidemiology*, 33, 587–95.

Demyttenaere, K., Bruffaerts, R., Posada-Villa, J., Gasquet, I., Kovess, V., Lepine, J. P., Angermeyer, M. C., Bernert, S., de Girolamo, G., Morosini, P., Polidori, G., Kikkawa, T., Kawakami, N., Ono, Y., Takeshima, T., Uda, H., Karam, E. G., Fayyad, J. A., Karam, A. N., Mneimneh, Z. N., Medina-Mora, M. E., Borges, G., Lara, C., de Graaf, R., Ormel, J., Gureje, O., Shen, Y., Huang, Y., Zhang, M., Alonso, J., Haro, J. M., Vilagut, G., Bromet, E. J., Gluzman, S., Webb, C., Kessler, R. C., Merikangas, K. R., Anthony, J. C., Von Korff, M. R., Wang, P. S., Brugha, T. S., Aguilar-Gaxiola, S., Lee, S., Heeringa, S., Pennell, B. E., Zaslavsky, A. M., Üstün, T. B. & Chatterji, S. (2004). Prevalence, severity, and unmet need for treatment of mental disorders in the World Health Organization World Mental Health Surveys. *Journal of the American Medical Association*, 291, 2581–90.

Efron, B. (1988). Logistic regression, survival analysis, and the Kaplan-Meier curve. *Journal of the American Statistical Association*, 83, 414–25.

ESEMeD/MHEDEA 2000 Investigators (2004a). Prevalence of mental disorders in Europe: Results from the European Study of the Epidemiology of Mental Disorders (ESEMeD) project. *Acta Psychiatrica Scandinavica*, 109, 21–7.

ESEMeD/MHEDEA 2000 Investigators, European Study of the Epidemiology of Mental Disorders (ESEMeD) Project (2004b). Use of mental health services in Europe: Results from the European Study of the Epidemiology of Mental Disorders (ESEMeD) project. *Acta Psychiatrica Scandinavica*, 420, 47–54.

Giuffra, L. A. & Risch, N. (1994). Diminished recall and the cohort effect of major depression: A simulation study. *Psychological Medicine*, 24, 375–83.

Gureje, O. (2000). Psychological disorders and symptoms in primary care: Association with disability and service use after 12 months. *Social Psychiatry and Psychiatric Epidemiology*, 37, 220–4.

Gureje, O. & Alem, A. (2000). Mental health policy developments in Africa. *Bulletin of the World Health Organization*, 78, 475–82.

Gureje, O., Kola, L. & Afolabi, E. (2007). Epidemiology of major depressive disorder in elderly Nigerians: A community survey. *Lancet*, 370, 957–64.

Gureje, O. & Lasebikan, V. O. (2006). Use of mental health services in a developing country: Results from the Nigerian survey of mental health and well-being. *Social Psychiatry and Psychiatric Epidemiology*, 41, 44–9.

Gureje, O., Lasebikan, V. O., Ephraim-Oluwanuga, O., Olley, B. O. & Kola, L. (2005). Community study of knowledge of and attitude to mental illness in Nigeria. *British Journal of Psychiatry*, 186, 436–41.

Gureje, O., Obikoya, B. & Ikuesan, B. A. (1992). Prevalence of specific disorders in an urban primary care setting. *East African Medical Journal*, 69, 282–7.

Gureje, O., Odejide, A. O., Olatawura, M. O., Ikuesan, B. A., Acha, R. A., Bamidele, R. W. & Raji, S. O. (1995). *Mental illness in general health care: Results from the Ibadan Centre*. London: John Wiley & Sons.

Hosmer, D. W. & Lemeshow, S. (2000). *Applied logistic regression*. New York: John Wiley & Sons.

Kessler, R. C. (2003). Epidemiology of women and depression. *Journal of Affective Disorders*, 74, 5–13.

Kessler, R. C., Berglund, P., Demler, O., Jin, R., Koretz, D., Merikangas, K. R., Rush, A. J., Walters, E. E. & Wang, P. S. (2003). The epidemiology of major depressive disorder. *Journal of the American Medical Association*, 289, 3095–105.

Kessler, R. C., Berglund, P., Demler, O., Jin, R. & Walters, E. E. (2005). Lifetime prevalence and age-of-onset distributions of DSM-IV disorders in the National Comorbidity Survey Replication. *Archives of General Psychiatry*, 62, 593–602.

Kessler, R. C., Haro, J. M., Heeringa, S. G., Pennell, B.-E. & Üstün, T. B. (2006). The World Health Organization World Mental Health Survey Initiative [editorial]. *Epidemiologia e Psichiatria Sociale*, 15, 161–6.

Kessler, R. C., McGonagle, K. A., Zhao, S., Nelson, C. B., Hughes, M., Eshleman, S., Wittchen, H.-U. & Kendler, K. S. (1994). Lifetime and 12-month prevalence of DSM-III-R psychiatric disorders in the United States: Results from the National Comorbidity Survey. *Achives of General Psychiatry*, 51, 8–19.

Kessler, R. C., Olfson, M. & Berglund, P. (1998). Patterns and predictors of treatment contact after first onset of psychiatric disorders. *American Journal of Psychiatry*, 155, 62–9.

Kessler, R. C. & Üstün, T. B. (2004). The World Mental Health (WMH) Survey Initiative version of the World Health Organization (WHO) Composite International Diagnostic Interview (CIDI). *International Journal of Methods in Psychiatric Research*, 13, 93–121.

Kish, L. (1965). *Survey sampling*. New York: John Wiley & Sons.

Narrow, W. E., Rae, D. S., Robins, L. N. & Regier, D. A. (2002). Revised prevalence estimates of mental disorders in the United States: Using a clinical significance criterion to reconcile 2 surveys' estimates. *Archives of General Psychiatry*, 59, 115–23.

Oakley-Browne, M. A., Wells, J. E., McGee, M. A. for the New Zealand Mental Health Survey Research Team (2006). Twelve-month and lifetime health service use in Te Rau Hinengaro: The New Zealand Mental Health Survey. *Australian and New Zealand Journal of Psychiatry*, 40, 855–64.

Odejide, A. O., Ohaeri, J. U., Adelekan, M. & Ikuesan, B. A. (1987). Drinking behaviour and social change among youths in Nigeria: A study of two cities. *Drug and Alcohol Dependence*, 20, 227–33.

Patel, V. & Kleinman, A. (2003). Poverty and common mental disorders in developing countries. *Bulletin of the World Health Organization*, 81, 609–15.

Regier, D. A., Kaelber, C. T., Rae, D.S., Farmer, M. E., Knauper, B., Kessler, R. C. & Norquist, G. S. (1998). Limitations of diagnostic criteria and assessment instruments for mental disorders: Implications for research and policy. *Archives of General Psychiatry*, 55, 109–15.

Regier, D. A., Narrow, W. E., Rupp, A. & Kaelber, C. T. (2000). The epidemiology of mental disorder treatment need: Community estimates of medical necessity. In *Unmet need in psychiatry*, ed. G. Andrews & S. Henderson. New York: Cambridge University Press. pp. 41–58.

Research Triangle Institute (2002). *SUDAAN: Professional software for survey data analysis 8.01*. Research Triangle Park, NC: Research Triangle Institute.

Robins, L. N. & Regier, D. A. (1991). *Psychiatric disorders in America: The Epidemiologic Catchment Area Study*. New York: Free Press.

Sheehan, D. V., Harnnet-Sheehan, K. & Raj, B. A. (1996). The measurement of disability. *International Clinical Psychopharmacology*, 11, 89–95.

Spitzer, R. L. (1998). Diagnosis and the need for treatment are not the same. *Archives of General Psychiatry*, 55, 120.

Wang, P. S., Lane, M., Olfson, M., Pincus, H. A., Wells, K. & Kessler, R. C. (2005a). Failure and delay in initial treatment contact after first onset of mental disorders in the National Comorbidity Survey Replication. *Archives of General Psychiatry*, 62, 629–40.

Wang, P. S., Lane, M., Olfson, M., Pincus, H. A., Wells, K. & Kessler, R. C. (2005b). Twelve-month use of mental health services in the United States: Results from the National Comorbidity Survey Replication. *Archives of General Psychiatry*, 62, 617–27.

WHO International Consortium in Psychiatric Epidemiology (2000). Cross-national comparisons of the prevalences and correlates of mental disorders. *Bulletin of the World Health Organization*, 78, 475–82.

World Health Organization (WHO) (2005). Health futures. Retrieved November 30, 2005, from http://www.who.int/hpr/expo1999.

# 11 The South African Stress and Health Study (SASH): A Foundation for Improving Mental Health Care in South Africa

ALLEN A. HERMAN, DAVID WILLIAMS, DAN J. STEIN, SORAYA SEEDAT,
STEVEN G. HEERINGA, AND HASHIM MOOMAL

## ACKNOWLEDGMENTS

The South African Stress and Health study is carried out in conjunction with the World Health Organization (WHO) World Mental Health (WMH) Survey Initiative. We thank the WMH staff for assistance with instrumentation, fieldwork, and some of the data analyses. These activities were supported by the U.S. National Institute of Mental Health (R01MH070884), the John D. and Catherine T. MacArthur Foundation, the Pfizer Foundation, the U.S. Public Health Service (R13-MH066849, R01-MH069864, and R01 DA016558), the Fogarty International Center (FIRCA R03-TW006481), the Pan American Health Organization, Eli Lilly and Company Foundation, Ortho-McNeil Pharmaceutical, GlaxoSmithKline, and Bristol-Myers Squibb. The South Africa Stress and Health study was funded by grant R01-MH059575 from the U.S. National Institute of Mental Health and the U.S. National Institute of Drug Abuse, with supplemental funding from the South African Department of Health and the University of Michigan. A complete list of WMH publications can be found at http://www.hcp.med.harvard.edu/wmh/.

## 1. INTRODUCTION

Apartheid has had a major effect on the mental health of all South Africans (de Beer 1977, 1980; Dommisse 1986; Hirschovitz & Orkin 1997). Psychological trauma was emblematic of South Africa before the 1994 election because the core philosophical principles of apartheid and legislative actions that resulted from those principles led to fundamental, society-wide human rights abuses. Additionally, mental health services for most South Africans were plagued by a dizzying array of public and contracted private service providers and characterized by a hierarchical racist system that added to the psychological trauma for the mentally ill. The health care system was fragmented and inadequate for the burdens of disease (Gillis 1977; Dommisse 1987; Freeman & de Beer 1992). This situation of the large burden of mental illness coupled with poor-quality mental health care is not unique to South Africa (Kessler & Frank 1997; Wang, Berglund & Kessler 2000). A final complication of the context of mental health in South Africa was that most mental health care was (and still is) provided through the complex lens of translating the many languages of South Africa into English and Afrikaans. This further impoverished the mental health care provided for the majority of South Africans. Linguistic diversity in South Africa is coupled with the absence of formal translation services in the health-care system and a reliance on ad hoc methods of cross-cultural communications with patients (Drennan, Levett & Swartz 1991; Drennan 1996; Swartz & Drennan 2000; Drennan & Swartz 2002).

At the end of the apartheid era, the African National Congress (ANC) formulated a broad policy framework that forms the basis for the current enabling health-care legislation. The ANC government developed a health-care delivery policy based on the district health system that is designed to extend the availability of appropriate health care (South African Department of Health 1997). The initial policy documents of the African National Congress were translated into the National Health Act of 2003 (Republic of South Africa 2003) and the Mental Health Act of 2002 (Republic of South Africa 2002). These policies place most of the public mental health care within an integrated primary health-care system. To achieve the goals of these two acts the South African government requires population-based data that identifies the prevalence of mental health disorders, the reasons for these disorders, patterns of treatment, barriers to treatment, and the potential approaches to improving care.

The South African Stress and Health Study (SASH) is the first large mental health epidemiological survey in South Africa (Williams et al. 2004). The SASH is carried out as part of the World Health Organization World Mental Health (WMH) Survey Initiative (Kessler et al. 2006). The SASH should be placed within the historical context of early postapartheid South Africa, where communities are still sharply divided by racial/ethnic and national identities and seemingly immutable socioeconomic contexts (Christopher 2004; Bornman 2006). This chapter describes some of these contexts and places our findings within the framework of the larger global mental health picture that is being drawn by the WMH surveys (Demyttenaere et al. 2004). Our exploration of the impact of the racial, ethnic, and political identities of South Africans and the human rights violations that defined apartheid South Africa and affected the lives of ordinary South Africans makes the SASH doubly unique. In this chapter, we describe the 12-month and lifetime prevalence of mental health disorders and the impact of context and individual socioeconomic status on the 12-month and lifetime distributions of mental health and the 12-month treatment use.

## 2. SAMPLING METHODS AND SAMPLE SIZE

The SASH sample is a three-stage, area probability sample of 4351 adults (18+ years old) of all races and ethnic groups living in households and single-sex migrant-laborer group quarters (hostels) in South Africa. Sample selection and data collection were completed from 2003 to 2004.

Within each of South Africa's nine provinces, neighborhoods were stratified into ten categories: (1) rural-commercial agricultural areas, (2) rural-traditional subsistence areas, (3) black low-cost housing townships, (4) informal urban or peri-urban slum areas, (5) single-sex hostels and other collective dwellings within black communities (these were included to maximize sample coverage of young working-age men), (6) Coloured low-cost housing townships, (7) Indian low-cost housing townships, (8) general metropolitan residential areas, (9) general large metropolitan residential areas, and (10) domestic servant accommodation in urban areas. The SASH survey population did not include individuals living in prisons, hospitals, and mental institutions. Members of the military who resided on military bases were also not included in the SASH survey population.

### 2.1. Primary-stage Sample

The SASH sampling is a stratified first-stage sample of South Africa's 2001 Census enumeration areas (EAs) followed by a second-stage sample of dwelling units from each sample EA and finally a third-stage random selection of a single adult respondent in each selected sample dwelling unit. The SASH primary-stage sampling units (PSUs) are EA units defined for the 2001 Census of South Africa. South Africa's land area is divided into 85,783 geographic EA units. Prior to the first stage of sample selection, each of these EAs was assigned to one of 53 strata based on the province in which it was located, its urban/rural status and the majority population group in the EA (African, Coloured, Indian, and white). A total primary stage sample size of 960 EA units was allocated to the 53 strata approximately in proportion to the total number of Census EAs in the stratum. Within each stratum, the allocated sample of EAs was selected with probability proportionate to the total 2001 Census count of adult population for the EA. Table 11.1 summarizes each of the 53 primary-stage strata in the SASH sampling design by province.

Table 11.1 also shows the racial stratification of South Africa. Although black EAs are present

**Table 11.1.** Sampled enumeration areas (EAs) by province and housing type

| EA housing type | | WC | EC | NC | FS | KZN | NWP | GP | MPL | LP | Total |
|---|---|---|---|---|---|---|---|---|---|---|---|
| | | | | | | **Province** | | | | | |
| Black rural | Total | 27 | 11,082 | 120 | 1739 | 6473 | 4773 | 573 | 3877 | 10,044 | 38,708 |
| | Sampled | 1 | 66 | 6 | 31 | 61 | 55 | 13 | 52 | 63 | 348 |
| | Percentage | 3.7 | 0.6 | 5.0 | 1.8 | 0.9 | 1.2 | 2.3 | 1.3 | 0.6 | 0.9% |
| Black urban | Total | 1842 | 3535 | 399 | 3092 | 4799 | 2053 | 11,362 | 1729 | 971 | 29,782 |
| | Sampled | 29 | 36 | 13 | 36 | 55 | 27 | 85 | 28 | 19 | 328 |
| | Percentage | 1.6 | 1.0 | 3.3 | 1.2 | 1.1 | 1.3 | 0.7 | 1.6 | 2.0 | 1.1% |
| Coloured rural | Total | 712 | 113 | 404 | 18 | 0 | 0 | 0 | 0 | 0 | 1247 |
| | Sampled | 13 | 6 | 12 | 1 | 0 | 0 | 0 | 0 | 0 | 32 |
| | Percentage | 1.3 | 5.3 | 3.0 | 5.6 | 0.0 | 0.0 | 0.0 | 0.0 | 0.0 | 2.6% |
| Coloured urban | Total | 2587 | 620 | 396 | 85 | 165 | 54 | 334 | 16 | 4 | 4261 |
| | Sampled | 32 | 13 | 12 | 5 | 5 | 4 | 8 | 2 | 1 | 82 |
| | Percentage | 1.2 | 2.1 | 3.0 | 5.9 | 3.0 | 7.4 | 2.4 | 12.5 | 25.0 | 1.9% |
| White rural | Total | 48 | 47 | 0 | 0 | 0 | 52 | 126 | 49 | 83 | 405 |
| | Sampled | 1 | 1 | 0 | 0 | 0 | 1 | 1 | 3 | 1 | 8 |
| | Percentage | 2.1 | 2.1 | 0.0 | 0.0 | 0.0 | 1.9 | 0.8 | 6.1 | 1.2 | 2.0% |
| White urban | Total | 1742 | 816 | 203 | 601 | 1241 | 424 | 3973 | 499 | 167 | 9666 |
| | Sampled | 18 | 4 | 6 | 14 | 20 | 10 | 36 | 10 | 4 | 122 |
| | Percentage | 1.0 | 0.5 | 3.0 | 2.3 | 1.6 | 2.4 | 0.9 | 2.0 | 2.4 | 1.3% |
| Indian urban | Total | 25 | 21 | 0 | 0 | 1359 | 23 | 257 | 19 | 10 | 1714 |
| | Sampled | 2 | 2 | 0 | 0 | 26 | 2 | 6 | 1 | 1 | 40 |
| | Percentage | 8.0 | 9.5 | 0.0 | 0.0 | 1.9 | 8.7 | 2.3 | 5.3 | 10.0 | 2.3% |
| All EAs | Total | 6983 | 16,234 | 1522 | 5535 | 14,037 | 7379 | 16,625 | 6189 | 11279 | 85,783 |
| | Sampled | 96 | 128 | 49 | 87 | 167 | 99 | 149 | 96 | 89 | 960 |
| | Percentage | 1.4 | 0.8 | 3.2 | 1.6 | 1.2 | 1.3 | 0.9 | 1.6 | 0.8 | 1.1% |

WC = Western Cape; EC = Eastern Cape; NC = Northern Cape; FS = Free State; KZN = KwaZulu-Natal; NWP = Northwest Province; GP = Gauteng Province; MPL = Mpumalanga; LP = Limpopo.

in all provinces of South Africa, they are more prevalent in those provinces that housed the segregated tribal/ethnic homelands. These homelands (10 self-governing territories for different ethnic groups were established as part of the policy of apartheid. Four were granted independence by South Africa (recognized only by South Africa and one another) ceased to exist on April 27, 1994, and were reincorporated into the nine new South African provinces. The distribution of the former homelands is:

1. Eastern Cape: Transkei and Ciskei
2. Kwazulu-Natal: Kwazulu
3. North West Province: Bophuthatswana
4. Mpumalanga: Kangwane, Lebowa

5. Limpopo: Venda, Gazankulu, KwaNdebele

Coloured EAs are found mostly in the Western Cape, Indian EAs are found mostly in Kwazulu-Natal, and white EAs are found throughout the country. The seeming anomaly of zero white EAs in rural Free State, Northern Cape, and Kwazulu-Natal is a function of the distribution of large-scale commercial farming in these provinces (Statistics South Africa 2002).

## 2.2. Second-stage Sample of Dwellings

Prior to the second stage of sample selection, an enumerative list of dwelling units was prepared using Census information and aerial photographs of more remote EA locations. When

**Table 11.2.** Sample sizes and final dispositions for the SASH study

| | |
|---|---|
| Sampled households | 5089 |
| Designated adult responders | 5089 |
| Initial interviews from field | 4434 |
| Interview cooperation rate | 87.1% |
| Final SASH cases for analysis | 4351 |
| Complete data interview rate | 98.1% |

interviewing teams first visited a sampled EA, the list of dwellings and Census maps were updated to include missed units. A random sample of five dwelling units in each EA was selected on the basis of the updated lists and maps.

## 2.3. Third-stage Selection of the SASH Respondent

SASH interviewers contacted each household in the sample of dwelling units and selected a single adult respondent at random using the Kish procedure for objective respondent selection (Kish 1949). If the household or the selected respondent refused to be interviewed for SASH, a random replacement was drawn from the enumerative listing for the EA. This procedure of randomly replacing nonrespondent sample units implicitly introduces an adjustment for nonresponse. Because the sample selections for individuals will vary, unbiased estimation and inference from the SASH sample to the South African survey population requires a case-specific sample selection weight factor.

## 2.4. Sample Outcomes

Table 11.2 provides a summary of the SASH sample dispositions and interview outcomes. A total sample of 5089 households was selected. Field interviews were obtained from 4433 (87.1%) of the designated respondents selected at random from the eligible persons in each sample household. On the basis of quality-control criteria, including completion of critical sections in the SASH questionnaire, a total of 4351 (98.1%) of the field interviews were retained for use in analysis.

## 3. MEASURES

### 3.1. Diagnostic Assessment of Lifetime and 12-month DSM-IV Disorders

DSM-IV diagnoses were made using Version 3.0 of the World Health Organization (WHO) Composite International Diagnostic Interview (CIDI) (Kessler & Üstün 2004); a fully structured lay-administered diagnostic interview that generates diagnoses according to the definitions and criteria of both the ICD-10 (World Health Organization 1991) and DSM-IV (American Psychiatric Association 1994) diagnostic systems. As the content of the CIDI is reviewed in detail in Chapter 4 of this volume, only a brief listing of the disorders assessed in the SASH is presented here. The disorders included in the SASH are anxiety disorders (panic disorder [PD], agoraphobia without panic [AG], social phobia [SoP], generalized anxiety disorder [GAD], and posttraumatic stress disorder [PTSD]); mood disorders (major depressive episode [MDE]); impulse control disorders (intermittent explosive disorder [IED]); and substance use disorders (alcohol abuse [AA], alcohol dependence [AD], substance abuse [SA], substance dependence [SD]). Lifetime prevalence, age of onset and 12-month prevalence were assessed separately for each disorder. All diagnoses are considered with organic exclusions and without diagnostic hierarchy rules. Bipolar disorders, oppositional-defiant disorder, conduct disorder, attention-deficit/hyperactivity disorder, obsessive compulsive disorder, specific phobia, and separation anxiety disorder were not assessed in the SASH. Twelve-month cases were classified by severity using a system described in detail elsewhere (Kessler et al. 2006) as serious, moderate, or mild.

### 3.2. 12-month Use of Mental Health Services

All respondents were asked whether they had ever received treatment for mental health problems or for problems associated with alcohol or drug use. Separate assessments were made for different types of professionals, support groups, self-help groups, mental health crisis hotlines (assumed to be visits with nonpsychiatrist mental health specialists), CAM therapies, and use of other treatment settings, including admissions to hospitals and other facilities. Follow-up questions asked about age at first and most recent contacts as well as number and duration of visits in the past 12 months.

In parallel with the coding scheme used in other WMH surveys, reports of 12-month service use were classified into the following categories in the SASH sample: psychiatrist; nonpsychiatrist mental health specialist (psychologist or other nonpsychiatrist mental health professional in any setting, mental health nurse, social worker or counselor in a mental health specialty setting, use of a mental health hotline); general medical provider (primary care doctor, other general medical doctor); nurse (excluding mental health nurses), and any other health professional not previously mentioned); human services professional (religious or spiritual advisor, social worker or counselor in any setting other than a specialty mental health setting); and complementary alternative medicine (CAM) professional (any other type of healer such as traditional healers, participation in an Internet support group, participation in a self-help group). Psychiatrist and nonpsychiatrist specialist categories were combined into a broader mental health specialty (MHS) category; MHS was also combined with general medical (GM) into an even broader health-care (HC) category. Human services (HS) and CAM were combined into a non–health-care (NHC) category.

### 3.3. Predictor Variables

Predictor variables in analyses of lifetime data include age of onset (AOO) of the focal disorder (coded into the categories 0–12, 13–19, 20–29, and 30+ years of age), cohort (defined by age at interview in the categories 18–29, 30–44, 45–59, 60+), sex, race (black, Coloured, white, Indian), education (categorized as either current students or nonstudents with 0–11, 12, 13–15, or 16+ years of education), and marital status (categorized as either currently married/cohabiting,

previously married, or never married). The last two of these predictors vary within a given individual over time. Information was obtained in the SASH on timing of marital histories (i.e., ages of marriage and marital dissolution), allowing marital status to be coded for each year of each respondents' lives. Information on years of education was also coded as a time-varying predictor by assuming an orderly educational history for each respondent in which eight years of education corresponds to being a student up to age 14 and other lengths of education are associated with ages consistent with this benchmark (e.g., 12 years of education is assumed to correspond to being a student up to age 18). Variables in analyses of 12-month data included sex, race, cohort, education, and marital status (all categorized as described previously). In addition, family income (categorized as low, low average, high average, and high) and urban or rural status were also included.

### 3.4. Analysis Procedures

The data were weighted to adjust for differential probabilities of selection of respondents within households and differential nonresponse as well as to adjust for residual differences between the sample and the South Africa population on the cross-classification of sociodemographic variables. An additional weight was used to adjust for differences in probability of selection into that sample. Simple cross-tabulation methods were used to estimate prevalence. AOO distributions were generated from retrospective AOO reports using the actuarial method (Halli & Rao 1992). Discrete-time survival analysis with person-year the unit of analysis (Efron 1988) was used to study predictors of lifetime risk. Logistic regression analysis (Hosmer & Lemeshow 1989) was used to study correlates of treatment.

### 4. RESULTS

### 4.1. South African Census Data

Compared to the 2001 South African census, females, Coloureds, Indians and individuals

**Table 11.3.** Comparison of the sociodemographic distributions of the SASH sample to the 2001 South African census

| Variables | SASH sample Unweighted | SASH sample Weighted | 2001 Census |
|---|---|---|---|
| **Gender** | | | |
| Male | 39.8 | 46.3 | 46.8 |
| Female | 60.2 | 53.7 | 53.2 |
| **Age (years)** | | | |
| 20–34 | 47.1 | 47.2 | 45.5 |
| 35–49 | 31.2 | 30.4 | 30.5 |
| 50–64 | 15.8 | 16.9 | 15.3 |
| 65+ | 5.9 | 5.5 | 8.7 |
| **Race** | | | |
| Black | 76.2 | 76.2 | 79.0 |
| Coloured | 12.9 | 10.4 | 8.9 |
| Indian or Asian | 3.7 | 3.4 | 2.5 |
| White | 7.2 | 10.0 | 9.6 |
| **Province** | | | |
| Eastern Cape | 14.2 | 13.1 | 13.3 |
| Free State | 9.7 | 6.2 | 6.2 |
| Guateng | 13.6 | 23.0 | 22.2 |
| Kwazulu-Natal | 17.2 | 19.5 | 20.2 |
| Limpopo | 9.6 | 10.5 | 10.5 |
| Mpumalanga | 9.5 | 6.6 | 6.6 |
| Northern Cape | 5.4 | 1.9 | 1.3 |
| North West | 10.4 | 8.3 | 8.3 |
| Western Cape | 10.3 | 11.1 | 10.8 |

residing in the Free State, Mpumalanga, Northern Cape, and North West Province were oversampled, whereas blacks, whites, and individuals living in Gauteng Province were undersampled (Table 11.3). A poststratification weight was used to adjust for these differences in the distribution of the sample compared to the population, so as to make the sample representative of the population in terms of race-ethnicity and geography.

## 4.2. Lifetime Prevalence of DSM-IV Mental Disorders

Table 11.4 shows the lifetime prevalence of mental disorders. The lifetime prevalence for any disorder is 30.3%; 11.2% of respondents had two or more lifetime disorders and 3.5% had three or more lifetime disorders. The most preva-

lent class of lifetime disorders is anxiety disorders (15.8%), followed by substance use disorders (13.3%) and mood disorders (9.8%). The most prevalent individual lifetime disorders are alcohol abuse (11.4%), major depressive disorder (9.8%), and agoraphobia without panic (9.8%).

Significant differences in lifetime prevalence of mental disorders occur across the nine provinces, with Western Cape having the highest rate at 42% compared to the lowest rate in the Northern Cape of 29%. Western Cape and Free State had prevalence rates that were significantly higher that the countrywide rates, and Eastern Cape and Northern Cape had rates that were significantly lower (Table 11.5). These provincial differences held for all mental disorders except impulse disorders, where the lowest provincial rates were found in Mpumalanga (0.2%) and the Eastern Cape (0.1%). Significant differences in prevalence with age occur with panic disorder and generalized anxiety disorder (showing a general monotonic increase in rates with age); and drug abuse and drug dependence (showing a tendency to peak at 35 to 49 years). There is a marginally significant increase in the rate of mood disorders with increasing age.

## 4.3. Distributions of the AOO of Mental Disorders

Table 11.6 shows the distributions of cumulative lifetime risk estimates of mental disorders that have been standardized for fixed percentiles. Median ages of onset (50th percentile of the age of onset AOO distribution) are earlier for substance use disorders (24 years) than for most anxiety disorders (32 years: 17–35 years) and mood disorders (37 years). The age of onset of anxiety disorders occurs over a wide range, with an interquartile range (IQR) from 16 years to 57 years. Social phobia (19 years) and agoraphobia without panic (18 years) have a median AOO during late adolescence and relatively narrow interquartile ranges. Major depressive disorder occurs over a wide age range (IQR 30 years: 23–53). Drug use disorders occur over a narrower age range of 11 years, and alcohol use disorders over an age range of 20 years.

**Table 11.4.** SASH sample estimates of lifetime prevalence of DSM-IV/CIDI disorders (by age category)

| Disorders | Total | Prevalence, % (se) | | | | | $\chi^2_3$ |
|---|---|---|---|---|---|---|---|
| | | All ages | 18y–34y | 35y–49y | 50y–64y | 65+y | |
| **Anxiety disorders** | | | | | | | |
| Panic disorder | 57 | 1.2 (0.2) | 0.6 (0.2) | 1.9 (0.4) | 1.9 (0.7) | 1.3 (0.9) | 10.0* |
| Agoraphobia without panic | 435 | 9.8 (0.6) | 10.5 (1.0) | 10.0 (1.0) | 8.1 (1.4) | 7.2 (1.7) | 4.7[NS] |
| Social phobia | 116 | 2.8 (0.4) | 2.7 (0.5) | 3.5 (0.7) | 2.5 (0.9) | 1.3 (0.8) | 3.7[NS] |
| Generalized anxiety disorder | 124 | 2.7 (0.3) | 1.2 (0.2) | 3.7 (0.4) | 4.1 (1.0) | 7.2 (2.5) | 40.5[†] |
| Posttraumatic stress disorder | 91 | 2.3 (0.2) | 1.8 (0.3) | 2.4 (0.5) | 2.7 (0.7) | 4.4 (2.9) | 1.5[NS] |
| Any anxiety disorder | 695 | 15.8 (0.8) | 14.7 (1.1) | 17.6 (1.1) | 15.9 (2.0) | 17.0 (3.3) | 3.6[NS] |
| **Mood disorders** | | | | | | | |
| Major depressive disorder | 439 | 9.8 (0.7) | 8.9 (0.8) | 11.9 (1.3) | 10.0 (1.3) | 6.5 (1.6) | 8.2[‡] |
| Any mood disorder | 439 | 9.8 (0.7) | 8.9 (0.8) | 11.9 (1.3) | 10.0 (1.3) | 6.5 (1.6) | 8.2[‡] |
| **Substance use disorders** | | | | | | | |
| Alcohol abuse | 435 | 11.4 (0.8) | 11.1 (1.1) | 12.8 (1.5) | 10.0 (1.8) | 10.3 (3.3) | 2.2[NS] |
| Alcohol dependence | 95 | 2.6 (0.4) | 2.3 (0.5) | 3.5 (0.8) | 1.9 (0.9) | 2.5 (1.4) | 2.3[NS] |
| Drug abuse | 139 | 3.9 (0.4) | 4.6 (0.6) | 4.2 (0.8) | 2.0 (0.7) | 1.6 (0.9) | 12.0* |
| Drug dependence | 19 | 0.6 (0.2) | 0.8 (0.3) | 0.5 (0.3) | 0.2 (0.2) | 0.0 (0.0) | 11.1* |
| Any substance use | 505 | 13.3 (0.9) | 13.5 (1.2) | 14.7 (1.6) | 11.0 (1.9) | 11.0 (3.3) | 3.5[NS] |
| **Any disorder** | | | | | | | |
| Any disorder | 1290 | 30.3 (1.1) | 29.4 (1.4) | 33.6 (2.0) | 28.3 (2.6) | 27.9 (3.4) | 6.1[NS] |
| Two or more disorders | 456 | 11.2 (0.8) | 10.4 (1.0) | 12.8 (1.2) | 11.2 (1.7) | 9.6 (3.0) | 3.1[NS] |
| Three or more disorders | 139 | 3.5 (0.5) | 3.2 (0.6) | 4.8 (0.8) | 2.5 (0.9) | 2.8 (2.1) | 5.1[NS] |

[NS] $p > 0.05$; * $0.01, p < 0.05$; [†] $p < 0.001$; [‡] $0.05 < p < 0.10$.

## 4.4. Projected Lifetime Risk of Mental Disorders

On the basis of the AOO distributions shown in Table 11.6, the projected lifetime risk of any mental disorders of 47.5% is higher than the lifetime prevalence of 30.3%. The greatest difference between projected risk and prevalence is observed for anxiety disorders (30.1% vs. 15.8%, difference of 14.3%), followed by major

**Table 11.5.** Provincial lifetime prevalence estimates (%) of DSM-IV/CIDI disorders by province

| Province | All disorders | Specific disorders (grouped) | | | | Sample size (n) |
|---|---|---|---|---|---|---|
| | | Anxiety | Mood | Substance Use | Impulse | |
| Western Cape | 39.4* | 18.9 | 13.7 | 20.6* | 4.5* | 448 |
| Free State | 37.5 | 21.5* | 14.6* | 15.5 | 3.3 | 421 |
| North West | 34.0 | 17.2 | 8.1 | 16.2 | 1.7 | 453 |
| Limpopo | 30.8 | 16.3 | 6.3* | 13.5 | 2.6 | 420 |
| Kwazulu-Natal | 28.0 | 12.9 | 9.0 | 12.8 | 2.1 | 749 |
| Gauteng | 29.8 | 15.7 | 10.2 | 12.3 | 5.4* | 593 |
| Mpumalanga | 29.2 | 16.0 | 9.0 | 9.1 | 0.1* | 415 |
| Eastern Cape | 25.7* | 13.3 | 8.3 | 8.5* | 1.1 | 619 |
| Northern Cape | 28.7 | 15.0 | 7.7 | 13.8 | 3.8* | 233 |
| South Africa | 30.8 | 15.8 | 9.7 | 13.3 | 3.0 | 4351 |

* $p < 0.05$ in contrasting province with South Africa as a whole.

**Table 11.6.** Ages at selected percentiles on the standardized age of onset distributions of DSM-IV/CIDI disorders with projected lifetime risk at age 75 years

| Disorders | Risk* % | (SE) | Age at age of onset percentiles 5 | 10 | 25 | 50 | 75 | 90 | 95 | 99 |
|---|---|---|---|---|---|---|---|---|---|---|
| **Anxiety disorder** | | | | | | | | | | |
| Panic disorder | 2.6 | (0.8) | 13 | 14 | 26 | 46 | 57 | 57 | 57 | 57 |
| Generalized anxiety disorder | 13.0 | (4.5) | 17 | 22 | 37 | 72 | 72 | 73 | 73 | 73 |
| Social phobia | 3.4 | (0.5) | 7 | 13 | 14 | 19 | 31 | 41 | 43 | 48 |
| Agoraphobia without panic | 12.7 | (0.8) | 6 | 11 | 13 | 18 | 35 | 51 | 59 | 65 |
| Posttraumatic stress disorder | 4.6 | (0.8) | 17 | 20 | 27 | 36 | 50 | 54 | 69 | 69 |
| Any anxiety disorder | 30.1 | (4.4) | 9 | 13 | 16 | 32 | 57 | 72 | 73 | 73 |
| **Mood disorders** | | | | | | | | | | |
| Major depressive disorder | 20.0 | (2.4) | 14 | 16 | 23 | 37 | 53 | 67 | 71 | 71 |
| Any mood disorder | 20.0 | (2.4) | 14 | 16 | 23 | 37 | 53 | 67 | 71 | 71 |
| **Substance use disorders** | | | | | | | | | | |
| Alcohol abuse | 15.3 | (1.1) | 17 | 19 | 21 | 26 | 31 | 41 | 46 | 59 |
| Alcohol dependence | 4.4 | (0.7) | 17 | 19 | 23 | 31 | 46 | 51 | 61 | 61 |
| Drug abuse | 4.9 | (0.5) | 15 | 16 | 19 | 21 | 30 | 41 | 54 | 54 |
| Any substance use disorder | 17.5 | (1.2) | 16 | 18 | 20 | 24 | 31 | 41 | 46 | 59 |
| Any disorder | 47.5 | (3.7) | 11 | 13 | 18 | 26 | 44 | 69 | 72 | 73 |

* Projected lifetime risk at age 75.

depressive disorder. The smallest difference between lifetime risk and prevalence is observed for substance use disorders (17.5% vs. 13.3%, difference of 3.2%). Disorders with a later AOO had a greater difference between projected risk and prevalence.

### 4.5. Cohort Effects in Lifetime Risk of Mental Disorders

Table 11.7 shows the results of discrete-time survival analysis used to predict lifetime risk of mental disorders for 18- to 34-year-olds; 35- to 49-year-olds; 50- to 64-year-olds, and those respondents older than 64 years. These groups correspond to cohorts born in the years 1975+, 1955–1969, to 1940–1954, and earlier than 1940. With the exception of generalized anxiety disorder and social phobia, there were significant positive associations between recency of cohorts and risk of mental disorders, risks increasing with decreasing age. The largest effects were seen for major depressive disorder, followed by drug and alcohol use disorders, agoraphobia without panic, and posttraumatic stress disorder.

One explanation for these apparent cohort effects is that lifetime risks are constant across cohorts but only appear to vary because onset of disorders is earlier in younger cohorts. A second explanation is that mortality may have an increasing impact on sample selection bias as age increases. Table 11.8 summarizes these variations in three broad cohorts (early, middle, and late). Total sample models evaluated the significance of interactions between cohort and person-year. Anxiety and major depressive disorders showed more significant associations with age in the middle and late cohorts, and substance use disorders had their greatest age effect in the earliest age cohort. The cohort effect in the middle and late cohorts was more striking for major depressive disorder than for the anxiety disorders.

### 4.6. Prevalence and Severity of 12-month Disorders

Table 11.9 shows the 12-month prevalence of mental disorders. Among the broad classes of disorders, anxiety disorders are the most prevalent

**Table 11.7.** Cohort (age at interview) as a predictor of lifetime risk of DSM-IV/CIDI disorders in the SASH

| Disorders | Odds ratios (CIs) for lifetime risk by age at interview, younger cohorts compared with 65+ y | | | |
|---|---|---|---|---|
| | 18–34 y $\psi$ (95% CI) | 35–49 y $\psi$ (95% CI) | 50–64 y $\psi$ (95% CI) | $\chi^2$ (3 df) |
| **Anxiety disorders** | | | | |
| Panic disorder | 3.0 (0.4–20.2) | 5.0 (0.8–30.2) | 2.2 (0.4–13.5) | 7.6* |
| Generalized anxiety disorder | 0.8 (0.2–3.1) | 1.2 (0.4–4.0) | 1.0 (0.3–3.1) | 2.8 |
| Social phobia | 3.2 (0.7–14.8) | 3.1 (0.6–15.2) | 2.0 (0.6–7.3) | 2.4 |
| Agoraphobia without panic | 2.5 (1.4–4.5)[†] | 1.9 (1.1–3.4)[†] | 1.3 (0.6–2.5) | 19.1[‡] |
| Posttraumatic stress disorder | 2.2 (0.4–11.0) | 1.0 (0.3–3.4) | 0.7 (0.2–2.6) | 12.4[‡] |
| Any anxiety disorder | 2.3 (1.3–4.0)[†] | 1.8 (1.1–3.1)[†] | 1.3 (0.8–2.1) | 16.5[‡] |
| **Mood disorders** | | | | |
| Major depressive disorder | 9.6 (5.5–16.7)[†] | 5.5 (3.1–9.9)[†] | 2.5 (1.4–4.4)[†] | 95.6[§] |
| Any mood disorder | 9.6 (5.5–16.7) | 5.5 (3.1–9.9)[†] | 2.5 (1.4–4.4)[†] | 95.6[§] |
| **Substance use disorders** | | | | |
| Alcohol abuse | 2.4 (1.1–5.1)[†] | 1.4 (0.7–2.7) | 1.0 (0.5–1.9) | 21.6[§] |
| Alcohol dependence | 3.7 (1.2–11.9)[†] | 2.3 (0.7–7.1) | 0.9 (0.2–3.7) | 13.1[‡] |
| Drug abuse | 5.4 (1.5–19.0)[†] | 3.1 (0.9–10.2) | 1.3 (0.3–5.3) | 18.4[§] |
| Any substance use disorder | 2.6 (1.3–5.4)[†] | 1.5 (0.8–2.9) | 1.0 (0.6–1.9) | 29.1[§] |
| Any disorder | 3.0 (2.1–4.2)[†] | 2.0 (1.5–2.7)[†] | 1.3 (0.9–1.8) | 76.4[§] |

* $0.05 < p < 0.10$; [†] $p < 0.05$; [‡] $0.0001 < p < 0.05$; [§] $p < 0.0001$.

**Table 11.8.** Variations in the effects of cohort (age-at-interview) on lifetime risk of DSM-IV/CIDI disorders

| Age at interview (years) | Lifetime risk by age at interview (y), $\psi$ (95% CI) | | |
|---|---|---|---|
| | Early | Middle | Late |
| **Anxiety disorders (reference: 65+ y)** | | | |
| 18 to 34 | 1.1 (0.5–2.4) | 3.0 (1.2–7.9)* | 3.1 (1.5–6.4)* |
| 35 to 49 | 0.8 (0.4–1.9) | 2.1 (0.8–5.7) | 3.3 (1.8–5.8)* |
| 50 to 64 | 0.5 (0.2–1.1) | 1.2 (0.4–3.6) | 2.2 (1.2–4.1)* |
| $\chi_3^2$ | 8.8* | 14.6[‡] | 18.0[‡] |
| Global $\chi_6^2$ | | 17.6y | |
| **Mood disorders (reference: 65+ y)** | | | |
| 18 to 34 | 5.5 (1.8–16.2)* | 18.1 (2.4–138.2)* | 11.3 (3.8–33.8)* |
| 35 to 49 | 2.8 (0.9–8.9) | 10.9 (1.4–85.9)* | 6.2 (2.6–14.9)* |
| 50 to 64 | 1.7 (0.4–7.9) | 4.5 (0.6–31.7) | 2.9 (1.4–6.1)* |
| $\chi_3^2$ | 26.7[‡] | 26.0[‡] | 25.9[‡] |
| Global $\chi_6^2$ | | 2.6[NS] | |
| **Substance use disorders (reference: 65+ y)** | | | |
| 18 to 34 | 11.6 (1.5–90.6)* | 2.0 (0.5–8.1) | 1.5 (0.6–4.0) |
| 35 to 49 | 3.7 (0.5–29.7) | 1.5 (0.4–5.4) | 1.5 (0.7–3.2) |
| 50 to 64 | 2.7 (0.3–26.0) | 0.9 (0.3–3.1) | 1.0 (0.4–2.3) |
| $\chi_3^2$ | 24.1[‡] | 9.9* | 2.8[NS] |
| Global $\chi_6^2$ | | 13.9* | |

* $p < 0.05$; [†] $0.05 < p < 0.01$; [‡] $p < 0.0001$.

*Note:* All models include time intervals and gender.

**Table 11.9.** 12-month prevalence and severity of DSM-IV/CIDI disorders (severity prevalence rates calculated from 4351 individuals and sum to 100% across rows)

| | | | | Severity | | | | | |
| | | | | Mild | | Moderate | | Severe | |
| | | Total | | | | | | | |
| Disorder | *n* | % | (se) | % | (se) | % | (se) | % | (se) |
|---|---|---|---|---|---|---|---|---|---|
| **Anxiety disorder** | | | | | | | | | |
| Panic disorder | 37 | 0.8 | (0.2) | 19.7 | (6.6) | 14.6 | (6.2) | 65.7 | (8.5) |
| Generalized anxiety disorder | 67 | 1.4 | (0.2) | 23.1 | (5.6) | 48.1 | (6.9) | 28.8 | (6.6) |
| Social phobia | 85 | 1.9 | (0.3) | 10.9 | (3.4) | 46.4 | (5.9) | 42.7 | (5.7) |
| Agoraphobia without panic | 215 | 4.8 | (0.4) | 44.1 | (3.2) | 28.3 | (3.1) | 27.7 | (3.0) |
| Posttraumatic stress disorder | 27 | 0.6 | (0.1) | 39.4 | (12.1) | 24.2 | (8.5) | 36.4 | (10.4) |
| Any anxiety disorder | 367 | 8.1 | (0.5) | 35.1 | (2.4) | 34.4 | (2.2) | 30.5 | (2.4) |
| **Mood disorder** | | | | | | | | | |
| Major depressive disorder | 223 | 4.9 | (0.4) | 20.3 | (3.5) | 45.4 | (4.0) | 34.3 | (3.3) |
| Any mood disorder | 223 | 4.9 | (0.4) | 20.3 | (3.5) | 45.4 | (4.0) | 34.3 | (3.3) |
| **Impulse disorder** | | | | | | | | | |
| Intermittent explosive disorder | 67 | 1.8 | (0.3) | 29.9 | (10.5) | 40.9 | (12.2) | 29.2 | (7.4) |
| Any impulse-control disorder | 52 | 1.9 | (0.3) | 21.8 | (6.2) | 42.9 | (11.5) | 35.3 | (10.2) |
| **Substance use disorder** | | | | | | | | | |
| Alcohol abuse | 167 | 4.5 | (0.4) | 61.5 | (4.1) | 11.6 | (2.9) | 26.9 | (4.6) |
| Alcohol dependence | 46 | 1.2 | (0.2) | 0.0 | (0.0) | 5.2 | (3.6) | 94.8 | (3.6) |
| Drug abuse | 50 | 1.4 | (0.2) | 54.1 | (8.5) | 14.4 | (5.3) | 31.6 | (7.5) |
| Drug dependence | 5 | 0.1 | (0.1) | 0.0 | (0.0) | 18.2 | (17.1) | 81.8 | (17.1) |
| Any substance use disorder | 211 | 5.8 | (0.5) | 56.7 | (3.8) | 12.5 | (2.6) | 30.9 | (4.3) |
| **All disorders** | | | | | | | | | |
| Any | 709 | 16.5 | (0.9) | 42.7 | (2.2) | 31.1 | (2.1) | 26.2 | (1.8) |
| 1 disorder | 496 | 11.3 | (0.7) | 54.1 | (3.1) | 32.1 | (3.2) | 13.8 | (1.6) |
| 2 disorders | 157 | 3.9 | (0.3) | 21.7 | (3.6) | 31.4 | (3.7) | 46.8 | (4.1) |
| 3+ disorders | 56 | 1.4 | (0.2) | 7.5 | (4.3) | 21.9 | (8.4) | 70.7 | (9.2) |

(8.1%), followed by substance use disorders (5.8%) and mood disorders (4.5%). The most common disorders are major depressive disorder (4.9%), agoraphobia without panic (4.8%), and alcohol abuse (4.5%). Seventeen percent of the respondents had one or more 12-month mental disorder; among these, more than half of cases had only one disorder (11%), with smaller proportions having two (3.9%) or more (1.4%).

Of the 12-month prevalence cases, 26% were classified as severe, 31% as moderate, and 43% as mild. A severe disorder was strongly associated with comorbidity, with 14% of respondents with severe disorders having one diagnosis, 47% having two, and 71% having three or more. The proportion of severe disorders was similar in the four broad groups of disorders. The anxiety disorder with the greatest proportion of severe cases was panic disorder (66%), followed by social phobia (43%) and posttraumatic stress disorder (36%). Slightly more than one-third of individuals with major depressive episode had a severe disorder. Alcohol (95%) and drug (82%) disorders tended to be severe diagnoses.

The provincial rates of 12-month prevalence showed the same significant excess in Western Cape and Free State (as seen in the lifetime prevalence rates) as compared to the rest of the country (Table 11.10). Much of the excess was reflected in an increase in moderate disorders in Western Cape and Free State and an excess in serious disorders in Western Cape (Table 11.11).

**Table 11.10.** Provincial 12-month prevalence estimates (%) of DSM-IV/CIDI disorders

| Province | All disorders | Specific disorders (grouped) | | | | |
| | | Anxiety | Mood | Substance use | Impulse | n |
| --- | --- | --- | --- | --- | --- | --- |
| Western Cape | 22.7* | 8.9 | 7.5 | 8.6* | 3.3* | 448 |
| Free State | 24.3* | 13.8* | 8.1* | 8.0 | 2.5 | 421 |
| North West | 16.7 | 8.4 | 2.5* | 7.1 | 0.8 | 453 |
| Limpopo | 17.3 | 10.1 | 2.8* | 5.9 | 1.2 | 420 |
| Kwazulu-Natal | 13.9 | 4.9* | 4.9 | 5.3 | 1.4 | 749 |
| Gauteng | 16.6 | 9.2 | 4.6 | 5.8 | 3.2* | 593 |
| Mpumalanga | 13.7 | 8.6 | 3.9 | 2.7 | 0.1* | 415 |
| Eastern Cape | 12.0* | 5.9* | 4.5 | 3.0 | 0.4 | 619 |
| Northern Cape | 19.2 | 11.0 | 6.0 | 7.5 | 2.3 | 233 |
| South Africa | 16.6 | 8.2 | 4.8 | 5.7 | 1.8 | 4351 |

* $p < 0.05$ in contrasting province with South Africa as a whole.

## 4.7. Prevalence and Severity of 12-month Disorders in the WMH

South Africa has a high 12-month prevalence of anxiety and mood disorders as compared to the other 16 countries in the WMH Survey, as is shown in Chapter 26 of this volume. Belgium, France, Germany, New Zealand, the Netherlands, Colombia, Lebanon, and the United States have higher rates of anxiety disorders, and Belgium, Lebanon, Colombia, the Netherlands, France, Ukraine, Israel, New Zealand, and the United States have higher rates of mood disorders. Twenty-six percent of DSM-IV disorders in

**Table 11.11.** Severity of 12-month DSM-IV/CIDI disorders by province

| Province | Severity of disorder | | | |
| | Mild | Moderate | Severe | n |
| --- | --- | --- | --- | --- |
| Western Cape | 8.5% | 6.9%* | 6.5%* | 448 |
| Free State | 7.3% | 11.8%* | 5.7% | 423 |
| North West | 7.5% | 3.1%* | 5.3% | 453 |
| Limpopo | 7.1% | 5.2% | 3.3% | 420 |
| Kwazulu-Natal | 6.1% | 4.3% | 4.1% | 749 |
| Gauteng | 6.3% | 5.3% | 4.7% | 591 |
| Mpumalanga | 8.2% | 3.6%* | 1.2%* | 415 |
| Eastern Cape | 4.9% | 4.0%* | 3.6% | 619 |
| Northern Cape | 7.3% | 6.0% | 4.3% | 233 |
| South Africa | 6.8% | 5.4% | 4.3% | 4351 |

* $p < 0.05$.

South Africa are considered severe, with only Belgium, Israel, and the Netherlands having higher rates of severe DSM-IV disorders.

There are only two African countries that participated in the WMH Survey: South Africa and Nigeria. The Nigerian Survey of Mental Health and Well-Being was conducted in five of six of the geopolitical regions of that country, see Chapter 10 of this volume for more description. Only one in 17 Nigerians had a DSM disorder in the preceding 12 months, and only one in five months. Only one in ten Nigerians had a lifetime DSM disorder, compared to one in three South Africans. Twice as many South Africans had lifetime anxiety disorders, four times as many had lifetime mood disorders, and almost six times as many had substance use disorders, as compared to Nigerians.

## 4.8. Bivariate Analyses of 12-month Comorbidity

Table 11.12 shows the tetrachoric correlations between hierarchy-free 12-month disorders. Only two are positively correlated and significant at $p < 0.05$ (AG × SoP and AA × AD), with 23 (42%) of the remainder being positively correlated and marginally significant ($0.05 < p < 0.10$). Drug dependence had a strong negative association with agoraphobia, social phobia, posttraumatic stress disorder, major depressive

**Table 11.12.** Tetrachoric correlations among hierarchy-free 12-month DSM-IV/CIDI disorders and factor loadings from a principal axis factor analysis of the correlation matrix

| Disorders | PD | AG | SoP | GAD | PTSD | MDE | IED | AA | AD | DA | DD |
|---|---|---|---|---|---|---|---|---|---|---|---|
| **Anxiety disorders** | | | | | | | | | | | |
| Panic disorder | 1.0 | | | | | | | | | | |
| Agoraphobia | 0.4 | 1.0 | | | | | | | | | |
| Social phobia | 0.5* | 0.6† | 1.0 | | | | | | | | |
| Generalized anxiety disorder | 0.4 | 0.3* | 0.5* | 1.0 | | | | | | | |
| Posttraumatic stress disorder | 0.2 | −0.1 | − | 0.4 | 1.0 | | | | | | |
| **Mood disorders** | | | | | | | | | | | |
| Major depressive episode | 0.3* | 0.3* | 0.3* | 0.4* | 0.4* | 1.0 | | | | | |
| **Impulse-control disorders** | | | | | | | | | | | |
| Intermittent explosive disorder | 0.3 | 0.3* | 0.3* | 0.4* | 0.1 | 0.4* | 1.0 | | | | |
| **Substance use disorders** | | | | | | | | | | | |
| Alcohol abuse | −0.1 | 0.2* | 0.3* | 0.2* | 0.0 | 0.1* | 0.5* | 1.0 | | | |
| Alcohol dependence | 0.4 | 0.2* | 0.3 | 0.3 | 0.2 | 0.2* | 0.3 | 0.8† | 1.0 | | |
| Drug abuse | 0.3 | 0.2* | 0.0 | 0.1 | 0.3 | 0.2* | 0.2 | 0.5* | 0.5* | 1.0 | |
| Drug dependence | 0.5 | −0.9† | −0.8† | 0.4 | −0.7† | −0.9† | −0.8† | 0.5 | 0.5 | 1.0† | 1.0 |
| Factor 1 | 0.4 | 0.3 | 0.4 | 0.3 | 0.1 | 0.3 | 0.2 | 0.0 | 0.1 | 0.0 | 0.0 |
| Factor 2 | 0.0 | 0.0 | 0.1 | 0.2 | 0.0 | 0.0 | 0.2 | 0.6 | 0.5 | 0.3 | 0.2 |

* $0.05 < p < 0.10$; † $p < 0.05$.

*Note:* Empty cells due to insufficient numbers for the estimate.

disorder, and intermittent explosive disorder. Major depressive episode was marginally correlated with all other disorders.

## 4.9. Sociodemographic Correlates of 12-month Disorders and Treatment

Being female was associated with increased severity of mental disorders. Compared to individuals aged 65 and older, there was an increased prevalence of any disorders in 35- to 49-year-olds. There was an increasing trend of treatment with increasing age to 64 years. Individuals with a low-average income had a decreased risk of disorders compared to individuals with high incomes. Individuals who were separated, widowed, or divorced had an increased risk of any disorder and more severe disorders compared to married individuals (Table 11.13).

Mood and anxiety disorders were more common among women, and substance use disorders were more common among men. Mood disorders and impulse-control disorders were disorders of younger individuals; substance use dis-

orders were most common among 35- to 49-year-olds. Mood disorders were more frequent among separated, widowed, and divorced individuals and among people with only an elementary school education (Table 11.14). Anxiety disorders were associated with being female (except among those older than 65 years; and those with an elementary education (especially among 35- to 49-year-olds). Mood disorders were associated with being female among 18- to 34-year-olds and individuals with an elementary and high school education (especially among 18- to 34-year-olds). Substance use disorders were more frequent among men (of all ages except 65+-year-olds) and individuals with more than a high school education (compared to those who were still students). There were no interactions between age and education and age and sex for specific disorders (Table 11.15).

## 4.10. Probability of 12-month Service Use

Table 11.16 shows the health-care and non–health-care use patterns of respondents in the

**Table 11.13.** Demographic correlates of 12-month DSM-IV/CIDI disorders, severity of disorders and treatment (evaluated on 4351 individuals): Odds ratios and 95% CI

| Variables | Disorder | Severity | Any treatment |
|---|---|---|---|
| **Gender (reference: male)** | | | |
| Female | 1.1 (0.9–1.4) | 1.8 (1.2–2.7)[‡] | 1.2 (0.9–1.5) |
| $\chi_1^2$ | 1.2 | 8.8* | 1.5 |
| **Age (reference: 65+y)** | | | |
| 18–34 | 1.4 (0.9–2.3) | 2.3 (0.9–5.8) | 0.9 (0.5–1.7) |
| 35–49 | 1.8 (1.2–2.7)[‡] | 2.1 (0.9–5.0) | 1.4 (0.8–2.2) |
| 50–64 | 1.4 (0.8–2.3) | 2.4 (1.0–6.0) | 1.6 (0.8–2.8) |
| $\chi_3^2$ | 9.23* | 3.7 | 8.0* |
| **Income (reference: high)** | | | |
| Low | 0.8 (0.7–1.1) | 1.0 (0.7–1.3) | 1.4 (1.0–2.1) |
| Low average | 0.7 (0.5–0.9)[‡] | 1.3 (0.7–2.5) | 1.4 (1.0–2.1) |
| High average | 1.1 (0.7–1.6) | 1.0 (0.4–2.2) | 1.6 (1.0–2.5) |
| $\chi_3^2$ | 9.3* | 1.4 | 5.7 |
| **Marital status (reference: married/cohabiting)** | | | |
| Separated/widowed/divorced | 1.5 (1.1–2.0)[‡] | 1.9 (1.1–3.6)[‡] | 0.9 (0.6–1.3) |
| Never married | 1.2 (1.0–1.5) | 0.8 (0.5–1.3) | 0.8 (0.5–1.1) |
| $\chi_2^2$ | 11.0[†] | 7.2[†] | 3.1 |
| **Education (reference: postsecondary education)** | | | |
| Low | 1.0 (0.6–1.8) | 1.0 (0.4–2.5) | 0.7 (0.4–1.2) |
| Low average | 1.4 (0.9–2.0) | 1.4 (0.6–2.9) | 0.8 (0.5–1.2) |
| High average | 1.0 (0.7–1.3) | 1.2 (0.7–2.0) | 0.8 (0.5–1.1) |
| $\chi_3^2$ | 8.9[†] | 1.7 | 2.6 |
| Overall $\chi_{13}^2$ | 780.2[§] | 46.2[§] | 905.3[§] |

* $p < 0.05$; [†] $0.001 < p < 0.05$; [‡] $0.0001 < p < 0.001$; [§] $p < 0.0001$.

year before the study. In the prior year, 15.4% of respondents used mental health services, including 25.5% of those with DSM-IV disorders and 13.4% of those without. The proportion of cases in treatment ranged from a low of 16.6% for alcohol dependence to a high of 39.7% for social phobia. Forty-two percent of those with any anxiety disorders were treated by non-health-care providers (of these 45% received their care from CAM health providers) and 50% of individuals with mood and substance use disorders were treated by non-health-care providers (of these 58% received their care from CAM health providers). Only 20.5% of individuals in the health-care group received their care from psychiatrists, 15% from nonphysician mental health care professionals (mostly mental health nurses in primary health care centers), 29% from other

mental health care providers (psychologists and social workers), and the remainder from general medical practitioners.

Almost 28% of individuals with severe or moderate disorders received some treatment; 24.4% of those with a mild disorder received treatment and 13.8% with no disorder received treatment. Overall, 15.9% of people with any disorder received treatment (Table 11.17).

## 4.11. Predictors of 12-month Service Use

Table 11.18 shows the association between specific disorders and sociodemographic variables and 12-month service use in the SASH. Specific disorders are not associated with service use and younger people are more likely to use health services (compared to those aged 65 and older).

**Table 11.14.** Demographic correlates of specific 12-month DSM-IV/CIDI disorders evaluated on 4351 individuals

| Variables | Mood OR (95% CI) | Anxiety OR (95% CI) | Impulse control OR (95% CI) | Substance use OR (95% CI) |
|---|---|---|---|---|
| **Gender (reference: male)** | | | | |
| Female | 2.0 (1.3–3.0)* | 2.1 (1.6–2.9)* | 1.0 (0.5–2.0) | 0.3 (0.2–0.4)* |
| $\chi_1^2$ | 11.3[†] | 26.6[§] | 0.0 | 39.3[§] |
| **Age (reference: 65+ y)** | | | | |
| 18–34 | 2.6 (1.3–5.5)* | 0.9 (0.5–1.8) | 7387.6 (2857.2–19102.0)[§] | 2.6 (0.9–7.5) |
| 35–49 | 2.2 (1.1–4.4)* | 1.3 (0.8–2.2) | 7075.0 (2906.2–17224.0)[§] | 3.6 (1.2–10.5)* |
| 50–64 | 2.0 (1.0–4.2) | 1.1 (0.6–2.0) | 1.2 (0.8–1.7) | 2.7 (0.8–9.6) |
| $\chi_3^2$ | 7.1 | 5.5 | 1044.5[§] | 7.3 |
| **Income (reference: high income)** | | | | |
| Low | 0.8 (0.5–1.2) | 0.9 (0.6–1.2) | 0.5 (0.2–1.1) | 0.9 (0.6–1.5) |
| Low average | 0.9 (0.5–1.4) | 0.7 (0.5–1.1) | 0.3 (0.1–1.0)* | 0.6 (0.3–1.0) |
| High average | 0.6 (0.3–1.2) | 1.0 (0.6–1.8) | 0.7 (0.2–3.2) | 1.1 (0.5–2.6) |
| $\chi_3^2$ | 3.3 | 2.6 | 6.0 | 5.0 |
| **Marital status (reference: married/cohabiting)** | | | | |
| Separated/widowed/divorced | 2.2 (1.4–3.5)* | 1.5 (1.0–2.2) | 2.7 (0.8–9.2) | 1.2 (0.6–2.6) |
| Never married | 0.7 (0.5–1.1) | 1.3 (1.0–1.6) | 2.1 (0.9–5.2) | 1.5 (1.0–2.1) |
| $\chi_3^2$ | 12.3[†] | 5.2 | 4.5 | 4.6 |
| **Education (reference: high education)** | | | | |
| Low | 0.6 (0.2–1.8) | 1.2 (0.6–2.4) | 1.1 (0.2–6.7) | 1.0 (0.5–2.1) |
| Low–Average | 2.1 (1.0–4.3)* | 1.4 (0.8–2.5) | 0.8 (0.2–2.7) | 0.7 (0.4–1.2) |
| High–Average | 1.0 (0.5–1.9) | 1.3 (0.8–2.1) | 0.8 (0.2–2.8) | 0.8 (0.5–1.3) |
| $\chi_3^2$ | 16.0[†] | 2.0 | 0.5 | 2.1 |
| Overall $\chi_{13}^2$ | 1278.3[§] | 1539.4[§] | 1930000.0[§] | 1570.2[§] |

* $p < 0.05$; [†] $0.001 < p < 0.05$; [‡] $0.0001 < p < 0.001$; [§] $p < 0.0001$.

Table 11.19 shows the association between race and type of care accessed. Whites, Coloureds and Indians are significantly more likely to access psychiatric care (compared to blacks) or any mental health care. Coloureds are significantly less likely to use CAM (compared to blacks).

## 4.12. Prevalence of Treatment in WMH Countries

Compared to the 16 other countries in the WMH, South Africa is among the bottom 4 in providing treatment for a diagnosis of moderate or severe DSM-IV disorder (27.6% for South Africans with either moderate or severe mental disorders compared to 58.7% for severe and 37.4% for mod-erate disorders among Spaniards). South Africa ranks first among the 16 countries that treat those with no mental disorder (13.4% of South Africans with no mental disorder receive mental health care, compared to 1% of Nigerians; see Chapter 27 of this volume).

There are two tiers of treatment coverage for WMH survey countries: those countries where 50% or more of people with severe disorders and 30% or more of people with moderate disorders receive care, and those countries where 25% or fewer of persons with moderate or severe mental disorders receive treatment. The first tier is made up of the United States and the developed countries of Western Europe, and the second tier includes Japan among the developing countries.

**Table 11.15.** Variation across cohorts in the association of education and gender with first age of onset of DSM-IV/CIDI disorders

| Predictors | All age groups OR (95% CI) | Age group | | | |
|---|---|---|---|---|---|
| | | 18y–34y OR (95% CI) | 35y–49y OR (95% CI) | 50y–64y OR (95% CI) | 65+y OR (95% CI) |
| **Anxiety disorders** | | | | | |
| **Education (reference: postsecondary education)** | | | | | |
| Student | 1.1 (0.6–1.8) | 1.3 (0.6–2.9) | 2.0 (0.4–9.2) | 0.5 (0.6–4.5) | 1.1 (0.1–12.9) |
| Low | 1.3 (0.6–2.7) | 0.5 (0.1–1.8) | 3.4 (0.7–16.4) | 0.8 (0.1–6.9) | 2.3 (0.4–14.9) |
| Low/medium | 1.5 (1.0–2.3)[†] | 1.0 (0.6–1.8) | 4.3 (1.2–16.0)[†] | 0.9 (0.1–6.7) | 3.2 (0.5–21.9) |
| Medium | 1.3 (0.8–2.0) | 1.0 (0.6–1.9) | 3.1 (0.8–12.5) | 1.0 (0.1–6.9) | 1.0 (1.0–1.0) |
| $\chi_4^2$ | 9.7* | 2.7 | 18.6[†] | 1.2 | 2.1 |
| **Gender (reference: male)** | | | | | |
| Female | 1.7 (1.4–2.1)[†] | 1.8 (1.4–2.4)[†] | 1.5 (0.9–2.5) | 2.4 (1.0–5.5)[†] | 1.0 (0.3–3.0) |
| $\chi_1^2$ | 24.6[‡] | 16.8[‡] | 2.0 | 4.3* | 0.0 |
| **Age (reference: 65+)** | | | | | |
| 18–34 | 2.0 (1.1–3.6)[†] | | | | |
| 35–49 | 1.4 (0.8–2.6) | | | | |
| 50–64 | 0.8 (0.4–1.4) | | | | |
| $\chi_3^2$ | 24.2[‡] | | | | |
| Age × education $\chi_{11}^2$ | 12.8 | | | | |
| Age × gender $\chi_3^2$ | 2.1 | | | | |
| **Major depression** | | | | | |
| **Education (reference: postsecondary education)** | | | | | |
| Student | 1.0 (0.4–2.3) | 1.3 (0.5–3.5) | 0.6 (0.1–3.3) | 0.8 (0.1–3.4) | |
| Low | 0.8 (0.3–2.1) | 0.3 (0.0–2.0) | 0.8 (0.1–5.1) | 0.9 (0.2–4.1) | 0.1 (0.1–1.4) |
| Low/medium | 2.6 (1.4–4.9) | 2.6 (1.3–5.4) | 2.9 (0.7–11.9) | 1.1 (0.4–3.5) | 1.0 (1.0–1.0) |
| Medium | 1.9 (1.0–3.8) | 1.7 (0.8–3.7) | 2.6 (0.6–10.2) | 1.0 (1.0–1.0) | |
| $\chi_4^2$ | 28.9[‡] | 13.2* | 20.8[‡] | 0.1 | 2.9 |
| **Gender (reference: male)** | | | | | |
| Female | 1.7 (1.1–2.6)[†] | 1.8 (1.2–2.9)[†] | 1.3 (0.7–2.5) | 1.9 (0.6–6.3) | 3.0 (0.3–31.5) |
| $\chi_1^2$ | 5.4* | 7.0[†] | 0.5 | 1.0 | 0.9 |
| **Age (reference: 65+)** | | | | | |
| 18–34 | 10.5 (3.9–28.0)[†] | | | | |
| 35–49 | 5.2 (1.8–15.1)[†] | | | | |
| 50–64 | 2.4 (0.8–7.5) | | | | |
| $\chi_3^2$ | 77.5[‡] | | | | |
| Age × education $\chi_8^2$ | 7.3 | | | | |
| Age × gender $\chi_3^2$ | 1.8 | | | | |
| **Substance use disorders** | | | | | |
| **Education (reference: postsecondary education)** | | | | | |
| Student | 0.3 (0.2–0.6)[†] | 0.3 (0.1–0.7)[†] | 0.1 (0.0–0.7)[†] | 1.6 (0.1–33.9) | |
| Low | 0.7 (0.4–1.3) | 0.3 (0.1–1.0) | 0.4 (0.1–1.4) | 2.7 (0.2–29.5) | 0.6 (0.0–6.6) |
| Low/medium | 0.8 (0.5–1.3) | 0.8 (0.4–1.8) | 0.8 (0.3–1.8) | 1.7 (0.2–18.7) | 0.3 (0.0–3.0) |
| Medium | 1.2 (0.7–1.8) | 1.1 (0.6–2.0) | 1.0 (0.5–2.0) | 2.7 (0.3–23.9) | 1.1 (0.1–14.1) |
| $\chi_4^2$ | 42.4[‡] | 27.9[‡] | 17.2[‡] | 2.1 | 2.6 |

| Predictors | All age groups OR (95% CI) | Age group | | | |
|---|---|---|---|---|---|
| | | 18y–34y OR (95% CI) | 35y–49y OR (95% CI) | 50y–64y OR (95% CI) | 65+y OR (95% CI) |
| Gender (reference: male) | | | | | |
| Female | 0.3 (0.2–0.4)[†] | 0.3 (0.2–0.4)[†] | 0.3 (0.2–0.4)[†] | 0.3 (0.1–0.5)[†] | 0.6 (0.1–2.6) |
| $\chi_1^2$ | 74.9[‡] | 42.4[‡] | 34.2[‡] | 12.5[‡] | 0.6 |
| Age (reference: 65+) | | | | | |
| 18–34 | 2.7 (1.2–6.3)[†] | | | | |
| 35–49 | 1.5 (0.7–3.2) | | | | |
| 50–64 | 1.2 (0.6–2.5) | | | | |
| $\chi_3^2$ | 23.9[‡] | | | | |
| Age × education $\chi_8^2$ | 6.2 | | | | |
| Age × gender $\chi_3^2$ | 1.0 | | | | |

* $0.01 < p < 0.05$; [†] $0.0001 < p < 0.01$; [‡] $p < 0.0001$.

# 5. DISCUSSION

## 5.1. Limitations of the SASH Findings

The interpretation of our results should take into account those limitations that are specific to the SASH and common across WMH surveys:

- We did not assess a number of key DSM-IV disorders; therefore, some individuals who were assessed as having no disorder and being in treatment may have had a clinical disorder not evaluated in the SASH.
- Homeless and institutionalized persons were excluded.
- Although the SASH had a relatively high response rate, the biases that are common with nonresponse errors, errors in recall, nonreporting, and diagnostic errors will likely lead to an underestimation of prevalence and unmet treatment needs.
- The SASH is a lay-administered interview, which may lead to systematic error.
- Health service use is commonly systematically over- or understated in interview data.

## 5.2. Historical Context of Mental Health Care in South Africa

The first center to cater to mentally ill patients in South Africa was an apartment in the Cape Hospital in the Cape of Good Hope in 1711. The first asylum for mentally ill patients was opened in the Old Somerset Hospital in the Cape of Good Hope in 1818 (Emsley 2001). Over the ensuing two centuries, the provision of mental health care was increasingly defined by the policies of racism that defined the South African state. To understand the evolution of psychiatry and mental health care in South Africa, one must appreciate the role of colonialism and apartheid in defining the African as an inferior other. Before 1948, successive colonial administrations saw the African as the primitive inferior other, with Coloureds and Indians occupying that vague eugenic middle ground between the advanced white and the primitive savage African. After the electoral success of the National Party in 1948 and with the advent of apartheid, the racial other was further characterized within the context of psychiatry as mentally primitive and emotionally immature.

Diagnostic rate ratios from government mental hospitals during this period reflected a hierarchy of diagnoses with the more advanced white patient being at greater risk of a more refined diagnosis like depression or anxiety and the less advanced and more primitive black patient being more likely to be diagnosed as having a less refined diagnoses (that commonly reject a distortion of reality) like schizophrenia and paranoia. This pattern can be seen in the prevalence rate ratios for the major psychiatric diagnostic categories in hospital data during the period from 1962 to 1968. Almost 70% of patients in government

**Table 11.16.** Prevalence of 12-month health service use in separate service sector by 12-month DSM-IV/CIDI disorders

| Disorders | Health care | | | | | Non–health-care | | | Any treatment | n_w |
| --- | --- | --- | --- | --- | --- | --- | --- | --- | --- | --- |
| | Mental health | | | General medical | Any health care | Human services | CAM[c] | Any non–health-care | | |
| | Psychiatrist | Other[a] | Any[b] | | | | | | | |
| **Anxiety disorders** | | | | | | | | | | |
| GAD | 6.7 (2.8) | 9.2 (3.7) | 11.3 (4.0) | 22.9 (5.9) | 28.6 (5.5) | 3.9 (2.3) | 4.4 (2.2) | 6.1 (2.8) | 31.8 (5.5) | 83 |
| Panic disorder | 2.6 (2.7) | 4.8 (4.6) | 7.4 (5.4) | 13.5 (6.7) | 13.5 (6.7) | 8.8 (6.5) | 5.9 (4.3) | 12.3 (7.3) | 25.8 (9.4) | 34 |
| Agoraphobia | 1.6 (1.1) | 1.5 (0.9) | 2.4 (1.2) | 19.2 (3.2) | 19.5 (3.2) | 4.3 (1.7) | 5.3 (1.5) | 9.6 (2.2) | 23.4 (3.4) | 205 |
| Social phobia | 3.6 (2.4) | 7.9 (3.6) | 9.6 (3.8) | 28.3 (5.7) | 32.8 (5.5) | 14.6 (5.7) | 8.9 (3.7) | 22.6 (6.1) | 39.7 (6.1) | 81 |
| Any anxiety | 3.7 (1.1) | 4.0 (1.2) | 6.2 (1.7) | 20.1 (2.5) | 22.5 (2.7) | 6.6 (1.7) | 5.4 (1.3) | 11.5 (2.0) | 27.2 (3.0) | 360 |
| **Mood disorders** | | | | | | | | | | |
| Major depressive | 4.0 (1.7) | 4.4 (1.6) | 6.8 (2.6) | 11.0 (2.4) | 15.1 (3.0) | 5.5 (1.6) | 6.6 (2.0) | 11.3 (2.5) | 22.6 (3.6) | 209 |
| Any mood | 4.2 (1.7) | 4.4 (1.6) | 6.8 (2.6) | 11.0 (2.4) | 15.1 (3.0) | 5.5 (1.6) | 6.6 (2.0) | 11.3 (2.5) | 22.6 (3.6) | 209 |
| **Substance use disorders** | | | | | | | | | | |
| Alcohol abuse | 5.0 (2.2) | 1.4 (0.7) | 6.0 (2.3) | 15.4 (3.7) | 18.2 (3.8) | 6.0 (2.5) | 5.2 (2.1) | 11.2 (3.3) | 25.3 (4.3) | 196 |
| Alcohol dependence | 2.2 (2.2) | 0.0 (0.0) | 2.2 (2.2) | 7.1 (4.9) | 9.3 (5.3) | 2.7 (2.7) | 9.2 (5.5) | 11.9 (6.0) | 16.6 (6.6) | 50 |
| Drug abuse | 3.7 (2.9) | 2.0 (1.5) | 4.9 (3.1) | 28.0 (6.7) | 28.7 (6.8) | 11.2 (4.6) | 15.4 (6.5) | 24.6 (6.4) | 43.1 (8.5) | 61 |
| Any substance | 4.4 (2.0) | 1.4 (0.6) | 5.5 (2.0) | 16.4 (3.0) | 19.1 (3.2) | 6.2 (2.1) | 7.9 (2.2) | 13.6 (2.8) | 27.6 (4.0) | 249 |
| **Composite** | | | | | | | | | | |
| Any disorder | 3.9 (1.0) | 2.9 (0.7) | 5.6 (1.3) | 16.6 (1.8) | 19.0 (2.0) | 6.6 (1.4) | 5.9 (1.0) | 12.0 (1.7) | 25.5 (2.5) | 690 |
| No disorder | 1.3 (0.3) | 0.8 (0.2) | 1.9 (0.3) | 9.0 (0.8) | 10.1 (0.8) | 3.1 (0.4) | 3.2 (0.3) | 5.7 (0.5) | 13.4 (0.9) | 3,625 |
| Part 2 rates | 1.7 (0.3) | 1.1 (0.2) | 2.5 (0.4) | 10.2 (0.8) | 11.5 (0.8) | 3.7 (0.4) | 3.7 (0.3) | 6.7 (0.6) | 15.4 (1.0) | 4,315 |

*Note:* PTSD ($n = 25$), dysthymia ($n = 2$), and drug dependence ($n = 5$) were excluded because of small numbers. $n_w$ = weighted number of respondents meeting criteria for each 12-month DSM-IV/CIDI disorder.

[a] Other mental health professional (mental health nurse, psychologist, social worker).

[b] Any mental health care provider.

[c] Complementary and alternative medicine (usually traditional healer).

**Table 11.17.** Severity of disorder by type of treatment

| Treatment | Moderate–severe % | (se) | Mild % | (se) | None % | (se) | Any disorder % | (se) |
|---|---|---|---|---|---|---|---|---|
| General medical | 19.4 | (2.5) | 14.6 | (2.2) | 9.3 | (0.8) | 10.6 | (0.8) |
| Mental health | 7.2 | (1.8) | 4.0 | (1.6) | 2.1 | (0.4) | 2.7 | (0.5) |
| Other health care | 22.1 | (2.7) | 17.0 | (2.3) | 10.4 | (0.9) | 12.0 | (0.9) |
| Non–health-care | 12.9 | (2.2) | 11.6 | (2.1) | 5.9 | (0.7) | 7.0 | (0.6) |
| Any treatment | 27.6 | (3.0) | 24.4 | (3.3) | 13.8 | (0.9) | 15.9 | (1.0) |
| No treatment | 72.4 | (3.0) | 75.6 | (3.3) | 86.2 | (0.9) | 84.1 | (1.0) |

**Table 11.18.** Sociodemographic and DSM-IV/CIDI disorder predictors of 12-month service use in the SASH (odds ratios and 95% CI for any given treatment)

| Predictors | $\psi$ (95% CI) | Wald $\chi^2$ |
|---|---|---|
| **Anxiety (reference: no disorder)** | | |
| Any anxiety disorder | 1.4 (0.9–2.2) | 2.2 |
| **Mood (reference: no disorder)** | | |
| Any mood disorder | 0.9 (0.5–1.6) | 0.2 |
| **Substance use (reference: no disorder)** | | |
| Any substance use disorder | 1.8 (0.9–3.3) | 3.3* |
| **Age (reference: 65+)** | | |
| 18 years to 34 years | 8.2 (1.5–46.1) | 7.3* |
| 35 years to 49 years | 8.8 (1.7–45.0) | |
| 50 years to 64 years | 8.7 (1.6–46.3) | |
| **Education (reference: 13+ years)** | | |
| Elementary school: 0 to 6 years | 1.5 (0.5–4.1) | 3.5 |
| Middle school: 7 to 9 years | 1.0 (0.5–2.3) | |
| High school: 10 to 12 years | 0.8 (0.4–1.5) | |
| **Income (reference: high income)** | | |
| Low | 1.2 (0.7–2.2) | 1.5 |
| Low average | 0.9 (0.5–2.0) | |
| High average | 1.3 (0.6–2.9) | |
| **Marital status (reference: married/cohabiting)** | | |
| Never married | 0.6 (0.3–1.1) | 7.3† |
| Separated/widowed/divorced | 1.6 (0.8–3.5) | |
| **Gender (reference: female)** | | |
| Male | 0.7 (0.4–1.1) | 2.9* |
| **Race (reference: black)** | | |
| White | 1.2 (0.6–2.6) | 1.5 |
| Coloured | 0.6 (0.3–1.1) | |
| Indian | 0.8 (0.3–2.3) | |

* $0.05 < p < 0.10$; † $p < 0.05$.

**Table 11.19.** 12-month service use by race (reference: black)

| Race | Health care | | | | |
|---|---|---|---|---|---|
| | Psychiatrist OR (95% CI) | Other mental health care OR (95% CI) | Any mental health care OR (95% CI) | General practitioner OR (95% CI) | Any health care OR (95% CI) |
| White | 14.3 (4.7–43.6)* | 5.2 (2.2–9.4)* | 11.2 (4.7–26.7)* | 0.9 (0.5–1.5) | 1.7 (0.9–3.0) |
| Coloured | 5.2 (1.6–17.6)* | 1.7 (0.4–7.6) | 3.0 (1.1–8.3)* | 0.6 (0.3–1.6) | 0.8 (0.3–1.8) |
| Indian | 7.8 (1.2–48.2)* | | 3.9 (0.7–21.6) | 1.1 (0.4–3.2) | 1.0 (0.3–2.9) |

| Race | Non–health care | | |
|---|---|---|---|
| | Human services OR (95% CI) | CAM OR (95% CI) | Any non–health care OR (95% CI) |
| White | 0.4 (0.0–2.3) | 0.2 (0.0–1.1) | |
| Coloured | 0.5 (0.1–1.6) | 0.0 (0.0–0.3)* | 0.2 (0.1–0.8)* |
| Indian | 2.1 (0.5–9.4) | 0.2 (0.0–1.6) | 1.1 (0.3–4.3) |

* $p < 0.05$.

mental health hospitals during that time with a diagnosis of defective mental development (an organic psychosis that was associated with insufficient development of the brain but did not include senile or atherosclerotic psychosis, toxic psychosis, or psychosis caused by syphilis) were white; 50% of patients with a diagnosis of manic-depressive psychosis were white, but only 20% of patients with schizophrenia and paranoia were white. Even when confronted by the same mental health outcomes in different races (e.g., suicide), the causes of such outcomes were usually ascribed to the refinement of the individual in the case of whites and the lack of refinement of the person when such a person is black (Jones 2000). A more modern version of the racial other was enunciated by Pretorius (1995) in his apologia for the poverty of mental health services for blacks in South Africa. He suggested that:

- 80% of blacks see a traditional healer before or after consulting a Western health-care provider.
- Blacks regard illness, particularly mental illness as the material sign of lack of harmony between a person and his social environment.
- Blacks have a distinction between natural and supernatural causes of disease.
- Blacks do not distinguish between physical and psychological illness.

## 5.3. Long-term Policy Analysis

Apartheid policies formed the basis of all health care before 1992, and these policies divided the health sector into 14 racially independent health departments with each homeland (i.e., quasi-independent state within South Africa), duplicating the services of provincial administrations. The 1913 Native Land Act and the related Natives Trust and Land Act of 1936 provided for 15.1 million hectares of land (13%) to be designated as native reserves in South Africa. Black people were often forcibly removed to these areas, which became known as the homelands or independent states. Additionally, black people were denied the right to own land outside of these reserves. With the new dispensation, these homelands were incorporated into the nine provinces. Additionally, each of the 400 local authorities had health departments (Bloom & McIntyre 1998). South Africa had many Health Rendering Authorities (HRAs) responsible for health service delivery. Although the vertical structure of the health-care system (with the hospital at the apex of a community health care system) has its foundation in the 1944 Gluckman Report, the horizontal (racial and regional) structure arises out of the apartheid policies that became firmly established after the 1948 election. Additionally, the health-care system was centered around the hospital, and as

Petersen and her colleagues argue, (Petersen 2000; Petersen & Swartz 2002), this has made it difficult to implement a comprehensive district-based, primary health-care system. They suggest that primary mental health care is not possible without integrating nonbiomedical approaches into the health-care system. Pillay and colleagues have demonstrated a lack of adequate mental health services and a lack of access to those services particularly to those in rural areas and to children (Pillay & Lockhat 1997; Pillay & Kriel 2006).

Although race and cultural identity played an important role in the provision of health care during the twentieth century, the policies that governed mental health care in South Africa also rejected the changing political landscape of the country, the substantial changes in psychiatry and mental health care in the twentieth century, and the changing role of race in the South African society. The key events that defined the legislative and policy contexts of mental health care over the past century are the following:

**1.** The end of the second South African War in 1910 and the creation of the Union of South Africa heralded a number of critical changes in the legislative and policy context of mental health in South Africa. In 1914, the Lunacy and Leprosy Laws of the Union were amended to ensure cross-provincial certification of mental illness and leprosy. In 1916, the Mental Disorders Act (No. 38) was enacted (adapted from Britain's Mental Disorders Act) to unify the mental health services under the custodial care of a commissioner of mental hygiene in the Department of Interior.

**2.** In 1944, during a period of critical transformation in health care, the Mental Disorders Act of 1916 was amended following a Commission of Inquiry into the Mental Disorders Act. This amendment heralded a change from custodial to therapeutic care and the introduction of community mental health care. As a reflection of this change, mental health care policy and decision making was moved from the Department of Interior to the Department of Health and mental asylums were renamed "mental hospitals."

**3.** Between 1948 and 1950, a number of key apartheid laws were enacted: (a) the Mixed Marriages Act, prohibiting marriage across racial lines, (b) the Group Areas Act, restricting racial groups to specific geographies, (c) the Population Registration Act, defining racial groups, (d) Immorality Act, prohibiting sexual relations across racial lines, and (e) Native Laws Amendment Act, mostly restricting the mobility of black South Africans. These laws redefined the nature of race and identity in South Africa and greatly influenced the changes that would take place in mental health care provision in the latter half of the twentieth century.

**4.** In 1967, the Prime Minister of South Africa was assassinated and the Rump Commission of Inquiry that investigated the role of psychiatry and the existing legal statutes regulating the responsibility of mentally deranged persons further separated the custodial and therapeutic aspects of existing mental health care. Coincident with the Rump Commission, a second commission (headed by Supreme Court Judge J. T. van Wyk) examined the existing legal regulations concerning psychiatric services. Both commissions resulted in the 1973 Mental Health Act.

**5.** The current Health and Mental Health Acts are designed to lead to the destigmatization of mental health, the deinstitutionalization of long-term residents of psychiatric hospitals, the expansion of primary mental health care and the integration of mental health care into the primary health-care setting. This process has been difficult, in part because of the paucity of well-trained health-care professionals with adequate training in mental health care.

## 5.4. Mental Health Care Facilities in Twentieth-Century South Africa

In 1910, there were 8 government mental health institutions with 3,624 inpatients; by 1965, there were 15 government mental health institutions with 8,747 beds for 13,979 black, Coloured, and Indian patients and 8,662 beds for 8,054 white patients. The government was not inclined to increase the capacity of mental health care for blacks, Coloureds and Indians, as such an increase would directly contradict the policies of apartheid where the responsibility for the care of individuals rested with defined racial communities. In 1962, Alistair Lamont, the then Commissioner of Mental Hygiene requested that Smith Mitchell & Company (now called Lifecare Inc.) provide temporary psychiatric beds for black patients. The company transformed mining hostels and tuberculosis facilities into mental health hospitals. The resulting institutions, referred to as Smith Mitchell institutions, became a permanent fixture of mental health care over the subsequent three decades. Government ministers and members of the ruling Nationalist Party profited from their associations with the company. The Department of Health appointed Smith Mitchell staff and most patients were transferred from government mental hospitals to the Smith Mitchell facilities. Between 1963 and 1985, Smith Mitchell increased the total number of beds to 11,972. Of these, 1102 beds were for white patients, 750 beds were for Coloured and Indian patients, and the remaining beds were for black patients.

Conditions for most patients in these institutions were appalling. Wards housed between 40 and 250 patients. Patients did not have their own beds and mostly slept on mattresses on the floor of the wards. Many black patients were not provided with bedding. Clothing was inadequate. Heating during winter was usually insufficient and bathing facilities were poor, mostly without hot water and privacy. Treatment was frequently nonexistent and most patients worked in on-site factories or in the hospitals. Some patients were hired out to local farmers or businesses and their income from these occupations were, for the most part, used to augment the income of Smith Mitchell & Company. Among those patients who were paid, blacks were paid less than one-third the income of whites and mental health patients were paid half the income paid to tuberculosis (TB) patients (also housed by Smith Mitchell & Company). Often Smith Mitchell mental health facilities and TB sanatoriums were in close proximity to each other, and mental health patients often worked in TB sanatoriums. Physical and

sexual abuse was common and rarely investigated. Women patients were sterilized or given some form of birth control. The physical and sexual abuse of psychiatric inpatients is still prevalent. Lucas and Stevenson (2006) reported abuse rates of 52.7% among 127 inpatients interviewed in 2005. Of the abuse, 38.8% was patient-on-patient violence, with 28.4% staff-on-patient violence and 32.8% of the patients reporting staff- and patient-on-patient violence. Medical care was poor and psychiatric care was almost nonexistent. Psychiatrists, almost always associated with academic institutions, usually served multiple institutions and rarely worked full-time for the Smith Mitchell institutions. All general practitioners and psychiatrists serving the patients before 1985, with the exception of one Indian doctor, were white. Diagnostic approaches were for the most part primitive, and patients were categorized into four groups depending on the amount of effort a patient was to staff:

1. "A" patients showed no sign of psychosis.
2. "B" patients were not obviously psychotic but needed help with some activities of daily living.
3. "C" patients looked mentally disturbed and were not as aware of their surroundings.
4. "D" patients required specialized nursing

Few of the men (and all site superintendents were white men) who supervised these institutions had any mental health training and acted mostly as custodians of the patients in their care. Most of the nurses were black women, and they held the most difficult position within Smith Mitchell institutions of having to deal with the often-conflicting and contradictory pronouncements of the state, company, superintendents, general practitioners, and psychiatrists, while trying at the same time to cope with the demands of their patients (Jones 2000). Starting in 1974, a number of lay and professional investigations took place that examined the care of patients in the Smith Mitchell institutions. South African media (most notably the *Sunday Times* newspaper, *Scope* magazine, and the *Rand Daily Mail* newspaper), international newspapers (e.g., the *Observer* in London, *Dagens Nyheter* of Sweden, and the *Village Voice* in New York), and the Church of Scientology all described the care received by patients at the Smith Mitchell institutions. All these reports describe a mental health care system that:

1. Was segregated by race and overcrowded for blacks.
2. Was mostly custodial in nature, with minimal psychiatric care and treatment.
3. Used its patients as paid laborers to increase profits of Smith Mitchell & Company.

This generated debate in the South African parliament and led to the enactment of the Mental Health Amendment Act that prohibited the publication of any photographs, sketches, or information regarding mental patients or institutions. Paradoxically, the South African government and the Smith Mitchell institutions invited the WHO and the International Committee of the Red Cross to investigate the conditions of mental health care in South Africa. The WHO did not do an *in situ* investigation but published a scathing report on the atrocious conditions of custodial mental health care in South Africa. It pointed out that the mental health institutions were open to abuse and were manifestations of apartheid. Not much was done in response to the 1977 WHO Report and criticism continued. In 1978, Smith Mitchell invited the American Psychiatric Association to investigate both government and Smith Mitchell institutions. The association reported evidence of high death rates in hospitals, unsatisfactory care, abusive practices, deficiency of professional staff, improper use of drugs, and general exploitation of patient labor. In response to this report, David Tabatznik, chief executive officer of Smith Mitchell, with the help of his brother Bernard Tabatznik, a cardiologist living in Maryland, recruited Stanley Platman, then assistant secretary of mental health for the state of Maryland, to conduct a review of the Smith Mitchell Institutions. Stanley Platman and his wife, Vera (a South African–born midwife) conducted their first review in 1981 and were given relatively full access to all parts of the institutions. Although much was done to improve the general quality of life for patients in response to the investigations of the Platmans, by 1998 the Centre for Health Policy at the University of

the Witwatersrand reported that mental health institutions were mostly custodial institutions for control and were producing low-quality care at low costs.

Currently, there are 24 registered public psychiatric hospitals in South Africa, accommodating more than 14,000 acute- and long-term-care patients. In 2001, the bed occupancy rate for the country was 83% (provincial range: 63%–109%); the annual rate of admission into psychiatric inpatient facilities was 150 per 100,000 population (provincial range: 33–300); the average length of stay of mental health patients was 219 days in psychiatric hospitals, 11 days in general hospitals, and 7 days in district hospitals; and 11% of psychiatric patients who attended ambulatory care services on a monthly basis failed to keep their appointments (Lund & Flisher 2001).

Most of the community health centers and primary health-care clinics have adequate but poorly maintained physical infrastructure. Water supply, electricity, communications, transportation, and security levels are poor and inadequate for the majority of the community-based health centers. Referral policies and protocols are adequate and, for the most part, work well, and patients are regularly referred from the primary health clinic to the community health center and hospital. Access to most community health centers and primary health-care clinics is poor, especially in the rural provinces of Limpopo, Eastern Cape, and Kwazulu-Natal. For those individuals who manage to get to these facilities, physician care is generally considered fair to good (except in the rural provinces). Surprisingly, nursing services, administrative services, and clinical support services are mostly considered fair to poor. Most community health centers and primary health-care clinics in the urban centers have at least five visits per week from a mental health professional (mostly a psychologist or a social worker, rarely a psychiatrist). For the most part, mental health policies and protocols are adequately implemented. The level of mental health training among the staff and provider-patient interaction in these community health settings is poor to fair. In general, access to specialist mental health care is poor (Herman, personal communication).

**Table 11.20.** Public service health professionals (2000–2005)

| Health professionals | South Africa | Province | Provincial Range |
|---|---|---|---|
| Clinical psychologists* | 0.7 to 1.0 | Eastern Cape | 0.4 to 0.6 |
| | | Gauteng | 2.1 to 1.7 |
| Medical practitioners* | 21.9 to 21.9 | | |
| Medical specialists* | 11.2 to 8.8 | Eastern Cape | 2.6 to 2.3 |
| | | Gauteng | 32.4 to 18.3 |
| Primary health care[†] | 23.5 to 29.4 | | |

* Per 100,000 population.
[†] Patients per nurse, per day.

## 5.5. Staffing Levels

From 1935 to 1965, the number of medical staff at mental hospitals increased from 45 to 73. Most of the staff was not trained in mental health. The number of registered psychiatrists increased from 26 in 1940 to 86 in 1964. The paucity of psychiatrists in South Africa is a reflection of the training of psychiatrists at South African medical schools. Psychiatry emerges as an independent discipline in 1922 with the initiation of teaching of medical students at the Valkenberg Mental Hospital in Western Cape. Blacks, Coloureds, and Indians gained increased access to medical education in 1951 with the creation of a medical school exclusively for blacks, Indians, and Coloureds at the University of Natal. It took an additional five years before psychiatric training was initiated for these students at Fort Napier Mental Hospital. In 1959 and 1961, full-time departments of psychiatry were established at the Universities of the Witwatersrand and Cape Town. These developments saw an almost four-fold increase in the number of registered psychiatrists in the decades after 1965. Because of the lag in the training of black, Coloured, and Indian medical practitioners, black, Coloured, and Indian psychiatrists are still a small fraction of the registered psychiatrists. Lund and Flisher describe rates of 17% of psychiatric public service staff located in community settings (provincial range: 3%–56%) and 66% (provincial range: 44%–93%) of patient contacts with mental health services that occur in ambulatory care service settings. They describe a wide variation in

health services use among the nine provinces. Their data reflect low use rates as compared to developed countries (Lund & Flisher 2003). In a second study, Lund and Flisher describe a distribution of clinical staff that indicates a focus on centralized hospital-based care coupled with inadequate community-based care (Lund & Flisher 2003).

Most of the public community health centers and district hospitals provide some level of mental health care, but access to care in the rural areas and blighted urban areas is poor. With a population of more than 45 million and slightly more than 400 registered psychiatrists (56% are in private practice and the remaining number work mostly in urban areas); much of the mental health care is provided by mental health nurses. The basic training of nurses in South Africa includes mental health nursing. Primary mental health care within the community health-care setting is mostly follow-up care of the discharged mental patient (Uys, Subedar & Lewis 1995). Additionally, the mental health nurse is being recast in a role that focuses on violence prevention, HIV/AIDS voluntary counseling, and testing service provision and substance abuse prevention rather than psychiatric care (Swartz & MacGregor 2002). Table 11.20 shows the extent to which nurses in the public sector primary health-care setting are overburdened. The absolute number of nurses in the public sector increased by 5% (41,734 to 43,660) from 2000 to 2005; however the workload of these nurses increased by 20% (23.5 to 29.4 patients per day) over the same period. Peterson

(2000) has pointed out that although the primary health-care nurse often replaces the doctor within the community health-care setting, nurses are not trained to provide comprehensive mental health care within this setting. In addition to the expanded clinical role, nurses are, and have been, cultural brokers for physicians and other health-care workers. There is a substantial unmet need within the public sector, particularly in the community health service sector. Given that the health policies of the postapartheid governments have emphasized community-based health care, this disjunction between policy and services presents a serious problem to the government. Kohn and colleagues (2004) describe postapartheid psychiatric services as deteriorating and a continuation of racial inequality and state that mental health care for black South Africans has been particularly deficient.

## 6. SURVEYS OF MENTAL HEALTH IN SOUTH AFRICA

Mental health research in South Africa prior to 1980 was largely ad hoc and idiosyncratic. The research reflected the personal interests of a small number of academic psychiatrists. The South African Medical Research Council established a clinical psychiatry research unit in 1980. Early research focused on mental illness in the elderly and the high readmission rates of psychiatric patients. This focus on readmission rates reflected ongoing deinstitutionalization of mental health patients and a movement away from custodial care to community care. Deinstitutionalization lagged by more than a decade in South Africa. Between 1964 and 1976, there was a 27% decline in inpatient psychiatric admissions and an 834% increase in outpatient visits. There was a decrease of more than 8000 inpatient beds between 1961 and 1989 (Jones 2000).

A number of mental health surveys were conducted among children and adolescents. Robertson and Juritz (1988) described rates of behavior disorders among 10- and 13-year-olds as between 10% and 20% (teacher assessment vs. parent assessment). Flisher and colleagues (1993) reported rates of attempted suicide of 7.8% and

suicide ideation of 19% among high school students. These rates were similar to those described by Mhlongo and Peltzer (1999) and Wild and colleagues (Wild, Flisher & Lombard 2004). Tobacco, drug, and alcohol use disorders are prevalent among adolescents (Flisher et al. 2003; Brook et al. 2006) and adults (Michalowsky, Wicht & Moller 1989; London 2000; Parry et al. 2002) in South Africa. Seedat and colleagues (2004), in a comparative study of posttraumatic stress disorder among grade 10 schoolchildren in Kenya and South Africa, reported similar rates of exposure to both more than one trauma and three traumas (83%, 85% and 44%, 45%) but very different rates of full symptom posttraumatic stress disorder among South African (22%) and Kenyan 5%) adolescents. In a comprehensive study of anxiety disorders among adolescents, Muris and colleagues (2002) described the following rates:

- DSM-IV anxiety disorders: 31.9% (females: 34.8%, males: 28.7%)
- DSM-IV panic disorder: 8.8% (females: 9.6%, males: 8%)
- DSM-IV generalized anxiety disorder (females: 8%, males: 6.5%)
- DSM-IV separation anxiety disorder (females: 7.7%, males: 6.2%)
- DSM-IV social phobia (females: 7.2%, males: 5.9%)
- DSM-IV school phobia (females: 2.3%, males: 2%)

Pillay and Kriel (2006) examined the use patterns of women in a district-level clinical psychology service provided at community mental health clinics, district general hospitals, and a primary health-care center serving a population of slightly more than 500,000 people. They reported 21% depression, 14% suicidal behavior, and 9.5% anxiety among women attending the service. Triant (2002) reported rates of depression of 32% and major depression of 13%; Bhagwanjee and colleagues (1998) reported a combined rate of generalized anxiety disorder and depression of 23.9%; Cooper and colleagues (1999) reported a rate of 34.7% of postpartum depression; and Carey and colleagues (2003) reported rates of 19.9% for posttraumatic stress disorder, 37% for depression, and 18.4% for somatization disorder among community health-care center attendees.

Most of the studies described in this section are clinic- or hospital-based studies or studies of children within a high school setting. These data reflect variation in rates of mental illness but emphasize a large burden of mental health disease. The SASH is the first large-scale study of the descriptive epidemiology of mental health in South Africa and gives us opportunities to describe the distributions of general mental health and the particular mental health disorders that contribute to the wellness of a society; the geographic, community, social, economic, and individual factors that influence these distributions; the susceptibility and resiliencies of individuals to these disorders; and the potential public health responses to mental health disorders.

The SASH study shows rates that are among the highest in the WMH series. What is remarkable are the stark differences in both 12-month and lifetime prevalence rates between South Africa and the only other African country in the survey, Nigeria. Nigerian rates may be much lower than South African rates because of (1) real differences in AOO of mental disorders between the two groups; (2) the differential effects of colonialism on the two countries; (3) the effect of apartheid and state-mandated racism in South Africa; (4) the differences in the age distributions of the populations in the studies; (5) the racial and ethnic differences between the two populations; and (6) the differential resiliency of the two populations.

The geographic differences in 12-month and lifetime prevalence rates across provinces are striking and could be explained by a number of sampling and contextual reasons. Western Cape was the first region of South Africa colonized by Europeans and has the longest period of colonial rule. It is also the province with a high level of urbanization, which may have an effect on the awareness of psychiatric morbidity among the people of the province. Free State is the province where apartheid was most strongly implemented. This province was the seat of the old Afrikaner

republic and during the years of apartheid the movement of blacks and Coloureds was severely restricted, and Indians were not permitted to stay for more than 24 hours in the province. The provinces also have very different age, sex, race and ethnic distributions. Finally, rural provinces like Eastern Cape, Northern Cape, Mpumalanga, and Limpopo all show much lower rates. It is also likely that the very different levels of participation in antiapartheid political activity across the provinces resulted in differences in resilience.

## REFERENCES

American Psychiatric Association (1994). *Diagnostic and statistical manual*, 4th ed. Washington, DC: American Psychiatric Association Press.

Bhagwanjee, A., Parekh, A., Paruk, Z., Petersen, I. & Subedar, H. (1998). Prevalence of minor psychiatric disorders in an adult African rural community in South Africa. *Psychological Medicine*, 28, 1137–47.

Bloom, G. & McIntyre, D. (1998). Towards equity in health in an unequal society. *Social Science and Medicine*, 47, 1529–38.

Bornman, E. (2006). National symbols and nation-building in the post-apartheid South Africa. *International Journal of Intercultural Relations*, 30, 383–99.

Brook, J. S., Morojele, N. K., Pahl, K. & Brook, D. W. (2006). Predictors of drug use among South African adolescents. *Journal of Adolescent Health*, 38, 26–34.

Carey, P. D., Stein, D. J., Zungu-Dirwayi, N. & Seedat, S. (2003). Trauma and posttraumatic stress disorder in an urban Xhosa primary care population: Prevalence, comorbidity, and service use patterns. *Journal of Nervous and Mental Disease*, 191, 230–6.

Christopher, A. J. (2004). Linguistic segregation in urban South Africa, 1996. *Geoforum*, 35, 145–56.

Cooper, P. J., Tomlinson, M., Swartz, L., Woolgar, M., Murray, L. & Molteno, C. (1999). Post-partum depression and the mother-infant relationship in a South African peri-urban settlement. *British Journal of Psychiatry*, 175, 554–8.

de Beer, J. (1977). Apartheid and mental health care. *Lancet*, 2, 1222–3.

de Beer, J. (1980). The tripartite system in mental health services. *South African Medical Journal*, 57, 433.

Demyttenaere, K., Bruffaerts, R., Posada-Villa, J., Gasquet, I., Kovess, V., Lepine, J. P., Angermeyer, M. C., Bernert, S., de Girolamo, G., Morosini, P.,

Polidori, G., Kikkawa, T., Kawakami, N., Ono, Y., Takeshima, T., Uda, H., Karam, E. G., Fayyad, J. A., Karam, A. N., Mneimneh, Z. N., Medina-Mora, M. E., Borges, G., Lara, C., de Graaf, R., Ormel, J., Gureje, O., Shen, Y., Huang, Y., Zhang, M., Alonso, J., Haro, J. M., Vilagut, G., Bromet, E. J., Gluzman, S., Webb, C., Kessler, R. C., Merikangas, K. R., Anthony, J. C., Von Korff, M. R., Wang, P. S., Brugha, T. S., Aguilar-Gaxiola, S., Lee, S., Heeringa, S., Pennell, B. E., Zaslavsky, A. M., Üstün, T. B. & Chatterji, S. (2004). Prevalence, severity, and unmet need for treatment of mental disorders in the world health organization world mental health surveys. *Journal of the American Medical Association*, 291, 2581–90.

Dommisse, J. (1986). The psychological effects of apartheid psychoanalysis: Social, moral and political influences. *International Journal of Social Psychiatry*, 32, 51–63.

Dommisse, J. (1987). The state of psychiatry in South Africa today. *Social Science and Medicine*, 24, 749–61.

Drennan, G. (1996). Counting the cost of language services in psychiatry. *South African Medical Journal*, 86, 343–5.

Drennan, G., Levett, A. & Swartz, L. (1991). Hidden dimensions of power and resistance in the translation process: A South African study. *Culture, Medicine and Psychiatry*, 15, 361–81.

Drennan, G. & Swartz, L. (2002). The paradoxical use of interpreting in psychiatry. *Social Science and Medicine*, 54, 1853–66.

Efron, B. (1988). Logistic regression, survival analysis, and the Kaplan-Meier curve. *Journal of the American Statistical Association*, 83, 414–25.

Emsley, R. (2001). Focus on psychiatry in South Africa. *British Journal of Psychiatry*, 178, 382–6.

Flisher, A. J., Parry, C. D., Evans, J., Muller, M. & Lombard, C. (2003). Substance use by adolescents in Cape Town: Prevalence and correlates. *Journal of Adolescent Health*, 32, 58–65.

Flisher, A. J., Ziervogel, C. F., Chalton, D. O., Leger, P. H. & Robertson, B. A. (1993). Risk-taking behaviour of Cape Peninsula high-school students. Part VIII. Sexual behaviour. *South African Medical Journal*, 83, 495–7.

Freeman, M. & de Beer, C. (1992). Viewing primary mental health care at a time of social transition in South Africa. *International Journal of Health Services*, 22, 339–48.

Gillis, L. S. (1977). Mental-health care in South Africa. *Lancet*, 2, 920–1.

Halli, S. S. & Rao, K. V. (1992). *Advanced techniques of population analysis*. New York: Plenum Press.

Hirschovitz, R. & Orkin, M. (1997). Trauma and mental health in South Africa. *Social Indicators Research*, 41, 169–82.

Hosmer, D. W. & Lemeshow, S. (1989). *Applied logistic regression*. New York: John Wiley & Sons.

Jones, T. F. (2000). Contradictions and constructions: Psychiatric perceptions in apartheid South Africa, 1948–1979. Master's thesis, Dalhousie University.

Kessler, R. C. & Frank, R. G. (1997). The impact of psychiatric disorders on work loss days. *Psychological Medicine*, 27, 861–73.

Kessler, R. C., Haro, J. M., Heeringa, S. G., Pennell, B. E. & Üstün, T. B. (2006). The World Health Organization World Mental Health Survey Initiative. *Epidemiologia e Psichiatria Sociale*, 15, 161–6.

Kessler, R. C. & Üstün, T. B. (2004). The World Mental Health (WMH) Survey Initiative version of the World Health Organization (WHO) Composite International Diagnostic Interview (CIDI). *International Journal of Methods in Psychiatric Research*, 13, 93–121.

Kish, L. (1949). A procedure for objective respondent selection within the household. *Journal of the American Statistical Association*, 44, 380–7.

Kohn, R., Szabo, C. P., Gordon, A. & Allwood, C. W. (2004). Race and psychiatric services in post-apartheid South Africa: A preliminary study of psychiatrists' perceptions. *International Journal of Social Psychiatry*, 50, 18–24.

London, L. (2000). Alcohol consumption amongst South African farm workers: A challenge for post-apartheid health sector transformation. *Drug and Alcohol Dependence*, 59, 199–206.

Lucas, M. & Stevenson, D. (2006). Violence and abuse in psychiatric in-patient institutions: A South African perspective. *International Journal of Law and Psychiatry*, 29, 195–203.

Lund, C. & Flisher, A. J. (2001). South African mental health process indicators. *Journal of Mental Health Policy and Economics*, 4, 9–16.

Lund, C. & Flisher, A. J. (2003). Community/hospital indicators in South African public sector mental health services. *Journal of Mental Health Policy and Economics*, 6, 181–7.

Mhlongo, T. & Peltzer, K. (1999). Parasuicide among youth in a general hospital in South Africa. *Curationis*, 22, 72–6.

Michalowsky, A. M., Wicht, C. L. & Moller, A. T. (1989). The psychosocial effects of living in an isolated community. A community health study. *South African Medical Journal*, 75, 532–4.

Muris, P., Schmidt, H., Engelbrecht, P. & Perold, M. (2002). DSM-IV-defined anxiety disorder symptoms in South African children. *Journal of the American Academy of Child and Adolescent Psychiatry*, 41, 1360–8.

Parry, C. D., Bhana, A., Myers, B., Pluddemann, A., Flisher, A. J., Peden, M. M. & Morojele, N. K. (2002). Alcohol use in South Africa: Findings from the South African Community Epidemiology Network on Drug Use (SACENDU) project. *Journal of Studies on Alcohol*, 63, 430–5.

Petersen, I. (2000). Comprehensive integrated primary mental health care for South Africa. Pipedream or possibility? *Social Science and Medicine*, 51, 321–34.

Petersen, I. & Swartz, L. (2002). Primary health care in the era of HIV/AIDS. Some implications for health systems reform. *Social Science and Medicine*, 55, 1005–13.

Pillay, A. L. & Kriel, A. J. (2006). Mental health problems in women attending district-level services in South Africa. *Social Science and Medicine*, 63, 587–92.

Pillay, A. L. & Lockhat, M. R. (1997). Developing community mental health services for children in South Africa. *Social Science and Medicine*, 45, 1493–501.

Pretorius, H. W. (1995). Mental disorders and disability across cultures: A view from South Africa. *Lancet*, 345, 534.

Republic of South Africa (2002). Mental Health Care Act, Act 17 of 2002. Available at http://www.info.gov.za/gazette/acts/2002/a17-02.pdf.

Republic of South Africa (2003). National Health Act, Act 61 of 2003. Available at http://www.info.gov.za/gazette/acts/2003/a61-03.pdf.

Robertson, B. A. & Juritz, J. M. (1988). Behavioural screening of 10- and 13-year-old pupils in selected schools in the Cape Peninsula. *South African Medical Journal*, 73, 24–5.

Seedat, S., Nyamai, C., Njenga, F., Vythilingum, B. & Stein, D. J. (2004). Trauma exposure and post-traumatic stress symptoms in urban African schools. Survey in Capetown and Nairobi. *British Journal of Psychiatry*, 184, 169–75.

South African Department of Health (1997). White paper for the transformation of the health system in South Africa. Technical report no. 382:1790.

Available at http://www.info.gov.za/whitepapers/1997/health.htm.

Statistics South Africa (2002). *Census of commercial agriculture: 2002 financial and production statistics*. Pretoria: Statistics South Africa. Available at http://www.statsonline.gov.za/publications/Report-11-02-01/CorrectedReport-11-02-01.pdf.

Swartz, L. & Drennan, G. (2000). Beyond words: Notes on the "irrelevance" of language to mental health services in South Africa. *Transcultural Psychiatry*, 37, 185–201.

Swartz, L. & MacGregor, H. (2002). Integrating services, marginalizing patients: Psychiatric patients and primary health care in South Africa. *Transcultural Psychiatry*, 39, 155–72.

Triant, V. A. (2002). The recognition and determinants of depression at a South African primary care clinic. Ph.D. dissertation, Yale University School of Medicine.

Uys, L. R., Subedar, H. & Lewis, W. (1995). Educating nurses for primary psychiatric care: A South African perspective. *Archives of Psychiatric Nursing*, 9, 348–53.

Wang, P. S., Berglund, P. & Kessler, R. C. (2000). Recent care of common mental disorders in the United States: Prevalence and conformance with evidence-based recommendations. *Journal of General Internal Medicine*, 15, 284–92.

Wild, L. G., Flisher, A. J. & Lombard, C. (2004). Suicidal ideation and attempts in adolescents: Associations with depression and six domains of self-esteem. *Journal of Adolescence*, 27, 611–24.

Williams, D. R., Herman, A., Kessler, R. C., Sonnega, J., Seedat, S., Stein, D. J., Moomal, H. & Wilson, C. M. (2004). The South Africa Stress and Health Study: Rationale and design. *Metabolic Brain Disease*, 19, 135–47.

World Health Organization (WHO) (1991). *International Classification of Diseases (ICD-10)*. Geneva: World Health Organization.

# 12 Mental Disorders and War in Lebanon

ELIE G. KARAM, ZEINA N. MNEIMNEH, AIMEE N. KARAM,
JOHN A. FAYYAD, SOUMANA C. NASSER, HANI DIMASSI,
AND MARIANA M. SALAMOUN

## ACKNOWLEDGMENTS

The LEBANON is carried out in conjunction with the World Health Organization World Mental Health (WMH) Survey Initiative. We thank the WMH staff for assistance with instrumentation, fieldwork, and data analysis. These activities were supported by the U.S. National Institute of Mental Health (R01MH070884), the John D. and Catherine T. Mac Arthur Foundation, the Pfizer Foundation, the U.S. Public Health Service (R13-MH066849, R01-MH069864, and R01 DA016558), the Fogarty International Center (FIRCA R03-TW006481), the Pan American Health Organization, Eli Lilly and Company Foundation, Ortho-McNeil Pharmaceutical, GlaxoSmithKline, and Bristol-Myers Squibb. A complete list of WMH publications can be found at http://www.hcp.med.harvard.edu/wmh/.

In addition, the LEBANON was partially supported by the Lebanese Ministry of Public Health, Fogarty International, anonymous private donations to IDRAAC, Lebanon (http://www.idraac.org), the World Health Organization (WHO, Lebanon), NAAMA, Act 4 Lebanon, and unrestricted grants from Janssen Cilag, Eli Lilly and Company Foundation, GlaxoSmithKline, Roche, and Novartis.

We would like to thank Ms. Yasmine Chatila for her work in supervising the fieldwork and data cleaning, Mrs. Caroline Cordahi-Tabet and Ms. Lilian Ghandour for their work in training and adaptation of the CIDI 3.0.

None of the authors have any conflict of interest with the institutions that have given unrestricted grants to the not-for-profit Institute for Development, Research Advocacy and Applied Care (IDRAAC), which conducted the LEBANON study.

## I. INTRODUCTION

Increasingly mental health disorders have proved to account for a significant portion of the global burden of disease in both developed and developing countries (Murray & Lopez 1996; World Health Organization 2001). Consequently, large-scale psychiatric epidemiologic studies have been conducted in the more industrialized world (Robins & Regier 1991; Kessler et al. 1994; Bijl, Ravelli & Zessen 1998; Henderson, Andrew & Hall 2000; Jenkins et al. 2003; ESEMeD 2004a; Kessler et al. 2005). In parallel, the past three decades have witnessed major advances in psychological and pharmacological treatments. Such advances have been brought to the Arab world mostly by Western mental health specialists trained in the West, who have implemented their expertise not only in the delivery of effective treatment interventions but also in conducting scientific research. Although clinical services in many centers in the Arab region meet the world's standards, research is still in its early stages (Okasha & Karam 1998). The starting point is to map out the needs: How common are psychiatric disorders? Are people who need care seeking help? Do mental disorders in Lebanon carry the same burden, and do these disorders evolve in Lebanon (and by extension in the Arab region) as they do in other regions of the world (economically and culturally different)? These and a multitude of questions will best be answered through international collaboration, using identical methodology, coupled with a common resolve on an international level to pool the existing expertise for consultation and consequent proper action.

Studies on mental disorders in the Arab world to date have either focused on single disorders (e.g., posttraumatic stress disorder [PTSD]) (Al-Hammadi et al. 1994), subpopulations (Ghubash, Hamdi & Bebbington 1992), or specific cities or areas (Okasha et al. 1988; Rahim & Cederblad, 1989; Abou Saleh, Daradkeh & Ghubash 2001). Nevertheless, among these studies, one used an approach that, if replicated in large communities, would add a lot to our knowledge in this part of the world. This study was carried out in Al Ain Community (United Arab Emirates [UAE]) and used the World Health Organization (WHO) Composite International Diagnostic Interview (CIDI), the most widely used structured interview to diagnose DSM disorders. The incidence of psychiatric disorders was 10.2% over a 12-month period, with 37% seeking treatment from psychiatric services (Daradkeh, Ghubash & Abou-Saleh 2000). The remaining published studies that looked at treatment in the Arab region focused on treatment referral patterns and types of services used among psychiatric patients in clinical settings, and thus do not fully represent the studied communities (El-Islam & Abu Dagga 1990; Houssein 1991; Al-Subaie 1994; Al-Jaddou et al. 1997; AbuMadini & Rahim 2002).

Lebanon is a small, mountainous country (area of 10,452 square kilometers) situated on the Mediterranean with a long history of various cultural influences, having started with its original seafaring Phoenicians and later colonized by all the major powers of the times. Lebanon gained its independence as a democratic republic in 1943. Its borders with Syria to the east and north and Israel to the south, its diverse population, and its geopolitical connections to the Arab world have been the source of various military conflicts that affected the population of around 4.2 million. War has been an ongoing challenge and has jeopardized the mental health and well-being of people for the past three decades. Consequently, most psychiatric epidemiologic studies in Lebanon so far have focused on mental disorders in communities exposed to war (Cross-National Collaborative Group 1992; Karam et al. 1998; Karam et al. 2000; Cordahi-Tabet et al. 2002; Farhood 2006; Karam 2006).

To address the aforementioned problems, the Institute for Development, Research, Advocacy and Applied Care (IDRAAC), in association with the Department of Psychiatry and Clinical Psychology at Balamand University and St. George Hospital University Medical Center, conducted the Lebanese Evaluation of the Burden of Ailments and Needs Of the Nation (LEBANON) study (Karam et al. 2006; 2008). This study is part of the WHO World Mental Health (WMH) Survey Initiative (Kessler et al. 2006). This chapter presents results on the prevalence, age of onset, and treatment of mental disorders, as well as the differential effect of war on first onset of these disorders from the LEBANON survey.

## 2. METHODS

### 2.1. Sample

A nationally representative multistage clustered area probability household sample of uninstitutionalised adults (ages 18+) was recruited for the LEBANON study ($n = 2857$). The response rate was 70.0% (ranging from 86.7% in the Bekaa region to 60.0% in Beirut). The first stage was constituted of 342 primary sampling units (PSUs) that were selected from each of the five region strata (North, South, Bekaa, Mount Lebanon, Beirut) with probabilities proportional to estimated size. A probability sample of households was selected from each PSU. The Kish selection method was then used to select one adult in each sample household (Kish 1967). In a random sample of 10% of the married couples, the spouse of a respondent was also selected for an interview. Further details on the sample design are presented in Chapter 2. Survey procedures were approved by the Balamand University Medical School Ethics committee.

## 2.2. Interviews

Interviewer training lasted for six days and was conducted by two trainers who had previously been certified by the WMH Data Collection Coordination Centre. Three hundred five interviewers were trained, and only 116 with the best performance were recruited. The survey was carried out between September 2002 and September 2003. Interviews were administered face-to-face in two parts. All respondents completed Part 1 for a core diagnostic assessment ($n = 2857$). Part 2 (which included correlates of disorders) was given to all Part 1 respondents who met lifetime criteria for any core disorder plus a probability subsample of the other respondents ($n = 1031$). Part 1 was weighted for differential probability of selection and was poststratified to government population data on sociodemographic and geographic variables (Central Administration for Statistics 1998). Part 2 was additionally weighted for differential probability of selection from the Part 1 sample. Further details on construction of analysis weights are found in Chapter 2.

## 2.3. Measures

### 2.3.1. 12-month Diagnoses

Version 3.0 of the CIDI (Kessler & Üstün 2004; see also Chapter 4), a fully structured lay-administered interview was used to generate both ICD-10 and DSM-IV diagnoses. DSM-IV criteria were used for this current analysis. The 12-month disorders included anxiety disorders, mood disorders, impulse-control disorders, and substance use disorders (Demyttenaere et al. 2004). Childhood disorders (conduct disorder and attention-deficit/hyperactivity disorder) were limited to respondents in the age range of 18–44 years to minimize recall bias among older respondents. The prevalence of any impulse-control disorder was estimated in that age range (Demyttenaere et al. 2004). DSM-IV organic exclusion and diagnostic hierarchy rules were used in making diagnoses other than substance use disorders (abuse was defined with or without dependence

in recognition of abuse often being a stage in the progression to dependence).

### 2.3.2. Instrument

As detailed by Haro and his colleagues in Chapter 6 of this volume, the CIDI showed good concordance with the Structured Clinical Interview for DSM-IV (SCID) in the four WMH countries where clinical reappraisal studies were carried out. Validation of the Arabic version of CIDI 3.0 has not yet been carried out. Translation of CIDI 3.0 into Arabic was undertaken by a five-step process of forward translation, back-translation, resolution of discrepancies between translation and back-translation, pilot testing, and final revision (Karam et al. 2006).

### 2.3.3. Disorder Severity

Following standard WMH coding procedures, 12-month cases were classified as serious if they had bipolar I disorder, substance dependence with a physiological dependence syndrome, 12-month suicide attempt, severe role impairment in at least two areas of role functioning assessed in the Sheehan Disability Scales (SDS) (Leon et al. 1997), or role functioning at a level consistent with a Global Assessment of Functioning (Endicott et al. 1976) score of 50 or less. Moderate cases had either substance dependence without a physiological dependence syndrome or at least moderate role impairment in two or more SDS domains. Remaining cases were classified as mild.

### 2.3.4. Sociodemographic Correlates

Sociodemographic correlates included age, sex, education (none or only primary, complementary or some secondary, completed secondary without university degree, and university degree), marital status (married, previously married, never married), and family income (defined using standard international welfare economics methods, with household income divided by number of family members to create income per family member). Age was linked to information collected on age of onset of disorders to define historical periods of time prior to the war years (before 1975), the years of war (1975–1989), and the postwar years (1990–2003) (Karam et al. 2006). To predict lifetime disorders using discrete-time survival analysis age was categorized into four groups (18–34, 35–49, 50–64, and 65 years and older) corresponding to cohorts born in the years 1969–1985, 1954–1968, 1939–1953, and 1938 or earlier.

### 2.3.5. Exposure to War-related Traumatic Events

War-related traumatic events included: being a combatant, a refugee, or civilian in a region of war or terror; witnessing atrocities or witnessing dead or injured bodies; being a peace worker in a war zone; being kidnapped or mobbed or threatened by a weapon; and having a loved one die or having other trauma occur to a loved one.

### 2.3.6. Use of Mental Health Services

Information on contact with health-care professionals was assessed in each diagnostic section of the CIDI along with the age the respondent initiated the first contact. Part 2 respondents also answered questions related to type of professionals they ever sought for emotional problems or alcohol/drug use. Twelve-month treatment was classified into three categories: mental health specialist (psychiatrist, psychologist, other mental health professional), general medical (general medical doctor, nurse, other health professional not in a mental health setting), non–health care (religious or spiritual advisor, herbalists, fortune-teller, or counselor not in a mental health setting).

### 2.3.7. Minimally Adequate Treatment

Consistent with the definitions used across all WMH surveys, minimally adequate treatment was defined as making four or more visits to any type of professional for emotional or substance problems, making two or three visits and receiving medication, or having recently started treat-

ment and still being in treatment (Wang et al. 2005).

### 2.4. Analysis Methods

Prevalence and severity were estimated by calculating means. Sociodemographic correlates were examined using logistic regression (Hosmer & Lemeshow 1989), with coefficients exponentiated and interpreted as odds ratios (ORs). Projected lifetime risk to age 75 was estimated using retrospective age of onset reports to estimate conditional probability of first onset at each year of life up to and including age 74. The actuarial method was used to cumulate these conditional probability estimates (Halli & Rao 1992). Predictors of first onset were studied with discrete-time survival analysis with person-year the unit of analysis (Efron 1988). Survival coefficients were exponentiated and are reported as ORs for ease of interpretation. Standard errors and 95% confidence intervals were obtained using the Taylor series method to adjust for the weighting and clustering of the sample design using SUDAAN software and SAS version 9.1 (SAS Institute 2001; Research Triangle Institute 2002). The standard errors of the estimates of projected lifetime risk were obtained from simulations using the method of jackknife repeated replications. Statistical significance was evaluated using two-sided, design-based 0.05-level tests.

## 3. RESULTS

### 3.1. Characteristics of the Sample

About two-thirds of the respondents were younger than 50 years, with 47.7% younger than 35 years. Of the sample, 49.5% were males, and about 57.2% of the sample was married or living with someone, whereas 37.4% had never been married. The educational level of 58.3% of the sample had incomplete secondary education, and 18.5% had completed college.

### 3.2. Prevalence of Mental Disorders

About one-fourth of the Lebanese sample met criteria for one of the DSM-IV disorders at some

**Table 12.1.** Lifetime and 12-month prevalence of disorders*

| | Lifetime prevalence[a] | | | 12-month prevalence[a,b] | | |
|---|---|---|---|---|---|---|
| | n[c] | % | (se)[d] | n | % | (se)[d] |
| **Anxiety disorder** | | | | | | |
| Panic disorder | 16 | (0.5%) | (0.1) | 7 | (0.2%) | (0.1) |
| Generalized anxiety disorder | 61 | (2.0%) | (0.3) | 37 | (1.3%) | (0.3) |
| Specific phobia | 202 | (7.1%) | (0.5) | 119 | (8.2%) | (1.0) |
| Social phobia | 52 | (1.9%) | (0.4) | 21 | (1.1%) | (0.4) |
| Agoraphobia without panic | 13 | (0.5%) | (0.1) | 6 | (0.3%) | (0.1) |
| Posttraumatic stress disorder[e] | 70 | (3.4%) | (0.6) | 29 | (2.0%) | (0.6) |
| Any anxiety disorder[e] | 282 | (16.7%) | (1.6) | 179 | (11.2%) | (1.1) |
| **Mood disorder** | | | | | | |
| Major depressive disorder | 283 | (9.9%) | (0.9) | 128 | (4.9%) | (0.7) |
| Dysthymia | 34 | (1.1%) | (0.2) | 19 | (0.8%) | (0.2) |
| Bipolar I–II disorders | 61 | (2.4%) | (0.4) | 34 | (1.5%) | (0.3) |
| Any mood disorder | 352 | (12.6%) | (0.9) | 165 | (6.6%) | (0.8) |
| **Impulse-control disorder** | | | | | | |
| Conduct disorder[f] | 13 | (1.0%) | (0.4) | 3 | (0.2%) | (0.2) |
| ADHD[f] | 20 | (1.5%) | (0.4) | 11 | (0.9%) | (0.3) |
| Intermittent explosive disorder | 43 | (1.7%) | (0.5) | 18 | (0.8%) | (0.2) |
| Any impulse-control disorder[f] | 53 | (4.4%) | (0.9) | 30 | (2.2%) | (0.5) |
| **Substance abuse disorder** | | | | | | |
| Alcohol abuse | 38 | (1.5%) | (0.3) | 9 | (1.2%) | (0.8) |
| Alcohol dependence with abuse | 9 | (0.4%) | (0.2) | 5 | (0.3%) | (0.2) |
| Drug abuse[e] | 6 | (0.5%) | (0.2) | 4 | (0.2%) | (0.1) |
| Drug dependence with abuse[e] | 3 | (0.1%) | (0.1) | 3 | (0.1%) | (0.1) |
| Any substance use disorder[c] | 27 | (2.2%) | (0.8) | 12 | (1.3%) | (0.8) |
| **Any disorder[e]** | 491 | (25.8%) | (1.9) | 308 | (17.0%) | (1.6) |

[a] The prevalence was estimated in the Part 1 sample ($n = 2857$) for all disorders other than those noted in notes e and f, where the samples reported there were used.

[b] The prevalence was estimated in the Part 2 sample ($n = 1031$) for all disorders other than those noted in note f, where the samples reported were used.

[c] The reported numbers of respondents with the individual disorders are unweighted numbers, which is why the ratios of these numbers to the total number of respondents in the survey do not equal the prevalence estimates.

[d] se: standard error.

[e] Estimated in the Part 2 sample ($n = 1031$), as posttraumatic stress, drug, and substance use disorders were assessed only in this sample.

[f] Estimated among respondents aged 18–44 in the Part 2 sample ($n = 595$), as conduct disorder and ADHD were estimated only in this subsample.

* Adapted from Karam et al. 2006; 2008.

point in their lives, and 17% had so in the past year of the study (Karam et al. 2006; 2008). Among disorders in the past year, 27.0% were classified as serious, 36.0% as moderate, and 37.0% as mild. Although anxiety disorders were the most common in Lebanon, a lower proportion of them were classified as serious as compared to mood, impulse, and substance use disorders (Tables 12.1 and 12.2).

## 3.3. Age Difference and Age of Onset of Mental Disorders

The median age of onset for having any disorder in an individual's life was 19 years (ranging from 13 years for any anxiety to 31 years for any mood disorder). The youngest median age of onset was for having specific phobia (median: 11 years) and the highest was for generalized anxiety

**Table 12.2.** 12-month severity of disorders[†]

| | Conditional prevalence* | | | | | | | | |
|---|---|---|---|---|---|---|---|---|---|
| | Serious | | | Moderate | | | Mild | | |
| | $n^a$ | $\%^b$ | $(se)^c$ | $n^a$ | $\%^b$ | $(se)^c$ | $n^a$ | $\%^b$ | $(se)^c$ |
| **Anxiety disorder** | | | | | | | | | |
| Panic disorder | 6 | (79.4%) | (14.4) | 0 | (0.0%) | (0.0) | 2 | (20.6%) | (14.4) |
| Generalized anxiety disorder | 8 | (24.4%) | (9.5) | 19 | (54.5%) | (10.4) | 10 | (21.1%) | (8.6) |
| Specific phobia | 30 | (18.4%) | (4.9) | 41 | (39.2%) | (7.0) | 48 | (42.4%) | (8.0) |
| Social phobia | 12 | (63.9%) | (15.1) | 7 | (29.7%) | (12.4) | 2 | (6.4%) | (6.3) |
| Agoraphobia without panic | 3 | (45.7%) | (24.3) | 2 | (47.2%) | (25.4) | 1 | (7.2%) | (7.5) |
| Posttraumatic stress disorder[d] | 14 | (25.7%) | (11.2) | 5 | (14.0%) | (12.6) | 10 | (60.3%) | (14.4) |
| Obsessive-compulsive disorder[d] | 1 | (9.0%) | (10.4) | 1 | (68.3%) | (27.4) | 1 | (22.8%) | (23.5) |
| Any anxiety disorder[d] | 49 | (19.7%) | (4.0) | 61 | (36.7%) | (6.0) | 69 | (43.6%) | (6.8) |
| **Mood disorder** | | | | | | | | | |
| Major depressive disorder | 56 | (42.5%) | (5.2) | 58 | (49.3%) | (4.8) | 14 | (8.2%) | (2.4) |
| Dysthymia | 9 | (35.7%) | (14.8) | 7 | (43.6%) | (13.5) | 3 | (20.7%) | (12.0) |
| Bipolar I–II disorder | 34 | (100.0%) | (0.0) | 0 | (0.0%) | (0.0) | 0 | (0.0%) | (0.0) |
| Any mood disorder | 90 | (54.9%) | (4.9) | 59 | (37.3%) | (4.4) | 16 | (7.8%) | (2.3) |
| **Impulse-control disorder** | | | | | | | | | |
| Conduct disorder[e] | 1 | (15.1%) | (18.2) | 1 | (36.4%) | (7.8) | 1 | (48.5%) | (10.4) |
| ADHD[e] | 6 | (60.3%) | (18.1) | 2 | (20.7%) | (14.1) | 3 | (19.0%) | (14.9) |
| Intermittent explosive disorder | 6 | (46.6%) | (11.9) | 9 | (36.5%) | (10.7) | 3 | (16.9%) | (10.4) |
| Any impulse-control disorder[e] | 12 | (50.4%) | (11.4) | 12 | (32.4%) | (8.7) | 6 | (17.1%) | (8.0) |
| **Substance use disorder** | | | | | | | | | |
| Alcohol abuse | 6 | (32.6%) | (22.3) | 1 | (4.2%) | (4.8) | 2 | (63.3%) | (24.5) |
| Alcohol dependence with abuse | 5 | (100.0%) | (0.0) | 0 | (0.0%) | (0.0) | 0 | (0.0%) | (0.0) |
| Drug abuse[d] | 2 | (61.8%) | (24.5) | 1 | (24.2%) | (21.7) | 1 | (14.0%) | (14.1) |
| Drug dependence with abuse[d] | 2 | (71.8%) | (25.1) | 1 | (28.2%) | (25.1) | 0 | (0.0%) | (0.0) |
| Any substance use disorder[d] | 7 | (32.8%) | (20.9) | 2 | (6.8%) | (6.0) | 3 | (60.3%) | (24.2) |
| **Any disorder**[d] | 108 | (27.0%) | (3.6) | 112 | (36.0%) | (4.5) | 88 | (37.0%) | (6.0) |
| **Total sample**[f] | 109 | (4.6%) | (0.7) | 112 | (6.1%) | (1.0) | 88 | (6.3%) | (1.2) |

* The conditional prevalence of severity was estimated in the Part 2 sample ($n = 1031$) for all disorders other than those noted in notes d and e, where the samples reported there were used.

[a] The reported numbers of respondents with the individual disorders are unweighted numbers, which is why the ratios of these numbers to the total number of respondents in the survey do not equal the prevalence estimates.

[b] Percentages are calculated across the row within disorders.

[c] se: standard error.

[d] Estimated in the Part 2 sample ($n = 1031$), as posttraumatic stress, obsessive-compulsive, drug, and substance use disorders were assessed only in this sample.

[e] Estimated among respondents aged 18–44 in the Part 2 sample ($n = 595$), as conduct disorder and ADHD were estimated only in this subsample.

[f] Results in this row describe prevalence estimates in the total sample; that is, 4.6% of all respondents are estimated to have a serious disorder, 6.1% moderate, and 6.3% mild, summing to 17.0% with any disorder reported at the bottom of the first column.

[†] Adapted from Karam et al. 2006.

**Table 12.3.** Cohort as a predictor of lifetime risk of disorders[†]

| | Cohort (years) | | | | | | | | |
| --- | --- | --- | --- | --- | --- | --- | --- | --- | --- |
| | 18–34 | | 35–49 | | 50–64 | | 65+ | | |
| | OR | (95% CI) | OR | (95% CI) | OR | (95% CI) | OR | (95% CI) | P |
| **Anxiety disorder**[a] | | | | | | | | | |
| Generalized anxiety disorder | 7.0* | (2.5, 19.2) | 2.2 | (0.9, 5.6) | 0.6 | (0.2, 2.0) | 1.0 | (1.0, 1.0) | <0.001 |
| Specific phobia | 2.2* | (1.1, 4.6) | 1.8 | (0.8, 4.1) | 1.2 | (0.5, 2.8) | 1.0 | (1.0, 1.0) | 0.018 |
| Social phobia | 8.3* | (1.8, 39.2) | 4.3 | (1.0, 18.8) | 2.9 | (0.5, 17.9) | 1.0 | (1.0, 1.0) | 0.001 |
| Posttraumatic stress disorder[b] | 4.9* | (1.5, 15.5) | 2.3 | (0.9, 6.0) | 1.7 | (0.6, 4.3) | 1.0 | (1.0, 1.0) | 0.040 |
| Adult separation anxiety[c] | 4.5* | (1.4, 13.9) | 2.5 | (0.7, 9.5) | 0.7 | (0.2, 2.7) | 1.0 | (1.0, 1.0) | <0.001 |
| Any anxiety disorder[b] | 3.2* | (1.6, 6.2) | 2.5* | (1.2, 5.1) | 1.0 | (0.5, 2.1) | 1.0 | (1.0, 1.0) | <0.001 |
| **Mood disorder** | | | | | | | | | |
| Major depressive disorder | 4.7* | (2.2, 10.1) | 2.8* | (1.2, 6.3) | 1.5 | (0.8, 3.0) | 1.0 | (1.0, 1.0) | <0.001 |
| Dysthymia | 1.6 | (0.2, 10.3) | 2.5 | (0.5, 12.8) | 2.1 | (0.4, 9.7) | 1.0 | (1.0, 1.0) | 0.64 |
| Bipolar I–II disorder | 41.4* | (6.6, 261) | 10.6* | (1.9, 58.6) | 3.2 | (0.5, 19.8) | 1.0 | (1.0, 1.0) | <0.001 |
| Any mood disorder | 6.2* | (3.0, 12.8) | 3.1* | (1.4, 6.7) | 1.7 | (0.8, 3.2) | 1.0 | (1.0, 1.0) | <0.001 |
| **Impulse-control disorder**[a] | | | | | | | | | |
| Intermittent explosive disorder | 8.1* | (1.1, 58.7) | 2.7 | (0.5, 16.1) | 0.5 | (0.2, 1.3) | 1.0 | (1.0, 1.0) | <0.001 |
| Any impulse-control disorder[c] | 1.4 | (0.6, 3.3) | 1.0 | – | – | – | 1.0 | (1.0, 1.0) | 0.36 |
| **Substance-abuse disorder**[a] | | | | | | | | | |
| Alcohol abuse | 6.9* | (2.3, 20.7) | 2.1 | (0.6, 7.6) | 1.5 | (0.4, 5.9) | 1.0 | (1.0, 1.0) | <0.001 |
| **Any disorder**[a] | 4.5* | (2.3, 8.7) | 3.0* | (1.5, 5.7) | 1.7 | (0.9, 3.4) | 1.0 | (1.0, 1.0) | <0.001 |

* $p$-value $< 0.05$.

[a] Panic, agoraphobia without panic, conduct disorder, alcohol dependence with abuse, drug abuse, drug dependence with abuse not calculated as cell size $\leq 30$ is too small to be estimated.

[b] Estimated in the Part 2 sample ($n = 1031$), as posttraumatic stress, obsessive-compulsive, and substance use disorders were assessed only in this sample.

[c] Estimated among respondents aged 18–44 in the Part 2 sample ($n = 595$), as conduct disorder, adult separation anxiety, and ADHD were estimated only in this subsample.

[†] Based on discrete-time survival models with person-year as the unit of analysis.

disorder (median: 39 years). Of all respondents, 32.9% are expected to meet criteria for any lifetime mental disorder by age 75 years. The highest projected lifetime risks were for mood disorders (20.1%) and anxiety disorders (20.2%) (Karam et al. 2008).

Age cohort effects were statistically significant for all the disorders except for PTSD, dysthymia, and any impulse-control disorder. The cohort effects for anxiety disorders were mainly because the 18–34 cohort had a higher risk then the 65+ years, and mainly in social phobia and general anxiety disorder (OR = 8.3 and OR = 7.0 respectively). The risk for bipolar-broad disorder (bipolar I, bipolar II, or subthreshold bipolar) was 40 times greater in the youngest cohort

and ten times in the subsequent cohort group (as compared to those born before 1939). The youngest cohorts (18–35 years) had a higher risk of having any disorder (Table 12.3).

### 3.4. Sociodemographic Correlates for Mental Disorders

Several factors were related to having mental disorder in the past year of the study period. The correlates of having a mood disorder were being a female (OR = 1.9, CI: 1.2–3.2), middle-aged versus 65 years and more (35–49 years: OR = 2.8, CI: 1.2–6.5; 50–64 years: OR = 2.4, CI: 1.3–4.7), and never married (OR = 2.3, CI: 1.3–4.0). The correlates of having anxiety disorders included being

**Table 12.4.** Sociodemographic predictors of lifetime risk of disorders

| | Lifetime risk[a] | | Any impulse control[c] OR (95% CI) | Alcohol abuse[d] OR (95% CI) |
|---|---|---|---|---|
| | Any anxiety[b] OR (95% CI) | Any mood OR (95% CI) | | |
| **Sex** | | | | |
| F | 3.0 (2.0–4.7)* | 1.6 (1.2–2.0)* | 0.7 (0.3–1.8) | 0.2 (0.0–0.9) |
| M | 1.0    – | 1.0    – | 1.0    – | 1.0    – |
| $\chi_1^2$ | 26.7 | 10.6 | 0.7 | 4.6 |
| **Education** | | | | |
| Student | 17.4 (1.8–172.3)* | 4.9 (1.6–14.9)* | 0.3 (0.0–4.4) | 0.2 (0.0–0.6)* |
| Low | 11.0 (1.1–108.6)* | 4.5 (1.6–12.6)* | 0.4 (0.0–4.1) | 0.7 (0.2–2.9) |
| Low medium | 17.3 (2.0–150.0)* | 4.4 (1.6–11.6)* | 0.0 (0.0–0.1)* | 0.4 (0.1–2.3) |
| Medium | 9.7 (1.2–80.2)* | 2.3 (0.6–8.6) | 0.1 (0.0–0.8)* | 1.0    – |
| High | 1.0    – | 1.0    – | 1.0    – | – |
| $\chi_4^2$ | 8.8 | 17.7 | 18.6 | 9.1 |
| **Age groups** | | | | |
| 18–34 | 2.7 (1.3–5.7)* | 5.9 (2.7–12.6)* | 1.6 (0.7–3.8) | 11.2 (2.2–57.0)* |
| 35–49 | 2.2 (1.0–4.7)* | 2.9 (1.2–6.8)* | 1.0 | 2.8 (0.5–15.3) |
| 50–64 | 0.9 (0.4–2.2) | 0.9 (0.4–1.8) | – | 1.2 (0.1–9.4) |
| 65+ | 1.0    – | 1.0    – | – | 1.0    – |
| $\chi_3^2$ | 13.8 | 65.2 | 1.3 | 22.9 |

* $p < 0.05$.
[a] Based on discrete–time survival models with person–year as the unit of analysis.
[b] Estimated in the Part 2 sample ($n = 1031$), as posttraumatic stress and obsessive–compulsive disorders were assessed only in this sample.
[c] Estimated among respondents aged 18–44 in the Part 2 sample ($n = 595$), as conduct disorder and ADHD were estimated only in this subsample.
[d] Alcohol abuse with/without dependence included instead of any substance because any substance has fewer than 30 cases.

female (OR = 7.0, CI: 4.4–11.1) and never married (OR = 1.7, CI: 1.0–2.9). Substance use was highly correlated with young age (18–34 years: OR = 14.5, CI: 1.7–127.6) and never married (OR = 6.4, CI: 1.7–23.7) (Karam et al. 2006). Predictors of lifetime risk of mood, anxiety, and alcohol abuse disorders are shown in Table 12.4.

### 3.5. Exposure to War-related Traumatic Events and Mental Health

War-related traumatic events (being a combatant, a civilian in area of heavy fighting, being displaced by the war, a refugee, witnessing people being killed, seeing dead bodies, having a loved one die, and sustaining a life-threatening war-related injury) were analyzed to explore their effects on 12-month prevalence of mental disor-

ders long after war had ended. A significant dose-response relationship was identified between number of war-related traumas and mood, anxiety, and impulse-control disorders. Respondents who were exposed to two or more war events were more likely to have any mood disorder (2 events: OR = 3.1, CI: 1.5–6.5; at least 3 events: OR = 4.9, CI: 2.2–10.8) and any impulse control disorder (2 events: OR = 3.6, CI: 1.4–9.5; at least 3 events: OR = 9.1, CI: 2.5–33.4) in the past 12-months (Karam et al. 2006).

Predictors of first onset of new disorders in an individual's lifetime were examined across three sets of years of the Lebanon wars: before (before 1975), during (1975–1989), and after (1990–2003). Four types of ten war-related traumatic events were included in the analysis: Type I (refugee/civilian in region of war or terror), Type II (witnessed atrocities/witnessed dead or injured bodies/peace worker), Type III (kidnapped/mobbed/threatened by weapon), and Type IV (death of loved one/other trauma occurred to loved one). Specific war traumas had differential effects on first onset of disorders. The risk for first onset of these disorders not only increased during the years of war but also continued to do so for mood and impulse-control disorders long after war had ended. Conversely, individuals with prewar impulse control disorders were more likely to have been exposed to specific war traumas (Table 12.5).

### 3.6. Use of Services and Treatment of Mental Disorders

Among respondents who met criteria for a DSM-IV disorder, only one out of ten sought any type of treatment. Treatment was more common for mood disorders (19.3%) than anxiety disorders (6.5%). Numbers were too small for impulse control and substance use to be analyzed. Among those who sought treatment, two-thirds did so in the general medical sector (2.9% of the general population), and only few (23.4%) were treated by mental health specialists (1% of the general population). Treatment rates were higher among severe to moderate cases (14%) than mild cases (4.8%). Health-care treatment was rated at least minimally adequate in 80.2% of those seeking treatment. Treatment in the past year was significantly more common among females than males, was positively related to family income, and was significantly but monotonically related to education (Karam et al. 2006).

Lifetime disorders such as specific phobia, major depression, and dysthymia were treated more often in younger cohorts. The median delay between age of onset and seeking treatment among those who had a lifetime mood disorder was 6 years, versus 9 and 28 years for substance use and anxiety disorders, respectively. The majority of people suffering from a mental disorder did not seek help in the year of onset of the disorder. Only 12.3% of those suffering from any mood disorder and 3.2% of those who had any anxiety disorder reported seeking treatment

in the first year of onset. However, about half of those with any mood disorder and 37.3% of those with any anxiety disorder eventually sought treatment within 50 years of onset. As for alcohol abuse, 35.4% of alcohol abusers will seek treatment within 50 years of onset, knowing that only 0.9% reported seeking treatment within the first year (Table 12.6) (Karam et al. 2008).

### 4. DISCUSSION

The LEBANON study is the first study in the Arab world to present data on the national prevalence of a wide array of psychiatric disorders. To our knowledge, only one previously published survey in the Arab world looked at the prevalence of mental disorders in a representative community sample, but it was restricted to one city (Abou Saleh, Daradkeh & Ghubash 2001). Our results show that one-quarter of the total Lebanese population has had at least one mental disorder, and this rate is expected to reach one-third as the Lebanese population ages. These estimates are sufficient to place mental disorders among the most commonly occurring health problems in Lebanon, leading to important implications on the social and economic fronts.

The main limitations of this study include recall bias, sampling design that excluded institutionalized respondents, and underreporting due to social desirability. Taking these limitations into consideration, the results are probably an underestimate of the true 12-month and lifetime prevalence of psychiatric disorders in Lebanon.

The LEBANON study has confirmed general findings in the literature that war indeed not only is deleterious to the economy and physical health but also seems to carry huge consequences on the mental health of individuals. It is evident that there is selective exposure to trauma, and research on this subject is ongoing around the world. We have found on a national level that people who were exposed to three or more war events were nine times more likely to have 12-month impulse-control disorders after war exposure. When exposed to specific trauma, there is a surge in new first time onsets of anxiety and mood disorders, which we know are

**Table 12.5.** War exposure predictors of lifetime risk of disorder by war period[a]

| | Lifetime risk, OR (95% confidence interval)[b] | | | | | | | | |
|---|---|---|---|---|---|---|---|---|---|
| | Any mood disorder[c] | | | Any anxiety disorder[d] | | | Any impulse-control disorder[e] | | |
| War period | Pre | During | Post | Pre | During | Post | Pre | During | Post |
| **Type of war exposure** | | | | | | | | | |
| Type I[g]. Refugee/residing in war area | 3.2* (1.2–8.4) | 1.5 (1.7–3.2) | 2.0** (1.3–3.1) | 1.6 (0.4–5.4) | 3.2 (0.8–12.4) | 1.0 (0.4–2.4) | 0.7 (0.2–3.3) | 8.1* (1.0–64.3) | 4.1 (0.8–21.5) |
| Type II[h]: Witnessed atrocities | 1.8 (0.9–3.9) | 0.9 (0.4–1.9) | 1.2 (0.7–1.9) | 0.8 (0.2–3.1) | 0.7 (0.3–1.6) | 1.7 (0.8–3.8) | 0.4 (0.1–1.1) | 2.1 (0.6–7.2) | 5.4* (1.1–27.4) |
| Type III: Kidnapped/ threatened by weapon | 1.4 (0.3–6.1) | 2.8* (1.2–6.2) | 1.1 (0.5–2.6) | 1.1 (0.2–6.2) | 5.2** (1.7–15.4) | 1.1 (0.2–5.0) | 7.8** (0.2–24.6) | 2.2 (0.3–15.4) | 2.1 (0.1–56.4) |
| Type IV: Trauma/death of a loved one | 1.3 (0.6–2.9) | 2.5** (1.4–4.6) | 1.0 (0.5–1.7) | 0.9 (0.3–2.8) | 1.1 (0.6–2.4) | 1.0 (0.3–3.1) | 0.4 (0.1–3.2) | 2.7 (0.7–9.9) | 1.9 (0.1–25.7) |
| Any type[f] | 1.7** (1.2–2.4) | 1.7** (1.3–2.3) | 1.3** (1.1–1.6) | 1.1 (0.6–1.8) | 1.6** (1.2–2.0) | 1.2 (0.8–1.7) | 0.5 (0.3–1.0) | 3.0** (1.3–6.8) | 4.5** (2.1–9.7) |

[a] Based on discrete-time survival models with person-year as the unit of analysis. Lebanese war period defined as 1975–1990. Models included sex, education, marital status, and cohort with nesting of each when there is a significant interaction. Results of the demographics are shown in text.

[b] $p$-value based on the Wald Chi-square test.

[c] Person-years below 12 years of age censored.

[d] Excluding specific and social phobia disorders, person-years above 58 years of age censored.

[e] Person-years above 20 years of age censored, age at interview less or equal to 44 years.

[f] Separate models with war exposure entered as any war type. Model for impulse control disorder excluded Type 3 from any war type.

[g] Type I (refugee/civilian in war region/civilian in terror region).

[h] Type II (witnessed atrocities/witnessed dead or injured bodies/peace worker).

\* $p$-value $< 0.05$; \*\* $p$-value $< 0.01$.

**Table 12.6.** Proportional treatment contact in the year of disorder onset and median duration of delay among cases that subsequently made treatment contact[a,b]

|  | % making treatment contact in year of onset | % ever making treatment contact | Median duration of delay (years) | n |
|---|---|---|---|---|
| Any anxiety disorder[c] | 3.2 | 37.3 | 28 | 299 |
| Any mood disorder | 12.3 | 49.2 | 6 | 349 |
| Any impulse-control disorder[c] | 3.8 | 15.1 | 3 | 53 |
| Any substance disorder | 0.9 | 35.4 | 9 | 38 |

[a] Adapted from Karam et al. 2008.

[b] Disorder hierarchy is not used in these diagnoses.

[c] Assessed in the Part 2 sample ($n = 1031$).

recurrent by nature and thus will have a life of their own even if there is no re-exposure to war (Karam et al. 2006; 2008).

Moreover, exposure to war continues to exert its effect not only shortly after war exposure or in the recurrence of mental disorders that started anew with it but also on new onsets of disorders several years after exposure. This could be due to a combination of factors, among them the "other" consequences of the specific type of exposure under study. For example, being displaced permanently from the original area of residence in Lebanon, which has an intricate web of social support/status that is rather independent of economic status, might erode the pride and the role of many individuals, who will only suffer many years after the war is over when worries of bare economic and physical survival have been already put to rest.

Compared to Western Europe, the prevalence of any lifetime disorder in Lebanon is estimated to be quite similar, but it is lower than in the United States (ESEMeD 2004a; Kessler et al. 2005). The highest lifetime prevalence was for anxiety and mood disorders (major depression: 9.9%). The difference in lifetime prevalence between these two classes dissipates in their high projected lifetime risk: mood disorders have a later age of onset than anxiety disorders (Karam et al. 2008). This high prevalence in Lebanon (as compared to other developing countries) could be related to the Western style of stressors that Lebanon would share with the more developed countries; on the other hand, the positive role of the social support that Lebanon continues to

enjoy might be counterbalanced by exposure to war and political instability. Add to this an ever-increasing younger population that has been shown repeatedly to be more prone to all mental disorders, the reasons of which are still under debate internationally (Cross-National Collaborative Group 1992; Weissman et al. 1996).

The lifetime PTSD rates (3.4%) were surprisingly low (even lower than U.S. rates) (Karam et al. 2008; Kessler et al. 2005), in spite of the high exposure to war traumas in Lebanon. One explanation is that our study reflects rates of disorders in the general population and not only in the heavily war affected areas. Our previous studies on samples of adults, adolescents, and children in these war-affected areas showed higher rates of PTSD (10.3% and 20.7% respectively) (Karam et al. 1998; Fayyad et al. 2003). Most of these PTSD episodes, however, dwindled within a few months. If these findings are reliable, it is very probable that war-related PTSD, when mild, will be remembered with difficulty by respondents several years later, in a country where intrusive ideation and decreased hope are a common occurrence and are normalized in an atmosphere of generalized alertness for several weeks after exposure to intense bombardments. On the other hand, the median age of onset for PTSD was higher than that of the U.S. population. One possible explanation for this difference could be war exposure: first, the median age of onset for PTSD was close to that of depression, which is a disorder related to war exposure; second, the prevalence of PTSD in the youngest group is lower than any other group, an age group that, in most areas of Lebanon and until July 2006, had not witnessed acts of war. A prospective follow-up study focusing on the influence of the environment on the progress of PTSD (duration and intensity) induced by rarer war events would be interesting.

There is an underreporting of alcohol and drug use across the world as a result of social desirability. In Lebanon, this holds true as well and is evident by the low rates of substance abuse disorders, as compared to previous data from our group, albeit on different populations and using different methodology (Karam et al. 2003; Karam, Maalouf & Ghandour 2004). The fact that psychiatric disorders, and some more than others, are still considered taboo topics in Lebanon leads to the underreporting and underestimation of the lifetime prevalence of psychiatric disorders. This might be even truer in view of the presence in Lebanon of not only Christians, but also Muslims who might have been reluctant (especially the older generation) to open up about use to an interviewer who is a stranger to them, especially when alcohol use is prohibited by religious faith. More focused analysis is needed to attempt to resolve this issue. As stated earlier, alcohol abuse/dependence in our previous studies that focused on the academic sectors in Lebanon (Karam, Maalouf & Ghandour 2004) had yielded higher prevalence, albeit in a higher-risk subgroup.

The proportion of cases in treatment was found to be much lower than in industrialized countries (Bijl et al. 2003; ESEMeD 2004b). Though treatment seeking rates were low, interestingly, delay among those who sought treatment was similar to industrialized countries (Karam et al. 2006; 2008; Wang et al. 2005). Some possible reasons contributing to the low treatment rates are the taboos surrounding mental health, lack of awareness in the community, and most important, the lack of private and public insurance to cover the high expenses of treating mental disorders. Whereas privately bought insurances cover a wide array of medical problems, still any treatment of mental disorders, as of the date of this writing, is nonexistent. Only the government-backed insurance covers some inpa-tient treatment (in specific facilities and quite restricted in the university medical centers), and about 30% of the cost of medication and ambulatory care (the rates of which are similar to Europe). More than 80% of health-care treatment of mental disorders in Lebanon was classified using WMH guidelines as at least minimally adequate. However, there is a need to validate this across Arab guidelines, which are not available at the present time.

In conclusion, this study has important implications for clinicians and policy makers alike, especially in the Middle East, where armed conflicts have taken place for decades. Given the high prevalence of these disorders, their young age of onset during the early formative and productive years, their strong relationship to war, and evidence of their equal (if not greater) burden on "physical" conditions, particular attention should be given to their early identification, treatment, and efforts to raise awareness about mental health.

## REFERENCES

Abou Saleh, M. T., Daradkeh, T. K. & Ghubash, R. (2001). Al Ain Community Psychiatric Survey I. Prevalence and socio Demographic correlates. *Social Psychiatry & Psychiatric Epidemiology*, 36, 20–8.

AbuMadini, M. & Rahim, S. (2002). Psychiatric admission in a general hospital: Patients profile and patterns of service utilization over a decade. *Saudi Medical Journal*, 23, 44–50.

Al-Hammadi, A., Behbehani, J., Staehr, A., Aref, M. & Al-Asfour, A. (1994). *The traumatic events and mental health consequences resulting from the Iraqi Invasion and occupation of Kuwait*. Kuwait: Al Riggae Specialized Center.

Al-Jaddou, H. & Malkawi, A. (1997). Prevalence, recognition and management of mental disorders in primary health care in Northern Jordan. *Acta Psychiatrica Scandinavica*, 96, 1, 31–5.

Al-Subaie, A. (1994). Traditional healing experiences in patients attending a university outpatient clinic. *Arab Journal of Psychiatry*, 5, 83–91.

Bijl, R. V., de Graaf. R., Hiripi, E., Kessler, R. C., Kohn, R., Offord, D. R., Üstün, T. B., Vicente, B., Vollebergh, W. A. M., Walters, E. E. & Wittchen, H.-U. (2003). The prevalence of treated and untreated mental disorders in five countries. *Health Affairs (Milwood)*, 22, 3, 122–33.

Bijl, R. V., Ravelli, A. & Zessen, G. (1998). Prevalence of psychiatric disorder in the general population: Results of the Netherlands Mental Health survey and Incidence Study (NEMESIS). *Social Psychiatry and Psychiatric Epidemiology*, 33, 587–95.

Central Administration for Statistics (1998). *Conditions de vie des ménages 1997*. Beirut: Central Administration for Statistics.

Cordahi-Tabet, C., Karam, E. G., Nehmé, G., Fayyad, J., Melhem, N. & Rashidi, N. (2002). Les orphelins de la guerre experience Libanaise et méthodologie d'un suivi prospectif. *Stress et Trauma*, 2, 227–35.

Cross-National Collaborative Group. (1992). The changing rate of major depression: Cross-national comparisons. *Journal of the American Medical Association*, 268, 3098–105.

Daradkeh, T. K., Ghubash, R. & Abou-Saleh, M. T. (2000). Al Ain community survey of psychiatric morbidity III: The natural history of psychopathology and the utilization rate of psychiatric services in Al Ain. *Social Psychiatry and Psychiatric Epidemiology*, 35, 548–53.

Demyttenaere, K., Bruffaerts, R., Posada-Villa, J., Gasquet, I., Kovess, V., Lepine, J. P., Angermeyer, M. C., Bernert, S., Girolamo, G., Morosini, P., Polidori, G., Kikkawa, T., Kawakami, N., Ono, Y., Takeshima, T., Uda, H., Karam, E. G., Fayyad, J. A., Karam, A. N., Mneimneh, Z. N., Medina-Mora, M. E., Borges, G., Lara, G., de Graaf, R., Ormel, J., Gureje, O., Shen, Y., Huang, Y., Zhang, M., Alonso, J., Haro, J. M., Vilagut, G., Bromet, E. J., Gluzman, S., Webb, C., Kessler, R. C., Merikangas, K. R., Anthony, J. C., Korff, M. R. V., Wang, P. S., Alonso, J., Brugha, T. S., Aguilar-Gaxiola, S., Lee, S., Heeringa, S., Pennell, B. E., Zaslavsky, A. M., Üstün, T. B. & Chatterji, S. (2004). Prevalence, severity and unmet need for treatment of mental disorders in the World Health Organization World Mental Health Surveys. *Journal of the American Medical Association*, 291, 2581–90.

Efron, B. (1988). Logistic regression, survival analysis, and the Kaplan-Meier curve. *Journal of the American Statistical Association*, 83, 414–25.

El-Islam, M. F. & Abou-Dagga, S. I. (1990). Illness behavior in mental ill-health in Kuwait. *Scandinavian Journal of Social Medicine*, 18, 195–201.

Endicott, J., Spitzer, R. L., Fleiss, J. L. & Cohen, J. (1976). The global assessment scale: A procedure for measuring overall severity of psychiatric disorders. *Archives of General Psychiatry*, 33, 766–71.

ESEMeD/MHEDEA investigators 2000. (2004a). Prevalence of mental disorders in Europe: results from the European Study of the Epidemiology of Mental Disorders (ESEMeD) project. *Acta Psychiatrica Scandinavica*, 109, 21–7.

ESEMeD/MHEDEA investigators 2000. (2004b). Use of mental health services in Europe: Results from the Study of the Epidemiology of Mental Disorders (ESEMeD) project. *Acta Psychiatria Scandinavica*, 109, 47–54.

Farhood, L. (2006). The WHO experience. Paper presented at the 3d Annual Mental Health Day of the Lebanese Psychiatric Society (LPS), Beirut.

Fayyad, J., Karam, E., Karam, A. N., Tabet, C. C., Mneimneh, Z. N. & Bou Ghosn, M. (2003). PTSD in children and adolescents following war. In *Posttraumatic stress disorders in children and adolescents*, ed. R. R. Silva, pp. 306–52. New York: W. W. Norton.

Ghubash R., Hamdi, E. & Bebbington. P. (1992). The Dubai community psychiatric survey: I. Prevalence and sociodemographic correlates. *Social Psychiatry*, 27, 53–61.

Halli, S. S. & Rao, K. V. (1992). *Advanced techniques of population analysis*. New York: Plenum Press.

Henderson, S., Andrew, G. & Hall, W. (2000). Australia's mental health: An overview of the general population survey. *Australian and New Zealand Journal of Psychiatry*, 34, 197–205.

Hosmer, D. W. & Lemeshow, S. (1989). Applied logistic regression. New York: John Wiley & Sons.

Houssein, F. M. (1991). A Study of the role of unorthodox treatments of psychiatric illnesses. *Arab Journal of Psychiatry* 2 (2), 170–84.

Jenkins, R., Lewis, F., Bebbington, P., Brugha, T., Farrell, M., Gill, B. & Meltzer, H. (2003). The National Psychiatric Morbidity Surveys of Great Britain: Initial findings from the household survey. *International Review of Psychiatry*, 15, 29–42.

Karam, E. G. (2006). Mental health disorders and war: National data. Paper presented at the 3d Annual Mental Health Day of the Lebanese Psychiatric Society (LPS), Beirut.

Karam E. G., Ghandour, L., Maalouf, W. & Yamout, K. (2003). Substance use and misuse in Lebanon: The Lebanon Rapid Situation Assessment & Responses Study. In *Technical reports on drugs and crime in North Africa and the Middle East*. United Nations Office on Drugs and Crime, Beirut-Lebanon.

Karam, E. G., Howard, D. B., Karam, A. N., Ashkar, A., Shaaya, M., Melhem, N. & El-Khoury N. (1998). Major depression and external stressors: The Lebanon Wars. *Europe Archives of Psychiatry & Clinical Neuroscience*, 248, 225–30.

Karam, E. G., Karam, A., Cordahi-Tabet, C., Fayyad, J., Melhem, N., Mneimneh, Z., Zebouni, V., Kayali, G., Yabroudi, P., Rashidi, N. & Dimasi, H. (2000). Community group treatment and outcome of war trauma in children. Paper presented at the 47th annual meeting of the American Academy of Child and Adolescent Psychiatry, New York.

Karam, E. G., Maalouf, W. & Ghandour, L. (2004). Alcohol use among university students in Lebanon: Prevalence, trends and risk factors. The IDRAC

University Substance Use Monitoring Study (1991 and 1999). *Drug and Alcohol Dependence*, 76, 273–86.

Karam, E. G., Mneimneh, Z. N., Fayyad, J. A., Dimassi, H., Karam, A. N., Nasser, S. C., Chatterji, S., Kessler, R. C. (2008). Lifetime prevalence of mental disorders: First onset, treatment and exposure to war. *PLoS Medicine*, 5, e61.

Karam, E. G., Mneimneh, Z. N., Karam, A. N., Fayyad, J. A., Nasser, S. C., Chatterji, S. & Kessler, R. C. (2006). 12-Month prevalence and treatment of mental disorders in Lebanon: A national epidemiological survey. *Lancet*, 367, 1000–6.

Kessler, R. C., Berglund, P. A., Demler, O., Jin, R., Walters, E. E. (2005). Lifetime prevalence and age of onset distributions of DSM-IV disorders in the National Comorbidity Survey Replication. *Archives of General Psychiatry*, 62, 593–602. Erratum in *Archives of General Psychiatry*, 62, 768.

Kessler, R. C., Haro, J. M., Heeringa, S. G., Pennell, B.-E. & Üstün, T. B. (2006). The World Health Organization World Mental Health Survey Initiative. *Epidemiologia e Psichiatria Sociale*, 15, 161–6.

Kessler, R. C., McGonagle, K. A., Zhao, S., Nelson, C. B., Hughes, M., Eshleman, S., Wittchen, H.-U., & Kendler, K. S. (1994). Lifetime and 12-month prevalence of DSM III-R psychiatric disorders in the United States. *Archives of General Psychiatry*, 51, 8–19.

Kessler, R. C. & Üstün, T. B. (2004). The World Mental Health (WMH) survey initiative version of the WHO-CIDI. *International Journal of Methods in Psychiatric Research*, 13, 95–121.

Kish, L. (1967). *Survey sampling.* New York: John Wiley & Sons.

Leon, A. C., Olfson, M., Portera, L., Farber, L. & Sheehan, D. V. (1997). Assessing psychiatric impairment in primary care with the Sheehan Disability Scale. *International Journal of Psychiatry in Medicine*, 27, 93–105.

Murray, C. J. L. & Lopez, A. D. (1996). *The global burden of disease.* Geneva: World Health Organization.

Okasha, A. & Karam, E. (1998). Mental health services and research in the Arab world. *Acta Psychiatrica Scandinavica*, 98, 406–13.

Okasha A., Khalil, A. H., El Fiky, M. R., Ghanem, M. & El Hakeem, R. (1988). Prevalence of depressive disorders in a sample of rural and urban Egyptian communities. *Egyptian Journal of Psychiatry*, 11, 167–81.

Rahim, S. I. & Cederblad, M. (1989). Epidemiology of mental disorders in young adults of a newly urbanized area in Khartoum, Sudan. *British Journal of Psychiatry*, 155, 44–7.

Research Triangle Institute (2002). *SUDAAN: Professional software for survey data analysis 8.01.* Research Triangle Park, NC: Research Triangle Institute.

Robins, L. N. & Regier, D. A. (1991). *Psychiatric disorders in America: The Epidemiologic Catchment Area Study.* New York: Free Press.

SAS Institute (2001). *SAS/STAT Software: Changes and enhancements, Release 8.2.* Cary, NC: SAS Publishing.

Wang, P. S., Lane, M., Kessler, R. C., Olfson, M., Pincus, H. A. & Wells, K. B. (2005). Twelve-month use of mental health services in the United States. *Archives of General Psychiatry*, 62, 629–40.

Weissman, M. M., Bland, R. C., Canino, G. J., Faravelli, C., Greenwald, S., Hwu, H. G., Joyce, P. R., Karam, E. G., Lee, C. K., Lellouch, J., Lépine, J. P., Newman, S. C., Rubio-Stipec, M., Wells, J. E., Wickramaratne, P. J., Wittchen, H. & Yeh, E. K. (1996). Cross-national epidemiology of major depression and bipolar disorders. *Journal of the American Medical Association*, 276, 293–9.

World Health Organization (WHO) (2001). *World health report: Mental health, new understanding, new hope.* Geneva: World Health Organization.

# 13 Mental Health in Belgium: Current Situation and Future Perspectives

RONNY BRUFFAERTS, ANKE BONNEWYN, AND KOEN DEMYTTENAERE

## ACKNOWLEDGMENTS

The ESEMeD project is funded by the European Commission (Contracts QLG5-1999-01042; SANCO 2004123), the Piedmont Region (Italy), Fondo de Investigación Sanitaria, Instituto de Salud Carlos III, Spain (FIS 00/0028), Ministerio de Ciencia y Tecnología, Spain (SAF 2000-158-CE), Departament de Salut, Generalitat de Catalunya, Spain, Instituto de Salud Carlos III (CIBER CB06/02/0046, RETICS RD06/0011 REM-TAP), and other local agencies, and by an unrestricted educational grant from GlaxoSmithKline. ESEMeD is carried out in conjunction with the World Health Organization World Mental Health (WMH) Survey Initiative. We thank the WMH staff for assistance with instrumentation, fieldwork, and data analysis. These activities were supported by the U.S. National Institute of Mental Health (R01MH070884), the John D. and Catherine T. MacArthur Foundation, the Pfizer Foundation, the U.S. Public Health Service (R13-MH066849, R01-MH069864, and R01 DA016558), the Fogarty International Center (FIRCA R03-TW006481), the Pan American Health Organization, Eli Lilly and Company Foundation, Ortho-McNeil Pharmaceutical, GlaxoSmithKline, and Bristol-Myers Squibb. A complete list of WMH publications can be found at http://www.hcp.med.harvard.edu/wmh/.

Portions of this chapter, including tables and figures, appeared previously in: Bruffaerts, R., Bonnewyn, A. & Demyttenaere, K. (2007). Delays in seeking treatment for mental disorders in the Belgian general population. Social Psychiatry and Psychiatric Epidemiology, 42(11), 937–44 and Bonnewyn, A., Bruffaerts, R., Vilagut, G., Almansa, J., & Demyttenaere, K. (2007). Lifetime risk and age of onset of mental disorders in the Belgian general population. Social Psychiatry and Psychiatric Epidemiology, 42(7), 522–9.

## I. INTRODUCTION

In an era in which people's health is no longer exclusively judged in terms of mortality statistics, mental health plays a central role in determining the health status of a population. In the Global Burden of Disease report by the World Health Organization (WHO) (Murray & Lopez 1996), mental illness has emerged as a highly significant feature of people's health status, accounting for more than 15% of the burden of disease in established market economies, even more than the disease burden caused by all cancers. Given that an optimal mental health policy aims to treat existing cases of mental illness and reduce future cases by means of early treatment, early detection, and prevention, it is mandatory to gain knowledge on the prevalence of mental disorders in the society.

Over the past decade, a number of surveys investigating the prevalence of mental disorders in the general population have been carried out in Europe, the Americas, and Australia (Kessler et al. 1994; Bijl, Ravelli & van Zessen 1998; Henderson, Andrews & Hall 2000; Jenkins et al. 2003; Kessler et al. 2003). From these studies, the first conclusion is that mental disorders are common disorders in the general populations of the countries where these studies took place. Depending on case definitions and instruments used, between one in four and one in ten persons meets the criteria for any mood or anxiety disorder throughout their life. A second conclusion is that the use of services by persons with mental disorders is suboptimal. By and large, about one person in three with a mental disorder seeks professional help for mental health reasons, despite that mental disorders have a dramatic impact on daily functioning (Alonso et al. 2004; Wang et al. 2005).

Although existing studies show that mental disorders are common and that the use of services is suboptimal, we should be cautious in generalizing and interpreting international data in a country-specific context. After all, we may assume that there are country-specific factors and cultural values that may influence the prevalence of mental disorders (Kleinman 1995). Moreover, countries also differ in their provision and organization of (mental) health services (e.g., the number of inpatient and outpatient facilities), and we may assume that these factors influence the course of the mental illness.

The present chapter describes the current situation and future perspective on mental health and mental health care in Belgium. Belgium is a small (11,730 square miles and approximately 10.5 million inhabitants) constitutional monarchy, since 1830, bordered by the Netherlands, Germany, and France. Today, Belgium is a high-income federal state, reorganized into three regions (Flanders, Wallonia, and Brussels Capital) and three communities (French-, Dutch-, and German-speaking populations), each with its own legislative and executive power (WHO 2005). French and Dutch are the main national languages. In addition, the first language of about 1% of Belgium's population is German. The life expectancy is about 75 years for male and 82 years for female inhabitants, with healthy life expectancies of 69 years for men and 73 years for women, respectively (WHO 2005).

## 2. THE BELGIAN MENTAL HEALTH CARE DELIVERY SYSTEM

Belgium has universal health insurance covering mental health and substance abuse treatment. There are no limits on the number of contacts with primary care physicians or mental health specialists (including medical doctors and psychologists). Moreover, there are no limits concerning the number of medications prescribed by medical doctors. Consumers have up to 80% public coverage of mental health treatment, psychotherapy, and medication consumption provided or prescribed by medical doctors (Lassey, Lassey & Jinks 1997). In descending order, the primary sources of financing mental health treatment are universal health insurance, private insurance, and out-of-pocket expenditures by the patient (WHO 2005). It is only recently that policy makers focused more attention on rising health-care costs (Kesteloot 2001).

Mental health treatment is part of both the primary care and the specialized care delivery system. Effective treatment of acute and/or severe mental disorders is available at the primary care level. Moreover, continuous trainings are carried out for primary care physicians concerning mental health issues (WHO 2005). Although the primary care physician takes a crucial role in detecting, referring, and treating patients with mental disorders, those seeking help have no constraints on access to any level of care. Indeed, patients may follow direct pathways from the community to a primary care physician, a psychiatrist, a psychologist, a hospital, a community service, or a combination of these services.

Contrary to the Americas and most of the European countries, the deinstitutionalization of mental health care in Belgium did not start before the mid-1970s. Consequently, in current Belgian mental health care, there are still a considerable number of inpatient facilities. There are about 22.1 psychiatric beds per 10,000 inhabitants (WHO 2005). Compared to other countries, the Belgian mental health care system peaks in the number of inpatient facilities (Bruffaerts, Bonnewyn & Demyttenaere 2006).

In addition to the overall high availability of psychiatric beds, many outpatient mental health providers also exist: per 10,000 inhabitants there are 1.4 psychiatrists, 3.2 psychologists, and 15.3 general practitioners (Bruffaerts et al. 2006). Details on the number of psychiatric nurses or social workers are not provided here because these care providers in Belgium are, contrary to other European countries, not entitled to provide mental health care unless they work within a hospital-based setting. There are also numerous subsidized community care facilities serving outpatient care. By and large, there is approximately one community center per 10,000 inhabitants, providing specialized outpatient treatment and counseling for mental disorders, drug related disorders, and psychosocial problems (Fondation Julie Renson 2005). One of the newest additions in the field of mental health care is the implementation of a full psychiatric staff in the emergency room, serving specialized care for persons with either acute mental illness or substance use disorders (Bruffaerts & Demyttenaere 2005). These services are provided 24 hours a day in 10 hospital sites in Belgium.

Taken together, the Belgian health-care system is a therapist-rich environment with many providers (both outpatient and inpatient, both general and mental health specialists) that could provide mental health care for persons with anxiety, mood, and alcohol use disorders. Persons seeking help have almost no constraints on accessing high-quality (mental) health care.

## 3. WHAT IS KNOWN OF THE EPIDEMIOLOGY OF MENTAL DISORDERS IN BELGIUM?

In Belgium, epidemiological mental health data are still limited in their completeness and comparability. It is only in response to the formulation of a national mental health care policy and mental health program in 1990 that policy makers gained more interest in the magnitude of mental disorders and mental health problems in Belgium's general population. This makes the collection of adequate general population mental health data a very recent phenomenon in Belgium. To our knowledge, there are three main sources of epidemiological information on the prevalence of mental disorders in Belgium: (1) a number of studies that were specifically designed to estimate the prevalence of mental disorders, (2) the Health Interview Surveys, and (3) the Panel Study on Belgian Households. There are

no studies investigating the prevalence of mental health problems in the general population younger than 15 years (Danckaerts in press).

### 3.1. Mental Health Surveys in Belgium

The first study that indicated that mental disorders were common among noninstitutionalized persons was the study by Baruffol and Thilmany (1993). In their relatively small regional study ($n = 240$), performed in 1992, point prevalence rates of anxiety, mood, and alcohol disorders (according to the Diagnostic and Statistical Manual, third edition [DSM-III], and assessed with the Diagnostic Interview Schedule Screening Interview [DISSI]) were estimated at 17%, 13%, and 9%, respectively. Lifetime prevalence rates were estimated at 29%, 27%, and 17%, respectively. The Depression Research in European Society (DEPRES) survey, with data gathered data in the mid-1990s using the Mini International Neuropsychiatric Interview (MINI), estimated the six-month prevalence of mood disorders (both major depressive episode and dysthymia) at 12% of the general population (Lepine et al. 1997; Tylee et al. 1999). The epidemiological studies carried out in the provinces of Luxembourg (Ansseau, Reggers & Nickels 1999) and Liège (Ansseau & Reggers 1999) were restricted to lifetime estimates of DSM-IV mental disorders as assessed with the Composite International Diagnostic Interview (CIDI-2.1): mood (24% and 34%, respectively), anxiety (24% and 29%, respectively), and alcohol disorders (both 30%).

Among these studies, there is only one that reports on treatment contacts. Ansseau and colleagues (1999) reported that, within a 12-month perspective, 37.1% of those with a disorder made at least one contact with a health-care professional because of a mental disorder. Contact rates varied by mental disorders, with highest rates for mood disorders (72.6%), followed by anxiety disorders (21.0%), and alcohol disorders (10.2%).

### 3.2. The Health Interview Surveys

The second source of information that contains data on the prevalence of mental disorders in

Belgium is the three-wave Health Interview Survey (HIS), a population-based survey conducted by the federal government in 1997 ($n = 10,221$ [Kittel, Ribourdouille & Dramaix 1997; Bietlot et al. 2000]), 2001 ($n = 12,111$ [Demarest et al. 2002]), and 2004 ($n = 12,945$ [Bayingana et al. 2006]). The HIS was specifically designed to assess general health issues of the Belgian general population (Van Oyen et al. 1997). In these surveys, the General Health Questionnaire (Goldberg 1972; Koeter & Ormel 1991) and the depression subscale of the Symptom Checklist-90 (Derogatis, Lipman & Covi 1973; Arrindell, Ettema & SCL-90 1986) were used to gather information on (12-month prevalence estimates of) depression and (point prevalence estimates of) anxiety symptoms. There are three main conclusions that emerge from the HIS: (1) the estimates of either anxiety or depression have a high degree of cross-temporal stability, (2) approximately 5%–6% of the general population met criteria for a 12-month depression, and (3) approximately 6% experienced anxiety symptoms the day before the interview took place.

The HIS of 1997, 2001, and 2004 also provide information on treatment contact rates for persons with 12-month mood disorders. The reports estimated the proportions of persons seeking help in primary or specialized care. Between 59.5% and 67.5% of the Belgian population with a mood disorder reported that it has made contact with a primary care physician because of depression, whereas between 33.0% and 38.7% of these made at least one contact with specialized mental health care.

### 3.3. The Panel Study of Belgian Households

The third source of information is the Panel Study of Belgian Households (PSBH), a longitudinal nine-wave survey ($n = 11,565$) on socioeconomic and family-related factors of the Belgian general population. In this survey, depression is measured by a shortened version of the Global Depression Scale of the Daily Living Form (Moos, Cronkite & Finney 1982). To our knowledge, there were no assessments of anxiety disorders or anxiety-related symptoms.

The 12-month estimates of depression assessed in 1992, 1993, and 1994 were centered around 15%–16% of the general population (Ansseau 1996). Against the background of the longitudinal character of this survey, attempts have been made to point out the course of depression over a longer period (1992–1999). Using latent variable growth curve modeling, Wauterickx and Bracke (2005) found an increased prevalence of depression in the Belgian general population. According to their results, the average respondent is expected to realize a linear 4% increase on the Global Depression Scale over an eight-year period. Moreover, female respondents were found to have a greater (i.e., 1.6 times) increase in depression rates than their male counterparts.

### 3.4. Limitations of Existing Studies

Although there is consistent evidence to conclude that mental disorders are common phenomena in Belgium, studies are not conclusive relative to the prevalence of mental disorders and their treatment in the Belgian general population. From all surveys that provide data of the prevalence of mental disorders, only a minority (three out of eight: Baruffol & Thilmany 1993; Ansseau & Reggers 1999; Ansseau et al. 1999) were developed to measure the prevalence of mental disorders. However, they only provide estimates for specific regions in Belgium (i.e., the small urban region of Wavre and the provinces of Liège and Luxembourg). The DEPRES study was the only psychiatric epidemiological survey using general population samples, but it only measured the prevalence of depression. Although the remainder of the surveys (Ansseau 1996; Kittel et al. 1997; Bietlot et al. 2000; Demarest et al. 2002; Bracke & Wauterickx 2003; Bayingana et al. 2006) were based on population-representative samples, they were not developed to assess mental health as such, and, consequently, they did not use standardized psychiatric interviews but rather psychiatric symptom rating scales to assess mental health. Another apparent finding is that the majority of the surveys almost exclusively reported on prevalence estimates of mental disorders or emotional problems. There seems to be a lack of studies that use population-representative samples to gather information on service use and patterns that lead persons with mental disorders to professional health care. The two reports that provide treatment rates were limited because they used data from nonrepresentative samples (Ansseau et al. 1999) or because they focused only on one disorder (Kittel et al. 1997; Bietlot et al. 2000; Demarest et al. 2002; Bayingana et al. 2006).

## 4. MATERIALS AND METHODS

### 4.1. Sample

The Belgian survey targeted the noninstitutionalized adult population (aged 18 years or older), representing a total of 7,900,000 inhabitants. Interviews were performed between April 2001 and June 2002. A stratified, multistage, clustered area, probability sample design was used. The initial response rate in Belgium was 50.7%.

Internal subsampling was used to reduce respondent burden by dividing the interview into two parts. Part 1 included the core diagnostic assessment of mental disorders. Part 2 included additional information relevant to a wide range of survey aims, including assessment of chronic physical conditions. Details of the subsampling are described elsewhere (Kessler & Üstün 2004). All respondents completed Part 1. All Part 1 respondents ($n = 2419$) who met criteria for any mental disorder and a probability sample of other respondents were administered Part 2. Part 2 ($n = 1043$) respondents were weighted by the inverse of their probability of selection for Part 2 of the interview to adjust for differential sampling. Analyses provided here were based on the weighted Part 2 sample.

### 4.2. Training and Field Procedures

The survey was carried out by the Scientific Institute of Public Health (IPH), a scientific institute of the federal Belgian state. With its main mission to carry out scientific research to inform federal health policies, IPH plays an important role in gathering survey data for Belgium.

The central World Mental Health (WMH) staff trained bilingual supervisors in Belgium. The WHO translation protocol was used to translate instruments and training materials. Interviews were carried out by professional lay interviewers (provided by the IPH) in Dutch and French. Standardized descriptions of the goals and procedures of the study, data use and protection, and the rights of respondents were provided in both written and verbal forms to all potentially eligible respondents before obtaining verbal informed consent for participation in the survey. Quality-control protocols, described in more detail elsewhere (Kessler & Üstün 2004), were standardized across countries to check interviewer accuracy and to specify data-cleaning and coding procedures. The institutional review board of the IPH approved and monitored compliance with procedures for obtaining informed consent and protecting human subjects. More information on training and field procedures is provided in Chapter 3 of this volume.

## 5. MEASURES

### 5.1. Mental Disorders

As described earlier in Chapter 4, data were gathered by using version 3.0 of the Composite International Diagnostic Interview (CIDI 3.0) of the World Health Surveys (WMH) of the World Health Organization (Kessler & Üstün 2004), which was developed and adapted by the WHO Coordinating Committee for the WMH initiative. The questionnaire consisted of a screening section that was given at the beginning of the questionnaire to each respondent. All participants responding positively to a specific screening question were eligible to complete the corresponding sections of the questionnaire. Lifetime and 12-month estimates were determined by whether respondents' symptomatology met the lifetime or 12-month diagnostic criteria, respectively, for the disorder. Lifetime risk of mental disorders was assessed using retrospective age-of-onset reports. The sequence of questions started with a question designed to emphasize the importance of accurate responses: "Can you remember your exact age the very first time you had the syndrome?" Respondents who were not able to answer this question were subsequently probed for a bound of uncertainty by moving up the age range incrementally (i.e., "Was it before you first started school?" or "Was it before you became a teenager?").

Mental disorders were assessed using the criteria of the *Diagnostic and Statistical Manual of Mental Disorders*, 4th edition (DSM-IV) (American Psychiatric Association 1994). Mental disorders included mood disorders (major depressive episode [MDE], dysthymia), anxiety disorders (generalized anxiety disorder [GAD], social phobia, specific phobia, posttraumatic stress disorder [PTSD], agoraphobia, panic disorder), impulse-control disorders (oppositional-defiant disorder, conduct disorder, and attention-deficit/hyperactivity disorder), and alcohol disorders (alcohol abuse, alcohol dependence). CIDI 3.0 organic exclusion rules were imposed in making all diagnoses. Methodological evidence collected in the WHO CIDI 3.0 field trials and later clinical calibration studies showed that all the disorders considered herein were associated with acceptable reliability and validity both in the original CIDI (Wittchen 1994) and in the original version of the CIDI 3.0 (Kessler & Üstün 2004).

## 5.2. Seriousness of Mental Disorders

Mental disorders were classified as serious, moderate, or mild. Respondents were categorized as having a serious mental disorder if they (1) had attempted suicide in the past 12 months and had any 12-month disorder, or (2) had substance dependence with physiological symptoms, or (3) or had more than one 12-month diagnosis and a high level of impairment on the Sheehan scales. Among those who are not categorized as serious, respondents were categorized as having a moderate mental disorder if they had at least one disorder and a moderate level of impairment or they had substance dependence without physiological signs. The remaining respondents with any 12-month disorder were categorized as mild.

## 5.3. 12-month and Lifetime Service Use for Mental Disorders

The use of services was assessed by asking respondents whether they ever saw any of the following types of professionals, either as an outpatient or inpatient, for problems with emotions, nerves, mental health, or use of alcohol: (1) mental health professionals (e.g., psychiatrist, psychologist), (2) general medical professionals (i.e., general practitioner), and (3) other health-care professionals. Follow-up questions asked about age at first and most recent contacts, as well as number and duration of visits in the past 12 months.

Twelve-month service use was classified into two broad groups of service providers: the health-care sector and the non–health-care sector. The health-care sector consisted of mental health care (e.g., psychiatrist, psychologist, other mental health professional in any setting, social worker or counselor in a mental health specialty setting, or use of a mental health hotline) and general medical health care (e.g., primary care doctor, other general medical doctor, or any other health professional not previously mentioned). The non–health-care sector consisted of human services (e.g., religious or spiritual adviser, social worker or counselor in any setting other than a specialty mental health setting) and complementary and alternative medicine (CAM) (i.e., any other type of healer such as chiropractors, participation in an Internet support group, or participation in a self-help group).

## 5.4. Treatment Adequacy

Respondents' service use in the prior year was categorized using two definitions of adequacy. The first broad definition (definition 1) defined those with "minimally adequate treatment" as meeting at least one of the following three criteria: (1) at least four visits in the prior year to any type of provider (e.g., CAM, human services, general medical), (2) at least two visits and any type of medication (including medications that are known to be inappropriate for the assessed disorder), or (3) respondent is still in treatment at the time of interview.

A second stricter definition (definition 2) identified those who may have received "adequate treatment" when meeting at least one of the following two criteria: (1) eight or more visits to any professional in the past 12 months (e.g., CAM, human services, general medical), or (2) four or more visits to any professional in the past 12 months plus 30 days or more on any medication (including medications that may be inappropriate for the assessed disorder).

Household income was included as a correlate of treatment adequacy. Income was defined as the sum of all pretax income in the past 12 months, including salaries earned by all members of the household plus all sources of other income (e.g., government transfers, pensions, investment income). Per capita income was then calculated for each household by dividing the household income by the number of people in the household as reported in the household listing. To compare income across countries, we created a four-category income scale. A respondent was assigned a category on this scale on the basis of the per capita income of the respondent's household divided by the median income for the country. Categories were based on ratio and included low (0.5 or less), low-average (0.5–1.0), high-average (1.0–2.0), and high (2.0).

## 6. ANALYSIS PROCEDURES

Twelve-month and lifetime prevalence estimates and treatment rates are provided and expressed in absolute numbers ($N$) and percentages (%) with standard errors (se). We also provide the mean ($M$) number of visits in those persons who reported the use of services in the past 12 months. Correlates of mental disorders were investigated by binary logistic regression analyses. The statistical significance of each independent variable to the predictive model was determined by Wald $\chi^2$ statistics and expressed in odds ratios (OR) and according to 95% confidence intervals (95% CI).

Projected lifetime risk as of age 75 years was estimated with survival curves, using the two-part actuarial method (Hall & Rao 1992). The cumulative risks estimates were standardized and analyzed for fixed percentiles (pc 5, 10, 25, 50, 75, 90, 95, 99). We also provide interquartile ranges (IQR) (i.e., the number of years between the 25th and 75th percentile of the age of onset distributions) as a measure of the spread of the ages of onset of mental disorders. Providing IQRs enables us to identify a critical age range in which a specific disorder may develop.

Cumulative lifetime probabilities for lifetime treatment contact were also estimated using the two-part actuarial method. Survival curves were used to make two estimates: (1) the proportion of cases that made treatment contact by 50 years from the year of first onset of the disorder, and (2) the duration of the delay in initial treatment contact was defined as the median number of years between disorder onset and the first treatment contact among those persons that eventually made contact. The cumulative probabilities were standardized and analyzed for fixed years since onset of the disorder. Correlates of treatment contact were investigated by using discrete-time survival analysis with person-year as the unit of analysis. Predictors included age of onset of disorders, cohort, and gender. We included only these three variables as a result of sparse data and small cell sizes for the remaining variables (i.e., number of years since the onset of the disorder, education, and marital status). The latter variables were included as controls in the prediction model. We used Wald $\chi^2$ tests to detect significance in the discrete-time survival analyses using Taylor series design-based coefficient variance-covariance matrices.

All analyses were performed using version 8 of the SAS System for Windows (SAS Institute 2001) and SUDAAN, a statistical package used to analyze data from complex sample surveys (i.e., multistage, stratified, unequally weighted, or clustered). Standard errors of ratio estimates, means, regression coefficients and other statistics were estimated taking into account the sample design, by using the Taylor series linearization method implemented in SUDAAN, version 8.01 (Shah & Barnwell 1997). Statistical significance was set at 0.05, with two-sided tests.

A number of estimates could not be calculated. For instance, it was not possible to calculate lifetime prevalence and lifetime risk estimates for some disorders because there were too many missing values in the age of onset for the disorder. We do not provide estimates for these outcome measures. This was also the case when there were too few cases per cell. In cells where there were fewer than 30 respondents, outcome measures were not provided. However, the broad disorder categories (any anxiety, any mood, any alcohol disorder) include these disorders on condition that the total number of disorders in the broad category is greater than or equal to 30.

## 7. RESULTS

### 7.1. Sociodemographic Description of the Sample

The average age of respondents who participated in the Belgian WMH study was 47 years, with the majority of the respondents (28%) between 35 and 49 years old. Males represented 48% of the sample. Approximately 57% were married or living with someone, 77% lived in midsize urban areas, and 47% of the sample had more than 13 years of full-time education. The majority was in paid employment at the time of the interview (53%).

### 7.2. Prevalence Estimates of Mental Disorders in Belgium

#### 7.2.1. Lifetime and 12-month Mental Disorders

Tables 13.1 and 13.2 show that 29% of respondents reported lifetime presence of any mental disorder, with nearly 12.7% experiencing a mental disorder in the past 12 months. Of respondents, 14.1% reported a lifetime history of any mood disorder, 13.1% any anxiety disorder, and 8.3% a lifetime history of any alcohol disorder. Impulse-control disorders were much less common in the Belgian general population, with a lifetime estimate of 5.2%. Within the 12 months preceding the interview, 12.7% of the respondents met the criteria for any mental disorder.

Among those with a mental disorder, anxiety disorders were most common (7.6%), followed by mood disorders (5.3%). Alcohol and impulse-control disorders had similar prevalence estimates: 1.8% and 1.7%, respectively. MDE and specific phobia were the most common mental disorders in both lifetime and 12-month perspective, followed by alcohol abuse. Table 13.2 illustrates the distribution of the lifetime prevalence estimates and shows that mood disorders were more common among the cohort between 50 and 64, and that alcohol disorders were more common among the cohorts younger than 65.

Lifetime comorbidity is a common condition. Although 29.1% of the Belgian population met criteria for at least one lifetime mental disorder, slightly more than 10% of the Belgian population met criteria for at least two lifetime disorders and almost 4% met criteria for at least three lifetime disorders.

Table 13.1 presents disorder severity distributions. Most of the disorders (38.1%) were classified as moderate, one in three disorders was serious, and the remainder (28.7%) were classified as mild. However, there were disorder-specific differences in severity: mood and alcohol disorders were mostly classified as serious (43.7% and 51.2%, respectively), whereas anxiety disorders were mostly moderate (41.9%) and impulse-control disorders were mostly classified as mild disorders (55.8%).

#### 7.2.2. Projected Lifetime Risk of Mental Disorders at Age 75

The projected lifetime risk of mental disorders at age 75 based on the age of onset distributions (Table 13.3) was 37.1% for any mental disorder, 15.7% for anxiety disorders, 22.8% for mood disorders, 10.5% for alcohol disorders, and 5.2% for impulse-control disorders. If we compare lifetime prevalence estimates with the projected lifetime risk estimates, we see that, in absolute percentages, the projected lifetime prevalence risk for any mental disorder increased by 8.0% (29.1% to 37.1%), with the most notable increase in mood disorders (8.7%). Thus, the prevalence

**Table 13.1.** Belgium 12-month prevalence and severity prevalence of DSM-IV disorders

| Diagnosis | 12-Month % | (se) | Serious % | (se) | Moderate % | (se) | Mild % | (se) |
|---|---|---|---|---|---|---|---|---|
| **Anxiety disorder** | | | | | | | | |
| Panic disorder | 0.9 | (0.3) | 37.7 | (7.8) | 25.4 | (13.3) | 36.9 | (12.1) |
| Generalized anxiety disorder with hierarchy | 0.6 | (0.2) | 40.0 | (16.3) | 50.9 | (17.2) | 9.2 | (5.5) |
| Specific phobia | 4.4 | (0.6) | 30.4 | (7.5) | 40.9 | (5.8) | 28.6 | (8.2) |
| Social phobia | 1.1 | (0.2) | 33.6 | (13.0) | 55.4 | (14.1) | 11.0 | (6.6) |
| Agoraphobia without panic | 0.4 | (0.2) | 92.7 | (7.8) | 7.3 | (7.8) | 0.0 | (0.0) |
| Posttraumatic stress disorder | 0.7 | (0.1) | 55.1 | (16.0) | 35.8 | (16.0) | 9.1 | (6.5) |
| Adult separation anxiety | 0.1 | (0.1) | 0.0 | (0.0) | 100.0 | (0.0) | 0.0 | (0.0) |
| Any anxiety disorder | 7.6 | (1.4) | 31.8 | (3.3) | 41.9 | (5.0) | 26.2 | (5.8) |
| **Mood disorder** | | | | | | | | |
| Major depressive disorder with hierarchy | 5.0 | (0.5) | 47.9 | (6.8) | 36.2 | (6.1) | 15.8 | (4.7) |
| Dysthymia without hierarchy | 1.1 | (0.3) | 32.6 | (10.2) | 29.4 | (12.3) | 37.9 | (10.5) |
| Any mood disorder | 5.3 | (0.5) | 43.7 | (6.1) | 36.8 | (6.0) | 19.4 | (5.0) |
| **Impulse disorder** | | | | | | | | |
| Oppositional-defiant disorder | 0.4 | (0.3) | 90.9 | (11.7) | 9.1 | (11.7) | 0.0 | (0.0) |
| Conduct disorder | 0.7 | (0.6) | 0.0 | (0.0) | 0.0 | (0.0) | 100.0 | (0.0) |
| Attention-deficit/hyperactivity disorder | 1.1 | (0.5) | 32.4 | (24.7) | 36.2 | (20.7) | 31.4 | (17.8) |
| Intermittent explosive disorder with hierarchy | – | – | – | – | – | – | – | – |
| Any impulse-control disorder | 1.7 | (1.0) | 19.9 | (9.7) | 24.3 | (18.3) | 55.8 | (10.9) |
| **Alcohol disorder** | | | | | | | | |
| Alcohol abuse | 1.7 | (0.4) | 41.1 | (15.1) | 9.1 | (6.0) | 49.8 | (16.3) |
| Alcohol dependence | 0.3 | (0.1) | 100.0 | (0.0) | 0.0 | (0.0) | 0.0 | (0.0) |
| Any alcohol disorder | 1.8 | (0.4) | 51.2 | (15.4) | 7.6 | (41.3) | 41.3 | (15.7) |
| **Any disorder** | 12.7 | (1.5) | 33.1 | (4.1) | 38.1 | (28.7) | 28.7 | (4.8) |

of any mental disorder is expected to increase by about one-fourth. If we consider the relative change in the most common disorders (MDE, alcohol disorders, and specific phobia), the highest increase is expected in MDE (61.7%), next is alcohol abuse disorders (34.6%), and then specific phobia (26.5%). There is no increase between lifetime prevalence and lifetime risk for impulse-control disorders. Both are estimated at 5.2%.

### 7.2.3. Age of onset Distributions

The median age of onset of mental disorders is approximately 24 years old, with considerable disorder-specific variations (Table 13.3). Mood disorders were found to have the latest median age of onset (38 years), and alcohol disorders gen-

erally started around 23 years. Impulse-control and anxiety disorders generally developed very early in life (with median ages of onset of 9 and 14, respectively). This implies that 75% of people who will ever have an anxiety disorder will have it by the age of 34. This finding is even more pronounced for impulse-control disorders: 75% of those who will eventually have this disorder will have it by the age of 15. Interestingly, there were considerable intradisorder differences in the age of onset of anxiety disorders: the median age of onset of PTSD was 54 years and 37 years for GAD, whereas panic disorder (26 years), social phobia (13 years), and specific phobia (9 years) start much earlier in life. Both mood and anxiety disorders tend to develop within a relatively broad age range (IQRs between 23 and 27 years, respectively) whereas impulse-control and

**Table 13.2.** Lifetime prevalence for Part 1 and Part 2 samples of DSM-IV disorders

| | Total | | Age group | | | | | | | $\chi^2$ | DF | *p*-value |
|---|---|---|---|---|---|---|---|---|---|---|---|---|
| | | | 18–34 | | 35–49 | | 50–64 | | 65+ | | | | |
| | % | (se) | % | (se) | % | (se) | % | (se) | % | (se) | | | |
| **Anxiety disorder** | | | | | | | | | | | | | |
| Panic disorder | 1.6 | (0.3) | 2.5 | (1.0) | 1.6 | (0.5) | 2.0 | (0.7) | 0.0 | (0.0) | 36.2 | 3 | <0.001 |
| Generalized anxiety disorder with hierarchy | 1.9 | (0.4) | 1.4 | (0.5) | 2.6 | (0.7) | 2.3 | (0.7) | 1.4 | (0.8) | 2.9 | 3 | 0.42 |
| Specific phobia | 6.8 | (1.0) | 8.8 | (1.9) | 4.9 | (1.0) | 6.2 | (1.2) | 7.4 | (2.0) | 3.4 | 3 | 0.35 |
| Social phobia | 2.0 | (0.4) | 2.2 | (0.8) | 3.1 | (1.0) | 1.9 | (0.8) | 0.3 | (0.3) | 23.3 | 3 | 0.001 |
| Agoraphobia without panic | 0.9 | (0.2) | 0.5 | (0.5) | 1.3 | (0.5) | 1.3 | (0.8) | 0.3 | (0.3) | 3.0 | 3 | 0.42 |
| Posttraumatic stress disorder | 2.6 | (0.5) | 1.2 | (0.8) | 3.7 | (0.7) | 2.4 | (1.2) | 3.1 | (1.7) | 8.7 | 3 | 0.06 |
| Adult separation anxiety | 1.0 | (0.5) | 1.2 | (0.8) | 0.8 | (0.2) | – | – | – | – | 0.3 | 1 | 0.62 |
| Any anxiety disorder | 13.1 | (1.9) | 15.8 | (3.6) | 13.0 | (1.3) | 12.2 | (2.6) | 10.5 | (3.3) | 2.3 | 3 | 0.53 |
| **Mood disorder** | | | | | | | | | | | | | |
| Major depressive disorder with hierarchy | 14.1 | (1.0) | 12.8 | (1.8) | 15.4 | (1.6) | 19.9 | (2.8) | 8.4 | (1.3) | 26.1 | 3 | <0.001 |
| Any mood disorder | 14.1 | (1.0) | 12.8 | (1.8) | 15.4 | (1.6) | 19.9 | (2.8) | 8.4 | (1.3) | 26.1 | 3 | <0.001 |
| **Impulse disorder** | | | | | | | | | | | | | |
| Oppositional-defiant disorder | 1.2 | (0.5) | 1.3 | (0.7) | 1.0 | (0.5) | – | – | – | – | 0.2 | 1 | 0.66 |
| Conduct disorder | 3.1 | (1.3) | 3.9 | (2.0) | 2.0 | (1.2) | – | – | – | – | 0.7 | 1 | 0.42 |
| Attention-deficit/hyperactivity disorder | 2.9 | (1.1) | 3.8 | (1.7) | 1.7 | (0.9) | – | – | – | – | 1.2 | 1 | 0.28 |
| Any impulse-control disorder | 5.2 | (1.4) | 5.8 | (2.0) | 4.2 | (1.3) | – | – | – | – | 0.6 | 1 | 0.46 |
| **Alcohol disorder** | | | | | | | | | | | | | |
| Alcohol abuse | 7.8 | (0.9) | 8.5 | (1.6) | 9.7 | (1.1) | 8.9 | (1.7) | 3.4 | (0.9) | 20.9 | 3 | 0.002 |
| Alcohol dependence | 1.7 | (0.5) | 1.5 | (1.0) | 2.4 | (0.8) | 2.6 | (0.8) | 0.2 | (0.2) | 7.6 | 3 | 0.08 |
| Any alcohol use disorder | 8.3 | (0.9) | 9.4 | (1.8) | 10.0 | (1.2) | 9.0 | (1.7) | 3.6 | (1.1) | 17.1 | 3 | 0.005 |
| **Any disorder** | 29.1 | (2.3) | 34.1 | (4.6) | 29.4 | (2.7) | 31.5 | (4.1) | 19.7 | (4.5) | 7.8 | 3 | 0.08 |
| 2+ disorder | 10.3 | (1.5) | 12.5 | (3.2) | 11.7 | (1.3) | 11.0 | (1.9) | 4.5 | (1.7) | 19.3 | 3 | 0.003 |
| 3+ disorder | 3.6 | (0.7) | 4.7 | (1.8) | 3.7 | (0.9) | 3.4 | (0.9) | 2.0 | (1.4) | 2.0 | 3 | 0.59 |

**Table 13.3.** Ages at selected percentiles on the standardized age-of-onset distributions of DSM-IV disorders with projected lifetime risk at age 75

| | Projected lifetime risk at age 75 | | Ages at selected age-of-onset percentiles | | | | | | | |
|---|---|---|---|---|---|---|---|---|---|---|
| | % | (se) | 5 | 10 | 25 | 50 | 75 | 90 | 95 | 99 |
| **I. Anxiety disorders** | | | | | | | | | | |
| Panic disorder | 2.2 | (0.5) | 7 | 10 | 19 | 25 | 33 | 48 | 60 | 60 |
| Specific phobia | 8.0 | (1.4) | 5 | 5 | 5 | 9 | 18 | 51 | 65 | 72 |
| Social phobia | 2.2 | (0.4) | 5 | 5 | 7 | 13 | 17 | 25 | 36 | 36 |
| Generalized anxiety disorder | 3.4 | (0.9) | 14 | 17 | 26 | 37 | 50 | 63 | 63 | 63 |
| Posttraumatic stress disorder | 6.7 | (3.5) | 8 | 15 | 26 | 54 | 69 | 69 | 69 | 69 |
| Any anxiety disorder | 15.7 | (2.5) | 5 | 5 | 7 | 14 | 34 | 54 | 63 | 72 |
| **II. Mood disorders** | | | | | | | | | | |
| Major depressive disorder | 22.8 | (1.7) | 17 | 19 | 26 | 38 | 49 | 63 | 64 | 69 |
| Any mood disorder | 22.8 | (1.7) | 17 | 19 | 26 | 38 | 49 | 63 | 64 | 69 |
| **III. Impulse-control disorders** | | | | | | | | | | |
| Oppositional-defiant disorder | 1.2 | (0.5) | 5 | 6 | 6 | 7 | 9 | 11 | 18 | 18 |
| Conduct disorder | 3.1 | (1.3) | 7 | 7 | 8 | 14 | 15 | 16 | 16 | 17 |
| Attention-deficit/hyperactivity disorder | 2.9 | (1.1) | 6 | 6 | 7 | 7 | 9 | 11 | 19 | 19 |
| Any impulse-control disorder | 5.2 | (1.4) | 6 | 6 | 7 | 9 | 15 | 16 | 16 | 19 |
| **IV. Alcohol disorders** | | | | | | | | | | |
| Alcohol abuse | 10.0 | (1.0) | 17 | 18 | 20 | 23 | 36 | 44 | 51 | 56 |
| Alcohol dependence | 2.4 | (0.7) | 19 | 19 | 21 | 31 | 37 | 43 | 43 | 52 |
| Any alcohol disorder | 10.5 | (1.1) | 17 | 18 | 20 | 23 | 31 | 44 | 51 | 56 |
| **V. Any disorder** | | | | | | | | | | |
| Any | 37.1 | (3.0) | 5 | 6 | 13 | 24 | 41 | 52 | 63 | 69 |

alcohol disorders tend to develop within a much smaller age range (IQRs between 8 and 11 years, respectively).

### 7.2.4. Cohort Effects in the Prevalence of Mental Disorders

Considering the projected lifetime risks in the different cohorts (Table 13.4), two main findings emerge. First, the youngest cohort (i.e., respondents between 18 and 34 years) showed the highest risk for lifetime mental disorders for the majority of disorders included in the WMH analyses (with ORs all in the 2.6–20.6 range). Second, for anxiety, mood, and alcohol disorders, there was a linear increase in the risk of a lifetime mental disorder in younger cohorts, compared to the oldest cohort. Although this trend was found for the broad group of anxiety disorders, only GAD and social phobia accounted for this significant trend.

## 7.3. Service Use and Delays in Seeking Professional Care for Mental Disorders in Belgium

### 7.3.1. 12-month Treatment for Mental Disorders

Table 13.5 shows that an average of 39.5% of the respondents with a 12-month mental disorder consulted a formal health service for their mental health problems in the previous 12 months. Among these, health-care services were most often contacted (38.7%) and non–health-care services were rarely contacted to treat persons with mental disorders (2.1%). As expected, treatment contact rates were higher for respondents with mood disorders (50.9%) than for those with either anxiety (37.5%) or alcohol disorders (21.4%).

Those persons with mental disorders who were treated in health-care sectors were most

**Table 13.4.** Cohort as a predictor of lifetime risk of DSM-IV disorders

| | Age group | | | | | | | | | | | |
|---|---|---|---|---|---|---|---|---|---|---|---|---|
| | 18–34 | | 35–49 | | 50–64 | | 65+ | | | | |
| | OR | (95% CI) | OR | (95% CI) | OR | (95% CI) | OR | (95% CI) | $\chi^2$ | DF | $p$-value |
| **Anxiety disorder** | | | | | | | | | | | |
| Panic disorder | 2.8 | (0.9–8.3) | 1.0 | (0.3–2.9) | 1.0 | (1.0–1.0) | – | – | 4.0 | 2 | 0.13 |
| Generalized anxiety disorder with hierarchy | 5.2* | (1.5–17.6) | 4.4* | (1.4–14.0) | 2.1 | (0.7–6.5) | 1.0 | (1.0–1.0) | 9.9 | 3 | 0.020 |
| Specific phobia | 1.4 | (0.8–2.6) | 0.7 | (0.4–1.3) | 0.9 | (0.5–1.6) | 1.0 | (1.0–1.0) | 4.5 | 3 | 0.21 |
| Social phobia | 7.3* | (1.6–34.1) | 9.3 | (0.8–10.4) | 5.4 | (0.6–48.3) | 1.0 | (1.0–1.0) | 9.3 | 3 | 0.026 |
| Posttraumatic stress disorder | 2.5 | (0.3–19.6) | 5.1* | (1.1–23.6) | 1.7 | (0.4–8.2) | 1.0 | (1.0–1.0) | 8.1 | 3 | 0.044 |
| Any anxiety disorder | 2.6* | (1.3–5.0) | 1.6 | (0.8–3.2) | 1.3 | (0.6–2.6) | 1.0 | (1.0–1.0) | 14.2 | 3 | 0.003 |
| **Mood disorder** | | | | | | | | | | | |
| Major depressive disorder with hierarchy | 11.3* | (6.1–20.9) | 4.9* | (3.2–7.5) | 3.6* | (2.0–6.4) | 1.0 | (1.0–1.0) | 87.3 | 3 | <0.001 |
| Any mood disorder | 11.3* | (6.1–20.9) | 4.9* | (3.2–7.5) | 3.6* | (2.0–6.4) | 1.0 | (1.0–1.0) | 87.3 | 3 | <0.001 |
| **Impulse disorder** | | | | | | | | | | | |
| Any impulse-control disorder | 1.4 | (0.6–3.4) | 1.0 | (1.0–1.0) | 1.0 | (1.0–1.0) | 1.0 | (1.0–1.0) | 0.6 | 1 | 0.42 |
| **Alcohol disorder** | | | | | | | | | | | |
| Alcohol abuse | 4.9* | (2.6–9.2) | 3.7 | (1.9–7.1) | 2.7* | (1.4–5.4) | 1.0 | (1.0–1.0) | 27.4 | 3 | <0.001 |
| Alcohol dependence | 20.6* | (1.9–21.8) | 13.9 | (1.3–14.9) | 12.4* | (1.4–112) | 1.0 | (1.0–1.0) | 7.1 | 3 | 0.07 |
| Any alcohol disorder | 5.0* | (2.6–9.8) | 3.6* | (1.7–7.3) | 2.6* | (1.2–5.4) | 1.0 | (1.0–1.0) | 26.7 | 3 | <0.001 |
| **Any disorder** | | | | | | | | | | | |
| Any | 4.7* | (2.6–8.7) | 2.5* | (1.3–4.6) | 2.0* | (1.2–3.3) | 1.0 | (1.0–1.0) | 37.2 | 3 | <0.001 |

* indicates $p < 0.01$.

**Table 13.5.** 12-month service usage in Belgium: Percentage treated by health-care professionals among people with a mental disorder

| | Type of professional | | | | | | | | |
|---|---|---|---|---|---|---|---|---|---|
| | Psychiatrist | Other mental health care | Any mental health care | General medicine | Any health care | Human service | CAM | Any non–health-care | Any treatment |
| | % (se) | % (se) | % (se) | % (se) | % (se) | % (se) | % (se) | % (se) | % (se) |
| Any anxiety disorder | 9.1 (3.1) | 12.1 (2.6) | 17.1 (2.9) | 29.6 (3.8) | 37.3 (3.3) | 1.4 (1.1) | 0.9 (0.7) | 2.4 (1.4) | 37.5 (3.3) |
| Any mood disorder | 18.0 (5.5) | 17.6 (3.2) | 29.2 (4.4) | 42.9 (6.5) | 49.6 (5.8) | 1.6 (1.3) | 2.3 (1.2) | 3.9 (1.9) | 50.9 (5.8) |
| Any alcohol use disorder | 15.5 (7.1) | 12.0 (6.7) | 19.7 (9.4) | 14.9 (6.9) | 21.4 (9.7) | 3.9 (3.9) | 0.0 (0.0) | 3.9 (3.9) | 21.4 (9.7) |
| Any disorder | 10.2 (3.0) | 14.3 (2.8) | 21.0 (2.8) | 31.6 (5.0) | 38.7 (4.1) | 0.9 (0.7) | 1.2 (0.6) | 2.1 (1.0) | 39.5 (4.1) |
| No disorder | 1.8 (0.4) | 1.5 (0.4) | 2.9 (0.5) | 4.8 (1.0) | 6.4 (1.1) | 0.3 (0.2) | 0.6 (0.3) | 0.9 (0.4) | 6.7 (1.1) |

often treated by general medicine (31.6%), followed by those treated in mental health care sectors (21.0%). However, this was only the case for anxiety and mood disorders, not for alcohol disorders (Table 13.5). Indeed, 19.7% of the general population meeting criteria for an alcohol disorder (or 92% of those who are in treatment) were treated by mental health care, compared to 14.9% (or 70% of those in treatment) by general medicine. In contrast, among those with an anxiety disorder, 29.6% (or 79% of those in treatment) received services from general health care compared to 17.1% (or 46% of those in treatment) receiving services from mental health care.

Interestingly, among those respondents without a DSM-IV disorder, 6.7% reported the use of services in the past year (as in previous communication of this study [Demyttenaere et al. 2004]), this group will be referred to as "subthreshold

cases"). The general medicine sector was the most important sector where persons without mental disorders sought professional help: 4.8% of the general population received treatment from general medicine (or 72% of those seeking any treatment), 1.8% received treatment from a psychiatrist, and 1.5% from another mental health care professional.

### 7.3.2. Mean Number of Visits Per Year

Among individuals with a 12-month mental disorder consulting health services, the mean number of visits per year approximated 12 (M = 12.6, SE = 3.3), with slightly more contacts for those with a mood disorder (M = 16.7, SE = 4.7) than for those with an anxiety disorder (M = 13.0, SE = 5.4; Table 13.6). Persons treated in mental health care sectors were more likely to have more treatment contacts than those in general

**Table 13.6.** 12-month service usage in Belgium: Mean number of visits in the past year

| | Type of professional | | | | | | | | |
|---|---|---|---|---|---|---|---|---|---|
| | Psychiatrist | Other mental health care | Any mental health care | General medicine | Any health care | Human service | CAM | Any non–health-care | Any treatment |
| | % (se) | % (se) | % (se) | % (se) | % (se) | % (se) | % (se) | % (se) | % (se) |
| Any anxiety disorder | – | – | – | 5.3 (1.2) | 12.7 (5.3) | – | – | – | 13.0 (5.4) |
| Any mood disorder | – | – | 19.5 (7.5) | 6.1 (1.5) | 16.8 (4.7) | – | – | – | 16.7 (4.7) |
| Any impulse-control disorder | | | | | | | | | |
| Any alcohol use disorder | – | – | – | – | – | – | – | – | – |
| Any disorder | – | 8.5 (1.9) | 15.0 (5.9) | 5.5 (1.1) | 12.6 (3.3) | – | – | – | 12.6 (3.3) |
| No disorder | – | – | 8.2 (1.9) | 3.9 (0.6) | 6.6 (1.1) | – | – | – | 6.9 (1.1) |

**Table 13.7.** 12-month service usage in Belgium: Severity by treatment

| Treatment | Serious % | (se) | Moderate % | (se) | Mild % | (se) | None % | (se) | Any % | (se) |
|---|---|---|---|---|---|---|---|---|---|---|
| General medical | 48.8 | (8.5) | 30.9 | (7.1) | 11.2 | (4.6) | 4.8 | (1.0) | 8.2 | (1.3) |
| Mental health | 36.4 | (8.5) | 18.7 | (4.7) | 5.3 | (2.4) | 2.9 | (0.5) | 5.2 | (0.7) |
| Health care | 60.2 | (9.0) | 38.4 | (8.3) | 12.4 | (4.5) | 6.4 | (1.08) | 10.5 | (1.4) |
| Non–health care | 6.1 | (3.2) | 0.0 | (0.0) | 0.4 | (0.3) | 0.9 | (0.4) | 1.1 | (0.4) |
| Any treatment | 62.1 | (9.3) | 38.4 | (8.3) | 12.7 | (4.6) | 6.8 | (1.1) | 10.9 | (1.1) |
| No treatment | 37.9 | (9.3) | 61.6 | (8.3) | 87.3 | (4.6) | 93.2 | (1.1) | 89.1 | (1.2) |

medicine sectors (M = 15.0, SE = 5.9 vs. M = 5.5, SE = 1.1, respectively). Subthreshold cases reported about seven visits per year, with more visits if they received services from mental health care (M = 8.2, SE = 1.9) than general medicine (M = 3.9, SE = 0.6).

If we look at disorder-specific variation in the mean number of visits per year, persons with a mood disorder who were treated in mental health care sectors had most visits per year: almost 20 (M = 19.5, SE = 7.5). By contrast, persons with a mood disorder who were treated in general medicine sectors reported only six visits per year (M = 6.1, SE = 1.5).

### 7.3.3. Treatment Rates by Seriousness

Table 13.7 shows that treatment rates varied by disorder severity: the more serious the disorder, the higher the probability that persons sought professional care. This is a consistent finding for all the general and mental health care sectors

included in this study. Slightly more than 62% of those persons with a serious mental disorder received any treatment, compared to only 38% of those with a moderate disorder and 13% of those with a mild disorder.

### 7.3.4. Adequacy of Treatment

Among persons receiving treatment for their mental disorder, the vast majority (all in the 69%–89% range) received minimally adequate treatment (Table 13.8), regardless of the sector from which they received treatment. The probability of receiving minimally adequate care was highest in the mental health care sector. Regardless of the sectors from which persons received treatment, persons with anxiety disorders (compared to those with mood disorders) were less likely to have minimally adequate treatment.

However, if we use the definition of adequate treatment, a quite different picture emerges (Table 13.9). Regardless of the sectors where these

**Table 13.8.** 12-month service usage in Belgium: Percentage receiving minimally adequate treatment among people seeing professionals

| | Type of professional | | | | | | | | |
|---|---|---|---|---|---|---|---|---|---|
| | Psychiatrist | Other mental health care | Any mental health care | General medicine | Any health care | Human service | CAM | Any non–health care | Any treatment |
| | % (se) | % (se) | % (se) | % (se) | % (se) | % (se) | % (se) | % (se) | % (se) |
| Any anxiety disorder | – | – | – | 73.6 (8.7) | 70.0 (8.8) | – | – | – | 69.7 (8.8) |
| Any mood disorder | – | – | 89.7 (6.7) | 82.4 (6.9) | 81.5 (6.5) | – | – | – | 80.4 (6.3) |
| Any alcohol use disorder | – | – | – | – | – | – | – | – | – |
| Any disorder | – | 85.2 (11.8) | 80.0 (5.5) | 70.7 (7.6) | 70.2 (6.8) | – | – | – | 69.2 (7.0) |
| No disorder | – | – | 89.1 (5.9) | 72.9 (8.3) | 74.7 (6.0) | – | – | – | 75.9 (5.6) |

**Table 13.9.** 12-month service usage in Belgium: Percentage receiving adequate treatment among people seeing professionals

| | Type of professional | | | | | | | | |
|---|---|---|---|---|---|---|---|---|---|
| | Psychiatrist | Other mental health care | Any mental health care | General medicine | Any health care | Human service | CAM | Any non–health care | Any treatment |
| | % (se) | % (se) | % (se) | % (se) | % (se) | % (se) | % (se) | % (se) | % (se) |
| Any anxiety disorder | – | – | – | 31.4 (8.9) | 30.1 (7.5) | – | – | – | 30.0 (7.5) |
| Any mood disorder | – | – | 77.2 (7.9) | 51.1 (10.0) | 54.5 (8.9) | – | – | – | 53.2 (9.0) |
| Any alcohol disorder | – | – | – | – | – | – | – | – | – |
| Any disorder | – | 56.1 (10.7) | 58.4 (7.5) | 37.8 (8.4) | 39.4 (6.8) | – | – | – | 38.7 (6.8) |
| No disorder | – | – | 47.6 (8.9) | 28.9 (7.5) | 30.9 (6.2) | – | – | – | 29.4 (6.2) |

persons were treated, our data indicate that the majority of those with mood disorders received adequate treatment (with proportions between 51.1% and 77.2%), whereas the vast majority of the anxiety disorders did not meet criteria for this definition (with proportions between 30.0% and 31.4%). The probability of receiving adequate care was highest (i.e., 77%) for persons with a mood disorder who were receiving treatment from mental health care sectors. Our data also suggest that treatment in mental health care sectors is more often adequate than the treatment provided in general medicine sectors (58.4% vs. 37.8%, respectively).

The only predictors of minimally adequate treatment that yielded statistical significance were sociodemographic characteristics (Table 13.10). Anxiety, mood, and alcohol disorders were not related to receiving minimally adequate treatment. By contrast, minimally adequate treatment was related to age (with lowest rates in the youngest cohort), educational attainment (with lowest rates in persons with either some secondary or secondary education), and income (with lowest rates in the lowest income group).

### 7.3.5. Lifetime Treatment and Duration of Delay

The results of the survival curves investigating lifetime treatment and duration of delay could be summarized in three main findings (Table 13.11). First, most persons with DSM-IV

disorders eventually seek treatment: 93.7% for mood disorders, 84.5% for anxiety, and 61.2% for alcohol disorders. Within the group of anxiety disorders, panic disorder, GAD, and social phobia had markedly higher lifetime treatment rates (between 81.6% and 91.0%) compared to specific phobias (65.9%). Second, relatively few persons with DSM-IV disorders seek help in the first year of the disorder onset: 47.8% for mood disorders, 19.8% for anxiety disorders, and 12.8% for alcohol disorders. There were also considerable differences in individual anxiety disorders: persons with either panic disorder or GAD were much more likely to make treatment contact within the first year of onset of these disorders (56.4% and 46.8%, respectively) than were persons with either specific or social phobia (5.4% and 0%, respectively). Third, the median duration between disorder onset and first treatment contact varies widely: 18 years in persons with alcohol disorders, 16 years in persons with anxiety disorders, and only 1 year for mood disorders (Figure 13.1). Moreover, within the category of anxiety disorders, panic disorders and GAD had a rather low duration of delay (1 year) whereas median delays in specific and social phobias were rather high (21 and 23 years, respectively).

### 7.3.6. Predictors of Lifetime Treatment

Cohort and age of onset were consistent predictors of lifetime treatment (Table 13.12). For the majority of disorders assessed, we found a dominant pattern that the odds of lifetime treatment

**Table 13.10.** 12-month service usage in Belgium: Sociodemographic and disorder type predictors of any and minimally adequate treatment

| Model effect | Effect level | Minimally adequate treatment given any treatment and 12-month disorder OR (95% CI) |
|---|---|---|
| Age | 18–34 | 0.1 (0.0–3.0) |
| | 35–49 | 0.4 (0.0–13.8) |
| | 50–64 | 9.8 (0.3–382.9) |
| | 64+ | 1.0 (ref) |
| | Overall test of effect | $\chi^2(3) = 9.3$, $p = 0.025$ |
| Any anxiety disorder | Yes | 3.6 (0.2–56.2) |
| | No | 1.0 (ref) |
| | Overall test of effect | $\chi^2(1) = 0.9$, $p = 0.34$ |
| Any mood disorder | Yes | 4.5 (0.4–46.7) |
| | No | 1.0 (ref) |
| | Overall test of effect | $\chi^2(1) = 1.8$, $p = 0.18$ |
| Any alcohol disorder | Yes | 3.9 (0.1–201.2) |
| | No | 1.0 (ref) |
| | Overall test of effect | $\chi^2(1) = 0.5$, $p = 0.48$ |
| Education | None/primary | 3.7 (0.2–54.8) |
| | Some secondary | 0.3 (0.0–2.9) |
| | Secondary | 0.6 (0.1–2.8) |
| | Any postsecondary | 1.0 (ref) |
| | Overall test of effect | $\chi^2(3) = 9.1$, $p = 0.028$ |
| Income | Low | 0.0 (0.0–0.2) |
| | Low average | 0.1 (0.0–2.6) |
| | High average | 0.2 (0.0–5.1) |
| | High | 1.0 (ref) |
| | Overall test of effect | $\chi^2(3) = 14.1$, $p = 0.003$ |
| Marital status | Never married | 1.2 (0.1–17.0) |
| | Separated/widowed/divorced | 1.6 (0.0–10.5) |
| | Married/cohabiting | 1.0 (ref) |
| | Overall test of effect | $\chi^2(2) = 0.4$, $p = 0.83$ |
| Sex | Male | 0.1 (0.0–1.6) |
| | Female | 1.0 (ref) |
| | Overall test of effect | $\chi^2(1) = 2.8$, $p = 0.09$ |

**Table 13.11.** Proportional treatment contact in the year of disorder onset and median duration of delay among cases that subsequently made treatment contact

| | % Making treatment contact in year of onset | % Making treatment contact by 50 years | Median duration of delay (years) |
|---|---|---|---|
| **Anxiety disorder** | | | |
| Panic disorder | 56.4 | 91.0 | 1 |
| Generalized anxiety disorder (with hierarchy) | 46.8 | 81.6 | 1 |
| Specific phobia | 5.4 | 65.9 | 21 |
| Social phobia | 0.0 | 81.6 | 23 |
| Any anxiety disorder | 19.8 | 84.5 | 16 |
| **Mood disorder** | | | |
| Major depressive disorder (with hierarchy) | 47.8 | 93.7 | 1 |
| Any mood disorder | 47.8 | 93.7 | 1 |
| **Alcohol disorder** | | | |
| Alcohol abuse | 13.4 | 58.0 | 18 |
| Alcohol dependence | – | – | – |
| Any alcohol disorder | 12.8 | 61.2 | 18 |

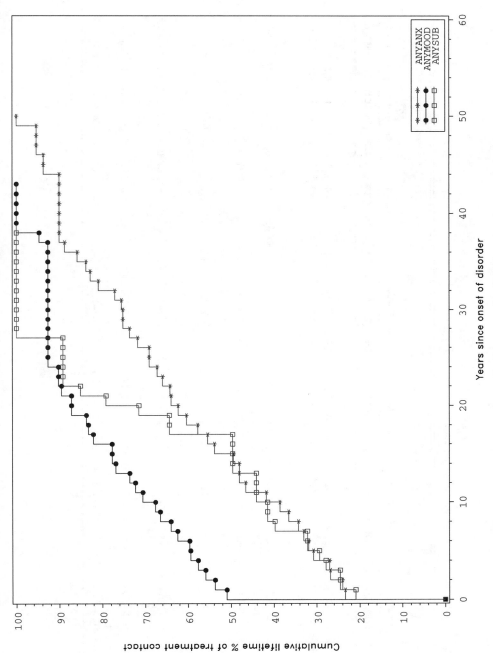

**Figure 13.1.** Cumulative lifetime % of tx contact for ANY disorders from year of onset.

Table 13.12. Sociodemographic predictors of lifetime treatment contact for specific DSM-IV disorders

| | Female | | χ² | Age 18–34 | | Age 35–49 | | Age 50–64 | | χ² | Early onset disorder | | Early onset average disorder | | Late onset average disorder | | χ² |
|---|---|---|---|---|---|---|---|---|---|---|---|---|---|---|---|---|---|
| | OR | (95% CI) | | OR | (95% CI) | OR | (95% CI) | OR | (95% CI) | | OR | (95% CI) | OR | (95% CI) | OR | (95% CI) | |
| **Anxiety disorder** | | | | | | | | | | | | | | | | | |
| Panic disorder | 0.7 | (0.1–3.3) | 0.2 | 2.3 | (0.5–12.0) | 1.1 | (0.3–3.3) | 1.0 | – | 1.2 | 0.1* | (0.0–0.7) | 0.3 | (0.0–4.7) | 0.7 | (0.1–5.5) | 17.2* |
| Generalized anxiety disorder with hierarchy | 1.5 | (0.7–2.9) | 1.3 | 1.5 | (0.2–10.3) | 3.3 | (0.9–13.0) | 1.4 | (0.3–5.8) | 4.5 | 0.4 | (0.0–3.1) | 1.0 | (0.3–3.6) | 0.8 | (0.1–6.2) | 4.6 |
| Specific phobia | 1.2 | (0.5–3.0) | 0.2 | 3.3 | (0.9–12.2) | 2.8 | (0.8–10.5) | 0.7 | (0.2–2.8) | 17.5* | 0.3* | (0.1–0.9) | 0.4 | (0.2–1.1) | 0.2* | (0.1–0.6) | 9.3* |
| Social phobia | 1.3 | (0.4–4.2) | 0.2 | 4.1 | (0.7–24.3) | 4.1 | (0.7–24.3) | 1.0 | – | 2.6 | 0.3* | (0.1–0.8) | 0.1* | (0.0–0.7) | 0.4* | (0.2–0.8) | 10.3* |
| Any anxiety disorder | 1.2 | (0.7–2.1) | 0.4 | 4.7* | (1.6–13.6) | 3.0* | (1.5–10.5) | 1.3 | (0.6–2.8) | 14.8* | 0.1* | (0.0–0.3) | 0.1* | (0.0–0.3) | 0.2* | (0.1–0.5) | 63.5* |
| **Mood disorder** | | | | | | | | | | | | | | | | | |
| Major depressive disorder with hierarchy | 1.4 | (0.9–2.1) | 2.5 | 3.9* | (1.2–12.5) | 3.9* | (1.5–10.5) | 1.7 | (0.7–4.0) | 14.5* | 0.2* | (0.1–0.6) | 0.4* | (0.2–0.9) | 0.6* | (0.4–0.9) | 14.2* |
| Any mood disorder | 1.4 | (0.9–2.1) | 2.5 | 3.9* | (1.2–12.5) | 3.9* | (1.5–10.5) | 1.7 | (0.7–4.0) | 14.5* | 0.2* | (0.1–0.6) | 0.4* | (0.2–0.9) | 0.6* | (0.4–0.9) | 14.2* |
| **Alcohol disorder** | | | | | | | | | | | | | | | | | |
| Alcohol abuse | 0.8 | (0.1–11.9) | 0.0 | 36.2* | (1.0–1312.5) | 36.2* | (1.0–1312.5) | 36.2* | (1.0–1312.5) | 4.3* | 0.1* | (0.0–0.2) | 0.1* | (0.0–0.2) | 0.1* | (0.0–0.2) | 18.8* |
| Alcohol dependence | – | | | – | | – | | – | | | – | | – | | – | | – |
| Any alcohol disorder | 0.7 | (0.1–8.3) | 0.1 | 35.9* | (1.1–1163.4) | 35.9* | (1.1–1163.4) | 35.9* | (1.1–1163.4) | 4.5* | 0.1* | (0.0–0.2) | 0.1* | (0.0–0.2) | 0.1* | (0.0–0.2) | 25.7* |

* indicates $p < 0.01$.

increase in more recent cohorts. Similarly, the association between the odds of lifetime treatment and age of onset shows that a higher age of onset was consistently related to higher odds of lifetime treatment. The only disorder for which lifetime treatment could not be predicted by cohort or age of onset was GAD. Furthermore, women did not have higher odds of treatment contact in any disorder assessed.

## 8. DISCUSSION

### 8.1. The Prevalence of Mental Disorders in Belgium

#### 8.1.1. 12-month Mental Disorders

Mental disorders are common in the Belgian general population: 13% met criteria for a DSM-IV disorder in the past year, whereas 29% met criteria for a lifetime mental disorder. Mood and anxiety disorders are the most common disorders in the population. An interesting addition from this study is that it provides 12-month and lifetime estimates of impulse-control disorders: these were estimated at 1.7% and 5.2%, respectively. The prevalence of these disorders (i.e., oppositional-defiant disorder, conduct disorder, and attention-deficit/hyperactivity disorder) is all in the range of the prevalence of separate anxiety disorders. Although the majority of previous studies have mentioned the high prevalence of anxiety, mood, and alcohol disorders, it is of crucial importance that impulse-control disorders are as common as anxiety disorders.

We can make only tentative and preliminary comparisons between our data and data from previous studies because of difficulties in conceptualizing and measuring mental disorders in previous surveys. Notwithstanding this, a few important findings warrant attention. For all disorders assessed, the present prevalence estimates are generally lower than those found in previous studies carried out in Belgium. For instance, our estimate that about 14% of the Belgian general population meets criteria for a 12-month mood disorder differs considerably from the 16% to 34% in previous surveys assessing DSM mood

disorders (Baruffol & Thilmany 1993; Ansseau & Reggers 1999; Ansseau et al. 1999; Bracke & Wauterickx 2003). When we compare the current prevalence rates with international prevalence rates from the WMH Survey Initiative (Demyttenaere et al. 2004; Kessler et al. 2006), we see that 12-month prevalence of mental disorders in Belgium is the median value within the European countries.

#### 8.1.2. Lifetime Risks of Mental Disorders

An important addition of this study is that it provides projections relative to the proportion of persons who will eventually develop a mental disorder. Lifetime risk of mental disorders in the general population of Belgium was estimated at 37%. This means that, in absolute terms, 37% (i.e., 8% more than the actual estimate of 29%) of respondents will ever have a mental disorder by the (theoretical) age of 75. The lifetime risks of anxiety and alcohol disorders approximate the lifetime prevalence estimates: the risks for these disorders were only 2.5% to 2.6% greater than prevalence estimates. This reflects their early ages of onset (Christie et al. 1988; WHO International Consortium Psychiatric Epidemiology 2000). This is even more pronounced in impulse-control disorders: lifetime prevalence estimates and lifetime risk estimates were exactly the same at 5.2%. Of particular importance is that the number of persons who will meet criteria for a mood disorder is expected to increase. Lifetime risk for mood disorders was considerably higher (8.7%) than the prevalence rate. Most probably, this is because we found both a late age of onset and a large IQR for mood disorders.

#### 8.1.3. Implications

If we compare our findings with those assessing ages of onset and lifetime risks of somatic diseases, there are two striking differences between mental and somatic disorders: (1) mental disorders have relatively early ages of onset with a strong foothold in youth and (2) the risk of ever developing a mental disorder seems to mature out once persons pass the critical high-risk age.

In combining Belgian WMH data, clinicians and policy makers may be more able to promote public interest in preventing, screening, and treating mental disorders. There are some important issues that emerge. First, our data enable us to put more emphasis on the early age at which most disorders develop. People with mental disorders seem to have these disorders in their prime of life. Moreover, mental disorders, and more specifically mood and alcohol disorders, were more common in persons from younger cohorts. These findings raise the question of whether there is a need for more screening and treatment interventions for children and adolescents to prevent undiagnosed and untreated disorders from progressing later life. This seems especially important with regard to impulse-control and anxiety disorders because these start in childhood and early adolescence. Second, our findings also enable us to identify the group of disorders with narrow IQRs: impulse-control and alcohol disorders. The time range in which they develop is quite narrow: 8 to 11 years (compared to 23 years in mood, and 27 years in anxiety disorders). Our data suggest that childhood and early adolescence (roughly between the ages of 9 and 16) is a critical high-risk period for impulse-control disorders. Similarly, young adulthood (roughly the ages between 20 and 31) appears to be a critical high-risk period for alcohol disorders. Third, our data also highlight the late onset of mood disorders, together with the broad age range in which these disorders develop. These findings suggest that the onset of mood disorders is generally not concentrated in a high-risk period. An important implication is that preventative or screening approaches will be far more difficult.

## 8.2. The Use of Services and Received Treatment for Mental Disorders

### 8.2.1. First Treatment Contacts

Our data confirm the common finding that the use of services for mental disorders is suboptimal, at least if we consider 12-month treatment rates: four in ten persons with mental disorders made

a first treatment contact with professional health care. Twelve-month treatment was related to disorder severity: severe disorders were more likely to receive treatment (i.e., 6 in 10) than moderate (4 in 10) and mild disorders (1 in 10). The proportions of persons with a mental disorder seeking professional care are quite comparable to earlier reported treatment rates in Belgium (Ansseau & Reggers 1999; Ansseau et al. 1999). They are also concordant with treatment rates in the Netherlands (Bijl & Ravelli 2000) and the United States (Wang et al. 2005), but higher than the average use of services in six European countries (Alonso et al. 2004). If we consider lifetime treatment rates, then a quite different conclusion can be drawn: the vast majority of persons with lifetime mental disorders in Belgium eventually make a first treatment contact. About nine in ten of those with a mood disorder, eight in ten of those with an anxiety disorder, and six in ten with an alcohol disorder. Mental disorders, and especially anxiety and mood disorders, were treated mostly within general medicine sectors, reflecting the crucial role of the general practitioner in the health-care system (Goldberg & Huxley 1980).

### 8.2.2. Follow-up after First Treatment Contact

Upon entering treatment, the average person made approximately 13 visits in the past year, with highest rates in mental health care (about 15) and in those persons with mood disorders (about 17). Persons treated in general medicine sectors received about six sessions in the past 12 months, features consistent with U.S. estimates (Kessler et al. 1999). Moreover, most persons in treatment receive only minimally adequate treatment. Thus, once persons have entered professional health care, the treatment is suboptimal when compared to minimal standards of treatment adequacy (Agency for Health Care Policy and Research 1993; American Psychiatric Association 1998; Bech 1999; Rush & Thase 1999). In a previous report, we found that up to one in five persons who sought professional help did not receive any follow-up treatment (Bruffaerts et al. 2004), with the highest rates for lack of any follow-up (i.e., 25%) in anxiety disorders. Our data do not allow us to draw direct conclusions, but they indicate that receiving minimal adequate treatment is linked with age (especially ages between 35 and 64), high education, and high-income.

### 8.2.3. Subthreshold Cases Seeking Treatment

Almost 7% of persons without 12-month mental disorders (or the subthreshold cases) received treatment. Although this seems a relatively low percentage, the vast majority of the general population (i.e., 87.3%) comprises persons without mental disorders. This implies that there is a meaningful fraction of the general population receiving treatment without meeting criteria for a 12-month DSM-IV mental disorder. These persons had an average of seven visits per year. Against the rising health-care expenditures in Belgium (Kesteloot 2001), this begs the question why persons without mental disorders receive treatment. One reason they were being treated may be that they have a lifetime disorder in partial or full remission, without, however, meeting enough diagnostic criteria for a 12-month DSM-IV disorder. It may also be that these persons may meet a few criteria for a mental disorder, without, however, reaching the diagnostic threshold. From a preventative viewpoint, it could be argued that subthreshold cases may benefit from treatment, in protecting further deterioration of the patient's condition (Kessler et al. 2003). Moreover, in light of the fact that the total disease burden of DSM-IV MDE may be reduced by only 50% under adequate treatment (Andrews et al. 2000), the importance of implementing preventative interventions for subthreshold cases should be stressed (Smit et al. 2006).

### 8.2.4. Mediators of Lifetime Treatment

Persons from more recent cohorts systematically had higher odds for lifetime treatment, suggesting that help-seeking behavior for a broad range

of mental disorders has improved in the recent past. Especially in the light of the organization of the Belgian mental health care delivery system, our findings are important because it may be that younger persons are more aware of the possible pathways that could lead them to professional care for emotional problems.

The likelihood of first treatment contact was lowest in persons with early-onset disorders, a pattern that is more or less consistent with established literature (Kessler, Olfson & Berglund 1998; Olfson et al. 1998). This is a finding with considerable implications because many mental disorders, especially anxiety disorders, have their onset in childhood or adolescence. Minors could therefore be less likely to receive timely treatment because those with early-onset disorders may not interpret emotional problems or disturbances as emotionally deviating, or because the recognition of a disorder may depend on proxies (Kessler et al. 2005).

### 8.2.5. Delays in Treatment

We found a low proportion of persons making treatment contact in the same year of the onset of the disorder (roughly between 13% and 48%) and impressive median durations of delay (between 1 and 18 years) from the onset of the disorder to the first treatment contact. This was especially the case for persons with either anxiety or alcohol disorders. One explanation for the finding that only one in five persons with an anxiety disorder made a first treatment contact in the year of the onset of the disorder could be that these disorders have their onset in childhood or adolescence (Kessler et al. 2005). This could imply, for example, that persons with an anxiety disorder are less likely to interpret their emotional problems in mental health terms. Following the early age of onset, anxious behavior can thus be interpreted as a normal behavioral standard with, accordingly, a very low need for treatment. Low treatment rates for alcohol disorders could possibly be explained by the fact that consuming alcohol is a socially accepted behavior that generally correlates with low perceived need for treatment (Zimberg 1994). Nevertheless, our findings demonstrate that most persons with mental disorders eventually seek treatment. Thus, from a general health perspective, the major concern is not the lack of seeking treatment as such, but rather the low proportion of persons seeking help in due time, and, consequently, the impressive delays in doing so. One possible implication for further research is to understand these factors that explain this enormous duration of delay between the disorder onset and the first treatment contact.

### 8.2.6. Interdisorder Variation in Service Use

Considerable interdisorder variation in lifetime treatment, duration of delay, and the proportion of persons making contact in the year of the onset of the disorder were observed. These variations were more or less consistent with existing studies (Kessler et al. 1998; Wang et al. 2004; Wang et al. 2005). Persons with either MDE or panic disorders were most likely (i.e., in more than 91% of cases) to receive lifetime treatment. One explanation may be that, at least for MDE, this disorder yields a high personal and social burden (Bonnewyn et al. 2005). It may also be that higher treatment rates for depression may be due to the recent public attention for this disorder. Another explanation may be that public beliefs tend to be milder for persons with depression than for persons with other disorders (Angermeyer & Dietrich 2006). One explanation for the high lifetime treatment estimates for panic disorders, compared to the other anxiety disorders, may be that this disorder is characterized by pronounced somatic symptoms, such as heart palpitations, racing heart, shortness of breath, nausea, shaking, and so on (American Psychiatric Association 1994).

### 8.2.7. Implications

Taken together, policy makers should gain awareness of the specificity of the mental health care delivery system in Belgium. Given the high accessibility of the system, the low out-of-pocket expenses, and the overall high density of inpatient and outpatient services, we expected that these features would lead to a higher proportion of persons seeking help for their mental disorders within a short-term perspective. However, the treatment rates in Belgium are not consistent with the hypothesis that countries with a higher provision of mental health services would show a higher probability of service use for mental reasons (Alonso et al. 2004). Indeed, 12-month and lifetime treatment rates for mental disorders in Belgian are quite comparable to those of other European and even non-European countries, even when those countries have considerably fewer treatment facilities (Bruffaerts et al. 2004). These findings suggest that other factors may explain these barriers to care. One explanation may also be that stigma plays a more crucial role in seeking professional help for mental disorders than does availability or accessibility of services. Another explanation could be that not all persons with mental disorders experience a need for treatment within the short term (i.e., 12-month), and that disorder severity may moderate the process of seeking help. Indeed, data indicate that treatment rates vary by disorder severity: the more severe the disorder, the higher is the probability of treatment. The finding that most of the persons with a disorder eventually make a treatment contact may indicate that, within the long term, most persons with mental disorders experience a certain need for treatment that drives them to contact a health-care professional. Given these findings, two major challenges in further thoughts of treating mental disorders in Belgium are essential: (1) how to reduce the impressive delays in making a first treatment contact with professional care, and (2) how to ensure adequate treatment when persons have finally entered the health-care system. To date, there are no obvious mechanisms by which these two challenges can be met. More research is needed to identify factors that may enhance help-seeking processes in a provider-rich environment.

## 9. CONCLUSIONS

The originality and enduring significance of this survey deserve some attention. This study is the first population-representative study in Belgium that has pointed to prevalence estimates of and treatment patterns for mental disorders. To investigate this, well-validated and structured instruments were used to diagnose mental disorders and to assess treatment contacts. Advanced statistical methods were used to calculate the proportion of persons who will eventually make treatment contact for their mental disorder. A major improvement in this study is that it focuses on lifetime treatment contact, whereas the majority of published studies focus on 12-month treatment for mental disorders.

Our data show that approximately 37% of the Belgian population will have had a mental disorder by the age of 75, with mood disorders being the most prevalent class of disorders (23%). Projected lifetime risks were 8% greater than lifetime prevalence estimates. Mental disorders start early in life: median age of onset was lowest for anxiety disorders (14 years) and highest for mood disorders (38 years). Mental disorders appeared to be more common among younger cohorts than among older cohorts. Although our observations are explorative and require more systematic study in the future, from a public health perspective they draw attention to preventive and curative initiatives that could be implemented in late childhood or early adolescence.

We also found that the majority of persons with a mental disorder will eventually get treated, but with dramatic delays between the disorder onset and the first treatment contact. This is even more pronounced against the background that the Belgian mental health care system is a provider-rich environment, with a high density of primary care and specialized services. Indeed, it is an interesting and challenging finding that both the number of persons seeking professional help in the first year of disorder and the delays in first treatment contact approximate those of the United States, despite the fact that there are considerably fewer treatment facilities in the United States. This suggests that factors other than those related to the availability and accessibility of treatment facilities explain the delays in seeking professional help.

## REFERENCES

Agency for Health Care Policy and Research (1993). *Depression Guideline Panel, Vol. 2: Treatment of major depression, Clinical Practice Guideline, No 5.* Rockville, MD: U.S. Department of Health and Human Services, Public Health Service, Agency for Health Care Policy and Research.

Alonso, J., Angermeyer, M. C., Bernert, S., Bruffaerts, R., Brugha, T. S., Bryson, H., de Girolamo, G., de Graaf, R., Demyttenaere, K., Gasquet, I., Haro, J. M., Katz, S. J., Kessler, R. C., Kovess, V., Lepine, J. P., Ormel, J., Polidori, G., Russo, L. J., Vilagut, G., Almansa, J., Arbabzadeh-Bouchez, S., Autonell, J., Bernal, M., Buist-Bouwman, M. A., Codony, M., Domingo-Salvany, A., Ferrer, M., Joo, S. S., Martinez-Alonso, M., Matschinger, H., Mazzi, F., Morgan, Z., Morosini, P., Palacin, C., Romera, B., Taub, N. & Vollebergh, W. A. (2004). Disability and quality of life impact of mental disorders in Europe: Results from the European Study of the Epidemiology of Mental Disorders (ESEMeD) project. *Acta Psychiatrica Scandinavica Supplement*, 38–46.

American Psychiatric Association (1994). *Diagnostic and Statistical Manual, 4th edition.* Washington, DC: American Psychiatric Association Press.

American Psychiatric Association (1998). *Practice guidelines for treatment of patients with panic disorder.* Washington, DC: American Psychiatric Association Press.

Andrews, G., Sanderson, K., Corry, J. & Lapsley, H. M. (2000). Using epidemiological data to model efficiency in reducing the burden of depression. *Journal of Mental Health Policy and Economics*, 3, 175–86.

Angermeyer, M. C. & Dietrich, S. (2006). Public beliefs about and attitudes towards people with mental illness: A review of population studies. *Acta Psychiatrica Scandinavica*, 113, 163–79.

Ansseau, M. (1996). *Epidemiologie van depressie in België: Socio-economische aspecten van depressie in België.* Brussel: Belgische Liga voor Depressie.

Ansseau, M. & Reggers, J. (1999). *Epidémiologie des troubles psychiatriques dans la province de Liège et leur prise en charge.* Liège: Plate-forme Psychiatrique Liégeoise.

Ansseau, M., Reggers, J. & Nickels, J. (1999). *Epidémiologie des troubles psychiatriques dans la province de Luxembourg.* Luxembourg: Plate-forme de concertation psychiatrique dans la province de Luxembourg.

Arrindell, W. A., Ettema, J. H. M. & SCL-90 (1986). *Handleiding bij een multidimensionele psychopahologie-indicator.* Lisse: Swets Publishers.

Baruffol, E. & Thilmany, M. C. (1993). Anxiety, depression, somatization and alcohol abuse:

Prevalence rates in a general Belgian community sample. *Acta Psychiatrica Belgica*, 93, 136–53.

Bayingana, K., Demarest, S., Gisle, L., Hesse, E., Miermans, P. J., Tafforeau, J. & Van Der Heyden, J. (2006). Gezondheidsenquête door middel van Interview, België, 2004. IPH/EPI Reports No. 2006-035. Wetenschappelijk Instituut Volksgezondheid, Afdeling Epidemiologie, Brussels.

Bech, P. (1999). Pharmacological treatment of depressive disorders. In *WPA Series Evidence and Experience in Psychiatry*, ed. M. Maj & N. Sartorius, pp. 89–127. New York: Wiley.

Bietlot, M., Demarest, S., Tafforeau, J. & Van Oyen, H. (2000). Enquête de santé 1997: La santé en Belgique, ses communautés et ses regions. Brussels: F-Twee Uitgeverij.

Bijl, R. V. & Ravelli, A. (2000). Psychiatric morbidity, service use, and need for care in the general population: Results of the Netherlands Mental Health Survey and Incidence Study. *American Journal of Public Health*, 90, 602–7.

Bijl, R. V., Ravelli, A. & van Zessen, G. (1998). Prevalence of psychiatric disorder in the general population: Results of the Netherlands Mental Health Survey and Incidence Study (NEMESIS). *Social Psychiatry and Psychiatric Epidemiology*, 33, 587–95.

Bonnewyn, A., Bruffaerts, R., Van Oyen, H., Demarest, S. & Demyttenaere, K. (2005). The impact of mental disorders on daily functioning in the Belgian community. Results of the study European Study on Epidemiology of Mental Disorders (ESEMeD). *Revue Medicale de Liege*, 60, 849–54.

Bracke, P. & Wauterickx, N. (2003). Complaints of depression in a representative sample of the Belgian population. *Archives of Public Health*, 61, 223–47.

Bruffaerts, R., Bonnewyn, A. & Demyttenaere, K. (2006). De geestelijke gezondheidszorg in België: Situatieschets en toekomstperspectieven. *Acta Hospitalia*, 46, 7–23.

Bruffaerts, R., Bonnewyn, A., Van Oyen, H., Demarest, S. & Demyttenaere, K. (2004). Patterns of service use for mental health disorders in Belgium: Results of the European Study on Epidemiology of Mental Disorders (ESEMeD). *Revue medicale de Liege*, 59, 136–44.

Bruffaerts, R. & Demyttenaere, K. (2005). Psychiatric emergency services in Belgium. *Emergency Psychiatry*, 11, 16–9.

Christie, K. A., Burke, J. D., Jr., Regier, D. A., Rae, D. S., Boyd, J. H. & Locke, B. Z. (1988). Epidemiologic evidence for early onset of mental disorders and higher risk of drug abuse in young adults. *American Journal of Psychiatry*, 145, 971–5.

Danckaerts, M. (in press). Ontwikkelingen en noden op vlak van de geestelijke gezondheidszorg voor kinderen en jongeren. *Acta Hospitalia*.

Demarest, S., Van Der Heyden, J., Gisle, L., Buziarist, J., Meirmans, P. J., Sartor, F., Van Oyen, H. & Tafforeau, J. (2002). Gezondheidsenquête door middel van Interview, België, 2001. IPH/EPI Reports No. 2002-25. Wetenschappelijk Instituut Volksgezondheid, Afdeling Epidemiologie, Brussels.

Demyttenaere, K., Bruffaerts, R., Posada-Villa, J., Gasquet, I., Kovess, V., Lepine, J. P., Angermeyer, M. C., Bernert, S., de Girolamo, G., Morosini, P., Polidori, G., Kikkawa, T., Kawakami, N., Ono, Y., Takeshima, T., Uda, H., Karam, E. G., Fayyad, J. A., Karam, A. N., Mneimneh, Z. N., Medina-Mora, M. E., Borges, G., Lara, C., de Graaf, R., Ormel, J., Gureje, O., Shen, Y., Huang, Y., Zhang, M., Alonso, J., Haro, J. M., Vilagut, G., Bromet, E. J., Gluzman, S., Webb, C., Kessler, R. C., Merikangas, K. R., Anthony, J. C., Von Korff, M. R., Wang, P. S., Brugha, T. S., Aguilar-Gaxiola, S., Lee, S., Heeringa, S., Pennell, B. E., Zaslavsky, A. M., Üstün, T. B. & Chatterji, S. (2004). Prevalence, severity, and unmet need for treatment of mental disorders in the World Health Organization World Mental Health Surveys. *Journal of the American Medical Association*, 291, 2581–90.

Derogatis, L. R., Lipman, R. S. & Covi, L. (1973). SCL-90: An outpatient psychiatric rating scale-preliminary report. *Psychopharmacology Bulletin*, 9, 13–28.

Fondation Julie Renson (2005). *Mémento de la santé mentale*. Brussels: Fondation Julie Renson.

Goldberg, D. P. (1972). *The detection of psychiatric illness by questionnaire: A technique for the identification and assessment of non-psychotic psychiatric illness*. London: Oxford University Press.

Goldberg, D. P. & Huxley, P. (1980). *Mental illness in the society: The pathways to psychiatric care*. London: Tavistock.

Hall, S. & Rao, K. (1992). *Advanced techniques of population analysis*. New York: Plenum.

Henderson, S., Andrews, G. & Hall, W. (2000). Australia's mental health: An overview of the general population survey. *Australian and New Zealand Journal of Psychiatry*, 34, 197–205.

Jenkins, R., Lewis, G., Bebbington, P., Brugha, T., Farrell, M., Gill, B. & Meltzer, H. (2003). The National Psychiatric Morbidity Surveys of Great Britain: Initial findings from the household survey. *International Review of Psychiatry*, 15, 29–42.

Kessler, R. C., Berglund, P., Demler, O., Jin, R., Koretz, D., Merikangas, K. R., Rush, A. J., Walters, E. E. & Wang, P. S. (2003). The epidemiology of major depressive disorder: Results from the National Comorbidity Survey Replication (NCS-R).

*Journal of the American Medical Association*, 289, 3095–105.

Kessler, R. C., Berglund, P., Demler, O., Jin, R., Merikangas, K. R. & Walters, E. E. (2005). Lifetime prevalence and age-of-onset distributions of DSM-IV disorders in the National Comorbidity Survey Replication. *Archives of General Psychiatry*, 62, 593–602.

Kessler, R. C., Haro, J. M., Heeringa, S. G., Pennell, B. E. & Üstün, T. B. (2006). The World Health Organization World Mental Health Survey Initiative. *Epidemiologia E Psichiatria Sociale*, 15, 161–6.

Kessler, R. C., McGonagle, K. A., Zhao, S., Nelson, C. B., Hughes, M., Eshleman, S., Wittchen, H. U. & Kendler, K. S. (1994). Lifetime and 12-month prevalence of DSM-III-R psychiatric disorders in the United States: Results from the National Comorbidity Survey. *Archives of General Psychiatry*, 51, 8–19.

Kessler, R. C., Merikangas, K. R., Berglund, P., Eaton, W. W., Koretz, D. S. & Walters, E. E. (2003). Mild disorders should not be eliminated from the DSM-V. *Archives of General Psychiatry*, 60, 1117–22.

Kessler, R. C., Olfson, M. & Berglund, P. A. (1998). Patterns and predictors of treatment contact after first onset of psychiatric disorders. *American Journal of Psychiatry*, 155, 62–9.

Kessler, R. C. & Üstün, T. B. (2004). The World Mental Health (WMH) Survey Initiative Version of the World Health Organization (WHO) Composite International Diagnostic Interview (CIDI). *International Journal of Methods in Psychiatric Research*, 13, 93–121.

Kessler, R. C., Zhao, S., Katz, S. J., Kouzis, A. C., Frank, R. G., Edlund, M. & Leaf, P. (1999). Past-year use of outpatient services for psychiatric problems in the National Comorbidity Survey. *American Journal of Psychiatry*, 156, 115–23.

Kesteloot, K. (2001). Hervormingen in de gezondheidszorg. Economische achtergrond en ethische implicaties. In *Moeten, mogen, kunnen: Lessen voor de éénentwintigste eeuw*, ed. B. Raymaekers, A. Van De Putte & G. Van Riel, pp. 159–85. Leuven: Universitaire Pers Leuven.

Kittel, F., Ribourdouille, M. & Dramaix, M. (1997). Mental health data analysis from the National Health Survey, Belgium 1997. *Archives of Public Health*, 50, 347–57.

Kleinman, A. (1995). Do psychiatric disorders differ in different cultures? The methodological questions. In *The culture and psychology reader*, ed. N. R. Goldberger & J. B. Veroff, pp. 631–51. New York: New York University Press.

Koeter, M. W. J. & Ormel, J. (1991). *General health questionnaire: Nederlandse bewerking*. Handleiding: Lisse, Swets & Zeitlinger.

Lassey, M. L., Lassey, W. R. & Jinks, M. J. (1997). *Health care systems around the world: Characteristics, issues, reforms*. Upper Saddle River, NJ: Prentice Hall.

Lepine, J. P., Gastpar, M., Mendlewicz, J. & Tylee, A. (1997). Depression in the community: The first pan-European study DEPRES (Depression Research in European Society). *International Clinical Psychopharmacology*, 12, 19–29.

Moos, R. H., Cronkite, R. C. & Finney, J. W. (1982). *Health and daily living form manual*. Palo Alto, CA: Mind Garden.

Murray, C. J. L. & Lopez, A. D. (1996). *The global burden of disease: A comprehensive assessment of mortality and disability from diseases, injuries and risk factors in 1990 and projected to 2020*. Cambridge, MA: Harvard University Press.

Olfson, M., Kessler, R. C., Berglund, P. A. & Lin, E. (1998). Psychiatric disorder onset and first treatment contact in the United States and Ontario. *American Journal of Psychiatry*, 155, 1415–22.

Rush, A. J. & Thase, M. (1999). Psychotherapies for depressive disorders: A review. In *WPA series evidence and experience in psychiatry*, ed. M. Maj & N. Sartorius, pp. 161–206. New York: Wiley.

SAS Institute (2001). *SAS/STAT software: Changes and enhancements, Release 8.2*. Cary, NC: SAS Publishing.

Shah, B. V. & Barnwell, B. G. (1997). *SUDAAN User's Manual Release 8.0.1*. Research Triangle Park, NC: Research Triangle Institute.

Smit, F., Ederveen, A., Cuijpers, P., Deeg, D. & Beekman, A. (2006). Opportunities for cost-effective prevention of late-life depression: An epidemiological approach. *Archives of General Psychiatry*, 63, 290–6.

Tylee, A., Gastpar, M., Lepine, J. P. & Mendlewicz, J. (1999). Identification of depressed patient types in the community and their treatment needs: Findings from the DEPRES II (Depression Research in European Society II) survey. *International Clinical Psychopharmacology*, 14, 153–65.

Van Oyen, H., Tafforeau, J., Hermans, H., Quataert, P., Schiettecatte, E., Lebrun, L. & Belameret, L. (1997). The Belgian Health Interview Survey. *Archives of Public Health*, 55, 1–13.

Wang, P. S., Berglund, P. A., Olfson, M. & Kessler, R. C. (2004). Delays in initial treatment contact after first onset of a mental disorder. *Health Services Research*, 39, 393–415.

Wang, P. S., Lane, M., Olfson, M., Pincus, H. A., Wells, K. B. & Kessler, R. C. (2005). Twelve-month use of mental health services in the United States: Results from the National Comorbidity Survey

Replication. *Archives of General Psychiatry*, 62, 629–40.

Wauterickx, N. & Bracke, P. (2005). Unipolar depression in the Belgian population: Trends and sex differences in an eight-wave sample. *Social Psychiatry and Psychiatric Epidemiology*, 40, 691–9.

WHO International Consortium Psychiatric Epidemiology (2000). Cross-national comparisons of the prevalences and correlates of mental disorders. *Bulletin of the World Health Organization*, 78, 413–23.

World Health Organization (WHO) (2005). *World mental health atlas*. Geneva: World Health Organization.

Zimberg, S. (1994). Psychotherapy with alcoholics. In *Specialized techniques for specific clinical problems in psychotherapy*, ed. T. B. Karasu & L. Bellak, pp. 382–99. London: Jason Aronson.

# 14 The Prevalence of Mental Disorders and Service Use in France: Results from a National Survey 2001–2002

SAENA ARBABZADEH-BOUCHEZ, ISABELLE GASQUET, VIVIANNE
KOVESS-MASFETY, LAURENCE NEGRE-PAGES, JEAN-PIERRE LÉPINE

## ACKNOWLEDGMENTS

The ESEMeD project is funded by the European Commission (Contracts QLG5-1999-01042; SANCO 2004123), the Piedmont Region (Italy), Fondo de Investigación Sanitaria, Instituto de Salud Carlos III, Spain (FIS 00/0028), Ministerio de Ciencia y Tecnología, Spain (SAF 2000-158-CE), Departament de Salut, Generalitat de Catalunya, Spain, Instituto de Salud Carlos III (CIBER CB06/02/0046, RETICS RD06/0011 REM-TAP), and other local agencies, and by an unrestricted educational grant from GlaxoSmithKline. ESEMeD is carried out in conjunction with the World Health Organization World Mental Health (WMH) Survey Initiative. We thank the WMH staff for assistance with instrumentation, fieldwork, and data analysis. These activities were supported by the U.S. National Institute of Mental Health (R01MH070884), the John D. and Catherine T. MacArthur Foundation, the Pfizer Foundation, the U.S. Public Health Service (R13-MH066849, R01-MH069864, and R01 DA016558), the Fogarty International Center (FIRCA R03-TW006481), the Pan American Health Organization, Eli Lilly and Company Foundation, Ortho-McNeil Pharmaceutical, GlaxoSmithKline, and Bristol-Myers Squibb. A complete list of WMH publications can be found at http://www.hcp.med.harvard.edu/wmh/.

## I. DESCRIPTION OF THE COUNTRY

### 1.1. Sociodemographic Description

According to the last population census, 59.3 million individuals lived in mainland France, to which must be added 1.7 million inhabitants from the four overseas departments (Guadeloupe, French Guiana, Martinique, and Réunion). France is the third most populated European country after Germany and the United Kingdom. Four climatic types prevail in metropolitan France: a temperate climate in the west, near the coast; a midlatitude continental climate in the interior of the country, a mountain climate in the high-altitude areas, and a Mediterranean-type climate along the southern coast. From an organizational point of view, French territory is administered through three main metropolitan units of government: 22 regions, to which the central government is increasingly transferring authority, 96 (plus 4 overseas) departments, and 36,565 municipalities.

The age pyramid in France is fairly typical of rich developed countries, with an increasingly broad top and a narrow base over the past 30 years (see Table 14.1). According to Organisation of Economic Co-operation (OECD) and INSEE (National Institute for Statistics and Economic Studies) projections, the percentage of individuals older than 60 should rise up to 26% in 2025 and 35% in 2050.

The population distribution is fairly irregular across the territory of 549,000 square kilometers. According to official INSEE criteria, more than 45 millions citizens dwell in urban areas (representing 75% of the total population). Average density range from 30 and 50 inhabitants/km$^2$ in the rural Corse and Auvergne regions, up to 322 and 912 inhabitants/km$^2$ in the industrialized and urbanized Nord-Pas-de-Calais and Île-de-France regions, respectively. About 42% of the population and an even higher share

**Table 14.1.** Population age distribution in France from 1970 to 2001

| Age (years) | 1970 | 1980 | 1990 | 2001 |
|---|---|---|---|---|
| Younger than 20 | 33.1 | 30.6 | 27.8 | 25.3 |
| 20–59 | 48.8 | 52.4 | 53.2 | 54.1 |
| 60 and older | 18.0 | 17.0 | 19.0 | 20.6 |

of total economic activity are located in the four largest conurbations (Paris, Lyon, Marseille/Aix-en-Provence, and Lille) and their respective regions (Île-de-France, Rhône-Alpes, Provence-Alpes–Côte d'Azur, Nord-Pas-de-Calais).

Migration represents about one-fifth of the population growth, which is less than other E.U. countries, partly because of a relatively high birth rate (French natural growth rate is only second to Ireland in the European Union). The number of foreign-born residents equals 7.4% of the total population. In 2000, only 16% of individuals obtaining French citizenship were born in other E.U. countries, as opposed to 48% in North Africa (Algeria, Morocco, and Tunisia).

The evolution of data concerning marital status follows the general European trend: marriages decrease whereas divorces increase. There are on average 6.2 weddings and 1.5 divorces per year per 1000 inhabitants in France (corresponding respectively to the 8th and 9th rank among E.U. countries). The percentage of couples without children rose from 23.7% in 1990 to 27.5% in 2001, whereas couples with children fell from 36.4% to 32.3%. A slight decrease is observed in the proportion of single-parent families (7.1% in 1999), yet there is a growing number of individuals living alone: figures for males rise from 10.1% (1990) to 12.5% (2001) of the total population, and from 17.1% to 18.7% for females.

The French gross domestic product (GDP) totalled EUR 1404 billion for the year 2002. Considered together with population figure, GDP per capita was above EUR 23,000 per year, corresponding to the 19th rank among OECD countries in 2001. Industrial activity is quite diversified in France. Agriculture and the related

industries represent a large share of economic activity compared to many other Western European countries: in 2000, these two sectors accounted for around 6% of total value added in the economy and for some 10% of total goods exports. Much of the output from these two sectors supplies the country's vast number of restaurants and hotels. Tourist-related economic activities – many involving gastronomy – play a significant role in the tertiary sector. The predominance of the services sector in the economy is considerable, accounting for 72% of GDP and 73% of employment. In addition, even in decline, the leading role of the state in the service sector should be mentioned, not only in the health-care and education domains but also in telecommunications and transport.

In spite of its strengths, the French economy fails to provide employment to each of its residents. After four promising years of decline, since 2001, the unemployment rate has consistently been on the rise, totaling 8.9% of the labor force in 2002. Unemployment affects females more severely (10.1%) as well as the younger population (20.2% of those aged 18–25).

## 1.2. Health-care System

Health-care expenditure amounts to 9.5% of the GDP in France, the fourth highest rate among the OECD countries. Average expenditure per year per capita increased from US$1517 in 1990 to US$2349 in 2000. Inpatient care accounts for 43% of the total health-care consumption, whereas pharmaceutical and other nondurables represent 20% of the total. According to a WHO study analyzing the performances of the health systems of its 191 members, France obtained the best overall health-care ranking.

Medical services in France are provided by public institutions (hospitals), private institutions (private hospitals or clinics), and private providers (doctors and other medical and paramedical professionals). The health system is being placed under the responsibility of the state, through the Health Ministry. Since 1996, the legislative body decides annually the health objectives as well as the financing of the social coverage system. The French medical system can be considered state-subsidized; the development of a comprehensive Social Security system began after World War II. In 1945, the General Scheme (Régime Général) was created, with the goal of rapidly covering the entire population. However, supplements to Social Security schemes were being developed and special independent schemes were being maintained or created. Health insurance has been constantly extended over the years to new categories of people. In 2000, universal medical coverage was implemented as a final step in this direction.

Today, Social Security schemes represent approximately 97% of public expenditures on health. Yet one can observe that out-of-pocket spending has increased in the past decade: on average, personal health expenses represented US$174 in 1990 and US$240 in 2000.

Public hospitals are financed through annual budgets by local hospital agencies (ARH, Agences Régionales de l'Hospitalisation). These agencies dispatch the regional budget among the different institutions. Payments for private hospitals are made on a fee-for-service basis, as a schedule of fees is defined each year. The ARH also monitor the activity of the medical institutions operating in their region, setting objectives and granting authorization for creation or expansion of medical departments and acquisition of major pieces of equipment. Following consultation with experts and providers, the government defines the prices of reimbursable drugs and other medical goods. Nonreimbursable drugs are priced by the pharmaceutical companies. Medical practitioners and workers are paid on a fee-for-service basis. Fees are part of periodic agreements (conventions) signed by professional associations and the three national health insurance funds (*Caisse Nationale de l'Assurance Maladie (CNAM), Mutualité Sociale Agricole (MSA) and Caisse d'Assurance Maladie des Professions Indépendantes (CANAM)*), supervised by the state.

The number of practicing physicians per 1000 inhabitants is quite stable (3.1 in 1990 vs. 3.3 in 2000), partly due to a system of quotas, which restricts the number of students allowed to enter the different disciplines. Public hospitals account for about three-quarters of the overall number of hospital beds. Since the mid-1970s, a series of reforms have been implemented in an attempt to slow the growth of the health-care expenditure and reduce the deficit. This, together with better medical techniques and the development of alternatives to regular hospitalisation, have led, for instance, to a decrease in the number of acute-care beds (6.2 per 1000 inhabitants in 1980 vs. 4.2 in 2000) and in the average length of stay in this type of units (9.9 days in 1980 vs. 5.5 days in 2000) (OECD data). On the other hand, beds in long-term-care institutions have increased in recent years, partly in response to the needs of a growing number of dependent elderly people (10% of the total number of hospital beds in 1987 vs. 17% in 1997).

## 2. THE MENTAL HEALTH SYSTEM

The mental health care system belongs to the general health system. As with other disabled individuals, those with mental illness can have access to disability pensions. As we will detail below, both public and private structures are available to treat the mentally ill.

### 2.1. Public Structures

Since 1972, public service psychiatry has been divided geographically into sectors, associated with public health hospitals (97 specialized in psychiatry plus 151 psychiatry departments operating within general hospitals). In 1997, there were 829 psychiatry sectors for adults (one for 54,000 inhabitants), 321 psychiatry sectors for children and adolescents (one for 49,000 inhabitants), as well as 26 sectors devoted to the prisoner population. Sectors may have at their disposal different types of facilities to perform the treatments. However, each sector does not always have all the existing facilities at its disposal. For long-lasting pathologies, the mental health care system provides about 57,000 beds in full-time confinement. Part-time hospitalization is also available (approximately 24,000 beds). Next, medical psychological centers (centres médico-psychologiques) provide outpatient consultations. These 2100 treatment centers are the basis of operations for coordinated actions. A total of 1400 part-time therapeutical centres are also available for less serious cases.

## 2.2. Private Structures

First, various private structures are also able to provide psychiatric beds: in 1997, there were 152 clinics for mental health, 27 institutions devoted to psychiatric aftercare, and 74 day-care hospitals run by nonprofit private associations. As a whole, these private structures manage a total of 14,000 hospital beds and 3000 beds for part-time hospitalisation. Next, there were 532 medical psychological educational centers (CMPP: centres médico-psycho-pédagogiques), run by associations. The CMPP have done pioneering work, particularly in ambulatory treatments of children with psychological disorders and difficulties in school. Last, specialized practitioners belong to the private health system. There were 6342 psychiatrists working in the private sector in 1998, to whom must be added a larger number of psychologists (10,000–15,000). Unlike psychiatrists' consultation, care provided by psychologists is not reimbursed in France by the Social Security scheme.

## 3. PREVIOUS MENTAL HEALTH EPIDEMIOLOGICAL STUDIES

Since 1985, a few mental health general population surveys have been conducted in France, some in national samples and others in regional or community samples. Some have focused on specific diagnoses and others on a larger range of disorders. We briefly review these previous studies in this section of the chapter.

## 3.1. DEPRES

Depression Research in European Society (DEPRES) was the first nationally representative study of mental health disorders in France (Lepine et al. 1997). DEPRES was a large, in-depth European survey of depression designed

to estimate the prevalence of depression in the general population, to evaluate the treatment needs, and to assess the consequences of depression for individuals and society at large. This two-phase study was conducted in six European countries: Belgium, France, Germany, the Netherlands, Spain, and the United Kingdom. The sample was designed to match the population in each country as closely as possible by taking into account sex, age, region, and other demographic factors such as employment. Interviews were conducted from April 1995 to July 1995.

Phase 1 of the study (DEPRES I) had three main objectives: (1) assess the six-month prevalence of depression in the community, (2) determine the extent to which persons suffering from depression sought treatment, and (3) assess the impact of depression related among other variables to the number of working days lost due to depression. In this first phase, subjects were evaluated by the depression section of the Mini-International Neuropsychiatric Interview (MINI). Questions concerning the health-care consultation, drug prescription, and days of work lost due to depression were also included.

A total of 13,359 of the 78,463 adults who participated in the DEPRES telephone screening interviews were identified as suffering or having suffered from any type of depression in the previous six months; thus, the six-month prevalence of any type of depression in the community was estimated at 17%.

A substantial proportion (43%) of the DEPRES respondents suffering from depression did not seek any treatment. Most of those who did seek care consulted a primary care physician. Patients with more severe depression were more likely to seek care. However, even among those suffering from major depression, 31% did not consult a physician.

Approximately 70% of the depressed patients who presented to a health-care professional did not receive any medication for their symptoms. Given that most health-care consultations were made by subjects with the most severe and disabling depressive symptoms, it is striking that 59% of the patients suffering from major

**Table 14.2.** Prevalence of mood and anxiety disorders according to DSM-III in Savigny

| | 12-month prevalence | | Lifetime prevalence | |
|---|---|---|---|---|
| | Men (%) (n = 658) | Women (%) (n = 1088) | Men (%) (n = 658) | Women (%) (n = 1088) |
| Major depression | 3.4 | 6.0 | 10.7 | 22.4 |
| Panic disorder | 0.5 | 1.9 | 1.4 | 3.3 |
| Generalized anxiety | 3.7 | 6.6 | 6.6 | 12.2 |
| Agoraphobia | – | – | 3.7 | 9.9 |
| Social phobia | – | – | 2.1 | 5.4 |
| Simple phobia | – | – | 10.5 | 23.2 |
| All phobias | 7.9 | 16.0 | 12.5 | 28.9 |

*Source:* Lépine et al. 1993.

depression were not prescribed any form of treatment. Overall, 25% of depressed subjects taking a medication were receiving antidepressant therapy; thus, only about 8% of all depressed subjects received an antidepressant. There was a widespread use of tranquilizers, and in most countries a higher proportion of depressed subjects were prescribed tranquilizers rather than antidepressants.

Compared with subjects who were not depressed, those with major depression lost four times as many working days over a six-month period.

## 3.2. CREDES Study

Using the MINI, the CREDES study (Le Pape & Lecomte 1999) in 1997–1999 assessed a random sample of French residents covered by health insurance. It is worth noting that health insurance coverage in France is almost universal.

The 12-month prevalence of depression was found to be 12% after assessment by MINI as compared with 6.3% based on self-declaration; the estimate was 6.8% when patients taking an antidepression medication the day before the survey were also included.

At several time points during the survey, questions were asked regarding the clinical management of patients. More than 40% of those with self-declared depression had at least one episode of care (visit) during a one-month period, and more than half took a psychoactive medica-tion the day before the survey. Patients with self-declared depression and positive response to MINI (or, identified as depressed by MINI) appeared to have a somewhat higher use of care. In contrast, patients with depression identified by MINI only had little access and/or use of care for symptoms related to their depression (about 8% during a one-month period). Regarding type of treatment, about 10% of patients treated, received a hypnotic agent or a tranquilizer, whereas only 3% took an antidepressant the day before the survey.

## 3.3. Savigny: A Community Survey

In the late 1980s, a survey was conducted in the general population of a new town in the Parisian suburbs to investigate the prevalence and risk factors arising from anxious and depressive states (Lepine et al. 1993). In the survey, 1746 subjects were assessed using the Diagnostic Interview Schedule (DIS), a structured interview developed for use by lay interviewers or clinicians in subjects in community or in clinical samples. DIS generates current and lifetime diagnoses according to DSM-III criteria. Anxiety and depression were common traits in this population (see Table 14.2). Furthermore, there was a significant comorbidity between anxiety and mood disorders. Identified risk factors for depression were separation, important family conflicts, a child's death, important professional conflicts, health problems, and financial problems.

## 3.4. Two Regional Studies: Parisian Area and Basse Normandie

Two regional studies have been conducted on representative adult samples of the Île-de-France (Kovess-Masféty, Gysens & Chanoit 1993) and Basse-Normandie regions (Kovess-Masféty & Delavelle 1998). Comparing prevalence between the two regions was made possible because similar methods and instruments were used in both studies, a simplified version of the WHO Composite International Diagnostic Interview (CIDIS) (Kovess- Masféty, Lecoutour & Delavelle 2005). Twelve-month prevalence for major depression was estimated to be slightly lower in the mostly urban Île-de-France region (5.9%) than in the more rural Basse-Normandie region (7.2%). Panic attacks were estimated to be rare in both regions, affecting only 0.3% and 0.4% of the population in the Île-de-France and Basse-Normandie regions, respectively. Prevalences for diagnosed paroxystic anxiety were much higher but did not significantly differ between regions (5.3% for Île-de-France and 4.7% for Basse-Normandie). On the contrary, phobias were estimated to be significantly more common in Île-de-France (3.4%) than in the Basse-Normandie region (1.4%). Finally, a contrast between regions was found regarding alcohol dependence and/or abuse (only 0.4% in Île-de-France but 1.4% in Basse-Normandie).

## 3.5. A Recent Four-region, 20,000-person, General Population Survey

More recently, in 2005, a four-region study was completed on 22,099 random persons by telephone (2000 for those having mobile only), and the participation rate was 65.5% (from 56.3% in Île-de-France to 66.5% in Lorraine). This study was a replication of the Ciarlo and Tweed study in Colorado looking for mental health indicators applicable for mental health planning purposes (Kovess-Masféty & Carmona 2006).

The short-form version of the CIDI (CIDI-SF; Kessler et al. 1998) was used to assess prevalence. CIDI-SF results were compared to those obtained with blinded clinical reappraisal interviews in a probability subsample of 150 primary health-care subjects in an effort to validate the CIDI-SF. Results show little differences across regions, although there are larger differences in health territories designed for mental health planning purposes (Table 14.3).

## 3.6. The French WMH Survey

The French WMH survey was administered as part of the European Study of the Epidemiology of Mental Disorders (ESEMeD; Alonso, Angermeyer & Lepine 2004), a coordinated series of nationally representative psychiatric epidemiological surveys carried out as part of the WMH Survey Initiative in six Western European countries. The six ESEMeD studies use comparable design and standardized field methods aimed at allowing valid comparisons to be made across participating countries in the prevalence and correlates of mental health disorders. All ESEMeD surveys focus on the noninstitutionalized household population ages 18 and older. In France, the survey was carried out between 2001 and 2003 and completed 2894 interviews.

## 4. METHODS

### 4.1. Sampling Frame for the Study Population in France

The principles of the study design (random sampling, nationally representative data, strict inclusion and exclusion criteria, standardized questionnaires and methods of data collection, centralized database, and quality control) for the survey in France were the same as those for the other ESEMeD surveys with the exception of the construction of the sampling frame. The sampling frame in France was constructed on the basis of a random list of telephone numbers generated for the country. The list of telephone numbers was then linked with the list of addresses associated with those telephone numbers to identify the households to be sampled. This procedure differed from that used in any other WMH country. This procedure was used in France because of limits in other potential sources of data. The census (INSEE) data for 1999 were not accessible. The same was true for

**Table 14.3.** Twelve-month prevalence of DSM–IV diagnoses in different regions of France

| | Île-de-France (n = 5413) | | Haute-Normandie (n = 5650) | | Lorraine (n = 5736) | | Rhône-Alpes (n = 5551) | |
|---|---|---|---|---|---|---|---|---|
| | % | (95 CI) | % | (95 CI) | % | (95 CI) | % | (95 CI) |
| MDD | | | | | | | | |
| Total | 10.7 | (9.9–11.5) | 8.4 | (7.7–9.2) | 10.2 | (9.4–11.0) | 8.4 | (7.7–9.1) |
| Mild | 1.3 | (1.0–1.6) | 1.3 | (1.0–1.6) | 1.2 | (0.9–1.5) | 1.0 | (0.8–1.3) |
| Moderate | 7.4 | (6.7–8.1) | 5.6 | (5.0–6.2) | 6.8 | (6.1–7.5) | 5.4 | (4.8–6.0) |
| Severe | 1.4 | (1.1–1.7) | 1.0 | (0.8–1.3) | 1.5 | (1.1–1.8) | 1.3 | (1.0–1.6) |
| Social phobia | 5.7 | (5.1–6.3) | 5.6 | (5.0–6.2) | 5.1 | (4.5–5.7) | 5.4 | (4.8–6.0) |
| Specific phobia | 7.3 | (6.6–8.0) | 7.4 | (6.7–8.1) | 8.3 | (7.6–9.0) | 7.5 | (6.8–8.3) |
| Agoraphobia without panic disorder | 2.5 | (2.1–2.9) | 2.7 | (2.3–3.1) | 2.6 | (2.2–3.1) | 2.7 | (2.3–3.1) |
| Panic disorder | | | | | | | | |
| Without agoraphobia | 0.5 | (0.3–0.7) | 0.4 | (0.2–0.5) | 0.5 | (0.3–0.7) | 0.3 | (0.2–0.5) |
| With agoraphobia | 2.0 | (1.7–2.4) | 2.1 | (1.7–2.5) | 1.9 | (1.6–2.3) | 2.0 | (1.6–2.4) |
| OCD | 3.3 | (2.8–3.7)* | 2.6 | (2.2–3.0)* | 3.4 | (3.0–3.9)* | 2.9 | (2.5–3.3)* |
| PTSD | 4.8 | (4.3–5.4) | 4.7 | (4.2–5.3) | 5.0 | (4.4–5.6) | 5.0 | (4.5–5.6) |
| GAD | 4.0 | (3.4–4.6) | 3.9 | (3.4–4.4) | 3.9 | (3.4–4.4) | 3.8 | (3.3–4.3) |
| Alcohol use | | | | | | | | |
| Abuse | 1.5 | (1.2–1.9)* | 1.4 | (1.1–1.7)* | 1.2 | (0.9–1.5)* | 2.2 | (1.6–2.4)* |
| Dependency | 2.3 | (1.9–2.7) | 1.6 | (1.3–2.0) | 1.9 | (1.5–2.2) | 1.9 | (1.6–2.3) |
| Illicit drug use | | | | | | | | |
| Abuse | 1.5 | (1.2–1.8)* | 1.4 | (1.1–1.8)* | 1.7 | (1.4–2.1)* | 1.7 | (1.4–2.0)* |
| Dependency | 1.6 | (1.3–1.9) | 1.0 | (0.8–1.3) | 1.4 | (1.1–1.7) | 1.7 | (1.4–2.1) |

* $p \leq 0.05$.
*Source:* Kovess et al. 2005.

a comprehensive household mailing address list. The electoral lists are, in general, not complete. A telephone frame was consequently considered the best feasible option.

A randomly generated list of telephone numbers, stratified by region and city size, was constructed to have a sample size proportional to the population in each region and to obtain a representative sample of households in France. An initial list including 1500 numbers was selected on the basis of data from France-Telecom. Unlisted (red/orange) numbers were not included in this initial list. The last two digits of each telephone number in this list were then modified at random to obtain seven new telephone numbers, thus generating 10,500 new numbers. This second list, which could include both listed and unlisted numbers, was then used to construct the list of addresses for the households to be contacted. Nonresponders and those who refused to participate were not replaced. The acceptance rate was estimated at 65%, which suggested that approximately 7000 individuals could be included. Next, using a telephone directory, the list of household addresses was established using the list of telephone numbers. Those numbers that did not correspond to private home addresses (e.g., fax, taxi cabs, public telephone, companies), as well as numbers that were not attributed, were deleted from the list. The final list of numbers was used to contact households to verify their eligibility. In each eligible household, an individual was selected and invited to participate in the study.

### 4.2. Measures: Diagnostic Assessment of Lifetime and 12-month DSM-IV Disorders

As with all WMH surveys, diagnoses were made using Version 3.0 of the WHO's CIDI (Kessler & Üstün 2004) a fully structured lay-administered diagnostic interview that generates diagnoses according to the definitions and criteria of both the ICD-10 (WHO 1991) and DSM-IV (American Psychiatric Association 1994) diagnostic systems. DSM-IV criteria are used in analyses for this chapter. As a detailed discussion of the instrument is presented in Chapter 4 of this volume, we only note here that the French WMH survey included the same assessments of mood disorders, anxiety disorders, impulse-control disorders, and substance disorders as the other ESEMeD surveys. As noted in Chapter 13 of this volume, this assessment excluded some of the disorders included in other WMH surveys. All diagnoses were made with organic exclusions and without diagnostic hierarchy rules. As described in Chapter 6 of this volume, a blinded clinical reappraisal study using the Structured Clinical Interview for DSM-IV (SCID) (First et al. 2002) showed generally good concordance between DSM-IV diagnoses based on the CIDI and independent diagnoses based on clinical assessments for anxiety, mood, and substance disorders. The CIDI diagnoses of impulse-control disorders have not been validated.

## 4.3. Other Measurement Issues

All other measurement issues were handled consistently in the ESEMeD surveys. Age of onset of disorders was assessed retrospectively. Twelve-month cases were classified by severity into serious, moderate, and mild cases on the basis of a complex classification scheme that was described by Bruffaerts and colleagues (see Chapter 13) in their description of the Belgium WMH survey. Lifetime treatment contact, 12-month service use, and minimally adequate treatment were also classified in the same way in France as in the other ESEMeD surveys. Predictor variables, finally, were the same as in the other ESEMeD countries.

## 4.4. Analysis Procedures

As noted previously, the data were weighted to adjust for differential probabilities of selection of respondents within households and differen-

tial nonresponse as well as to adjust for residual differences between the sample and the French population on the cross-classification of sociodemographic variables. An additional weight was used in the Part 2 sample to adjust for differences in probability of selection into that sample. Simple cross-tabulation was used to estimate prevalence and distributions of treatment. Survival analysis was used to make estimated projections of cumulative lifetime probability of disorders and treatment contact from year of onset using the actuarial method (Halli & Rao 1992). Discrete-time survival analysis (Efron 1988) with person-year as the unit of analysis was used to examine correlates of disorders and treatment contact. Logistic regression analysis (Hosmer & Lemeshow 1989) was used to study sociodemographic predictors of 12-month disorders, receiving treatment for these disorders, and treatment adequacy. Standard errors were estimated using the Taylor series method as implemented in SUDAAN (Research Triangle Institute 2002). Multivariate significance tests were made using Wald $\chi^2$ tests based on coefficient variance-covariance matrices that were adjusted for design effects using the Taylor series method. Statistical significance was evaluated using two-sided design-based tests and the 0.05 level of significance.

## 5. RESULTS

### 5.1. Participation Rate

The response rate was 46% for France, the lowest of any WMH surveys. We attribute this low participation rate to the fact that the necessary use of the telephone sampling frame added an extra layer of difficulty in contacting and establishing rapport with respondents that did not exist in other countries. In light of this difficulty, it would be most desirable for future related studies in France to address the problem of the sampling frame in creative ways, such as establishing a collaboration with a government agency that could provide access to voting registry or working with government mail lists or combinations of commercial mailing lists that might provide more comprehensive coverage and all direct household sampling rather than first-stage telephone recruitment.

Subsequently, we discuss some of the preliminary descriptive results obtained in the first phase of the analysis of the French data. These results include estimates of the overall lifetime prevalence of the mental health disorders assessed in the study, as well as their relation to sociodemographic factors including age, sex, marital status, income, and birth cohort.

## 5.2. Prevalence and the Sociodemographic Correlates of DSM-IV Disorders

Table 14.4 shows the overall lifetime prevalence of the mental health disorders assessed in the study and their relations with age, whereas Table 14.5 presents the relation between the 12-month prevalence of specific disorders and the subjects' age groups using odds ratios (ORs) as the measure of association.

Overall, 37.9% (95% CI, 34.6–41.2) of patients had a diagnosis of a mental health disorder during their lifetime (Table 14.4); 14.8% (95% CI, 12.6–17.0) had two or more diagnoses, and 6.2% (95% CI, 4.8–7.6) had three or more. As a group, anxiety and mood disorders had the highest lifetime prevalences: 22.3% (95% CI, 19.6–25.0) and 21.0% (95% CI, 18.8–23.2), respectively. Impulse-control and substance abuse disorders had comparable prevalences of 7.6% (95% CI, 5.1–10.1) and 7.1% (95% CI, 6.1–8.1), respectively.

Among anxiety disorders, specific phobia had the highest lifetime prevalence (10.7%), followed by GAD with hierarchy (4.9%) and social phobia (4.3%). MDE had a prevalence of 21.0% (95% CI, 18.8–23.2). Among impulse-control disorders, the most prevalent was attention-deficit/hyperactivity disorder (ADHD) (4.7%). Oppositional Defiant Disorder (ODD) and Conduct Disorder (CD) had comparable prevalences of 2.0% and 2.5%, respectively. The lifetime prevalence of alcohol abuse was 6.7% and that of any substance abuse was 7.1%.

There was a statistically significant association ($p = 0.006$) between the lifetime prevalence of a mental health disorder (any diagnosis) and age. The prevalence tended to be stable until 50 years, with decreases thereafter. This was also true for the 12-month prevalence of mental health disorders (any diagnosis) with about a 1.6- to 2-fold increase in the odds of a mental health disorder for subjects aged 18–34 years (OR 1.6, 95% CI, 1.0–2.7) and aged 35–49 years (OR 2.0, 95% CI, 1.3–2.9), as compared with those aged 65 years and older.

A statistically significant association was also noted between age and the lifetime prevalence of three or more diagnoses of mental health disorders, with a substantially lower prevalence for older subjects. Specifically, those 65 years and older had about a fourfold lower prevalence (1.7%) for three or more diagnoses as compared with those aged 18–34 years (9.6%) and 35–49 years (7.0%); subjects aged 50–64 years also had about a twofold lower prevalence (4.3%) than younger subjects.

Age was found to be related to the prevalence of several disorders but not others. Disorders significantly associated with subject's age included panic, social phobia, anxiety and mood disorders, and alcohol and other substance abuse. The lifetime prevalence of panic disorders was relatively stable until 50 years of age and decreased thereafter ($p = 0.055$). The prevalence was 2.5%–2.8% for subjects younger than 50 as compared with 1.5% for those aged 50–64 and 0.9% for those 65 years and older.

Lifetime prevalence of social phobia decreased (monotonically) with age ($p = 0.01$) with the highest prevalence (6.0%) for those aged 18–34 years and the lowest for those 65 years and older (1.6%). The lifetime prevalence of anxiety disorders (any) was relatively stable until 50 years of age with decreases thereafter; the prevalence decreased from about 25%–29% for subjects younger than 50 years to 18.7%, and 12.7% for those aged 50–64 and 65 years or older, respectively ($p = 0.024$). The 12-month prevalence of anxiety disorders was also higher for subjects younger than 50 years with about a twofold increase in the odds of anxiety disorders for subjects younger than 50 years as compared with those 65 years and older (Table 14.5).

**Table 14.4.** Overall lifetime prevalence of the mental health disorders in France

| Disorder group | Disorder | Age (years) 18–34 | | 35–49 | | 50–64 | | 65+ | | $\chi^2$ | All n | % | (95% CI) |
|---|---|---|---|---|---|---|---|---|---|---|---|---|---|
| | | % | (95% CI) | % | (95% CI) | % | (95% CI) | % | (95% CI) | | | | |
| Anxiety | Panic | 2.5 | (1.3–3.7) | 2.8 | (1.6–4.0) | 1.5 | (0.9–2.1) | 0.9 | (0.9–0.9) | 8.6 | 56 | 2.1 | (1.5–2.7) |
| | GAD with hierarchy | 5.1 | (3.1–6.9) | 4.6 | (3.0–6.2) | 5.7 | (3.9–7.5) | 3.9 | (3.9–3.9) | 1.9 | 142 | 4.9 | (3.9–5.9) |
| | Social phobia | 6.0 | (4.0–8.0) | 5.4 | (3.2–7.6) | 3.0 | (1.6–4.4) | 1.6 | (1.6–1.6) | 13.2* | 124 | 4.3 | (3.3–5.3) |
| | Specific phobia | 10.2 | (8.0–12.4) | 11.5 | (8.6–14.4) | 10.6 | (8.2–13.0) | 10.1 | (10.1–10.1) | 0.7 | 312 | 10.7 | (9.5–11.9) |
| | Agoraphobia without panic | 0.6 | (0.0–1.2) | 1.2 | (0.4–2.0) | 1.5 | (0.3–2.7) | 0.7 | (0.7–0.7) | 2.3 | 36 | 1.0 | (0.6–1.4) |
| | PTSD | 4.4 | (2.0–6.8) | 3.5 | (2.1–4.9) | 4.5 | (1.2–7.8) | 2.8 | (2.8–2.8) | 1.5 | 96 | 3.9 | (2.7–5.1) |
| | SAD/ASA | 3.1 | (0.7–5.5) | 2.4 | (0.6–4.2) | – | | – | | 0.2 | 31 | 2.8 | (1.2–4.4) |
| | Any anxiety | 24.8 | (18.5–31.1) | 29.0 | (22.3–35.7) | 18.7 | (14.0–23.4) | 12.7 | (12.7–12.7) | 11.0* | 445 | 22.3 | (19.6–25.0) |
| Mood | MDE | 23.6 | (19.7–27.5) | 21.2 | (17.3–25.1) | 21.8 | (18.5–25.1) | 16.1 | (16.1–16.1) | 7.6 | 648 | 21.0 | (18.8–23.2) |
| | Any mood | 23.6 | (19.7–27.5) | 21.2 | (17.3–25.1) | 21.8 | (18.5–25.1) | 16.1 | (16.1–16.1) | 7.6 | 648 | 21.0 | (18.8–23.2) |
| Impulse | ODD with hierarchy | 2.0 | (0.4–3.6) | 2.0 | (0.0–4.4) | – | | – | | 0.0 | 24 | 2.0 | (0.6–3.4) |
| | CD | 3.3 | (0.4–6.2) | 1.3 | (0.5–2.1) | – | | – | | 2.2 | 23 | 2.5 | (0.5–4.5) |
| | ADHD | 5.6 | (1.7–9.5) | 3.3 | (1.3–5.3) | – | | – | | 1.0 | 38 | 4.7 | (2.3–7.1) |
| | Any impulse | 8.7 | (4.8–12.6) | 5.9 | (3.2–8.6) | – | | – | | 1.2 | 71 | 7.6 | (5.1–10.1) |
| Substance | Alcohol abuse | 8.4 | (6.4–10.4) | 7.6 | (5.4–9.8) | 7.0 | (4.5–9.5) | 2.6 | (1.2–4.0) | 35.6* | 189 | 6.7 | (5.7–7.7) |
| | Alcohol dependence with abuse | 2.5 | (1.3–3.7) | 1.2 | (0.6–1.8) | 1.6 | (0.2–3.0) | 0.7 | (0.0–1.7) | 12.2* | 47 | 1.6 | (1.0–2.2) |
| | Any substance | 9.0 | (6.8–11.2) | 8.0 | (5.8–10.2) | 7.0 | (4.5–9.5) | 3.0 | (1.6–4.4) | 36.7* | 202 | 7.1 | (6.1–8.1) |
| All | Any DX | 40.4 | (33.7–47.1) | 44.8 | (38.1–51.5) | 37.6 | (33.5–41.7) | 24.4 | (17.7–31.1) | 15.4* | 847 | 37.9 | (34.6–41.2) |
| | 2+ | 18.0 | (13.5–22.5) | 14.6 | (11.5–17.7) | 14.5 | (10.0–19.0) | 10.3 | (5.4–15.2) | 4.2 | 384 | 14.8 | (12.6–17.0) |
| | 3+ | 9.6 | (5.5–13.7) | 7.0 | (4.8–9.2) | 4.3 | (2.5–6.1) | 1.7 | (0.3–3.1) | 36.5* | 165 | 6.2 | (4.8–7.6) |

* Significant at the 0.05 level, double-sided test.

**Table 14.5.** Demographic correlates of 12-month health-care treatment using Part 2 weights after stratification

|  | OR | (95% CI) |
|---|---|---|
| **Sex** |  |  |
| Male | 1.0 | – |
| Female | 1.3 | (0.7–2.6) |
| $\chi^2$ |  | 0.7 |
| **Age** |  |  |
| 18–34 | 0.9 | (0.6–1.5) |
| 35–49 | 1.4 | (0.7–2.5) |
| 50–64 | – | – |
| 65+ | 1.0 |  |
| $\chi^2$ |  | 1.2 |
| **Income** |  |  |
| Low | 0.8 | (0.4–1.5) |
| Low-average | 1.3 | (0.7–2.5) |
| High-average | 1.3 | (0.8–2.0) |
| High | 1.0 | – |
| $\chi^2$ |  | 4.2 |
| **Marital status** |  |  |
| Married/cohabiting | 1.0 | – |
| Separated/widowed/divorced | 1.1 | (0.6–1.8) |
| Never married | 0.9 | (0.5–1.7) |
| $\chi^2$ |  | 0.2 |
| **Severity** |  |  |
| Severe | 11.9 | (5.9–24.2) |
| Moderate | 5.4 | (3.1–9.4) |
| Mild | 3.4 | (1.8–6.3) |
| None | 1.0 | – |
| $\chi^2$ |  | 64.6* |

* Significant at the 0.05 level, double-sided test.

The lifetime prevalence of mood disorders was relatively stable for subjects aged 18–64 years and appeared to decrease thereafter; however, differences across age groups were not statistically significant at 0.05 level ($p = 0.08$). The 12-month prevalence of mood disorders was also not significantly associated with subjects' age; however, point estimates again suggested a lower odds for subjects 65 years and older.

Both the lifetime and 12-month prevalence estimates of alcohol and other substance abuse were significantly associated with age ($p < 0.001$). The lifetime prevalence of alcohol abuse was somewhat higher for subjects aged 18–34 years as compared with those aged 50–64 years; prevalence rates were 8.0% and 7.0%, respec-

tively. Thereafter, the prevalence of alcohol abuse decreased more than threefold for those aged 65 years and older (2.6%) as compared with younger subjects. The prevalence rates for alcohol dependence with substance abuse and that of any substance abuse were also relatively stable or decreased slightly between 18 and 64 years with substantial decreases for subjects 65 years of age and older.

In contrast, we did not find statistically significant associations between age and several other disorders, including Generalized Anxiety Disorder (GAD) with hierarchy, specific phobia, agoraphobia without panic, posttraumatic stress disorder, Separation Anxiety Disorder (SAD), Adult Separation Anxiety (ASA), or impulse control disorders; the latter comprised the following categories: ODD with hierarchy, CD, ADHD, and any impulse-control disorder. It should be noted, however, that for SAD/ASA and impulse-control disorders, only subjects aged 18–44 years were included.

Table 14.6 shows the relation between sex, marital status, and income with the 12-month prevalence of a selected set of disorders. Sex was significantly associated with mood, anxiety, and substance abuse. Women had about a twofold higher odds of a mood disorder (OR 1.8, 95% CI, 1.2–2.7), and more than a threefold higher odds of an anxiety disorder (OR 3.4, 95% CI, 2.1–5.4). In contrast, women had about a tenfold lower odds of substance abuse (OR 0.1, 95% CI, 0.0–0.4).

Marital status was significantly associated with substance abuse but not with either the overall prevalence or the specific prevalence of mood, anxiety, or impulse-control disorders. In particular, there was more than a fourfold (OR, 4.5, 95% CI, 1.6–12.3) increase in the odds of substance abuse. In contrast, income was not found to be significantly associated with the overall prevalence of mental health disorders or the specific prevalence of mood, anxiety, impulse-control, or substance abuse disorders.

We also found a cohort effect (Tables 14.7 and 14.8) for several disorders. For most disorders, the younger birth cohorts tended to have substantially higher prevalence rates than did older

**Table 14.6.** Demographic correlates of 12-month DSM-IV disorders using Part 2 weights after stratification

| | Mood | | Anxiety | | Impulse control | | Substance | |
|---|---|---|---|---|---|---|---|---|
| | OR | (95% CI) | OR | (95% CI) | OR | (95% CI) | OR | (95% CI) |
| **Sex** | | | | | | | | |
| Male | 1.0 | – | 1.0 | – | 1.0 | – | 1.0 | – |
| Female | 1.8 | (1.2–2.7) | 3.4 | (2.1–5.4) | 0.4 | (0.1–1.4) | 0.1 | (0.0–0.4) |
| $\chi^2$ | | 9.3* | | 27.7* | | 2.2 | | 12.4* |
| **Age** | | | | | | | | |
| 18–34 | 1.5 | (0.9–2.5) | 1.7 | (0.9–3.0) | 1.5 | (0.6–3.4) | 2.2 | (0.4–10.4) |
| 35–49 | 1.3 | (0.9–1.8) | 2.3 | (1.4–3.9) | – | – | 1.2 | (0.3–4.4) |
| 50–64 | – | – | – | – | – | – | – | – |
| 65+ | 1.0 | – | 1.0 | – | 1.0 | – | 1.0 | – |
| $\chi^2$ | | 3.9 | | 10.7* | | 0.9 | | 1.7 |
| **Income** | | | | | | | | |
| Low | 1.7 | (0.7–4.3) | 1.2 | (0.5–2.9) | 2.1 | (0.2–27.2) | 3.2 | (0.4–26.6) |
| Low average | 1.3 | (0.7–2.4) | 0.9 | (0.4–2.0) | 0.7 | (0.1–4.9) | 2.9 | (0.5–18.9) |
| High average | 1.3 | (0.6–2.7) | 0.7 | (0.4–1.3) | 0.5 | (0.1–3.0) | 3.5 | (0.6–19.7) |
| High | 1.0 | – | 1.0 | – | 1.0 | – | 1.0 | – |
| $\chi^2$ | | 1.8 | | 3.3 | | 6.3 | | 2.4 |
| **Marital Status** | | | | | | | | |
| Married/cohabiting | 1.0 | – | 1.0 | – | 1.0 | – | 1.0 | – |
| Separated/widowed/divorced | 1.6 | (1.0–2.5) | 1.6 | (1.0–2.6) | 0.9 | (0.1–6.8) | 1.7 | (0.2–15.4) |
| Never married | 1.5 | (0.8–2.9) | 1.1 | (0.6–2.0) | 1.1 | (0.2–5.5) | 4.5 | (1.6–12.3) |
| $\chi^2$ | | 6.7* | | 4.1 | | 0.0 | | 9.4* |

* Significant at the 0.05 level, double-sided test.

cohorts. Specifically, a significant cohort effect was found for the following disorders: panic, GAD with hierarchy, social phobia, PTSD, SAD/ASA, anxiety disorders (any), mood, and substance abuse. In contrast, no significant cohort effect was observed for specific phobias, agoraphobia without panic, or any of the impulse-control disorders.

The odds of panic disorder with more than a sixfold increase (OR 6.1, 95% CI, 1.6–23.5) for the youngest cohort, and almost a fourfold increase (OR 3.7, 95% CI, 1.2–11.1) for the cohort of subjects aged 35–49 years as compared with the oldest cohort (older than 65 years). The odds of PTSD increased more than eight-fold (OR 8.3, 95% CI, 3.2–21.3), and those of SAS/ASA tenfold (OR 10.0, 95% CI, 1.6–61.1) for the youngest compared to the oldest cohort.

The odds of a mood disorder were also highest for the youngest cohort (OR 9.0, 95% CI, 6.0–

13.5). Similarly, the odds of alcohol and, more so, alcohol dependence with substance abuse, were substantially higher for the youngest cohort, with almost a sixfold increase (OR 5.9, 95% CI, 3.210.9) for alcohol abuse and a 12-fold increase for alcohol dependence with substance abuse (OR 12.0, 95% CI, 2.9–49.7).

There were statistically significant variations across the life course in the associations between cohorts and lifetime risk of mental health disorders (Table 14.7). More specifically, there were significant interactions between the age of onset of anxiety, mood and substance abuse disorders, and the cohort effects. Impulse disorders were not included in this set of analyses, as by far the majority of these disorders have an age of onset in a narrow interval.

For anxiety disorders (Table 14.8) with a late age of onset the younger cohorts (younger than 50 years) had a substantially higher odds of

**Table 14.7.** Cohort as a predictor of lifetime risk of DSM-IV disorders

| Disorder | Age group | | | | | | | | | | | | χ² | DF | p |
|---|---|---|---|---|---|---|---|---|---|---|---|---|---|---|---|
| | 18–34 | | | 35–49 | | | 50–64 | | | 65+ | | | | | |
| | OR | LCL | UCL | OR | LCL | UCL | OR | LCL | UCL | OR | LCL | UCL | | | |
| Panic DX | 6.1* | 1.6 | 23.5 | 3.7* | 1.2 | 11.1 | 1.7 | 0.6 | 5.0 | 1.0 | 1.0 | 1.0 | 17.6* | 3 | 0.001 |
| GAD with hierarchy | 4.1* | 1.8 | 9.2 | 1.9 | 0.8 | 4.5 | 1.7 | 0.8 | 3.7 | 1.0 | 1.0 | 1.0 | 23.0* | 3 | 0.000 |
| Social phobia | 4.9* | 1.5 | 15.6 | 3.8* | 1.1 | 13.5 | 2.0 | 0.6 | 6.1 | 1.0 | 1.0 | 1.0 | 11.5* | 3 | 0.009 |
| Specific phobia | 1.1 | 0.7 | 1.9 | 1.2 | 0.6 | 2.2 | 1.1 | 0.6 | 1.8 | 1.0 | 1.0 | 1.0 | 1.0 | 3 | 0.80 |
| Agoraphobia without panic | 2.0 | 0.4 | 8.6 | 2.4 | 0.6 | 9.1 | 2.4 | 0.7 | 8.5 | 1.0 | 1.0 | 1.0 | 2.2 | 3 | 0.53 |
| PTSD | 8.3* | 3.2 | 21.3 | 2.8* | 1.0 | 7.7 | 2.4 | 1.0 | 6.0 | 1.0 | 1.0 | 1.0 | 21.8* | 3 | <.001 |
| SAD/ASA | 10.0* | 1.6 | 61.1 | 5.8* | 1.1 | 31.8 | 1.0 | 1.0 | 1.0 | – | – | – | 6.8* | 2 | 0.033 |
| Any anxiety | 3.1* | 1.5 | 6.4 | 3.2* | 1.5 | 6.7 | 1.6 | 0.8 | 3.3 | 1.0 | 1.0 | 1.0 | 21.3* | 3 | <.001 |
| MDE | 9.0* | 6.0 | 13.5 | 3.0* | 2.2 | 4.2 | 1.8* | 1.2 | 2.6 | 1.0 | 1.0 | 1.0 | 146.4* | 3 | <.001 |
| Any mood | 9.0* | 6.0 | 13.5 | 3.0* | 2.2 | 4.2 | 1.8* | 1.2 | 2.6 | 1.0 | 1.0 | 1.0 | 146.4* | 3 | <.001 |
| ODD with hierarchy+ | – | | | | | | | | | | | | | | |
| CD+ | | | | | | | | | | | | | | | |
| ADHD | 1.8 | 0.6 | 5.0 | 1.0 | 1.0 | 1.0 | 1.0 | 1.0 | 1.0 | 1.0 | 1.0 | 1.0 | 1.2 | 1 | 0.28 |
| Any impulse | 1.5 | 0.7 | 3.2 | 1.0 | 1.0 | 1.0 | 1.0 | 1.0 | 1.0 | 1.0 | 1.0 | 1.0 | 1.3 | 1 | 0.25 |
| Alcohol abuse | 5.9* | 3.2 | 10.9 | 3.5* | 2.0 | 6.3 | 2.8* | 1.5 | 5.1 | 1.0 | 1.0 | 1.0 | 36.5* | 3 | <.001 |
| Alcohol dependency with abuse | 12.0* | 2.9 | 49.7 | 2.8 | 0.4 | 18.2 | 2.6 | 0.5 | 14.5 | 1.0 | 1.0 | 1.0 | 35.7* | 3 | <.001 |
| Any substance | 5.8* | 3.3 | 10.0 | 3.3* | 2.0 | 5.7 | 2.5* | 1.4 | 4.2 | 1.0 | 1.0 | 1.0 | 44.1* | 3 | <.001 |
| Any DX | 4.2* | 2.5 | 7.1 | 3.3* | 2.0 | 5.3 | 1.9* | 1.2 | 2.9 | 1.0 | 1.0 | 1.0 | 44.8* | 3 | <.001 |

Based on discrete-time survival models with person-year as the unit of analysis.

Controls are time intervals.

* Significant at the 0.05 level.

+ = Cell size < = 30 cases, too small to estimate.

**Table 14.8.** Variation across the life course in the association of cohort in predicting lifetime risk of anxiety disorders

| | | Age of onset | | | | | | | | |
| | | Early | | | Middle | | | Late | | |
| Disorder | Ages | OR | LCL | UCL | OR | LCL | UCL | OR | LCL | UCL |
|---|---|---|---|---|---|---|---|---|---|---|
| Anxiety | 18–34 | 2.4 | 0.9 | 6.6 | 2.5 | 0.9 | 6.9 | 7.3* | 3.3 | 16.3 |
| | 35–49 | 3.0* | 1.1 | 8.2 | 3.2* | 1.4 | 7.3 | 3.5* | 1.7 | 7.2 |
| | 50–64 | 1.3 | 0.6 | 2.9 | 1.5 | 0.5 | 4.3 | 2.2 | 1.0 | 4.9 |
| | 65+ | 1.0 | 1.0 | 1.0 | 1.0 | 1.0 | 1.0 | 1.0 | 1.0 | 1.0 |
| | $\chi^2$/DF/$p$-value | 10.5 | 3 | 0.015 | 10.3 | 3 | 0.016 | 27.1 | 3 | <0.001 |
| | | – | – | – | | – | – | | – | – |

$\chi^2 = 9.3$, DF = 6, $p = 0.16$.

* Significant at the 0.05 level.

*Notes:* Model includes time intervals and sex as controls. Impulse disorders not included because the vast majority of such disorders have onsets in a very narrow time window.

having the disorder than did the oldest cohort. The youngest (18–34 years) cohort had more than a sevenfold (OR 7.3, 95% CI, 3.3–16.3) increase in the odds of an anxiety disorder with a late age of onset, and the 35–49 year age group had more than a threefold increase (OR 3.5, 95% CI, 1.7–7.2) in the odds of an anxiety disorder with a late age of onset, as compared with the oldest cohort. In general, the aged 18–34 cohort had about a threefold increase in the odds of an anxiety disorder for all three categories of age of onset as compared with the oldest cohort.

For mood disorders (Table 14.9), the youngest cohort had more than a 13-fold increase (OR 13.4, 95% CI, 6.7–26.8) in the odds of a mood disorder with a middle age of onset, and about a 6.5-fold increase (OR 6.5, 95% CI, 3.3–13.1) in the odds of a mood disorder with an early age of onset, as compared with the oldest cohort. The aged 35–49 cohort had higher odds of a mood disorder than did the oldest cohort, regardless of the age of onset. The greatest increase was for mood disorders with a middle age of onset (OR 4.6, 95% CI, 2.2–9.6). The aged 50–64 cohort also had higher odds of a mood disorder with a middle (OR 2.6, 95% CI, 1.0–6.5) or late (OR 2.1, 95% CI, 1.2–3.4) age of onset than did the oldest cohort.

**Table 14.9.** Variation across the life course in the association of cohort in predicting lifetime risk of mood disorders

| | | Age of onset | | | | | | | | |
| | | Early | | | Middle | | | Late | | |
| Disorder | Age group | OR | LCL | UCL | OR | LCL | UCL | OR | LCL | UCL |
|---|---|---|---|---|---|---|---|---|---|---|
| Mood | 18–34 | 6.5* | 3.2 | 13.1 | 13.4* | 6.7 | 26.8 | 1.0 | 1.0 | 1.0 |
| | 35–49 | 2.0* | 1.1 | 3.5 | 4.6* | 2.2 | 9.6 | 3.2* | 1.9 | 5.4 |
| | 50–64 | 1.2 | 0.5 | 3.0 | 2.6* | 1.0 | 6.5 | 2.1* | 1.2 | 3.4 |
| | 65+ | 1.0 | 1.0 | 1.0 | 1.0 | 1.0 | 1.0 | 1.0 | 1.0 | 1.0 |
| | $\chi^2$/DF/$p$-value | 90.2 | 3 | <0.001 | 125.7 | 3 | <0.001 | 21.7 | 2 | <0.001 |
| | | – | – | – | | – | – | | – | – |

Global $\chi^2 = 5.5$, DF = 5, $p = 0.36$.

* Significant at the 0.05 level.

*Notes:* Model includes time intervals and sex as controls. Impulse disorders not included because the vast majority of such disorders have onsets in a very narrow time window.

**Table 14.10.** Variation across the life course in the association of cohort in predicting lifetime risk of substance disorders

| | | Age of onset | | | | | | | | |
|---|---|---|---|---|---|---|---|---|---|---|
| | | Early | | | Middle | | | Late | | |
| Disorder | Age group | OR | LCL | UCL | OR | LCL | UCL | OR | LCL | UCL |
| Substance | 18–34 | 5.6* | 1.8 | 17.9 | 4.1* | 1.1 | 15.4 | 2.6* | 1.0 | 7.0 |
| | 35–49 | 3.3* | 1.1 | 9.3 | 3.2 | 0.9 | 11.3 | 1.4 | 0.6 | 3.0 |
| | 50–64 | 1.0 | 1.0 | 1.0 | 1.8 | 0.5 | 6.6 | 2.0* | 1.1 | 3.8 |
| | 65+ | – | – | – | 1.0 | 1.0 | 1.0 | 1.0 | 1.0 | 1.0 |
| | $\chi^2$/DF/$p$-value | 9.5 | 2 | 0.009 | 6.0 | 3 | 0.11 | 8.0 | 3 | 0.045 |
| | | – | – | – | – | – | – | – | – | – |

Global $\chi^2 = 15.2$, DF $= 5$, $p = 0.009$.

* Significant at the 0.05 level.

*Notes:* Model includes time intervals and sex as controls. Impulse disorders not included because the vast majority of such disorders have onsets in a very narrow time window.

For substance abuse disorders (Table 14.10), the youngest cohort had higher odds regardless of the age of onset. The greatest increase was for substance abuse disorders with an early (OR 5.6, 95% CI, 1.8–17.9) or middle (OR 4.1, 95% CI, 1.1–15.4) age of onset. The aged 35–49 cohort also had a significant increase (OR 3.3, 95% CI, 1.1–9.3) in the odds of a substance abuse disorder with an early age of onset. In contrast, the aged 50–64 cohort had a significant increase (OR 2.0,

95% CI, 1.1–3.8) in the odds of a substance abuse disorder with a late age of onset than did the oldest cohort.

## 5.3. Use of Care

Table 14.11 shows the disorder-specific percentages of respondents who made treatment contact during the year of onset or by 50 years of age, as well as median duration of delay. For

**Table 14.11.** Proportional treatment contact in the year of disorder onset and median duration of delay among cases that subsequently made treatment contact

| | % Making treatment contact in year of onset | % Making treatment contact by 50 years | Median duration of delay (years) | n |
|---|---|---|---|---|
| **I. Anxiety disorders** | | | | |
| Panic disorder | 62.9 | 98.5 | 1 | 55 |
| GAD | 39.4 | 83.0 | 2 | 190 |
| Specific phobia | 4.6 | 83.6 | 27 | 309 |
| Social phobia | 1.7 | 73.8 | 22 | 121 |
| Any anxiety disorders | 16.1 | 93.3 | 18 | 545 |
| **II. Mood disorders** | | | | |
| Major depressive episode | 42.7 | 98.6 | 3 | 644 |
| **III. Substance disorders** | | | | |
| Alcohol abuse | 17.5 | 62.3 | 13 | 66 |
| Alcohol abuse with dependence[a] | – | – | – | – |
| Any substance disorders | 15.7 | 66.5 | 13 | 73 |

[a] Disorder was omitted due to insufficient $n < 30$ but will be included as one of the disorders in "Any" category.

anxiety disorders, overall, 16% of people who met lifetime criteria for such a disorder made treatment contact within a year from onset and 93% by 50 years. The median duration of delay was 18 years. There was substantial variations across specific anxiety disorders. The majority of subjects (62%) made treatment contact within a year from onset and essentially all (99%) by 50 years. The median duration of delay was one year. In contrast, less than 2% of subjects with social phobia and less than 5% of those with specific phobias made treatment contact within one year; however, by far, the majority of these subjects, 74% and 84%, respectively, made treatment contact by 50 years. The median duration of delay was 22 and 27 years for social and specific phobias, respectively. For generalized anxiety disorders, about 40% made treatment contact within a year and 83% by 50 years with a median duration of delay of two years.

Approximately 40% of subjects with a major depressive episode made treatment contact within a year of onset and essentially all (99%) by 50 years with a median duration of delay of three years. For substance abuse disorder, less than 20% of those with alcohol or any substance abuse made treatment contact within a year from onset and about two-thirds by 50 years. The median duration of delay was 13 years.

Table 14.12 shows sociodemographic correlates of lifetime treatment contact for each disorder. Women were significantly more likely (OR 1.5, 95% CI, 1.1–2.1) to seek treatment for anxiety disorders. Subjects from younger cohorts (younger than 50 years) were substantially more likely to make treatment contact for anxiety disorders. The youngest cohort had about a 4.5-fold increase (OR 4.5, 95% CI, 2.5–8.1) in the odds of lifetime treatment for anxiety disorders (any). This was generally true for specific anxiety disorders; however, the estimates did not reach statistical significance for generalized anxiety disorders and social phobia. The aged 35–49 cohort had substantially increased odds of treatment contact for panic disorder (OR 5.1, 95% CI, 1.9–13.4) and, to a lesser degree, for anxiety disorders in general (i.e., any). For age of onset, in general, earlier ages of onset were associated with sub-

stantially lower odds of treatment contact. This was particularly the case for panic disorder but was generally true for all anxiety disorders.

For a major depressive episode, there was no statistically significant correlation between sex and treatment contact. Younger cohorts were substantially more likely to make treatment contact, particularly for cohorts younger than 50 years old. The 18–34 cohort had about a 5.7-fold increase (OR 5.7, 95% CI, 3.1–10.5) and the 35–49 year cohort more than a 4-fold increase (OR 4.4, 95% CI, 2.4–8.0) in the odds of lifetime treatment contact than did the oldest cohort.

We found no significant sex, cohort, or age of onset associations with the odds of lifetime treatment contact. This was probably at least in part due to limited precision of estimates, which was related to small sample sizes for this set of disorders. The point estimates suggested lower odds of treatment contact for women, younger cohorts, and earlier ages of onset. However, the confidence intervals were wide; thus, the results were not statistically significant.

Table 14.13 shows the sociodemographic and disorder-type correlates of any and minimally adequate therapy. For any treatment given, marital status was the most important predictor of treatment after adjustment for other sociodemographic factors and type of disorder. Subjects never married had odds of treatment that were approximately threefold lower (OR 0.3, 95% CI, 0.2–0.7) than for those married or living in cohabitation. Subject's age, sex, and income were not independently associated with odds of any treatment.

Type of disorder was the most significant predictor of treatment. The greatest increase in the odds of treatment was related to mood disorders, with more than a 5-fold increase (OR 5.2, 95% CI, 2.7–10.1) in the odds of treatment when a mood disorder was identified. Anxiety disorder was also associated with higher odds (OR 3.1, 95% CI, 1.3–7.4) of any treatment. In contrast, presence of a substance abuse disorder did not significantly increase the odds of treatment (OR 1.6, 95% CI, 0.3–8.7).

The relations between sociodemographic factors and type of disorder with minimally

**Table 14.12.** Sociodemographic predictors of lifetime treatment contact for specific DSM-IV/CIDI disorders

| | Sex | | | Cohort (age at interview) | | | | | | | Age of onset | | | | | | |
| | Female | | | Age 18–34 | | Age 35–49 | | Age 50–64 | | | Early | | Early average | | Late average | | |
| | OR | (95% CI) | $\chi^2_1$ | OR | (95% CI) | OR | (95% CI) | OR | (95% CI) | $\chi^2_{2-3}$ | OR | (95% CI) | OR | (95% CI) | OR | (95% CI) | $\chi^2_{1-3}$ |
|---|---|---|---|---|---|---|---|---|---|---|---|---|---|---|---|---|---|
| **I. Anxiety disorders** | | | | | | | | | | | | | | | | | |
| Panic disorder | 1.5 | (0.3–6.6) | 0.3 | 4.6* | (0.9–22.5) | 5.1* | (1.9–13.4) | 1.0 | — | 12.2* | **0.1*** | **(0.0–0.7)** | **0.1*** | **(0.0–0.7)** | **0.1*** | **(0.0–0.7)** | 5.6* |
| Generalized anxiety disorder | 1.4 | (0.8–2.4) | 1.7 | 1.8 | (0.6–5.2) | 1.7 | (0.7–4.2) | 0.9 | (0.4–2.2) | 2.9 | **0.3*** | (0.1–0.8) | 0.9 | (0.3–3.0) | 0.6 | (0.2–1.6) | 10.9* |
| Specific phobia | 1.0 | (0.7–1.4) | 0.0 | 3.2* | (1.1–9.0) | 2.1 | (0.8–5.1) | 1.7 | (0.6–5.3) | 6.6 | 0.4 | (0.2–0.8) | 0.6 | (0.2–1.3) | 0.5 | (0.2–1.1) | 7.5 |
| Social phobia | 2.3 | (0.9–6.1) | 3.0 | 2.7 | (0.7–10.8) | 0.8 | (0.2–2.7) | 0.3* | (0.1–1.1) | 12.7* | **0.2*** | (0.1–0.9) | **0.2*** | (0.0–0.5) | 0.7 | (0.3–2.0) | 14.6* |
| Any anxiety disorders | 1.5* | (1.1–2.1) | 8.8* | 4.5* | (2.5–8.1) | 2.3* | (1.3–4.2) | 1.3 | (0.7–2.5) | 52.2* | **0.2*** | (0.1–0.3) | **0.2*** | (0.1–0.3) | **0.3*** | (0.2–0.5) | 82.4* |
| **II. Mood disorders** | | | | | | | | | | | | | | | | | |
| Major depressive episode | 1.3 | (0.9–1.8) | 2.9 | 5.7* | (3.1–10.5) | 4.4* | (2.4–8.0) | 2.0* | (1.1–3.5) | 44.3* | **0.2*** | (0.1–0.4) | **0.4*** | (0.2–0.8) | 0.6 | (0.3–1.2) | 54.9* |
| **III. Substance disorders** | | | | | | | | | | | | | | | | | |
| Alcohol abuse | 0.5 | (0.0–4.6) | 0.5 | 0.2 | (0.0–3.5) | 0.5 | (0.1–4.0) | 1.0 | — | 1.5 | **0.3** | **(0.1–2.2)** | **0.3** | **(0.1–2.2)** | **0.3** | **(0.1–2.2)** | 1.5 |
| Alcohol abuse with dependence | _a | _a | _a | _a | _a | _a | _a | _a | _a | _a | _a | _a | _a | _a | _a | _a | _a |
| Any substance disorders | 0.8 | (0.2–3.2) | 0.2 | 0.2 | (0.0–3.2) | 0.7 | (0.1–4.8) | 1.0 | — | 2.1 | **0.4** | **(0.1–2.6)** | **0.4** | **(0.1–2.6)** | **0.4** | **(0.1–2.6)** | 1.0 |

*Note:* Bold numbers indicate that groups were collapsed. Thus, the degree of freedom for each chi-square is based on the number of group available in each main category.

[a] Disorder was omitted due to insufficient lifetime cases ($n < 30$), but will be included as one of the disorders in "Any" category.

* Significant at the 0.05 level, two-sided test.

**Table 14.13.** Sociodemographic and disorder-type predictors of any and minimally adequate treatment with 12-month service usage

| Model effect | Effect level | Any treatment given any 12-month disorder OR (95% CI) | Minimally adequate treatment given any treatment and 12-month disorder OR (95% CI) |
|---|---|---|---|
| Age | 18–34 | 1.9 (0.5, 6.5) | – |
| | 35–49 | 1.1 (0.3, 4.1) | – |
| | 50–64 | 2.4 (0.6, 8.9) | – |
| | 65+ | 1.0 (1.0, 1.0) | – |
| | Overall test of effect | Wald-Chi 3 df = 4.7, $p$-value = 0.19 | |
| Age | 18–34 | | 0.1 (0.0, 0.4) |
| | 35–49 | | 0.1 (0.0, 0.4) |
| | 50+ | | 1.0 (1.0, 1.0) |
| | | | Wald-Chi 2 df = 16.3*, $p$-value = <0.001 |
| Any anxiety | Yes | 3.1 (1.3, 7.4) | 3.4 (1.0, 11.2) |
| | No | 1.0 (1.0, 1.0) | 1.0 (1.0, 1.0) |
| | Overall test of effect | Wald-Chi 1 df = 7.0*, $p$-value = 0.008 | Wald-Chi 1 df = 4.3*, $p$-value = 0.039 |
| Any mood | Yes | 5.2 (2.7, 10.1) | 2.3 (0.7, 8.1) |
| | No | 1.0 (1.0, 1.0) | 1.0 (1.0, 1.0) |
| | Overall test of effect | Wald-Chi 1 df = 26.1*, $p$-value = <0.001 | Wald-Chi 1 df = 2.0, $p$-value = 0.16 |
| Any substance | Yes | 1.6 (0.3, 8.7) | 2.9 (0.1, 86.6) |
| | No | 1.0 (1.0, 1.0) | 1.0 (1.0, 1.0) |
| | Overall test of effect | Wald-Chi 1 df = 0.3, $p$-value = 0.58 | Wald-Chi 1 df = 0.4, $p$-value = 0.53 |
| Income | Low | 1.2 (0.5, 3.0) | 1.3 (0.1, 11.3) |
| | Low average | 1.6 (0.8, 2.9) | 0.4 (0.1, 2.6) |
| | High average | 1.6 (0.9, 3.0) | 1.5 (0.2, 14.2) |
| | High | 1.0 (1.0, 1.0) | 1.0 (1.0, 1.0) |
| | Overall test of effect | Wald-Chi 3 df = 4.1, $p$-value = 0.26 | Wald-Chi 3 df = 7.0, $p$-value = 0.07 |
| Marital status | Never married | 0.3 (0.2, 0.7) | 0.8 (0.2, 3.3) |
| | Separated/widowed/divorced | 1.3 (0.5, 3.1) | 0.4 (0.1, 1.5) |
| | Married/cohabiting | 1.0 (1.0, 1.0) | 1.0 (1.0, 1.0) |
| | Overall test of effect | Wald-Chi 2 df = 10.3*, $p$-value = 0.006 | Wald-Chi 2 df = 2.4, $p$-value = 0.29 |
| Sex | Male | 1.7 (0.8, 3.6) | 0.9 (0.3, 3.0) |
| | Female | 1.0 (1.0, 1.0) | 1.0 (1.0, 1.0) |
| | Overall test of effect | Wald-Chi 1 df = 2.1, $p$-value = 0.15 | Wald-Chi 1 df = 0.0, $p$-value = 0.83 |

* Significant at the 0.05 level, two-sided test.

**Table 14.14.** Severity by treatment

| Treatment | Severe | | Moderate | | Mild | | None | | Any | |
|---|---|---|---|---|---|---|---|---|---|---|
| | % | (se) | % | (se) | % | (se) | % | (se) | % | (se) |
| General medical | 33.8 | (4.2) | 24.4 | (3.8) | 15.9 | (2.4) | 5.6 | (1.0) | 8.8 | (0.9) |
| Mental health | 23.9 | (6.2) | 9.9 | (2.7) | 7.6 | (1.7) | 2.8 | (0.6) | 4.4 | (0.5) |
| Health care | 45.4 | (6.9) | 27.7 | (3.8) | 20.1 | (3.1) | 6.6 | (1.0) | 10.6 | (0.8) |
| Non–health-care | 3.8 | (2.0) | 2.0 | (1.3) | 2.6 | (1.6) | 0.5 | (0.3) | 0.9 | (0.3) |
| Any treatment | 48.0 | (6.4) | 29.4 | (4.0) | 22.4 | (3.4) | 7.0 | (1.1) | 11.3 | (1.0) |
| No treatment | 52.0 | (6.4) | 70.6 | (4.0) | 77.6 | (3.4) | 93.0 | (1.1) | 88.7 | (1.0) |

*Note:* Non–health-care includes human services and CAM.

adequate treatment were, in general, not the same as those observed for any treatment. Younger subjects had almost a 10-fold lower odds of treatment (OR 0.1, 95% CI, 0.0–0.4), whereas the effect of marital status was no longer significant. Sex and level of income were not significantly associated with the odds of minimal treatment.

Type of disorder had a significant association with the odds of minimally adequate treatment for anxiety disorders but not others. The odds of minimally adequate treatment was about 3.4-fold (OR 3.4, 95% CI, 1.0–11.2) increased for anxiety disorders, which was similar to the estimate obtained for any treatment. In contrast, for mood disorders, the odds for minimally adequate treatment was about 2-fold lower for minimally adequate treatment than for any treatment, and were no longer statistically significant; the ORs for minimally adequate and any treatment were 2.3 (95% CI, 0.7–8.1) and 5.2 (95% CI, 2.7–10.1), respectively.

Table 14.14 shows the relation between severity and the probability, as well as type of health provider prescribing treatment. In general, patients with more severe illness were substantially more likely to be treated. However, even for the most severe category, almost half of patients (48.0%) were not treated. Overall, about 11.3% of subjects received treatment. Among those treated, by far the majority of subjects were treated by health-care providers rather than by the non–health-care sector (the latter included human services and CAM). Among health-care providers, generalists were much more likely to be the provider who prescribed treatment; how-

ever, this was much less the case when the disorder was severe. For moderate and mild disorders, more than two-thirds of the patients did not receive any treatment.

Figures 14.1, 14.2, 14.3, and 14.4 show the cumulative probability of treatment contact by type of disorder for those who were eventually treated. Overall, about 20% of patients with anxiety disorders (any) who were eventually treated received their treatment shortly after the onset; 30% after about 10 years and 50% after about 20 years. It took about 30 years after the onset for 80% of the patients treated to receive their treatment.

Patients with panic disorder had the highest probability of treatment (approximately 65%) shortly after the onset of disorder. This percentage increased to approximately 70% and 80% 2 and 15 years, respectively, after the onset of the disorder. Of patients, 90% were treated by 30 years after the onset of the disorder and all by about 32 years.

For GAD, there was almost a linear increase in the cumulative probability of treatment. Initially after the onset, about 50% of patients were treated, and about 70% after ten years. Thereafter, the rate of increase slowed somewhat with about 80% of patients treated by 25 years and all by 30 years.

For social and specific phobias, a small percentage of patients received treatment shortly after the onset. Moreover, only 20% of patients with social phobia and less than 10% with specific phobias received treatment by five years after the onset. It took about 25 years after the onset for

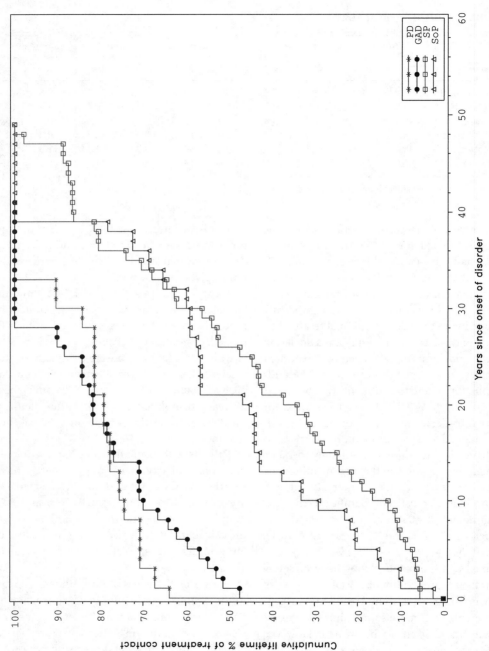

**Figure 14.1.** Cumulative lifetime % of treatment contact for anxiety disorders from year of onset.

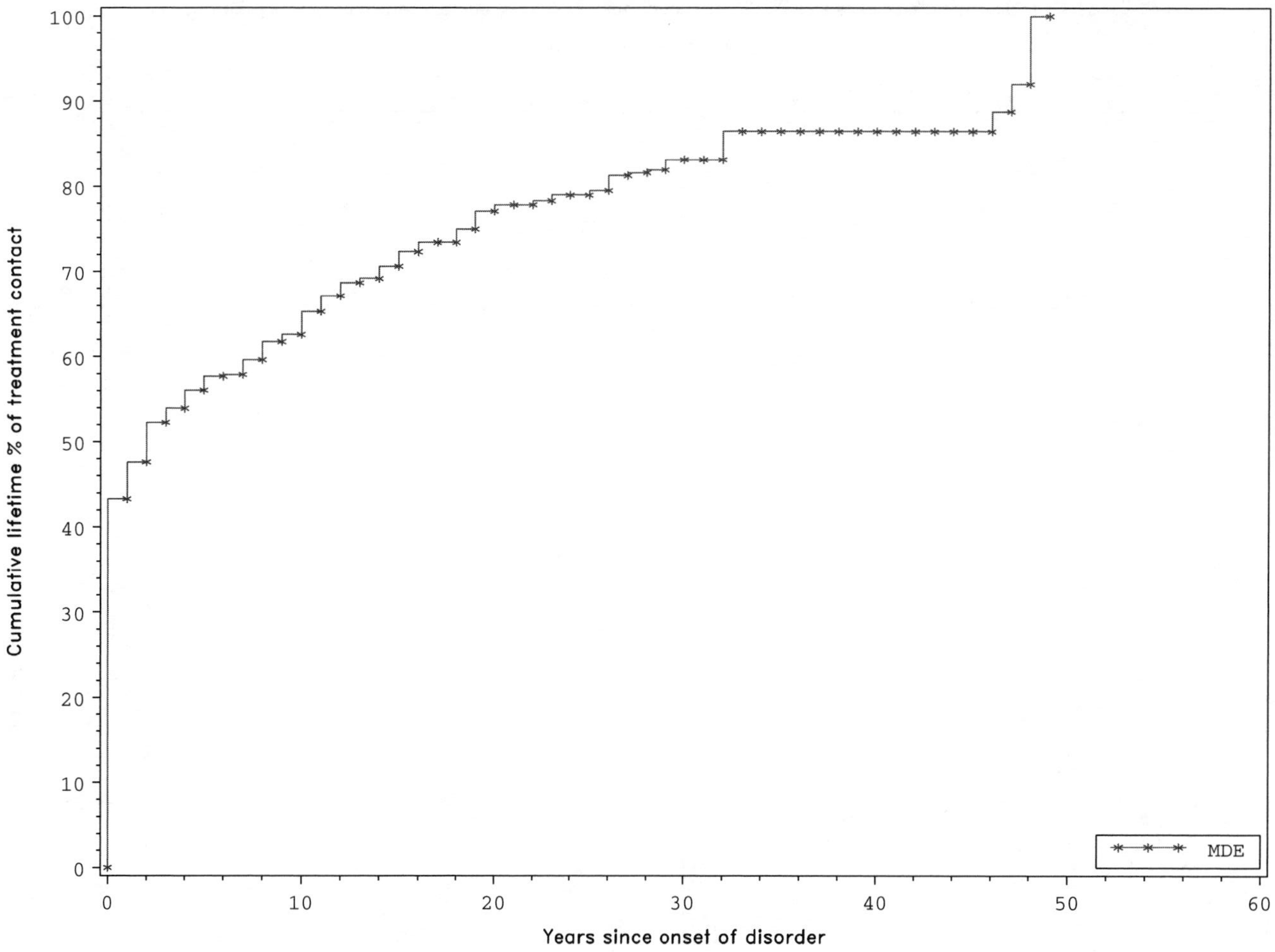

**Figure 14.2.** Cumulative lifetime % of treatment contact for mood disorders from year of onset.

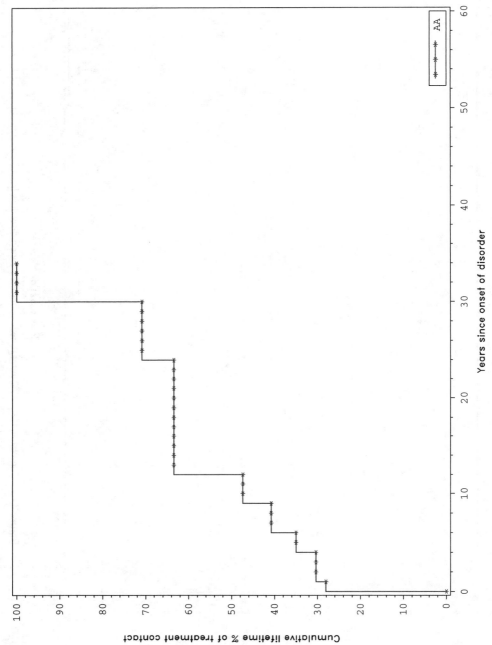

**Figure 14.3.** Cumulative lifetime % of treatment contact for substance disorders from year of onset.

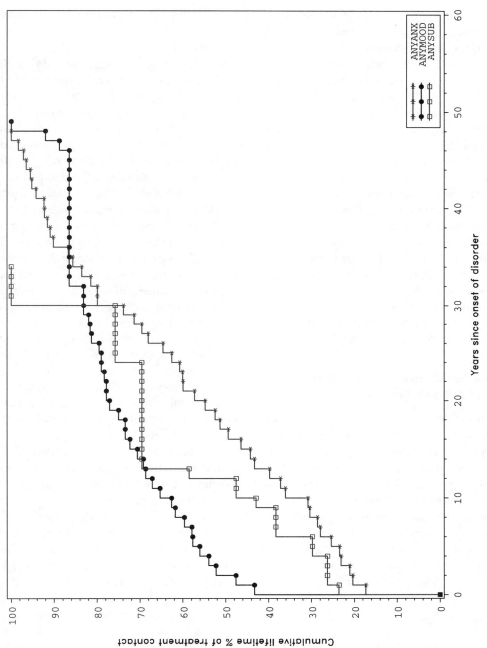

**Figure 14.4.** Cumulative lifetime % of treatment contact for ANY disorders from year of onset.

50% of patients with social phobias (who eventually received treatment) to be treated and about 30 years for those with specific phobias.

For mood disorders, about 45% of patients who were eventually treated received their treatment shortly after the onset. Nevertheless, it took about 20 years after the onset for 75% of the patients to receive treatment and almost 30 years after onset for 80% of the patients treated to receive their treatment.

As a group, for patients with substance abuse disorders (any) who were eventually treated, about 25% received their treatment shortly after the onset with 30% five years after and 40% ten years after the onset. It took about 20 years after the onset for 70% of the patients to receive their treatment and almost 40 years for 80%. For alcohol abuse, about 30% of patients received their treatment shortly after the onset. By about 15 years after the onset, 50% of patients treated received their treatment and 70% by 30 years.

## 5.4. General Practitioner (GP) Referrals to Mental Health Professionals

French subjects were referred to mental health specialists by their GPs in only 22.2% of cases, which is a rather low percentage and this applies for any diagnostic group category (Kovess-Masféty et al. 2006). The low level of relationship between GPs and psychiatrists on the one hand and nonmedical providers such as psychologists, whose costs are mainly paid out of pocket on the other hand is one of the characteristics of the French system that may contribute to the high psychotropic drug consumption rate.

## 6. CONCLUSIONS

The results of the current survey are important in light of the fact that they provide representative data from a large sample that is representative of the French population. Importantly, the standardized methods of assessment used here are the same as those in the other ESEMeD surveys in all respects other than sampling and are very similar to those in the other WMH surveys with the exception of the deletion of several

disorders. These similarities provide an unprecedented opportunity for cross-national comparison of results.

In summary, results suggest that almost 40% of adults in the French sampling frame had a diagnosis of at least one of the DSM-IV disorders assessed in the CIDI at some time in their life and about 15% two or more diagnoses. Anxiety and mood disorders had the highest prevalence, with estimates of approximately 22% each. Impulse-control and substance abuse disorders had a similar prevalence of about 7%. Among anxiety disorders, specific phobias had the highest lifetime prevalence and among impulse-control disorders ADHD had the highest lifetime prevalence.

Overall, the prevalence of mental health disorders increased until the age of about 50 years and decreased thereafter. Disorders that were significantly associated with age included panic, social phobia, anxiety and mood disorders, and alcohol and other substance abuse. Sex was significantly associated with mood, anxiety, and substance abuse disorders, with women having two- to threefold higher odds of mood and anxiety disorders but substantially lower odds of substance abuse. In general, younger cohorts had a higher prevalence of mental health disorders.

For anxiety disorders, approximately 15% of subjects made treatment contact within a year from onset and 93% by 50 years of age. The median duration of delay was 18 years. There were substantial variations in speed of treatment contact across specific anxiety disorders. Overall, more than 60% of patients made treatment contact within a year and the median duration of delay was one year. However, less than 2% of patients with social phobia, and less than 5% of those with specific phobias, made treatment contact within a year from onset. The median duration of delay for specific and social phobias was 22 and 27 years, respectively. About 40% of patients with a major depressive episode made treatment contact within a year and less than 20% of those with substance abuse. Median duration of delay was 3 years for a major depressive episode and 13 years for substance abuse disorders. These results show that significant pockets of long-term unmet need for treatment exist for particular disorders, which could possibly be the focus of public education outreach efforts.

Women and younger cohorts of patients were more likely to seek treatment whereas the most important predictor of receiving (any) treatment was marital status. In contrast, marital status was not a significant predictor of minimally adequate treatment and younger patients were much less likely to receive adequate treatment.

Type of disorder was the most significant predictor of treatment. Mood and anxiety disorders had the highest odds of treatment, whereas the presence of a substance abuse disorder did not significantly increase the odds of treatment. Type of disorder had a significant association with the odds of minimally adequate treatment for anxiety disorders but not for others; however, this was in part a result of limited precision of estimates, as mood disorder also appeared to be associated with higher odds of minimally adequate treatment.

Overall, about 11% of people with a 12-month DSM-IV/CIDI disorder were treated in the year of interview. Those with more severe disorders were much more likely to be treated. Nevertheless, even in the most severe category, almost half of the patients were left untreated. The GPs were much more likely to be the provider who prescribed treatment, and only 22% of patients were referred to a mental health specialist by a GP. This was less so, however, for more severe disorders.

These findings highlight the importance of mental health disorders as a public health problem. They also underscore the need for initiatives designed to reduce unmet need for treatment of mental disorders. Although the results reported in this chapter documented the existence of high unmet need in the year before interview and presented some information about the disorders least likely to be treated and the sociodemographic characteristics of the people who were not treated, no information was provided on reasons for not seeking treatment or modifiable barriers to treatment, which could be the focus of future public health initiatives. This further investigation has to be a high priority of the next phase of WMH research activity, as the high magnitude of the problem is clear but the action implications for addressing the problem are obscure. Improvements in the diagnosis and adequate treatment of mental health disorders must rely on better communication between GPs and mental health care specialists and more optimal referral patterns, but there are doubtlessly also important barriers to be discovered that concern inability of people with emotional disorders to recognize their problems as indicative of a mental illness and reluctance on the part of those people to seek help when they suspect that they have such a disorder. The WMH surveys include useful information on all these issues, which will be the focus of investigation in the next phase of the initiative.

## REFERENCES

Alonso, J., Angermeyer, M. C. & Lepine, J. P. (2004). The European Study of the Epidemiology of Mental Disorders (ESEMeD) project: An epidemiological basis for informing mental health policies in Europe. *Acta Psychiatrica Scandinavica*, 109 (suppl. 420), 5–7.

American Psychiatric Association (1994). *Diagnostic and Statistical Manual of Mental Disorders (DSM-IV)*, 4th ed. Washington, DC: American Psychiatric Association.

Efron, B. (1988). Logistic regression, survival analysis, and the Kaplan-Meier curve. *Journal of the American Statistical Association*, 83, 414–25.

First, M. B., Spitzer, R. L., Gibbon, M. & Williams, J. B. W. (2002). *Structured Clinical Interview for DSM-IV Axis I Disorders, Research Version, Nonpatient Edition (SCID-I/NP)*. New York: Biometrics Research, New York State Psychiatric Institute.

Halli, S. S. & Rao, K. V. (1992). *Advanced techniques of population analysis*. New York: Plenum Press.

Hosmer, D. W. & Lemeshow, S. (1989). *Applied logistic regression*. New York: John Wiley & Sons.

Kessler, R. C., Andrews, G., Mroczek, D., Üstün, T. B. & Wittchen, H. U. (1998). The World Health Organization Composite International Diagnostic Interview Short Form (CIDI-SF). *International Journal of Methods in Psychiatric Research*, 7, 171–85.

Kessler, R. C. & Üstün, T. B. (2004). The World Mental Health (WMH) Survey Initiative Version of the World Health Organization (WHO) Composite International Diagnostic Interview (CIDI). *International Journal of Methods in Psychiatric Research*, 13, 93–121.

Kovess-Masféty, V., Alonso, J., Brugha, T. S., Angermeyer, M. C., Haro, J. M., Sevilla-Dedieu, C. & the

ESEMeD/MHDEA 2000 Investigators (2006). Differences in the lifetime use of services for mental health problems in six European countries: Results of the ESEMeD project. *Psychiatric Services*, 58, 213–20.

Kovess-Masféty, V. & Carmona, E. (2006). Toward a regional mental health policy: Results from population mental health surveys in four French regions. 13th Association of European Psychiatrists (AEP) symposium. Association of European Psychiatrists section epidemiology and social psychiatry. Bordeaux, France.

Kovess-Masféty, V. & Delavelle, S. (1998). La Santé mentale des Bas-Normands in La Basse Normandie face à sa santé. *INSEE*, 21–37.

Kovess-Masféty, V., Gysens, S. & Chanoit, P. F. (1993). Une enquête de santé mentale: L'enquête de santé des franciliens. *Annales Médico-Psychologiques*, 151, 624–8.

Kovess-Masféty, V., Lecoutour, X. & Delavelle, S. (2005). Mood disorders and urban/rural settings: Comparisons between two French regions. *Social Psychiatry and Psychiatric Epidemiology*, 40, 613–8.

Le Pape, A. & Lecomte, T. (1999). Prévalence et prise en charge médicale de la dépression: France 1996–1997. *CREDES*, Report No. 1277.

Lépine, J. P., Gastpar, M., Mendlewicz, J. & Tylee, A. (1997). Depression in the community: The first pan-European study DEPRES (Depression Research in European Society). *International Clinical Psychopharmacology*, 12, 19–29.

Lépine, J. P., Lellouch, J., Lovell, A., Téhérani, M. & Pariente, P. (1993). L'épidémiologie des troubles anxieux et dépressifs dans une population générale Française. *Confrontations Psychiatriques*, 35, 139–61.

Research Triangle Institute (2002). *SUDAAN: Professional software for survey data analysis 8.01*. Research Triangle Park, NC: Research Triangle Institute.

World Health Organization (WHO) (1991). *International Classification of Diseases (ICD-10)*. Geneva: World Health Organization.

# 15 Prevalence and Treatment of Mental Disorders in Germany: Results from the European Study of the Epidemiology of Mental Disorders (ESEMeD) Survey

JORDI ALONSO AND RONALD C. KESSLER

## ACKNOWLEDGMENTS

The ESEMeD project is carried out in conjunction with the World Health Organization World Mental Health (WMH) Survey Initiative. We thank the WMH staff for assistance with instrumentation, fieldwork, and data analysis. These activities were supported by the U.S. National Institute of Mental Health (R01MH070884), the John D. and Catherine T. MacArthur Foundation, the Pfizer Foundation, the U.S. Public Health Service (R13-MH066849, R01-MH069864, and R01 DA016558), the Fogarty International Center (FIRCA R03-TW006481), the Pan American Health Organization, Eli Lilly and Company Foundation, Ortho-McNeil Pharmaceutical, GlaxoSmithKline, and Bristol-Myers Squibb. A complete list of WMH publications can be found at http://www.hcp.med.harvard.edu/wmh/. The ESEMeD project is funded by the European Commission (Contracts QLG5-1999-01042; SANCO 2004123), the Piedmont Region (Italy), Fondo de Investigación Sanitaria, Instituto de Salud Carlos III, Spain (FIS 00/0028), Ministerio de Ciencia y Tecnología, Spain (SAF 2000-158-CE), Departament de Salut, Generalitat de Catalunya, Spain, and other local agencies, and by an unrestricted educational grant from GlaxoSmithKline.

## 1. THE GERMAN HEALTH SYSTEM

Since the reunification of East and West Germany in 1990, the German health-care system has changed through a number of health-care reform legislations. In recent years, the structure of health-care systems and the supply of health-care resources in Germany have been discussed in terms of lacking or decreasing financial resources. A reform process was initiated that aimed to constrain the growing costs of health care and to increase its efficiency. The introduction of legally fixed budgets or spending caps for the major sectors of health care was only one key element of these reform efforts. In general, these reforms led to a shift from the former cost containment to an expansion of copayments (e.g., for inpatient care, ambulatory care, rehabilitative care, pharmaceuticals, and medical aids).

Health care in Germany is mainly covered by the statutory health insurance (SHI). For all employees whose gross income does not exceed a certain level, membership in such an insurance plan is mandatory. In the year 2000, 88% of the population was covered by SHI; 74% of adults and their dependents were mandatory members, and 14% of adults and their dependents were voluntary members. Of the population, 9% was covered by private health insurance, 2% by free governmental health care (i.e., police officers, soldiers, and those doing the civil alternative to military service), and only 0.1% not insured. Contributions to health insurance depend on a member's income, and these contributions are shared equally between the insured and his or her employer (i.e., if the contribution rate to health insurance is 12.5% of gross income, the employee and employer each pay equal shares of 6.25%). Included in the health-care benefits are services for the prevention, screening, and treatment of diseases. The total per capita expenditure on health care in the year 2000 was US$2365.

In Germany, health care is publicly provided. Primary and secondary ambulatory care are provided through office-based physicians, and hospital care is provided by a separate inpatient care system.

## 1.1. Mental Health Care

Since a parliamentary committee report in 1975 criticized the institutionalization and low quality of care for people with long-term mental illness, mental health care in the Federal Republic of Germany (FRG) shifted gradually to offer community-integrated services. During the process of dehospitalization, the number of beds for the mentally ill was reduced from 150,000 in the FRG in 1976 to 69,000 in Germany in 1995. During the same period, the duration of stay in psychiatric hospitals was decreased from an average of 152 days to 44 days. The situation of mental health care in the eastern part of Germany in 1990 was similar to conditions in the FRG before the psychiatric reforms of the 1970s. The lack of specialized community-integrated services was further aggravated by staff shortages. Thus, big institutions with 300 to 1800 beds provided relatively low-quality care. Of inpatients, 60% were judged as not needing hospital care in 1990. Consequently, local, state, and national funds promoted the provision of long-term-care homes and ambulatory services within communities, particularly in the eastern part of the country. However, social integration and access to services in the community are still judged to be inadequate, although currently Germany enjoys a favorable position by international comparison. In 1995, between 24% and 40% of the institutionalized mentally ill were still estimated to not need such a high level of institutionalized care. Ten thousand hospital patients could still be transferred into less restrictive homes for long-term care. The dehospitalization process led to an increase of homes for long-term mental care within the community, which are funded by sub-regional funds. There were as many as 250 ambulatory psychosocial services in 1992 that offered advice and therapy to 8000 mentally ill patients. The decentralization of care did not necessarily entail the decentralization of finance and planning. Thus, ambulatory services are characterized by substantial regional differences that depend largely on budgets and local community policies to contract with private deliverers. Public health offices deliver social-psychiatric services themselves for the most disadvantaged people among the mentally ill by offering home visits and counseling. There is a general lack of comprehensive community-based services. Day clinics, which are mostly attached to psychiatric departments of hospitals, are funded by sickness funds or by retirement funds as social rehabilitation; however, not all patients are entitled to these benefits. Hospitals also offer flexible services for crisis intervention, which are usually paid by health insurance or public assistance. Ambulatory care for the mentally ill is also supported by the increasing number of psychiatrists, neurologists, and psychotherapists working in the ambulatory care sector. In addition the process of dehospitalization for psychiatric patients was accompanied by an increasing number of private hospitals that offer short-term-care and/or rehabilitative care for patients with addiction problems and psychosomatic disturbances (which lie outside the Länder hospital plans).

## 2. PREVIOUS PSYCHIATRIC EPIDEMIOLOGICAL RESEARCH

Epidemiological research of mental disorders has had a long tradition in Germany. In 1855, one of the first community surveys ever undertaken was conducted in the city of Lübeck to assess the prevalence of mental disorders in an effort to decide whether the mental health service system provided by the state was sufficient for the number of mentally ill people in this region (Eschenburg 1855). Cases were identified by relying on the information of key informants and agency records. Following the definition by Dohrenwend (1990), this example of assessing mental disorders in the community could be regarded as a first-generation study of mental disorders.

By contrast, the second-generation studies of mental disorders relied on face-to-face interviews with all subjects, interviewed mainly by psychiatrists. An example of second-generation studies in Germany is the baseline assessment of the longitudinal Upper Bavarian Study (Dilling, Weyerer & Fichter 1989; Weyerer & Dilling 1984). With the development of widely accepted and reliable diagnostic systems (DSM-III and ICD-10), a new era of community surveys in psychiatric research began. On the basis of these modern diagnostic systems, formal semistructured clinician-administered interviews (e.g., Present State Examination [PSE], Schedule for Affective Disorders and Schizophrenia [SADS]) were developed for the assessment of mental disorders.

To fulfill the criteria of a third-generation survey, research must use a structured clinical interview with explicit diagnostic criteria to identify cases. To date, a number of community surveys have been conducted to assess the spread of mental disorders in the population, but only a few fulfilled criteria of third-generation studies (for a more detailed overview of epidemiological surveys in Germany after 1980, see Riedel-Heller, Luppa & Angermeyer 2004).

The following third-generation studies have been carried out in Germany. First, the Early Developmental Stages of Psychopathology Study (EDSP)(Wittchen, Nelson & Lachner 1998) was conducted among young adults and adolescents (14–24 years old) in Munich. Mental disorders were assessed by using the Munich version of the Composite International Diagnostic Interview (M-CIDI) (Wittchen et al. 1998). Second, the Dresden Predictor Study (DPS)(Becker et al. 2000; Hoyer, Becker & Margraf 2002) was conducted to assess the prevalence and risk factors of mental disorders among young women ($n =$ 2064). A representative sample, aged 18–24 years, from the city of Dresden was interviewed with a modified version of the Diagnostisches Interview für Psychische Störungen – Forschungsversion (F-DIPS). Third, the Transitions in Alcohol Consumption and Smoking (TACOS) study was carried out in the city of Lübeck and its surrounding communities. A random sample of adults (18–64 years, $n =$ 4075) drawn from the resident registers were interviewed using the Munich version of the CIDI (M-CIDI). Although this study focused on smoking and alcohol consumption,

it also provided lifetime prevalence estimates of mental disorders (Meyer et al. 2000). Fourth, in 1997, a nationwide study was conducted as part of the German National Health Survey. The Mental Health Supplement of this survey studied a subsample of the nationally representative German National Health Interview and Examination Survey (GNHIES, $n =$ 7124). The mental health supplement of the GNHIES (GHS-MHS, $n =$ 4181) was the first nationwide survey that assessed mental disorders with a standardized diagnostic interview (M-CIDI). A total of 4181 individuals participated in this study (Wittchen et al. 1999; Jacobi et al. 2002).

## 3. THE GERMAN WMH SURVEY

The German WMH survey was administered as part of the European Study of the Epidemiology of Mental Disorders (ESEMeD; Alonso, Angermeyer & Lepine 2004), a coordinated series of nationally representative psychiatric epidemiological surveys carried out as part of the WMH Survey Initiative in six Western European countries. The six ESEMeD surveys use comparable design and standardized field methods aimed at allowing valid comparisons to be made across participating countries on the prevalence and correlates of mental disorders. All ESEMeD surveys focus on the noninstitutionalized household population aged 18 and older. This chapter presents the results of the German ESEMeD survey.

## 4. SUBJECTS AND METHODS

### 4.1. Sample

A total of 3555 persons participated in the German ESEMeD survey. The survey was fielded from August 2002 to July 2003 in a sample designed to represent all persons aged 18 years and older who resided in private households in the Federal Republic of Germany. Individuals were selected from the registers of residents' registration offices. Persons living in institutions and those who were not able to understand German were not eligible for the study. The

**Table 15.1.** Population and sample characteristics by age and gender

|  | Overall | Gender | | Age | | | | |
|---|---|---|---|---|---|---|---|---|
|  |  | Male n (%) | Female n (%) | 18–24 n (%) | 25–34 n (%) | 35–49 n (%) | 50–64 n (%) | 65+ n (%) |
| Population | 67,058,890 | 32,379,052 (48.3) | 34,679,838 (51.7) | 6,632,169 (9.9) | 11,170,785 (16.6) | 19,647,320 (29.3) | 15,542,894 (23.2) | 14,065,722 (21.0) |
| Sample | 3555 | 1660 (46.7) | 1895 (53.3) | 264 (7.4) | 551 (15.5) | 1180 (33.2) | 893 (25.1) | 667 (18.8) |
| Weighted sample | 3555 | 1711 (48.1) | 1844 (51.9) | 351.2 (9.9) | 593.9 (16.7) | 1044 (29.4) | 817.7 (23.0) | 747.8 (21.0) |

sample of German residents was drawn using a two-stage sampling procedure. In the first stage, a sample of 147 communities (primary sampling units) was drawn, in which the sample probability of the local communities was proportional to the extrapolated residential population. All the largest cities were included, sometimes as more than one primary sampling unit if they were very large, to account for the fact that the population could not have been represented adequately without these unique self-representing units. Smaller cities and areas other than cities, in comparison, were stratified samples according to the combination of districts and local community-size categories that guaranteed representativeness of the non–self-representing areas of the country (Behrens 1994). Allocation was optimized allowing for only the most minor deviations from the sample with respect to the federal state, administrative region, and local community category. In the second sampling stage, the same number of persons was randomly drawn in each primary sampling unit to create an equal-probability sample of the population (i.e., a sample in which each person in the population had the same probability of selection).

The survey was conducted by the staff of a private survey firm (Institut für angewandte Sozialforschung, infas GmbH) under close monitoring by the Department of Psychiatry at the University of Leipzig. The weighted response rate was 57.8% (ESEMeD 2004). Participation of eligible persons did not significantly differ with regard to age and sex. However, there was some variation with regard to other characteristics. Table 15.1

shows the demographic distribution of the sample compared to the total population in Germany. Of the interviewed sample, 46.7% were men and 53.3% were women; the mean age of the interviewed subjects was 48.1 years (standard of deviation [SD] = 16.4). The greatest differences between sample and population could be found in the group of those aged 35 to 49 years. This group of respondents was somewhat overrepresented in the unweighted sample. Survey sample weights were used to adjust for these discrepancies between the sample and the population.

## 4.2. Interview

As described in more detail in previous chapters (see especially Chapter 4), the Composite International Diagnostic Interview (CIDI) is a comprehensive, fully structured diagnostic interview for the assessment of mental disorders (Kessler & Üstün 2004). It provides, by means of computerized algorithms, lifetime and current (12 months and one month prior to the interview) diagnoses according to the definitions and criteria of the International Classification of Diseases (ICD-10) (WHO 1991), and the Diagnostic Statistical Manual for Mental Disorders (DSM-IV) (American Psychiatric Association 1994). The CIDI was developed for use by trained lay interviewers. Previous versions of the CIDI have been shown to be reliable and valid (Robins et al. 1988; Wittchen 1994; Wittchen et al. 1998). As noted in previous chapters, a new version of the instrument was administered, CIDI Version 3.0. This new version of CIDI was computerized to facilitate administration. It includes fully structured questions on presence, persistence, and intensity of clusters of psychiatric symptoms followed by probes for age of onset and lifetime course. CIDI 3.0 also gathers information on risk factors, symptoms, use of services, and use of medication. Also embedded in the CIDI 3.0 are sections that assess disability and dimensions of health-related quality of life as measured by the WHO Disablement Assessment Schedule II (WHO-DAS-II), the Short-Form-12 Health Survey (SF-12) (Ware, Kosinski & Keller 1995), and the EuroQol 5D (EQ-5D) (EuroQol Group 1990).

The translation and back-translation of the German version of CIDI 3.0 was carried out by scientists with outstanding English-language skills who had worked for several years as survey interviewers. All translators, whose mother tongue was German, were knowledgeable regarding American English and culture. An expert panel was consulted to discuss problems with regard to item wording, response categories, and adaptation to the German cultural context. The expert panel comprised two psychiatrists, one psychologist, one mental health service expert, one statistician, and one sociologist. Focus groups with individuals from the general population and patients were conducted to check comprehensibility of the interview schedule. Selection of participants in the groups was governed by the premise that the individuals selected are representative of the sampling population for the study. Attempts were made to reflect the structure of the general population in Germany as closely as possible. Finally, pilot interviews were conducted to serve as a test for the feasibility of the German instrument in an interview situation. These interviews were carried out by staff who had not otherwise been involved in the translation process. The final forward translation was translated back into English by an independent translator, whose mother tongue is American English. The translator had no knowledge of the questionnaire. Discrepancies between the forward translation and the back-translation were discussed by the German expert panel. All suggested changes were then implemented in the final version of the questionnaire.

Once the instrument was in final form and interviewers were trained, production interviews for the survey were conducted by lay interviewers using a Computer-Assisted Personal Interview (CAPI). Prior to the fieldwork, all interviewers received a three-day interviewer-training course to learn about the administration of the interview. Only those interviewers who passed this training course successfully were allowed to conduct interviews. A total of 198 interviewers conducted the interviews. The mean number of interviews completed by each interviewer was 18.0 (SD = 16.7). The work of all interviewers was carefully reviewed during the entire fieldwork period.

## 4.3. Measures

The German survey included the assessment of mood disorders, anxiety disorders, impulse-control disorders, and substance disorders, as did the other ESEMeD surveys. As noted in Chapter 13 of this volume, this assessment excluded some of the disorders included in other WMH surveys. All diagnoses were made with organic exclusions and without diagnostic hierarchy rules. As described by Haro and colleagues in Chapter 6 of this volume, a blinded clinical reappraisal study using the Structured Clinical Interview for DSM-IV (SCID) (First et al. 2002) showed generally good concordance between DSM-IV diagnoses based on the CIDI and independent diagnoses based on clinical assessments for anxiety, mood, and substance disorders. The CIDI diagnoses of impulse-control disorders have not been validated.

All other measurement issues were handled consistently in the ESEMeD surveys. Age of onset of disorders was assessed retrospectively. Twelve-month cases were classified by severity into serious, moderate, and mild cases on the basis of a complex classification scheme described by Bruffaerts and colleagues (see Chapter 13) in their description of the Belgium WMH survey. Lifetime treatment contact, 12-month service use, and minimally adequate treatment were also classified in the same way in France and in the other ESEMeD surveys. Predictor variables, finally, were the same as in the other ESEMeD countries.

## 4.4. Analysis Procedures

As noted previously, the data were weighted to adjust for differential nonresponse and for residual differences between the sample and the German population on a number of sociodemographic and geographic variables. An additional weight was used in the Part 2 sample to adjust for differences in probability of selection into that sample. Simple cross-tabulation was used to estimate prevalence and distributions of treatment. Survival analysis was used to make estimated projections of cumulative lifetime probability of disorders and treatment contact from year of onset using the actuarial method (Halli & Rao 1992). Discrete-time survival analysis (Efron 1988) with person-year as the unit of analysis was used to examine correlates of disorders and treatment contact. Logistic regression analysis (Hosmer & Lemeshow 1989) was used to study sociodemographic predictors of 12-month disorders, receiving treatment for these disorders, and treatment adequacy. Design-based standard errors were estimated using the STATA 8.2 software system (Stata Corporation 2003).

## 5. RESULTS

### 5.1. Lifetime and 12-month Prevalence Estimates

In Table 15.2, overall lifetime and 12-month prevalence estimates and standard errors are shown for each of ten DSM-IV mental disorders assessed in the survey. Lifetime prevalence is the proportion of individuals in the sample that fulfilled criteria of at least one mental disorder at some time in their life according to DSM-IV criteria as operationalized in the CIDI. Twelve-month prevalence rates refer to the 12 months prior to the interview.

The most prevalent lifetime disorders are estimated to be major depression (9.9%) and specific phobia (9.9%). The next most common lifetime disorder is alcohol abuse (6.3%). Far less

prevalent were dysthymia (2.7%), social phobia (2.5%), and panic disorder (1.1%). Twelve-month prevalence rates are highest for specific phobia (6.5%), followed by episodes of major depression (3.0%). The next most common disorders 12 months prior to the interview are social phobia (0.4%) and alcohol abuse (1.0%). Less prevalent are dysthymia (0.8%) and panic disorder (0.7%).

One in four respondents in the German survey reported having had one or more of the presented mental disorders at least once in his or her lifetime, and almost one in ten individuals fulfilled criteria for any mental disorder in the past 12 months prior to the interview. More than 14% fulfilled the criteria of any lifetime anxiety disorder assessed with the ESEMeD/MHEDEA 2000 interview, and 8% reported one of any anxiety disorder 12 months prior to the interview. Approximately one in ten respondents reported a lifetime history of at least one mood disorder, and 3.3% had a mood disorder in the past 12 months.

In accordance with other community surveys, the rates for any mental disorders reported in the bottom line of Table 15.2 are much smaller than the sum of the ten disorders in all presented columns. That is, a significant amount of respondents had more than one mental disorder at any time in their life or in the 12 months preceding the interview, respectively.

### 5.2. Demographic Correlates of 12-month Mental Disorders

In Table 15.3, the extent to which the 12-month disorders assessed in the survey are associated with sociodemographic variables is shown for different diagnostic groups (mood, anxiety, and alcohol-related disorders). Associations are reported by odds ratios (OR) with 95% confidence intervals (CIs). The logistic regression analysis for computing the ORs have been adjusted for sex and age.

### 5.3. Sex

The findings of the survey are consistent with previous epidemiological surveys in showing that

**Table 15.2.** Germany lifetime, 12-month and severity prevalence of DSM-IV disorders

| Diagnosis | Lifetime prevalence | | | 12-month prevalence | | | Severity prevalence of DSM-IV disorders | | | | | |
|---|---|---|---|---|---|---|---|---|---|---|---|---|
| | | | | | | | Serious | | Moderate | | Mild | |
| | n | % | (se) | n | % | (se) | % | (se) | % | (se) | % | (se) |
| **Anxiety disorder** | | | | | | | | | | | | |
| Panic disorder* | 58 | 1.6 | (0.2) | 28 | 0.7 | (0.2) | 24.2 | (8.9) | 35.0 | (11.9) | 40.8 | (10.5) |
| Generalized anxiety disorder with hierarchy* | 41 | 1.1 | (0.2) | 12 | 0.3 | (0.1) | 57.5 | (18.7) | 42.5 | (18.7) | 0.0 | (0.0) |
| Specific phobia* | 360 | 9.9 | (0.7) | 234 | 6.5 | (0.5) | 13.1 | (3.0) | 42.6 | (6.6) | 44.3 | (7.5) |
| Social phobia* | 92 | 2.5 | (0.3) | 55 | 1.4 | (0.2) | 14.7 | (7.0) | 52.5 | (10.0) | 32.8 | (10.4) |
| Agoraphobia without panic* | 19 | 0.5 | (0.1) | 12 | 0.3 | (0.1) | 30.1 | (24.8) | 45.2 | (12.8) | 24.7 | (18.9) |
| Posttraumatic stress disorder** | 52 | 1.6 | (0.3) | 24 | 0.7 | (0.2) | 28.4 | (10.2) | 59.4 | (11.3) | 12.2 | (5.5) |
| Adult separation anxiety*** | 21 | 2.0 | (0.6) | 3 | 0.2 | (0.1) | 81.0 | (18.9) | 0.0 | (0.0) | 19.0 | (18.9) |
| Any anxiety disorder** | 313 | 14.6 | (1.5) | 189 | 8.1 | (1.0) | 13.9 | (2.6) | 40.9 | (5.4) | 45.1 | (6.0) |
| **Mood disorder** | | | | | | | | | | | | |
| Major depressive disorder with hierarchy* | 372 | 9.9 | (0.6) | 109 | 3.0 | (0.3) | 23.6 | (5.8) | 32.4 | (5.7) | 43.9 | (6.2) |
| Dysthymia without hierarchy* | 94 | 2.7 | (0.3) | 25 | 0.8 | (0.2) | 20.7 | (9.6) | 46.9 | (12.2) | 32.5 | (10.8) |
| Any mood disorder* | 398 | 10.7 | (0.7) | 120 | 3.3 | (0.3) | 21.9 | (5.6) | 34.5 | (5.7) | 43.6 | (6.0) |
| **Impulse disorder** | | | | | | | | | | | | |
| Oppositional-defiant disorder*** | 5 | 0.4 | (0.3) | 2 | 0.3 | (0.2) | 0.0 | (0.0) | 22.6 | (24.7) | 77.4 | (24.7) |
| Conduct disorder*** | 10 | 1.3 | (0.6) | 0 | 0.0 | (0.0) | – | | – | | – | |
| Attention-deficit/ hyperactivity disorder*** | 20 | 1.8 | (0.7) | 9 | 0.6 | (0.3) | 32.1 | (15.9) | 23.0 | (16.3) | 44.9 | (22.3) |
| Intermittent explosive disorder with hierarchy* | – | – | – | – | – | – | – | | – | | – | |
| Any impulse-control disorder*** | 31 | 3.1 | (0.8) | 9 | 0.6 | (0.3) | 32.1 | (15.9) | 23.0 | (16.3) | 44.9 | (22.3) |
| **Substance disorder** | | | | | | | | | | | | |
| Alcohol abuse* | 224 | 6.3 | (0.5) | 42 | 1.0 | (0.2) | 7.4 | (3.1) | 30.9 | (19.9) | 61.8 | (18.8) |
| Alcohol dependence* | 44 | 1.5 | (0.3) | 10 | 0.3 | (0.1) | 9.2 | (9.2) | 90.8 | (9.2) | 0.0 | (0.0) |
| Any substance use disorder* | 228 | 6.5 | (0.6) | 45 | 1.1 | (0.2) | 8.4 | (3.5) | 32.8 | (18.8) | 58.8 | (17.6) |
| **Any disorder** | | | | | | | | | | | | |
| Any** | 587 | 25.5 | (2.0) | 264 | 10.9 | (1.3) | 11.7 | (2.2) | 37.6 | (4.0) | 50.8 | (4.5) |
| **Total sample** | | | | | | | | | | | | |
| Total sample** | – | – | – | 1323 | – | – | 1.3 | (0.3) | 4.1 | (0.6) | 5.7 | (0.8) |

*Note:* Severity calculated using Part 2 weights.

* Part 1 sample, prevalence calculated using Part 1 weights.

** Part 2 sample, prevalence calculated using Part 2 weights.

*** Part 2 sample (age ≤44), prevalence and severity calculated using Part 2 weights for ages ≤44.

**Table 15.3.** Demographic correlates of 12-month DSM-IV disorder groups in Germany

| Demographic factor | Any mood disorder OR (95% CI) | Any anxiety disorder OR (95% CI) | Any alcohol OR (95% CI) | Any mental disorder OR (95% CI) |
|---|---|---|---|---|
| Overall | | | | |
| **Sex** | | | | |
| Male | 1.0 | 1.0 | 1.0 | 1.0 |
| Female | 1.8 (1.2–2.8)* | 1.7 (1.2–2.3)* | 0.2 (0.1–0.4)* | 1.4 (1.1–1.8)* |
| **Age** | | | | |
| 18–24 | 3.1 (1.3–7.1)* | 4.5 (2.3–8.7)* | 14.0 (1.8–112.1)* | 3.7 (2.2–6.3)* |
| 25–34 | 2.5 (1.3–4.9)* | 2.3 (1.3–4.2)* | 17.5 (2.3–135.5)* | 2.5 (1.6–3.9)* |
| 35–49 | 1.5 (0.8–3.0) | 2.3 (1.4–4.0)* | 9.2 (1.2–69.9)* | 2.1 (1.4–3.2)* |
| 50–64 | 1.7 (0.8–3.3) | 2.3 (1.3–4.0)* | 2.4 (0.3–22.2) | 2.0 (1.2–3.0)* |
| 65+ | 1.0 | 1.0 | 1.0 | 1.0 |
| **Living situation** | | | | |
| Living with someone | 1.0 | 1.0 | 1.0 | 1.0 |
| Living alone | 2.7 (1.8–4.0)* | 1.4 (1.0–1.9)* | 1.9 (1.0–3.6)* | 1.5 (1.2–2.0)* |
| **Education** | | | | |
| 0–8 years | 1.0 | 1.0 | 1.0 | 1.0 |
| 9–11 years | 0.8 (0.5–1.5) | 1.3 (0.8–2.2) | 0.4 (0.2–1.2) | 1.1 (0.7–1.6) |
| 12+ years | 0.6 (0.3–1.1) | 1.6 (0.9–2.7) | 0.6 (0.2–1.5) | 1.1 (0.7–1.6) |
| **Employment status** | | | | |
| Paid employment | 1.0 | 1.0 | 1.0 | 1.0 |
| Unemployed | 7.2 (3.9–13.4)* | 1.8 (1.0–3.2)* | 6.1 (2.7–13.9)* | 3.0 (1.9–4.6)* |
| Retired | 1.1 (0.6–1.9) | 0.6 (0.4–0.9)* | 0.3 (0.1–1.1) | 0.7 (0.5–1.0)* |
| Homemaker | 2.0 (1.0–4.0) | 1.4 (0.7–2.5) | 0.2 (0.1–1.4) | 1.3 (0.8–2.2) |
| Student | 1.6 (0.5–5.1) | 1.1 (0.5–2.4) | 5.5 (2.1–14.0)* | 1.5 (0.8–2.8) |
| Other | 2.8 (1.5–5.3)* | 1.1 (0.7–1.9) | 2.2 (0.7–6.7) | 1.6 (1.1–2.4)* |
| **Urbanity** | | | | |
| Rural | 1.0 | 1.0 | 1.0 | 1.0 |
| Midsize urban | 1.4 (0.7–2.7) | 1.0 (0.6–1.7) | 13.2 (1.7–99.7)* | 1.2 (0.8–1.8) |
| Large urban | 1.2 (0.6–2.5) | 1.0 (0.6–1.6) | 9.8 (1.3–73.7)* | 1.1 (0.7–1.6) |
| **East–West** | | | | |
| West | 1.0 | 1.0 | 1.0 | 1.0 |
| East | 0.9 (0.6–1.5) | 0.8 (0.5–1.3) | 2.5 (1.2–5.0)* | 1.0 (0.7–1.4) |

* $p < 0.05$.

women have significantly higher rates of mood and anxiety disorders, whereas men have higher rates of alcohol use disorders. Also, the grouping of "any mental disorder" shows significantly higher prevalence rates for women than men.

### 5.4. Age

The results in Table 15.3 show that the younger age groups have significantly higher 12-month prevalence of all grouped disorders than do older respondents. Highest prevalence rates are shown in the group of 18- to 24-year-old respondents, with the exception of alcohol use disorder. Alcohol use disorders are most prevalent in the group of 25- to 34-year-old respondents. The common pattern for the age groups is that prevalence rates decline with age.

### 5.5. Education

Education is examined here by distinguishing years of school completed. The patterns of association are variable for the different education groups. Mood disorders are higher in the lowest education group. A similar pattern is found in the group of alcohol use disorders. Anxiety disorders are somewhat higher in the higher education groups. From the lowest to the highest education groups, no significant coefficients were found in all disorder categories.

## 5.6. Employment

Unemployment is strongly and significantly associated with all disorder categories. Retired people report the lowest prevalence rates in three of four disorder groups (any mood, any anxiety, and any mental). It is noteworthy that students report significantly higher rates of alcohol abuse disorders than do any of the other occupational groups. Only the OR of unemployed people exceeded that of students.

## 5.7. Living Situation

Living without a partner is strongly associated with all disorder categories. Highest rates were found for mood disorders (OR = 2.7).

## 5.8. Urbanicity

Respondents living in rural regions, defined as regions with fewer than 5000 inhabitants, showed somewhat lower (but not significant) rates in mood disorders, anxiety disorders, and the overall disorder category. A strong association was found for alcohol disorders, with highest prevalence rates in midsize urban areas, followed by large urban areas.

## 5.9. Region

There is only one significant coefficient that indicates a higher risk of having a mental disorder in the eastern part of Germany. Only the coefficient for "any alcohol disorder" is significant at the 5% level (OR = 2.5), which means that there is a higher rate of alcohol use disorders in the eastern part of Germany than in the western part. Region was not a significant predictor for mood, anxiety, or any mental disorder.

## 6. TREATMENT OF MENTAL DISORDERS IN GERMANY

Table 15.4 presents the percentage of people who have visited a health service as a result of problems with their mental health in the past year. Results are presented by disorder and for each service provider used. The general practitioner (GP) was the most commonly used service provider among all disorder groups presented here. Highest rates of GP use were found for social phobia (27.9%) and for major depressive episodes (26.8%); lower treatment rates were found for specific phobia (15.9%). "Other mental health care" was the second most visited category of health service providers. Highest treatment rates for "other mental health care" were found for social phobia (24.6%) and lowest treatment rates for alcohol abuse (2.8%). The proportions of visits to a psychiatrists were highest for major depressive episodes (21.0%). In general, only a minority of respondents with a DSM-IV diagnosis reported having used any treatment because of their symptoms. In addition, among those who received treatment, a smaller fraction visited a mental health care specialist. Most people who reported having a mental disorder in the 12 months prior to the interview used "any other general health care" or "other types of services." Regardless of disorder, the majority of people with mental disorder did not receive any form of health care. The lowest treatment rates were found for substance abuse, leaving almost 90% of affected respondents untreated.

Treatment contact in the first year of the disorder and the delay of treatment are reported in Table 15.5. The rates for making treatment contact in the first year of disorder onset range from 58.6% for generalized anxiety disorder and 57.1% for panic disorder to 3.4% for specific phobia. Of respondents with major depression, 40.4% make their first treatment contact within the first year following onset. Median years of treatment delay differ greatly across disorders. Panic disorders and generalized anxiety disorders showed the least delay (both one year), whereas specific phobia (32 years) and social phobia (20 years) showed much higher treatment delays.

**Table 15.4.** 12-month service usage in Germany: Percentage treated by health-care professionals among people with mental disorders

| Disorder group | Mental disorder | Measure | Type of professional | | | | | | | | | Unweighted n with mental disorder | Weighted n with mental disorder |
| --- | --- | --- | --- | --- | --- | --- | --- | --- | --- | --- | --- | --- | --- |
| | | | Psychiatrist % (se) | Other mental health care % (se) | Any mental health care % (se) | General medical % (se) | Any health care % (se) | Human services % (se) | CAM % (se) | Any non–health care % (se) | Any treatment % (se) | | |
| Anxiety | Social phobia* | Percentage in treatment | 9.9 (5.1) | 24.6 (6.8) | 27.1 (7.0) | 27.9 (8.0) | 42.3 (7.7) | 2.4 (2.5) | 2.7 (1.8) | 5.1 (3.2) | 43.5 (7.9) | 55 | 51 |
| | | Unweighted n in treatment | 5 | 13 | 15 | 12 | 21 | 1 | 2 | 3 | 22 | | |
| | Specific phobia* | Percentage in treatment | 7.1 (1.7) | 9.4 (2.1) | 12.3 (2.2) | 15.9 (2.6) | 23.5 (3.0) | 0.8 (0.6) | 1.0 (0.6) | 1.8 (0.8) | 24.3 (3.1) | 234 | 230 |
| | | Unweighted n in treatment | 18 | 23 | 31 | 36 | 55 | 2 | 3 | 5 | 57 | | |
| | Any anxiety disorder** | Percentage in treatment | 7.6 (2.3) | 11.3 (2.4) | 13.6 (2.7) | 15.6 (2.8) | 23.1 (3.7) | 1.7 (0.8) | 1.1 (0.5) | 2.9 (0.9) | 24.1 (3.8) | 190 | 108 |
| | | Unweighted n in treatment | 24 | 32 | 41 | 38 | 62 | 5 | 4 | 9 | 65 | | |
| Mood | Major depressive episode* | Percentage in treatment | 21.0 (4.1) | 19.3 (4.5) | 29.8 (5.3) | 26.8(6.8) | 45.3 (7.0) | 4.7 (2.3) | 3.7 (1.8) | 8.4 (3.0) | 48.6 (6.5) | 109 | 107 |
| | | Unweighted n in treatment | 24 | 22 | 34 | 28 | 49 | 5 | 5 | 10 | 52 | | |
| | Any mood disorder* | Percentage in treatment | 20.1 (3.7) | 17.9 (4.1) | 27.9 (4.8) | 26.9(6.5) | 43.6 (6.7) | 4.7 (2.2) | 3.4 (1.6) | 8.1 (2.5) | 46.5 (6.2) | 120 | 118 |
| | | Unweighted n in treatment | 26 | 23 | 36 | 32 | 53 | 6 | 5 | 11 | 56 | | |
| Substance | Alcohol abuse* | Percentage in treatment | 4.0 (4.0) | 2.8 (2.8) | 6.8 (4.9) | 0.0 (0.0) | 6.8 (4.9) | 0.0 (0.0) | 0.0 (0.0) | 0.0 (0.0) | 6.8 (4.9) | 42 | 37 |
| | | Unweighted n in treatment | 1 | 1 | 2 | 0 | 2 | 0 | 0 | 0 | 2 | | |
| | Any substance* | Percentage in treatment | 3.6 (3.6) | 6.6 (4.7) | 10.2 (5.8) | 0.0 (0.0) | 10.2(5.8) | 0.0 (0.0) | 0.0 (0.0) | 0.0 (0.0) | 10.2 (5.8) | 45 | 41 |
| | | Unweighted n in treatment | 1 | 2 | 3 | 0 | 3 | 0 | 0 | 0 | 3 | | |
| Composite | Any disorder** | Percentage in treatment | 8.3 (1.9) | 9.9 (1.9) | 13.6 (2.4) | 17.6 (2.7) | 24.6 (3.3) | 2.0 (0.8) | 1.2 (0.5) | 3.2 (0.8) | 26.0 (3.4) | 263 | 143 |
| | | Unweighted n in treatment | 35 | 40 | 56 | 60 | 89 | 8 | 6 | 14 | 94 | | |

*Note:* Values are percentages with standard errors in parentheses. Disorders with unweighted *n* less than 30 do not have percentages.

* Denotes Part I weight.  ** Denotes Part II weight.

**Table 15.5.** Proportional treatment contact in the year of disorder onset and median duration of delay among cases that subsequently made treatment contact

|  | % Making treatment contact in year of onset | % Making treatment contact by 50 yrs | Median duration of delay (years) | n |
|---|---|---|---|---|
| **I. Anxiety disorders** | | | | |
| Panic disorder | 57.1 | 96.1 | 1 | 58 |
| Generalized anxiety disorder | 58.6 | 94.8 | 1 | 58 |
| Specific phobia | 3.4 | 85.3 | 32 | 359 |
| Social phobia | 8.1 | 85.3 | 20 | 92 |
| Any anxiety disorders | 13.7 | 95.0 | 23 | 464 |
| **II. Mood disorders** | | | | |
| Major depressive episode | 40.4 | 89.1 | 2 | 371 |
| **III. Substance disorders** | | | | |
| Alcohol abuse | 14.8 | 82.4 | 12 | 53 |
| Alcohol abuse with dependence | –* | –* | –* | –* |
| Any substance disorders | 13.2 | 86.1 | 9 | 56 |

* Disorder was omitted due to insufficient $n < 30$, but it will be included as one of the disorders in "Any" category.

## 7. DISCUSSION

The German segment of the ESEMeD project is the first national representative study in Germany that allows for cross-national comparisons of prevalence rates, correlates, and treatment associated with mental disorders by virtue of the implementation of consistent instrument and field quality-control procedures in all countries of the ESEMeD consortium and close correspondence of these procedures with those used in the remainder of the larger WMH consortium.

### 7.1. Prevalence

The survey findings show that mental disorders are frequent in the adult population in Germany. More than 25% of the sample reported at least one of the assessed disorders at any time of their life. Twelve-month prevalence rates are somewhat lower but also show a remarkable number of people (10.9%) who reported a disorder 12 months prior to the interview. The results of the study confirm some of the prevalence patterns found in earlier European studies that used the CIDI as psychiatric interview (Bijl, Ravelli & van Zessen 1998; Wittchen et al. 1999; Kringlen, Torgersen & Cramer 2001). Major depressive disorder is the most common mental disorder, followed by specific phobia and then social phobia.

Men have significantly lower rates of anxiety and mood disorders than do women and higher rates of alcohol use disorders.

Comparing the current findings with the results of the TACOS study, we find nearly completely consistent lifetime prevalence rates (e.g., major depression: 10.0%; dysthymia: 2.5%). Twelve-month prevalence results have not yet been reported for the TACOS study. Quite the reverse is found when the results of the current survey are compared with those of the GHS-MHS (Wittchen et al. 1999; Wittchen et al. 2000; Wittchen & Jacobi 2002; Kruse, Schmitz & Thefeld 2003). The GHS-MHS rates are much higher than those in the current survey. Indeed, the GHS-MHS results exceed the rates in the current survey by up to three times (e.g., 12-month major depression: 8.3%; dysthymia: 4.5%). It follows from this that almost the same differences exist when comparing the results of TACOS with those of GHS-MHS. This is an interesting finding because the same questionnaire (M-CIDI) was used in both of the latter studies. In this context, it is noteworthy that, although the diagnostic instrument used in TACOS and GHS-MHS (the M-CIDI) is very similar to the instrument used in the WMH surveys (CIDI 3.0), there are some differences in wording, probing, and question order that might have an impact on the prevalence rate estimation. It must also be noted that the sampling frames used to choose eligible respondents differ among all the studies. Whereas the TACOS study used a comparable two-stage sampling design in a northern region in Germany, the GHS-MHS was administered to a subsample of the German Health Survey respondents. Furthermore, the studies differ with regard to the interviewers who conducted the interviews. Whereas the TACOS and ESEMeD interviewers were trained lay interviewers, most of the interviewer staff of the GHS-MHS were clinical psychologists. In addition, the disorder categories also differ from study to study. For example, the ESEMeD mood category includes only major depression and dysthymia. In other studies, bipolar disorders and subthreshold disorders are included in much broader categories of affective disorders. The same applies to the anxiety disorder category and, as a result of these categorizations, to the overall disorder category. Taking all this into account might help explain, to some extent, the differences across the studies. The international data of the ESEMeD survey reveal that prevalence estimates of mental disorders in Germany are ranked in the middle compared to other ESEMeD countries (Demyttenaere et al. 2004). Lifetime prevalence estimates in the ESEMeD data vary from a low of 18.1% in Italy to a high of 37.9% in France. In Germany, the overall prevalence of mental disorders is 25.2%. Lifetime prevalence rates of anxiety disorders range from a high of 22.0% in France to a low of 10.0% in Spain (Germany: 14.1%), mood disorders range from a high of 23.3% in France to a low of 10.2% in Italy (Germany: 10.9%), and alcohol use disorders range from a high of 8.7% in Belgium to a low of 1.2% in Italy (Germany: 6.3%). Minor differences of prevalence rates reported here as compared with those reported by Demyttenaere et al. (2004) are due to different weighting strategies and to the disorders included in the disorder categories.

## 7.2. Demographic Correlates of Mental Disorders

The correlates of mental disorders examined in this chapter show partly consistent patterns com-

pared with the TACOS project data and those of the GHS-MHS. The data for sex as a predictor of mental disorders are consistent with those reported in the TACOS project and the GHS-MHS study, in both of which women experienced considerably more affective and anxiety disorders and men showed much higher rates in alcohol use disorders.

For all disorder groupings, a decline of prevalence rates in the older cohorts could be found in the German ESEMeD survey. This pattern is consistent with the pattern of the TACOS data, although it is more pronounced in the ESEMeD data. With the exception of substance use disorders, no decline of mental disorders at later ages is reported for the GHS-MHS data. This finding is not consistent with findings of previous European studies (Bijl, Ravelli & van Zessen 1998; Kringlen, Torgersen & Cramer 2001).

Comparing the German ESEMeD data with the data of GHS-MHS for employment as a predictor of mental disorder, we find similar associations. Unemployment is a strong predictor for "any mental disorder" group in both studies. The TACOS project does not report results for employment as a predictor of mental disorders.

With the exception of anxiety disorders in the TACOS study, the associations found between living situation (or marital status) are consistent across all German surveys. Findings show that people who are living with someone or who are married are less prone, respectively, to have any mental disorder.

The rates of service use show that a considerable number of people classified with 12-month depressive disorder according to DSM-IV criteria do not receive treatment. This finding is consistent with previous studies on service use for mental disorders in Europe (Bijl & Ravelli 2000; Schmitz & Kruse 2002). Being diagnosed as having a mental disorder does not necessarily mean that treatment is needed, but previous studies indicate that mild and subthreshold mental disorders should receive treatment to prevent those disorders from becoming worse, becoming chronic, or causing other psychosocial disabilities (Kuhn et al. 2002; Kessler et al. 2003). Consistent with other surveys, the GP is the most commonly visited service provider for all disorder groups (Boerma & Verhaak 1999). In all disorder groups, "other mental health care" is the second most received type of health care, followed by visits to psychiatrists.

## 8. CONCLUSIONS

Despite the use of reliable and valid diagnostic instruments in recent epidemiological surveys in Germany, prevalence estimates vary substantially from survey to survey, even when the same diagnostic instrument is used. The differences across surveys can best be explained by differences in sampling methods, diagnostic instruments, and interviewer characteristics. Thus, comparisons across surveys require consistent sampling methods, diagnostic instruments, and qualifications of interviewers. The WMH surveys meet these requirements and are, therefore, useful tools for estimating prevalence rates of mental disorders across countries.

## 9. LIMITATIONS

It should be noted that there are some limitations. Certain groups of individuals (e.g., people without fixed addresses, those unable to understand the German language, those living in institutions) were not represented in the survey. In general, the impact of omitting these groups on the results presented here remains unclear. It is known that individuals who are hard to reach have somewhat higher rates of psychopathology (Kessler, Little & Groves 1995), especially in psychotic symptoms. Because we have only assessed mood, anxiety, and alcohol use disorders, we expect that prevalence rates were only slightly influenced by the omission of the previously mentioned groups. Moreover, having not assessed psychotic disorders is another limitation of the study.

## REFERENCES

Alonso, J., Angermeyer, M. C. & Lepine, J. P. (2004). The European Study of the Epidemiology of Mental Disorders (ESEMeD) project: An epidemiological basis for informing mental health policies in Europe. *Acta Psychiatrica Scandinavica*, 109, 5–7.

American Psychiatric Association (1994). *Diagnostic and statistical manual of mental disorders (DSM-IV)*, 4th ed. Washington, DC: American Psychiatric Association.

Becker, E. S., Türke, V., Neumer, S., Soeder, U., Krause, P. & Margraf, J. (2000). Incidence and prevalence of rates of mental disorders in a community sample of young women: Results of the Dresden study. In *Public health research and practice: Report of the Public Health Research Association Saxony*, Vol. 2, ed. R. Heeß-Erler, R. Manz & W. Kirch, pp. 259–92. Regensburg: Roderer.

Behrens, K. (1994). Schichtung und Gewichtung: Verbesserung der regionalen Repräsentanz. In *Schichtung und Gewichtung in der Umfragepraxis*, ed. S. Gabler, J. H. P. Hoffmeyer-Zlotnik & D. Krebs, pp. 27–41. Opladen: Westdeutscher Verlag.

Bijl, R. V. & Ravelli, A. (2000). Psychiatric morbidity, service use, and need for care in the general population: Results of the Netherlands Mental Health Survey and Incidence Study. *American Journal of Public Health*, 90, 602–7.

Bijl, R. V., Ravelli, A. & Van Zessen, G. (1998). Prevalence of psychiatric disorder in the general population: Results of the Netherlands Mental Health Survey and Incidence Study (NEMESIS). *Social Psychiatry and Psychiatric Epidemiology*, 33, 587–95.

Boerma, W. G. & Verhaak, P. F. (1999). The general practitioner as the first contacted health professional by patients with psychosocial problems: A European study. *Psychological Medicine*, 29, 689–96.

Demyttenaere, K., Bruffaerts, R., Posada-Villa, J., Gasquet, I., Kovess, V., Lepine, J. P., Angermeyer, M. C., Bernert, S., Girolamo, G., Morosini, P., Polidori, G., Kikkawa, T., Kawakami, N., Ono, Y., Takeshima, T., Uda, H., Karam, E. G., Fayyad, J. A., Karam, A. N., Mneimneh, Z. N., Medina-Mora, M. E., Borges, G., Lara, G., de Graaf, R., Ormel, J., Gureje, O., Shen, Y., Huang, Y., Zhang, M., Alonso, J., Haro, J. M., Vilagut, G., Bromet, E. J., Gluzman, S., Webb, C., Kessler, R. C., Merikangas, K. R., Anthony, J. C., Korff, M. R. V., Wang, P. S., Alonso, J., Brugha, T. S., Aguilar-Gaxiola, S., Lee, S., Heeringa, S., Pennell, B. E., Zaslavsky, A. M., Üstün, T. B., & Chatterji, S. (2004). Prevalence, severity and unmet need for treatment of mental disorders in the World Health Organization World Mental Health Surveys. *Journal of the American Medical Association*, 291, 2581–90.

Dilling, H., Weyerer, S. & Fichter, M. (1989). The Upper Bavarian studies. *Acta Psychiatrica Scandinavica*, 348, 113–39.

Dohrenwend, B. P. (1990). The problem of validity in field studies of psychological disorders' revisited. *Psychological Medicine*, 20, 195–208.

Efron, B. (1988). Logistic regression, survival analysis, and the Kaplan-Meier curve. *Journal of the American Statistical Association*, 83, 414–25.

Eschenburg, B. G. (1855). Die Irren-Statistik des Luebeckischen Staates. *Neue Luebeckische Blätter*, 21, 329–31.

ESEMeD/MHEDEA 2000 Investigators (2004). Sampling and methods of the European Study of the Epidemiology of Mental Disorders (ESEMeD) project. *Acta Psychiatrica Scandinavica*, 109 (suppl. 420), 8–20.

EuroQol Group (1990). EuroQol: A new facility for the measurement of health-related quality of life. *Health Policy*, 16, 199–208.

First, M. B., Gibbon, M., Spitzer, R. & Williams, J. B. W. (2002). *The Structured Clinical Interview for DSM-IV*. Washington, DC: American Psychiatric Press.

Halli, S. S. & Rao, K. V. (1992). *Advanced techniques of population analysis*. New York: Plenum Press.

Hosmer, D. W. & Lemeshow, S. (1989). *Applied logistic regression*. New York: John Wiley & Sons.

Hoyer, J., Becker, E. S. & Margraf, J. (2002). Generalized anxiety disorder and clinical worry episodes in young women. *Psychological Medicine*, 32, 1227–37.

Jacobi, F., Wittchen, H. U., Holting, C., Sommer, S., Lieb, R., Hofler, M. & Pfister, H. (2002). Estimating the prevalence of mental and somatic disorders in the community: Aims and methods of the German National Health Interview and Examination Survey. *International Journal of Methods in Psychiatric Research*, 11, 1–18.

Kessler, R. C., Little, R. J. A. & Groves, R. M. (1995). Advances in strategies for minimizing and adjusting for survey nonresponse. *Epidemiologic Reviews*, 17, 192–204.

Kessler, R. C., Merikangas, K. R., Berglund, P., Eaton, W. W., Koretz, D. & Walters, E. E. (2003). Mild disorders should not be eliminated from the DSM-V. *Archives of General Psychiatry*, 60, 1117–22.

Kessler, R. C. & Üstün, T. B. (2004). The World Mental Health (WMH) Survey Initiative Version of the World Health Organization (WHO) Composite International Diagnostic Interview (CIDI). *International Journal of Methods in Psychiatric Research*, 13, 93–121.

Kringlen, E., Torgersen, S. & Cramer, V. (2001). A Norwegian psychiatric epidemiological study. *American Journal of Psychiatry*, 158, 1091–8.

Kruse, J., Schmitz, N. & Thefeld, W. (2003). On the association between diabetes and mental disorders in a community sample: Results from the German national health interview and examination survey. *Diabetes Care*, 26, 1841–6.

Kuhn, K. U., Quednow, B. B., Barkow, K., Heun, R., Linden, M. & Maier, W. (2002). Chronic course and psychosocial disability caused by depressive illnesses in general practice patients during a one year period: Results of a study by the World Health Organization. *Nervenarzt*, 73, 644–50.

Meyer, C., Rumpf, H. J., Hapke, U., Dilling, H. & John, U. (2000). Lifetime prevalence of mental disorders in general adult population: Results of TACOS study. *Nervenarzt*, 71, 535–42.

Riedel-Heller, S. G., Luppa, M. & Angermeyer, M. (2004). Psychiatrische Epidemiologie in Deutschland. *Psychiatrische Praxis*, 31, 288–97.

Robins, L. N., Wing, J., Wittchen, H. U., Helzer, J. E., Babor, T. F., Burke, J., Farmer, A., Jablenski, A., Pickens, R., Regier, D. A., Sartorius, N. & Towle, L. H. (1988). The Composite International Diagnostic Interview: An epidemiologic instrument suitable for use in conjunction with different diagnostic systems and in different cultures. *Archives of General Psychiatry*, 45, 1069–77.

Schmitz, N. & Kruse, J. (2002). The relationship between mental disorders and medical service utilization in a representative community sample. *Social Psychiatry and Psychiatric Epidemiology*, 37, 380–6.

Stata Corporation (2003). *Stata Statistical Software: Release 8.2*. College Station, TX: Stata Corporation.

Ware, J. E., Kosinski, M. & Keller, S. D. (1995). *SF-12: How to score the SF-12 Physical and Mental Health Summary Scales*. Boston: The Health Institute, New England Medical Center.

Weyerer, S. & Dilling, H. (1984). Prevalence and treatment of psychiatric diseases in the general population: Results of a field study in 3 communities of Upper Bavaria. *Nervenarzt*, 55, 30–42.

Wittchen, H. U. (1994). Reliability and validity studies of the WHO-Composite International Diagnostic Interview (CIDI): A critical review. *Journal of Psychiatric Research*, 28, 57–84.

Wittchen, H. U., Carter, R. M., Pfister, H., Montgomery, S. A. & Kessler, R. C. (2000). Disabilities and quality of life in pure and comorbid generalized anxiety disorder and major depression in a national survey. *International Clinical Psychopharmacology*, 15, 319–28.

Wittchen, H. & Jacobi F. (2002). Die Versorgungssituation psychischer Störungen in Deutschland. *Psychotherapeutenjournal*, 6–15.

Wittchen, H. U., Lachner, G., Wunderlich, U. & Pfister, H. (1998). Test-retest reliability of the computerized DSM-IV version of the Munich-Composite International Diagnostic Interview (M-CIDI). *Social*

*Psychiatry and Psychiatric Epidemiology*, 33, 568–78.

Wittchen, H. U., Muller, N., Pfister, H., Winter, S. & Schmidtkunz, B. (1999). Affective, somatoform and anxiety disorders in Germany-initial results of an additional federal survey of "psychiatric disorders." *Gesundheitswesen*, 61, S216–S222.

Wittchen, H. U., Nelson, C. B. & Lachner, G. (1998). Prevalence of mental disorders and psychosocial impairments in adolescents and young adults. *Psychological Medicine*, 28, 109–26.

World Health Organization (WHO) (1991). *International Classification of Diseases (ICD-10)*. Geneva: World Health Organization.

# 16 The Prevalence of Mental Disorders and Service Use in Israel: Results from the National Health Survey, 2003–2004

DAPHNA LEVINSON, YAACOV LERNER, NELLY ZILBER, ITZHAK LEVAV, AND JACOB POLAKIEWICZ

## ACKNOWLEDGMENTS

The national health survey was funded by the Ministry of Health, with support from the Israel National Institute for Health Policy and Health Services Research and the National Insurance Institute of Israel.

Collaborating investigators include Daphna Levinson (principal investigator, Ministry of Health, Mental Health Services), Itzhak Levav (co–principal investigator, Ministry of Health), Alexander Grinshpoon (Ministry of Health), Ziona Haklai (Ministry of Health), Anat Shemesh (Ministry of Health), Gabi Bin Nun (Ministry of Health), Alexander Ponizovsky (Ministry of Health), Yaacov Lerner (Falk Institute), Nelly Zilber (Falk Institute and French Research Center of Jerusalem), Anneke Ifrah (Israel Center for Disease Control), Yehuda Neumark (Hebrew University–Hadassah, School of Public Health), Julia Mirsky (Ben Gurion University), Alean Al-Krenawi (Ben Gurion University), Haim Knobler (Hebrew University, Ben Gurion University), and Robert Kohn (Brown University).

The survey was carried out by the Israel Central Bureau of Statistics. We thank Ari Paltiel, Naama Rotem, Michal Nir, Yoel Domb, Tzufit Bartov, Rinat Rivlis Tzachi Makovki, and their staff for the skillful execution of the survey in the field. Nabil Geraisy and Razek Khwaled translated the questionnaires into Arabic, and Alexander Ponizovsky and Julia Mirsky into Russian.

The views and opinions expressed in this chapter are those of the authors and should not be construed to represent the views of any of the sponsoring organizations or of the government.

The IMHS is carried out in conjunction with the World Health Organization World Mental Health (WMH) Survey Initiative. We thank the staff of the WMH Data Collection and Data Analysis Coordination centers for assistance with instrumentation, fieldwork, and consultation on data analysis. These activities were supported by the National Institute of Mental Health (R01 MH070884), the John D. and Catherine T. MacArthur Foundation, the Pfizer Foundation, the U.S. Public Health Service (R13-MH066849, R01-MH069864, and R01 DA016558), the Fogarty International Center (FIRCA R03-TW006481), the Pan American Health Organization, Eli Lilly and Company Foundation, Ortho-McNeil Pharmaceutical, GlaxoSmithKline, and Bristol-Myers Squibb. A complete list of WMH publications can be found at http://www.hcp.med.harvard.edu/wmh/.

Portions of this chapter are based on two previously published articles: Levinson, D., Zilber, N., Lerner, Y., Grinshpoon, A., Levav, I. (2007). Prevalence of Mood and Anxiety Disorders in the Community: Results from the Israel National Health Survey. Israel Journal of Psychiatry, 44(2), 94–103; and Levinson, D., Lerner, Y., Zilber, N., Grinshpoon, A., Levav, I. (2007). Twelve-month Service Utilization Rates for Mental Health Reasons: Data from the Israel National Health Survey. Israel Journal of Psychiatry, 44(2), 114–125.

# I. INTRODUCTION

Israel is a multiethnic society. In January 2006, the Israeli population was estimated at about 7,000,000 people, of whom 76% were Jews and 24% non-Jews. Of the latter, the majority are Muslim Arabs (1,090,000), Christian Arabs (116,500), and Druze (111,900) (estimates are from 2004). The two official languages are Hebrew and Arabic.

The citizens of Israel are relatively young: 29% of the population is younger than the age of 15 and only 10% are older than the age of 64. The population density is among the highest in the West, with 288 people per square kilometer.

Immigration has played a critical role in the demography of the Israeli-Jewish sector. In the early years of the state, about three-quarters of the population comprised Jewish immigrants. They came mainly from Europe, many of them survivors of the Holocaust, and from Arab countries, many of them refugees. Immigration continued ever since, with two major waves from the Soviet Union, one during the 1970s and another one with almost 1 million new immigrants during the years 1990–2000.

## 1.1. Health Care in Israel

Health care in Israel is a publicly administered and financed system of managed care. Most curative care is delivered through four nonprofit health maintenance organizations (HMOs), which operate like the HMOs in the United States, in their own facilities or through contracted providers. On January 1, 1995, the National Health Insurance (NHI) Law came into effect, mandating compulsory health insurance for all Israeli permanent residents in an HMO of their choice. The law forbids making enrollment conditional on anything and also forbids HMOs from engaging in favorable selection of members. Each adult resident pays a health tax of 4.8% of monthly income. Revenues from the health tax, combined with direct government contributions, are distributed by the National Insurance Institute to the HMOs according to a risk-adjusted capitation formula. The law stipulates the bene-

fits package that HMOs are obliged to provide to their members. HMOs are also allowed to offer supplemental coverage of services not included in the basic basket mandated by law. Private insurers may also offer policies that cover both basic and additional services. The costs of most psychotropic medications are included in the basic basket of services. In 2003, the national expenditure on health care was about 8.5% of Israel's gross domestic product (Ministry of Health & Health Economics and Insurance Division 2006). Under the NHI law, all health services were transferred in 1995 from the government to the HMOs except for preventive, mental health, and geriatric care. Of the three, mental health is the more likely to be transferred to the HMOs in the near future.

## 1.2. Mental Health Care

Mental health care is delivered through a public system of psychiatric inpatient facilities (psychiatric hospitals or psychiatric departments in general hospitals), outpatient facilities (community mental health centers, outpatient clinics in hospitals), and rehabilitation services (housing, vocational rehabilitation, supported education, social and leisure-time activity, and more). The latter are granted by the Mentally Disabled Act of 2000.

In 2003, there were 5489 psychiatric beds in Israel, equivalent to 0.8 per 1000 persons (1.14 per 1000 aged 15 and older) (Ministry of Health, Mental Health Services & Department of Information and Evaluation 2004). Government policy aims to substantially reduce inpatient beds to a rate of 0.5 per 1000 persons and expand outpatient services. In 2004, the mental health budget was 6.2% of the total health budget (Ministry of Health et al. 2004).

The government mental health outpatient services operate as walk-in clinics and are provided free of charge to all residents. Individuals requesting service are screened by professionals who determine the urgency of each case. Waiting lists are common, as there is a shortage of human resources. Other public health agents, such as HMOs and government hospitals, provide mental health services for a subsidized fee. The professional staff in the community mental health centers includes licensed specialists in the field of mental health: psychiatrists, nurses, psychologists, social workers, and occupational therapists. Psychotherapy or any other type of mental health therapy is offered also by professionals who operate privately for a fee.

Outside the mental health sector, general primary care is highly accessible and is fully paid by the HMOs. Primary care doctors are trained during their residency to diagnose and treat common mental disorders. In a survey of primary care physicians (Rabinowitz et al. 1998), more than half reported treating depression by themselves, without making a referral to a specialist.

## 1.3. Mental Health Epidemiological Studies in Israel

This national health survey is the first general population study designed to estimate the prevalence of common mental disorders in Israel and of the use of health and other services by adults affected by mental problems. Surveys on both of these subjects were, until now, limited to population subgroups, to measures of nonspecific distress or to treated populations (Lerner 1992). There were two exceptions, but both provided only partial results.

The first of these two was an epidemiological study of mental disorders carried out during the 1980s (Dohrenwend et al. 1992; Levav et al. 1993) on a ten-year cohort based on a two-stage procedure. During the course of the study, 4914 Israel-born offspring of selected Jewish immigrants were examined. The respondents were screened with the Psychiatric Epidemiology Research Interview (PERI) (Dohrenwend et al. 1980), and all those screened positive along with a proportion of the screened negatives were interviewed by psychiatrists using a semistructured research diagnostic interview, a modified version of the SADS-L (Endicott & Spitzer 1978). The diagnoses included schizophrenia, major depression, antisocial personality, and substance abuse, among other disorders.

This study found a six-month prevalence rate of 27.9% of any disorder studied. The most

common disorder was generalized anxiety disorder (GAD) (6.6%), followed by phobic disorders (4.2%) and major depression (4.2%). Alcohol and drug abuse disorders were relatively rare (0.8% and 1.3%, respectively). Schizophrenia was found to have a prevalence of 0.7%. A main focus of the study was on the adjudication between two competing interpretations of the well-known inverse association between social class and mental illness. The findings of this survey, which compared this association separately among more and less socially advantaged ethnic segments of society, were used to argue for the greater importance of social selection (i.e., genetic and/or biological factors) than social causation factors in accounting for the inverse association of social class with schizophrenia, whereas social causation was argued to be more important in accounting for the inverse associations of social class with major depression among women and within antisocial personality and substance abuse disorders among men.

The second study was a national survey of mental health services, which was carried out during the last week of May 1986 among all inpatients and outpatients who were then cared for in public mental health facilities. The outpatient point prevalence rates of treated cases were then compared with those of a survey carried out in New York City using the same methodology. The rates per 1000 in New York City were higher both for males (5.7 vs. 3.8) and for females (6.0 vs. 3.8). The authors hypothesized that this pattern reflected the fact that stigma against the use of mental health services in Israel was higher than in New York City (Siegel et al. 1993). That same survey also showed that service use was positively related to being female or divorced or single and negatively related to being Arab or of older age (Feinson, Popper & Handelsman 1992).

Further analysis of that survey data using Laska's approach (Laska, Meisner & Siegel 1988) showed that about 2% of the population used specialized mental health services during one year and that about one-third of the users in each year belonged to the "severe mental illness" group (Levinson et al. 1996; Feinson et al. 1997). These results led to the conclusion that in Israel, as in other Western countries (Bebbington et al.

2000; Kohn et al. 2004; Kessler et al. 2005), most people with common mental health problems, such as anxiety or mood disorders, do not receive professional help from the public specialty services.

As noted previously, the Israel WMH survey is the first general population survey designed to estimate the prevalence of common mental disorders and substance abuse and to estimate the size of the population using any type of health, social, or other traditional service for the treatment of emotional or mental problems. Both estimates are of major importance, especially because of the pending inclusion of mental health services in the mandatory basket of services provided to all by the HMOs (Haver et al. 2005).

Although extrapolations from previous or foreign studies are feasible, the adult population of Israel differs from populations in most other countries with comparable populations by the relatively frequent exposure to wars and terror (Somer & Bleich 2005), the experience of dislocation or immigration (Lerner, Kertes & Zilber 2005), and the legacy of the Holocaust (Levav 1998). All these factors were assumed to increase the level of stress in daily life, which presumably manifests itself in an increased likelihood of mental health problems (World Health Organization 2001; Danieli, Brom & Sills 2005).

Joining the World Mental Health (WMH) Survey Initiative was the best strategy to obtain the needed national estimates using advanced psychiatric epidemiological methods (Kessler et al. 2006) and to check whether and to what extent Israel differs from other countries in view of the noted factors. This chapter presents descriptive data from the Israel WMH survey regarding the lifetime and 12-month prevalence rates of mood and anxiety disorders and the 12-month prevalence of service use. The discussion provides the main implications of the results with reference to service provision in Israel.

## 2. METHODS

### 2.1. Sample

The sample was extracted from the national population register (NPR) and was designed to reflect the distribution of sex, age, and population (Arabs, Immigrants: post-1990 immigrants from the former USSR; Jews and Others: born in Israel, pre-1990 immigrants or post-1990 immigrants from countries other than the former USSR) in the noninstitutionalized de jure residents of Israel aged 21 and older. The decision to sample persons aged 21 and older was made because the nonresponse among people aged 18–21 was expected to be very high as a result of the large numbers of that age group participating in the armed services. The interviewed sample was weighted back to the total population to compensate for unequal selection probabilities resulting from disproportionate stratification, clustering effects, and nonresponse. The weights were adjusted to make weighted sample totals conform to known population totals taken from reliable Central Bureau of Statistics (CBS) sources.

Face-to-face interviews were conducted in the homes of respondents from May 2003 through April 2004 in Arabic, Hebrew, and Russian. The survey was administered using laptop computer-assisted personal interview (CAPI) methods by professional survey interviewers trained and supervised by the CBS. A letter signed by the government statistician explaining the purpose of the survey and the rights of respondents was sent to each potential respondent a few days prior to the first contact attempt. Upon making in-person contact with the sampled respondent, the interviewer explained the survey again and obtained verbal informed consent.

Interviews took on average 60 minutes. The overall response rate was 73%: 88% among Arab-Israelis and 71% among Jewish-Israelis, totaling 4859 completed interviews. Sampling was done without replacements. A human subjects committee approved the study.

### 2.2. Measures

#### 2.2.1. Sociodemographic Characteristics

A standard questionnaire on sociodemographic variables (e.g., age, sex, employment status, education, income) was administered to all respondents.

## 2.2.2. Diagnostic Assessment

The diagnostic instrument used in the survey was the special version of the WHO Composite International Diagnostic interview (CIDI) that was developed for the WMH surveys (Kessler & Üstün 2004). The CIDI is a fully structured diagnostic instrument that assesses lifetime and recent prevalence of disorders according to both the ICD-10 and the DSM-IV psychiatric classification systems. DSM-IV criteria were used to generate the results reported herein.

The following disorders were assessed in the Israel WMH survey: anxiety disorders (panic disorder, generalized anxiety disorder, agoraphobia without panic disorder, and posttraumatic stress disorder [PTSD]); mood disorders (major depressive disorder, dysthymia, bipolar I and II disorders), and substance abuse disorders (which are not reported in this chapter). Note that anxiety disorders in this survey did not include the prevalent disorders of specific phobia or social phobia. Nor did we include an assessment of the impulse-control disorders that were included in the vast majority of other WMH surveys. Organic exclusion criteria were taken into account in the evaluation of the DSM-IV diagnoses. Lifetime and 12-month prevalence were assessed and age of onset was determined from retrospective reports.

## 2.2.3. Severity of Diagnosis

Respondents who had any mood or anxiety disorder (AMAD) in the past 12 months were grouped according to three levels of severity: Respondents were defined as having "severe" cases if they had either bipolar I disorder or substance dependence with a physiological dependence syndrome or admitted a suicide attempt in the past 12 months or reported at least two areas of role functioning with severe role impairment due to a mental disorder in the disorder-specific Sheehan Disability Scales (SDS) (Sheehan 1983) The SDS assessed disability in work-role performance, household maintenance, social life, and intimate relationships on 0–10 visual analogue scales with verbal descriptors and associated scale

scores of none, 0; mild, 1–3; moderate, 4–6; severe, 7–9; and very severe, 10. Other respondents were defined as having "moderate" cases of disorders if the interference due to a mental disorder was at least moderate or if they had substance dependence without physiological signs. All other respondents were classified as having "mild" cases of the disorders.

## 2.2.4. Consultation with Health Services

Respondents were asked whether they had visited any one of a list of professionals to talk about problems related to their mental or emotional health. The professionals included those in specialized mental health services (psychologists, psychiatrists, social workers), general medical professionals (e.g., general practitioners [GPs]), religious counselors (rabbis, sheikhs), and other healers (e.g., naturopathic practitioners). The questionnaire asked about consultation in the past 12 months and consultation "ever" in life, type of organization providing the service and number of visits per year, and satisfaction with services.

One of the main objectives of the present study was to determine the extent to which mental health professionals are consulted by those who need them most. This question assumes a clear hierarchy of expertise among the types of services used by the persons with a mental health disorder, with mental health services at the top. Any visit to a professional mental health worker likely implies awareness of a psychiatric problem by the user (e.g., a family member or a referring agent) as well as knowledge of the existence and the specific purpose of the mental health services.

A visit to general health or other types of services rather than mental health services for emotional and/or mental problems might indicate a lesser awareness of the psychiatric problem; a lesser willingness to get help from mental health professionals, possibly because of fear of stigma; or lack of access to mental health services or no referral by the GP to professional mental health services. Thus, the types of services used were divided into the following categories.

The first category consisted of specialty mental health treatment, which included: (1) consultation with a mental health professional in a public medical setting (e.g., mental health government clinic, HMO mental health clinic, or psychiatric hospital emergency department); (2) consultation with a mental health professional in the private clinic of a mental health professional; (3) consultation with a mental health professional in workplaces, welfare services, or other settings outside of the medical system.

The second category consisted of treatment in the general medical sector, including treatment for an emotional problem or substance problem by a GP or other doctor or other health professional who was not a mental health professional. The third category consisted of consultation with a religious leader or other traditional healer.

In a separate section of the interview, all respondents were asked whether they used "any type of prescription medicine in the past 12 months for problems with emotions, substance use, energy, concentration, sleep, or ability to cope with stress" and were instructed to report any medicines of this sort that they had used (even if they had used them only once) from a list of psychotropic medications presented to them. For each medicine mentioned, respondents were asked about the length of the period they took it and the dosage. For three medicines (randomly chosen from all medicines used by the respondent if given respondent used more than three), further treatment details were asked.

To remove respondents with primarily sleep problems, all those with the following characteristics were excluded: taking sedatives exclusively, having sleep problems (sleep information was obtained from another section of the interview), aged 65 or older, and not having any mood or anxiety disorder in the past 12 months. Note that having a CIDI diagnosis was not required in any of the "type of service" groups.

## 2.3. Categories of Impairment

As noted previously, the truncated version of the CIDI used in the Israel WMH survey did not assess phobic disorders, impulse-control disorders, schizophrenia, or other nonaffective psychotic disorders. Therefore, it was necessary to find a marker for those who did not meet criteria for any of the disorders assessed in the survey (i.e., mood and anxiety disorders) but who were nevertheless legitimate users of mental health services. It was decided to use responses to a question about employment limitations due to health (physical and/or mental) as a marker for those who might have had mental health problems not classified as an anxiety or mood disorder. This chapter reports, therefore, on two groups of subjects with impairment: those with mood or anxiety disorders and those who were not classified as having mood or anxiety disorder but who reported health-related (mental and/or physical) employment limitations.

## 2.4. Employment Limitations

All respondents were asked about their present and past employment: the length of time they were employed, the type of work they did, and if relevant, reasons for less-than-full employment. In that section of the survey, respondents were asked about physical or emotional limitations on employment, and whether they were out of the workforce, temporarily unemployed, or fully employed. On the basis of responses to these questions ("What was the main reason you were not working and also not looking for a job?" "Do you have any problems with your physical or emotional health that would prevent you from working for pay if you wanted to?" "Are you limited in the kind or amount of work you can do because of any problem with your physical or emotional health?"), the variable of employment limitations was created. This variable had four categories: (1) limitations due to physical health problems, (2) limitations due to mental health problems, (3) limitations due to physical and mental health problems, (4) no health limitations with regard to employment. Categories 2 and 3 were later combined to one "having limitation due to physical and mental health problems." Note that all those who stated that they did not work or were not looking for work because they had retired, were of old age, were homemakers, or because of any reason other than health were classified as having "no limitation due to physical or mental health problems."

## 2.5. Statistical Analysis

The data were weighted to adjust for differential probabilities of selection and nonresponse, and for the differences between the sample and the Israeli adult population. Prevalence estimates were calculated and are expressed as percentages with standard errors. Survival analysis was used to make estimated projections of cumulative lifetime probability of disorders and treatment contact from year of onset using the actuarial method (Halli & Rao 1992) implemented in SAS V8.2 (SAS Institute 2001). Discrete-time survival analysis (Efron 1988) with person-year as the unit of analysis was used to examine correlates of disorders and treatment contact. Models of lifetime treatment contact for particular disorders were estimated using survival analysis to estimate the typical time interval between age of onset and first contact with the treatment system for that disorder. Basic predictors of 12-month service use were examined with logistic regression analysis (Hosmer & Lemeshow 1989). Standard errors were estimated using the Taylor series method as implemented in SUDAAN (Research Triangle Institute 2002). Multivariate significance tests were made using Wald $\chi^2$ tests based on coefficient variance-covariance matrices that were adjusted for design effects using the Taylor series method. Statistical significance was evaluated using two-sided design-based tests and the 0.05 level of significance.

## 3. RESULTS

### 3.1. Sociodemographic Characteristics

The characteristics of the study sample in comparison to the general population are shown in Table 16.1. About half the respondents were younger than 50, and 35% were younger than 35. Of the sample, 13% consisted of Arab-Israelis and the rest were Jewish-Israelis and others. About 65% of the sample was married or living with

someone, and 19% had never been married. The educational level of 22% of the sample had incomplete secondary education, and 25% of the sample had completed college. At the time of the survey, 43% of the sample was working and 37% was out of the civilian workforce.

Differences in the sociodemographic composition of the sample and the general population are small and, especially in the education and employment distributions, can be explained by the fact that the general population data summarizes those aged 15 and older and therefore has lower rates of both workers and uneducated older persons.

### 3.2. Prevalence of Mood and Anxiety Disorders

Table 16.2 shows that almost one in five respondents (17.6%) reported a lifetime presence of AMAD, and nearly one in ten (9.7%) adults, or about 390,000 individuals, reported AMAD in the previous 12 months. Mood disorders were more than twice as common as anxiety disorders. A lifetime history of mood disorders was found in 10.7% of respondents, whereas only 5.2% had any anxiety disorder. In the 12 months prior to the interview, the figures were 6.4% for any mood disorder and 3.2% for any anxiety. Major depression was the most prevalent disorder (9.8% lifetime prevalence rate); next was generalized anxiety disorder (GAD) with 2.7%. Only 1.5% of the population passed the threshold for posttraumatic stress disorder (PTSD) in their lifetime and only 0.5% experienced it in the year prior to the survey.

Among all respondents with a disorder in the past 12 months, 37.5% were classified as severe, 34.3% as moderate, and 28.1% as mild. The distribution within each of the disorders, however, shows that in five of seven specific disorders, about 50% or more of the respondents were classified as severe cases. Those with bipolar disorders were all classified as severe cases as a result of the specific definition used (see Section 2). PTSD had the second greatest proportion of serious cases (70%), followed by dysthymia (53.7%), panic (52.8%), and agoraphobia without panic (49.7%). Respondents with

**Table 16.1.** Sociodemographic distribution of the IMHS sample compared to the Israeli population

| | IMHS unweighted | | IMHS weighted | | Israel population (*) | |
|---|---|---|---|---|---|---|
| | *n* | % | *n* | % | *n* | % |
| Gender[a] | | | | | | |
| Male | 2380 | 49 | 1,904,227 | 48 | 2,080,600 | 48 |
| Female | 2479 | 51 | 2,051,268 | 52 | 2,228,800 | 52 |
| Age[a] | | | | | | |
| >35 | 1585 | 33 | 1,382,896 | 35 | 1,585,500 | 37 |
| 35–49 | 1317 | 27 | 1,099,338 | 28 | 1,166,350 | 27 |
| 50–64 | 1080 | 22 | 848,732 | 21 | 881,750 | 20 |
| 65+ | 877 | 18 | 624,529 | 16 | 675,800 | 16 |
| Population group[a] | | | | | | |
| Jews and others | 4200 | 86 | 3,450,883 | 87 | 3,655,300 | 85 |
| Arabs | 659 | 14 | 504,612 | 13 | 654,100 | 15 |
| Family status[b] | | | | | | |
| Married/cohabiting | 3229 | 66 | 2,683,338 | 68 | 2,731,600 | 65 |
| Separated/widowed/divorced | 730 | 15 | 530,836 | 13 | 596,400 | 14 |
| Never married | 900 | 19 | 741,321 | 19 | 898,400 | 21 |
| Education[c] | | | | | | |
| None, some primary or secondary | 1068 | 22 | 857,141 | 22 | 1,225,620 | 18 |
| Complete secondary | 1728 | 36 | 1,458,883 | 37 | 2,859,780 | 42 |
| Postsecondary | 800 | 16 | 640,598 | 16 | 953,260 | 14 |
| Complete college | 1263 | 26 | 998,873 | 25 | 1,770,340 | 26 |
| Employment status[c] | | | | | | |
| Worked full-time | 2211 | 46 | 1,702,313 | 43 | 1,541,300 | 32 |
| Worked part-time | 472 | 10 | 372,808 | 9 | 703,500 | 14 |
| Temporarily absent from work | 174 | 4 | 144,691 | 4 | 156,100 | 3 |
| Worked in the past 12 months | 141 | 3 | 123,039 | 3 | 114,300 | 2 |
| Did not work in the past 12 months | 157 | 3 | 132,306 | 3 | 163,500 | 3 |
| Not in civilian workforce | 1704 | 35 | 1,480,338 | 37 | 2,197,500 | 45 |

(*) *Statistical Abstract of Israel 2005-No.56*, available at http://www1.cbs.gov.il/reader/shnatonenew_site.htm.
Including institutional population and Arab population of East Jerusalem.

[a] Average 2004, table 2-10 for age 20 and above.

[b] Average 2003, table 2-19 for age 20 and above.

[c] Average 2004, table 8-5 and table 12-01 for age 15 and above. Available at http://www1.cbs.gov.il/reader/shnaton/shnatone_new.htm?CYear=2005&Vol=56&CSubject=30.

major depression were almost equally divided into severe (41.1%) and moderate (43.1%) cases, and the rest were mild cases. In the case of GAD, 32.7% of the cases were severe, about 40% moderate, and about 25% mild.

More than 70% of those with AMAD in their lifetime or in the past 12 months (more than 80%) had only one diagnosis. Another 14% had two disorders and only 3.6% had three diagnoses or more. Severity was related to comorbidity. Of those with one diagnosis, only 32% were classi-

fied as severe, compared to 54.8% among those with two diagnoses and 84% among those with three or more diagnoses.

### 3.3. Age of Onset

The distributions of cumulative lifetime risk estimates were standardized and examined for fixed percentiles. One-quarter of those with AMAD had their first episode of the disorder before the age of 25. The median age of onset was 35, and

**Table 16.2.** Lifetime and 12-month prevalence rates and severity of DSM-IV/CIDI disorders

| | Lifetime prevalence | | | 12 months | | | | | | | | |
| | | | | Prevalence | | | Distribution of cases by severity | | | | | |
| | | | | | | | Mild | | Moderate | | Severe | |
| Diagnosis | n | % | (se) | n | % | (se) | % | (se) | % | (se) | % | (se) |
|---|---|---|---|---|---|---|---|---|---|---|---|---|
| Dysthymia | 46 | 0.9 | (0.1) | 30 | 0.6 | (0.1) | 12.6 | (6.4) | 33.7 | (8.8) | 53.7 | (9.5) |
| Major depressive disorder | 484 | 9.8 | (0.5) | 280 | 5.9 | (0.4) | 15.8 | (2.2) | 43.1 | (3.1) | 41.1 | (3.1) |
| Bipolar disorder | 32 | 0.7 | (0.1) | 22 | 0.5 | (0.1) | 0.0 | (0.0) | 0.0 | (0.0) | 100.0 | (0.0) |
| Any mood disorder | 524 | 10.7 | (0.5) | 303 | 6.4 | (0.4) | 14.5 | (2.1) | 39.4 | (3.0) | 46.1 | (3.1) |
| Panic disorder | 46 | 0.9 | (0.1) | 30 | 0.6 | (0.1) | 24.6 | (7.9) | 22.6 | (8.4) | 52.8 | (9.4) |
| Generalized anxiety disorder | 136 | 2.7 | (0.2) | 86 | 1.8 | (0.2) | 26.0 | (4.8) | 41.3 | (5.4) | 32.7 | (5.2) |
| Agoraphobia without panic | 27 | 0.6 | (0.1) | 17 | 0.4 | (0.1) | 15.0 | (8.8) | 35.3 | (11.9) | 49.7 | (12.6) |
| Posttraumatic stress disorder | 67 | 1.5 | (0.2) | 23 | 0.5 | (0.1) | 14.7 | (7.1) | 15.3 | (7.2) | 70.1 | (9.3) |
| Any anxiety disorder | 252 | 5.2 | (0.3) | 152 | 3.2 | (0.3) | 23.3 | (3.5) | 33.2 | (3.9) | 43.6 | (4.1) |
| AMAD(*) | 860 | 17.6 | (0.6) | 464 | 9.7 | (0.4) | 28.1 | (2.1) | 34.3 | (2.3) | 37.5 | (2.4) |

* Includes substance abuse disorders, which are not presented here.

by the age of 53, 75% of those with AMAD had already had their first episode of the disorder. For most (90%) of the individuals with AMAD, the first time they experienced the disorder happened before the age of 66. Disorders with the highest rate of severe cases (Table 16.2), namely PTSD and bipolar disorders, were among those with the earliest average age of onset. By the age of 46 to 48, the disorder was already present in 75% of all lifetime cases of bipolar or PTSD. The number of years between the 25th and 75th percentiles of the age of onset distributions was the highest for major depression (36 years) and the lowest for PTSD or GAD (23–25 years).

### 3.4. Projected Lifetime Risk

The lifetime risk estimates provide an indication of the proportion of the population expected to develop the disorders over the average life expectancy of the population. Compared with the lifetime prevalence rates presented in Table 16.2, the projected lifetime risk as of age 75 for the various disorders was almost 100% higher for all disorders. This result is another expression of the fact that the median onset of most disorders in Israel is in the 35–45 age group and that the adult population is relatively young, with 50% under the age of 50.

### 3.5. Use of Services

Overall, 20% of the total population reported that they had consulted a health professional or a traditional healer for their mental health problems at some point in their life, and 7.5% had done so in the previous 12 months. About 8% of the sample had used psychotropic medication under medical supervision during the past 12 months for problems with their "emotions, substance use, energy, concentration, sleep, or ability to cope with stress." In most cases, those who were prescribed psychotropic medications also reported consultation regarding "mental or emotional health" and are included in Table 16.3 under the service they had used.

There were, however, another 2.8% of the general adult population that was prescribed psychotropic medications for problems with their emotions and/or mental health but that apparently did not consider this type of visit as "consultation regarding emotions/mental health" and therefore skipped the main mental health services questionnaire. We nevertheless included them in Table 16.3 under "Consult general health professionals – psychotropic medication only," assuming (as shown in Table 16.5) that they either visited the doctor because of somatic reasons and minimized the importance of the underlying

**Table 16.3.** Use of professional and traditional services by types of users: Rates per 100 (se) and distribution of services

| | | 12 months | | | | | | | | | | Lifetime |
| | | Consult mental health professional | | | | Consult general health professionals | | | | | | |
| Diagnosis | n | Public clinic<br>% (se) | Private practice<br>% (se) | Non-health sector<br>% (se) | Total<br>% (se) | Doctor/other health prof.<br>% (se) | Psychotr. med. only<br>% (se) | Total<br>% (se) | Consult any prof. health services<br>% (se) | Consult religious/spiritual/alternat.<br>% (se) | Consult any prof.<br>% (se) | Consult any profess. (*)<br>% (se) |
|---|---|---|---|---|---|---|---|---|---|---|---|---|
| TOTAL | 4859 | 2.0 (0.2)<br>19% | 2.1 (0.2)<br>20% | 0.5 (0.1)<br>5% | 4.6 (0.3)<br>45% | 1.6 (0.2)<br>16% | 2.8 (0.2)<br>27% | 4.4 (0.3)<br>43% | 9.0 (0.4)<br>87% | 1.3 (0.2)<br>13% | 10.3 (0.4)<br>100% | 20 (0.6) |
| AMAD | 470 | 9.1 (1.4)<br>27% | 7.4 (1.3)<br>22% | 1.9 (0.6)<br>6% | 18.6 (1.9)<br>55% | 5.9 (1.3)<br>17% | 5.5 (1.0)<br>16% | 11.4 (1.6)<br>33% | 30.1 (2.2)<br>88% | 4.0 (0.9)<br>12% | 34.1 (2.3)<br>100% | 48 (2.4) |
| Serious | 168 | 13.5 (2.7)<br>28% | 9.4 (2.3)<br>19% | 2.9 (1.3)<br>6% | 26.5 (3.5)<br>54% | 11.8 (2.9)<br>24% | 6.1 (1.8)<br>13% | 17.9 (3.3)<br>37% | 44.4 (4.1)<br>91% | 4.4 (1.7)<br>9% | 48.8 (4.1)<br>100% | 57 (4.1) |
| Moderate | 166 | 8.5 (2.2)<br>25% | 8.3 (2.3)<br>25% | 1.8 (1.0)<br>5% | 18.6 (3.2)<br>56% | 3.4 (1.5)<br>10% | 5.1 (1.6)<br>15% | 8.5 (2.2)<br>25% | 27.1 (3.6)<br>81% | 6.4 (1.9)<br>19% | 33.5 (3.7)<br>100% | 45 (4.0) |
| Mild | 136 | 3.9 (1.7)<br>26% | 3.5 (1.7)<br>23% | 0.6 (0.6)<br>4% | 8.0 (2.5)<br>53% | 1.1 (0.8)<br>7% | 5.3 (1.9)<br>35% | 6.4 (2.0)<br>43% | 14.4 (3.1)<br>96% | 0.6 (0.6)<br>4% | 15.0 (3.1)<br>100% | 40 (4.4) |
| No AMAD | 4389 | 1.2 (0.2)<br>16% | 1.5 (0.2)<br>19% | 0.3 (0.0)<br>4% | 3.1 (0.3)<br>40% | 1.2 (0.2)<br>16% | 2.5 (0.2)<br>32% | 3.6 (0.3)<br>47% | 6.7 (0.4)<br>87% | 1.0 (0.2)<br>13% | 7.7 (0.4)<br>100% | 17 (0.6) |

* Excluding "psychotropic medication only" type of service.

emotional problems the doctor disclosed or presented themselves to the doctor with somatic symptoms because they believed that reporting somatic symptoms is a more appropriate route for seeking help from a primary care physician (Simon et al. 1999). In both cases, the patients did not think that they "talk about mental/emotional problems" even though they knew that they take medication purported to alleviate such problems. Thus, a total of 10.3% of the population had received some form of treatment for mental or emotional problems in the previous 12 months.

Table 16.3 shows the consultation rates for the entire population and for different groups of AMAD users. Overall, 4.6% of the general population consulted a mental health professional, another 4.4% visited general or other physicians, and 1.3% visited only traditional healers. About half of those consulting mental health professionals attended public mental health clinics (2%), and the other half met with therapists in private settings. A small minority (0.5%) discussed their problems with professionals in other social, nonhealth services.

Respondents with AMAD had, as expected, much higher consultation rates. Almost half (48%) had ever talked about their problem. In the past 12 months, 34.1% had done so: 18.6% had consulted mental health professionals, almost equally distributed between public (9.1%) and private (7.4%) settings, and another 1.9% had done so in nonhealth public settings. More than 10% of those with AMAD went to primary care or other physicians to consult or get medication, and 4% saw traditional healers only.

Altogether, 34.1% of those with AMAD received any type of treatment. For 22.8% of respondents with AMAD the treatment included psychotropic medication (not shown in the table).

## 3.6. Consultation Rates by Severity Levels of Impairment

Consultation rates and use of psychotropic medication were clearly related to the severity level of the impairment. Among more severe cases, 48.8% had some type of consultation in the past 12 months, and 32% had used psychotropic medication. Individuals with moderate or mild cases of AMAD had lower rates of consultation (33.5% and 15.0%, respectively) and lower rates of psychotropic drug use (21% and 13%, respectively). Among those who had sought any type of mental health treatment, there were very few differences in the preferred type of treatment. The highest proportion of consultation by respondents with all severity levels of impairment was with mental health professionals (53%–56%), with a slight preference for those in public settings (25%–28%).

The three severity groups differed in their use of general health services. The more severe cases used consultation with primary care doctors proportionally more than the less severe (moderate or mild) cases (24%, 10%, and 7%, respectively) and used the psychotropic medication much less than the mild group (13% compared with 35%) Those with moderate level of severity used the traditional healers proportionally more than the other groups (19%, 9%, and 4%)

## 3.7. Consultation Rates by Employment Limitations

Table 16.4 presents the consultation rates of respondents who did not have any anxiety or mood disorders in the past 12 months but admitted having employment limitations due to physical or mental reasons. Consultation patterns were related to the reason for the employment limitation. About half (47%) of those with "mental health" or both "physical and mental health" employment limitations had some type of consultation in their life compared to those with only physical limitation, who had consultation rates and patterns similar to or lower than the entire population (21%).

Altogether, 32.6% of respondents with some mental limitation had received some type of treatment in the 12 months prior to the interview, and 31% reported using psychotropic drugs. Most of those with some mental health–related

**Table 16.4.** Use of professional and traditional services by types of users: Rates per 100 and distribution of services

| Diagnosis | n | Consult mental health professional | | | | Consult general health professionals | | | | Consult any prof. health services % (se) | Consult religious/ spiritual/ alternat. % (se) | Consult any prof. % (se) | Lifetime Consult any profess. (*) % (se) |
| | | Public clinic % (se) | Private practice % (se) | Non– health sector % (se) | Total % (se) | Doctor/ other health prof. % (se) | Psychotr. med. only % (se) | Total % (se) | | | | |
|---|---|---|---|---|---|---|---|---|---|---|---|---|
| Total | 4859 | 2.0 (0.2) 19% | 2.1 (0.2) 20% | 0.5 (0.1) 5% | 4.6 (0.3) 45% | 1.6 (0.2) 16% | 2.8 (0.2) 27% | 4.4 (0.3) 43% | 9 (0.4) 87% | 1.3 (0.2) 13% | 10.3 (0.4) 100% | 20 (0.6 ) |
| No AMAD | | | | | | | | | | | | |
| Physical limitation | 542 | 1.3 (0.5) 12% | 0.8 (0.4) 7% | 0.2 (0.2) 2% | 2.3 (0.7) 21% | 3.1 (0.8) 29% | 4.1 (0.9) 38% | 7.2 (1.1) 67% | 9.5 (1.3) 89% | 1.2 (0.4) 11% | 10.7 (1.4) 100% | 21 (1.9) |
| Physical & mental limitation | 78 | 20.0 (4.7) 62% | 2.2 (1.5) 6% | – – | 22.3 (4.8) 68% | 4.0 (2.3) 12% | 5.2 (2.6) 16% | 9.2 (3.4) 28% | 31.5 (5.4) 97% | 1.1 (1.1) – | 32.6 (5.4) 100% | 47 (5.9) |

*Excluding "psychotropic medication only" type of service.

357

employment limitation (68%) had consulted with mental health specialists: 62% in public and 6% in private settings. Another 28% (12% and 16%) talked to doctors or had been prescribed psychotropic medication for their conditions.

In summary, the highest proportion of respondents in treatment was found among individuals with severe AMAD. Next was the group of individuals with a moderate severity level of AMAD and the group with no AMAD but that had employment limitations due to "mental or physical" reasons. The highest proportion of psychotropic medication use, without considering it consultation, was among respondents with mild cases of disorders and among those with physical health–related employment limitations. The use of public versus private mental health services differentiated between the severe cases of CIDI/DSM-IV mood or anxiety disorders and those with mental employment limitation. Of those with mental employment limitations, 62% used the public system versus only 28% of those with severe cases of AMAD.

Survival curves were used to project the proportion of cases that would eventually make treatment contact for each disorder assessed in the survey. These survival curves were used to estimate the proportion of persons who made treatment contact in the first year of onset of the disorder, within the first five years, and the median delay among those who eventually made treatment contact after the year of first onset.

The proportion of respondents who made treatment contact within the year of onset of the disorder ranged between 30% and 40% for any mood or anxiety disorders, yet was clearly higher in panic and bipolar disorders, where 57% and 50%, respectively, made treatment contact within the first year of onset. Within the first five years after onset, 50% to 60% of respondents made treatment contact for their disorder.

Apart from panic and bipolar disorders, the median duration of delay for anxiety disorders was three years and six years for mood disorders. That is, 50% of cases of with mood disorders would not seek treatment within the first six years after the first onset of the disorder. Com-

parison of the median duration to the proportion making treatment contact within the first year showed that unless the treatment contact was made within the first year, the likelihood of treatment diminishes steadily.

### 3.8. Type of Services: Rates of Usage

Table 16.5 shows, for each type of services, the proportion used by AMAD respondents and by those with mental and/or physical health–related employment limitations but not AMAD. In general, of those approaching any professional or traditional healers to talk about emotional or mental problems in the past year, more than half (51%) had neither AMAD nor health-related employment limitations. This proportion was smaller only in mental health public clinics (32%) and among those contacting GPs (39%). Among respondents taking psychotropic medications without a self-defined mental health consultation, the proportion of those with no AMAD or some health-related employment limitations was 61%.

### 3.9. Number of Visits in the Past 12 Months

Table 16.6 presents the number of visits made by those who reported talking to professionals about mental health problems in the past 12 months. The table presents separately the number of visits (means and medians) made by those talking to psychiatrists, psychologists, psychiatric social workers, or other mental health professionals, or to GPs and other nonpsychiatrist doctors. The visits to each type of professional include all those who visited that professional whether or not they had visited other types of professionals as well. The mean number of visits was always higher than the median, indicating a skewed distribution of visits. The smallest difference between the mean and median was in the visits to GPs, where more than 50% of respondents had only one visit. Those talking to psychologists or social workers had the highest number of visits, with a median of 5 visits compared to a median of 2.5 visits to psychiatrists and a median of one visit to

**Table 16.5.** Distribution (%) of users in the different types of services

| | | Consult mental health professional | | | | Consult general health professionals | | | Consult religious/ spiritual/ alternat. | Consult any prof. |
|---|---|---|---|---|---|---|---|---|---|---|
| | | Public clinic | Private practice | Non– health sector | Total | Doctor/ other health prof. | Psychotr. med. only | Total | | |
| N | 4859 | 96 | 102 | 24 | 225 | 76 | 154 | 230 | 60 | 515 |
| % | 100.0 | 100.0 | 100.0 | 100.0 | 100.0 | 100.0 | 100.0 | 100.0 | 100.0 | 100.0 |
| AMAD severity | % (se) | % (se) | % (se) | % (se) | % (se) | % (se) | % (se) | % (se) | % (se) | % (se) |
| Serious | 4 (0.3) | 25 (4.7) | 17 (4.0) | 22 (9.0) | 21 (3.0) | 27 (5.8) | 8 (2.3) | 15 (2.7) | 13 (4.5) | 17 (1.8) |
| Moderate | 3 (0.3) | 14 (3.5) | 14 (3.7) | 12 (7.0) | 14 (2.4) | 7 (3.1) | 6 (1.9) | 7 (1.7) | 17 (4.8) | 11 (1.4) |
| Mild | 3 (0.2) | – | – | – | 5 (1.5) | – | 5 (1.8) | 4 (1.3) | – | 4 (0.9) |
| No AMAD employment limitation | | | | | | | | | | |
| Physical limitation | 11 (0.5) | 7 (2.8) | – | – | 6 (1.7) | 21 (4.8) | 17 (3.3) | 18 (2.7) | 10 (4.0) | 12 (1.5) |
| Physical & mental limitation | 2 (0.2) | 17 (4.1) | – | – | 8 (2.0) | – | – | – | – | 5 (1.1) |
| No AMAD and no employment limitation | 77 (0.6) | 32 (4.6) | 59 (5.1) | 53 (10.6) | 47 (3.4) | 39 (5.8) | 61 (4.1) | 53 (3.4) | 58 (6.5) | 51 (2.3) |

* Unreliable values were omitted.

**Table 16.6.** Number of visits to health professionals in the past 12 months (median and mean)

| Mental disorder | | Psychiatrist | Type of professional | | |
|---|---|---|---|---|---|
| | | | Psychologist/ social worker/ other MH | Any mental health | Doctor/ other health prof. |
| Total | n | 107 | 139 | 215 | 169 |
| | Median | 2.6 | 5.3 | 4.7 | 1.4 |
| | (se) | (0.4) | (1.0) | (0.8) | (0.1) |
| | Mean | 8.3 | 14.3 | 13.6 | 3.0 |
| | (se) | (1.7) | (1.6) | (1.4) | (0.4) |
| AMAD | n | 56 | 47 | 83 | 77 |
| | Median | 2.7 | 5.2 | 4.5 | 1.4 |
| | (se) | (0.6) | (2.0) | (1.2) | (0.1) |
| | Mean | 8.7 | 14.9 | 14.6 | 2.5 |
| | (se) | (2.5) | (2.7) | (2.4) | (0.3) |
| No AMAD | n | 51 | 92 | 133 | 92 |
| | Median | 2.4 | 5.3 | 4.8 | 1.4 |
| | (se) | (0.6) | (1.2) | (0.9) | (0.1) |
| | Mean | 7.8 | 14.0 | 12.9 | 3.4 |
| | (se) | (2.1) | (1.9) | (1.7) | (0.8) |

*Note:* Values are medians with standard errors in parentheses.

the GP. The mean and the median number of visits to all types of professionals did not distinguish between those with or without AMAD.

### 3.10. Sociodemographic Correlates of Mental Disorders

The logistic regression of AMAD and of the level of clinical severity on the sociodemographic variables showed that women were only slightly more likely to have had any mood disorder in the past 12 months but were significantly more likely to have a more severe case of the disorder. Age groups did not predict either the frequency of disorders or the degrees of severity. The lowest income level (the income variable was divided into four categories based on the median per capita income) did not have significantly higher odds for having AMAD disorders but did have significantly higher odds of severe manifestations of them.

Family status was highly related to rates of disorders, particularly mood disorders, and to the severity with which they were expressed. Respondents who were separated, divorced, or widowed were twice as likely to have a disorder and 70% more likely to have severe cases than were those who were married. Respondents with less education had significantly higher odds of AMAD, particularly anxiety disorders, but did not differ from the others in their likelihood of severe manifestations of the disease.

The logistic regression of any use ("talk to any professional") in the past 12 months of health services for mental or emotional problems among individuals with AMAD on the sociodemographic variables showed that use of services was significantly more prevalent among the 35–64 age group but was not related to level of education or income, gender, or marital status.

### 4. DISCUSSION

The main factor urging the initiation of the present survey was the pending inclusion of mental health services in the basket of services provided to all residents by the HMOs. The worry that there are too many potential customers waiting to be admitted into the already-overcrowded public mental health clinics was possibly part of the reason for the ten years of delay in this reform.

The present survey shows that, contrary to expectations stemming from the unique conditions of the Israeli society (massive immigration and protracted Arab–Israeli conflict), the prevalence rates of mood or anxiety disorders in Israel and the annual service use for mental health reasons fall within the range of other Western countries (ESEMeD/MHEDEA 2000 Investigators 2004a; Kessler et al. 2005). However, because of the early age of onset of most disorders, their often-protracted course, and future modifications in the age pyramid, the total burden of mental disorders in forthcoming years might be higher than it is today.

The sociodemographic correlates of the 12-month prevalence rates of mood or anxiety disorders did not show the patterns that are typical of other large-scale cross-sectional surveys in other countries (Fryers, Melzer & Jenkins 2003). Being female (Gold 1998; Patel et al. 1999), middle-aged (Paykel, Brugha & Fryers 2005) or low income (Kessler et al. 1994; Kohn, Dohrenwend & Mirotznik 1998) was not related to higher odds of any mood or anxiety disorders but was related to higher odds of a more severe manifestation of the disorder once it exists. These results possibly reflect an interaction between sociodemographic variables and the three main population groups as defined earlier in Section 2.1. The question of whether the main sociodemographic risk factors for higher rates of common mental health disorders in Israel differ from other countries will have to await a more detailed comparison among the three population groups.

It was also found that about half the users contacted general health rather than mental health professionals: a finding that highlights the importance of family doctors in the provision of mental health care in Israel, as also reported in other countries (ESEMeD/MHEDEA 2000 Investigators 2004b). We do not know, however, why those who chose general health doctors did so or whether the level of care provided by them is adequate.

The survey also showed that there is only a partial overlap between respondents who use the services and those for which the services were intended. About two-thirds of those who used services did not have either a diagnosis of mood or anxiety disorder or some other mental health problem that limits their employment. On the other hand, only about one-third of those diagnosed with the CIDI/DSM-IV diagnosis of mood or anxiety disorders in the past 12 months had used any type of service to alleviate their condition, and they did not differ from the other two-thirds with respect to gender, family status, income level, or education level.

Therapists, in mental health services and primary care, viewed all those approaching the services as equal in their need for care and allocated the same number of visits to AMAD and non-AMAD patients (probably with Axis-2 or subthreshold disorders).

Thus, for service planning, the presence of a full clinical diagnosis cannot be used as the single parameter for estimating need. Therapists do not consider a full clinical diagnosis as the only indicator of need, and by contrast, not all untreated cases of AMAD necessarily represent unmet needs.

Finally, access to services among those with mood or anxiety disorders did not depend on any crude socioeconomic measure, as should have been expected by the fact that the provision of mental health care either by the government or HMO primary-care doctors is essentially free. However, as mentioned previously, only one-third of those with severe cases of AMAD approached any type of service. Further analysis should reveal whether language and/or cultural barriers or regional problems of availability prevent access from these individuals.

Before closing, it is important to recognize that the Israel WMH survey had limitations that should be considered when the results are being evaluated. For one, there might be a selection bias in the sample. Although the response rate was relatively high (72%) and only about 15% of the intended interviewees clearly refused to answer, refusal might be lower among the healthier. The prevalence estimates presented in this chapter and the service use rates should thus be considered conservative. In addition, it is important to bear in mind that the survey focused only on the most common mental health disorders. It did not cover the full spectrum of mental disorders or of subthreshold conditions. Calculation of the burden of mental health in Israel, based on our data, may therefore result in underestimation, even after the inclusion of those limited in their employment as a result of mental health problems.

The Israeli version of CIDI 3.0 was used for the first time in the present survey. For anonymity and economic reasons, a reappraisal study to corroborate diagnoses derived from the CIDI was not performed. In the reappraisal studies done in the United States and Western Europe, there was good individual-level concordance between the CIDI and blinded clinical reappraisal interviews (Haro et al. 2006; see Chapter 6 of this volume). Nonetheless, in the absence of a local study in Israel, confidence in these results depends on the extent to which the Israeli version of the CIDI is comparable to the language versions used in the countries where clinical reappraisal studies were carried out and the extent to which the Israeli respondents answered the CIDI questions with the same degree of care and honesty as those in the countries where the CIDI diagnoses obtained in WMH surveys were evaluated with clinical reappraisal interviews.

## REFERENCES

Bebbington, P. E., Brugha, T. S., Meltzer, H., Jenkins, R., Ceresa, C., Farrell, M. & Lewis, G. (2000). Neurotic disorders and the receipt of psychiatric treatment. *Psychological Medicine*, 30, 1369–76.

Danieli, Y., Brom, D. & Sills, J. (2005). *The trauma of terrorism: Sharing knowledge and shared care, an international handbook*. Binghamton, NY: Maltreatment & Trauma Press.

Dohrenwend, B. P., Levav, I., Shrout, P. E., Schwartz, S., Naveh, G., Link, B. G., Skodol, A. E. & Stueve, A. (1992). Socioeconomic status and psychiatric disorders: The causation-selection issue. *Science*, 255, 946–52.

Dohrenwend, B. P., Shrout, P. E., Egri, G. & Mendelsohn, F. S. (1980). Nonspecific psychological distress and other dimensions of psychopathology: Measures for use in the general population. *Archives of General Psychiatry*, 37, 1229–36.

Efron, B. (1988). Logistic regression, survival analysis and the Kaplan-Meier curve. *Journal of the American Statistical Association*, 83, 414–25.

Endicott, J. & Spitzer, R. L. (1978). A diagnostic interview: The schedule for affective disorders and schizophrenia. *Archives of General Psychiatry*, 35, 837–44.

ESEMeD/MHEDEA 2000 Investigators (2004a). Prevalence of mental disorders in Europe: Results from the European Study of the Epidemiology of Mental Disorders (ESEMeD) project. *Acta Psychiatrica Scandinavica Suppl.*, 420, 21–7.

ESEMeD/MHEDEA 2000 Investigators (2004b). Use of mental health services in Europe: Results from the European Study of the Epidemiology of Mental Disorders (ESEMeD) project. *Acta Psychiatrica Scandinavica Suppl.*, 420, 47–54.

Feinson, M. C., Lerner, Y., Levinson, D. & Popper, M. (1997). Ambulatory mental health treatment under universal coverage: Policy insights from Israel. *Milbank Quarterly*, 75, 235–60.

Feinson, M. C., Popper, M. & Handelsman, M. (1992). *Utilization of public ambulatory mental health services in Israel: A focus on age and gender patterns*. Jerusalem: Mental Health Services, Ministry of Health, JDC-Brookdale Institute of Gerontology and Human Development.

Fryers, T., Melzer, D. & Jenkins, R. (2003). Social inequalities and the common mental disorders: A systematic review of the evidence. *Social Psychiatry and Psychiatric Epidemiology*, 38, 229–37.

Gold, J. H. (1998). Gender differences in psychiatric illness and treatments: A critical review. *Journal of Nervous and Mental Disease*, 186, 769–75.

Halli, S. S. & Rao, K. V. (1992). *Advanced techniques of population analysis*. New York: Plenum Press.

Haro, J. M., Arbabzadeh-Bouchez, S., Brugha, T. S., de Girolamo, G., Guyer, M. E., Jin, R., Lepine, J.-P., Mazzi, F., Reneses, B., Vilagut, G., Sampson, N. A. & Kessler, R. C. (2006). Concordance of the Composite International Diagnostic Interview Version 3.0 (CIDI 3.0) with standardized clinical assessments in the WHO World Mental Health Surveys. *International Journal of Methods in Psychiatric Research*, 15, 167–80.

Haver, E., Shani, M., Kotler, M., Fast, D., Elizur, A. & Baruch, Y. (2005). Reform in mental health services: From whence and to where. *Harefuah*, 144, 327–31.

Hosmer, D. W. & Lemeshow, S. (1989). *Applied logistic regression*. New York: John Wiley & Sons.

Kessler, R. C., Demler, O., Frank, R. G., Olfson, M., Pincus, H. A., Walters, E. E., Wang, P., Wells, K. B. & Zaslavsky, A. M. (2005). Prevalence and treatment of mental disorders, 1990 to 2003. *New England Journal of Medicine*, 352, 2515–23.

Kessler, R. C., Haro, J. M., Heeringa, S. G., Pennell, B. E. & Üstün, T. B. (2006). The World Health Organization World Mental Health Survey Initiative. *Epidemiologia E Psichiatria Sociale*, 15, 161–6.

Kessler, R. C., McGonagle, K. A., Zhao, S., Nelson, C. B., Hughes, M., Eshleman, S., Wittchen, H. U. & Kendler, K. S. (1994). Lifetime and 12-month prevalence of DSM-III-R psychiatric disorders in the United States: Results from the National Comorbidity Survey. *Archives of General Psychiatry*, 51, 8–19.

Kessler, R. C. & Üstün, T. B. (2004). The World Mental Health (WMH) Survey Initiative Version of the World Health Organization (WHO) Composite International Diagnostic Interview (CIDI). *International Journal of Methods in Psychiatric Research*, 13, 93–121.

Kohn, R., Dohrenwend, B. P. & Mirotznik, J. (1998). Epidemiological findings on selected psychiatric disorders in the general population. In *Adversity, stress and psychopathology*, ed. B. P. Dohrenwend, pp. 235–84. New York: Oxford University Press.

Kohn, R., Saxena, S., Levav, I. & Saraceno, B. (2004). The treatment gap in mental health care. *Bulletin of the World Health Organization*, 82, 858–66.

Laska, E. M., Meisner, M. & Siegel, C. (1988). Estimating the size of a population from a single sample. *Biometrics*, 44, 461–72.

Lerner, Y. (1992). Psychiatric epidemiology in Israel. *Israel Journal of Psychiatry & Related Sciences*, 29, 218–28.

Lerner, Y., Kertes, J. & Zilber, N. (2005). Immigrants from the former Soviet Union, 5 years post-immigration to Israel: Adaptation and risk factors for psychological distress. *Psychological Medicine*, 35, 1805–14.

Levav, I. (1998). Individuals under conditions of maximum adversity: The Holocaust. In *Adversity, stress and psychopathology*, ed. B. P. Dohrenwend, pp. 13–33. New York: Oxford University Press.

Levav, I., Kohn, R., Dohrenwend, B. P., Shrout, P. E., Skodol, A. E., Schwartz, S., Link, B. G. & Naveh, G. (1993). An epidemiological study of mental disorders in a 10-year cohort of young adults in Israel. *Psychological Medicine*, 23, 691–707.

Levinson, D., Popper, M., Lerner, Y. & Feinson, M. C. (1996). *Patterns of ambulatory mental health services' utilization in Israel: Analysis of data from a national survey – 1986 and from a follow up – 1994*. Department of Information and Evaluation, Mental Health Services, Ministry of Health, and JDC-Israel Falk Institute for Mental Health and Behavioral Studies (in Hebrew).

Ministry of Health & Health Economics and Insurance Division (2006). *International comparisons of health systems: OECD countries and Israel 1980–2003*. Jerusalem: Ministry of Health & Health Economics and Insurance Division (in Hebrew).

Ministry of Health, Mental Health Services & Department of Information and Evaluation (2004). *Statistical Annual 2004*. Jerusalem: Ministry of Health, Mental Health Services & Department of Information and Evaluation (in Hebrew).

Patel, V., Araya, R., de Lima, M., Ludermir, A. & Todd, C. (1999). Women, poverty and common mental disorders in four restructuring societies. *Social Science & Medicine*, 49, 1461–71.

Paykel, E. S., Brugha, T. & Fryers, T. (2005). Size and burden of depressive disorders in Europe. *European Neuropsychopharmacology*, 15, 411–23.

Rabinowitz, J., Feldman, D., Gross, R. & Boerma, W. (1998). Which primary care physicians treat depression? *Psychiatric Services*, 49, 100–2.

Research Triangle Institute (2002). *SUDAAN: Professional software for survey data analysis 8.01*. Research Triangle Park, NC: Research Triangle Institute.

SAS Institute (2001). *SAS/STAT Software: Changes and enhancements, Release 8.2*. Cary, NC: SAS Publishing.

Sheehan, D. (1983). *The anxiety disease*. New York: Bantam Books.

Siegel, C., Handelsman, M., Haugland, G., Popper, M., Jouchovitzky, T. & Katz, S. (1993). A comparison of the mental health systems of New York State and Israel. *Israel Journal of Psychiatry & Related Sciences*, 30, 130–41.

Simon, G. E., VonKorff, M., Piccinelli, M., Fullerton, C. & Ormel, J. (1999). An international study of the relation between somatic symptoms and depression. *New England Journal of Medicine*, 341, 1329–35.

Somer, E. & Bleich, A. (2005). The stress of a population under a prolonged terror attack: Challenges in characterization, identification and response. In *Mental Health in Terror's Shadow: The Israeli experience*, ed. E. Somer & A. Bleich, pp. 9–26. Ramot: Tel Aviv University Press (in Hebrew).

World Health Organization (WHO) (2001). *The World Health Report 2001 – Mental health: New understanding, new hope*. Geneva: World Health Organization.

# 17 The Prevalence of Mental Disorders and Service Use in Italy: Results from the National Health Survey 2001–2003

GIOVANNI DE GIROLAMO, PIERLUIGI MOROSINI,
ANTONELLA GIGANTESCO, SARA DELMONTE, AND RONALD C. KESSLER

## ACKNOWLEDGMENTS

The Italian Mental Health Survey was carried out as part of the European Study of the Epidemiology of Mental Disorders (ESEMeD). ESEMeD is funded by the European Commission (Contracts QLG5-1999-01042; SANCO 2004123), the Piedmont Region (Italy), Fondo de Investigación Sanitaria, Instituto de Salud Carlos III, Spain (FIS 00/0028), Ministerio de Ciencia y Tecnología, Spain (SAF 2000-158-CE), Departament de Salut, Generalitat de Catalunya, Spain, and other local agencies and by an unrestricted educational grant from GlaxoSmithKline. ESEMeD is carried out in conjunction with the World Health Organization World Mental Health (WMH) Survey Initiative. We thank the WMH staff for assistance with instrumentation, fieldwork, and data analysis. These activities were supported by the U.S. National Institute of Mental Health (R01MH070884), the John D. and Catherine T. MacArthur Foundation, the Pfizer Foundation, the U.S. Public Health Service (R13-MH066849, R01-MH069864, and R01 DA016558), the Fogarty International Center (FIRCA R03-TW006481), the Pan American Health Organization, Eli Lilly and Company Foundation, Ortho-McNeil Pharmaceutical, GlaxoSmithKline, and Bristol-Myers Squibb. Thanks are due to the following collaborators of the Italian WMH survey, who gave an invaluable help at different stages of the project: Jordi Alonso, Francesca Falsirollo, Fausto Mazzi, Gabriella Polidori, Valeria Reda, Vilma Scarpino, Giulio Serra, Gemma Vilagut, and Giovanni Visonà.

## I. THE ITALIAN HEALTH-CARE SYSTEM

In 1978, Italy established the Italian National Health Service (NHS), or Servizio Sanitario Nazionale, which provides universal coverage free of charge at any point of service. The Ministry of Health oversees the system at the national level and is responsible for regulating the general objectives, overseeing the financial resources to be spent, and administering the health-care system itself. The regional governments then ensure delivery of benefits packages through the network of local health management organizations and public and private hospitals (referred to as local health units, or LHUs). The system was created with a structure of three levels of public authority: national, regional, and local. Through reforms in the early 1990s, the system has become very decentralized, giving most administrative, political, and financial responsibility to Italy's 21 regions. They, in turn, give much of the responsibilities to the LHUs, each of which takes care of a geographically defined catchment area (Maio & Manzoli 2002; de Girolamo et al. 2007). Italian universal coverage entitles all citizens equal access to necessary health care. Essential care is provided for free, or with a minimal fee, and includes general and pediatric services, drugs of proven effectiveness that are used for acute or chronic diseases, hospitalization, rehabilitation, and most services used in early diagnoses and preventive care.

## 1.1. Mental Health Care

The same year the NHS was established in Italy, the government passed Law 180, which concerns mental health care. This legislative change completely overhauled the Italian system for mental health services. There was a gradual closing down of all mental hospitals in the country and transfer of care for the mentally ill to a network of community-based mental health services. There are now in Italy 211 departments of mental health, based on geographically defined catchment areas, that are responsible for the full range of outpatient, inpatient, and residential care to people suffering from mental disorders. Hospitals are required to have acute inpatient units with a maximum of 15 psychiatric beds. However, most care for the mentally ill still falls on the individual and his or her family (Palermo 1991), although there are also private facilities in service. Because of the diverse nature of service providers and facilities within the 21 regions, there is great variation in the type and quality of care for the mentally ill (Piccinelli, Politi & Barale 2002; de Girolamo et al. 2007). Access to mental health services is, like general medical services, free of charge unless it involves some specific type of examination for which there may be a nominal fee. Medicines for mental illness are also generally free, with few exceptions (e.g., benzodiazepines, to prevent dependence), and the NHS also covers the fee for inpatient care when it is delivered in any of the 56 private inpatient facilities located in the country (this count does not include Sicily). The switch to community-based care seems to have had a positive effect on those patients who might not have sought care under the older asylum-based system (Piccinelli et al. 2002). Unfortunately, although the reform law set down the principles of care for the mentally ill, it did not provide a detailed framework as to its application. This means that the planning and definition of this framework was left to regional authorities. As a result, there is currently a marked variability

in a variety of quantitative and qualitative indicators of care for the mentally ill in Italy (Piccinelli et al. 2002; de Girolamo et al. 2007).

## 1.2. Previous Psychiatric Epidemiological Research

Few community epidemiological studies of psychiatric disorders have been conducted in Italy to date, and those that have been conducted are subject to certain limitations, such as the restriction of sampling to circumscribed geographic areas, which limits the possibility of generalizing results to the entire country (Zimmerman-Tansella 1994; Gigantesco et al. 2006). This is problematic, given the wide sociodemographic, economic, and cultural differences across different areas of Italy, which are reflected in the uneven composition and functioning of health and mental health services. The community survey with the most precise methodology was recently conducted in Sesto Fiorentino, in the suburbs of Florence (Faravelli et al. 2004a, 2004b). From the lists of 18 general practitioners (GPs), a random sample of 2500 people aged 14 and older was selected, of whom 2365 were evaluated by their own GP using the Mini International Neuropsychiatric Interview (MINI). Of those, 625 screened positive for a mental disorder, and 605, together with 123 screen-negative cases, were interviewed by psychiatrists using the Florence Psychiatric Interview.

The Italian WMH survey was carried out in the hopes of addressing this problem of limited epidemiological data on the prevalence and correlates of mental disorders in Italy. The survey was carried out as part of the European Study of the Epidemiology of Mental Disorders (ESEMeD) consortium of six Western European countries (ESEMeD/MHEDEA 2000 Investigators 2004), which is part of the WHO World Mental Health (WMH) Survey Initiative (Kessler et al. 2006). The Italian WMH survey is a cross-sectional, face-to-face, household survey of a probability sample of the adult population of Italy. It is the first Italian nationwide study to investigate the 1-month, 12-month, and lifetime prevalence rates and sociodemographic correlates of mood, anxiety, and alcohol disorders. It also assessed the levels of disability, the quality of life, the use of services, and the consumption of psychotropic medications by people with mental disorders. In this chapter, we present an overview of the initial results from the survey regarding prevalence and treatment of mental disorders.

## 2. SUBJECTS AND METHODS

### 2.1. Sample

The Italian Mental Health Survey is a nationally representative household survey of respondents ages 18 and older in Italy (de Girolamo et al. 2005). Face-to-face interviews were carried out with 4712 respondents between January 2001 and July 2003. Part 1 included a core diagnostic assessment administered to all respondents. Part 2 assessed risk factors, correlates, service use, and additional disorders and was administered to all Part 1 respondents with lifetime disorders as well as to a probability subsample of other respondents. The overall response rate was 71.3%. A more complete discussion of the sample design is presented elsewhere (de Girolamo et al. 2005).

### 2.2. Measures

DSM-IV diagnoses were made using Version 3.0 of the World Health Organization's (WHO) Composite International Diagnostic Interview (CIDI) (Kessler & Üstün 2004), a fully structured lay-administered diagnostic interview that generates diagnoses according to the definitions and criteria of both the ICD-10 (WHO 1991) and DSM-IV (American Psychiatric Association 1994) diagnostic systems. DSM-IV criteria are used in the analyses reported in this chapter. The disorders considered here are the same as in the other ESEMeD surveys: mood disorders (major depressive episode [MDE], anxiety disorders (panic disorder [PD], agoraphobia without panic [AG], specific phobia [SP], social phobia [SoP], generalized anxiety disorder [GAD], posttraumatic stress disorder [PTSD], and separation anxiety disorder [SAD]), substance disorders (alcohol abuse and dependence [AA, AD]), oppositional defiant disorder [ODD], and attention-deficit/hyperactivity disorder [ADHD]). Note that, unlike most other WMH surveys, we did not assess bipolar disorder, obsessive-compulsive disorder, or illicit drug disorders. Lifetime prevalence, age of onset, and 12-month prevalence were assessed separately for each disorder (de Girolamo et al. 2005). All diagnoses are considered with organic exclusions and without diagnostic hierarchy rules.

### 2.3. Severity of 12-month Cases

All measurement issues were handled consistently with the other WMH surveys. Age of onset of disorders was assessed retrospectively. Twelve-month cases were classified by severity into serious, moderate, and mild cases on the basis of a complex classification scheme that is as described in other chapters in this volume. Lifetime treatment contact, 12-month service use, and minimally adequate treatment were also classified in the same way as in the other WMH surveys. Predictor variables, finally, were the same as in the other surveys. Predictor variables in analyses of lifetime data include age of onset (AOO) of the focal disorder (coded into the categories early, middle, and late), cohort (defined by age at interview in the categories 18–34, 35–49, 50–64, 65+), gender, education (categorized as primary, secondary, high school, or some college), and marital status (categorized as currently married or cohabiting, previously married, or never married).

### 2.4. Analysis Procedures

The data were weighted to adjust for differential probabilities of selection of respondents within households and differential nonresponse as well as to adjust for residual differences between the sample and the Italian population on the cross-classification of sociodemographic variables. An additional weight was used in the Part 2 sample to adjust for differences in probability of selection into that sample. Cumulative probability of lifetime treatment contact curves were estimated using survival analysis and were used to make estimated projections of cumulative lifetime probability of treatment contact from year of onset. The typical duration of delay in initial treatment contact was defined on the basis of the curves as the median number of years from disorder onset to first treatment contact among cases that eventually made treatment contact.

Discrete-time survival analysis (Efron 1988) with person-year as the unit of analysis was used to examine correlates of disorders and treatment contact. Models of treatment contact were estimated for a given disorder among respondents with a history of the disorder to study the predictors of ever making a treatment contact. Basic patterns of 12-month disorders and service use were examined by computing proportions, means, and medians. Logistic regression (Hosmer & Lemeshow 1989) analysis was used to study sociodemographic predictors of having 12-month disorders, receiving any 12-month treatment in the total sample, receiving treatment in particular sectors among those receiving any treatment, and receiving treatment that met criteria for being minimally adequate. Standard errors were estimated using the Taylor series method as implemented in SUDAAN (Research Triangle Institute 2002). Multivariate significance tests were made using Wald $\chi^2$ tests based on coefficient variance-covariance matrices that were adjusted for design effects using the Taylor series method. Statistical significance was evaluated using two-sided design-based tests and the 0.05 level of significance.

## 3. RESULTS

### 3.1. Lifetime Prevalence of DSM-IV Mental Disorders

Table 17.1 shows the estimated lifetime prevalence of mental disorders in the survey. Lifetime prevalence of any DSM-IV/CIDI disorder is estimated at 18.1%, with 6.3% of respondents having two or more lifetime disorders and 1.7% having three or more. Anxiety disorders make up the most prevalent class of disorders (11.0%),

followed by mood disorders (9.9%), impulse-control disorders (1.7%), and substance disorders (1.3%). The most prevalent individual lifetime disorders are MDE (9.9%) and SP (5.4%).

Significant differences in lifetime prevalence with age occur only for four of the disorders considered here: PD, SoP, PTSD, and MDE. Two of these four (PD and PTSD) have a general increase across the age range, while the other two have their lowest prevalence in the oldest age group of the sample. The prevalence of PD and PTSD is lowest in the youngest age group (18–34), the prevalence of SoP is lowest in the oldest age group (65+), and the prevalence of MDE is lowest in both youngest and oldest groups.

### 3.2. Distributions of the Age of Onset of Mental Disorders

Table 17.2 presents the distributions of cumulative lifetime risk estimates that have been standardized and examined for fixed percentiles. Median ages of onset (i.e., the 50th percentile on the AOO distribution) are earliest for impulse-control disorders (age 9), somewhat later for anxiety disorders (age 16), and later for substance (age 28) and mood (age 37) disorders. Age of onset has a wide age range for most classes of disorder, with an interquartile range (IQR) (i.e., the number of years between the 25th and 75th percentiles of the AOO distributions) of 15 years (ages 20–35) for substance use disorders, 31 years (ages 25–56) for mood disorders, and 32 years (ages 7–39) for anxiety disorders. However, the IQR for impulse-control disorders is quite narrow (4 years, ages 7–11).

### 3.3. Projected Lifetime Risk of Mental Disorders

On the basis of the AOO distributions shown in Table 17.2, the projected lifetime risk of mental disorders as of age 75 was estimated to be 25% higher than the lifetime prevalence estimates for anxiety disorders, 75% higher for mood disorders, and 44% higher for any disorder. Not surprisingly, the greatest differences between lifetime prevalence and projected lifetime risk were

**Table 17.1.** Lifetime prevalence of DSM-IV/CIDI disorders in the total WMH/WHO Italian sample and by age

| | Total | | 18–34 | | 35–49 | | 50–64 | | 65+ | | $\chi^2_3$ |
|---|---|---|---|---|---|---|---|---|---|---|---|
| | % | (se) | % | (se) | % | (se) | % | (se) | % | (se) | |
| **I. Anxiety disorders** | | | | | | | | | | | |
| Panic disorder | 1.5 | (0.2) | 0.8 | (0.3) | 1.7 | (0.3) | 2.3 | (0.4) | 1.5 | (0.5) | 13.4** |
| Agoraphobia without panic | 0.8 | (0.2) | 1.0 | (0.3) | 1.1 | (0.3) | 0.4 | (0.2) | 0.6 | (0.4) | 3.1 |
| Specific phobia | 5.4 | (0.5) | 4.9 | (0.8) | 5.5 | (0.7) | 6.5 | (0.8) | 4.6 | (0.8) | 4.0 |
| Social phobia | 1.8 | (0.2) | 2.4 | (0.5) | 2.0 | (0.4) | 2.1 | (0.5) | 0.6 | (0.3) | 12.2* |
| Generalized anxiety disorder | 1.4 | (0.2) | 1.0 | (0.3) | 1.7 | (0.4) | 1.4 | (0.4) | 1.3 | (0.4) | 2.7 |
| Posttraumatic stress disorder[a] | 2.3 | (0.5) | 0.7 | (0.2) | 2.1 | (0.6) | 3.5 | (1.3) | 3.3 | (1.1) | 8.9* |
| Separation anxiety disorder[b] | 1.4 | (0.6) | 1.8 | (0.8) | 0.7 | (0.5) | – | –[b] | – | –[b] | 1.4[d] |
| Any anxiety disorder[c] | 11.0 | (0.9) | 9.3 | (1.6) | 12.4 | (1.4) | 12.3 | (1.7) | 10.4 | (2.2) | 3.5 |
| **II. Mood disorders** | | | | | | | | | | | |
| Major depressive episode | 9.9 | (0.5) | 8.5 | (0.6) | 11.6 | (1.0) | 11.4 | (1.1) | 8.4 | (1.1) | 17.5** |
| Any mood disorder | 9.9 | (0.5) | 8.5 | (0.6) | 11.6 | (1.0) | 11.4 | (1.1) | 8.4 | (1.1) | 17.5** |
| **III. Impulse-control disorders** | | | | | | | | | | | |
| Oppositional-defiant disorder | 0.8 | (0.3) | 0.6 | (0.3) | 1.1 | (0.5) | – | –[b] | – | –[b] | 1.1[d] |
| Conduct disorder | 0.3 | (0.2) | 0.1 | (0.1) | 0.5 | (0.5) | – | –[b] | – | –[b] | 0.6[d] |
| Attention-deficit/hyperactivity disorder | 0.9 | (0.2) | 0.9 | (0.3) | 0.9 | (0.4) | – | –[b] | – | –[b] | 0.0[d] |
| Any impulse-control disorder | 1.7 | (1.4) | 1.5 | (0.4) | 2.1 | (0.7) | – | –[b] | – | –[b] | 0.8[d] |
| **IV. Substance disorders** | | | | | | | | | | | |
| Alcohol abuse | 1.2 | (0.2) | 1.1 | (0.3) | 1.5 | (0.4) | 1.4 | (0.4) | 0.9 | (0.3) | 1.9 |
| Alcohol dependence | 0.3 | (0.1) | 0.3 | (0.2) | 0.3 | (0.2) | 0.7 | (0.3) | 0.1 | (0.1) | 6.4 |
| Any substance disorder | 1.3 | (0.2) | 1.2 | (0.3) | 1.5 | (0.4) | 1.4 | (0.4) | 0.9 | (0.3) | 1.8 |
| **V. Any disorder** | | | | | | | | | | | |
| Any[c] | 18.1 | (1.1) | 15.7 | (1.6) | 20.1 | (1.6) | 20.2 | (2.2) | 16.5 | (2.6) | 6.6 |
| Two or more disorders[c] | 6.3 | (0.5) | 4.4 | (0.7) | 7.3 | (0.8) | 7.5 | (1.1) | 6.2 | (1.6) | 9.1* |
| Three or more disorders[c] | 1.7 | (0.2) | 2.3 | (0.5) | 2.3 | (0.5) | 1.5 | (0.3) | 0.6 | (0.3) | 15.7** |
| **VI. Sample sizes** | | | | | | | | | | | |
| Part 1 | (4712) | | | | | | | | | | |
| Part 2 | (1779) | | | | | | | | | | |

[a] Posttraumatic stress disorder was assessed only in the Part 2 sample ($n = 1779$).

[b] Separation anxiety disorder, oppositional-defiant, disorder, conduct disorder, and attention-deficit/hyperactivity disorder were assessed only among Part 2 respondents aged 18–44 years ($n = 853$).

[c] These summary measures were analyzed in the full Part 2 sample ($n = 1779$). Separation anxiety disorder, oppositional-defiant disorder, conduct disorder, and attention-deficit/hyperactivity disorder were coded as absent among respondents who were not assessed for these disorders.

[d] The $\chi^2$ test evaluates statistical significance of age-related differences in estimated prevalence: $\chi^2$ is evaluated with one degree of freedom for separation anxiety disorder, oppositional-defiant, disorder, conduct disorder, and attention-deficit/hyperactivity disorder.

* Significant age difference at the 0.05 level. ** Significant age difference at the .01 level.

**Table 17.2.** Ages at selected percentiles on the standardized age of onset distributions of DSM-IV/CIDI disorders with projected lifetime risk at age 75

| | Projected lifetime risk at age 75 | | Ages at selected age of onset percentiles | | | | | | | |
|---|---|---|---|---|---|---|---|---|---|---|
| | % | (se) | 5 | 10 | 25 | 50 | 75 | 90 | 95 | 99 |
| I. Anxiety disorders | | | | | | | | | | |
| Panic disorder | 2.3 | (0.4) | 5 | 14 | 23 | 39 | 57 | 61 | 70 | 70 |
| Agoraphobia without panic | 1.0 | (0.2) | 7 | 8 | 15 | 31 | 36 | 66 | 66 | 66 |
| Specific phobia | 5.7 | (0.5) | 5 | 5 | 5 | 8 | 14 | 28 | 44 | 61 |
| Social phobia | 2.0 | (0.3) | 5 | 7 | 13 | 15 | 20 | 28 | 36 | 56 |
| Generalized anxiety disorder | 2.0 | (0.3) | 13 | 18 | 26 | 38 | 51 | 61 | 70 | 70 |
| Posttraumatic stress disorder[a] | 4.0 | (1.0) | 16 | 16 | 32 | 41 | 59 | 64 | 64 | 64 |
| Separation anxiety disorder[b] | 1.0 | (0.6) | 5 | 5 | 5 | 8 | 8 | 15 | 15 | 15 |
| Any anxiety disorder[c] | 13.7 | (1.2) | 5 | 5 | 7 | 16 | 39 | 55 | 61 | 66 |
| II. Mood disorders | | | | | | | | | | |
| Major depressive episode | 17.3 | (1.2) | 15 | 18 | 25 | 37 | 56 | 69 | 71 | 73 |
| Any mood disorder | 17.3 | (1.2) | 15 | 18 | 25 | 37 | 56 | 69 | 71 | 73 |
| III. Impulse-control disorders | | | | | | | | | | |
| Oppositional-defiant disorder[b] | 0.8 | (0.3) | 5 | 8 | 8 | 13 | 13 | 14 | 14 | 14 |
| Conduct disorder[c] | 0.3 | (0.2) | 9 | 9 | 9 | 9 | 14 | 24 | 24 | 24 |
| Attention-deficit/hyperactivity disorder[b] | 0.9 | (0.2) | 5 | 5 | 7 | 8 | 9 | 11 | 11 | 12 |
| Any impulse-control disorder[b] | 1.7 | (0.4) | 5 | 5 | 7 | 9 | 11 | 14 | 14 | 24 |
| IV. Substance disorders | | | | | | | | | | |
| Alcohol abuse[a] | 1.6 | (0.3) | 17 | 19 | 21 | 31 | 36 | 41 | 48 | 55 |
| Alcohol dependence[a] | 0.5 | (0.2) | 15 | 19 | 27 | 33 | 36 | 55 | 55 | 55 |
| Any substance use disorder[c] | 1.6 | (0.3) | 17 | 19 | 20 | 28 | 35 | 41 | 48 | 55 |
| V. Any disorder | | | | | | | | | | |
| Any[c] | 26.0 | (1.9) | 5 | 5 | 11 | 26 | 45 | 62 | 69 | 73 |

[a] Posttraumatic stress disorder and substance disorders were assessed only in the Part 2 sample ($n = 1779$).

[b] Separation anxiety disorder, oppositional-defiant, disorder, conduct disorder, and attention-deficit/hyperactivity disorder were assessed only among Part 2 respondents aged 18–44 years ($n = 853$).

[c] These summary measures were analyzed in the full Part 2 sample ($n = 1779$). Separation anxiety disorder, oppositional-defiant, disorder, conduct disorder, and attention-deficit/hyperactivity disorder were coded as absent among respondents who were not assessed for these disorders.

observed for disorders with late AOO distributions (e.g., MDE and PTSD). The order is reversed relative to lifetime prevalence estimates for anxiety disorders and mood disorders, with anxiety disorders having a higher prevalence (11.0% vs. 9.9%) and mood disorders having a higher projected risk (17.3% vs. 13.7%). The lowest project risk is for substance disorders (1.6%). Of projected new onsets, 29% are in people with existing disorders. This derives from the fact that the overall projected risk in the total sample is only 7.9% higher than the lifetime prevalence reported in Table 17.1 (26.0% vs. 18.1%).

This means that a substantial proportion of new onsets are predicted to be secondary comorbid disorders.

## 3.4. Cohort Effects in Lifetime Risk of Mental Disorders

Discrete-time survival analysis was used to predict lifetime risk of disorders in various age groups (i.e., 18–34, 35–49, 50–64, and 65+). Impulse-control disorders were excluded because of the restricted age range of the sample in which they were assessed and their restricted

**Table 17.3.** Cohort (age at interview) as a predictor of lifetime risk of DSM-IV/WMH-CIDI disorders in the WMH/WHO Italian sample[a]

| | Younger cohorts (age at interview) compared to respondents ages 65+ | | | | | | |
|---|---|---|---|---|---|---|---|
| | 18–34 | | 35–49 | | 50–64 | | |
| | OR | (95% CI) | OR | (95% CI) | OR | (95% CI) | $\chi^2_3$ |
| **I. Anxiety disorders** | | | | | | | |
| Panic disorder | 2.0 | (0.7–5.4) | 2.3* | (1.1–4.9) | 2.0 | (0.9–4.5) | 4.9 |
| Agoraphobia without panic | 4.1 | (0.6–26.5) | 2.4 | (0.5–10.6) | 0.9 | (0.2–4.5) | 5.3 |
| Specific phobia | 1.2 | (0.7–1.9) | 1.3 | (0.8–1.9) | 1.4 | (1.0–2.1) | 3.6 |
| Social phobia | 4.5* | (1.6–12.3) | 3.4* | (1.2–9.6) | 3.4* | (1.2–10.2) | 9.5** |
| Generalized anxiety disorder | 3.9* | (1.3–11.5) | 2.7* | (1.2–6.0) | 1.4 | (0.6–3.4) | 8.6** |
| Posttraumatic stress disorder[b] | 1.3 | (0.3–6.4) | 1.6 | (0.6–3.9) | 1.5 | (0.5–4.3) | 2.0 |
| Separation anxiety disorder[c+] | | | | | | | |
| Any anxiety disorder[b] | 1.5 | (0.7–3.0) | 1.6 | (0.9–2.8) | 1.3 | (0.8–2.2) | 3.3 |
| **II. Mood disorders** | | | | | | | |
| Major depressive episode | 5.7* | (3.8–8.4) | 3.6* | (2.6–5.0) | 2.3* | (1.6–3.3) | 91.3** |
| Any mood disorder | 5.7* | (3.8–8.4) | 3.6* | (2.6–5.0) | 2.3* | (1.6–3.3) | 91.3** |
| **III. Impulse-control disorders** | | | | | | | |
| Oppositional-defiant disorder[c+] | | | | | | | |
| Conduct disorder[c+] | | | | | | | |
| Attention-deficit/hyperactivity disorder[c+] | | | | | | | |
| Intermittent explosive disorder | | | | | | | |
| Any impulse-control disorder[c+] | | | | | | | |
| **IV. Substance use disorders** | | | | | | | |
| Alcohol abuse or dependence | 2.6 | (1.0–7.0) | 1.8 | (0.8–4.2) | 1.5 | (0.6–3.8) | 5.4 |
| Alcohol dependence[+] | | | | | | | |
| Any substance disorder | 2.6* | (1.0–6.7) | 1.8 | (0.8–4.1) | 1.6 | (0.6–3.9) | 5.5 |
| **V. Any disorder** | | | | | | | |
| Any[d] | 2.2* | (1.3–3.9) | 2.0* | (1.3–3.1) | 1.6 | (1.0–2.5) | 11.8** |

[a] Based on discrete-time survival models with person-year as the unit of analysis.

[b] Estimated in the Part 2 sample ($n = 1779$).

[c] Estimated among respondents aged 18–44 years in the Part 2 sample ($n = 853$).

[d] Estimated in the full Part 2 sample. Separation anxiety disorder, oppositional-defiant, disorder, conduct disorder, and attention-deficit/hyperactivity disorder were coded as absent among respondents who were not assessed for these disorders.

+ Cell size $\leq 30$ cases; too small to estimate.

* Significant difference compared to the 65+ year olds at the 0.05 level, two-sided test.

** Significant intercohort differences in global test.

AOO distribution. As shown in Table 17.3, the vast majority of the odds ratios (ORs) are greater than 1.0, indicating lowest risk in the oldest age group (respondents aged 65+). Several of these differences are statistically significant, and in all cases indicate higher risk in successively younger cohorts. The largest significant cohort effects were associated with MDE, SoP, and GAD.

An alternative explanation for these apparent cohort effects is that lifetime risk is actually constant across cohorts but appears to vary with cohort because onsets occur earlier in more recent than later cohorts (as might happen if there were secular changes in environmental triggers or to age-related differences in AOO recall accuracy). Another explanation might be that mortality has an increasing impact on sample

**Table 17.4.** Variations in the effects of cohort (age at interview) in predicting lifetime risk of DSM-IV/WMH-CIDI disorders[a]

| | Age of onset | | | | | |
| --- | --- | --- | --- | --- | --- | --- |
| | Early | | Middle | | Late | |
| | OR | (95% CI) | OR | (95% CI) | OR | (95% CI) |
| I. Anxiety disorders | | | | | | |
| 18–34 | 1.1 | (0.5–2.8) | 1.7 | (0.6–4.4) | 1.8 | (0.7–4.5) |
| 35–49 | 0.9 | (0.4–1.9) | 1.6 | (0.7–3.5) | 4.3* | (2.7–8.3) |
| 50–64 | 0.9 | (0.4–2.3) | 1.0 | (0.4–2.5) | 2.9* | (1.7–5.0) |
| 65+ | 1.0 | – | 1.0 | – | 1.0 | – |
| | $\chi^2_6 = 18.5^{***}$ | | $\chi^2_3 = 0.6$ | | $\chi^2_3 = 2.3$ | $\chi^2_3 = 29.3^{**}$ |
| II. Mood disorders | | | | | | |
| 18–34 | 4.2* | (2.2–7.8) | 7.8* | (3.0–20.0) | 1.0 | (6.1–13.9) |
| 35–49 | 2.2* | (1.2–4.1) | 5.3* | (2.2–12.7) | 4.5* | (2.8–7.1) |
| 50–64 | 1.6 | (0.8–3.0) | 3.4* | (1.2–9.1) | 2.2* | (1.4–3.6) |
| 65+ | 1.0 | – | 1.0 | – | 1.0 | – |
| | $\chi^2_3 = 5.4$ | | $\chi^2_3 = 45.3^{**}$ | | $\chi^2_3 = 33.3^{**}$ | $\chi^2_3 = 40.3^{**}$ |
| III. Substance disorders | | | | | | |
| 18–34 | 1.4 | (0.3–5.8) | 1.9 | (0.4–9.2) | 3.4 | (0.6–18.6) |
| 35–49 | 0.6 | (0.1–2.8) | 2.0 | (0.4–10.0) | 2.5 | (0.7–8.3) |
| 50–64 | 0.5 | (0.1–2.7) | 1.4 | (0.3–8.2) | 2.4 | (0.5–10.4) |
| 65+ | 1.0 | – | 1.0 | – | 1.0 | – |
| | $\chi^2_3 = 4.3$ | | $\chi^2_3 = 3.8$ | | $\chi^2_3 = 1.6$ | $\chi^2_3 = 3.0$ |

[a] Based on discrete-time survival models with person-year as the unit of analysis. Total-sample models evaluated the significance of interactions between cohort and person-year. This was not done for impulse-control disorders because the vast majority of such disorders have onsets in a very narrow time window. All analyses were carried out in the full Part 2 sample.

\* Significant difference compared with the age ≥65 years cohorts at the 0.05 level, two-sided test in the subsample of person-years defined by the column headings.

\*\* Significant intercohort differences in the global test in the subsample of person-years.

\*\*\* Significant interaction between cohort and age of onsets in the lives of respondents in the total sample.

selection bias as age increases. To study these possibilities, the cohort model was examined to determine whether intercohort differences decrease significantly with increasing age. Differences were examined separately for first onsets in the ranges early, middle, and late. Results in Table 17.4 show that there was no evidence of consistently decreasing cohort effects with increasing age for anxiety or mood disorders. Indeed, if anything, the pattern appears to be the opposite, although intercohort variation does not vary significantly by AOO of disorders either for mood disorders or for substance disorders. In the case of anxiety disorders, the cohort effect is significant only for late-onset disorders and the elevations appear in the middle cohorts rather than the youngest cohort. Patterns of this sort are unlikely to be due to age-related variation in recall bias.

### 3.5. Sociodemographic Predictors of Lifetime Risk of Mental Disorders

Table 17.5 presents sociodemographic predictors of lifetime risk of mental disorders identified in survival analyses that adjusted for cohort. Consistent with the results in many other surveys, women have significantly higher risk of anxiety and mood disorders, whereas men have significantly higher risk of alcohol use disorders. Level of education is unrelated to risk of anxiety, mood, or alcohol disorders. Age is inversely related to

**Table 17.5.** Sociodemographic predictors of lifetime risk of any DSM-IV/WMH-CIDI anxiety, mood, and substance use disorders

|  | Anxiety | | Mood | | Substance | |
|---|---|---|---|---|---|---|
|  | OR | (95% CI) | OR | (95% CI) | OR | (95% CI) |
| **I. Sex** | | | | | | |
| Female | 3.7* | (2.5–5.4) | 2.0* | (1.6–2.6) | 0.4* | (0.0–0.2) |
| Male | 1.0 | – | 1.0 | – | 1.0 | – |
| $\chi^2_1$ | | 52.0* | | 45.7* | | 22.9* |
| **II. Education** | | | | | | |
| Student | 1.8 | (0.4–7.3) | 1.5 | (0.8–2.8) | 1.7 | (0.2–12.8) |
| Low | 1.1 | (0.2–4.4) | 0.9 | (0.4–1.7) | 4.0 | (0.5–31.8) |
| Low-medium | 0.8 | (0.1–3.7) | 1.0 | (0.5–1.7) | 3.5 | (0.4–30.0) |
| Medium | 2.1 | (0.5–8.3) | 1.0 | (0.6–1.7) | 1.5 | (0.2–10.9) |
| High | 1.0 | – | 1.0 | – | 1.0 | – |
| $\chi^2_4$ | | 12.9 | | 4.5 | | 4.2 |
| **III. Age** | | | | | | |
| 18–34 | 1.1 | (0.5–2.3) | 4.0* | (1.9–8.3) | 2.7 | (0.9–7.7) |
| 35–49 | 1.1 | (0.6–1.9) | 2.3* | (1.1–4.6) | 1.6 | (0.5–4.7) |
| 50–64 | 1.0 | (0.5–1.7) | 1.6 | (0.8–3.3) | 0.9 | (0.3–2.8) |
| 65+ | 1.0 | – | 1.0 | – | 1.0 | – |
| $\chi^2_3$ | | 0.5 | | 42.2* | | 8.8 |

*Note:* Models include time intervals as controls. Person years are restricted to $\leq 29$ years.
* Significant at the 0.05 level.

risk of mood disorders, but not to either anxiety disorders or alcohol disorders.

To examine whether the increasing prevalence of disorders in recent cohorts is concentrated in certain subgroups, variation across cohorts in the association of sex and education with first AOO of disorders were studied (results are not shown but are available on request). Of note, sex differences in anxiety, mood, and alcohol disorders did not differ across cohort, but women with mood disorders were found to be more similar to men in the oldest cohort. Significant associations between lower education and anxiety disorders were observed only in the oldest cohort and between AOO and mood disorders only in recent cohorts.

### 3.6. Cumulative Lifetime Probabilities of Treatment Contact

Figure 17.1 presents survival curves showing the speed of initial treatment contact among respondents with specific anxiety disorders and major depression who will eventually make treat-

ment contact. More than two-thirds of eventual patients with panic disorder in Italy seek treatment in the year of onset of their first panic attack. Comparable percentages are 50% for GAD and 45% for MDE, but considerably lower (1%–16%) for phobias.

### 3.7. Duration of Delays in Initial Treatment Contact

The proportion of cases that made treatment contact in the year of first onset of the disorder is shown in Table 17.6, along with the median delay among people who eventually made treatment contact after the year of first onset. These results are estimates from survival curves estimated for each disorder, which are not shown. The proportion of cases making treatment contact in the year of disorder onset ranges from a high of 65.2% for panic disorders to a low of 0.5 for SP. The median duration of delay in seeking help also varies greatly across disorders, from low of 2 years for MDE to highs of 20–31 years for SoP and SP.

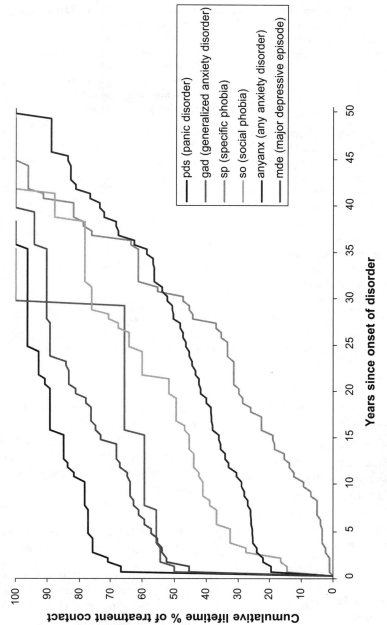

**Figure 17.1.** Cumulative lifetime percentage of treatment contact for anxiety and mood.

Legend:
- pds (panic disorder)
- gad (generalized anxiety disorder)
- sp (specific phobia)
- so (social phobia)
- anyanx (any anxiety disorder)
- mde (major depressive episode)

X-axis: Years since onset of disorder

Y-axis: Cumulative lifetime % of treatment contact

**Table 17.6.** Proportional treatment contact in the year of disorder onset and median duration of delay among cases that subsequently made treatment contact

|  | Treatment contact made in year of onset, % | Median duration of delay (years)[a] | n[b] |
|---|---|---|---|
| **I.  Anxiety disorders** |  |  |  |
| Panic disorder | 65.2 | 1 | 72 |
| Specific phobia | 0.5 | 31 | 253 |
| Social phobia | 8.2 | 20 | 91 |
| Generalized anxiety disorder | 31.0 | 2 | 100 |
| Any anxiety disorder | 17.1 | 28 | 429 |
| **II.  Mood disorders** |  |  |  |
| Major depressive episode | 28.8 | 2 | 449 |
| **III.  Substance disorders** |  |  |  |
| Alcohol abuse | –[c] | –[c] | –[c] |
| Alcohol dependence | –[c] | –[c] | –[c] |
| Any substance disorders | –[c] | –[c] | –[c] |

[a]  Projections based on time-to-contact survival curves in Figures 17.1–17.3.
[b]  Weighted number of respondents with a lifetime history of the disorder.
[c]  Disorder was omitted due to insufficient $n > 30$, but it will be included as one of the disorders in the "Any" category.

## 3.8. Predictors of Failure and Delay in Initial Treatment Contact

Table 17.7 displays predictors of lifetime treatment contact among respondents with lifetime disorders. Cohort and AOO are significantly related to lifetime treatment contact in panic disorder and any anxiety disorders. Moreover, AOO is significantly related to treatment contact in MDE. No differences exist between women and men.

## 3.9. Prevalence and Severity of 12-month Disorders

Table 17.8 shows the 12-month prevalence of disorders, with the most common being SP (3.5%) and MDE (3.0%). Among classes, anxiety disorders are the most prevalent (6.0%), followed by mood disorders (3.4%). The 12-month prevalence of any disorder is 8.4%.

Of 12-month cases, 16.5% were classified as serious, 46.4% as moderate, and 37.0% as mild. Among disorder classes, mood disorders have the

highest percentage of serious cases (30.4%) and anxiety disorders the lowest (15.4%). The anxiety disorder with the greatest proportion of serious cases is AG (47.0%), while MDE has the greatest proportion of serious case (34.2%) among mood disorders.

## 3.9. Sociodemographic Correlates of 12-month Mental Disorders

Correlates of being affected by anxiety or mood disorders include being female and, for anxiety disorders, never married (see Table 17.9). None of the associations was significant between sociodemographic variables and prevalence of impulse-control and alcohol disorders.

## 3.10. Probability of 12-month Service Use

A total of 4.3% of respondents used services for the treatment of a mental or alcohol disorder at some time in the year before interview (Table 17.10). This includes 27.3% of respondents with

**Table 17.7.** Sociodemographic predictors of lifetime treatment contact for specific DSM-IV/CIDI disorders

| | Anxiety disorders | | | | | | | | | | Mood disorders | | Substance disorders | | | | | |
| --- | --- | --- | --- | --- | --- | --- | --- | --- | --- | --- | --- | --- | --- | --- | --- | --- | --- | --- |
| | Panic disorder | | Generalized anxiety disorder | | Specific phobia | | Social phobia | | Any anxiety disorders | | Major depressive episode | | Alcohol abuse | | Alcohol abuse with dependence | | Any substance disorders | |
| | OR | (95% CI) | OR | (95% CI) | OR | (95% CI) | OR | (95% CI) | OR | (95% CI) | OR | (95% CI) | OR | (95% CI) | OR | (95% CI) | OR | (95% CI) |
| I. Cohort (age at interview) | | | | | | | | | | | | | | | | | | |
| 18–34 | 5.0* | (1.9–13.4) | 1.4 | (0.3–7.1) | 4.2* | (1.1–15.8) | 1.7 | (0.5–5.4) | 2.6* | (1.3–5.2) | 1.4 | (0.7–2.8) | –$^a$ | –$^a$ | –$^a$ | –$^a$ | –$^a$ | –$^a$ |
| 35–49 | 2.0 | (0.8–5.0) | 2.5 | (0.8–7.8) | 2.6 | (0.8–8.3) | 1.4 | (0.5–3.6) | 2.1* | (1.2–3.7) | 1.6 | (0.8–2.9) | –$^a$ | –$^a$ | –$^a$ | –$^a$ | –$^a$ | –$^a$ |
| 50–64 | 0.4 | (0.1–1.3) | 2.1 | (0.6–7.3) | 1.8 | (0.5–6.3) | 1.0 | – | 1.4 | (0.7–2.9) | 1.1 | (0.6–2.1) | –$^a$ | –$^a$ | –$^a$ | –$^a$ | –$^a$ | –$^a$ |
| $\chi_3^2$ | 16.0* | | 3.0 | | 5.6 | | 0.9 | | 16.0* | | 2.8 | | –$^a$ | | –$^a$ | | –$^a$ | |
| II. Age of onset | | | | | | | | | | | | | | | | | | |
| Early | 0.0* | (0.0–0.0) | 0.5 | (0.1–3.9) | 0.3* | (0.2–1.1) | 0.3* | (0.1–0.8) | 0.1* | (0.1–0.2) | 0.4* | (0.2–0.8) | –$^a$ | –$^a$ | –$^a$ | –$^a$ | –$^a$ | –$^a$ |
| Early-average | 0.1* | (0.0–0.7) | 1.1 | (0.3–4.2) | 0.3* | (0.1–0.9) | 0.4* | (0.1–0.7) | 0.1* | (0.1–0.2) | 0.8 | (0.4–1.6) | –$^a$ | –$^a$ | –$^a$ | –$^a$ | –$^a$ | –$^a$ |
| Late-average | 0.2 | (0.0–2.1) | 1.1 | (0.4–3.3) | 0.5* | (0.2–0.9) | 0.5 | (0.3–1.1) | 0.3* | (0.2–0.5) | 0.8 | (0.4–1.4) | –$^a$ | –$^a$ | –$^a$ | –$^a$ | –$^a$ | –$^a$ |
| $\chi_3^2$ | 37.4* | | 1.1 | | 7.2 | | 6.3 | | 101.8* | | 15.7* | | –$^a$ | | –$^a$ | | –$^a$ | |
| III. Sex | | | | | | | | | | | | | | | | | | |
| Female | 1.4 | (0.6–3.0) | 0.7 | (0.3–1.7) | 0.7 | (0.4–1.1) | 1.5 | (0.7–3.4) | 1.1 | (0.7–1.5) | 1.4 | (0.9–2.0) | –$^a$ | –$^a$ | –$^a$ | –$^a$ | –$^a$ | –$^a$ |
| $\chi_3^2$ | 0.6 | | 0.7 | | 2.7 | | 0.9 | | 0.1 | | 2.6 | | –$^a$ | | –$^a$ | | –$^a$ | |

$^a$ Disorder was omitted due to insufficient lifetime cases ($n < 30$), but it will be included as one of the disorders in the "Any" category.
* Significant at the 0.05 level, two-sided test.

**Table 17.8.** 12-month prevalence and severity of DSM-IV/CIDI disorders

| | Total | | Severity | | | | | |
| | | | Serious[b] | | Moderate[b] | | Mild[b] | |
| | % | (se) | % | (se) | % | (se) | % | (se) |
|---|---|---|---|---|---|---|---|---|
| **I. Anxiety disorders** | | | | | | | | |
| Panic disorder[a] | 0.7 | (0.1) | 29.9 | (8.8) | 53.9 | (8.3) | 16.1 | (6.9) |
| Agoraphobia without panic[a] | 0.4 | (0.1) | 47.0 | (18.9) | 33.7 | (17.8) | 19.2 | (10.7) |
| Specific phobia[a] | 3.5 | (0.3) | 11.6 | (3.6) | 47.7 | (7.4) | 40.7 | (7.4) |
| Social phobia[a] | 1.0 | (0.2) | 23.3 | (8.6) | 63.2 | (9.0) | 13.5 | (5.4) |
| Generalized anxiety disorder[a] | 0.4 | (0.1) | 26.8 | (12.6) | 38.8 | (15.0) | 34.4 | (16.7) |
| Posttraumatic stress disorder[b] | 0.7 | (0.2) | 24.2 | (10.3) | 67.0 | (11.4) | 8.8 | (5.2) |
| Separation anxiety disorder[c] | 0.0 | (0.0) | | | | | | |
| Any anxiety disorder[b] | 6.0 | (0.6) | 15.4 | (3.2) | 51.2 | (5.1) | 33.4 | (5.3) |
| **II. Mood disorders** | | | | | | | | |
| Major depressive disorder[a] | 3.0 | (0.2) | 34.2 | (4.7) | 40.8 | (4.5) | 25.0 | (3.0) |
| Dysthymia[a] | 0.9 | (0.1) | 30.9 | (6.3) | 27.5 | (6.0) | 41.6 | (7.1) |
| Bipolar I-II disorders[a] | | | | | | | | |
| Any mood disorder[c] | 3.4 | (0.2) | 30.4 | (4.4) | 38.6 | (4.0) | 31.0 | (3.3) |
| **III. Impulse-control disorders** | | | | | | | | |
| Oppositional-defiant disorder[c] | 0.1 | (0.1) | 43.4 | (34.7) | 0.0 | (0.0) | 56.6 | (34.7) |
| Conduct disorder[c] | 0.0 | (0.0) | 100.0 | (0.0) | 0.0 | (0.0) | 0.0 | (0.0) |
| Attention-deficit/hyperactivity disorder[a] | 0.3 | (0.1) | 0.0 | (0.0) | 45.2 | (25.2) | 54.8 | (25.2) |
| Intermittent explosive disorder[a] | | | | | | | | |
| Any impulse–control disorder[c] | 0.4 | (0.2) | 19.0 | (14.5) | 31.7 | (18.5) | 49.3 | (19.0) |
| **IV. Substance disorders** | | | | | | | | |
| Alcohol abuse[a] | 0.2 | (0.1) | 29.6 | (29.5) | 0.0 | (0.0) | 70.4 | (29.5) |
| Alcohol dependence[a] | 0.1 | (0.0) | 100.0 | (0.0) | 0.0 | (0.0) | 0.0 | (0.0) |
| Drug abuse[b] | | | | | | | | |
| Drug dependence[b] | | | | | | | | |
| Any substance disorder[a] | 0.2 | (0.1) | 29.6 | (29.5) | 0.0 | (0.0) | 70.4 | (29.5) |
| **V. Any disorder** | | | | | | | | |
| Any[b] | 8.4 | (0.7) | 16.5 | (2.8) | 46.4 | (3.9) | 37.0 | (4.0) |
| **VI. Total sample** | | | | | | | | |
| Total sample[b] | | | 1.4 | (0.2) | 3.9 | (0.5) | 3.1 | (0.5) |

[a] Part 1 sample ($n = 4712$); prevalence calculated using Part 1 weights.

[b] Part 2 sample ($n = 1779$); prevalence calculated using Part 2 weights.

[c] Part 2 sample among respondents aged 18–44 years ($n = 853$); prevalence and severity calculated using Part 2 weights for age $\leq 44$.

a 12-month DSM-IV disorder and 2.2% of those without such a disorder. The highest proportion of cases in treatment is for PD (65.7%). Most of those treated receive services in health-care sectors (4.1% of respondents, representing 95.4% of those in treatment). Among those treated in health-care sectors, most received services in the general medical sector (3.0% of respondents, representing 69.8% of those in treatment).

### 3.11. Number of Visits in the Prior Year

The median number of 12-month visits among those receiving any treatment in the year before interview was 2.5 (Table 17.11). This number was higher among patients without (3.0) than with (1.9) DSM-IV/CIDI disorders. The median number of within-sector visits was fairly similar across sectors (ranging from 1.7 for

**Table 17.9.** Sociodemographic predictors of 12-month risk of any DSM-IV/CIDI mood, anxiety, impulse-control, substance use, and any disorder

| | Mood[a] | | Anxiety[a] | | Impulse control[b] | | Substance[a] | | Any[a] | |
|---|---|---|---|---|---|---|---|---|---|---|
| | OR | (95% CI) | OR | (95% CI) | OR | (95% CI) | OR | (95% CI) | OR | (95% CI) |
| **I. Sex** | | | | | | | | | | |
| Female | 2.3* | (1.5–3.5) | 4.4* | (2.9–6.5) | 0.7 | (0.1–3.9) | 1.0 | – | 3.1* | (2.3–4.3) |
| Male | 1.0 | – | 1.0 | – | 1.0 | – | – | – | 1.0 | – |
| $\chi^2_1$ | 16.8* | | 55.3* | | 0.2 | | – | | 51.4* | |
| **II. Age** | | | | | | | | | | |
| 18–34 | 0.7 | – | 0.8 | (0.3–1.8) | 0.7 | (0.1–3.2) | – | – | 0.7 | (0.4–1.4) |
| 35–49 | 0.7 | (0.6–0.9) | 0.9 | (0.4–1.9) | 1.0 | – | – | – | 0.8 | (0.4–1.4) |
| 50–64 | 1.1 | (0.6–0.9) | 0.7 | (0.4–1.6) | – | – | – | – | 0.8 | (0.4–1.5) |
| 65+ | 1.0 | (0.9–1.5) | 1.0 | – | – | – | 1.0 | – | 1.0 | – |
| $\chi^2_3$ | 10.2* | | 1.2 | | 0.3 | | – | | 1.0 | |
| **III. Education** | | | | | | | | | | |
| Primary | – | – | – | – | – | – | – | – | – | – |
| Secondary | 1.0 | (0.6–1.8) | 1.1 | (0.6–2.0) | 0.6 | (0.1–5.0) | – | – | 0.9 | (0.6–1.5) |
| High school | 0.8 | (0.5–1.5) | 1.5 | (0.8–2.8) | 1.3 | (0.5–3.4) | – | – | 1.2 | (0.7–1.9) |
| Some college | 1.0 | – | 1.0 | – | 1.0 | – | 1.0 | – | 1.0 | – |
| $\chi^2_3$ | 0.6 | | 1.8 | | 0.6 | | – | | 1.2 | |
| **IV. Marital status** | | | | | | | | | | |
| Married–cohabiting | 1.0 | – | 1.0 | – | 1.0 | – | 1.0 | – | 1.0 | – |
| Previously married | – | – | – | – | – | – | – | – | – | – |
| Never married | 1.5 | (0.7–1.3) | 0.6* | (0.4–0.8) | 0.8 | (0.1–5.4) | – | – | 0.8 | (0.6–1.1) |
| $\chi^2_2$ | 4.4* | | 9.8* | | 0.1 | | – | | 1.5 | |
| **V. Income** | | | | | | | | | | |
| Low | 1.1 | (0.5–2.5) | 0.7 | (0.3–1.5) | 1.9 | (0.1–39.2) | – | – | 0.7 | (0.4–1.4) |
| Low-average | 1.3 | (0.7–2.5) | 0.7 | (0.3–1.6) | 1.4 | (0.1–19.7) | – | – | 0.8 | (0.4–1.5) |
| High-average | 0.8 | (0.4–1.4) | 1.0 | (0.5–2.2) | 0.8 | (0.1–7.5) | – | – | 0.8 | (0.4–1.7) |
| High | 1.0 | – | 1.0 | – | 1.0 | – | 1.0 | – | 1.0 | – |
| $\chi^2_3$ | 5.4 | | 2.8 | | 0.6 | | – | | 0.9 | |
| (n) | (1779) | | (1779) | | (853) | | (1779) | | (1779) | |

[a] Based on the Part 2 sample ($n = 1779$). In the case of any anxiety disorder, obsessive-compulsive disorder was coded as absent among respondents who were not assessed for this disorder.
[b] Based on Part 2 respondents aged 18–44 years ($n = 853$).
* Significant at the 0.05 level, two-sided test.

general medical to 2.6 for any mental health specialty).

Mean numbers of visits are consistently higher than the median (results are not shown but are available on request). For example, among patients receiving any treatment the median was 2.5 versus a mean of 7.2. Patients with and without disorders made similar mean visits (7.1 and 7.4). Mean within-sector visits were lowest for general medical (3.8) and higher for any mental health specialty (8.7) (no estimate was made for human services and complementary and alternative medicine [CAM] because the number of

patients who were treated in the sector was fewer than 30). The greater magnitude of means than medians implies that a relatively small number of patients receive a disproportionately high share of all visits.

### 3.12. Minimally Adequate Treatment in the Prior Year

Among patients with DSM-IV/CIDI disorders who were in treatment at some time in the past 12 months, 82.7% were classified as receiving at least minimally adequate treatment (Table 17.12).

**Table 17.10.** Prevalence of 12-month mental health service use in separate service sectors by 12-month DSM-IV/CIDI disorders

| Disorder group | Measure | Health care — Mental health specialty — Psychiatrist % | (se) | Nonpsychiatrist[b] % | (se) | Any % | (se) | General medical[d] % | (se) | Any % | (se) | Non-health care — Human services[d] % | (se) | CAM[e] % | (se) | Any % | (se) | Any service use % | (se) | Unweighted N with mental disorder | Weighted N with mental disorder |
|---|---|---|---|---|---|---|---|---|---|---|---|---|---|---|---|---|---|---|---|---|---|
| **I. Anxiety disorder** | | | | | | | | | | | | | | | | | | | | | |
| GAD* | Percentage in treatment | – | (–) | – | (–) | – | (–) | – | (–) | – | (–) | – | (–) | – | (–) | – | (–) | – | (–) | | |
| | Unweighted N in treatment | 1 | | 2 | | 3 | | 14 | | 15 | | 1 | | 2 | | 2 | | 15 | | 28 | 29 |
| Panic disorder* | Percentage in treatment | 19.4 | (7.1) | 6.7 | (4.6) | 22.4 | (8.6) | 62.1 | (7.4) | 65.7 | (7.1) | 0 | | 2.8 | (2.8) | 2.8 | (2.8) | 65.7 | (7.1) | | |
| | Unweighted N in treatment | 6 | | 2 | | 7 | | 18 | | 19 | | 0 | | 1 | | 2 | | 19 | | 30 | 31 |
| Agoraphobia without panic* | Percentage in treatment | – | (–) | – | (–) | – | (–) | – | (–) | – | (–) | – | (–) | – | (–) | – | (–) | – | (–) | | |
| | Unweighted N in treatment | 1 | | 2 | | 2 | | 6 | | 7 | | 0 | | 0 | | 0 | | 7 | | 16 | 20 |
| Social phobia* | Percentage in treatment | 5.1 | (3.6) | 3.5 | (3.3) | 8.6 | (4.7) | 20.1 | (5.8) | 28.6 | (7.4) | 1.4 | (1.4) | 0 | | 1.4 | (1.4) | 28.6 | (7.4) | | |
| | Unweighted N in treatment | 2 | | 1 | | 3 | | 10 | | 13 | | 1 | | 0 | | 1 | | 13 | | 49 | 48 |
| Specific phobia* | Percentage in treatment | 3.6 | (1.6) | 3.1 | (1.5) | 4.8 | (1.8) | 17.3 | (3.0) | 18.7 | (3.2) | 1.3 | (0.9) | 0.6 | (0.6) | 1.9 | (1.4) | 20.5 | (3.5) | | |
| | Unweighted N in treatment | 6 | | 5 | | 8 | | 27 | | 29 | | 2 | | 1 | | 3 | | 32 | | 161 | 164 |
| Adult separation anxiety disorder** | Percentage in treatment | – | (–) | 0 | (–) | – | (–) | – | (–) | – | (–) | – | (–) | – | (–) | – | (–) | – | (–) | | |
| | Unweighted N in treatment | 0 | | 0 | | 0 | | 0 | | 0 | | 0 | | 0 | | 0 | | 0 | | 0 | 0 |
| Posttraumatic stress disorder** | Percentage in treatment | – | (–) | – | (–) | – | (–) | – | (–) | – | (–) | – | (–) | – | (–) | – | (–) | – | (–) | | |
| | Unweighted N in treatment | 1 | | 0 | | 1 | | 8 | | 9 | | 0 | | 0 | | 0 | | 9 | | 24 | 13 |
| Any** | Percentage in treatment | 6.4 | (2.4) | 4.6 | (2.0) | 8.7 | (2.8) | 26.1 | (3.4) | 29.4 | (3.7) | 1.4 | (0.7) | 0.9 | (0.5) | 2 | (1.0) | 30.5 | (3.7) | | |
| | Unweighted N in treatment | 13 | | 9 | | 18 | | 58 | | 65 | | 4 | | 3 | | 6 | | 68 | | 183 | 109 |

| | | | | | | | | | | | | | | | | | | | | | |
|---|---|---|---|---|---|---|---|---|---|---|---|---|---|---|---|---|---|---|---|---|---|
| **II. Mood disorder** | | | | | | | | | | | | | | | | | | | | | |
| Major depressive episode* | Percentage in treatment | 12.3 | (3.9) | 7 | (2.7) | 14.5 | (4.4) | 35.6 | (5.4) | 38.9 | (5.7) | 1.8 | (1.1) | 1.3 | (0.9) | 2.4 | (1.2) | 39.5 | (5.5) | 129 | 141 |
| | Unweighted *N* in treatment | 15 | | 8 | | 19 | | 45 | | 50 | | 3 | | 2 | | 4 | | 51 | | | |
| Dysthymia* | Percentage in treatment | 8.7 | (2.8) | 6.8 | (3.9) | 12.8 | (3.8) | 24.3 | (6.2) | 27.5 | (6.5) | 1.6 | (1.6) | 0 | 0 | 1.6 | (1.6) | 27.5 | (6.5) | 43 | 44 |
| | Unweighted *N* in treatment | 4 | | 3 | | 6 | | 11 | | 13 | | 1 | | 0 | | 1 | | 13 | | | |
| Any* | Percentage in treatment | 10.8 | (3.5) | 6.7 | (2.5) | 13.7 | (4.0) | 32.4 | (4.7) | 35.8 | (5.1) | 1.6 | (0.9) | 1.2 | (0.8) | 2.1 | (1.1) | 36.3 | (4.9) | 148 | 160 |
| | Unweighted *N* in treatment | 15 | | 9 | | 20 | | 47 | | 53 | | 3 | | 2 | | 4 | | 54 | | | |
| **III. Substance disorder** | | | | | | | | | | | | | | | | | | | | | |
| Alcohol disorder* | Percentage in treatment | – | (–) | – | (–) | – | (–) | – | (–) | – | (–) | – | (–) | – | (–) | – | (–) | – | (–) | 7 | 8 |
| | Unweighted *N* in treatment | 0 | | 0 | | 0 | | 1 | | 1 | | 0 | | 0 | | 0 | | 1 | | | |
| Alcohol abuse with dependence* | Percentage in treatment | – | (–) | – | (–) | – | (–) | – | (–) | – | (–) | – | (–) | – | (–) | – | (–) | – | (–) | 4 | 4 |
| | Unweighted *N* in treatment | 0 | | 0 | | 0 | | 1 | | 1 | | 0 | | 0 | | 0 | | 1 | | | |
| Any* | Percentage in treatment | – | (–) | – | (–) | – | (–) | – | (–) | – | (–) | – | (–) | – | (–) | – | (–) | – | (–) | 7 | 8 |
| | Unweighted *N* in treatment | 0 | | 0 | | 0 | | 1 | | 1 | | 0 | | 0 | | 0 | | 1 | | | |
| **IV. Composite** | | | | | | | | | | | | | | | | | | | | | |
| Any disorder** | Percentage in treatment | 6.6 | (2.1) | 4.3 | (1.5) | 9 | (2.4) | 23 | (2.7) | 26.3 | (2.9) | 1.3 | (0.6) | 0.7 | (0.4) | 1.7 | (0.7) | 27.3 | (2.9) | 270 | 148 |
| | Unweighted *N* in treatment | 20 | | 13 | | 28 | | 72 | | 83 | | 5 | | 3 | | 7 | | 87 | | | |
| No disorder** | Percentage in treatment | 0.9 | (0.2) | 0.6 | (0.3) | 1.4 | (0.3) | 1.2 | (0.3) | 2.1 | (0.4) | 0.3 | (0.1) | 0 | 0 | 0.3 | (0.1) | 2.2 | (0.4) | 1509 | 1631 |
| | Unweighted *N* in treatment | 20 | | 12 | | 27 | | 35 | | 49 | | 10 | | 1 | | 10 | | 54 | | | |
| Total Part 2 sample** | Percentage in treatment | 1.4 | (0.2) | 0.9 | (0.3) | 2 | (0.3) | 3 | (0.3) | 4.1 | (0.4) | 0.4 | (0.1) | 0.1 | 0 | 0.4 | (0.1) | 4.3 | (0.4) | 1779 | 1779 |
| | Unweighted *N* in treatment | 40 | | 25 | | 55 | | 107 | | 132 | | 15 | | 4 | | 17 | | 141 | | | |
| | Weighted *N* in treatment | 24 | | 16 | | 36 | | 54 | | 73 | | 7 | | 1 | | 8 | | 76 | | | |

*Note:* Disorders with unweighted *n* less than 30 do not have percentages.

[a] Nonpsychiatrist is defined as psychologist or other nonpsychiatrist mental health professional in any setting, social worker or counselor in a mental health specialty setting, use of a mental health hotline.

Table 17.11. Median number of visits in separate service sectors among patients treated in those sectors by 12-month DSM-IV/CIDI disorder[a]

| | Health care | | | | | Non-health care | | | Any service use |
|---|---|---|---|---|---|---|---|---|---|
| | Mental health specialty | | | General medical[c] | Any | Human services[d] | CAM[e] | Any | |
| | Psychiatrist | Nonpsychiatrist[b] | Any | | | | | | |
| I. Any anxiety disorder** | – | – | – | 1.6 (0.1) | 1.8 (0.6) | – | – | – | 1.9 (0.6) |
| II. Any mood disorder* | – | – | – | 1.8 (0.5) | 1.9 (0.7) | – | – | – | 1.9 (0.9) |
| III. Any substance disorder* | – | – | – | – | – | – | – | – | – |
| IV. Composite | | | | | | | | | |
| Any disorder** | – | – | – | 1.7 (0.1) | 1.9 (0.6) | – | – | – | 1.9 (0.6) |
| No disorder** | – | – | – | 1.8 (0.3) | 2.8 (0.5) | – | – | – | 3.0 (0.5) |
| Total Part 2 sample** | 1.9 (1.4) | – | 2.6 (0.8) | 1.7 (0.1) | 2.3 (0.5) | – | – | – | 2.5 (0.5) |

[a] Values are medians with standard errors in parentheses. Missing cell entries indicate that the number of patients with the disorder who were treated in the sector was less than 30, in which case no estimate was made.

[b] Nonpsychiatrist is defined as psychologist or other nonpsychiatrist mental health professional in any setting, social worker or counselor in a mental health specialty setting, use of a mental health hotline.

[c] General medical is defined as primary care doctor, other general medical doctor, nurse, any other health professional not previously mentioned.

[d] Human services professional defined as religious or spiritual advisor, social worker, or counselor in any setting other than a specialty mental health setting.

[e] CAM is defined as any other type of healer, participation in an Internet support group, or participation in a self-help group.

* Denotes Part 1 weight.

** Denotes Part 2 weight.

**Table 17.12.** Percentage of patients who received at least minimally adequate treatment in those sectors by 12-month DSM-IV/CIDI disorder[a]

| | | Health care | | | | | | | | | Non–health care | | | | | | Any service use | | Unweighted N with mental disorder | Weighted N with mental disorder |
|---|---|---|---|---|---|---|---|---|---|---|---|---|---|---|---|---|---|---|---|---|---|
| | | Mental health specialty | | | | | | General medical[c] | | Any | | Human services[d] | | CAM[e] | | Any | | | | | |
| Disorder group | Measure | Psychiatrist % | (se) | Nonpsychiatrist[b] % | (se) | Any % | (se) | % | (se) | % | (se) | % | (se) | % | (se) | % | (se) | % | (se) | | |
| I. Any anxiety disorder** | % getting minimally adequate treatment | – | – | – | – | – | – | 81.1 | (6.2) | 82.1 | (5.6) | – | – | – | – | – | – | 82.8 | (5.5) | 183 | 109 |
| | Unweighted N in treatment | 13 | | 9 | | 18 | | 58 | | 65 | | 4 | | 3 | | 6 | | 68 | | | |
| II. Any mood disorder* | % getting minimally adequate treatment | – | – | – | – | – | – | 86.3 | (5.7) | 86.1 | (5.6) | – | – | – | – | – | – | – | – | 148 | 160 |
| | Unweighted N in treatment | 15 | | 9 | | 20 | | 11 | | 13 | | 1 | | 0 | | 1 | | 13 | | | |
| III. Any substance disorder* | % getting minimally adequate treatment | – | – | – | – | – | – | – | – | – | – | – | – | – | – | – | – | – | – | 7 | 8 |
| | Unweighted N in treatment | 0 | | 0 | | 0 | | 1 | | 1 | | 0 | | 0 | | 0 | | 1 | | | |
| IV. Composite Any disorder** | % getting minimally adequate treatment | – | – | – | – | – | – | 82.5 | (5.6) | 82.9 | (5.2) | – | – | – | – | – | – | 82.7 | (5.0) | 270 | 148 |
| | Unweighted N in treatment | 20 | | 13 | | 28 | | 72 | | 83 | | 5 | | 3 | | 7 | | 87 | | | |
| V. Composite No disorder** | % getting minimally adequate treatment | – | – | – | – | – | – | 88.6 | (5.3) | 90.6 | (3.4) | – | – | – | – | – | – | 91.0 | (3.2) | 1509 | 1631 |
| | Unweighted N in treatment | 20 | | 12 | | 27 | | 35 | | 49 | | 10 | | 1 | | 10 | | 54 | | | |
| Total Part 2 sample** | % getting minimally adequate treatment | 96.3 | (2.3) | – | – | 95.5 | (2.0) | 84.8 | (4.2) | 86.5 | (3.3) | – | – | – | – | – | – | 86.6 | (3.2) | 1779 | 1779 |
| | Unweighted N in treatment | 40 | | 25 | | 55 | | 107 | | 132 | | 15 | | 4 | | 17 | | 141 | | | |
| | Weighted N in treatment | 24 | | 16 | | 36 | | 54 | | 73 | | 7 | | 1 | | 8 | | 76 | | | |

[a] Missing cell entries indicate that the number of patients with the disorder who were treated in the sector was less than 30, in which case no estimate was made.

[b] Nonpsychiatrist defined as psychologists or other nonpsychiatrist mental health professional in any setting, social worker or counselor in a mental health specialty setting. Use of a mental health hotline removed from definition as it is not considered adequate treatment.

[c] General medical defined as primary care doctor, other general medical doctor, nurse, any other health professional not previously mentioned.

[d] Human services professional defined as religious or spiritual advisor, social worker, or counselor in any setting other than a specialty mental health setting.

* Denotes Part 1 weight.   ** Denotes Part 2 weight.

## 3.13. Sociodemographic and Disorder-type Predictors of any 12-month Treatment

As shown in Table 17.13, receiving any 12-month health treatment is significantly related to having any anxiety or mood disorders. No significant sociodemographic correlates were found.

## 4. DISCUSSION

The results of this survey suggest that roughly one out of every five Italians has experienced a DSM-IV common mental disorder at some time in his or her life, and that roughly one person out of every 12 has had an episode of such a disorder in the prior year. Major depression and specific phobias were estimated to be the most common individual disorders, as they were in many other WMH countries. Roughly one out of every ten Italians was estimated to have an episode of major depression at some time in his or her life and 3% in the past year. Nearly 6% of subjects met criteria for a specific phobia at some time in their life and 3.5% in the past year. In our sample, the risk of any common mental disorder was almost three times greater among women than among men.

The low estimated prevalence of alcohol use disorders (0.2%, 1-month and 12-month prevalence; 1.3%, lifetime) requires discussion, as it seems too low on an intuitive basis as well as considering that mortality from cirrhosis during the period 1997–2001 was substantial in Italy, 26.5 per 100,000 for men and 12.2 per 100,000 for women (Leon & McCambridge 2006). To check the accuracy of this estimate, a random sample of 315 spouses was interviewed. Among the spouses interviewed, two spouses responded that the subject had "often" drunk alcohol to excess in the prior year, two reported "sometimes," and five "rarely," but in none of these cases did the information provided by the main respondent meet criteria for alcohol use disorder. The frequency of spouses' responses that the subject "often" drank to excess (0.6%) was higher than the 12-month prevalence estimate of self-reported alcohol disorder (0.1%), although the number of cases is too small to draw any firm conclusions. A number of other observations place in question the accuracy

**Table 17.13.** Demographic and disorder-type predictors of any 12-month service use

|  | Any treatment given for any 12-month disorder | |
| --- | --- | --- |
|  | OR | (95% CI) |
| **I. Age** | | |
| 18–34 | 0.5 | (0.2–1.8) |
| 35–49 | 0.9 | (0.3–2.4) |
| 50–64 | 2.0 | (0.8–5.1) |
| 65+ | 1.0 | – |
| $\chi^2_3$ | 6.6 | |
| **II. Sex** | | |
| Female | 1.0 | (0.3–1.7) |
| Male | 0.7 | – |
| $\chi^2_1$ | 0.6 | |
| **III. Education** | | |
| Primary | 0.3 | (0.1–1.2) |
| Secondary | 0.7 | (0.2–2.0) |
| High school | 0.4 | (0.1–1.4) |
| Some college | 1.0 | – |
| $\chi^2_3$ | 3.5 | |
| **IV. Marital status** | | |
| Married-cohabiting | 1.0 | – |
| Previously married | 1.2 | (0.4–3.4) |
| Never married | 2.0 | (1.0–4.1) |
| $\chi^2_2$ | 4.1 | |
| **V. Family income** | | |
| Low | 2.1 | (0.8–5.8) |
| Low-average | 0.7 | (0.2–2.1) |
| High-average | 0.8 | (0.3–2.6) |
| High | 1.0 | – |
| $\chi^2_3$ | 5.5 | |
| **VI. Any anxiety** | | |
| Yes | 7.5* | (3.6–15.7) |
| No | 1.0 | – |
| $\chi^2_1$ | 30.8* | |
| **VII. Any mood** | | |
| Yes | 5.6* | (2.4–12.9) |
| No | 1.0 | – |
| $\chi^2_1$ | 17.3* | |
| **VIII. Any substance** | | |
| Yes | 1.8 | (0.3–10.6) |
| No | 1.0 | – |
| $\chi^2_1$ | 0.5 | |

* Significant at the 0.05 level, two-sided test.

of the finding of very low rates of alcohol use disorder in Italy.

Other data suggesting that the estimate of alcohol disorder in our survey is too low come from a recent study of drinking habits and physical health of the adult inhabitants of two northern Italian towns that found that 3.9% of the sample consumed more than 90 grams of alcohol (more than a bottle of wine) a day and that 3.7% of the sample showed persistent signs of alcohol-related liver damage (Bellentani et al. 1997). A similar study of adult subjects selected at random from the population of the Lazio Region established that 8.3% of men and 2.6% of women exceeded the daily alcohol consumption recommended by the Italian Society for Human Nutrition (60 grams a day for men and 40 grams for women) (Scafato et al. 1999). Another survey of alcohol use, this one conducted in a northern Italian rural area, estimated the 12-month prevalence of alcohol-related problems to be 1.9% in those older than age 15 (Corrao et al. 2000). All of these studies, which focused specifically on alcohol consumption, reported substantially higher prevalence rates of excess consumption and alcohol-related problems, and suggest that the 12-month prevalence rate of 0.2% for alcohol use disorder found in our survey is likely to be an underestimate. On the other hand, the recent survey carried out in Sesto Fiorentino (near Florence) using the MINI to investigate rates of common mental disorder, and not focusing solely on alcohol abuse/dependence, found low rates of substance use disorder, similar to our finding, with a combined 12-month prevalence of any alcohol and drug use disorders of 0.2% and a lifetime prevalence of 0.7% (Faravelli et al. 2004a, 2004b). It seems unlikely, therefore, that the low rate of alcohol use disorder detected in our study was a consequence of the survey instrument used, the CIDI, especially because all the other European countries surveyed in the ESEMeD-WMH study using this instrument recorded significantly higher 12-month (0.3%–3.0%) prevalence rates of any alcohol use disorder than did Italy.

A possible conclusion to draw from these findings is that the social acceptance of the consumption of substantial amounts of alcohol in Italy discourages subjects from reporting their use pattern as being problematic in a general psychiatric survey, and that interview techniques specifically focused on alcohol use are necessary to gather accurate information on this subject in this cultural context. An alternate explanation is that, while the prevalence of excessive use of alcohol and its health-related effects, such as cirrhosis, are high in Italy, the pattern of alcohol use is such that it produces less social harm. This might be true, for example, if the common use pattern in Italy were consistent daily consumption of substantial amounts of wine rather than the binge consumption of excessive quantities of spirits. Such differences in the use of alcohol between northern Europe and the wine-producing countries of southern Europe have previously been noted (Rehm et al. 2005; Leon & McCambridge 2006) and may help explain the general finding that the countries with the lowest detected rates of alcohol use disorder in the ESEMeD series (i.e., Italy, Spain, and France) have relatively high rates of cirrhosis compared to other European countries (Leon & McCambridge 2006). Consistent with this possibility, Rehm and colleagues (2005) observed that the national prevalence of alcohol use disorder in Europe is negatively correlated with per capita alcohol consumption rates but positively correlated with the Hazardous Drinking Score, a measure of binge drinking. The low Italian prevalence of alcohol use disorder in the present study appears to fit this pattern.

## 5. THE 12-MONTH PREVALENCE OF MENTAL DISORDERS IN ITALY COMPARED TO OTHER EUROPEAN COUNTRIES

The estimated 12-month prevalence of any mental disorder, any mood disorder, any anxiety disorder, and any alcohol use disorder in our survey are lower than in any of the other European countries surveyed as part of the ESEMeD project. The 12-month prevalence estimates in every category of mental disorder were more than twice as high in France and close to twice as high in the Netherlands as in Italy. A recent meta-analysis of 27 epidemiological studies conducted in

16 European countries revealed average prevalence rates of each category of mental disorder to
be at least twice as high across Europe as in this
Italian sample (Wittchen & Jacobi 2005).

What are the possible explanations of this
finding? Nonresponse rates do not appear to
explain the difference in prevalence. Many researchers argue that community survey subjects
who refuse to be interviewed or are untraceable
have a greater probability of suffering from a
mental disorder than do survey participants (de
Graaf et al. 2000). In the ESEMeD series, though,
the highest prevalence estimates of DSM-IV disorders were found in France and the Netherlands,
the countries with the lowest rates of subject
participation.

It is possible that the number of subjects
excluded because they were institutionalized or
without a fixed address affected the prevalence
rates detected. However, the small number of
such subjects renders this possibility unlikely.
According to the Italian governmental database
(ISTAT 1999), the number of people aged 18 or
older who were institutionalized in 1999 totaled
only 0.6% of the Italian population (301,904, of
whom 263,084 were residents of nursing homes
or similar facilities and of whom 38,820 were in
jail). Also excluded from the Italian sample were
immigrants, a group that is larger than the institutionalized population and that may have a
higher prevalence of common mental disorders.
To explore the effect of the exclusion of this group
further, it would be necessary to conduct epidemiological studies of mental disorders in different ethnic immigrant groups.

A common explanation for variations in
prevalence among different studies has to do
with different assessment instruments used (Patten 2003). This explanation does not apply to
the ESEMeD-WMH study, as the same diagnostic instruments were employed in all countries.
Another possible explanation is national differences in the propensity for individuals to reveal
details of their personal and emotional lives,
which might well be influenced by differences
in the degree of stigma attached to mental disorders (WHO International Consortium in Psychiatric Epidemiology 2000; Patten 2003). At least
some of the difference in prevalence rates for

common mental disorders described in various
reviews of population studies (Kohn, Dohrenwend & Mirotznik 1998; de Girolamo & Bassi
2003; Patten 2003) is likely to be due to real differences in the frequency of occurrence of these disorders, in turn related to interactions among the
environment, biological factors, lifestyle, interpersonal relationships, and socioeconomic factors. Interestingly, the prevalence rates of nonmental disorders similarly appear to vary quite
substantially from country to country. A recent
review of prevalence rates of 17 chronic physical illnesses in eight European nations (including all the European countries participating in
the ESEMeD project, except Germany) revealed
marked differences in all prevalence rates among
countries, in some cases as great as 20 to 1
(Dalstra et al. 2005).

Comparisons of the results reported here with
those in previous Italian epidemiological studies must be made with caution, as each previous study used a somewhat different method of
sample selection and different assessment instrument. The prevalences estimated in our survey
are generally similar to those found in the recent
study in Sesto Fiorentino mentioned previously
(Faravelli et al. 2004a, 2004b). The 12-month
prevalence estimate of all mental disorders was
7.3% in our survey, compared to 8.6% in that
in Sesto Fiorentino. The 12-month prevalence
of all mental disorders in the two sexes was also
similar: 3.9% among men and 10.4% in women
in our survey versus 5.4% and 12.1%, respectively, in the Sesto Fiorentino survey. The lifetime prevalence estimates for all mental disorders combined were also similar: 7.2% of men
and 14.9% of women were estimated to have a
lifetime depressive disorder in our survey, compared to 6.5% of men and 15.8% of women in the
Sesto Fiorentino survey. In our survey, 5.5% of
men and 16.2% of women were estimated to have
a lifetime history of any anxiety disorder, compared to 7.0% of men and 14.9% of women in the
Sesto Fiorentino survey. The 12-month prevalence estimate of any anxiety disorder was somewhat greater among men in our survey (3.9%)
than in the Sesto Fiorentino survey (2.2%), but
the prevalence estimate among women was very
similar (roughly 8%) in the two surveys.

The prevalence estimates in the current study are also similar to those observed in the two studies conducted recently in Jesi (Gigantesco et al. 2006), the first using the PSE-9 and the second using the CIDI. This consistency suggests that the comparatively low prevalence estimates found in our survey relative to those in the WMH surveys in other Western European countries reflects a genuinely lower prevalence of psychopathology in Italy than in these other countries. To confirm this suspicion, more detailed clinical reappraisal studies are needed in future rounds of the Western European WMH surveys than were carried out in the current surveys.

The associations of sociodemographic variables with mental disorders in our survey are in many ways similar to that observed in previous research. Overall prevalence of mental disorder is commonly found to be higher in women than men, and this is almost always true for the gender difference in depression (Bebbington 1988). In general, the elevated risk of depressive disorder in women lies between 1.0 and 3.0, with a range from 1.4 to 2.7 (Kessler 2003). A meta-analysis of European studies conducted using the General Health Questionnaire or the CIDI concluded that the risk of depressive disorder was twice as great in women as in men (Fryers et al. 2004). Men and women have comparable prevalence of the functional psychoses, schizophrenia, and bipolar disorder (Warner & de Girolamo 1995; Tsuchiya, Byrne & Mortensen 2003). Men have a higher prevalence than women of alcohol and substance abuse/dependence (Day & Homish 2002) and antisocial personality disorder (de Girolamo & Reich 1993).

In our survey, no substantial differences were observed in the distribution of different mental disorders across the age range of the sample, or by education, income, or to a lesser degree, marital status, although never married people had a significantly higher prevalence of anxiety disorders than did other respondents. This generally nonsignificant pattern of associations means that even though mental disorders have a relatively low prevalence in Italy compared to other Western European countries, they are widely distributed in the population on the basis of sociodemographic characteristics rather than highly concentrated in any one segment of society.

The comparatively low rate of treatment for mental disorders among young people in the current survey is worrisome, as our data show that most of the common mental disorders begin relatively early in life. There is some reason to believe that lack of timely treatment can lead to self-medication and substance use disorders. Among individuals with a formal diagnosis of a mental disorder, primary care consultation for mental problems is the most commonly reported modality of use of health services (more than two-thirds of individuals), which indicates that the GP still has the predominant role in managing formal mental disorders in Italy. The fact that young people are not frequent users of primary care services in general might help account for the low rate of treatment among young Italians with a mental disorder.

Particularly noteworthy is the significantly lower probability of use of mental health services among people with mental disorders in Italy than in the other ESEMeD countries. Possible reasons for this pattern might be lower provision of mental health services in Italy than other developed European countries, underrecognition, and poor liaison between primary care and mental health specialized care providers. Other possible reasons may be stigma, denial, and failure to perceive need for services. Further research is needed to improve our understanding of the relative importance of these factors in an effort to target modifiable barriers to treatment that could be the focus of intervention efforts. The adoption of formal recommendations for recognition and treatment of mental disorders needs to be considered. The importance of the review of Italian health system in eliciting psychiatric symptoms should receive emphasis in clinical training.

## REFERENCES

American Psychiatric Association (1994). *Diagnostic and statistical manual of mental disorders (DSM-IV)*, 4th ed. Washington, DC: American Psychiatric Association.

Bebbington, P. E. (1988). The social epidemiology of clinical depression. In *Handbook of social psychiatry*, ed. A. S. Henderson & G. D. Burrows, pp. 87–102. Amsterdam: Elsevier.

Bellentani S., Saccoccio, G., Costa, G., Tiribelli, C., Manenti, F., Sodde, M., Saveria Croce, L., Sasso, F., Pozzato, G., Cristianini, G. & Brandi, G. (1997). Drinking habits as cofactors of risk for alcohol induced liver damage: The Dionysos Study Group. *Gut*, 41, 845–50.

Corrao, G., Bagnardi, V., Vittadini, G. & Favilli, S. (2000). Capture-recapture methods to size alcohol related problems in a population. *Journal of Epidemiology and Community Health*, 54, 603–10.

Dalstra, J. A., Kunst, A. E., Borrell, C., Breeze, E., Cambois, E., Costa, G., Geurts, J. J., Lahelma, E., Van Oyen, H., Rasmussen, N. K., Regidor, E., Spadea, T. & Mackenbach, J. P. (2005). Socioeconomic differences in the prevalence of common chronic diseases: An overview of eight European countries. *International Journal of Epidemiology*, 28, 316–26.

Day, N. L. & Homish, G. G. (2002). The epidemiology of alcohol use, abuse, and dependence. In *Textbook in psychiatric epidemiology*, 2d ed., ed. M. T. Tsuang & M. Tohen, pp. 459–77. Chichester, UK: John Wiley & Sons.

de Girolamo, G. & Bassi, M. (2003). Community surveys of mental disorders: Recent achievements and works in progress. *Current Opinion in Psychiatry*, 16, 403–11.

de Girolamo, G., Bassi, M., Neri, G., Ruggeri, M., Santone, G. & Picardi, A. (2007). The current state of mental health care in Italy: Problems, perspectives, and lessons to learn. *European Archives of Psychiatry and Clinical Neuroscience*, 257, 83–91.

de Girolamo, G., Polidori, G., Morosini, G., Scarpino, V., Reda, V., Serra, G., Mazzi, F., Visonà, G., Falsirollo, F. & Rossi, A. (2005). Prevalenza dei disturbi mentali in Italia, fattori di rischio, stato di salute ed uso dei servizi sanitari: Il progetto ESEMeD-WMH. *Epidemiologia e Psichiatria Sociale*, suppl. 8, 1–100.

de Girolamo, G. & Reich, J. (1993). *Personality disorders*, WHO Series on Epidemiology of Mental Disorders and Psychosocial Problems, Vol. 1. Geneva: World Health Organization.

de Graaf, R., Bijl, R. V., Smit, F., Ravelli, A. & Vollebergh, W. A. (2000). Psychiatric and sociodemographic predictors of attrition in a longitudinal study: The Netherlands Mental Health Survey and Incidence Study (NEMESIS). *American Journal of Epidemiology*, 152, 1039–47.

Efron, B. (1988). Logistic regression, survival analysis, and the Kaplan-Meier curve. *Journal of the American Statistical Association*, 83, 414–25.

ESEMeD/MHEDEA 2000 investigators (2004). Sampling and methods of the European Study of the Epidemiology of Mental Disorders (ESEMeD) project. *Acta Psychiatrica Scandinavica*, 109, 8–20.

Faravelli, C., Abrardi, L., Bartolozzi, D., Cecchi, C., Cosci, F., D'Adamo, D., Lo Iacono, B., Ravaldi, C., Scarpato, M. A., Truglia, E. & Rosi, S. (2004a). The Sesto Fiorentino Study: Background, methods and preliminary results; Lifetime prevalence of psychiatric disorders in an Italian community sample using clinical interviewers. *Psychotherapy and Psychosomatics*, 73, 216–25.

Faravelli, C., Abrardi, L., Bartolozzi, D., Cecchi, C., Cosci, F., D'Adamo, D., Lo Iacono, B., Ravaldi, C., Scarpato, M. A., Truglia, E., Rossi Prodi, P. M. & Rosi, S. (2004b). The Sesto Fiorentino study: Point and one-year prevalences of psychiatric disorders in an Italian community sample using clinical interviewers. *Psychotherapy and Psychosomatics*, 73, 226–34.

Fryers, T., Brugha, T., Morgan, Z., Smith, J., Hill, T., Carta, M., Lehtinen, V. & Kovess, V. (2004). Prevalence of psychiatric disorder in Europe: The potential and reality of meta-analysis. *Social Psychiatry and Psychiatric Epidemiology*, 39, 899–905.

Gigantesco, A., Palumbo, G., Mirabella, F., Pettinelli, M. & Morosini, P. (2006). Prevalence of psychiatric disorders in an Italian town: Low prevalence confirmed with two different interviews. *Psychotherapy and Psychosomatics*, 75, 170–6.

Hosmer, D. W. & Lemeshow, S. (1989). *Applied logistic regression*. New York: John Wiley & Sons.

Kessler, R. C. (2003). The epidemiology of women and depression. *Journal of Affective Disorders*, 74, 5–13.

Kessler, R. C., Haro, J. M., Heeringa, S. G., Pennell, B.-E. & Üstün, T. B. (2006). The World Health Organization World Mental Health Survey Initiative. *Epidemiologia e Psichiatria Sociale*, 15, 161–6.

Kessler, R. C. & Üstün, T. B. (2004). The World Mental Health (WMH) Survey Initiative Version of the World Health Organization (WHO) Composite International Diagnostic Interview (CIDI). *International Journal of Methods in Psychiatric Research*, 13, 93–121.

Kohn, R., Dohrenwend, B. & Mirotznik, J. (1998). Epidemiological findings on selected psychiatric disorders in the general population. In *Adversity, stress and psychopathology*, ed. B. P. Dohrenwend, pp. 235–84. Cambridge, UK: Cambridge University Press.

ISTAT (Istituto Nazionale di Statistica) (1999). *La situazione del paese nel 1999*. Rome: ISTAT.

Leon, D. A. & McCambridge, J. (2006). Liver cirrhosis mortality rates from Britain, 1950 to 2002: An analysis of routine data. *Lancet*, 367, 52–6.

Maio, V. & Manzoli, L. (2002). The Italian health care system: WHO ranking versus public perception. *Pharmacy and Therapeutics*, 27, 301–8.

Palermo, G. B. (1991). The 1978 Italian mental health law – a personal evaluation: A review. *Journal of the Royal Society of Medicine*, 84, 99–102.

Patten, S. B. (2003). International differences in major depression prevalence: What do they mean? *Journal of Clinical Epidemiology*, 56, 711–6.

Piccinelli, M., Politi, P. & Barale, F. (2002). Focus on psychiatry in Italy. *British Journal of Psychiatry*, 181, 538–44.

Rehm, J., Room, R., van den Brink, W. & Jacobi, F. (2005). Alcohol use disorders in EU countries and Norway: An overview of the epidemiology. *European Neuropsychopharmacology*, 15, 377–88.

Research Triangle Institute (2002). *SUDAAN: Professional software for survey data analysis 8.01.* Research Triangle Park, NC: Research Triangle Institute.

Scafato, E., Attili A. F., Farchi, R., Capocaccia, R., Giampaoli, S., Giorni Rossi, A. & Capocaccia, L. (1999). Alcohol consumption and drinking patterns in an Italian general population survey: The CO.A.L.A. project (alcohol consumption in the Latium region). *Alcologia*, 11, 121–34.

Tsuchiya, K. J., Byrne, M. & Mortensen, P. B. (2003). Risk factors in relation to an emergence of bipolar disorder: A systematic review. *Bipolar Disorders*, 5, 231–42.

Warner, R. & de Girolamo, G. (1995). *Schizophrenia: Epidemiology of mental disorders and psychosocial problems*, Vol. 3. Geneva: World Health Organization.

WHO International Consortium in Psychiatric Epidemiology (2000). Cross-national comparisons of the prevalences and correlates of mental disorders. *Bulletin of the World Health Organization*, 78, 413–26.

Wittchen, H.-U. & Jacobi, F. (2005). Size and burden of mental disorders in Europe: A critical review and appraisal of 27 studies. *European Neuropsychopharmacology*, 15, 357–76.

World Health Organization (WHO) (1991). *International Classification of Diseases (ICD-10)*. Geneva: World Health Organization.

Zimmermann-Tansella, C. (1994). Epidemiologia dei disturbi psichiatrici nella popolazione generale: Le esperienze e i risultati italiani. *Epidemiologia e Psichiatria Sociale*, 3, 5–14.

# 18 Mental Disorders and Service Use in the Netherlands: Results from the European Study of the Epidemiology of Mental Disorders (ESEMeD)

RON DE GRAAF, JOHAN ORMEL, MARGREET TEN HAVE, HUIBERT BURGER, AND MARTINE BUIST-BOUWMAN

## ACKNOWLEDGMENTS

This study is part of the European Study on the Epidemiology of Mental Disorders (ESEMeD). This project was funded by the European Commission (Contract QLG5-1999-01042), the Piedmont Region (Italy), Fondo de Investigación Sanitaria, Instituto de Salud Carlos III, Spain (FIS 00/0028; Red Temática RIRAG 03/061), Ministerio de Ciencia y Tecnología, Spain (SAF 2000–158-CE), Departament de Salut, Generalitat de Catalunya, Spain, and other local agencies and by an unrestricted educational grant from GlaxoSmithKline. The ESEMeD project is carried out in conjunction with the World Health Organization World Mental Health (WMH) Survey Initiative. We thank the staff of the WMH Data Collection and Data Analysis Coordination Centres for assistance with instrumentation, fieldwork, and consultation on data analysis. These activities were supported by the National Institute of Mental Health (R01 MH070884), the John D. and Catherine T. MacArthur Foundation, the Pfizer Foundation, the U.S. Public Health Service (R13-MH066849, R01-MH069864, and R01 DA016558), the Fogarty International Center (FIRCA R03-TW006481), the Pan American Health Organization, Eli Lilly and Company Foundation, Ortho-McNeil Pharmaceutical, GlaxoSmithKline, and Bristol-Myers Squibb.

## 1. INTRODUCTION

The Dutch system of health care makes services for mental disorders much more readily available than in many other countries around the world (Stolk & Rutten 2005). Previous cross-national research has shown that a comparatively high proportion of Dutch people with mental disorders seek treatment compared to people with the same disorders in other countries (Bijl et al. 2003). Financial barriers to seeking treatment for mental disorders have also been shown to be lower in the Netherlands than other countries in comparative analyses of epidemiological data (Alegria et al. 2000). However, these results are now well more than a decade old, and it is not clear that such differences continue. A survey of the Netherlands was included in the European Study of the Epidemiology of Mental Disorders (ESEMeD/MHEDEA 2000 Investigators 2004a) to provide up-to-date data on this matter and to expand the investigation of the prevalence and consequences of mental disorders.

## 2. PREVIOUS PSYCHIATRIC EPIDEMIOLOGICAL STUDIES

In 1996, for the first time in the Netherlands, accurate general population data on mental disorders and service use were collected in the Netherlands Mental Health Survey and Incidence Study (NEMESIS) (Bijl et al. 1998b). Before that time, only regional data on the mental health status of the Dutch population were available, based on older instruments (Hodiamont 1986; van Limbeek et al. 1994). Nowadays, few people realize that before 1996 there was no accurate information about the prevalence of mental disorders in the general population of our country and of many other countries as well. So, gathering this type of data is a fairly recent phenomenon (Vollebergh et al. 2003). Indeed, psychiatric epidemiology lags behind most somatic branches of epidemiology. Although information from registries of service use can give useful information, general population data can give good insight into the determinants of use and unmet need, because both users and nonusers of mental health services are included in the study (ten Have 2004).

The first survey in the world employing modern methods with specific diagnostic criteria and reliable instruments to identify mental disorders was the Epidemiologic Catchment Area (ECA) study, conducted in the United States in the 1980s (Robins & Regier 1991). The ECA was followed by the National Comorbidity Survey (NCS) (Kessler et al. 1994). The ECA, NCS, and NEMESIS surveys showed that high lifetime and 12-month mental disorders are prevalent in the community and that unmet needs for services are widespread.

To shed light on the impacts of mental disorders and to provide up-to-date data on the care of mental disorders in Western Europe, ESEMeD was undertaken as part of the larger World Health Organization (WHO) World Mental Health (WMH) Survey Initiative (Kessler et al. 2006). This chapter describes data from the Dutch study regarding lifetime prevalence of mental disorders, lifetime service use, delay in initial treatment seeking, 12-month prevalence of disorders, 12-month service use, and their correlates. We refer the reader for more detailed information to recent publications, based on the data of all six countries of ESEMeD, on the methods of ESEMeD (ESEMeD/MHEDEA 2000 Investigators 2004a), and on the results on prevalence (ESEMeD/MHEDEA 2000 Investigators 2004b), psychiatric and somatic comorbidity (ESEMeD/MHEDEA 2000 investigators 2004c; Demyttenaere et al. 2006), functioning (ESEMeD/MHEDEA 2000 Investigators 2004d, 2006), and service use (ESEMeD/MHEDEA 2000 Investigators 2004e, 2004f; Kovess-Masfety et al. 2007).

## 3. METHODS

### 3.1. Sample

The Dutch substudy of ESEMeD is a nationally representative household survey of respondents aged 18 and older (ESEMeD/MHEDEA 2000 Investigators 2004a). Face-to-face interviews were carried out with 2372 respondents between December 2001 and August 2003. The sample frame was postal registries. The sampling frame had two stages. First, a random sample of addresses of households was selected, with an equal probability, from postal registries. Second, a random selection of the respondent in each of these households was made. Institutionalized individuals (i.e., those living in prisons, hospitals, hotels, or other institutions), as well as those not able to understand the Dutch language, were excluded from the study.

As the end of the data collection approached, to minimize nonresponse, the individuals who either had been difficult to reach or had refused to perform the interview were identified. A random subsample of individuals within these groups was approached to ask again for participation with a financial incentive for doing so. In the analysis, the results from the interviews obtained from this approach were weighted by the inverse of their probability of selection, to restore artificially the representation of the hard-to-reach segment of the population to the full sample (ESEMeD/MHEDEA 2000 Investigators 2004a). The overall weighted response rate was 56.4%. The recruitment, consent, and field procedures were approved by the ethics committee of the Netherlands Institute of Mental Health and Addiction, Utrecht, the Netherlands. A more detailed discussion of the sample design is presented elsewhere (ESEMeD/MHEDEA 2000 Investigators 2004a).

### 3.2. Measures

#### 3.2.1. Diagnostic Assessment of Lifetime and 12-Month DSM-IV Disorders

As discussed in Chapter 4 of this volume, DSM-IV diagnoses were made using Version 3.0 of the World Health Organization (WHO) Composite International Diagnostic Interview (CIDI) (Kessler & Üstün 2004), a fully structured lay-administered diagnostic interview that generates diagnoses according to the definitions and criteria of both the ICD-10 (World Health Organization 1991) and the DSM-IV (American Psychiatric Association 1994) diagnostic systems. DSM-IV criteria are used in analyses for this chapter.

The CIDI Version 3.0 was first produced in English and underwent a rigorous process of adaptation following guidelines recommended by the WHO to obtain a conceptually and cross-culturally comparable version in Dutch. This process included forward and back-translations, a review by a panel of experts, pretest using cognitive interview, and debriefing techniques (ESEMeD/MHEDEA 2000 Investigators 2004a).

To optimize the interviewing process and costs, a two-phase interview procedure was used. The first phase was administered to all respondents and contained the diagnostic assessment of the most common mood and anxiety disorders, health-related quality of life, health services use, and main demographic characteristics (Part 1). Only those who exceeded a number of symptoms of specific mood or anxiety disorders and a random 25% of the remainder entered the second phase, which included, among other information, an interview about additional mental disorders, chronic physical conditions, and risk factors (Part 2).

The disorders assessed in the first and second phase included mood disorders (major depressive episode and dysthymia [information on lifetime dysthymia is not presented as a result of skip problems in the ESEMeD questionnaire for the age of onset]), anxiety disorders (panic disorder, agoraphobia without panic, specific phobia, social phobia, generalized anxiety disorder [GAD], posttraumatic stress disorder [PTSD], and adult separation anxiety disorder), alcohol use disorders (alcohol abuse with or without dependence, and alcohol dependence with or without abuse), and impulse-control disorders (also often called externalizing disorders) (oppositional-defiant disorder, conduct disor-

der, and attention-deficit/hyperactivity disorder [ADHD]). Unfortunately, drug abuse and dependence could not be evaluated as substance use disorders as a result of problems in the skip logic of this section of the questionnaire. For reasons of accurate recall, separation anxiety disorder and the impulse-control disorders were assessed among subjects aged 18–44 years only. Lifetime prevalence, age of onset, and 12-month prevalence were assessed separately for each disorder (ESEMeD/MHEDEA 2000 Investigators 2004b, 2004c). All diagnoses are considered with organic exclusions and with diagnostic hierarchy rules. As described in Chapter 6 of this volume (Haro et al. 2006), a blinded clinical reappraisal study using the Structured Clinical Interview for DSM-IV (SCID) (First et al. 2002) showed generally good concordance between DSM-IV diagnoses based on the CIDI and the SCID for anxiety, mood, and substance disorders. The CIDI diagnoses of impulse-control disorders have not been validated, except for ADHD (Kessler et al. 2006).

### 3.2.2. Severity of 12-month Cases

Individuals with at least one 12-month mental disorder were classified in three severity groups (severe, moderate, or mild) according to the following criteria. Individuals were classified as severe if they fulfilled any of the following conditions: (1) attempted suicide within the past 12 months; (2) alcohol dependence with physiological dependence syndrome; (3) severe role impairment (scores from eight to ten) in at least two areas of the Sheehan Disability Scales (SDS) (Leon et al. 1997). Cases not defined as severe were defined as moderate if they had moderate role impairment in at least one domain of the SDS (i.e., score greater than four) or if they had alcohol dependence disorder without physiological dependence. All other individuals with mental disorders were classified as mild. As a result of an error in the CAPI program, some of the respondents with a major depressive episode were not assessed using the SDS. SDS values for those individuals were imputed using polytomous logistic regression models obtained from the available information to obtain a probability distribution and, based on that, a likely approximation of the unobserved scores. This classification scheme of severity reported here is somewhat more refined than the previously published one used in comparative analyses of all WMH surveys (Demyttenaere et al. 2004).

### 3.2.3. Initial Lifetime Treatment Contact

Near the end of each CIDI diagnostic section, respondents were asked whether they had ever in their life "talked to a medical doctor or other professional" about the disorder under investigation (ESEMeD/MHEDEA 2000 Investigators 2004d). In asking this question, the interviewer clarified that the term "other professional" was meant to apply broadly to include "psychologists, counselors, spiritual advisors, herbalists, acupuncturists, and any other healing professionals." Respondents who reported ever having talked to any of these professionals about the disorder in question were then asked how old they were the first time they did so. The response to this question was used to define age of first treatment contact.

### 3.2.4. Twelve-month Use of Mental Health Services

In addition to service use questions in each CIDI diagnostic section, a section on general service use was administered. All Part 2 respondents were asked whether they had ever received treatment for any "problems with your emotions or nerves or your use of alcohol or drugs." Separate assessments were made for different types of services. Follow-up questions asked about age at first and most recent contacts. Reports of 12-month service use were classified into the following categories: psychiatrist; nonpsychiatrist mental health specialist (psychologist or other nonpsychiatrist mental health professional in any setting, social worker or counselor in a mental health specialty setting, use of a mental health hotline); general medical provider (primary-care doctor, other general medical doctor, nurse, any other health professional not previously mentioned); human services professional (religious or spiritual advisor, social worker or counselor in any setting other than a specialty mental health setting); and complementary and alternative medicine (CAM) professional (any other type of healer such as chiropractors, participation in an Internet support group, participation in a self-help group). Psychiatrist and nonpsychiatrist specialist categories were combined into a broader category: the mental health specialty sector.

### 3.2.5. Predictor Variables

Predictor variables in the analyses of the lifetime prevalence and service use data include age of onset of the disorder (coded into four categories: 0–12, 13–19, 20–29, and 30+ years of age), age (defined by age at interview in the categories 18–34, 35–49, 50–64, 65+), sex, and education (four categories). Variables used in the analysis of 12-month data were age (defined the same as described previously), sex, per capita income of the respondent's household divided by the median income (four categories: low ≤0.5; low-average = 0.5–1.0; high-average = 1.0–2.0; high ≥2.0), partner status (married or cohabiting, previously married, never married), and education (none or some primary, complete primary, secondary, college).

### 3.3 Analysis Procedures

In the analyses, individuals were weighted to account for the different probabilities of selection within a household and among hard to reach individuals, as well as to restore age and sex of the Dutch general population. An additional weight was used in the Part 2 sample to adjust for differences in probability of selection into that sample.

When we compare the unweighted sociodemographic distributions with the weighted distributions (the latter representing population distributions), differences are found for sex and age. Males are underrepresented: 43.5% of the sample was male, while this figure is 49.1% in the population. Younger people aged 18–24 are also underrepresented: they consist of 5.6% of the sample, and 14.6% of the population, while people aged 50–64 and 65+ are overrepresented, consisting of 26.4% and 19.1%, respectively, of the sample, and 21.5% and 16.7%, respectively, of the population. The weights correct for these discrepancies between the sample and the population distributions.

Basic patterns of 12-month disorders were examined by computing proportions, means, and medians. Logistic regression analyses were used to study sociodemographic predictors of having 12-month disorders and of receiving any 12-month treatment in the total sample. Survival analysis was used to make estimated projections of cumulative lifetime probability of disorders and treatment contact from year of onset. The actuarial method implemented in SAS 8.2 (SAS Institute 2001) was used. To obtain projections of lifetime risk of specific mental disorders at the age of 75 years old, the Kaplan–Meier methodology implemented in SUDAAN V9.0 (Research Triangle Institute 2002) was used. Discrete-time survival analysis with person-year as the unit of analysis was used to examine correlates of lifetime disorder and lifetime treatment contact (Efron 1988).

Data were analyzed using SAS 8.2 for UNIX. The standard errors of ratio estimates, means, regression coefficients, and other statistics were estimated taking into account the sample design by using the Taylor series linearization method implemented in SUDAAN 9.0. Multivariate significance tests were made using Wald $\chi^2$ tests based on coefficient variance-covariance matrices that were adjusted for design effects using the Taylor series method. Statistical significance was evaluated using two-sided design-based tests and the 0.05 level of significance.

## 4. RESULTS

### 4.1. Lifetime Prevalence of DSM-IV Mental Disorders

Table 18.1 shows the lifetime prevalence of mental disorders. Almost one in three respondents reported a lifetime presence of any disorder

(31.7%). Of all respondents, 12.0% had two or more lifetime disorders, and 4.9% had three or more. Thus, among those subjects with a lifetime disorder, comorbidity is found among a substantial proportion (37.9%). Mood disorders (here, major depression only) (17.9%) and anxiety disorders (15.9%) are the most prevalent classes of disorders, followed by alcohol use disorders (8.9%) and impulse-control disorders (4.7%). The most common individual lifetime disorders are major depression (17.9%), alcohol abuse (8.4%), and specific phobia (7.6%). Lifetime PTSD is prevalent in 4.0% of the subjects.

### 4.2. Sociodemographic Correlates of Lifetime Mental Disorders

Table 18.1 shows that significant differences in lifetime prevalence among age groups occur for the any disorder category and for all classes of disorders, except impulse-control disorders (note that because the disorders were measured among subjects aged 18–44 years only, age differences were more difficult to find for this class). Any disorders were highest in the 35–49 (41.5%) and 50–64 (34.1%) age groups, lower in the youngest (18–34) age group (29.3%), and lowest in the oldest (65+) age group (16.6%). Any anxiety disorders were also highest in the 35–49 (21.7%) and 50–64 (18.6%) age groups, lower in the youngest (18–34) age group (13.2%), and lowest in the oldest (65+) age group (8.2%). A similar pattern was found for mood disorders. The pattern of alcohol use disorders shows a different picture: the prevalence is almost similar among the three youngest age groups (9.2%–11.1%), but the prevalence is very low among the oldest age group (1.9%).

Sex and educational level as correlates of lifetime risk of mental disorders are identified in survival analyses that adjusted for cohort effects (data not presented). Compared to male respondents, females have twice as high a risk for any anxiety disorder (OR = 2.3; 95% CI = 1.4–3.9) and mood disorder (OR = 2.3; 95% CI = 1.4–3.8). In contrast, females are at decreased risk for any alcohol use disorder (OR = 0.2; 95% CI = 0.2–0.4). No differences are found for any

**Table 18.1.** Lifetime prevalence of DSM-IV/CIDI disorders, by age

| | Total | | 18–34 | | 35–49 | | 50–64 | | 65+ | | $\chi_3^2$ |
|---|---|---|---|---|---|---|---|---|---|---|---|
| | % | (se) | % | (se) | % | (se) | % | (se) | % | (se) | |
| **I. Anxiety disorders** | | | | | | | | | | | |
| Panic disorder | 3.0 | (0.4) | 2.3 | (0.8) | 5.9 | (1.1) | 1.4 | (0.5) | 1.5 | (0.7) | 10.8* |
| Agoraphobia without panic | 0.6 | (0.2) | 0.1 | (0.1) | 1.4 | (0.6) | 0.6 | (0.3) | 0.0 | – | 11.5* |
| Specific phobia | 7.6 | (0.7) | 7.6 | (1.5) | 7.9 | (1.3) | 8.3 | (1.2) | 6.3 | (1.2) | 2.1 |
| Social phobia | 2.6 | (0.4) | 3.4 | (0.9) | 2.7 | (0.7) | 2.6 | (0.9) | 0.7 | (0.5) | 15.5* |
| Generalized anxiety disorder | 2.6 | (0.4) | 1.7 | (0.5) | 3.0 | (0.6) | 4.5 | (1.0) | 0.8 | (0.3) | 16.1* |
| Posttraumatic stress disorder[a] | 4.0 | (0.7) | 1.5 | (0.4) | 5.4 | (1.2) | 7.6 | (2.5) | 1.9 | (0.9) | 9.6* |
| Separation anxiety disorder[b] | 2.9 | (0.9) | 2.6 | (1.1) | 3.4 | (1.5) | – | –[b] | – | –[b] | 0.2[d] |
| Any anxiety disorder[c] | 15.9 | (1.1) | 13.2 | (2.4) | 21.7 | (2.1) | 18.6 | (2.2) | 8.2 | (1.4) | 38.7* |
| **II. Mood disorders** | | | | | | | | | | | |
| Major depressive disorder | 17.9 | (1.0) | 16.7 | (1.8) | 22.9 | (1.5) | 18.9 | (1.9) | 10.2 | (1.8) | 33.4* |
| **III. Impulse-control disorders** | | | | | | | | | | | |
| Oppositional-defiant disorder[b] | 2.5 | (1.0) | 3.2 | (1.3) | 1.3 | (0.8) | – | –[b] | – | –[b] | 1.6[d] |
| Conduct disorder[b] | 1.3 | (0.5) | 1.6 | (0.6) | 0.9 | (0.8) | – | –[b] | – | –[b] | 0.4[d] |
| Attention-deficit/hyperactivity disorder[b] | 2.9 | (0.9) | 3.3 | (1.2) | 2.2 | (1.4) | – | –[b] | – | –[b] | 0.3[d] |
| Any impulse-control disorder[b] | 4.7 | (1.1) | 5.0 | (1.5) | 4.1 | (1.7) | – | –[b] | – | –[b] | 0.1[d] |
| **IV. Alcohol use disorders** | | | | | | | | | | | |
| Alcohol abuse | 8.4 | (0.9) | 10.8 | (1.9) | 8.3 | (1.3) | 10.1 | (1.7) | 1.7 | (0.6) | 78.2* |
| Alcohol dependence | 1.5 | (0.3) | 0.7 | (0.3) | 2.3 | (0.6) | 2.3 | (1.0) | 0.5 | (0.3) | 7.8 |
| Any alcohol use disorder | 8.9 | (0.9) | 10.9 | (1.9) | 9.2 | (1.2) | 11.1 | (2.0) | 1.9 | (0.6) | 77.7* |
| **V. Any disorder** | | | | | | | | | | | |
| Any[c] | 31.7 | (2.0) | 29.3 | (3.5) | 41.5 | (4.0) | 34.1 | (3.3) | 16.6 | (2.1) | 47.5* |
| Two or more disorders[c] | 12.0 | (1.0) | 12.4 | (1.9) | 16.1 | (2.1) | 11.2 | (1.5) | 5.2 | (1.2) | 29.1* |
| Three or more disorders[c] | 4.9 | (0.8) | 6.5 | (1.8) | 6.3 | (1.2) | 4.3 | (1.2) | 0.1 | (0.1) | 64.6* |

[a] Posttraumatic stress disorder was assessed only in the Part 2 sample ($n = 1094$).

[b] Separation anxiety disorder, oppositional-defiant disorder, conduct disorder, and attention-deficit/hyperactivity disorder were assessed only among Part 2 respondents aged 18–44 years ($n = 516$).

[c] These summary measures were analyzed in the full Part 2 sample ($n = 1094$). Separation anxiety disorder, oppositional-defiant disorder, conduct disorder, and attention-deficit/hyperactivity disorder were coded as absent among respondents who were not assessed for these disorders.

[d] The $\chi^2$ test evaluates statistical significance of age-related differences in estimated prevalence: $\chi^2$ is evaluated with one degree of freedom for separation anxiety disorder, oppositional-defiant disorder, conduct disorder, attention-deficit/hyperactivity disorder, and any impulse-control disorder.

* Significant age difference at the 0.05 level.

impulse-control disorder (OR = 1.4, 95% CI = 0.5–3.4). These sex differences for anxiety, mood, and alcohol use disorders are consistent across age groups, with the exception of anxiety disorder in the 65+ age group, where the sex imbalance is much higher (OR = 7.40; 95% CI = 1.70–32.31), and with the exception of alcohol use disorders, where the sex imbalance is not as high in the youngest age cohort of 18–34 years (OR = 0.4;

95% CI = 0.2–0.8). Educational level is not associated with the different disorder classes.

## 4.3. Distributions of the Age of Onset of Mental Disorders

Table 18.2 shows the distributions of cumulative lifetime risk estimates that have been standardized and examined for fixed percentiles (eight

**Table 18.2.** Ages at selected percentiles on the standardized age of onset distributions of DSM-IV/CIDI disorders with projected lifetime risk at age 75

| | Projected lifetime risk at age 75 | | Ages at selected age of onset percentiles | | | | | | | |
|---|---|---|---|---|---|---|---|---|---|---|
| | % | (se) | 5 | 10 | 25 | 50 | 75 | 90 | 95 | 99 |
| **I. Anxiety disorders** | | | | | | | | | | |
| Panic disorder | 5.2 | (1.0) | 13 | 15 | 24 | 33 | 48 | 71 | 71 | 71 |
| Agoraphobia without panic | —[a] | | | | | | | | | |
| Specific phobia | 8.1 | (0.7) | 5 | 5 | 6 | 8 | 13 | 26 | 36 | 59 |
| Social phobia | 3.1 | (0.5) | 5 | 7 | 11 | 17 | 29 | 41 | 49 | 52 |
| Generalized anxiety disorder | 4.3 | (0.7) | 14 | 19 | 25 | 40 | 49 | 55 | 56 | 63 |
| Posttraumatic stress disorder[b] | 6.1 | (1.2) | 10 | 16 | 20 | 34 | 55 | 67 | 74 | 74 |
| Separation anxiety disorder[c] | —[a] | | | | | | | | | |
| Any anxiety disorder[d] | 21.4 | (1.8) | 5 | 6 | 8 | 21 | 42 | 59 | 67 | 74 |
| **II. Mood disorders** | | | | | | | | | | |
| Major depressive disorder | 28.9 | (1.9) | 13 | 16 | 25 | 36 | 50 | 61 | 71 | 75 |
| **III. Impulse-control disorders** | | | | | | | | | | |
| Oppositional-defiant disorder[c] | —[a] | | | | | | | | | |
| Conduct disorder[c] | —[a] | | | | | | | | | |
| Attention-deficit/hyperactivity disorder[c] | —[a] | | | | | | | | | |
| Any impulse-control disorder[c] | 4.8 | (1.1) | 5 | 5 | 7 | 10 | 13 | 16 | 29 | 29 |
| **IV. Alcohol use disorders** | | | | | | | | | | |
| Alcohol abuse | 10.6 | (1.1) | 16 | 17 | 18 | 21 | 31 | 46 | 57 | 64 |
| Alcohol dependence | 2.3 | (0.5) | 19 | 21 | 26 | 36 | 43 | 47 | 47 | 60 |
| Any alcohol use disorder[d] | 11.4 | (1.2) | 16 | 17 | 19 | 21 | 36 | 47 | 52 | 64 |
| **V. Any disorder** | | | | | | | | | | |
| Any[d] | 42.9 | (2.5) | 5 | 7 | 14 | 26 | 43 | 58 | 63 | 72 |

[a] Cell size too small to estimate for this individual disorder. This disorder is included in the class of disorders.

[b] Posttraumatic stress disorder was assessed only in the Part 2 sample ($n = 1094$).

[c] Separation anxiety disorder, oppositional-defiant disorder, conduct disorder, attention-deficit/hyperactivity disorder, and any impulse-control disorder were assessed only among Part 2 respondents aged 18–44 years ($n = 516$).

[d] These summary measures were analyzed in the full Part 2 sample ($n = 1094$). Separation anxiety disorder, oppositional-defiant disorder, conduct disorder, and attention-deficit/hyperactivity disorder were coded as absent among respondents who were not assessed for these disorders.

rightmost columns). Median ages of onset (i.e., the 50th percentile on the age of onset distribution) are earlier for the classes of anxiety disorders (age 21), impulse-control disorders (age 10), and alcohol use disorders (age 21) than for mood disorders (age 36). Of the individual anxiety disorders, median ages of onset are earlier for specific phobia (age 8) and social phobia (age 17) than for panic disorder (age 33), GAD (age 40), and PTSD (age 34). Median ages of onset are concentrated in a very narrow age range for some disorders, with interquartile ranges (i.e., the number of years between the 25th and 75th

percentiles of the median age of onset distributions) of only six years (ages 7–13) for impulse-control disorders and 17 years (ages 19–36) for alcohol use disorders, compared to 25 years (ages 25–50) for mood disorders and 34 years (ages 8–42) for anxiety disorders.

## 4.4. Projected Lifetime Risk of Mental Disorders

On the basis of the age of onset distributions, the projected lifetime risk of mental disorders at the age of 75 is calculated. The difference

**Table 18.3.** Proportional treatment contact in the year of disorder onset and median duration of delay among cases that subsequently made treatment contact

| | Treatment contact made in year of onset, % | Treatment contact by 50 years, % | Median duration of delay (years)[a] | n[b] |
|---|---|---|---|---|
| **I. Anxiety disorders** | | | | |
| Panic disorder | 56.4 | 97.5 | 1 | 75 |
| Specific phobia | 3.1 | 95.8 | 28 | 196 |
| Social phobia | 16.7 | 55.0 | 12 | 68 |
| Generalized anxiety disorder | 68.2 | 82.9 | 1 | 110 |
| Any anxiety disorder | 28.0 | 91.1 | 10 | 360 |
| **II. Mood disorders** | | | | |
| Major depressive episode | 52.1 | 96.9 | 1 | 475 |
| **III. Alcohol use disorders** | | | | |
| Alcohol abuse | 18.4 | 65.6 | 9 | 58 |
| Alcohol dependence | —[c] | —[c] | —[c] | —[c] |
| Any alcohol use disorder | 15.5 | 66.6 | 9 | 59 |

[a] Projections based on time-to-contact survival curves.
[b] Weighted number of respondents with a lifetime history of the disorder.
[c] Disorder was omitted as a result of insufficient cases; it is included as one of the disorders in "any alcohol use disorder."

between lifetime prevalence, as presented previously, and projected lifetime risk is as follows: lifetime risk is the prevalence of a disorder until the respondent's age at interview, whereas the projected lifetime prevalence is an estimation of the prevalence at the end of the respondent's lives. The projected lifetime risk is 35% higher than the lifetime prevalence estimates for anxiety disorders, 61% higher for mood disorders, 2% higher for impulse-control disorders, 28% higher for alcohol use disorders, and 35% higher for any disorder (Table 18.2, Column 1, compared to the figures of Table 18.1, Column 1; for example, the projected lifetime risk of any disorder is 42.9%, and the lifetime prevalence is 31.7%; thus, the projected risk is (42.9–31.7)/31.7 = 35.3% higher than the lifetime prevalence). The greatest differences between lifetime prevalence and projected lifetime risk were observed for late-onset disorders, such as major depression, GAD, and PTSD.

## 4.5. Cumulative Lifetime Probabilities of Treatment Contact

On the basis of survival curves of the proportion of cases with disorders that will eventu-

ally make treatment contact, the percentages of those estimated to make treatment contact by 50 years are calculated. These figures are presented in the second column of Table 18.3. Agoraphobia, PTSD, separation anxiety disorder, and all impulse-control disorders are not included in this table because of the small numbers of people with the disorder of interest. The proportion of lifetime cases with anxiety disorders making treatment contact within 50 years after the disorder onset is 91.1%. For mood disorders and alcohol use disorders, these figures are 96.9% and 66.6%, respectively. Of all individual anxiety disorders, social phobia has the lowest proportion of cases making treatment contact by 50 years (55.0%).

## 4.6. Duration of Delays in Initial Treatment Contact

The proportion of cases that made treatment contact in the year of first onset of the disorder and the median delay among people who eventually made treatment contact after the year of first onset are shown in the first and third column of Table 18.3. Proportions of cases making treatment contact in the year of disorder onset is 52.1% for mood disorders, 28.0% for any anxiety disorders, and 15.5% for any alcohol use disorders. The figures of the individual anxiety disorders range from 3.1% for specific phobia to 68.2% for GAD. The median years of delay also differ greatly, from a low of 1 year for major depression, panic disorder, and GAD, to highs of 9 years for alcohol abuse, 12 years for social phobia, and 28 years for specific phobia.

## 4.7. Sociodemographic Correlates of Lifetime Treatment Contact

Sociodemographic correlates of failure to ever make a treatment contact among respondents with lifetime disorders were studied (data not presented in table). Women have no significantly higher odds of treatment contact than do men for anxiety, mood, and alcohol use disorders. Subjects with younger age have a significantly higher chance of treatment contact than do older subjects for anxiety disorders (ages 18–34: OR = 3.0; 95% CI = 1.8–5.1; ages 35–49 years: OR = 2.5; 95% CI = 1.6–3.7; reference = 50+), and mood disorders (ages 18–34: OR = 3.9; 95% CI = 1.7–8.9; ages 35–49 years: OR = 2.7; 95% CI = 1.6–4.4; reference = 50+), but not for alcohol use disorders. Thus, generally monotonic relationships between being in younger cohorts and higher probability of initial treatment contact are found for anxiety and mood disorders. Cases with earlier ages of onset of their anxiety disorders (early: OR = 0.1; 95% CI = 0.0–0.2; early-average: OR = 0.1; 95% CI = 0.1–0.3; late-average: OR = 0.4; 95% CI = 0.2–0.7; reference = late) and mood disorders (early: OR = 0.1; 95% CI = 0.0–0.3; early-average: OR = 0.3; 95% CI = 0.1–0.6; late-average: OR = 0.5; 95% CI = 0.3–0.8; reference = late) are significantly less likely to make treatment contact, but no relationship has been found for alcohol use disorders.

Educational level as predictor could not be studied as a result of small cell sizes.

## 4.8. Prevalence and Severity of 12-month Disorders

The 12-month prevalence estimates are presented in Table 18.4. The 12-month prevalence of any disorder is 13.4%. Thus, of those respondents with any lifetime disorder (31.7%), 42.3% (still) have the disorder in the past year. Anxiety disorders are the most prevalent class of disorders (8.6%), followed by mood disorders (5.1%), impulse-control disorders (1.9%), and substance disorders (1.9%). The most prevalent individual disorders are specific phobia (5.2%) and major depressive disorder (4.9%). Note that these disorders are also the most common lifetime disorders, besides alcohol abuse. The fact that 12-month alcohol abuse is not highly prevalent while lifetime alcohol abuse is signifies that, in many cases, this disorder does not have a chronic course.

Of those subjects with any 12-month disorder, 30.8% were classified as serious, 31.0% as moderate, and 38.2% as mild. Among the different disorder classes, mood disorders have the highest percentage of serious cases (54.9%), followed by anxiety disorders (29.9%). The lowest percentages are found for impulse-control disorders (21.0%) and alcohol use disorders (23.9%). The anxiety disorders with the greatest proportion of serious cases are social phobia (75.8%) and GAD (73.4%). Major depression has the greatest proportion of serious cases (57.0%) among the mood disorders, and, not surprisingly, alcohol dependence has the highest (67.0%) among alcohol use disorders.

## 4.9. Sociodemographic Correlates of 12-month Mental Disorders

Age, sex, income, partner status, and educational level were studied as correlates of 12-month mental disorders (data not presented). Lower age (18–34 and 35–49) is associated with alcohol use disorders (OR = 8.3; 95% CI = 2.1–31.8 and OR = 5.4; 95% CI = 1.2–24.5, respectively; reference = 65+). Lower age (18–34) is also associated with impulse-control disorders (OR = 16.6; 95% CI = 2.3–120.8; reference = 35–49). Compared to male respondents, females are more likely to have any anxiety disorders (OR = 4.4; 95% CI = 2.3–8.2), mood disorders (OR = 2.6; 95% CI = 1.7–4.1), and impulse-control disorders (OR = 5.1; 95% CI = 1.4–18.4). Females are not at decreased risk for alcohol use disorders,

**Table 18.4.** 12-month prevalence and severity of DSM-IV/CIDI disorders

| | Total | | Serious | | Moderate | | Mild | |
|---|---|---|---|---|---|---|---|---|
| | % | (se) | % | (se) | % | (se) | % | (se) |
| **I. Anxiety disorders** | | | | | | | | |
| Panic disorder | 1.3 | (0.3) | 44.1 | (11.7) | 28.1 | (12.1) | 27.7 | (10.4) |
| Agoraphobia without panic | 0.3 | (0.1) | —[e] | | —[e] | | —[e] | |
| Specific phobia | 5.2 | (0.6) | 17.0 | (5.6) | 33.0 | (4.9) | 50.1 | (6.1) |
| Social phobia | 1.3 | (0.3) | 75.8 | (8.6) | 15.3 | (6.7) | 8.9 | (4.9) |
| Generalized anxiety disorder | 0.6 | (0.2) | 73.4 | (12.2) | 18.4 | (10.8) | 8.2 | (8.9) |
| Posttraumatic stress disorder[b] | 2.5 | (0.7) | 36.9 | (10.0) | 37.9 | (12.4) | 25.2 | (15.5) |
| Separation anxiety disorder[c] | 0.6 | (0.4) | —[e] | | —[e] | | —[e] | |
| Any anxiety disorder[b] | 8.6 | (1.0) | 29.9 | (4.6) | 33.1 | (4.8) | 37.0 | (6.2) |
| **II. Mood disorders** | | | | | | | | |
| Major depressive disorder | 4.9 | (0.5) | 57.0 | (6.9) | 26.9 | (4.0) | 16.0 | (5.3) |
| Dysthymia | 1.6 | (0.3) | 45.2 | (11.9) | 50.4 | (12.3) | 4.4 | (2.1) |
| Any mood disorder | 5.1 | (0.5) | 54.9 | (6.8) | 29.2 | (4.3) | 15.9 | (5.1) |
| **III. Impulse-control disorders** | | | | | | | | |
| Oppositional-defiant disorder[c] | 0.9 | (0.5) | —[e] | | —[e] | | —[e] | |
| Conduct disorder[c] | 0.4 | (0.3) | —[e] | | —[e] | | —[e] | |
| Attention-deficit/hyperactivity disorder[c] | 1.0 | (0.4) | —[e] | | —[e] | | —[e] | |
| Any impulse-control disorder[c] | 1.9 | (0.7) | 21.0 | (9.3) | 26.1 | (16.7) | 52.9 | (16.8) |
| **IV. Alcohol use disorders** | | | | | | | | |
| Alcohol abuse | 1.8 | (0.3) | 17.3 | (6.9) | 32.1 | (17.6) | 50.6 | (16.0) |
| Alcohol dependence | 0.4 | (0.1) | 67.0 | (20.8) | 33.0 | (20.8) | 0.0 | (0.0) |
| Any alcohol use disorder | 1.9 | (0.3) | 23.9 | (8.7) | 29.5 | (16.6) | 46.6 | (14.7) |
| **V. Any disorder** | | | | | | | | |
| Any[d] | 13.4 | (1.0) | 30.8 | (3.5) | 31.0 | (3.7) | 38.2 | (4.7) |

[a] Percentages in the three severity columns are repeated as proportions of all cases and sum to 100% across each row.

[b] Assessed in the Part 2 sample ($n = 1094$).

[c] Assessed in the Part 2 sample among respondents aged 18–44 years ($n = 516$).

[d] Estimated in the Part 2 sample. No adjustment is made for the fact that one or more disorders in the category were not assessed for all Part 2 respondents.

[e] Estimates could not be made as figures were too low. These disorders are included in the class of disorders.

as was found for lifetime alcohol use disorders. Anxiety disorders are somewhat more common among respondents with a low-medium level of income than among those with a high income (OR = 2.0; 95% CI = 1.2–3.5). Mood disorders are more common among the never married than among those married or cohabiting (OR = 2.5; 95% CI = 1.1–5.6), and impulse-control disorders are more common among those separated/divorced or widowed than among those married or cohabiting (OR = 22.4; 95% CI = 4.3–116.5). Impulse-control disorders are more common among those subjects with a low-medium level of education (complete primary) than among those with a high level of education (secondary college) (OR = 7.8; 95% CI = 1.4–42.9).

## 4.10. 12-month Service Use

In the year before the interview, 10.9% of all respondents used any mental health services (mental health specialty, general medical, human services, and/or alternative sources), including

30.3% of those with 12-month DSM-IV disorders (the anxiety, mood, or alcohol use disorders from Table 18.4) and 8.0% of those without these disorders (data not presented). Most of those treated received services in the general medical sector (7.7% of respondents, representing 71.2% of those in treatment) and in the mental health specialty sector (5.5% of respondents, representing 51.0% of those in treatment). Of all respondents, 0.6% (or 5.4% of those in treatment) received care from human services and 1.5% from alternative sources (13.5% of those in treatment).

In the year before the interview, 30.6% of respondents with any anxiety disorders, 50.2% of respondents with any mood disorders, and 18.3% of respondents with any alcohol use disorders received any mental health services. For the following individual disorders, the numbers are not too small to present these figures: social phobia (40.5%), specific phobia (25.3%), PTSD (39.1%), major depression (52.2%), dysthymia (37.0%), and alcohol abuse (14.2%).

A clear monotonic relationship exists between the severity of the disorder and the probability of service use: 49.2% of the cases classified as severe received any mental health services, compared to 31.3% of the moderate cases, 16.1% of the mild cases, and 7.7% of those without apparent disorders, as assessed in ESEMeD. The last group makes up the vast majority of the population; therefore, these cases are a substantial proportion of all people in treatment. Among those respondents receiving any mental health services, 66.9% of severe cases received this in the mental health specialty sector; for moderate cases this figure is 45.2%, and for those without apparent disorders it is 47.5% (the number of treated mild cases was too low to estimate this figure).

### 4.11. Sociodemographic Predictors of 12-month Service Use

Among all respondents, the sociodemographic predictors of any mental health service use have been studied. Receiving any 12-month mental health services is significantly related to sex: women are more likely to receive treatment than men (OR = 2.2; 95% CI = 1.1–4.7). Those subjects with the highest level of education are also more likely to receive any treatment than those with the lowest level of education (OR = 2.7; 95% CI = 1.1–6.8). Age, partner status, and income are not related to service use.

Looking only to those respondents with any 12-month mental disorder, the sociodemographic predictors of any service use are being 35–49 years of age compared to 65+ (OR = 6.6; 95% CI = 1.5–29.2), high level compared to low-medium level of education (OR = 5.0; 95% CI = 2.0–10.0), and being separated/divorced or widowed compared to being married or cohabiting. Among subjects with mental disorders, sex and income are not related to service use.

## 5. DISCUSSION

### 5.1. Limitations

These results should be interpreted with the following limitations in mind. First, for a psychiatric epidemiological survey, this study has a relatively low number of respondents as a result of limited financial resources for the fieldwork of this study. Because of the low prevalences of some disorders, these figures should be considered with caution. For this reason, lifetime and 12-month service use and severity by 12-month prevalence could not be presented for all disorders.

Second, the response in this study was low compared to the previous Dutch study NEMESIS (response: 69.7%), performed in 1996 (Bijl, van Zessen & Ravelli 1998a; Bijl et al. 1998b) and to other studies like the NCS-R (response: 70.9%) (Kessler et al. 2005a). A possible explanation is that in the past decade in the Netherlands commercial surveys have tried to contact people with a high frequency, which may have had a negative effect on the public's willingness to participate. Economic incentives for respondents, which may increase response rate, were not given, except for the hard-to-reach cases at the end of the data collection phase. Systematic survey nonresponse could lead to bias in the estimates of disorder prevalence or service use. People with mental disorders tend to have a higher survey refusal rate than those without disorders (Allgulander 1989; Eaton et al. 1992; Turner et al. 1998; de Graaf et al. 2000); therefore, it is likely that disorder prevalences and unmet needs for treatment have been underestimated. The youngest age group was underrepresented in the study. This was also the case in the first wave of NEMESIS (Bijl et al. 1998a; Bijl et al. 1998b) and in its loss to follow-up (de Graaf et al. 2000) and in other studies (Ribisl et al. 1996). Nonresponse among young adults can be a particular source of bias with respect to problems such as substance use disorder, which are much more common in this age group (Bijl et al. 1998a; Bijl et al. 1998b). In future research, special efforts should be made to recruit young adults.

Third, as mentioned in the "Methods" section, there were a number of skip problems in the questionnaire. For example, it was not possible to generate the prevalence of drug abuse and dependence, the age of onset of dysthymia, and the score on the Sheehan Disability Scale for all subjects with major depression. Because the ESEMeD countries were the first countries in the field using the CIDI 3.0, these countries encountered the most problems. Countries that entered the field later had the benefit that these problems had been solved.

Fourth, this study excludes people who are not able to understand the Dutch language well and people that are homeless or institutionalized. As such people make up only a small proportion of the Dutch population, the results presented here apply to the vast majority of the population.

Fifth, diagnoses were made using fully structured diagnostic interviews administered by lay interviewers, which might not match the accuracy of diagnoses made by clinicians. However, a clinical reappraisal study using the SCID (First et al. 2002) found generally good individual-level concordance between the CIDI and the SCID and conservative estimates of prevalence compared to the SCID (Haro et al. 2006). Furthermore, the data were based on retrospective recall. This can be a source of considerable recall bias in recording lifetime disorders (Blazer et al. 1994; Kessler et al. 1996) but is less probable for the 12-month disorders.

## 5.2. Lifetime Prevalence Findings

The estimates in this study of the lifetime prevalence of mental disorders are broadly consistent with those found in NEMESIS, the first wave of which was conducted in the Netherlands in 1996 (Bijl et al. 1998a, 1998b). About one-third of the general population has met criteria for one or more mental disorders at some time in their lives. In the current study, this was 31.7% and in NEMESIS 41.2%. In part, these differences can probably be explained by the previously mentioned differences in response rate between the two studies. Note that these figures are not completely comparable as a result of different disorders under study, different diagnostic classifications used to define disorders (this study: DSM-IV; NEMESIS: DSM-III-R), different age ranges of the populations studied (this study: 18+; NEMESIS: 18–65), and different measures (this study: CIDI version 3.0; NEMESIS: CIDI version 1.1). In both studies, anxiety disorders and mood disorders are the most common classes of disorders. In both studies, lifetime major depression is prevalent in one out of six respondents (this study: 17.9%; NEMESIS: 15.4%). Also in both studies, specific phobia is the most common individual lifetime anxiety disorder (this study: 7.6%; NEMESIS: 10.1%), and alcohol abuse is the most common individual lifetime substance use disorder (this study: 8.4%; NEMESIS: 11.7%). The lower prevalence of alcohol use disorders in this study was expected (8.9% vs. 18.2%), as the DSM-IV criteria for substance use disorders are stricter than the DSM-III-R criteria, especially in requiring criterion A symptoms to cluster in a single year of life (Kessler et al. 2005a). Although DSM-III-R lifetime alcohol use disorders are very high among young people (e.g., for males aged 18–25 years this was 29.0% in NEMESIS) and show a clear decline in older cohorts (Verdurmen et al. 2003), both are not the case in the current study for DSM-IV alcohol use disorders. The stricter definition of substance use seems useful, given that DSM-III-R alcohol abuse overestimates cases in younger age groups (given the very high percentage of young people with this disorder) (Bijl et al. 1998a; Bijl et al. 1998b), is not strongly associated with other mental disorders (de Graaf et al. 2002a), and is not associated with functional disabilities (Bijl & Ravelli 2000a). In DSM-III-R alcohol abuse, we probably are not dealing with psychopathology but with behavior specific to a particular phase of early adulthood (de Graaf et al. 2002a). The remarkable lower prevalence of social phobia in this study (2.6%) compared to that in NEMESIS (7.8%) is difficult to explain and was not found in the NCS-R (12.1%) (Kessler et al. 2005a) as compared to the NCS (13.3%) (Kessler et al. 1994).

For the first time in the Netherlands, information on a range of impulse-control disorders has been gathered in the general population of adults, although only among a subsample of respondents aged 18–44 years ($n = 516$). The lifetime prevalence of any impulse-control disorder is 1 out of 20 respondents (4.7%). Also for the first time in the Netherlands, information on PTSD has been gathered in the general population, among a subsample of 1094 respondents. The lifetime prevalence of PTSD is 1 out of 25 respondents (4.0%).

Comorbidity is high: of those with a lifetime disorder, 38% have two or more disorders, which means that the burden of disorders is concentrated in a relatively small group with multiple disorders.

Like in many other studies, women are more at risk for anxiety and mood disorders than are men, but they are less at risk for alcohol use disorders (Bijl et al. 1998a; Bijl et al. 1998b). No differences are found for any impulse-control disorder, which is striking because in all other countries in the WMH, except for Germany, males are more at risk (Kessler et al. 2006). For anxiety disorders, it was found that in the 65+ age group many more women than men were diagnosed with this disorder than in younger age groups. This sex difference might be partly explained by the fact that there are more women in the older age group who have lost their partner at older age, thereby inducing an anxiety disorder. The sex imbalance for alcohol use disorders is not as high in the youngest age cohort of 18–34 years, which can be explained by fewer differences in alcohol con-

sumption between the sexes in younger cohorts. This adolescent phenomenon has recently been reported in the Netherlands.

From the age of onset distributions of mental disorders, it can be concluded that these disorders are concentrated in the first two decades of life. Consistent with previous studies (de Graaf et al. 2003; WHO International Consortium in Psychiatric Epidemiology 2000), anxiety and alcohol use disorders have earlier ages of onset than mood disorders. As a result, mood disorders largely occur as temporally secondary comorbid conditions (de Graaf et al. 2003) and are more common as comorbid conditions than as pure conditions compared to anxiety and alcohol use disorders (de Graaf et al. 2002b). Furthermore, it must be noted that within the anxiety disorders, there are substantial differences in the age of onset, with specific phobia and social phobia having much earlier onsets than GAD, PTSD, and panic disorder.

The projected lifetime risk of any mental disorder at the age of 75 (43%) is much higher than the estimated lifetime prevalence to the date of interview (32%). Thus, between one-third and one-half of the Dutch population will eventually suffer from a mental disorder at some time during their lives.

## 5.3. 12-month Prevalence Findings

The results show that episodes of DSM-IV disorders are prevalent during the prior year among one in seven persons of the Dutch population (13.4%). This is somewhat lower than in NEMESIS (Bijl et al. 1998a, 1998b), but this difference should not be overinterpreted because of the previously mentioned differences in study design between the two studies. Anxiety disorders are the most prevalent class of disorder (8.6%), followed by mood disorders (5.1%), which is consistent with findings in other studies (Bijl et al. 1998a; Bijl et al. 1998b; Bijl et al. 2003; Demyttenaere et al. 2004). The most prevalent individual disorders are specific phobia (5.2%) and major depressive disorder (4.9%). Many cases are moderate or serious cases. Mood disorders have the highest proportion of serious cases, followed by anxiety disorders, alcohol use disorders, and impulse-control disorders.

The sociodemographic correlates of having 12-month disorders are broadly consistent with previous surveys: lower age (for any alcohol use and impulse-control disorders); being female (for any anxiety and mood disorders), being unmarried (for mood disorders); being separated, divorced, or widowed (for impulse-control disorders); and having low-medium income (for anxiety disorders) (Lépine et al. 1989; Bijl et al. 1998a; Bijl et al. 1998b; WHO International Consortium in Psychiatric Epidemiology 2000; Demyttenaere et al. 2004). The finding that impulse-control disorders are more prevalent among women than among men was an unexpected one. Additional analyses on sex differences, separately for ADHD, conduct disorder, and oppositional-defiant disorder, show that ADHD and conduct disorder are not significantly more common among men or women, but oppositional-defiant disorder is significantly more common among women (OR = 3.3; 95% CI = 1.0–10.0).

## 5.4. Lifetime Service Use Findings

The vast majority of lifetime cases eventually seek help, especially cases of anxiety and mood disorders. This is less true for alcohol use disorders, for which nearly 35% of all lifetime cases failed to ever make any treatment contact. Although previous research focused on treatment of current cases (e.g., Leaf et al. 1988; Bijl & Ravelli 2000b), the new trend in general population psychiatric research is to study treatment delays. We found that the delay among those who eventually seek help, is large for some disorders, but not for all disorders. Panic disorder, GAD, and major depression have a relatively short duration of delay. When we compare the Dutch figures on delay with those of the United States, for most disorders the delay is shorter in the Netherlands. This can probably be explained by differences in the systems of health insurance between Netherlands and the United States, with better

access to mental health services for residents of the Netherlands (for a discussion regarding the U.S. health-care system, see Chapter 9 of this volume).

There is considerable variation among disorders in the probability of eventually making treatment contact, in the probability of making treatment contact in the year of onset, and in durations of delay. For major depression and some anxiety disorders (e.g., panic disorder and GAD), lifetime treatment contact and treatment contact by age 50 are high, and the average duration of delay is short. Larger failure and delays are found for specific and social phobia, as well as for alcohol abuse. Disorders with higher impairment and disorders that have a later onset had higher initial treatment contact rates and shorter delays (Leaf et al. 1988; Wang et al. 2004). Previous research has shown that cases with substance use disorders often do not perceive a need for treatment (Bijl & Ravelli 2000b; Mojtabai, Olfson & Mechanic 2002).

Sociodemographic and clinical correlates of failure in making initial treatment contact are older age (for anxiety and mood disorders) and earlier age of onset of the disorder (for anxiety and mood disorders). Sex is not associated. It is likely that older people more often have negative attitudes toward mental health service use, have financial barriers, and/or have been less exposed to programs that increase awareness of mental illness.

## 5.5. 12-month Service Use Findings

The majority of cases did not receive any mental health care in the year before the interview. Thirty percent of those with any anxiety, mood, or alcohol use disorder, 30.6% of those with anxiety disorders, 50.2% of those with mood disorders, and 18.3% of those with alcohol use disorders received care. The NEMESIS project reported treatment rates to be 33.9%, 40.5%, 63.8%, and 17.5%, respectively, in 1996 (Bijl & Ravelli 2000b). The current study was not designed to make a comparison with the findings on service use of NEMESIS. As a result of different disorders being under study, different questionnaires on care settings, and a different age range of the respondents, it is difficult to compare these figures. Nevertheless, the clear increase in the rate of mental health service use that was found in the NCS-R compared to the NCS a decade earlier (Kessler et al. 2005b; Wang et al. 2005b), was not found in the Netherlands. It might be that the shorter time frame between the two Dutch studies, five to six years, was too short to find a clear difference.

A considerable amount of mental health services are being provided to respondents without apparent disorders or to respondents with mild disorders: 7.7% of those cases classified as without apparent disorders and 16.1% of those classified as having mild disorders received services. Although respondents without disorders are less likely to receive treatment, they make up such a large majority of the population (86.6%), that they account for a substantial proportion of all people treated. As mentioned by others before (Wang et al. 2005b), certainly some services are being used appropriately to treat disorders not assessed in this study (e.g., personality disorders), to treat subthreshold symptoms, as secondary prevention of lifetime disorders, and even as primary prevention of disorders. However, it remains concerning that such a high proportion of treatment resources are being potentially diverted to individuals without mental disorders when unmet needs among people with well-defined disorders are so great (Narrow et al. 2002; Wang et al. 2005b).

The sociodemographic predictors of 12-month service use shows that treatment is seen less often among males and those with a low educational level, as was previously found in the Netherlands (Bijl & Ravelli 2000b).

## 6. CONCLUSIONS AND FUTURE DIRECTIONS

This chapter has shown that the use of the CIDI 3.0, which was produced for the WHO WMH Survey Initiative, can provide much up-to-date and detailed data on the enormous societal burdens that mental disorders impose in the Netherlands. The information that the CIDI 3.0 gener-

ates is more detailed than the CIDI version used in the previous Dutch study NEMESIS (CIDI 1.1). For example, in the current study, information is gathered about failure to make prompt initial treatment contact, which is a pervasive aspect of unmet need for mental health care (Wang et al. 2005a). For some disorders, it is typical for delays to persist for years and sometimes for decades. From these data it is possible to conclude that to reduce the burden of untreated disorders, more effort is needed to increase the speed of initial help seeking and to prompt initial treatment contact (Wang et al. 2005a).

As mentioned before, this study has a number of limitations, including the number of respondents and the relatively low response rate. This is due, in large part, to limited financial resources. Because of the low prevalence of some disorders and the broad confidence interval of the prevalence rate, the findings should be considered with caution. As readers may have noticed, many estimates could not be presented on several disorders, as a result of very low rates of prevalence or service use. For example, because of the low prevalence of impulse-control disorders, it was not possible to study treatment contact for such disorders. Thus, future studies, though expensive because of the high costs of fieldwork, should include more respondents.

The use of the CIDI 3.0 has the potential to become a powerful tool in the future, in new studies, like the second NEMESIS study, which is currently in the process of being fielded. Examination of temporal trends between these studies is important so that change in disorder prevalence and change in use of mental health services can be studied. Using consistent methodology in these studies is important; for example, the questions on service use must be the same in order to make comparisons. Population-based surveys can become uniquely powerful if applied longitudinally; as such, the course, incidence, and risk factors of mental disorders can be studied.

## REFERENCES

Alegria, M., Bijl, R. V., Lin, E., Walters, E. E. & Kessler, R. C. (2000). Income differences in persons seeking outpatient treatment for mental disorders: A comparison of the United States with Ontario and The Netherlands. *Archives of General Psychiatry*, 57, 383–91.

Allgulander, C. (1989). Psychoactive drug use in a general population sample, Sweden: Correlates with perceived health, psychiatric diagnoses, and mortality in an automated record-linkage study. *American Journal of Public Health*, 79, 1006–10.

American Psychiatric Association (1994). *Diagnostic and statistical manual of mental disorders (DSM-IV)*, 4th ed. Washington, DC: American Psychiatric Association.

Bijl, R. V., de Graaf, R., Hiripi, E., Kessler, R. C., Kohn, R., Offord, D. R., Üstün, T. B., Vicente, B., Vollebergh, W. A., Walters, E. E. & Wittchen, H.-U. (2003). The prevalence of treated and untreated mental disorders in five countries. *Health Affairs (Millwood)*, 22, 122–33.

Bijl, R. V. & Ravelli, A. (2000a). Current and residual functional disability associated with psychopathology. *Psychological Medicine*, 30, 657–68.

Bijl, R. V. & Ravelli, A. (2000b). Psychiatric morbidity, service use, and need for care in the general population: Results of the Netherlands Mental Health Survey and Incidence study. *American Journal of Public Health*, 90, 602–7.

Bijl, R. V., van Zessen, G. & Ravelli, A. (1998a). Prevalence of psychiatric disorder in the general population: Results of the Netherlands Mental Health Survey and Incidence Study (NEMESIS). *Social Psychiatry and Psychiatric Epidemiology*, 33, 587–95.

Bijl, R. V., van Zessen, G., Ravelli, A., de Rijk, C. & Langendoen, Y. (1998b). The Netherlands Mental Health Survey and Incidence Study (NEMESIS): Objectives and design. *Social Psychiatry and Psychiatric Epidemiology*, 33, 581–6.

Blazer, D. G., Kessler, R. C., McGonagle, K. A. & Swartz, M. S. (1994). The prevalence and distribution of major depression in a national community sample: The National Comorbidity Survey. *American Journal of Psychiatry*, 151, 979–86.

de Graaf, R., Bijl, R. V., Ravelli, A., Smit, F. & Vollebergh, W. A. M. (2002a). Predictors of first incidence of DSM-III-R psychiatric disorders in the general population: Findings from the Netherlands Mental Health Survey and Incidence Study. *Acta Psychiatrica Scandinavica*, 106, 303–13.

de Graaf, R., Bijl, R. V., Smit, F., Ravelli, A. & Vollebergh, W. A. M. (2000). Psychiatric and sociodemographic predictors of attrition in a longitudinal study: The Netherlands Mental Health Survey and Incidence Study (NEMESIS). *American Journal of Epidemiology*, 152, 1039–47.

de Graaf, R., Bijl, R. V., Smit, F., Vollebergh, W. A. M. & Spijker, J. (2002b). Risk factors for 12-month comorbidity of mood, anxiety and substance use

disorders: Findings from the Netherlands Mental Health Survey and Incidence Study. *American Journal of Psychiatry*, 159, 620–9.

de Graaf, R., Bijl, R. V., Vollebergh, W. A. M. & Spijker, J. (2003). Temporal sequencing of lifetime mood disorders in relation to comorbid anxiety and substance use disorders: Findings from the Netherlands Mental Health Survey and Incidence Study. *Social Psychiatry and Psychiatric Epidemiology*, 38, 1–11.

Demyttenaere, K., Bonnewyn, A., Bruffaerts, R., Brugha, T., de Graaf, R. & Alonso, J. (2006). Comorbid painful physical symptoms and depression: Prevalence, work loss, and help seeking. *Journal of Affective Disorders*, 92, 185–93.

Demyttenaere, K., Bruffaerts, R., Posada-Villa, J., Gasquet, I., Kovess, V., Lepine, J. P., Angermeyer, M. C., Bernert, S., Girolamo, G., Morosini, P., Polidori, G., Kikkawa, T., Kawakami, N., Ono, Y., Takeshima, T., Uda, H., Karam, E. G., Fayyad, J. A., Karam, A. N., Mneimneh, Z. N., Medina-Mora, M. E., Borges, G., Lara, G., de Graaf, R., Ormel, J., Gureje, O., Shen, Y., Huang, Y., Zhang, M., Alonso, J., Haro, J. M., Vilagut, G., Bromet, E. J., Gluzman, S., Webb, C., Kessler, R. C., Merikangas, K. R., Anthony, J. C., Korff, M. R. V., Wang, P. S., Alonso, J., Brugha, T. S., Aguilar-Gaxiola, S., Lee, S., Heeringa, S., Pennell, B.-E., Zaslavsky, A. M., Üstün, T. B. & Chatterji, S. (2004). Prevalence, severity and unmet need for treatment of mental disorders in the World Health Organization World Mental Health Surveys. *Journal of the American Medical Association*, 291, 2581–90.

Eaton, W. W., Anthony, J. C., Tepper, S. & Dryman, A. (1992). Psychopathology and attrition in the Epidemiologic Catchment Area Study. *American Journal of Epidemiology*, 135, 1051–9.

Efron, B. (1988). Logistic regression, survival analysis, and the Kaplan-Meier curve. *Journal of the American Statistical Association*, 83, 414–25.

ESEMeD/MHEDEA 2000 Investigators (2004a). Sampling and methods of the European Study of the Epidemiology of Mental Disorders (ESEMeD) Project. *Acta Psychiatrica Scandinavica*, 109, 8–20.

ESEMeD/MHEDEA 2000 Investigators (2004b). Prevalence of mental disorders in Europe: Results from the European Study of the Epidemiology of Mental Disorders (ESEMeD) Project. *Acta Psychiatrica Scandinavica*, 109, 21–7.

ESEMeD/MHEDEA 2000 Investigators (2004c). 12-month comorbidity patterns and associated factors in Europe: Results from the European Study of the Epidemiology of Mental Disorders (ESEMeD) Project. *Acta Psychiatrica Scandinavica*, 109, 28–37.

ESEMeD/MHEDEA 2000 Investigators (2004d). Disability and quality of life impact of mental disorders in Europe: Results from the European Study of the Epidemiology of Mental Disorders (ESEMeD) Project. *Acta Psychiatrica Scandinavica*, 109, 38–46.

ESEMeD/MHEDEA 2000 Investigators (2004e). Use of mental health services in Europe: Results from the European Study of the Epidemiology of Mental Disorders (ESEMeD) Project. *Acta Psychiatrica Scandinavica*, 109, 47–54.

ESEMeD/MHEDEA 2000 Investigators (2004f). Psychotropic drug utilisation in Europe: Results from the European Study of the Epidemiology of Mental Disorders (ESEMeD) Project. *Acta Psychiatrica Scandinavica*, 109, 55–64.

ESEMeD/MHEDEA 2000 Investigators (2006). Functional disability of mental disorders and comparison with physical disorders: A study among the general population of six European countries. *Acta Psychiatrica Scandinavica*, 113, 492–500.

First, M. B., Spitzer, R. L., Gibbon, M. & Williams, J. B. W. (2002). *Structured Clinical Interview for DSM-IV-TR axis I disorders, research version, non-patient edition (SCID-I/NP): User's guide and interview, research version.* New York: Biometrics Research, New York State Psychiatric Institute.

Haro, J. M., Arbabzadeh-Bouchez, S., Brugha, T. S., de Girolamo, G., Guyer, M. E., Jin, R., Lepine, J.-P., Mazzi, F., Reneses, B., Vilagut, G., Sampson, N. A. & Kessler, R. C. (2006). Concordance of the Composite International Diagnostic Interview Version 3.0 (CIDI 3.0) with standardized clinical assessments in the WHO World Mental Health Surveys. *International Journal of Methods in Psychiatric Research*, 15, 167–80.

Hodiamont, P. P. G. (1986). Searching sick souls: A study on diagnostics, epidemiology and help seeking behaviour in the context of social psychiatry. Dissertation, Katholieke Universiteit Nijmegen, Nijmegen, The Netherlands.

Kessler, R. C., Adler, L., Barkley, R., Biederman, J., Conners, C. K., Demler, O., Faraone, S. V., Greenhill, L. L. & Howes, M. J. (2006). The prevalence and correlates of adult ADHD in the United States: Results from the National Comorbidity Survey Replication. *American Journal of Psychiatry*, 163, 716–23.

Kessler, R. C., Berglund, P., Demler, O., Jin, R. & Walters, E. E. (2005a). Lifetime prevalence and age-of-onset distributions of DSM-IV disorders in the National Comorbidity Survey Replication. *Archives of General Psychiatry*, 62, 593–602.

Kessler, R. C., Demler, O., Frank, R. G., Olfson, M., Pincus, H. A., Walters, E. E., Wang, P. S., Wells, K. B. & Zaslavsky, A. M. (2005b). Prevalence and treatment of mental disorders, 1990 to 2003. *New England Journal of Medicine*, 352, 2515–23.

Kessler, R. C., Haro, J. M., Heeringa, S. G., Pennell, B.-E. & Üstün, T. B. (2006). The World Health Organization World Mental Health Survey Initiative. *Epidemiologia e Psichiatria Sociale*, 15, 161–6.

Kessler, R. C., McGonagle, K. A., Zhao, S., Nelson, C. B., Hughes, M., Eshleman, S., Wittchen, H.-U. & Kendler, K. S. (1994). Lifetime and 12-month prevalence of DSM-III-R psychiatric disorders in the United States: Results from the National Comorbidity Survey. *Archives of General Psychiatry*, 51, 8–19.

Kessler, R. C., Nelson, C. B., McGonagle, K. A., Liu, J., Swartz, M. & Blazer, D. G. (1996). Comorbidity of DSM-III-R major depressive disorder in the general population: Results from the U.S. National Comorbidity Survey. *British Journal of Psychiatry*, 168, 17–30.

Kessler, R. C. & Üstün, T. B. (2004). The World Mental Health (WMH) survey initiative version of the World Health Organization (WHO) Composite International Diagnostic Interview (CIDI). *International Journal of Methods in Psychiatric Research*, 13, 93–121.

Kovess-Masfety, V., Alonso, J., Brugha, T., Angermeyer, M. C., Haro, J. M. & Sevilla-Dedieu, C., on behalf of the ESEMeD/MHEDEA 2000 Consortium (2007). Differences in the lifetime use of services for mental health problems in six European countries. *Psychiatric Services*, 58, 213–20.

Leaf, P. J., Bruce, M. L., Tischler, G. L., Freeman, D. H., Weissman, M. M. & Myers, J. K. (1988). Factors affecting the utilization of specialty and general medical mental health services. *Medical Care*, 26, 9–26.

Leon, A. C., Olfson, M., Portera, L., Farber, L. & Sheehan, D. V. (1997). Assessing psychiatric impairment in primary care with the Sheehan Disability Scale. *International Journal of Psychiatry in Medicine*, 27, 93–105.

Lépine, J.-P., Lellouch, J., Lovell, A., Teherani, M., Ha, C., Verdier-Taillefer, M. G., Rambourg, N. & Lempérière, T. (1989). Anxiety and depressive disorders in a French population: Methodology and preliminary results. *Psychiatric Psychobiology*, 4, 267–74.

Mojtabai, R., Olfson, M. & Mechanic, D. (2002). Perceived need and help-seeking in adults with mood, anxiety, or substance use disorders. *Archives of General Psychiatry*, 59, 77–84.

Narrow, W. E., Rae, D. S., Robins, L. N. & Regier, D. A. (2002). Revised prevalence estimates of mental disorders in the United States: Using a clinical significance criterion to reconcile 2 surveys' estimates. *Archives of General Psychiatry*, 59, 115–23.

Research Triangle Institute (2002). *SUDAAN: Professional software for survey data analysis 8.01.* Research Triangle Park, NC: Research Triangle Institute.

Ribisl, K. M., Walton, M. A., Mowbray, C. T., Luke, D. A., Davidson, W. S. & Bootsmiller, B. J. (1996). Minimizing participant attrition in panel studies through the use of effective retention and tracking strategies: Review and recommendations. *Evaluation and Program Planning*, 19, 1–25.

Robins, L. N. & Regier, D. A. (1991). *Psychiatric disorders in America: The Epidemiologic Catchment Area Study*. New York: Free Press.

SAS Institute (2001). *SAS/STAT software: Changes and enhancements, Release 8.2*. Cary, NC: SAS Publishing.

Stolk, E. A. & Rutten, F. F. (2005). The "health benefit basket" in The Netherlands. *European Journal of Health Economics*, 53–7.

ten Have, M. L. (2004). Care service use for mental health problems in the general population: Trends and expectations. Dissertation, University of Groningen, The Netherlands.

Turner, C. F., Ku, L., Rogers, S. M., Lindberg, L. D., Pleck, J. H. & Sonenstein, F. L. (1998). Adolescent sexual behavior, drug use, and violence: Increased reporting with computer survey technology. *Science*, 280, 867–73.

van Limbeek, J., van den Berg, C. E. A., Sergeant, J. A., Geerlings, P. J. & Fransman, J. M. L. (1994). Patient, disorder and care: A study on prevalence, course of illness and recognition of mental disorder in East and South East Amsterdam. Amsterdam: GG&GD and University of Amsterdam.

Verdurmen, J., Monshouwer, K., van Dorsselaer, S. & de Graaf, R. (2003). *Bovenmatig drinken in Nederland: Uitkomsten van de "Netherlands Mental Health Survey and Incidence Study" (Nemesis): Achtergrondstudie Nationale Drugmonitor (NDM)*. Utrecht: Bureau of the National Drug Monitor.

Vollebergh, W. A. M., de Graaf, R., ten Have, M., Schoemaker, C. G., van Dorsselaer, S., Spijker, J. & Beekman, A. T. F. (2003). Psychische stoornissen in Nederland: Overzicht van de resultaten van NEMESIS. Utrecht: Trimbos-instituut.

Wang, P. S., Berglund, P. A., Olfson, M. & Kessler, R. C. (2004). Delays in initial treatment contact after first onset of a mental disorder. *Health Services Research*, 39, 393–415.

Wang, P. S., Berglund, P. A., Olfson, M., Pincus, H. A., Wells, K. B. & Kessler, R. C. (2005a). Failure and delay in initial treatment contact after first onset of mental disorders in the National Comorbidity Survey Replication. *Archives of General Psychiatry*, 62, 603–13.

Wang, P. S., Lane, M., Olfson, M., Pincus, H. A., Wells, K. B. & Kessler, R. C. (2005b). Twelve-month use of mental health services in the United States. *Archives of General Psychiatry*, 62, 629–40.

WHO International Consortium in Psychiatric Epidemiology (2000). Cross-national comparisons of the prevalences and correlates of mental disorders. *Bulletin of the World Health Organization*, 78, 413–26.

World Health Organization (WHO) (1991). *International classification of diseases (ICD-10)*. Geneva: World Health Organization.

# 19 The Epidemiology of Mental Disorders in the General Population of Spain

JOSEP MARIA HARO, JORDI ALONSO, ALEJANDRA PINTO-MEZA,
GEMMA VILAGUT SAIZ, ANA FERNÁNDEZ, MIQUEL CODONY,
MONTSERRAT MARTÍNEZ, ANTONIA DOMINGO, JUAN
VICENTE TORRES, JOSUÉ ALMANSA, SUSANA OCHOA,
AND JAUME AUTONELL

## ACKNOWLEDGMENTS

The ESEMeD project is funded by the European Commission (Contracts QLG5-1999-01042; SANCO 2004123), the Piedmont Region (Italy), Fondo de Investigación Sanitaria, Instituto de Salud Carlos III, Spain (FIS 00/0028), Ministerio de Ciencia y Tecnología, Spain (SAF 2000-158-CE), Departament de Salut, Generalitat de Catalunya, Spain, Instituto de Salud Carlos III (CIBER CB06/02/0046, RETICS RD06/0011 REM-TAP), and other local agencies, and by an unrestricted educational grant from GlaxoSmithKline. ESEMeD is carried out in conjunction with the World Health Organization World Mental Health (WMH) Survey Initiative. We thank the WMH staff for assistance with instrumentation, fieldwork, and data analysis. These activities were supported by the U.S. National Institute of Mental Health (R01MH070884), the John D. and Catherine T. MacArthur Foundation, the Pfizer Foundation, the U.S. Public Health Service (R13-MH066849, R01-MH069864, and R01 DA016558), the Fogarty International Center (FIRCA R03-TW006481), the Pan American Health Organization, Eli Lilly and Company Foundation, Ortho-McNeil Pharmaceutical, GlaxoSmithKline, and Bristol-Myers Squibb. A complete list of WMH publications can be found at http://www.hcp.med.harvard.edu/wmh/.

## I. INTRODUCTION

### I.I. The Spanish Health-Care System

The Spanish National Health System (SNHS) was established in 1986, promoting decentralized health care. Responsibility was transferred from central administration to the 17 regional governments, although, until recently, only seven had obtained full powers. The National Health Institute, INSALUD, managed most health services in the remaining regions until 2004. The SNHS is financed by general taxes, with almost universal coverage for all citizens. Provision is mostly publicly owned and managed. Most taxes are centrally raised, as regional and local governments have limited fiscal autonomy. An exception for the coverage of the population is civil servants, who may choose between the SNHS or another health system, which is a mutual fund roughly similar to health maintenance organizations in the United States. Overall, of the total Spanish population, 94.6% are covered by the SNHS and the remaining 4.6% are civil servants and their dependants covered by the mutual funds (Rico & Sabés 2000). Besides the universal coverage, a small proportion of the population (approximately 10%), usually upper classes, have double health insurance: besides the SNHS they have private health insurance, which covers outpatient care and low-complexity hospital services.

Benefits covered by the SNHS include: (1) primary health care, which includes medical and pediatric health care, prevention of disease, health promotion, and rehabilitation; (2) specialized health care, in the form of outpatient and inpatient care, which covers all medical and surgical specialties in acute care; and (3) pharmaceutical and complementary benefits such as prostheses or orthopedic products. The package does not include social care, and the main benefit historically excluded is dental care. For the working population a copayment for medication is applied. Mental health care was integrated within the general health care system in 1986 and submitted to structural reform. Psychiatric reform has had an uneven development among regions and there are difficulties coordinating health and social services in this area (Rico & Sabés 2000). Given that psychiatric outpatient care is not well developed in many regions, psychiatrists working in private settings provide outpatient services on fee-per-service basis or through private health insurance companies. They are outside the public system but cover a significant part of mental health care.

The health-care system is still centered around hospitals rather than around primary health care. Organization and planning is regionally based. Most hospitals are publicly owned and the majority of the staff is salaried. Alongside the hospital system there is an extensive network of outpatient ambulatory centers (Rico & Sabés 2000).

The level of total health-care expenditure is below the European Union (EU) average for the period 1990–1997. Per capita expenditure represents 75% of the EU average, and the same is true for public health-care expenditure (Rico & Sabés 2000).

Core national programs are epidemiological surveillance and AIDS. The National Epidemiological Surveillance Network was created in 1996 and the Ministry of Health is the key sponsor of the National Plan against AIDS. There is also a national antidrug program, run through the Ministry of the Interior, as drug addiction is a major problem in Spain (Rico & Sabés 2000).

## 1.2. Psychiatric Epidemiology in Spain

At the end of the 1970s and during the 1980s, with double-phase studies, an important advance was made within European psychiatric epidemiology. This research strategy was particularly appropriate for measuring mental illness in the general population, as it allowed for standardized systems of evaluating psychiatric symptoms to be incorporated into the study of large populations with a reasonable degree of reliability. In the first phase of double-phase studies, the population under study is classified (by means of a screening questionnaire) in terms of the probable presence or absence of psychiatric pathology. In the second, a proportion of such probable cases and, many times, a proportion of noncases is examined by a mental health professional (by means of a standardized psychiatric interview) to establish a definitive diagnosis (Vázquez-Barquero et al. 1986). However, double-phase epidemiological designs in which the diagnostic instrument is restricted to the second phase have limitations, such as prevalence estimates usually being limited to the time of assessment (point prevalence, instead of 12-month or lifetime prevalence) or, given that the second-phase questionnaire is administered to a reduced part of participants, prevalence estimates being biased.

The introduction of new assessment instruments such as the Diagnostic Interview Schedule (DIS) (Robins et al. 1981) or the consecutive versions of the Composite International Diagnostic Interview (CIDI) (Robins et al. 1988) allowed for researchers to make diagnoses linked to international classification systems such as ICD-10 (World Health Organization [WHO] 1992) and DSM-IV (American Psychiatric Association 2000) in one-phase studies. These instruments can be administered by lay interviewers, which opens the door to large, population-based epidemiological surveys. The DIS and the CIDI have improved the standardization, reliability, and meaningfulness of system and diagnostic rating. The most recent epidemiological research, belonging to the so-called third-generation epidemiological studies, makes use of these standardized interviews and better techniques for sampling large community populations.

In Spain, several double-phase studies have been carried out during the past decades. In a study conducted in the Baztan Valley in 1975 (mostly a rural community situated on the French border of the northwestern part of the province of Navarre), a total of 1156 persons were assessed in a first-phase screen with the General Health Questionnaire (GHQ). In the second phase, all participants considered as "potential positives" for a psychiatric disorder according to GHQ, plus randomly selected potential negatives were assessed by means of a psychiatric interview (Goldberg's Clinical Interview Schedule: CIS [Goldberg et al. 1970]). The point prevalence of psychiatric disorders (including neuroses, functional psychoses, organic psychoses, personality disorders, addictions, dementia, subnormality, and other psychiatric diagnosis) was 19.2% for men and 28.3% for women (23.8% for both sexes) (Vázquez-Barquero, Muñoz & Madoz Jáuregui 1982). Prevalence figures were markedly different from those reported in a contemporary study carried out in Cantabria (three adjoining counties located on the eastern border of the bay of Santander, representing the nonurban coastal zone), evaluating 1223 persons using the GHQ and the 9th 140-item version of the Present State Examination (PSE). The second instrument was administered to 452 persons (50% higher than and 50% lower than GHQ cutoff score for a possible psychiatric case). The point prevalence of psychiatric disorders was 8.1% for men and 20.6% for women (14.7% for both sexes) (Vázquez-Barquero et al. 1987a). The disorders included were anxiety neurosis, phobic neurosis, obsessive neurosis, depressive neurosis, manic depressive psychosis, paranoid schizophrenia, reactive psychosis, and unspecified psychosis, which were classified using the International Classification of Mental and Behavioral Disorders, 9th edition (ICD-9) (WHO 1987).

More recently, in a study carried out in Reus (a city in Catalonia, a northeastern autonomous community in Spain), it was found that point prevalence of psychiatric disorders was 14.5% for men and 24.9% for women (20.6% for both sexes). The disorders included were mood, anxiety, eating, psychotic, sleep, adjustment, somatoform, substance use, and others according to the third revised version of the Diagnostic and Statistical Manual of Mental Disorders: DSM-III-R. Sleep (13.4%), mood (11.7%), and anxiety (9.0%) disorders were the most prevalent (Canals et al. 1997). The study included only 290 participants who were evaluated in one single phase with the Schedules for Clinical Assessment in Neuropsychiatry (SCAN). These results should be interpreted with caution given the small sample size. This study is atypical given that studies using the SCAN are usually double phase.

Although these previous studies found diverse prevalence rates, they agreed in reporting significant differences in point prevalence between sexes (higher for women in all three). A study carried out in Formentera (a small island located at the south of the Balearic Islands) reported no sex differences. A total of 697 participants were assessed in the first phase with the GHQ-28 and in the second with SCAN (50% of above and 50% of below GHQ cutoff score for possible psychiatric case, for 282 subjects). Point prevalence of psychiatric disorders (mood, nonorganic sleep, neurotic and somatoform, substance use, eating, and organic disorders, plus schizophrenia and psychosis) was 22.9% for men and 21.2% for women (21.8% for both sexes). Substance-related (6.1%), neurotic and somatoform (5.7%), and nonorganic sleep (3.7%) disorders were among the most prevalent. Unfortunately, the use of the category of neurotic disorder makes it hard to compare results with studies using DSM categories (Gili et al. 1998).

Among studies assessing specific subpopulations, a double-phase study using the GHQ-28 and the CIS evaluated 400 participants older than 15 years old from a health area of Valdefierro in Zaragoza. The point prevalence of psychiatric disorders was 11% (Lou Arnal et al. 1990). In primary care, a double-phase study using the GHQ-28 and the SCAN evaluated 823 participants from four urban primary care centers in northern

Spain. Point prevalence of psychiatric disorders was 22.3% for men and 36.7% for women (31.5% for both sexes) (Vázquez-Barquero et al. 1997). Among 293 elderly participants from an urban area from Aragon, the point prevalence of psychiatric disorders was 14.7%. Although in the first phase participants were assessed with the GHQ-28, in the second phase the CIS was administered (Seva Díaz et al. 1992).

Another prevalence study examined mental disorders in the elderly population in Galicia (Mateos et al. 2000). In this project, a sample of 3580 people older than 60 years of age was interviewed at home with the 60-item version of the GHQ. In the second phase, all the traced subjects with high GHQ scores (532 participants) and a representative sample (149 individuals) of people below the cutoff point, were interviewed at home using the third version of the DIS.

In Spain, two epidemiological surveys have been carried out using the DIS or the CIDI (Vázquez, Muñoz & Sanz 1997; Arillo Crespo, Aguinaga Ontoso & Guillén Grima 1998). The first one, which used the DIS, estimated the prevalence of mental pathology in a sample of 237 women between 18 and 70 years old in a health district of Pamplona. The 12-month prevalence of psychiatric disorders was 33.3% (95% CI 27.5%–39.5%) and lifetime prevalence was 49.3% (95% CI 43.0%–55.7%). Depression and phobias were the most prevalent disorders both for 12-month and lifetime periods. Psychiatric disorders were more prevalent among women between 21 and 30 years old (Arillo Crespo et al. 1998). The second study, using the CIDI, assessed 261 homeless individuals from Madrid between November 1993 and April 1994, reporting 12-month prevalences of 28% for alcohol abuse or dependence, 13% for major depression, and 2% for schizophrenia (Vázquez et al. 1997). Unfortunately, these data belong to a very specific population, which makes it impossible to generalize results to the general population of Spain.

Although these studies are very heterogeneous, most of them suggest that depressive disorders are among the most frequently observed in the general population and that women tend to have a higher prevalence than men (Vázquez-Barquero et al. 1982, 1986, 1987a, 1997; Seva Díaz et al. 1992; Canals et al. 1997). They also produced prevalence estimates somewhat lower than those found in most comparable surveys in other developed countries. The evidence that prevalence of mental disorders might be lower in Spain than in other developed countries also emerges in a recent epidemiological study carried out in a number of European countries and aimed to address depressive disorders. The point prevalence among participants from urban areas in Santander was 2.6% (95% CI 1.7%–4.0%), the lowest among countries involved (e.g., Ireland: 12.3% [95% CI 5.7%–26.3%]; Norway: 8.8% [95% CI 6.1%–12.9%]). Point prevalence for DSM-IV major depressive episode, dysthymic disorder, and adjustment disorder were 1.8% (95% CI 1.1%–3.0%), 0.5% (95% CI 0.2%–1.2%), and 0.2% (95% CI 0.1%–0.5%), respectively (Ayuso-Mateos et al. 2001).

Taking all of these studies together, we can conclude that Spanish epidemiological studies have an important limitation: they have reported prevalence figures for relatively small geographical areas, not representing all Spanish sociodemographic environments. Moreover, important portions of the population have never been assessed (e.g., southern Spain, Canary Islands). Additionally, existing differences in reported prevalence estimates make it hard to determine true national psychiatric disorder prevalence. Thus, results have limited usefulness for estimating the prevalence and impact of mental disorders in the general population of the country.

The European Study of the Epidemiology of Mental Disorders-Spain (ESEMeD-Spain) is the largest epidemiological survey carried out in Spain. It is part of the ESEMeD project, involving six European countries (Belgium, Denmark, France, Italy, Netherlands, and Spain), and of the World Mental Health (WMH) Survey Initiative (Kessler et al. 2006). The aims of the ESEMeD-Spain study subject to discussion in this chapter were (1) estimation of lifetime and 12-month prevalence of the most common mental disorders in the general population and

(2) analysis of the treatments received by individuals meeting diagnostic criteria, their unmet needs of care, and the quality of the care received.

## 2. METHODS

The ESEMeD-Spain was a cross-sectional face-to-face household interview survey conducted on a probability sample of the general Spanish population aged 18 years or older living in private households. Institutionalized individuals (i.e., those living in prisons, hospitals, hotels, or other institutions) and those who are not able to understand the Spanish language were excluded from the study. The fieldwork was conducted between June 2001 and July 2002.

A stratified four-stage random sample without replacement was drawn. The population was stratified according to autonomous community and size of municipality (fewer than 10,000 inhabitants, from 10,000 to 50,000 inhabitants, from 50,001 to 250,000, and more than 250,000). The sampling units of the first stage were municipalities selected for each of the strata. The second stage consisted of the selection of census tracts within those municipalities. The third stage consisted of the systematic selection of households within each census tract. Because that information was not available, the interviewer had to make a list of all households in the census tract and systematically select six of them. The interviewer had to ask one person of the household to participate in the study and secure one interview in each household. If he or she was successful in all households, then the census tract was completed. Otherwise, if one household refused the interview, the interviewer had to select a new household following the same procedure. If two households refused, the interviewer had to select two new households. The maximum number of households to be selected for each census tract was nine. The fourth stage consisted on the random selection of one 18+ year old individual among all individuals living in that household. The selection of the individual to be interviewed within the household was automatically drawn from the computerized list of adult household members that the interviewer cre-

ated once one person of the household agreed to participate.

As the end of the data collection approached, to minimize nonresponse, the individuals who either had been difficult to reach or had refused to perform the interview were identified. A random selection of individuals within these groups was reapproached to ask again for participation. In the analysis, the interviews obtained from this approach were weighted by the inverse of their probability of selection, to restore their representation in the initial sample. Individuals who agreed to participate gave their written informed consent and all of them received an economic incentive of €12 (voucher or gift). Hard to reach individuals who were approached at the end of the fieldwork received an additional incentive. Methods of the ESEMeD study conducted in Spain are explained in detail elsewhere (Haro et al. 2003, 2006). Fieldwork was conducted by a private survey firm (IPSOS-Ecoconsulting). Interviews were conducted by professional interviewers that were contracted by the survey firm and received a 35-hour training course. They were mostly paid by interview and had an economic incentive for interviewing the hard-to-reach subjects selected at the end of the field period.

The final sample size was $n = 5473$. The initial sample size was lower, but funding from the Catalonian government allowed an oversampling of 886 additional interviews from the population of Catalonia, allowing for 1645 interviews in this autonomous community. These interviews were properly weighted to restore their representation in the whole Spanish sample. Weighted response rate was 78.6%.

Quality-control procedures were implemented across individuals, variables, and interviewers. Checks across individuals implied that each released sampled respondent was checked to verify completion of the interview, that the individual identifier was correct, that there was consistency across the questionnaire variables, and that the itinerary of the respondent was followed in a proper way. Variables were checked by analyzing frequency distributions. That is, all coded variables (variables with predesignated response categories) were checked to identify any out-of-range response values. Finally, checks across interviewers included the evaluation of the number of disorders screened positive and verification of interviews. For the first, a new variable was created that counted the number of sections an interviewee entered according to the responses to the corresponding variables in the screening section located at the beginning of the questionnaire. If the mean value of this variable for a specific interviewer was lower than the lower bound of the 90% confidence interval for all interviewers together, then details of the interviewer were sent to the survey firm so it could monitor him or her closely. For the second, telephone or mail verification of 10% of the interviews of each interviewer took place. In the case of the "suspect" interviewers found, a higher proportion of interviews were targeted for assessment. Concordance was evaluated with overall sensitivity for the entrance to the depression section, taking the verification interview as the gold standard (i.e., the proportion of individuals entering depression in the CIDI 3.0 questionnaire among those that also entered depression in the reinterview).

## 2.1. The Interview

The instrument used for this study was version 3.0 of the World Health Organization (WHO) Composite International Diagnostic Interview (CIDI), developed and adapted by the WHO to be used in the WMH surveys (Kessler & Üstün 2004; see also Chapter 4). The CIDI 3.0 is a comprehensive, fully structured lay-administered diagnostic interview for the assessment of mental disorders that provides lifetime, 12-month and 1-month prevalence of a number of mental disorders according to the definitions and criteria of the 10th version of the International Classification of Diseases (ICD-10) (WHO 1992), and the fourth edition of the Diagnostic and Statistical Manual for Mental disorders (DSM-IV) (American Psychiatric Association 2000). To facilitate administration, the CIDI was converted to a computer-assisted personal interview (CAPI) that was programmed centrally with the Blaise software system. The Blaise software is an interviewing application developed by Statistics Netherlands (Herleen, 1999).

CIDI 3.0 was first produced in English and underwent a rigorous process of adaptation following guidelines recommended by the WHO to obtain a conceptually and cross-culturally comparable version in Spanish. This process included forward and back-translations, a review by a panel of experts, and a pretest using cognitive interview and debriefing techniques. After the translation and adaptation was performed, an international harmonization panel group, which included investigators from the CIDI editorial committee and the other Spanish-speaking countries participating in the WMH initiative, reviewed the instrument and created a Spanish version that with minimal adaptations could be used in all Spanish-speaking countries in the WMH series (Haro et al. 2003).

To optimize the interviewing process and cost, the CIDI was divided into two parts for use in the WMH surveys. The first part was administered to all respondents and contained the diagnostic assessment of the most common mood and anxiety disorders, health-related quality of life, health services use, and main demographic characteristics. Only those who exceeded a number of symptoms of specific mood or anxiety disorders and a random 25% of the rest were asked to participate in the second phase, that included among other information, a detailed questionnaire about additional mental disorders, self-reported chronic physical conditions, and risk factors.

The mental disorders assessed in the ESEMeD surveys were a somewhat short series than in some of the other WMH surveys. The disorders included mood disorders (major depressive episode [MDE] and dysthymic disorder without hierarchy [DYS]), anxiety disorders (panic disorder [PD], generalized anxiety disorder with hierarchy [GAD], specific phobia [SP], social phobia [SO], agoraphobia without panic [AGP], posttraumatic stress disorder [PTSD], adult separation anxiety [ASA]), impulse-control disorders (oppositional-defiant disorder with hierarchy [ODD], conduct disorder [CD], attention-deficit/hyperactivity disorder [ADHD]) and alcohol-related disorders (alcohol abuse [ALA], alcohol dependence [ALD]). DSM-IV (American Psychiatric Association 2000) diagnostic criteria were used, taking into account organic exclusions. Compared to other WMH surveys, bipolar disorder and intermittent explosive disorder (IED) were not assessed in ESEMeD. Also, drug abuse, drug dependence, and obsessive-compulsive disorder were not analyzed as a result of an error in the ESEMeD questionnaire skips.

## 2.2. Severity of 12-month Cases

Individuals with at least one 12-month mental disorder were classified into three severity groups (severe, moderate, or mild) according to the following rules (individuals were classified as severe if they fulfilled any of the following conditions): (1) attempted suicide within the past 12 months; (2) ALD with physiological dependence syndrome; or (3) severe role impairment (scores from eight to ten) in at least two areas of the WMH adapted version of the Sheehan Disability Scales (SDS; Sheehan, Harnett-Sheehan & Raj 1996). Cases not defined as severe were defined as moderate if they had moderate role impairment in at least one domain of the SDS (i.e., a score greater than four), or if they had ALD disorder without physiological dependence. All other individuals with mental disorders were classified as mild.

Briefly, the WMH adapted version of the SDS evaluates current disability in four domains: home management, ability to work, ability to form and maintain close relationships, and social life. The domains can be scored using a Likert scale ranging from 0 ("no, not at all") to 10 ("severe"). It has been suggested that scores between 0 and 3 reveal mild disability; 4 to 6, moderate disability; and 7 to 10, severe disability (Sheehan et al. 1996).

Because of an error in the early version of the CAPI program that was used in all the ESEMeD countries, a subsample of the respondents with a major depressive episode were not assessed with the Sheehan Disability Scale. Sheehan Disability Scale values for those individuals were imputed

using polytomous logistic regression models that took into account the ratings of other disability and quality-of-life scales included in the CIDI.

## 2.3. Use of Health Services

All respondents were initially asked to delineate lifetime use of any service as a result of their "emotions or mental health problems." Individuals who reported use of services because of their "emotions or mental health problems" were then asked to select who they had seen with respect to those problems from a list of professionals: psychiatrist, nonpsychiatrist mental health specialist (i.e., psychologist, psychotherapist, social worker, or counselor), a general medical provider (i.e., general family doctor, any other doctor, any other health professional such as a nurse or nutritionist), human services professionals (a religious or spiritual advisor), and complementary and alternative medicine (CAM) professionals (any other healer such as an herbalist, chiropractor, or spiritualist).

For the analyses, psychiatrist and nonpsychiatrist specialist categories were combined into a broader mental health specialty (MHS) category; MHS was also combined with general medical (GM) into an even broader health-care (HC) category. Human services (HS) and CAM were also combined into a non–health-care (NHC) category.

For each of these providers, participants were asked about the age at first contact, whether last contact was within the previous 12 months, and if so, whether the last contact was within the previous 30 days. In addition, participants were asked about the number of visits they had made to these providers in the previous 12 months and their duration, whether they were still using the service or had stopped, and the type of treatment received.

In each of the questionnaire diagnostic sections about mental disorders, additional questions regarding the use of health services for those specific mental problems were asked. Twelve-month treatment variables for the analyses were created using a combination of the use of services information of the individual diagnostic sections and the responses to questions in the general services section.

## 2.4. Predictor Variables

Predictor variables in analysis of lifetime data included age of onset (AOO) of the disorder (coded into the categories early, middle, late), sex, cohort (defined by age at interview in the categories 18–34, 35–49, 50–64, 65+), and education (student or nonstudent with low, low/medium, medium, or high education level). This last variable was used as time-varying covariates (i.e., vary within a given individual over time). To code years of education as a time-varying predictor, an orderly correspondence between educational history and age was assumed for each respondent, in which it was considered that individuals started studying at the age of six.

Variables used in the analysis of 12-month data were sex, cohort in the same groups described previously, per capita income of the respondent's household divided by the median income for the country in a four-category scale (low $\leq 0.5$; low-average 0.5–1.0; high-average 1.0–2.0; high $\geq 2.0$), marital status (married or cohabiting, previously married, never married), and education (none or some primary, complete primary, secondary, college).

## 2.5. Analysis Procedures

Individuals were weighted to account for the different probabilities of selection within household and among hard to reach individuals, as well as to restore age, sex, and autonomous-community distribution of the Spanish general population. An additional weight was used in the Part 2 sample to adjust for differences in probability of selection into that sample.

Basic patterns of 12-month disorders were examined by computing proportions, means, and medians. Logistic regression analyses were used to study sociodemographic predictors of having 12-month disorders, severity of mental disorders, and receiving any 12-month treatment in the total sample.

The actuarial method implemented in SAS 8.0 (SAS Institute 1999) was used to obtain estimated projections of cumulative lifetime probability of disorders and treatment contact from year of onset. These values were then divided by the cumulative lifetime probability at 75 years old (standardization) to determine the age of onset percentiles. To obtain projections of lifetime risk and the corresponding standard error of specific mental disorders at the age of 75 years old, the Kaplan–Meier methodology implemented in SUDAAN V9.0 (Research Triangle Institute 2004) was used.

Discrete-time survival analysis with person-year as the unit of analysis was used to examine correlates of disorder and treatment contact (Efron 1988). Data were analyzed using SAS 8.0 for UNIX (SAS Institute 1999). The standard errors of ratio estimates, means, regression coefficients, and other statistics were estimated taking into account the sample design by using the Taylor series linearization method implemented in SUDAAN software V9.0 (Research Triangle Institute 2004). Multivariate significance tests were made using Wald $\chi^2$ tests based on coefficient variance-covariance matrices that were adjusted for design effects using the Taylor series method. Statistical significance was evaluated using two-sided design-based tests and the 0.05 level of significance.

## 3. RESULTS

Sociodemographic characteristics of respondents are presented in Table 19.1, both for Part 1 and Part 2 sample. Weighted proportions are compared to the Spanish general population based on the 2001 Census (Instituto Nacional de Estadística 2001). Nonweighted data showed a higher proportion of women and older individuals than in the general population of Spain, a common participation bias pattern in population-based studies. The weighted percentages of age groups, sex, and municipality size, both for the Part 1 and Part 2 samples, were very similar and, at the same time, very close to those for the general population. Of the sample, 55.8% were women, 67.1% were married or cohabiting,

**Table 19.1.** Sociodemographic characteristics of the Part 1 and Part 2 study sample of Spain

| | P1 unweighted | | P1 weighted | | P2 unweighted | | P2 weighted | | Census 2001[a] | |
|---|---|---|---|---|---|---|---|---|---|---|
| | n | % | n | % | n | % | n | % | n | % |
| Overall | 5473 | 100.0 | 5473 | 100.0 | 2121 | 100.0 | 2121 | 100.0 | 33,505,967 | 100.0 |
| Sex[b] | | | | | | | | | | |
| Male | 2421 | 44.2 | 2618.8 | 47.8 | 819 | 38.6 | 1031.8 | 48.6 | 16,243,472 | 48.5 |
| Female | 3052 | 55.8 | 2854.2 | 52.2 | 1302 | 61.4 | 1089.2 | 51.4 | 17,262,495 | 51.5 |
| Age categories[b] | | | | | | | | | | |
| 18–34 | 1567 | 28.6 | 1875.6 | 34.3 | 545 | 25.7 | 741.2 | 34.9 | 11,115,775 | 33.2 |
| 35–49 | 1431 | 26.2 | 1406.8 | 25.7 | 556 | 26.2 | 534.5 | 25.2 | 8,929,100 | 26.6 |
| 50–64 | 1024 | 18.7 | 1062.1 | 19.4 | 456 | 21.5 | 413.4 | 19.5 | 6,496,942 | 19.4 |
| 65+ | 1451 | 26.5 | 1128.5 | 20.6 | 564 | 26.6 | 431.9 | 20.4 | 6,964,267 | 20.8 |
| Inhabitants number | | | | | | | | | | |
| ≤10,000 | 1411 | 25.8 | 1399.6 | 25.6 | 520 | 24.5 | 565.1 | 26.6 | 7,994,646 | 23.9 |
| 10,000–50,000 | 1377 | 25.2 | 1348.6 | 24.6 | 544 | 25.6 | 508.6 | 24.0 | 8,435,169 | 25.2 |
| 50,000–100,000 | 1732 | 31.6 | 1793.1 | 32.8 | 664 | 31.3 | 707.2 | 33.3 | 11,175,976 | 33.4 |
| >500,000 | 953 | 17.4 | 931.7 | 17.0 | 393 | 18.5 | 340.1 | 16.0 | 5,900,176 | 17.6 |
| Per capita income | | | | | | | | | | |
| Low | 769 | 14.1 | 946.3 | 17.3 | 309 | 14.6 | 323.6 | 15.3 | | |
| Low-average | 1734 | 31.7 | 1793.9 | 32.8 | 721 | 34.0 | 766.3 | 36.1 | | |
| High-average | 1952 | 35.7 | 1869.3 | 34.2 | 716 | 33.8 | 718.1 | 33.9 | | |
| High | 1018 | 18.6 | 863.5 | 15.8 | 375 | 17.7 | 313.1 | 14.8 | | |
| Marital status categories | | | | | | | | | | |
| Married/cohabiting | 3674 | 67.1 | 3576.2 | 65.3 | 1398 | 65.9 | 1385.9 | 65.3 | 19,099,287 | 57.4 |
| Previously married | 722 | 13.2 | 490.1 | 9.0 | 350 | 16.5 | 196.9 | 9.3 | 3,808,346 | 11.5 |
| Never married | 1077 | 19.7 | 1406.7 | 25.7 | 373 | 17.6 | 538.2 | 25.4 | 10,356,334 | 31.1 |
| Education categories | | | | | | | | | | |
| None/some primary | 1545 | 28.2 | 1410.6 | 25.8 | 647 | 30.5 | 548.0 | 25.8 | | |
| Complete primary | 1747 | 31.9 | 1733.6 | 31.7 | 679 | 32.0 | 688.5 | 32.5 | | |
| Secondary | 857 | 15.7 | 894.5 | 16.3 | 317 | 14.9 | 326.4 | 15.4 | | |
| College | 1324 | 24.2 | 1434.3 | 26.2 | 478 | 22.5 | 558.2 | 26.3 | | |

[a] General population of Spain, 18 years or older (available at http://www.ine.es/censo/es/inicio.jspp, accessed September 12, 2006).
[b] Sociodemographic variables used in poststratification of weight. P1 = Part 1 sample, P2 = Part 2 sample.

45.2% of the sample were 50 years or older, and 67.4% of respondents were within the average range of income per capita (0.5–2.0 compared to the median income for the country).

## 3.1. Lifetime Prevalence of Mental Disorders

The most prevalent lifetime disorders (Table 19.2) were MDE (10.6%), specific phobia (4.8%), alcohol abuse (3.6%), and dysthymic disorder (3.6%). Mood disorders were the most prevalent class of disorders (11.6%), followed by any anxiety (9.9%), alcohol (3.6%), and impulse-control disorders (2.3%). The lifetime prevalence of any of the disorders analyzed was 20.2%, while 7.9% of respondents had two or more lifetime disorders and 3.0% had three or more.

The distributions of cumulative lifetime risk estimates were standardized and examined for fixed percentiles (Table 19.3). The lowest median AOO (i.e., 50th percentile on the AOO distribution) were found for SP (age 7) and SO (age 13). Although the median AOO of impulse-control

**Table 19.2.** Lifetime prevalence of DSM-IV/CIDI disorders in the adult Spanish population (Part I sample, $n = 5473$)

| Disorder class | Disorder | Total % (se) | 18–34 % (se) | 35–49 % (se) | 50–64 % (se) | 65+ % (se) | $\chi^2$ (df) |
|---|---|---|---|---|---|---|---|
| Anxiety | Panic | 1.2 (0.2) | 1.1 (0.3) | 1.9 (0.4) | 1.1 (0.3) | 0.7 (0.2) | 7.1 (3) |
| | GAD with hierarchy | 1.3 (0.2) | 1.2 (0.3) | 1.4 (0.3) | 1.6 (0.5) | 1.1 (0.2) | 1.2 (3) |
| | Social phobia | 1.2 (0.2) | 1.9 (0.4) | 1.4 (0.5) | 0.4 (0.2) | 0.4 (0.2) | 11.9 (3)* |
| | Specific phobia | 4.8 (0.4) | 5.1 (0.7) | 4.9 (0.7) | 4.8 (0.8) | 4.0 (0.5) | 2.5 (3) |
| | Agoraphobia without panic | 0.6 (0.1) | 0.7 (0.2) | 0.8 (0.3) | 0.5 (0.3) | 0.4 (0.1) | 2.8 (3) |
| | PTSD[a] | 2.0 (0.4) | 2.0 (0.5) | 2.1 (1.2) | 2.1 (0.5) | 1.9 (0.8) | 0.0 (3) |
| | SAD/ASA[b] | 1.1 (0.4) | 1.4 (0.6) | 0.5 (0.2) | – | – | 1.7 (1) |
| | Any anxiety[a] | 9.9 (1.1) | 12.0 (1.8) | 11.8 (2.3) | 7.1 (1.3) | 6.7 (1.2) | 10.9 (3)* |
| Mood | MDE | 10.6 (0.5) | 9.1 (0.8) | 11.9 (0.8) | 12.6 (1.0) | 9.8 (1.0) | 10.9 (3)* |
| | Dysthymic disorder | 3.6 (0.3) | 2.1 (0.4) | 3.8 (0.6) | 5.9 (0.9) | 4.0 (0.6) | 3.0 (3)* |
| | Any mood | 11.6 (0.5) | 9.4 (0.8) | 13.2 (0.8) | 13.8 (1.2) | 11.0 (1.0) | 19.1 (3)* |
| Impulse | ODD with hierarchy[b] | 0.5 (0.2) | 0.6 (0.3) | 0.4 (0.3) | – | – | 0.3 (1) |
| | CD[b] | 0.5 (0.2) | 0.7 (0.3) | 0.2 (0.1) | – | – | 1.6 (1) |
| | ADHD[b] | 1.8 (0.8) | 2.0 (1.2) | 1.4 (0.6) | – | – | 0.2 (1) |
| | Any impulse[b] | 2.3 (0.8) | 2.6 (1.2) | 1.7 (0.7) | – | – | 0.4 (1) |
| Alcohol | Alcohol abuse | 3.6 (0.4) | 5.0 (0.7) | 4.7 (0.8) | 1.9 (0.5) | 1.2 (0.6) | 31.0 (3)* |
| | Alcohol dependence | 0.6 (0.1) | 0.6 (0.2) | 1.0 (0.4) | 0.5 (0.3) | 0.1 (0.0) | 24.8 (3)* |
| | Any alcohol disorder | 3.6 (0.4) | 5.1 (0.7) | 4.8 (0.8) | 1.9 (0.5) | 1.2 (0.6) | 32.7 (3)* |
| All disorders | Any disorder[a] | 20.2 (1.5) | 22.0 (2.3) | 23.1 (2.6) | 17.7 (1.8) | 15.9 (1.8) | 10.8 (3)* |
| | 2+ disorders[a] | 7.9 (0.7) | 9.1 (1.5) | 8.7 (1.8) | 6.3 (0.8) | 6.4 (1.1) | 4.2 (3) |
| | 3+ disorders[a] | 3.0 (0.4) | 3.1 (0.5) | 4.2 (1.4) | 3.0 (0.6) | 0.2 (0.3) | 12.2 (3)* |

*Notes:* CIDI: World Mental Health Composite International Diagnostic Interview; GAD: generalized anxiety disorder; PTSD: posttraumatic stress disorder; SAD/ASA: separation anxiety disorder/adult separation anxiety; MDE: major depressive episode; ODD: oppositional-defiant disorder; CD: conduct disorder; ADHD: attention-deficit/hyperactivity disorder. Intermittent explosive disorder, drug abuse, drug dependence, and bipolar disorder were not assessed in Spain.

[a] Denotes Part 2 disorder (evaluated on $n = 2121$).

[b] Denotes disorder in Part 2 and age $\leq 44$ years (evaluated on $n = 960$).

* $p < 0.05$.

disorders (age 9) and anxiety disorders (age 19) were the lowest for class of disorders, it was substantially higher for mood disorders (age 43).

Interquartile ranges (IQR), that is, the number of years between the 25th and 75th percentiles of AOO distributions, were 30 years for both anxiety (7–37 years) and mood disorders (28–58 years). The IQR was substantially narrower for impulse-control disorders (8–11 years) than for alcohol disorders (20–35 years).

Projected lifetime risk at the age of 75 was higher for mood disorders (20.8%), followed by anxiety disorders (13.3%), alcohol disorders (4.6%), and impulse-control disorders (2.3%).

Projected lifetime risk for mental disorders at the age of 75 was 100% higher than the actual lifetime prevalence for mood disorders, 34% higher for anxiety disorders, 36% higher for alcohol disorders, and 50% higher for any mental disorder.

As it can be observed in Table 19.4, lifetime risk for mental disorders is much higher for the younger age cohorts. Although differences between individuals from 50 to 65 years old and 65 and older are small, subjects from 35 to 49 and mostly those younger than 35 showed a much higher risk of developing mental disorders at some time in their lives. The largest

**Table 19.3.** Percentiles of standardized age of onset distributions of mental disorders according to DSM-IV and projected lifetime risk at age 75 (general population of Spain)

| Disorder class | Disorder | Age of onset percentiles | | | | | | | | Projected lifetime risk at age 75 | |
|---|---|---|---|---|---|---|---|---|---|---|---|
| | | 5 | 10 | 25 | 50 | 75 | 90 | 95 | 99 | % | (se) |
| Anxiety | Panic | 14 | 17 | 24 | 33 | 47 | 60 | 64 | 65 | 2.1 | (0.3) |
| | GAD with hierarchy | 9 | 14 | 20 | 35 | 55 | 62 | 68 | 69 | 2.2 | (0.4) |
| | Social phobia | 5 | 5 | 9 | 13 | 19 | 22 | 48 | 48 | 1.3 | (0.2) |
| | Specific phobia | 5 | 5 | 5 | 7 | 16 | 43 | 56 | 66 | 5.5 | (0.5) |
| | Agoraphobia without panic | 11 | 11 | 20 | 39 | 47 | 61 | 73 | 73 | 1.0 | (0.3) |
| | PTSD | 10 | 20 | 23 | 34 | 54 | 70 | 75 | 75 | 4.4 | (1.4) |
| | SAD/ASA[a] | – | – | – | – | – | – | – | – | – | – |
| | Any anxiety | 5 | 5 | 7 | 19 | 37 | 60 | 66 | 71 | 13.3 | (1.4) |
| Mood | MDE | 16 | 19 | 28 | 43 | 58 | 69 | 73 | 75 | 20.8 | (1.2) |
| | Any mood | 16 | 19 | 28 | 43 | 58 | 69 | 73 | 75 | 20.8 | (1.2) |
| Impulse | ODD with hierarchy[a] | – | – | – | – | – | – | – | – | – | – |
| | CD[a] | – | – | – | – | – | – | – | – | – | – |
| | ADHD[a] | – | – | – | – | – | – | – | – | – | – |
| | Any impulse | 7 | 7 | 8 | 9 | 11 | 13 | 17 | 17 | 2.3 | (0.8) |
| Alcohol | Alcohol abuse | 17 | 18 | 20 | 23 | 35 | 41 | 43 | 56 | 4.6 | (0.5) |
| | Alcohol dependence | 17 | 18 | 20 | 23 | 36 | 39 | 43 | 43 | 0.7 | (0.2) |
| | Any alcohol disorder | 17 | 18 | 20 | 23 | 35 | 41 | 43 | 56 | 4.6 | (0.5) |
| All | Any disorder | 5 | 6 | 16 | 31 | 51 | 65 | 71 | 75 | 29.0 | (1.8) |

*Notes:* GAD: generalized anxiety disorder; PTSD: posttraumatic stress disorder; SAD/ASA: separation anxiety disorder/adult separation anxiety; MDE: major depressive episode; ODD: oppositional-defiant disorder; CD: conduct disorder; ADHD: attention-deficit/hyperactivity disorder. Dysthymic disorder omitted as a result of lack of age of onset data.

[a] Cell size ≤30 cases; too small to estimate.

cohort effects were observed for ALD, AGP, PD, and MDE. However, for this to be true, the AOO pattern of disorders should be maintained for the younger age cohorts: we should be observing an increase in the frequency of mental disorders and not purely a decrease in AOO.

Table 19.5 presents the association of education (analyzed as a time-varying covariate) and sex with the lifetime risk of the DSM-IV disorders broad categories (any mood, any anxiety, any alcohol, and any impulse) after adjusting by age cohort. The interactions between age cohorts and both education and sex were also tested (results not shown). Females had a statistically significant higher risk of mood and anxiety disorders and a lower risk for alcohol disorders. The interaction between study cohort and sex was statistically significant for anxiety and alcohol disorders, whereas the interaction between age cohort and

education was not significant in predicting the risk of any group of disorders.

### 3.2. 12-month Prevalence and Severity of Mental Disorders

The most prevalent 12-month mental disorders were MDE (4.0%), SP (3.6%), and DYS (1.5%) (Table 19.6). The most prevalent class of disorder was anxiety disorders (6.2%), followed by mood disorders (4.4%), alcohol disorders (0.7%), and impulse-control disorders (0.5%). The latter was almost entirely defined by the presence of ADD (0.4%). Overall, the 12-month prevalence of mental disorders was 9.3%.

Considering severity of disorders, among those with at least a 12-month mental disorder, 20.7% were classified as serious, 44.6% as moderate, and 34.8% as mild. The class of disorder

**Table 19.4.** Lifetime risk of DSM-IV mental disorders according to age cohort in the Spanish general population

| Disorder | Age group (reference = 65+) | | | $\chi^2$ (DF) | p-value |
| | 18–34 | 35–49 | 50–64 | | |
| | OR (95% CI) | OR (95% CI) | OR (95% CI) | | |
| --- | --- | --- | --- | --- | --- |
| Panic | 7.8* (2.7, 22.3) | 6.4* (3, 13.5) | 1.9 (0.8, 4.4) | 31.7 (3) | <0.001 |
| GAD with hierarchy | 3.7* (1.6, 8.5) | 2.7* (1.2, 5.9) | 2.1* (1.0, 4.2) | 11.4 (3) | 0.010 |
| Social phobia | 5.6* (1.8, 16.9) | 3.6* (1.1, 12.1) | 0.9 (0.2, 3.5) | 20.8 (3) | <0.001 |
| Specific phobia | 1.6* (1.1, 2.3) | 1.4 (0.9, 2.2) | 1.3 (0.8, 2.1) | 6.7 (3) | 0.08 |
| Agoraphobia without panic | 9.6* (3.6, 25.9) | 6.6* (1.9, 22.2) | 1.9 (0.5, 7.9) | 21.7 (3) | <0.001 |
| PTSD | 3.8 (0.7, 20.6) | 2.1 (0.3, 12.8) | 1.5 (0.4, 5.5) | 5.7 (3) | 0.13 |
| SAD/ASA[a] | – | – | – | – | – |
| Any anxiety | 3.8* (2.2, 6.5) | 2.8* (1.5, 5.2) | 1.3 (0.8, 2.2) | 28.7 (3) | <0.001 |
| MDE | 9.6* (6.6, 13.9) | 4.2* (3.0, 5.9) | 2.2* (1.6, 3.0) | 176.3 (3) | <0.001 |
| Any mood | 9.6* (6.6, 13.9) | 4.2* (3.0, 5.9) | 2.2* (1.6, 3.0) | 176.3 (3) | <0.001 |
| ODD with hierarchy[a] | – | – | – | – | – |
| CD[a] | – | – | – | – | – |
| ADHD[a] | – | – | – | – | – |
| Any impulse | 1.5 (0.5, 5.3) | 1.0 (1.0, 1.0) | 1.0 (1.0, 1.0) | 0.5 (1) | 0.48 |
| Alcohol abuse | 9.4* (3.6, 24.7) | 5.0* (1.8, 13.7) | 1.5 (0.6, 4.2) | 38.4 (3) | <0.001 |
| Alcohol dependence | 17.8* (4.7, 66.8) | 19.2* (4.3, 86.7) | 7.7* (1.4, 41.5) | 20.9 (3) | <0.001 |
| Any alcohol disorder | 9.3* (3.6, 24.2) | 5.0* (1.8, 13.7) | 1.5 (0.6, 4.2) | 38.1 (3) | <0.001 |
| Any disorder | 6.0* (3.9, 9.3) | 3.5* (2.2, 5.4) | 1.6* (1.1, 2.4) | 119.6 (3) | <0.001 |

*Notes:* GAD: generalized anxiety disorder; PTSD: posttraumatic stress disorder; SAD/ASA: separation anxiety disorder/adult separation anxiety; MDE: major depressive episode; ODD: oppositional-defiant disorder; CD: conduct disorder; ADHD: attention-deficit/hyperactivity disorder; OR: odds ratio; DF: degrees of freedom. Based on discrete-time survival models with person-year as the unit of analysis. Controls are time intervals.

[a] Cell size ≤30 cases; too small to estimate.

* Significant at the 0.05 level.

with the highest percentage of serious cases was mood disorders (33.8%), followed by impulse-control disorders (22.1%) and anxiety disorders (19.6%). People with ALA or ALD showed the lowest percentage of severe cases (4.2%). The disorder with the highest proportion of severe cases was ASA (73.7%), followed by PD (45.3%), and DYS (40.1%).

The only statistically significant sociodemographic predictor of having a 12-month mental disorder was sex, with women having an odds ratio for any 12-month mental disorder of 2.3 (CI 95%: 1.4–3.8) compared to men (Table 19.7). Other sociodemographic characteristics such as age, income, marital status, and education were not associated. Sex was a significant predictor of having a 12-month mental disorder, but it did not serve to distinguish severe or moderate cases from mild cases among those with at least one

mental disorder. Furthermore, no sociodemographic variable proved a significant predictor of severity among people with any 12-month mental disorder.

Sex, age, and severity of the 12-month mental disorders were significant predictors of the use of health-care treatment. Women showed an odds ratio of 1.8 (CI 95%: 1.1–3.0) compared to men, respondents younger than 35 years old showed an odds ratio of 0.3 (CI 95%: 0.2–0.5) compared to those older than 64 years old, and severe disorders had the highest odds ratio 41.1 (CI 95%: 20.7–81.4).

### 3.3. 12-month Treatment for Mental Disorders

Among individuals with 12-month mental disorders, 35.2% consulted any HC professional.

**Table 19.5.** Adjusted association of sex, education, and cohort with lifetime risk of DSM-IV mental disorders (general population of Spain)

| | | Disorder | | | |
|---|---|---|---|---|---|
| | | **Any anxiety** | **Any mood** | **Any impulse** | **Any alcohol** |
| | | OR (95% CI) | OR (95% CI) | OR (95% CI) | OR (95% CI) |
| Education | Student | 1.1 (0.3, 3.7) | 1.0 (0.4, 2.4) | 1.0 (0.0, 25.4) | 2.0 (0.6, 6.7) |
| | Low | 0.2* (0.1, 0.8) | 0.8 (0.4, 1.7) | 2.7 (0.0, 143.4) | 1.2 (0.3, 4.2) |
| | Low-medium | 1.0 (0.3, 3.9) | 1.2 (0.6, 2.5) | 1.0 (1.0, 1.0) | 2.1 (0.7, 6.5) |
| | Medium | 0.7 (0.2, 2.5) | 1.5 (0.8, 3.0) | –(–) | 1.2 (0.4, 4.0) |
| | High | 1.0 (1.0, 1.0) | 1.0 (1.0, 1.0) | –(–) | 1.0 (1.0, 1.0) |
| | $\chi^2$ | 27.2 (df = 4, $p$ < 0.001) | 7.7 (df = 4, $p$ = 0.10) | 1.8 (df = 2, $p$ = 0.40) | 5.2 (df = 4, $p$ = 0.26) |
| Sex | Male | 1.9* (1.1, 3.4) | 2.2* (1.6, 2.9) | 0.5 (0.2, 1.7) | 0.2* (0.1, 0.4) |
| | Female | 1.0 (1.0, 1.0) | 1.0 (1.0, 1.0) | 1.0 (1.0, 1.0) | 1.0 (1.0, 1.0) |
| | Chi-square | 4.9 (df = 1, $p$ = 0.026) | 26.4 (df = 1, $p$ < 0.001) | 1.2 (df = 1, $p$ = 0.28) | 30.7 (df = 1, $p$ < 0.001) |
| Age | 18–34 | 3.1* (1.6, 6.0) | 5.6* (3.1, 9.9) | 1.6 (1.4, 5.3) | 5.5* (1.4, 21.1) |
| | 35–49 | 2.2 (1.0, 5.0) | 2.2* (1.2, 4.0) | 1.0 (1.0, 1.0) | 2.5 (0.6, 10.3) |
| | 50–64 | 1.2 (0.6, 2.4) | 1.0 (0.5, 1.8) | –(–) | 0.8 (0.2, 3.5) |
| | 65+ | 1.0 (1.0, 1.0) | 1.0 (1.0, 1.0) | –(–) | 1.0 (1.0, 1.0) |
| | $\chi^2$ | 18.4 (df = 3, $p$ < 0.001) | 95.4 (df = 3, $p$ < 0.001) | 0.5 (df = 1, $p$ = 0.47) | 24.2 (df = 3, $p$ < 0.001) |

*Note:* OR: odds ratio; df: degrees of freedom. Models include time intervals as controls. Person-years are restricted to ≤29 years. Interactions of age with education and sex were tested. The interaction of age and gender was significant for anxiety and alcohol disorders; interaction between age and education was not significant in predicting the age of onset of any group of disorders.

* Significant at the 0.05 level.

**Table 19.6.** 12-month prevalence and severity of mental disorders (adult general population of Spain)

| Disorder | n | Total % (se) | Serious[b] % (se) | Moderate[b] % (se) | Mild[b] % (se) |
|---|---|---|---|---|---|
| **Anxiety disorders** | | | | | |
| Panic disorder[a] | 45 | 0.6 (0.1) | 45.3 (8.1) | 35.9 (8.7) | 18.8 (7.8) |
| Generalized anxiety disorder with hierarchy[a] | 36 | 0.5 (0.1) | 23.5 (8.0) | 44.0 (11.8) | 32.5 (12.9) |
| Specific phobia[a] | 195 | 3.6 (0.4) | 12.9 (3.6) | 52.2 (8.9) | 34.9 (9.5) |
| Social phobia[a] | 31 | 0.6 (0.1) | 38.8 (10.3) | 44.0 (10.6) | 17.1 (11.0) |
| Agoraphobia without panic[a] | 22 | 0.3 (0.1) | 25.6 (13.1) | 63.0 (13.0) | 11.3 (6.7) |
| Posttraumatic stress disorder[b] | 31 | 0.5 (0.1) | 39.5 (11.3) | 44.1 (11.6) | 16.4 (7.4) |
| Adult separation anxiety[c] | 4 | 0.2 (0.1) | 73.7 (23.3) | 26.3 (23.3) | 0.0 (0.0) |
| Any anxiety disorder[b] | 223 | 6.2 (0.8) | 19.6 (3.2) | 49.8 (6.1) | 30.6 (6.8) |
| **Mood disorders** | | | | | |
| Major depressive disorder with hierarchy[a] | 247 | 4.0 (0.3) | 36.2 (3.7) | 38 (2.9) | 25.9 (2.7) |
| Dysthymic disorder without hierarchy[a] | 91 | 1.5 (0.3) | 40.1 (5.6) | 27.8 (5.6) | 32.1 (5.9) |
| Any mood disorder[a] | 270 | 4.4 (0.3) | 33.8 (3.1) | 35.5 (3.0) | 30.7 (2.8) |
| **Impulse disorders** | | | | | |
| Oppositional-defiant disorder[c] | 1 | 0.0 (0.0) | 0.0 (0.0) | 100.0 (0.0) | 0.0 (0.0) |
| Conduct disorder[c] | 1 | 0.0 (0.0) | 100.0 (0.0) | 0.0 (0.0) | 0.0 (0.0) |
| Attention-deficit/hyperactivity disorder disorder[c] | 12 | 0.4 (0.2) | 15.7 (10.4) | 20.3 (13.8) | 64 (16.9) |
| Any impulse-control disorder[c] | 14 | 0.5 (0.2) | 22.1 (11.8) | 24.3 (13.3) | 53.6 (16.7) |
| **Alcohol disorders** | | | | | |
| Alcohol abuse[a] | 32 | 0.7 (0.2) | 4.2 (3.8) | 0.0 (0.0) | 95.8 (3.8) |
| Alcohol dependence[a] | 5 | 0.1 (0.1) | 100.0 (0.0) | 0.0 (0.0) | 0.0 (0.0) |
| Any alcohol disorder[a] | 32 | 0.7 (0.2) | 4.2 (3.8) | 0.0 (0.0) | 95.8 (3.8) |
| **Any disorder** [b] | 405 | 9.3 (0.8) | 20.7 (2.4) | 44.6 (4.1) | 34.8 (4.6) |
| Total sample[b] | 2121 | 9.8 (0.7) | 1.9 (0.2) | 4.2 (0.5) | 3.5 (0.6) |

*Note:* Severity calculated using Part 2 weights. Bipolar I/II/subthreshold, intermittent explosive disorder, drug abuse, and drug dependence were not assessed in Spain.

[a] Part 1 sample; prevalence calculated using Part 1 weights.

[b] Part 2 sample; prevalence calculated using Part 2 weights.

[c] Part 2 sample (age ≤44); prevalence and severity calculated using Part 2 weights for ages ≤44.

Mood disorders showed the highest consultation rates to HC professionals (56.0%). On the contrary, alcohol disorders showed the lowest consultation rates to HC professionals (1.2%). Moreover, participants with alcohol disorders only consulted psychiatrists. Among the persons not fulfilling any of the 12-month diagnosis assessed, 3.8% consulted any HC professional (Table 19.8).

Among those treated in the HC sector, the majority consulted the GM services (24% of those with 12-month mental disorders, representing 68% of those consulting HC services). Although those with anxiety disorders showed a consultation rate to GM professionals much higher than to MHS professionals (24.9% vs. 14.5%, respectively), those with mood disorders showed similar rates of consultation to GM and MHS professionals (37.5% vs. 35.8%, respectively). Exclusive use of NHC (HS or CAM) was very low, representing less than 2% of the overall consultation rate among those with any 12-month mental disorder.

The median number of 12-month visits among those receiving any treatment was 2.2 (standard error [se] = 0.2). This was slightly higher among those with any 12-month mental

**Table 19.7.** Association of sociodemographic variables with 12-month DSM-IV mental disorders in the Spanish general adult population

| | Any 12-month disorder | | Severity[a] | | Health-care treatment | |
|---|---|---|---|---|---|---|
| | OR | (95% CI) | OR | (95% CI) | OR | (95% CI) |
| **Sex** | | | | | | |
| Male | 1.0 | (1.0–1.0) | 1.0 | (1.0–1.0) | 1.0 | (1.0–1.0) |
| Female | 2.3 | (1.4–3.8) | 1.4 | (0.6–3.3) | 1.8 | (1.1–3.0) |
| $\chi^2$ | | 12.1[a] | | 0.8 | | 5.9[a] |
| **Age** | | | | | | |
| 18–34 | 1.4 | (0.9–2.1) | 0.9 | (0.4–2.4) | 0.3 | (0.2–0.5) |
| 35–49 | 1.4 | (0.8–2.2) | 0.9 | (0.4–2.0) | 0.9 | (0.5–1.7) |
| 50–64 | – | (–) | – | (–) | – | (–) |
| 65+ | 1.0 | (1.0–1.0) | 1.0 | (1.0–1.0) | 1.0 | (1.0–1.0) |
| $\chi^2$ | | 3.0 | | 0.1 | | 29.6[a] |
| **Income** | | | | | | |
| Low | – | (–) | – | (–) | – | (–) |
| Low-average | 1.2 | (0.7–2.0) | 1.0 | (0.5–2.1) | 0.8 | (0.6–1.1) |
| High-average | – | (–) | – | (–) | – | (–) |
| High | 1.0 | (1.0–1.0) | 1.0 | (1.0–1.0) | 1.0 | (1.0–1.0) |
| $\chi^2$ | | 0.5 | | 0.0 | | 1.7 |
| **Marital status** | | | | | | |
| Married/cohabiting | 1.0 | (1.0–1.0) | 1.0 | (1.0–1.0) | 1.0 | (1.0–1.0) |
| Separated/widowed/divorced | – | (–) | – | (–) | – | (–) |
| Never married | 1.2 | (0.7–2.1) | 0.8 | (0.4–1.5) | 1.4 | (1.0–2.2) |
| $\chi^2$ | | 0.4 | | 0.6 | | 3.3 |
| **Education** | | | | | | |
| None/some primary | 0.8 | (0.4–1.6) | 1.4 | (0.5–4.4) | 1.0 | (0.5–2.1) |
| Complete primary | – | (–) | – | (–) | – | (–) |
| Secondary | 1.0 | (0.6–1.9) | 1.5 | (0.6–4.0) | 0.7 | (0.4–1.2) |
| College | 1.0 | (1.0–1.0) | 1.0 | (1.0–1.0) | 1.0 | (1.0–1.0) |
| $\chi^2$ | | 2.1 | | 0.8 | | 4.8 |
| **Severity** | | | | | | |
| Severe | | | | | 41.1 | (20.7–81.4) |
| Moderate | | | | | 13.9 | (7.3–26.4) |
| Mild | | | | | 11.0 | (6.6–18.3) |
| None | | | | | 1.0 | (1.0–1.0) |
| $\chi^2$ | | | | | | 213.0[a] |

*Note:* Part 2 sample ($n = 2121$).
[a] Severity is a dichotomy: 1 = severe or moderate; 0 = mild, defined among those with a 12-month disorder.

disorder (2.7; se = 0.6) than among those without them (2.0; se = 0.2) (Table 19.9). Among respondents with a 12-month mental disorder, the median number of visits to the GM service (1.8; se = 0.2) was lower than those to the MHS (3.0; se = 0.5). No significant differences in the median number of visits were observed between participants with mood and anxiety disorders. The median number of visits to the GM service was the same for respondents with (1.8; se = 0.2) or without (1.8; se = 0.1) 12-month mental disorders. On the contrary, the median number

**Table 19.8.** Percentage of use of health-care services among individuals with 12-month mental disorder in the Spanish general population

| Disorder class | Mental disorder | Type of professional | | | | | | | | | Unweighted n with mental disorder | Weighted n with mental disorder |
| | | Psychiatrist % (se) | Other mental health care % (se) | Any mental health care % (se) | General medical % (se) | Any health care % (se) | Human services % (se) | CAM % (se) | Any non-health care % (se) | Any treatment % (se) | | |
|---|---|---|---|---|---|---|---|---|---|---|---|---|
| Anxiety | GAD[a] | 27.1 (6.0) | 9.9 (4.0) | 31.1 (7.0) | 48.4 (7.4) | 66.9 (6.3) | 2.5 (2.1) | 2.0 (1.4) | 3.5 (2.3) | 66.9 (6.3) | 59 | 45 |
| | Panic disorder[a] | 34.1 (8.8) | 13.2 (5.4) | 39.4 (9.4) | 53.9 (8.8) | 74.6 (7.6) | 3.3 (2.4) | 3.3 (2.4) | 3.3 (2.4) | 74.6 (7.6) | 45 | 33 |
| | Agoraphobia w/o panic[a] | –(–) | –(–) | –(–) | –(–) | –(–) | –(–) | –(–) | –(–) | –(–) | 22 | 19 |
| | Social phobia[a] | 20.7 (8.3) | 11.1 (4.2) | 24.3 (8.5) | 36.5 (10.9) | 45.8 (10.5) | 1.4 (1.4) | 1.4 (1.4) | 1.4 (1.4) | 45.8 (10.5) | 31 | 35 |
| | Specific phobia[a] | 3.4 (1.2) | 1.7 (0.8) | 4.7 (1.5) | 14.3 (3.4) | 17.6 (3.6) | 0.7 (0.5) | 0.5 (0.4) | 1.0 (0.6) | 17.9 (3.6) | 195 | 197 |
| | ASA[b] | –(–) | –(–) | –(–) | –(–) | –(–) | –(–) | –(–) | –(–) | –(–) | 4 | 2 |
| | PTSD[b] | 37.7 (11.4) | 20.6 (10.7) | 43.5 (11.8) | 55.0 (12.0) | 63.9 (11.8) | 3.6 (3.6) | 15.2 (10.3) | 16.9 (10.6) | 63.9 (11.8) | 31 | 11 |
| | Any anxiety disorder[b] | 13.2 (2.7) | 4.9 (1.4) | 14.5 (2.7) | 24.9 (3.6) | 31.3 (4.2) | 0.9 (0.4) | 1.5 (1.0) | 1.9 (1.0) | 31.3 (4.2) | 233 | 133 |
| Mood | Major depressive episode[a] | 34.1 (2.8) | 16.6 (2.6) | 37.9 (3.0) | 39.0 (3.6) | 58.7 (3.6) | 1.3 (0.7) | 3.3 (1.2) | 3.7 (1.3) | 59.1 (3.6) | 247 | 218 |
| | Dysthymic disorder[a] | 32.2 (5.8) | 16.2 (4.7) | 33.0 (6.0) | 42.3 (8.0) | 56.2 (7.4) | 1.3 (0.9) | 1.6 (1.1) | 1.6 (1.1) | 56.2 (7.4) | 91 | 82 |
| | Any mood disorder[a] | 32.3 (3.0) | 15.3 (2.3) | 35.8 (3.2) | 37.5 (3.6) | 56.0 (4.0) | 1.2 (0.7) | 3.0 (1.1) | 3.3 (1.2) | 56.4 (4.0) | 270 | 241 |
| Alcohol | Alcohol abuse[a] | 1.2 (1.2) | 0.0 (0.0) | 1.2 (1.2) | 0.0 (0.0) | 1.2 (1.2) | 0.0 (0.0) | 0.0 (0.0) | 0.0 (0.0) | 1.2 (1.2) | 32 | 38 |
| | Alcohol dependence[a] | –(–) | –(–) | –(–) | –(–) | –(–) | –(–) | –(–) | –(–) | –(–) | 5 | 5 |
| | Any alcohol disorder[a] | 1.2 (1.2) | 0.0 (0.0) | 1.2 (1.2) | 0.0 (0.0) | 1.2 (1.2) | 0.0 (0.0) | 0.0 (0.0) | 0.0 (0.0) | 1.2 (1.2) | 32 | 38 |
| Composite | Any disorder[b] | 18.8 (2.2) | 8.3 (1.3) | 20.9 (2.3) | 24.0 (2.6) | 35.2 (3.3) | 0.6 (0.3) | 1.6 (0.7) | 1.9 (0.7) | 35.5 (3.3) | 400 | 196 |
| | No disorder[b] | 1.4 (0.3) | 0.7 (0.2) | 1.8 (0.3) | 2.4 (0.4) | 3.8 (0.5) | 0.1 (0.0) | 0.1 (0.0) | 0.2 (0.1) | 3.9 (0.5) | 1,721 | 1,925 |
| | Total Part 2 sample[b] | 3.0 (0.3) | 1.4 (0.2) | 3.6 (0.4) | 4.4 (0.4) | 6.7 (0.5) | 0.1 (0.1) | 0.2 (0.1) | 0.4 (0.1) | 6.8 (0.5) | 2,121 | 2,121 |

*Note:* GAD: generalized anxiety disorder; ASA: adult separation anxiety; PTSD: posttraumatic stress disorder; CAM: complementary and alternative medicine. Values are percentages with standard errors in parentheses. Disorders with *n* less than 30 do not have percentages.

[a] Denotes Part 1 weight.
[b] Denotes Part 2 weight.

**Table 19.9.** Median number of visits in the past year (and standard error) among those receiving treatment

| Disorder group | Psychiatrist | Other mental health care | Any mental health care | General medical | Any health care | Human services | CAM | Any non–health care | Any treatment |
|---|---|---|---|---|---|---|---|---|---|
| Any anxiety disorder[b] | 2.6 (0.6) | – | 3.1 (0.7) | 1.8 (0.1) | 2.0 (0.5) | – | – | – | 2.0 (0.5) |
| Any mood disorder[a] | 2.5 (0.4) | 2.8 (0.7) | 3.2 (0.8) | 1.9 (0.3) | 3.0 (0.8) | – | – | – | 3.0 (0.6) |
| Any alcohol disorder[a] | – | – | – | – | – | – | – | – | – |
| Any disorder[b] | 2.6 (0.4) | 2.7 (0.7) | 3.0 (0.5) | 1.8 (0.2) | 2.7 (0.6) | – | – | – | 2.7 (0.6) |
| No disorder[b] | 1.4 (0.3) | – | 1.7 (0.4) | 1.8 (0.1) | 2.0 (0.2) | – | – | – | 2.0 (0.2) |
| Total Part 2 sample[b] | 1.8 (0.3) | 2.8 (0.6) | 2.4 (0.5) | 1.8 (0.1) | 2.3 (0.2) | – | – | – | 2.2 (0.2) |

*Notes:* CAM: complementary and alternative medicine. Non–health care includes human services and CAM.

[a] Denotes Part 1 weight.

[b] Denotes Part 2 weight.

of visits to MHS was lower for participants without 12-month mental disorders (1.7; se = 0.4 vs. 3.0; se = 0.5).

Table 19.10 presents the analysis of the relationship of disorder severity and use of services. We can observe that the frequency of treatment contact greatly increased with severity of the disorder: although 43% of individuals with a severe disorder consulted the GM sector and 38.4% the MHS sector, the percentages among those with mild disorders were 12.6% and 7.1%, respectively. We cannot observe a tendency for severe cases more frequently consulting the specialized

sector, as severe cases tended to use the GM sector more than the specialized one.

### 3.4. Lifetime Treatment for Mental Disorders

The percentage of individuals making a treatment contact during the year-of-onset of the disorder, among those who received care, varied substantially across mental disorders (Table 19.11). Respondents with SP (3.6%) and SO (10.5%) showed the lowest percentages, followed by respondents with ALA (17.1%). Almost 60%

**Table 19.10.** Percentage (se) of use of health-care services, according to severity of the disorder

| Treatment | Severe % (se) | Moderate % (se) | Mild % (se) | None % (se) | Any % (se) |
|---|---|---|---|---|---|
| General medical | 43.0 (4.8) | 22.9 (4.3) | 12.6 (3.8) | 2.4 (0.4) | 4.4 (0.4) |
| Mental health | 38.4 (5.0) | 23.0 (3.5) | 7.1 (2.1) | 1.8 (0.3) | 3.6 (0.4) |
| Health care | 58.4 (4.8) | 37.4 (5.0) | 16.9 (4.3) | 3.8 (0.5) | 6.7 (0.5) |
| Non–health care | 2.2 (1.4) | 2.4 (1.5) | 1.0 (0.6) | 0.2 (0.1) | 0.4 (0.1) |
| Any treatment | 58.7 (4.9) | 37.4 (5.0) | 17.3 (4.3) | 3.9 (0.5) | 6.8 (0.5) |
| No treatment | 41.3 (4.9) | 62.6 (5.0) | 82.7 (4.3) | 96.1 (0.5) | 93.2 (0.5) |

*Note:* Non–health care includes human services and complementary and alternative medicine.

**Table 19.11.** Percentage of treatment contact in the year of disorder onset and median duration of delay among cases that subsequently made treatment contact

| | % making treatment contact in year of onset | % making treatment contact by 50 years | Median duration of delay (years) | n |
|---|---|---|---|---|
| **Anxiety disorders** | | | | |
| Panic disorder | 59.3 | 91.9 | 1 | 87 |
| Generalized anxiety disorder | 51.2 | 89.3 | 1 | 131 |
| Specific phobia | 3.6 | 61.0 | 37 | 259 |
| Social phobia | 10.5 | 68.4 | 14 | 61 |
| Any anxiety disorder | 23.2 | 86.6 | 17 | 463 |
| **Mood disorders** | | | | |
| Major depressive episode | 48.5 | 96.4 | 1 | 665 |
| **Alcohol disorders** | | | | |
| Alcohol abuse | 17.1 | 38.9 | 6 | 49 |
| Alcohol dependence | —[a] | —[a] | —[a] | —[a] |
| Any alcohol disorder | 18.6 | 40.1 | 6 | 52 |

[a] Disorder was omitted as a result of insufficient ($n < 30$), but it will be included as one of the disorders in "Any" category. Posttraumatic stress disorder, agoraphobia without panic, and separation anxiety disorder/adult separation anxiety are not included in the table because of insufficient $n < 30$.

of the individuals with PD made a treatment contact within the year-of-onset of the disorder. This percentage was close to 50% for MDE and GAD. The median duration of delay among those who made treatment contact ranged from 1 year for PD, GAD, and MDE to 37 years for SO. The percentage of individuals making treatment contact by 50 years did also differ greatly, being highest for MDE (96.4%) and the lowest for ALA (38.9%).

Discrete-time survival analyses were conducted to evaluate the associations among sex, study cohort, and AOO of the disorders with lifetime treatment contact among respondents with lifetime disorders. As shown in Table 19.12, the AOO was significantly related to the lifetime treatment contact. Individuals with early or early-average AOO of the disorder presented lower odds of lifetime treatment contact for all the disorders evaluated. Sex was not found to be associated with lifetime treatment contact for any of the disorders. Younger individuals showed statistically significant higher odds of lifetime treatment contact than did older cohorts.

## 4. DISCUSSION

### 4.1. Mental Disorders in the General Population of Spain

Mental disorders are frequent in the general population of Spain. About one out of five persons showed a lifetime mental disorder. MDE, SP, and ALA were among the most frequent disorders, with lifetime prevalences ranging from 3.6% to 10.6%. Almost 10% of the population suffered from a 12-month mental disorder. MDE and SP were again the most prevalent disorders. Overall, severity of 12-month mental disorders was moderate. However, most of PD, SO, MDE, and DYS were serious. On the other hand, alcohol-related and impulse-control disorders were mostly mild.

The comparability of these results with previous Spanish studies is limited, as no prior study assessed mental disorders in a representative sample of the general population of Spain, and previous studies used different assessment procedures and different classification systems. However, in general, previous studies showed

**Table 19.12.** Sociodemographic predictors of lifetime treatment contact for specific mental disorders

| | Sex | Cohort (age at interview) | | | | Age of onset | | | |
| | Female | Age 18–34 | Age 35–49 | Age 50–64 | | Early | Early-average | Late-average | |
| | OR (95% CI) | OR (95% CI) | OR (95% CI) | OR (95% CI) | $\chi^2$ | OR (95% CI) | OR (95% CI) | OR (95% CI) | $\chi^2$ |
|---|---|---|---|---|---|---|---|---|---|
| **Anxiety disorders** | | | | | | | | | |
| Panic disorder | 0.7 (0.2–2.0) | 2.9 (0.5–16.7) | 3.1 (0.7–13.7) | 1.1 (0.2–5.4) | 4.9 | 0.2* (0.0–0.6) | 0.6 (0.1–2.7) | 0.6 (0.2–2.1) | 11.2* |
| Generalized anxiety disorder | 1.7 (0.9–3.3) | 1.6 (0.5–4.8) | 1.7 (0.6–4.4) | 0.5 (0.2–1.2) | 7.8* | 0.3* (0.1–0.9) | 0.5 (0.1–1.5) | 1.3 (0.5–3.3) | 8.8* |
| Specific phobia | 1.5 (0.6–3.5) | 1.2 (0.4–4.1) | 0.6 (0.2–1.6) | 0.5 (0.2–1.4) | 8.3* | 0.2* (0.1–0.5) | 0.8 (0.3–2.0) | 0.5 (0.2–1.3) | 12.0* |
| Social phobia | 0.3 (0.1–1.2) | 1.6 (0.5–5.5) | 1.2 (0.3–4.0) | 1.0 (0.1–16.3) | 0.8 | 0.2 (0.0–1.7) | 0.1* (0.0–0.9) | 0.3 (0.1–2.1) | 5.4 |
| Any anxiety disorder | 1.0 (0.7–1.6) | 3.3* (1.9–5.7) | 2.0* (1.1–3.7) | 0.8 (0.5–1.3) | 38.5* | 0.1* (0.0–0.1) | 0.1* (0.0–0.2) | 0.2* (0.1–0.4) | 96.2* |
| **Mood disorders** | | | | | | | | | |
| Major depressive episode | 1.2 (0.8–1.8) | 1.9 (0.9–3.8) | 2.7* (1.4–5.1) | 1.3 (0.8–2.1) | 11.3* | 0.4* (0.2–0.8) | 0.4* (0.2–0.9) | 0.7 (0.4–1.2) | 8.3* |
| **Alcohol disorders** | | | | | | | | | |
| Alcohol abuse | 1.5 (0.1–27.5) | 7.0* (1.3–36.4) | 1.0 (–) | 1.0 (–) | 5.6* | 0.0* (0.0–0.3) | 0.0* (0.0–0.5) | 0.2 (0.0–1.8) | 12.6* |
| Alcohol dependence | —[a] | —[a] | —[a] | —[a] | —[a] | —[a] | —[a] | —[a] | —[a] |
| Any alcohol disorder | 1.5 (0.1–41.2) | 8.1* (1.4–46.8) | 1.0 (–) | 1.0 (–) | 5.8* | 0.0* (0.0–0.1) | 0.0* (0.0–0.7) | 0.2 (0.0–1.7) | 16.0* |

*Note:* OR: odds ratio.

[a] Disorder was omitted as a result of insufficient lifetime cases ($n < 30$), but it will be included as one of the disorders in "Any" category.

* Significant at the 0.05 level, two-sided test.

higher prevalence figures of depression and over-all prevalence of mental disorders. For example, the study by Gaminde and colleagues (1993), which included participants between 18 and 65 years old, reported lifetime prevalence of depression of 20.6% for men and 36.7% for women, which represent higher figures than those presented here. Also, point prevalences reported by Vázquez-Barquero and colleagues (1987b) for depression (7.8% for women and 4.3% for men) and anxiety (20.6% for women and 8.1% for men) were higher than ours. Finally, Roca and colleagues (1999) reported a point prevalence of mental disorders of 21.4%. We found 12-month and lifetime prevalences of 9.3% and 20.2%, respectively, a lower prevalence than previous studies. Again, it is important to mention that these studies used different instruments (e.g., PSE and SCAN) and different classification systems (CATEGO, DSM-III, and ICD-10). On the other hand, the ODIN study carried out in Santander (Ayuso-Mateos et al. 2001) found a very low prevalence of current major depression.

Our prevalence figures are also lower than those reported by international epidemiological surveys. Although in the National Comorbidity Survey (NCS) (Kessler et al. 1994), its replication (Kessler et al. 2003), and the NEMESIS study (Bijl, Ravelli & Van Zessen 1998), lifetime prevalences of depression were higher than 20% for women and 10% for men, in our study, prevalences were much lower. Differences were similar for the 12-month figures, as these studies reported prevalences of depression between 10% and 13% for women, and between 5% and 8% for men (compared to 4.4% for both sexes in our study). The same differences are observed for anxiety disorders. For example, in the NCS, lifetime prevalence of PD was 5% for women and 2% for men; in the NEMESIS study, prevalence was 5.7% for women and 1.9% for men. According to our data, lifetime prevalence of PD was 1.2% for both sexes. It could be possible that differences emerged because of using a different version of the CIDI, which could reduce the estimation of false positive cases (Kessler et al. 2003). However, differences between NCS (Kessler et al. 1994) and

its replication (Kessler et al. 2003), where the new version of the CIDI was used, were minor compared to differences among NCS, NEMESIS, and our data.

A particular striking difference is for 12-month and lifetime prevalence of ALA (0.7% and 3.6%, respectively). This could be somehow explained because we used DSM-IV diagnostic criteria, which could be more restrictive than previous DSM versions (First 2002) and do not define abuse only on the basis of the quantity of alcohol consumed. Nevertheless, information bias (individuals denying their ALA) and selection bias (individuals rejecting the interview or absent from their homes) could be possible. Previous studies have related nonresponse to higher rates of mental disorders. However, findings are controversial (Kessler, Little & Groves 1995; De Graaf et al. 2000). In any case, CIDI has shown to be reliable for assessing dependence disorders, including ALD (Compton et al. 1996).

Two patterns emerged regarding the standardized AOO distributions of mental disorders. First, the median AOO was much earlier for anxiety disorders (19 years) and for alcohol disorders (23 years) than for mood disorders (43 years). Among anxiety disorders, the median AOO varied, with the earliest median age of onset for SP and SO (7 and 13 years, respectively), and the latest for AGP, GAD with hierarchy, and PTSD (39, 35, and 34 years, respectively). Second, AOO was concentrated in wide age ranges for most disorders, with IQRs of 30 years for anxiety disorders (7–37) and mood disorders (28–58), and 15 years for alcohol disorders (20–35) compared to three years (8–11) for impulse disorders. Compared to the NCS replication study figures (Kessler et al. 2005), in Spain the median AOO for anxiety (11 years vs. 19 years), mood (30 years vs. 43 years), and alcohol (20 years vs. 23 years) disorders was higher, and AOO ranges were markedly wider for most disorders (e.g., 6–21 years vs. 7–37 years for anxiety disorders, or 18–27 years vs. 20–35 years for alcohol disorders), except for impulse-control disorders (7–15 years vs. 8–11 years).

Among mental disorders, projected lifetime risk at the age of 75 years was the highest for mood disorders (which included only MDE) and anxiety disorders. These results are consistent with data from the NCS replication study. However, important differences were observed for the projected lifetime risk for any mental disorder. Although in Spain this risk was 50% higher than the current lifetime prevalence, in the United States the difference was 9% (Kessler et al. 2005). These large differences are attributed to a much higher increase in the prevalence of mental disorders in the younger age cohorts, which may imply that in the future the gap between the prevalence in Spain and in other Western countries such as the United States will diminish or disappear.

An important association was observed between recentness of age cohort and lifetime risk for mental disorders, especially for ALD, AGP, and MDE. Respondents born between 1966 and 1982 were at higher risk for these disorders than were respondents born before 1936. Consistently, in the NCS replication (Kessler et al. 2005) an important association was observed between recentness of age cohort and lifetime risk for mental disorders. However, the strongest associations were observed for drug use disorders and bipolar I and II disorders (not evaluated in our study: ESEMeD-Spain). Additionally, the strength of association was higher than those from the United States for ALD, AGP, and MDE. This increase is greatly important for the perspectives about the societal burden associated to mental disorders: if prevalence increases, the estimates of the burden of mental disorders will also increase in the future.

Consistent with previous surveys, our study revealed that being female was associated with 12-month prevalence of mental disorders (Kessler et al. 1994; Bijl et al. 1998; WHO International Consortium in Psychiatric Epidemiology 2000). However, these studies also suggested that divorced or widowed participants and some age groups are at higher risk of mental disorders. Our data do not support other sociodemographic predictors.

## 4.2. Lifetime and 12-month Treatment for Mental Disorders

Among respondents, 6.7% used services in the prior year, including 35.2% of those with a 12-month DSM-IV disorder (American Psychiatric Association 2000) and 3.8% of those without them. These figures are markedly lower than those reported in the NCS replication study, where 17.9% of respondents used services in the last 12 months, including 41.1% of those with a 12-month mental disorder and 10.1% of those without them (Wang et al. 2005). Use of services ranged from a high for PD (74.6%) to a low for ALA (1.2%), which presumably reflects the influence of greater distress and impairment on help seeking. The lower treatment rate for ALA may reflect diminished perceived need for treatment on the part of patients and tendencies for patients and providers to view this problem as social rather than medical (Kaskutas, Weisner & Caetano 1997; Mojtabai, Olfson & Mechanic 2002). Overall, most treatment occurred in the HC sector, with a substantial predominance of the GM sector in all mental disorders but ALA, where MHS predominated. Similarly, in the United States, general physicians were more frequently giving treatment for 12-month mental disorders, except for alcohol and mood disorders, where MHS was predominant. This situation is not surprising considering that, in Spain, general physicians are increasingly acting as gatekeepers responsible for initiating mental health treatments themselves and for deciding whom to triage for specialty care.

As shown, 12-month treatment data revealed serious problems in meeting the treatment needs of people with mental disorders in Spain. Use of services was strikingly low, with most respondents with at least one mental disorder not receiving any care in the past 12 months. Moreover, the median number of 12-month visits among those receiving any treatment was slightly higher among those with DSM-IV disorders (2.7) than among those without disorders (2.0). A close but less alarming situation was observed in the NCS replication study, where 58.9% of persons with any 12-month mental disorder did not use any treatment and statistically significant differences were observed in the median number of 12-month visits between those with disorders (4.5) and those without them (1.9) (Wang et al. 2005).

As it has been observed in many other countries (WHO World Mental Health Survey

Consortium 2004), health care was more frequently used by persons with severe mental disorders, followed by persons with moderate and mild cases. In fact, severity of disorder was a predictor of health-care use. However, about 41% of severe cases and 63% of moderate cases did not use any treatment, revealing important unmet health-care needs among the Spanish population. Also, 3.8% of those without a 12-month DSM-IV (American Psychiatric Association 2000) mental disorder used health care. These data might reflect the joint effects of the CIDI 3.0 not assessing all mental disorders, some true cases of the disorders being wrongly classified as noncases, and some persons in treatment not meeting the criteria of a DSM-IV disorder (American Psychiatric Association 2000). The fact that noncases make up the vast majority of the population means that noncases constitute a meaningful fraction of all people in treatment. If we add the fact that almost 17% of those with mild disorders did also use health care, we could state that treatment-planning efforts should be made regarding the provision and redirection of health care (this will be discussed in the next section).

Being male and younger age were associated with reduced use of health-care treatment among those with mental disorders during the past year. These data are consistent with prior research carried out in the United States (Kessler et al. 1999; Wang et al. 2005). The lower association of health-care treatment to male sex could be explained by the greater perceived stigma and women's greater abilities to translate nonspecific feelings of distress into conscious recognition of having a mental disorder (Kessler, Brown & Broman 1981; Williams et al. 1995). The same could be argued for the lower association of treatment with older age: it may be because of the greater perceived stigma of mental disorders among older people (Leaf et al. 1985).

A great variability was observed across diagnoses in the percentage of respondents making a treatment contact in the year-of-onset of the disorder. In general, mood and anxiety disorders showed the highest frequencies. However, among anxiety disorders, although almost 60% of respondents with PD made contact in the year of onset, only 3.6% of those with SP and 10.5% of those with SO made contact. Moreover, regarding SP, 37 years was the median duration of delay among cases that made treatment contact, the highest among mental disorders. Because the distress and impairment associated to SP is restricted to the phobic object/situation, presumably leaving general role functioning without major impairment, seeking help could be delayed or avoided.

Overall, the use of non–health-care treatment was rather low (close to 2%), except for PTSD (almost 17%). In this case, CAM played a major role. As Wang and colleagues (2005) have suggested, this represents a challenge for providers of conventional services who should ascertain why CAM has such great appeal for patients suffering PTSD and which aspects are related to this appeal (e.g., a greater orientation to patient-centered care) could be adopted by conventional health-care providers to increase the attractiveness of evidence-based treatments.

## 4.3. Implications for Treatment Planning Efforts in Spain

The main implications of these findings for service planning are that health services must be prepared to attend the growing burden that mental disorders represent in the population of Spain. Current prevalence is not only high but also growing in the younger cohorts. Moreover, unmet need for treatment is still very high.

One notable finding of our survey is that many services are being consumed by respondents without apparent disorders. Given the profound unmet need for mental health services among people with well-defined mental disorders, the use of treatment resources by individuals without mental disorders is concerning. A partial explanation of this finding is that individuals who previously suffered from a disorder could now be recovered and receiving maintenance care, thereby not fulfilling diagnostic criteria for a mental disorder. In addition, disorder severity was strongly associated with treatment, which suggests that demand for treatment is related to severity, presumably mediated by distress and impairment.

Some limitations should be acknowledged when evaluating these results. First, the ESEMeD-Spain was a cross-sectional population survey. As is commonly observed in this kind of study, a proportion of individuals reject responding to the interview. Thus, we do not know to what extent it is possible that nonrespondents could show differences in the prevalence of mental disorders compared to respondents. Also, the exclusion of institutionalized persons, despite the fact that they make up a small proportion of the population, should be taken into account. Second, mental disorders were diagnosed according to DSM-IV criteria, using CIDI 3.0 administered by lay interviewers and excluding some diagnoses (e.g., schizophrenia, bipolar disorders, nonalcohol, substance-related disorders). Despite the acceptable validity and reliability of this instrument (Wittchen et al. 1991; Haro et al. 2007), it is important to note that prevalence figures obtained using the CIDI differ from those obtained by means of clinical interviews. Limited diagnostic validity, especially for some particular diagnoses (Brugha et al. 1999), could be attributable to the instrument's structured and inflexible characteristics. Considering this, the present study collected information regarding diagnoses on which CIDI has shown better reliability. Third, the absence of previous Spanish data about treatment use does not allow comparisons within Spain regarding the validity of self-reported treatment use. A recent study of the Ontario Health Survey (Rhodes, Lin & Mustard 2002) suggested that self-reports of mental health service use overestimate the number of visits and services use among respondents with more distressing disorders.

In summary, the ESEMeD-Spain Study has provided for the first time countrywide estimates of the prevalence and treatment of mental disorders in Spain. We have reported here a summary of the main findings of the project, which will be followed by future analysis on specific topics.

## REFERENCES

American Psychiatric Association (2000). *Diagnostic and statistical manual of mental disorders*, 4th ed. Washington, DC: American Psychiatric Association.

Arillo Crespo, A., Aguinaga Ontoso, I. & Guillén Grima, F. (1998). Prevalencia de enfermedades mentales en mujeres de una zona urbana [Prevalence of mental disorders in women in an urban area]. *Atención Primaria*, 21, 265–9.

Ayuso-Mateos, J. L., Vázquez-Barquero, J. L., Dowrick, C., Lehtinen, V., Dalgard, O. S., Casey, P, Wilkinson, C., Lasa, L., Page, H., Dunn, G., Wilkinson, G. & ODIN Group (2001). Depressive disorders in Europe: Prevalence figures from the ODIN study. *British Journal of Psychiatry*, 179, 308–16.

Bijl, R., Ravelli, A. & Van Zessen, G. (1998). Prevalence of psychiatric disorder in the general population: Results of the Netherlands Mental Health Survey and Incidence Study. *Social Psychiatry and Psychiatric Epidemiology*, 33, 587–95.

Brugha, T. S., Bebbington, B. E., Jenkins, R., Meltzer, H., Taub, N., Janas, M. & Vernon, J. (1999). Cross-validation of a general population survey diagnostic interview: A comparison of CIS-R with SCAN ICD-10 diagnostic categories. *Psychological Medicine*, 29, 1029–42.

Canals, J., Domènech, E., Carbajo, G. & Blade, J. (1997). Prevalence of DSM-III-R and ICD-10 psychiatric disorders in a Spanish population of 18-year-olds. *Acta Psychiatrica Scandinavica*, 96, 287–94.

Compton, W. M., Cottler, L. B., Dorsey, K. B., Spitznagel, E. L. & Mager, D. E. (1996). Comparing assessments of DSM-IV substance dependence disorders using CIDI-SAM and SCAN. *Drug and Alcohol Dependence*, 41, 179–87.

de Graaf, R., Bijl, R. V., Smit, F., Ravelli, A. & Vollebergh, W. A. (2000). Psychiatric and sociodemographic predictors of attrition in a longitudinal study: The Netherlands Mental Health Survey and Incidence Study (NEMESIS). *American Journal of Epidemiology*, 152, 1039–47.

Efron, B. (1988). Logistic regression, survival analysis, and the Kaplan-Meier curve. *Journal of the American Statistical Association*, 83, 414–25.

First, M. B. (2002). DSM-IV and psychiatric epidemiology. In *Textbook in psychiatric epidemiology*, ed. M. T. Tsuang & M. Tohen, pp. 333–62. New York: John Wiley & Sons.

Gaminde, I., Uria, M., Padro, D., Querejeta, I. & Ozamiz, A. (1993). Depression in three populations in the Basque country: A comparison with Britain. *Social Psychiatry and Psychiatric Epidemiology*, 28, 243–51.

Gili, M., Ferrer, V., Roca, M. & Bernardo, M. (1998). Diferencias de género en un estudio epidemiológico de salud mental en la población general en la isla de Formentera [Gender differences in an epidemiological study of mental health in the general population of Formentera Island]. *Actas Luso-Españolas de Neurología, Psiquiatría y Ciencias Afines*, 26, 90–6.

Goldberg, D. P., Cooper, B., Eastwood, M. R., Kedward, H. B. & Shepherd, M. (1970). A standardized psychiatric interview for use in community surveys. *British Journal of Preventive and Social Medicine*, 24, 18–23.

Haro, J. M., Arbabzadeh-Bouchez, S., Brugha, T. S., de Girolamo, G., Guyer, M. E., Jin, R., Lepine, J. P., Mazzi, F., Reneses, B., Vilagut, G., Sampson, N. A. & Kessler, R. C. (2007). Concordance of the Composite International Diagnostic Interview Version 3.0 (CIDI 3.0) with standardized clinical assessments in the WHO World Mental Health Surveys. *International Journal of Methods in Psychiatric Research*, 15, 167–80.

Haro, J. M., Palacin, C., Vilagut, G., Martinez, M., Bernal, M., Luque, I., Codony, M., Dolz, M., Alonso, J. & Grupo ESEMeD-España (2006). Prevalence of mental disorders and associated factors: Results from the ESEMeD-Spain study. *Medicina Clínica*, 126, 445–51.

Haro, J. M., Palacin, C., Vilagut, G., Romera, B., Codony, M., Autonell, J., Ferrer, M., Ramos, J., Kessler, R. C. & Alonso, J. (2003). Epidemiology of mental disorders in Spain: Methods and participation in the ESEMeD-Spain project. *Actas Españolas de Psiquiatría*, 31, 182–91.

Instituto Nacional de Estadística (2001). Censos de población y viviendas 2001: Resultados definitivos. Available at http://www.ine.es/censo/es/inicio.jsp (accessed October 12, 2006).

Kaskutas, L. A., Weisner, C. & Caetano, R. (1997). Predictors of help seeking among a longitudinal sample of the general population. *Journal of Studies on Alcohol*, 58, 155–61.

Kessler, R. C., Berglund, P., Demler, O., Jin, R., Koretz, D., Merikangas, K. R., Rush, A. J., Walters, E. E. & Wang, P. S. (2003). The epidemiology of major depressive disorder: Results from the National Comorbidity Survey Replication (NCS-R). *Journal of the American Medical Association*, 289, 3095–105.

Kessler, R. C., Berglund, P., Demler, O., Jin, R. & Walters, E. E. (2005). Lifetime prevalence and age-of-onset distributions of DSM-IV disorders in the National Comorbidity Survey Replication. *Archives of General Psychiatry*, 62, 593–602.

Kessler, R. C., Brown, R. L. & Broman, C. L. (1981). Sex differences in psychiatric help-seeking: Evidence from four large-scale surveys. *Journal of Health and Social Behavior*, 22, 49–64.

Kessler, R. C., Haro, J. M., Heeringa, S. G., Pennell, B.-E. & Üstün, T. B. (2006). The World Health Organization World Mental Health Survey Initiative. *Epidemiologia e Psichiatria Sociale*, 15, 161–6.

Kessler, R. C., Little, R. J. & Groves, R. M. (1995). Advances in strategies for minimizing and adjusting for survey nonresponse. *Epidemiologic Reviews*, 17, 192–204.

Kessler, R. C., McGonagle, K. A., Zhao, S., Nelson, C. B., Hughes, M., Eshleman, S., Wittchen, H.-U. & Kendler, K. S. (1994). Lifetime and 12-month prevalence of DSM-III-R psychiatric disorders in the United States. *Archives of General Psychiatry*, 51, 8–19.

Kessler, R. C. & Üstün, T. B. (2004). The World Mental Health (WMH) Survey Initiative Version of the World Health Organization (WHO) Composite International Diagnostic Interview (CIDI). *International Journal of Methods in Psychiatric Research*, 13, 93–121.

Kessler, R. C., Zhao, S., Katz, S. J., Kouzis, A. C., Frank, R. G., Edlund, M. & Leaf, P. (1999). Past year use of outpatient services for psychiatric problems in the National Comorbidity Survey. *American Journal of Psychiatry*, 156, 115–23.

Leaf, P. J., Livingston, M. M., Tischler, G. L., Weissman, M. M., Holzer, C. E. & Myers, J. K. (1985). Contact with health professionals for the treatment of psychiatric and emotional problems. *Medical Care*, 23, 1322–37.

Lou Arnal, S., Magallón Botaya, R., Orozco González, F., Arto Serrano, A., Pons Pons, L., Betorz Latorre, J. J. & Ucar Hernández, F. (1990). Estudio epidemiológico en salud mental en una zona de salud [Mental health epidemiological study in a health area]. *Atención Primaria*, 7, 338–43.

Mateos, R., González, F., Páramo, M., García, M. C., Carollo, M. C. & Rodríguez-López, A. (2000). The Galicia study of mental health of the Elderly I: General description of methodology. *International Journal of Methods in Psychiatric Research*, 9, 165–73.

Mojtabai, R., Olfson, M. & Mechanic, D. (2002). Perceived need and help-seeking in adults with mood, anxiety, or alcohol disorders. *Archives of General Psychiatry*, 59, 77–84.

Research Triangle Institute (2004). *SUDAAN language manual, Release 9.0*. Research Triangle Park, NC: Research Triangle Institute.

Rhodes, A. E., Lin, E. & Mustard, C. A. (2002). Self-reported use of mental health services versus administrative records: Should we care? *International Journal of Methods in Psychiatric Research*, 11, 125–33.

Rico, A. & Sabés, R. (2000). *Health care systems in transition: Spain*. Copenhagen: WHO Regional Office for Europe on behalf of the European Observatory on Health Systems and Policies.

Robins, L. N., Helzer, J. E., Croughan, J. & Ratcliff, K. (1981). National Institute of Mental Health Diagnostic Interview Schedule: Its history, characteristics and validity. *Archives of General Psychiatry*, 38, 381–9.

Robins, L. N., Wing, J., Wittchen, H. U., Helzer, J. E., Babor, T. F., Burke, J., Farmer, A., Jablenski, A., Pickens, R. & Regier, D. A. (1988). The Composite International Diagnostic Interview: An epidemiologic instrument suitable for use in conjunction with different diagnostic systems and in different cultures. *Archives of General Psychiatry*, 45, 1069–77.

Roca, M., Gili, M., Ferrer, V., Bernardo, M., Montano, J. J., Salva, J. J., Flores, I. & Leal, S. (1999). Mental disorders on the island of Formentera: Prevalence in general population using the Schedules for Clinical assessment in Neuropsychiatry (SCAN). *Social Psychiatry and Psychiatric Epidemiology*, 34, 410–15.

SAS Institute (1999). *SAS Software, Version 8.0*, 4th ed. Cary, NC: SAS Publishing.

Seva Díaz, A., Sarasola, A., Merino, J. A. & Magallón, R. (1992). Trastornos psíquicos en ancianos de una población urbana aragonesa (España) y su relación con los determinantes de la salud [Mental disorders in elderly participants from an urban population from Aragon (Spain) and their relation to mental health determinants]. *Actas Luso-Españolas de Neurología, Psiquiatría y Ciencias Afines*, 20, 23–9.

Sheehan, D. V., Harnett-Sheehan K. & Raj, B. A. (1996). The measurement of disability. *International Clinical Psychopharmacology*, 11 (suppl. 3), 89–95.

Statistics Netherlands (1999). *Blaise developer's guide*. Herleen: Department of Statistical Informatics.

Vázquez, C., Muñoz, M. & Sanz, J. (1997). Lifetime and 12-month prevalence of the DSM-III-R mental disorders among the homeless in Madrid: A European study using the CIDI. *Acta Psychiatrica Scandinavica*, 95, 523–30.

Vázquez-Barquero, J. L., Díez-Manrique, J. F., Peña, C., Aldama, J., Samaniego Rodríguez, C., Menéndez Arango, J. & Mirapeix, C. (1987a). A community mental health survey in Cantabria: A general description of morbidity. *Psychological Medicine*, 17, 227–41.

Vázquez-Barquero, J. L., Diez-Manrique, J. F., Peña Martín, C., Luquerica Puente, J., Artal Simon, J. A., Liano Rincón, A. & Arenal, A. (1987b). Depresión y ansiedad: Perfiles sociodemográficos diferenciales en la población general [Depression and anxiety:

Differential sociodemographic profiles in the general population]. *Actas Luso-Españolas de Neurología, Psiquiatría y Ciencias Afines*, 15, 95–109.

Vázquez-Barquero, J. L., Díez-Manrique, J. F., Peña, C., Quintanal, R. G. & Labrador Lopez, M. (1986). Two stage design in a community survey. *British Journal of Psychiatry*, 149, 88–97.

Vázquez-Barquero, J. L., García, J., Artal Simón, J., Iglesias, C., Montejo, J., Herrán, A. & Dunn G. (1997). Mental health in primary care. *British Journal of Psychiatry*, 170, 529–35.

Vázquez-Barquero, J. L., Muñoz, P. E. & Madoz Jáuregui, V. (1982). The influence of the process of urbanization on the prevalence of neurosis. *Acta Psychiatrica Scandinavica*, 65, 161–70.

Wang, P. S., Lane, M., Olfson, M., Pincus, H. A., Wells, K. B. & Kessler, R. C. (2005). 12-month use of mental health services in the U.S.: Results from the National Comorbidity Survey Replication (NCS-R). *Archives of General Psychiatry*, 62, 629–40.

WHO International Consortium in Psychiatric Epidemiology (2000). Cross-national comparisons of the prevalences and correlates of mental disorders. *Bulletin of the World Health Organization*, 78, 413–26.

WHO World Mental Health Survey Consortium (2004). Prevalence, severity and unmet need for treatment of mental disorders in the World Health Organization World Mental Health Surveys. *Journal of the American Medical Association*, 291, 2581–90.

Williams, J. B., Spitzer, R. L., Linzer, M., Kroenke, K., Hahn, S. R., deGruy, F. V. & Lazev, A. (1995). Gender differences in depression in primary care. *American Journal of Obstetrics and Gynecology*, 173, 654–9.

Wittchen, H.-U., Robins, L. N., Cottler, L. B., Sartorius, N., Burke, J. D. & Regier D. (1991). Cross-cultural feasibility, reliability and sources of variance of the Composite International Diagnostic Interview (CIDI): The multicentre WHO/ADAMHA Field Trials. *British Journal of Psychiatry*, 159, 645–53.

World Health Organization (WHO) (1987). *The International classification of diseases, 9th revision, clinical modification: ICD-9-CM*. Geneva: World Health Organization.

World Health Organization (WHO) (1992). *The ICD-10 classification of mental and behavioral disorders: Clinical descriptions and diagnostic guidelines*. Geneva: World Health Organization.

# 20 The State of Mental Health and Alcoholism in Ukraine

EVELYN J. BROMET, SEMYON F. GLUZMAN, NATHAN L. TINTLE,
VOLODYMYR I. PANIOTTO, CHARLES P. M. WEBB, VICTORIA ZAKHOZHA,
JOHAN M. HAVENAAR, ZINOVIY GUTKOVICH, STANISLAV
KOSTYUCHENKO, AND JOSEPH E. SCHWARTZ

## ACKNOWLEDGMENTS

The Ukraine survey was funded by the U.S. National Institute of Mental Health (NIMH) (MH61905). We thank Valeriy Khmelko (Kiev International Institute of Sociology) and Julia Pievskaya (Ukrainian Psychiatric Association) for their invaluable assistance in conducting the fieldwork and providing information on the mental health service system; and Inna Korchak, Roksolana Mykhaylyk, Margaret Bloom, and Svetlana Stepukhovich for translating and back-translating the various components of the study. As part of the World Health Organization World Mental Health (WMH) Survey Initiative, we also thank the WMH staff for assistance with instrumentation, fieldwork, and data analysis. Their activities were supported by NIMH grant R01MH070884, the John D. and Catherine T. MacArthur Foundation, the Pfizer Foundation, the U.S. Public Health Service (R13-MH066849, R01-MH069864, and R01-DA016558), the Fogarty International Center (FIRCA R03-TW006481), the Pan American Health Organization, Eli Lilly and Company Foundation, Ortho-McNeil Pharmaceutical, GlaxoSmithKline, and Bristol-Myers Squibb. A complete list of WMH publications can be found at http://www.hcp.med.harvard.edu/wmh/.

## I. INTRODUCTION

This chapter describes the findings on mental health and alcoholism in Ukraine, a country that became independent in 1991 with the breakup of the Soviet Union. Ukraine is bordered by Russia to the east and northeast, Belarus to the North, Poland to the northwest, Moldova, Romania, and Slovakia to the west and southwest, and the Black Sea to the south. Its population of approximately 48 million makes it the second-largest country in Europe. The capital city is Kiev. Ethnic Ukrainians comprise about 75% of the population and ethnic Russians about 22%. The literacy rate is 98%. About one-fifth of the population is retired or receiving welfare (Mokhovikov & Donets 1996). Ukraine is rich in natural resources, including iron ore, coal, natural gas, oil, timber, and fertile land. Indeed, it is nicknamed "the breadbasket of Europe." Although part of the Soviet Union, Ukraine was one of the founding states of the United Nations.

Like other countries of the former Soviet Union, the public health conditions of Ukraine markedly deteriorated after 1991. Life expectancy declined (Shkolnikov, McKee & Leon 2001) and mortality increased, especially from cardiovascular disease, accidents, and other conditions related to heavy alcohol use and smoking (Perlman & Bobak 2008). The suicide rate of approximately 30 per 100,000 persons places Ukraine in the top ten countries worldwide (Mokhovikov & Donets 1996). Violence against women (Horne 1999), binge drinking (Webb et al. 2005), and nicotine addiction (Gilmore et al. 2001) are three principal public health problems. In addition, Ukrainian families carry painful intergenerational burdens, including the famine-genocide of the 1930s, the violent deaths, disappearances, and incarcerations during the Stalin era, mass destruction of human life during Nazi occupation, numerous industrial, mining, and transport accidents, poverty (World Bank 2003), a woefully inadequate infrastructure (e.g., water, roads, sewage), and widespread political and economic corruption. The accident at the Chernobyl nuclear power plant in April 1986 affected 19 of the 27 oblasts (states), and 350,000 people were permanently evacuated from contaminated areas around the plant. A recent comprehensive review by the World Health Organization (WHO) (2006) of the health effects of Chernobyl concluded that over the 20 years since the accident, the physical health effects were restricted to thyroid cancer, especially in children, but the mental health consequences were widespread and nonspecific, ranging from demoralization to depression, health-related anxiety (especially regarding potential genetic effects in children born after the catastrophe), posttraumatic stress symptoms, and even suicide among highly exposed cleanup workers (Rahu et al. 1997; Bromet et al. 2002). Indeed, the report maintained that the "mental health impact ... is the largest public health problem caused by the accident to date" (WHO 2006). These historical events shaped the environment of Ukraine and constitute the backdrop for Ukraine's joining the World Mental Health (WMH) Survey Initiative (Kessler et al. 2006).

The scientific context of the Ukraine WMH study with respect to epidemiology, psychiatry, and psychiatric epidemiology is equally important to describe. With regard to epidemiology, there were no population-based studies of health or mental health in Ukraine prior to the WMH survey, apart from government statistical reports about morbidity, such as infectious disease surveillance data (Farmer, Goodman & Baldwin et al. 1993). However, the potential for epidemiological research in Ukraine changed profoundly and irrevocably after the Chernobyl catastrophe of 1986 and the breakup of the Soviet Union. The two initial issues giving rise to modern epidemiology in Ukraine were the radiation exposure from Chernobyl and its impact on morbidity and mortality from cancer, as well as the decline in life expectancy in men. To address the former issue, Western investigators transferred basic epidemiological concepts to Ukraine,

Russia, Belarus, and other former Soviet countries; these concepts included fundamental principles of unbiased sampling, reliable and valid procedures for measuring clinical end points and risk factors, and comprehensive consideration of competing risk factors (e.g., Rahu et al. 2006). Our research on Chernobyl's mental health impact was the first basic epidemiological study of the mental health of women and children carried out in that context (Bromet et al. 2000). To address the decline in life expectancy, several social epidemiological surveys, particularly on stress, smoking, and drinking behaviors, were initiated throughout Eastern Europe by Western investigators, particularly the International Centre for Health and Society at University College London (e.g., Nicholson et al. 2005). In addition, the founding of the Ukrainian Psychiatric Association (UPA) with its mission of Western psychiatric diagnosis and treatment, and of the Kiev International Institute of Sociology (KIIS), modeled on the Institute for Social Research at the University of Michigan, provided infrastructures from which to launch epidemiological prevalence studies, such as the WMH survey.

With regard to psychiatry, in the twentieth century, medicine in the former Soviet Union evolved separately from the West, and the nosology and treatment of psychiatric patients took on its own character (Rezvyy et al. 2005). Moreover, psychiatry developed a very negative image because it was used by the authorities as a way to maintain social control over the population by punishment of political dissidents (Gluzman 1991). Thus, psychiatric disorders were and still are highly stigmatized (Schulman & Adams 2002). The main form of psychiatric treatment is hospitalization (McDaid et al. 2006). These services are by and large reserved for patients with psychosis and organic disorders, many of which are alcohol induced. Treatments for common mental disorders, such as anxiety and depression, are limited to the most severe cases. Although the economic and social costs of alcoholism are well known in Ukraine, efforts to curb the problem have been limited to controlling the sale and distribution of alcohol rather than to developing prevention and intervention programs. Thus, prior to 1991, there was no infrastructure or common language from which to launch clinical research. After 1991, however, with the founding of UPA and the introduction of Western concepts of diagnosis and treatment, a dialogue between psychiatrists in former Soviet countries and psychiatrists in the West was opened (Ougrin, Gluzman & Dratcu 2006). The UPA facilitated this transition by translating and disseminating European and North American textbooks and psychiatric journals and by accepting open and transparent clinical research collaborations with Western investigators. Our study of the mental health impact of Chernobyl, conducted with UPA, demonstrated the feasibility of implementing systematic epidemiological research on mental health (Bromet et al. 2000) and paved the road for the Ukraine WMH survey.

A handful of local community mental health surveys, mostly in circumscribed areas of Russia, were undertaken after 1991 and provided important insights for the development and interpretation of the Ukraine WMH survey. These surveys found unusually high rates of common mental disorders, heavy (mostly binge) drinking, smoking, and subjective reporting of poor health. For example, on the basis of the Munich checklist for DSM-III-R disorders, Havenaar and colleagues (1997) evaluated residents of a midsize town in Russia and found one-month prevalence rates of 12.8% for mood disorders, 18.5% for anxiety disorders, and 2.9% for alcohol disorders. A study of a rural region in Russia using the WHO's Composite International Diagnostic Interview (CIDI) found lifetime and 12-month rates of DSM-III-R mood disorders of 28.8% and 17.4% in men, respectively, and 53.4% and 40.5% in women (Pakriev et al. 1998a), respectively, and lifetime rates of ICD-10 alcohol dependence of 69.3% in men and 3.7% in women (Pakriev et al. 1998b). Surveys by the International Centre for Health and Society found that 31% of Russian men were monthly binge drinkers (Bobak et al. 1999), while 23% of adult men and 43.9% of women had high scores on a measure of depressive symptoms (Bobak et al. 2006). More broadly, a questionnaire survey in northwestern Russia in 1999 found that 32.3% of men and 68.7% of

women had significant symptoms of depression, sleep disorder, and anxiety (Averina et al. 2005). A Center for Disease Control and Prevention (CDC) survey found that one in five women in Ukraine was physically abused by her spouse, perhaps as a consequence of binge drinking (Ashford et al. 2003). The rate of current smoking is not only high (medians in 11 Eastern Bloc countries are 56.0% in men and 9.3% in women), but the rates in young women living in urban areas are rising dramatically (Gilmore et al. 2001; Webb et al. 2007). Last, in a national survey of Ukraine conducted by KIIS, 25% of men and 43% of women rated their health as poor or very poor (Gilmore, McKee & Rose 2002). Thus, the levels of morbidity described in Ukraine and neighboring countries far exceed those reported for European and other Western countries and demonstrate the critical importance of launching epidemiological research on health and mental health in Ukraine and other former Soviet settings.

As noted previously, the possible need for care for common mental disorders and alcoholism is not matched by service availability. Only 6% of the budget of the Ministry of Health is earmarked for mental health, and 89% of mental health monies are directed toward mental hospitals. There are 89 psychiatric hospitals, which primarily admit patients with schizophrenia, mental retardation, and organic mental disorders, such as epilepsy, but only 37 community-based inpatient units. Two-thirds of the psychiatrists in Ukraine are employed in the mental hospital system. The estimated rate of mental hospitalization is 86 per 10,000 population. The few outpatient programs that exist primarily treat patients with drug abuse, organic mental disorders, and mental retardation, and it is estimated that 25% of these clinics do not have access to medications, whereas 75% have access to one medication from each major class (antidepressant, antipsychotic, mood stabilizer, anxiolytic, and antiseizure). However, these medications are underused because they are extremely costly to consumers. There is no system of private insurance in Ukraine. The estimated rate of outpatient use is 473.5 per 10,000 population. Alcoholism is largely untreated, although public drunkenness can result in incarceration. Alcoholics Anonymous has not been successful to date. The general medical system is composed of local and regional polyclinics that contain a range of primary care and specialty doctors. However, these general practitioners and nurses have almost no training in psychiatry, and only a handful of psychologists, social workers, and occupational therapists work in this system. Thus, Ukraine has not yet articulated its mental health policy, and while there appears to be a huge gulf between the high levels of morbidity described previously and the availability of services to address these needs, the Ukraine WMH survey was the first systematic source of information that could be applied for this purpose.

This chapter describes the lifetime and 12-month prevalence and demographic correlates of psychiatric disorders including alcoholism in Ukraine. To provide a comprehensive picture of the current public mental health profile of Ukraine, the 12-month prevalence findings are supplemented by data on disorder severity as well as on cigarette smoking, heavy alcohol use, and spouse violence toward women. For further details, we refer readers to recent publications on the prevalence of mood, anxiety, and alcohol disorders (Bromet et al. 2005) and heavy alcohol use (Webb et al. 2005).

# 2. METHODS

## 2.1. Sample

The Ukraine WMH survey is a nationally representative survey of residents aged 18 and older from the 24 oblasts (states) and the autonomous republic of Crimea. The fieldwork was conducted from February to December 2002. The sampling design had four stages. First, 170 primary sampling units (PSUs) were selected from the cities, towns, and villages with probability proportional to size. That is, the PSUs were drawn such that each oblast, and the urban and rural populations in each oblast, were represented proportionally. Second, within the PSUs, postal districts were randomly selected. Third, within each postal district, streets were randomly selected; then buildings within streets; and last, apartments within buildings. Fourth, people 18 years and older were randomly selected within apartments.

The recruitment, consent, and field procedures were approved by the Human Subjects Committees of the State University of New York at Stony Brook, KIIS, and UPA. A total of 4725 adults participated in Part 1 of the survey and 1720 participated in Part 2. The response rate was 78.3%.

## 2.2. Measures

Prior to conducting the study, six discussion groups with recent immigrants from Ukraine were convened at the State University of New York as Stony Brook to evaluate the cultural and conceptual appropriateness of the major domains of the study and the procedure for obtaining informed consent. A pilot study of the SCID was also conducted by ZG in New York with 50 Russian immigrants. In addition, a pretest was conducted in the Kiev metropolitan area to evaluate the cross-cultural utility of the WMH interview schedule and the consent process. The results of all these activities led to refinements in specific sections of the interview, namely, alcohol consumption, treatment, employment, socioeconomic status, and types of traumatic events; more importantly, they established the cross-cultural suitability of these Western clinical instruments and the DSM-IV in Ukraine.

The paper-and-pencil version of the WHO Composite International Diagnostic Interview (CIDI; Kessler & Üstün 2004; see also Chapter 4) was used in the survey. This instrument was administered by 62 professional interviewers of KIIS, who were trained and monitored by VZ. In addition, a small clinical reappraisal study was conducted by 15 psychiatrists from Kiev, L'viv, and Donetsk who were trained in the SCID by ZG and closely monitored by SK. The findings support the overall validity of the CIDI assessments. The interviews were translated into Russian and Ukrainian following the WHO guidelines. The training manuals were translated only into Russian, as all interviewers were bilingual.

The disorders included in this chapter are anxiety disorders (panic disorder, agoraphobia without panic disorder, social phobia, generalized anxiety disorder, and posttraumatic stress disorder [PTSD]), depressive disorders (major depressive episode and dysthymia), impulse-control disorders (intermittent explosive disorder and conduct disorder), and substance use disorders (alcohol abuse with and without dependence, and other substances including illicit drugs and nonmedical use of prescription drugs). For PTSD, the most commonly reported traumatic exposures were the unexpected death of a loved one, witnessing someone dead or seriously hurt, having a life-threatening illness, and being in an automobile accident. Current smoking was determined from the screening item on tobacco use. Heavy alcohol use in the past 12 months was defined for men as consuming 80 grams or more of ethanol in a typical drinking day or consuming either 60 grams or more for three to four days per week or 40 grams or more nearly every day (Webb et al. 2005). For women, the dose criteria were reduced by 25%. Partner violence, assessed for the past 12 months in married respondents, was defined for males as ever having aggressed against their partner (i.e., pushed, grabbed, shoved, slapped, hit, or threw something at her) and for females as having ever been the target of aggression by her current partner.

The service providers enumerated in the Ukraine interview were as follows: psychiatrists or narcologists (alcohol or drug specialist); other mental health professionals (i.e., psychologists or psychotherapists); family doctors; other medical doctors; other health professionals (i.e., feldshers, who are comparable to nurse-practitioners in the United States); religious or spiritual advisors; and other healers, including herbalists, chiropractors, acupuncturists, spiritualists, psychic healers, telepathic healers, and faith healers.

Three demographic risk factors are examined in this chapter: age, sex, and education. Education is a time-varying predictor that is divided into five categories: current student, low (up to eight years of schooling), low-medium (9–10 years of schooling), medium (12–13 years,

including specialized secondary beyond high school), and high (at least 14 years of schooling).

## 2.3. Weighting

The sample was weighted by sex, age (six groups), region (five regions), and urbanity (urban vs. rural) using the 2001 census. The weighted sample was predominantly female (55%), older than 40 years old (60%), and had at least a high school education (90%). Table 20.1 shows the 2001 census findings for Ukraine, the actual sample distributions, and the weighted distributions.

## 3. RESULTS

### 3.1. Lifetime Prevalence of DSM-IV Disorders

Table 20.2 shows the lifetime prevalence of the DSM-IV psychiatric and substance use disorders assessed in the survey and operationalized by the CIDI. The estimated lifetime prevalence of any disorder is 36.1%; 14.1% of respondents had two or more lifetime DSM-IV/CIDI disorders, and 4.8% had three or more. The most prevalent class is depression (15.8%), followed by substance disorders (15.0%) and anxiety disorders (10.9%). The most prevalent individual lifetime disorders are major depression (14.6%) and alcohol abuse (13.5%). The least common disorders are agoraphobia without panic (0.3%) and drug abuse (0.5%).

The lifetime prevalence rates of each disorder differed significantly across the life span (Table 20.2). The rates of agoraphobia, social phobia, intermittent explosive disorder, and substance use disorders decreased with increasing age. In contrast, the rates of depression, dysthymia, panic, generalized anxiety disorder, and PTSD increased with increasing age. Indeed, one in five respondents age 65 or older met criteria for lifetime depression compared to one in ten in the age group 18–34.

The median ages of onset varied widely across the classes of disorders. Specifically, the median ages and interquartile ranges were 35 (18–51) for anxiety disorders, 40 (25–55) for depressive

**Table 20.1.** Demographic distribution of the 2002 Ukraine-WMH respondents compared with the general population of Ukraine

|  | General population | Weighted sample | Unweighted sample |
|---|---|---|---|
| Total | 48,457,100[a] | 4725 | 4725 |
|  | % | % | % (n) |
| **Sex** |  |  |  |
| Male | 45.0 | 45.0 | 38.0 (1793) |
| Female | 55.0 | 55.0 | 62.0 (2932) |
| **Age**[a] |  |  |  |
| Younger than 25 | 13.3 | 13.7 | 11.3 (533) |
| 25–34 | 17.4 | 16.6 | 14.0 (661) |
| 35–49 | 28.2 | 28.7 | 25.9 (1225) |
| 50+ | 41.1 | 41.0 | 48.8 (2306) |
| **Region**[a] |  |  |  |
| West | 21.8 | 21.8 | 22.1 (1046) |
| Central (excluding Kiev) | 25.4 | 25.6 | 25.4 (1202) |
| Kiev metropolitan area | 9.3 | 9.4 | 9.1 (432) |
| East | 43.4 | 43.2 | 43.3 (2045) |
| **Urbanity**[a] |  |  |  |
| Rural | 32.2 | 32.2 | 29.8 (1408) |
| Midsized urban | 32.7 | 34.9 | 36.2 (1711) |
| Large urban | 35.1 | 32.9 | 34.0 (1606) |
| **Marital status**[b] |  |  |  |
| Married | 60.1 | 59.8 | 59.7 (2820) |
| Never married | 14.2 | 15.4 | 12.8 (606) |
| Married before | 25.6 | 24.8 | 27.5 (1299) |
| **Education**[b] |  |  |  |
| Primary | 6.6 | 9.8 | 11.3 (535) |
| Secondary | 43.2 | 46.1 | 44.9 (2119) |
| Specialized secondary | 32.0 | 27.1 | 26.6 (1258) |
| Higher | 18.2 | 17.0 | 17.2 (812) |
| **Employment status**[b] |  |  |  |
| Employed | 46.3 | 48.2 | 46.7 (2062) |
| Unemployed | 10.6 | 11.3 | 9.9 (466) |
| Retired/disabled | 32.8 | 31.3 | 37.6 (1774) |
| Student | 4.4 | 3.6 | 3.0 (140) |
| Homemaker | 5.9 | 5.7 | 5.9 (280) |

[a] Population data from 2001 Ukrainian census.
[b] Population data from KIIS.

disorders, 15 (13–23) for impulse-control disorders, and 26 (21–30) for alcohol abuse with or without dependence (medians could not be calculated for drug disorders because of the small n). However, within classes of disorder, there was considerable variability. Among the anxiety disorders, for example, the average age of onset ranged from 14 for social phobia (interquartile range = 11–16) to 50 for PTSD (interquartile range = 34–63).

Table 20.3 shows the relationship of sex with onset of disorder. Consistent with other countries, women in Ukraine were 2 times as likely to develop a depressive disorder and more than 1.5 times as likely to develop an anxiety disorder. However, we note that before age 65, the odds

**Table 20.2.** Lifetime prevalence of DSM-IV/CIDI disorders in the total Ukraine sample, by age

| | Total | | 18–34 | | 35–49 | | 50–64 | | 65+ | | $\chi_3^2$ |
|---|---|---|---|---|---|---|---|---|---|---|---|
| | % | (se) | % | (se) | % | (se) | % | (se) | % | (se) | |
| **I. Anxiety disorders** | | | | | | | | | | | |
| Panic disorder | 2.2 | (0.3) | 1.6 | (0.4) | 1.9 | (0.4) | 2.3 | (0.6) | 3.2 | (0.6) | 11.0* |
| Agoraphobia without panic | 0.3 | (0.1) | 0.6 | (0.2) | 0.1 | (0.1) | 0.3 | (0.2) | 0.1 | (0.1) | 10.0* |
| Social phobia | 2.6 | (0.2) | 4.2 | (0.5) | 2.9 | (0.5) | 1.9 | (0.4) | 0.3 | (0.1) | 117.5*** |
| Generalized anxiety disorder | 2.0 | (0.2) | 1.1 | (0.3) | 1.4 | (0.3) | 3.0 | (0.6) | 3.0 | (0.6) | 10.4* |
| Posttraumatic stress disorder[a] | 4.8 | (0.6) | 2.3 | (0.7) | 3.5 | (1.1) | 5.3 | (1.0) | 10.0 | (1.8) | 24.4*** |
| Any anxiety disorder[a] | 10.9 | (0.8) | 8.9 | (1.4) | 8.9 | (1.6) | 12.6 | (1.8) | 15.0 | (2.2) | 9.4* |
| **II. Depression** | | | | | | | | | | | |
| Major depressive disorder | 14.6 | (0.7) | 10.4 | (0.8) | 12.5 | (0.9) | 17.3 | (1.4) | 21.3 | (2.0) | 30.9*** |
| Dysthymia | 3.0 | (0.3) | 1.1 | (0.3) | 2.8 | (0.5) | 3.6 | (0.5) | 5.6 | (0.9) | 47.7*** |
| Any depression | 15.8 | (0.8) | 10.7 | (0.8) | 13.9 | (0.9) | 18.8 | (1.3) | 23.4 | (2.0) | 47.4* |
| **III. Impulse-control disorders** | | | | | | | | | | | |
| Conduct disorder[a] | 3.4 | (0.8) | 3.2 | (0.9) | 4.1 | (2.1) | – | | – | | – |
| Intermittent explosive disorder | 4.3 | (0.3) | 6.1 | (0.8) | 4.9 | (0.7) | 2.8 | (0.5) | 1.6 | (0.4) | 32.3*** |
| Any impulse-control disorder[a] | 8.7 | (1.1) | 9.0 | (1.3) | 7.4 | (2.3) | – | | – | | – |
| **IV. Substance use disorders** | | | | | | | | | | | |
| Alcohol abuse w/without dependence | 13.5 | (0.8) | 16.2 | (1.4) | 17.3 | (1.7) | 12.5 | (1.2) | 4.6 | (0.7) | 102.1*** |
| Alcohol dependence w/abuse | 3.5 | (0.3) | 4.1 | (0.6) | 4.7 | (0.6) | 3.1 | (0.7) | 1.1 | (0.4) | 40.2*** |
| Drug abuse w/without dependence[a] | 0.9 | (0.2) | 2.2 | (0.7) | 0.7 | (0.4) | 0.0 | (0.0) | 0.0 | (0.0) | 14.1** |
| Drug dependence w/abuse[a] | 0.5 | (0.2) | 1.3 | (0.5) | 0.2 | (0.1) | 0.0 | (0.0) | 0.0 | (0.0) | 9.9* |
| Any substance[a] | 15.0 | (1.3) | 18.8 | (2.3) | 19.9 | (2.9) | 12.4 | (2.4) | 4.7 | (1.4) | 32.1*** |
| **V. Any disorder** | | | | | | | | | | | |
| Any[a] | 36.1 | (1.5) | 34.2 | (2.4) | 35.3 | (3.5) | 38.7 | (3.1) | 37.4 | (3.6) | 1.9 |
| Two or more disorders[a] | 14.1 | (1.0) | 13.5 | (1.5) | 16.0 | (2.3) | 14.4 | (1.5) | 13.4 | (1.7) | 1.3 |
| Three or more disorders[a] | 4.8 | (0.5) | 5.7 | (0.7) | 3.8 | (0.9) | 5.1 | (0.9) | 4.7 | (1.0) | 0.3 |

[a] Based on the Part 2 sample.

* $p < 0.05$. ** $p < 0.01$. *** $p < 0.001$.

**Table 20.3.** Variations across cohorts in the association of sex with onset of disorder

|  | Total | | 18–34 | | 35–49 | | 50–64 | | 65+ | |
|---|---|---|---|---|---|---|---|---|---|---|
|  | OR[a] | (95% CI) | OR[a] | (95% CI) | OR[a] | (95% CI) | OR[a] | (95% CI) | OR[a] | (95% CI) |
| Anxiety[b] | 1.6 | (0.9–2.9) | 2.9* | (1.1–7.3) | 1.4 | (0.6–3.4) | 1.1 | (0.5–2.1) | 1.2 | (0.6–2.5) |
| Depression | 2.1* | (1.7–2.6) | 2.4* | (1.6–3.4) | 2.5* | (1.4–4.5) | 2.4* | (1.4–4.1) | 1.4* | (1.0–1.9) |
| Impulse control | 0.7 | (0.4–1.4) | 0.8 | (0.4–1.8) | 0.3* | (0.1–0.8) | – | | – | |
| Substance | 0.1* | (0.1–0.2) | 0.2* | (0.1–0.3) | 0.3* | (0.0–0.1) | 0.0* | (0.0–0.1) | 0.1 | (0.0–0.4) |

[a] Males were the reference group.
[b] Based on the Part 2 sample.
* $p < 0.05$. ** $p < 0.01$. *** $p < 0.001$.

ratios (ORs) were somewhat higher, whereas after age 65, the increased risk was considerably smaller though still statistically significant. The sex imbalance for substance use disorders was more extreme than expected, with men being nine times as likely as women to develop a substance use disorder and seven times as likely to have an impulse-control disorder. Unlike anxiety and depressive disorders, these sex differences were consistent across the age groups.

Compared to respondents with the most education, those with the least amount of schooling were at increased risk for anxiety disorders (OR = 4.0; 95% CI = 1.1–15.5). Similarly, respondents with low-medium levels of schooling were at increased risk for depression (OR = 1.5; 95% CI = 1.0–2.2). Consistent with the age of onset distributions, students were at low risk for depression (OR = 0.6; 95% CI = 0.3–1.0) and at increased risk for impulse-control disorders (OR = 5.2, 95% CI = 1.1–25.5). There were no significant findings for substance use disorders.

### 3.2. Prevalence and Severity of 12-month Disorders

One-fifth of the sample (20.9%) had a diagnosable disorder in the 12 months preceding the interview (Table 20.4). This corresponds to slightly more than half of respondents with a lifetime disorder (57.9%). As was true for the lifetime prevalence rates, the two most common 12-month disorders were major depression (8.4%) and alcohol abuse (5.5%). Compared to men, women were significantly more likely to have 12-month depressive (OR = 1.5; 95% CI = 1.1–2.1) and anxiety (OR = 2.0; 95% CI = 1.2–3.5) disorders and considerably less likely to have a substance disorder (OR = 0.1; 95% CI = 0.0–0.2).

Additional analyses indicate that younger respondents and those with less education were more likely to have impulsive-control and substance disorders than were older and more educated respondents. Overall, older respondents and those with less education were more likely to have an episode of depression or anxiety in the past 12 months. Indeed, the 12-month prevalence rates of major depression in men and women over the age of 50 were 7.2% and 13.6%, respectively, whereas the rates for male and female respondents younger than age 25 were 2.7% and 7.8%, respectively.

Table 20.4 also shows, consistent with the U.S. findings, that 23.0% of the 12-month cases were classified as serious, 37.7% as moderate, and 39.4% as mild. Among the disorder categories, substance use disorders contained the largest percentage of serious cases (38.9%) and anxiety disorders the smallest (23.4%). Apart from substance dependence, the diagnoses with the greatest proportion of cases classified as serious were generalized anxiety disorder (42.6%), agoraphobia without panic (40.9%), and intermittent explosive disorder (37.6%). The disorders with the greatest percentage classified as mild were social phobia (44.4%), PTSD (40%), and conduct disorder (72.0%). Approximately half of respondents with a depressive disorder were classified as moderate. Overall, the degree of severity was not significantly associated with sex, age, or education.

**Table 20.4.** 12-month prevalence and severity of DSM-IV disorders

| Diagnosis | 12-month % | (se) | Serious[b] % | (se) | Moderate[b] % | (se) | Mild[b] % | (se) |
|---|---|---|---|---|---|---|---|---|
| **Anxiety disorder** | | | | | | | | |
| Panic disorder[a] | 1.4 | (0.3) | 26.7 | (5.0) | 55.0 | (5.5) | 18.3 | (4.5) |
| Generalized anxiety disorder[a] | 1.0 | (0.1) | 42.6 | (7.7) | 42.6 | (7.4) | 14.8 | (6.9) |
| Social phobia[a] | 1.5 | (0.2) | 17.0 | (4.0) | 38.7 | (8.1) | 44.4 | (9.1) |
| Agoraphobia without panic[a] | 0.2 | (0.1) | 40.9 | (16.0) | 45.6 | (19.7) | 13.6 | (9.6) |
| Posttraumatic stress disorder[b] | 2.8 | (0.5) | 27.3 | (6.1) | 32.5 | (5.6) | 40.2 | (7.0) |
| Any anxiety disorder[b] | 6.8 | (0.7) | 23.4 | (3.3) | 41.0 | (4.3) | 35.6 | (4.4) |
| **Depressive disorder** | | | | | | | | |
| Major depressive disorder[a] | 8.4 | (0.6) | 27.4 | (3.1) | 51.5 | (3.5) | 21.2 | (3.0) |
| Dysthymia[a] | 1.9 | (0.2) | 23.3 | (4.6) | 57.6 | (6.6) | 19.1 | (5.2) |
| Any depression[a] | 8.9 | (0.6) | 26.3 | (2.9) | 52.4 | (3.8) | 21.4 | (3.1) |
| **Impulse disorder** | | | | | | | | |
| Conduct disorder[c] | 1.1 | (0.6) | 24.0 | (16.9) | 4.0 | (4.5) | 72.0 | (18.5) |
| Intermittent explosive disorder[a] | 2.8 | (0.3) | 37.6 | (4.7) | 27.2 | (4.7) | 35.1 | (6.4) |
| Any impulse-control disorder[c] | 5.7 | (0.9) | 30.4 | (5.9) | 25.4 | (6.6) | 44.2 | (8.9) |
| **Substance disorder** | | | | | | | | |
| Alcohol abuse[a] | 5.5 | (0.5) | 34.3 | (5.7) | 10.6 | (3.1) | 55.2 | (6.9) |
| Alcohol abuse w/dependence[a] | 2.1 | (0.2) | 96.9 | (1.9) | 3.1 | (1.9) | 0.0 | (0.0) |
| Drug abuse[b] | 0.4 | (0.2) | 47.4 | (21.9) | 0.0 | (0.0) | 52.6 | (21.9) |
| Drug dependence[b] | 0.2 | (0.1) | 100.0 | (0.0) | 0.0 | (0.0) | 0.0 | (0.0) |
| Any substance use disorder[b] | 6.4 | (0.8) | 38.9 | (6.0) | 9.8 | (2.7) | 51.3 | (6.7) |
| **Any disorder[b]** | 20.9 | (1.3) | 23.0 | (1.8) | 37.7 | (2.7) | 39.4 | (3.0) |

*Note:* Severity calculated for Part 2 sample ($n = 1720$) using Part 2 weights.
[a] Part 1 sample; prevalence calculated using Part 1 weights.
[b] Part 2 sample; prevalence calculated using Part 2 weights.
[c] Part 2 sample (age ≤39); prevalence and severity calculated using Part 2 weights for ages ≤39.

To complete the clinical picture and provide a comprehensive perspective on the current state of public mental health in Ukraine, we also present descriptive data on heavy alcohol use, smoking, and spouse violence toward women. Overall, 22% of the sample engaged in heavy alcohol use (mostly binge drinking), 32.4% were current smokers, and 12.1% of women were physically assaulted in the past 12 months. As shown in Figure 20.1, alcohol and smoking were about five times more common in men than in women. Slightly more than one in ten men reported behaving aggressively toward their wives, and similarly slightly more than one in ten women reported that their husbands were physically aggressive toward them.

The highest rates of heavy drinking were found in men aged 35–49 (44.5%) and in women ages 18–34 (14.3%). The highest rates of smoking

occurred in men and women ages 18–34 (68.3% in men and 24.7% in women). The highest rates of domestic violence against women were reported by men aged 35–49 (14.5%) and women aged 18–34 (15.5%). All three sets of behaviors decreased with age, especially after age 65.

Heavy alcohol use and smoking were significantly elevated in men and especially in women with intermittent explosive disorder and substance use disorders, but contrary to Western studies, they were not significantly associated with depression or anxiety disorders. Specifically, for men, heavy alcohol users were 1.6 times as likely to have intermittent explosive disorder (95% CI = 1.0–2.6) and 6.1 times as likely to have a substance use disorder (95% CI = 3.1–12.4), and smokers were 4.6 times as likely to have a substance use disorder (95% CI = 2.5–8.4). For women, heavy alcohol users were 5.1

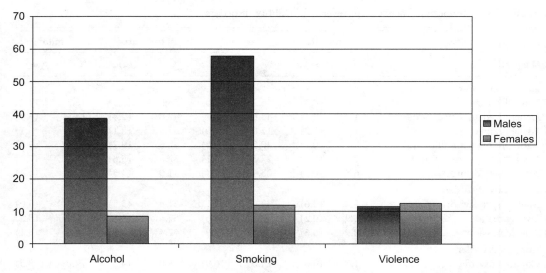

**Figure 20.1.** Rates of 12-month heavy alcohol use, current smoking, and 12-month spousal violence in Ukraine.

times as likely to have intermittent explosive disorder (95% CI = 2.9–9.0) and 47.3 times as likely to have a substance use disorder (95% CI = 14.9–150.1), and smokers were 2.8 times as likely to have intermittent explosive disorder (95% CI = 1.7–4.5) and 13.3 times as likely to have a substance use disorder (95% CI = 3.9–45.5).

Surprisingly, partner violence was not significantly associated with either depression or anxiety disorders, though as expected, it was positively associated with intermittent explosive disorder and substance disorder. Specifically, men who reported aggressive behavior were 4.3 times as likely to meet criteria for intermittent explosive disorder (95% CI = 1.3–13.9) and 5.7 times as likely to have a substance disorder (95% CI = 2.0–16.2). Similarly, women who reported being victimized were 4.2 times as likely to meet criteria for intermittent explosive disorder (95% CI = 1.6–10.8) and 20.5 times as likely to have a substance disorder (95% CI = 5.4–77.2).

### 3.3. 12-month Service Use

As noted in the introduction, outpatient mental health services are not generally available in Ukraine. Thus, only 1.2% of respondents used mental health services in the 12 months

preceding the interview, including 4% of those with 12-month DSM-IV disorders and 0.6% of those without. A larger percentage, 4.9%, accessed some type of medical care, including 14.2% of those with 12-month DSM-IV disorders and 2.6% of those without. Across all types of providers (psychiatric, general, human service, alternative sources), 7.2% of the sample received care, including 18.1% of those with a diagnosable disorder and 4.5% of those without. However, the median number of visits was less than 2.

Cases classified as moderate or severe were more likely to receive care from a mental health professional (5.6% of severe or moderate vs. <1% of mild cases). Moreover, 22.5% of severe cases received some form of general health care in the previous year compared to less than 10% of mild cases. Strikingly, when compared to respondents with no 12-month disorder, the severe cases were almost 13 times as likely to seek help (OR = 12.8; 95% CI = 7.3–22.4), the moderate cases were eight times as likely (OR = 8.1, 95% CI = 4.3–15.0), and respondents classified as having a mild episode were almost four times as likely to seek help (OR = 3.8; 95% CI = 1.6–9.0).

The disorder associated with the greatest likelihood of help seeking was panic disorder (44.6% sought some type of treatment), and the vast majority of these respondents sought care at a polyclinic (general medical provider). The second most common disorder leading to help seeking was generalized anxiety disorder, with 28.3% receiving some type of care, mostly from their polyclinic. Somewhat fewer respondents with depression (24%) sought help, though once again, most of them visited a polyclinic.

In contrast, respondents with alcohol abuse with and without dependence were least likely to receive any type of health care (8.1%); when they did receive care, they were less likely than depressed or anxious respondents to visit a polyclinic. Similarly, respondents who drank heavily (1.9% vs. 4.5% of normal drinkers) or smoked (1.4% vs. 5.3% of nonsmokers) were significantly less likely to visit a general practitioner (alcohol OR = 0.4; 95% CI = 0.2–0.7; smoking OR = 0.3; 95% CI = 0.1–0.7) or any health professional (alcohol OR = 0.3; 95% CI = 0.3–0.7; smoking OR = 0.5; 95% CI = 0.2–0.6) compared to nonusers and nonsmokers. However, the associations of partner violence with service use were small and nonsignificant.

## 4. DISCUSSION

The WMH Survey Initiative provides the first systematic, epidemiological data on the mental health of Ukraine. Some of the findings were expected, such as the high rates of alcoholism, binge drinking, smoking, and partner violence, and the very low rate of treatment. Other findings were not expected, including the high rate of major depression, especially in older men and women, and the lack of association of smoking and partner violence with depression and anxiety disorders. Overall, the prevalence and comorbidity findings present much needed empirical support for the development of mental health policy in Ukraine regarding types of services that are needed, high risk groups for various conditions, and the urgency of providing mental health training for primary care physicians and nurses.

The most relevant comparison for the Ukraine WMH survey findings are the European Study of the Epidemiology of Mental Disorders (ESEMeD) surveys (Alonso, Angermeyer

& Lépine 2004). For women, with one exception, the lifetime and 12-month prevalence rates are within two percentage points of one another. The exception is the 12-month prevalence rate of major depression in Ukrainian women (11.3%), which is double that reported for ESEMeD women (5.0%). Several explanations may be offered for this unusual finding, including loss of spouse, loss of income (pensions have not kept up with the rising cost of living), being used as free household labor (many older respondents live with their adult children and grandchildren and are expected to do the housekeeping and child rearing), and difficulty adjusting to the changing sociopolitical climate. For men, the lifetime and 12-month rates in Ukraine are also similar to those of ESEMeD with the exception of alcohol abuse/dependence, which has a lifetime rate that is threefold higher (26.5% vs. 9.3%) and a 12-month rate that is ninefold higher (11.5% vs. 1.7%). In fact, the rate of alcoholism in the Ukraine WMH survey was the highest of the countries included in the first cross-national comparison (Demyttenaere et al. 2004).

As a group, Ukrainian men minimize their drinking (Nemtsov 2003). Indeed, one interviewer described her encounter with a male respondent in a small village as follows: "I did the interview, and when I got to the alcohol questions, he did not acknowledge much drinking, and I sensed that he was being untruthful. So the next day, I went back to his flat and told him that we were going to do the interview again, and that it is really important that he answer all questions honestly." The respondent disclosed his heavy alcohol use and binge drinking at the second interview. Another interviewer also described that the wife of a respondent was present during the interview and confronted her husband about minimizing his drinking. Thus, as high as the rates of alcoholism and binge drinking may seem, they are undoubtedly underestimates of the true rates in the general population (Webb et al. 2005).

One in five respondents, representing half of all respondents with a lifetime disorder, experienced an episode in the year before interview. Furthermore, 23% of respondents with a recent episode experienced what is considered a serious condition. This means that 9.6 million adults in Ukraine experienced a disorder in the past year, and 2.3 million had a condition classified as serious. Only a minority of serious cases received care, primarily from general medical doctors with no training in mental health. Even psychiatrists, according to a survey by the UPA, are unable to make accurate diagnoses or provide adequate mental health treatment (Gluzman, Golovakha & Panina 1992). Thus, it is unlikely that any medical professional would have recognized the emotional component of the clinic visit.

When we complete the clinical picture and consider binge drinkers and smokers, the high rates translate into millions of people who could potentially benefit from interventions, but it appears that such individuals in fact avoid medical and mental health services. Men who were aggressive toward their wives and women who were the victims of domestic violence were also unlikely, and in some cases less likely, to seek medical attention. Thus, the Ukraine WMH survey underscores and quantifies the potential unmet need for mental health interventions among individuals with diagnosable mental disorders and with health behaviors that carry a high risk of morbidity and mortality.

The Ukraine WMH survey was conducted under less than ideal circumstances. Apartments where the interviews took place were small and overcrowded, making privacy at times impossible. The paper-and-pencil version of the CIDI was cumbersome and long, and thus taxing for respondents and interviewers alike. One question raised early on was whether the CIDI and DSM-IV disorders had the same integrity in Ukraine as in the West. The fact that the rates, age of onset curves, comorbidities, and demographic patterns, particularly the sex differences, largely mirrored those found in Western settings suggests that the enterprise produced meaningful data in Ukraine, as was the case with previous cross-national endeavors by the WHO (e.g., Simon et al. 2002). Moreover, as part of the Ukraine WMH survey, 15 psychiatrists received training in DSM-IV in preparation for learning to administer a semistructured diagnostic interview schedule. Any lingering concerns we might have had about overlooking culturally sanctioned idioms for expressing emotional problems were put to rest by this group who fully embraced the classification system and found it consistent with their own clinical experience. As the study progressed, the psychiatrists interviewed about 175 respondents. For the first time ever, they left their safe offices and went into the very environments that spawned these disorders, often traversing muddy roads en route to respondents living in impoverished rural villages or seedy sections of a city. Often a picture is worth a thousand words. These psychiatrists not only became emissaries for articulating the importance of Western nosology and of a psychiatric epidemiologic approach to understanding community mental health, but they developed a deeper appreciation and understanding of the roots of our study's findings.

In comparing the rates found for Ukraine with those of other settings, it is important to note some other limitations of our study. The sample excluded settings where conditions such as alcoholism and PTSD are probably more common, such as the military. The instrument did not include the specific phobia diagnosis module, thus decreasing the overall rate of anxiety disorders and increasing the average age of onset for this class of disorders. Last, the interviewers had never used an instrument of such complexity. Overall, these limitations would serve to underestimate the true rate of psychiatric morbidity in Ukraine.

As in other countries, the onset of several disorders occurred early in life. However, some disorders, such as PTSD and depression, had an older than expected age of onset. On the one hand, younger people in Ukraine are growing up under a new political order and are exposed to drugs, television, movies, and behavioral patterns that differ markedly from their parents' childhood experiences. Thus, they are now exposed to the same risk factors for poor mental health found in Western research, and one might have expected an inverse relationship between age and mental health. Their parents and grandparents, however, endured the Nazi occupation during World War II, the atrocities inflicted by Stalin, the Chernobyl nuclear power plant accident, and the havoc of major social and economic upheaval. The older segments of our sample thus have higher current rates of disorders, like depression and anxiety, which suggests that either the toxicity of their early life exposures had enduring consequences and/or their current living conditions, characterized for many by poverty and social isolation, have contributed to the higher rates. Our findings on higher 12-month rates of anxiety and depression are consistent with results from the Czech Republic (Hraba, Lorenz & Pechacova 1997) and Russia (Averina et al. 2005; Pakriev et al. 1998a). However, the rates of current heavy alcohol use and smoking are lower in the older members of the cohort. This is largely because alcoholism, heavy alcohol use, and smoking are associated with early mortality, and the study participants represent a biased sample of "healthy" survivors. Nevertheless, even with the unavoidable selection bias, our findings emphasize high risk groups that should be considered as a formal mental health policy is developed.

## 5. FUTURE DIRECTIONS

The Ukraine WMH survey is the first epidemiological study of its kind in a former Soviet country. Although knowledge about the rates and risk factors for alcoholism, drug abuse, and mental disorders and the use of services accumulated in Europe and North America, no comparable body of knowledge was acquired by Eastern Bloc countries. Thus, this study is the trailblazer for future research in Ukraine and other Soviet countries. Beyond providing the descriptive data needed for planning mental health services, the process of conducting the study showed that it is feasible to conduct Western-style psychiatric epidemiological research in a Slavic setting and that the concepts and procedures are appropriate and well tolerated. Furthermore, the Ukraine WMH survey aids in constructing a global portrait of mental health by addressing a society that had never been studied before. The Ministry of Health of Ukraine and UPA have available the first representative data on the magnitude and distribution of need for substance and mental health services. The 15 participating psychiatrists are now versed in the DSM-IV. The Ukraine WMH survey provides the seeds from which to grow analytic, longitudinal, and focused epidemiological research, and epidemiology provides the tools with which to develop and test interventions that are appropriate for that setting.

## REFERENCES

Alonso, J., Angermeyer, M. C. & Lépine, M. P. (2004). The European Study of the Epidemiology of Mental Disorders (ESEMeD) project. *Acta Psychiatrica Scandinavica Supplement*, 420, 5–64.

Ashford, L, Morris, L., Goldberg, H., Serbanescu, F., Sullivan, J., Lazear, M. J. & Micka, M. A. (2003). *Reproductive health trends in Eastern Europe and Eurasia*. Atlanta: Division of Reproductive Health, Centers for Disease Control and Prevention.

Averina, M., Nilssen, O., Brenn, T., Brox, J., Arkhipovsky, V. L. & Kalinin, A. G. (2005). Social and lifestyle determinants of depression, anxiety, sleeping disorders and self-evaluated quality of life in Russia: A population-based study in Arkhangelsk. *Social Psychiatry and Psychiatric Epidemiology*, 40, 511–8.

Bobak, M., McKee, M., Rose, R. & Marmot, M. (1999). Alcohol consumption in a national sample of the Russian population. *Addiction*, 94, 857–66.

Bobak, M., Pikhart, H., Pajak, A., Kubinova, R., Malyutina, S., Sebakova, H., Topor-Madry, T., Nikitin, Y. & Marmot, M. (2006). Depressive symptoms in urban population samples in Russia, Poland and the Czech Republic. *British Journal of Psychiatry*, 188, 359–65.

Bromet, E. J., Gluzman, S. F., Paniotto, V. I., Webb, C. P., Tintle, N. L., Zakhozha, V., Havenaar, J. M., Gutkovich, Z., Kostyuchenko, S. & Schwartz, J. E. (2005). Epidemiology of psychiatric and alcohol disorders in Ukraine: Findings from the Ukraine World Mental Health survey. *Social Psychiatry and Psychiatric Epidemiology*, 40, 681–90.

Bromet, E. J., Gluzman, S., Schwartz, J. E. & Goldgaber D. (2002). Somatic symptoms in women 11 years after the Chornobyl accident. *Environmental Health Perspectives*, 110 (suppl. 4), 625–9.

Bromet, E. J., Goldgaber, D., Carlson, G., Panina, N., Golovakha, E., Gluzman, S. F., Gilbert, T., Gluzman, D., Lyubsky, S. & Schwartz, J. E. (2000). Children's well-being 11 years after the Chernobyl catastrophe. *Archives of General Psychiatry*, 57, 563–71.

Demyttenaere, K., Bruffaerts, R., Posada-Villa, J., Gasquet, I., Kovess, V., Lepine, J. P., Angermeyer, M. C., Bernert, S., Girolamo, G., Morosini, P., Polidori, G., Kikkawa, T., Kawakami, N., Ono, Y., Takeshima, T., Uda, H., Karam, E. G., Fayyad, J. A., Karam, A. N., Mneimneh, Z. N., Medina-Mora, M. E., Borges, G., Lara, G., de Graaf, R., Ormel, J., Gureje, O., Shen, Y., Huang, Y., Zhang, M., Alonso, J., Haro, J. M., Vilagut, G., Bromet, E. J., Gluzman, S., Webb, C., Kessler, R. C., Merikangas, K. R., Anthony, J. C., Korff, M. R. V., Wang, P. S., Alonso, J., Brugha, T. S., Aguilar-Gaxiola, S., Lee, S., Heeringa, S., Pennell, B.-E., Zaslavsky, A. M., Üstün, T. B. & Chatterji, S. (2004). Prevalence, severity and unmet need for treatment of mental disorders in the World Health Organization World Mental Health surveys. *Journal of the American Medical Association*, 291, 2581–90.

Farmer, R. G., Goodman, R. A. & Baldwin, R. J. (1993). Health care and public health in the former Soviet Union, 1992: Ukraine – a case study. *Annals of Internal Medicine*, 119, 324–8.

Gilmore, A. B., McKee, M. & Rose, R. (2002). Determinants of and inequalities in self-perceived health in Ukraine. *Social Science & Medicine*, 12, 2177–88.

Gilmore, A. B., McKee, M., Telishevska, M. & Rose, R. (2001). Epidemiology of smoking in Ukraine, 2000. *Preventive Medicine*, 33, 453–61.

Gluzman, S. F. (1991). Abuse of psychiatry: Analysis of the guilt of medical personnel. *Journal of Medical Ethics*, 17 (suppl.), 19–20.

Gluzman, S. F., Golovakha, Y. I. & Panina, N. V. (1992). First Ukrainian psychiatry poll. *Psychiatric Times*, (May), 47–9.

Havenaar, J. M., Rumyantzeva, G. M., Vandenbrink, W., Poelijoe, N. W., Vandenbout, J., Vanengeland, H. & Koeter, M. W. J. (1997). Long-term mental health effects of the Chernobyl disaster: An epidemiologic survey in two former Soviet regions. *American Journal of Psychiatry*, 154, 1605–7.

Horne, S. (1999). Domestic violence in Russia. *American Psychologist*, 54, 55–61.

Hraba, J., Lorenz, F. O. & Pechacova, Z. (1997). Age and depression in the post-Communist Czech Republic. *Research on Aging*, 19, 442–61.

Kessler, R. C., Haro, J. M., Heeringa, S. G., Pennell, B.-E. & Üstün, T. B. (2006). The World Health Organization World Mental Health Survey Initiative. *Epidemiologia e Psichiatria Sociale*, 15, 161–6.

Kessler, R. C. & Üstün, T. B. (2004). The World Mental Health (WMH) Survey Initiative version of the World Health Organization (WHO) Composite International Diagnostic Interview (CIDI). *International Journal of Methods in Psychiatric Research*, 13, 93–121.

McDaid, D., Samyshkin, Y. A., Jenkins, R., Potasheva, A., Nikiforov, A. & Atun, R. A. (2006). Health system factors impacting on delivery of mental health services in Russia: Multi-methods study. *Health Policy*, 79, 144–52.

Mokhovikov, A. & Donets, O. (1996). Suicide in the Ukraine: Epidemiology, knowledge, and attitudes of the population. *Crisis*, 7, 128–34.

Nemtsov, A. (2003). Alcohol consumption level in Russia: A viewpoint on monitoring health conditions in the Russian federation (RLMS). *Addiction*, 98, 369–70.

Nicholson, A., Bobak, M., Murphy, M., Rose, R. & Marmot, M. (2005). Alcohol consumption and increased mortality in Russian men and women: A cohort study based on the mortality of relatives. *Bulletin of the World Health Organization*, 83, 812–9.

Ougrin, D., Gluzman, S. & Dratcu L. (2006). Psychiatry in post-communist Ukraine: Dismantling the past, paving the way for the future. *Psychiatric Bulletin*, 30, 456–9.

Pakriev, S., Vasar, V., Aluoja, A., Saarma, M. & Shlik, J. (1998a). Prevalence of mood disorders in the rural population of Udmurtia. *Acta Psychiatrica Scandinavica*, 97, 169–74.

Pakriev, S., Vasar, V., Aluoja, A. & Shlik, J. (1998b). Prevalence of ICD-10 harmful use of alcohol and alcohol dependence among the rural population in Udmurtia. *Alcohol and Alcoholism*, 33, 255–64.

Perlman, F. & Bobak, M. (2008). Socioeconomic and behavioral determinants of mortality in posttransition Russia: a prospective population study. *Annals of Epidemiology*, 18, 92–100.

Rahu, M., Rahu, K., Auvinen, A., Tekkel, M., Stengrevies, A., Hakulinen, A., Boice, J. D., Jr. & Inskip, P. D. (2006). Cancer risk among Chernobyl cleanup workers in Estonia and Latvia, 1986–1998. *International Journal of Cancer*, 119, 162–8.

Rahu, M., Tekkel, M., Veidebaum, T., Pukkala, T., Hakulinen, A., Auvinen, A., Rytomaa, T., Inskip, P. D. & Boice, J. D., Jr. (1997). The Estonian study of Chernobyl clean-up workers: II. Incidence of cancer and mortality. *Radiation Research*, 147, 653–7.

Rezvyy, G., Øiesvold, R., Parniakov, A. & Olstad, R. (2005). A comparative study of diagnostic practice in psychiatry in Northern Norway and Northwest Russia. *Social Psychiatry and Psychiatric Epidemiology*, 40, 316–23.

Shkolnikov, V., McKee, M. & Leon, D. A. (2001). Changes in life expectancy in Russia in the mid-1990s. *Lancet*, 357, 917–21.

Shulman, N. & Adams, B. (2002). A comparison of Russian and British attitudes towards mental health problems in the community. *International Journal of Social Psychiatry*, 48, 266–78.

Simon, G. E., Goldberg, D. P., Von Korff, M. & Üstün, T. B. (2002). Understanding cross-national differences in depression prevalence. *Psychological Medicine*, 32, 585–94.

Webb, C. P. M., Bromet, E. J., Gluzman, S., Tintle, N. L., Schwartz, J. E., Kostyuchenko, S. & Havenaar, J. M. (2005). Epidemiology of heavy alcohol use in Ukraine: Findings from the World Mental Health Survey. *Alcohol and Alcoholism*, 40, 327–35.

Webb, C. P. M., Bromet, E. J., Tintle, N. L., Schwartz, J. E., Gluzman, S., Kostyuchenko, S. & Havenaar, J. M. (2007). Smoking initiation and nicotine dependence symptoms in Ukraine: Findings from the World Mental Health Survey. *Public Health*, 121, 663–72.

World Bank (2003). *Ukraine country brief.* Available at http://web.worldbank.org/WBSITE/EXTERNAL/COUNTRIES/ECAEXT/UKRAINEEXTN/0, menuPK:328543~pagePK:141132~piPK:141107~theSitePK:328533,00.html#Economy (accessed October 31, 2007).

World Health Organization (WHO) (2006). *Health effects of the Chernobyl accident and special health care programmes.* Geneva: World Health Organization.

# 21 | Mental Disorders and Service Use in China

YUEQIN HUANG, ZHAORUI LIU, MINGYUAN ZHANG, YUCUN SHEN, CHEUK HIM ADLEY TSANG, YANLING HE, AND SING LEE

## ACKNOWLEDGMENTS

The WMH Survey Initiative in China is a community-based epidemiological survey using the CIDI. Approval from the Ministry of Health of China allowed the survey to be realized in two metropolitan areas: Beijing and Shanghai. Instrument development and training were carried out by the WMH Data Collection Coordination Centre at the Survey Research Center, at the University of Michigan, supported by the U.S. National Institute of Mental Health (R13 MH066849-02), the John D. and Catherine T. MacArthur Foundation, and the Pfizer Foundation. The Research Center for Contemporary China of Peking University conducted the field survey. WMH data were centrally processed by the WMH Data Analysis Coordination Centre at the Department of Health Care Policy, Harvard Medical School, and other U.S. institutions. The research fellows from Institute of Mental Health, Peking University, and Hong Kong Mood Disorder Center, the Chinese University of Hong Kong, Hong Kong Special Administrative Region, contributed their effort for data analysis and paper writing. All study subjects in Beijing and Shanghai participated with informed written consent.

## I. THE EXISTING TREATMENT SYSTEM FOR MENTAL DISORDERS IN CHINA

In China, the existing treatment systems for mental disorders are diverse, and access to care has been a problem following the country's economic reform (Lee & Kleinman 2000). The magnitude of the treatment gap for people with mental disorders in the community has not been studied until recently (Lee et al. 2007).

In the clinical setting, pharmacotherapy is the principal choice for most psychotic and nonpsychotic disorders. In keeping with American and European standards, the newest medications are widely available in China. Psychotherapy has become more popular in China in recent years, though the standard of professional training still needs to be improved. Alternative medicine, such as Chinese traditional medicine, is often administered in the clinical treatment of mental disorders. For psychotic disorders, hospitalization is the main form of treatment, whereas nonpsychotic disorders are mostly treated on an outpatient basis. Most people with nonpsychotic disorders avoid seeking help at psychiatric hospitals because of stigma or because they are not aware that they have a mental disorder. Physicians in general hospitals seldom refer patients with mental disorders to psychiatric hospitals because of their lack of sensitivity to psychiatric symptoms. Dissemination of information about mental health to the public and professionals is needed to overcome these problems.

By 2000, senior psychiatrists in China had seriously considered carrying out a new national survey on mental disorders because data from the two previous national surveys, which are discussed subsequently, might no longer apply. Consequently, when the World Mental Health (WMH) Survey Consortium sought collaborating country partners worldwide, some senior Chinese psychiatrists (Yucun Shen, Mingyuan Zhang, and Sing Lee) responded positively, which resulted in WMH surveys being carried out in Beijing and Shanghai (Kessler et al. 2006). Supported by the Ministry of Health of China, the field study was successfully conducted and the data were obtained. On the basis of the results of these surveys, WMH surveys have now been completed in other areas of China and their results will soon be available.

## 2. PREVIOUS PSYCHIATRIC EPIDEMIOLOGICAL STUDIES IN CHINA

### 2.1. Large-scale Epidemiological Surveys of Mental Disorders

In China, there have been two large-scale epidemiological surveys of mental disorders in the previous two decades. The first was conducted in 1982 in 12 regions and the second was conducted in 1993 in 7 regions. The 12-region survey, sponsored by the Ministry of Health of China and supported by the World Health Organization, was completed in 1982 and resulted from a large-scale collaborative effort among the psychiatric teams. The 12 units were chosen so as to represent different geographical regions and sociocultural groups of the country. Each center studied both a rural sample of 500 households and an urban sample of 500 households. The 12,000 households that comprised the total sample contained 51,982 persons (38,136 over the age of 15 years). A survey team was identified in each of the 12 units, which was composed of both senior and junior psychiatrists, general medical doctors, psychiatric nurses, and medical assistants. The survey instruments included the Psychosis Screening Schedule (10 items), the PSE-9 Neurosis Screening Schedule (12 items),

the PSE-9 (Chinese version), the Social Disability Screening Schedule (SDSS), the Household and Socio-demographic Information Schedule, the General Psychiatric Interview Schedule and Summary Form, and the Assessment Schedule for Children (ASC-40). Subjects aged over 14 years who gave a positive rating on either of the two questions in the Psychosis Screening Schedule were regarded as possible cases and were seen individually for a clinical assessment according to the criteria and definition of the ICD-9.

The survey estimated that the overall point prevalence rates of all mental disorders in the 12 study areas was 1.05%, and that the lifetime prevalence rate was 1.27%. The point prevalence rate of schizophrenia was 4.75 per 1000 people in the population and the lifetime prevalence was 5.69 per 1000. The point prevalence of schizophrenia in urban areas was 6.06 per 1000, which is higher than that in rural areas (3.42 per 1000). The point prevalence of manic-depressive psychosis was 0.37 per 1000 people and the lifetime prevalence was 0.76 per 1000. One-fifth of all survey respondents were screened for neurosis, which was estimated to have an overall prevalence of 2.22%, including the neurasthenic (1.30%), hysterical (0.36%), depressive (0.31%), anxiety (0.15%), phobic (0.06%), obsessive-compulsive (0.03%), and hypochondriacal (0.02%) subtypes. According to the government's needs, the survey was focused on prevalence of psychotic disorders and included moderate and severe mental retardation.

The survey also studied correlates of mental disorders and found, most notably, that schizophrenia was associated with substantial social disability. Despite the low rates, the results of the survey were of great importance for planning and developing national mental health services in China. Furthermore, carrying out the survey was instrumental in introducing the methodology of modern epidemiological psychiatry in community settings to Chinese psychiatrists (twelve collaborating units of epidemiological survey on mental disorders 1986a, 1986b; Cooper & Sartorius 1996).

Under the leadership of the Ministry of Health, the epidemiological survey of mental disorders was completed in 1993 in seven of the same 12 regions examined in 1982. This survey, like the earlier 1982 survey, was also supported by the WHO. The study methods and procedures were very similar to those of the first survey. However, several new instruments were added, including the Negative Symptom Assess Scale, the Wechsler Intelligence Scale for Children (WISC), the Adult Intelligence Disability Assessment Instrument, the Chinese Classification of Mental Disorders-Second Version (CCMD-2), the ICD-10, and the instruments and tables used in the International Collaboration Research for Schizophrenia.

As in the 1982 survey, each participating center studied both a rural sample of 500 households and an urban sample of 500 households. The 7000 households that comprised the total sample contained 23,333 persons. The results showed that the overall point prevalence of mental disorders (excluding neurosis by original design of the survey) in the seven study areas was 1.12%, and the lifetime prevalence was 1.35%. Of all the mental disorders, the prevalence of schizophrenia was the highest, with a point prevalence of 5.31 per 1000 population and a lifetime prevalence rate of 6.55 per 1000. The prevalence of mental retardation was 2.70 per 1000, the second most prevalent disorder studied, with manic-depressive psychosis ranking third (point prevalence 0.52 per 1000 and lifetime prevalence 0.83 per 1000). The prevalence of alcohol dependence (0.68 per 1000) was statistically higher than in the 12-region survey. The prevalence of Alzheimer's disease was 0.36 per 1000 (Zhang et al. 1998).

## 2.2. Regional Epidemiological Surveys of Mental Disorders in China

### 2.2.1. Epidemiological Surveys of Mental Disorders in Shandong Province

Two provincial surveys of mental disorders were carried out in 1984 and 1994 in Shandong Province by the Shandong Center for Mental Health. The surveys used the same instruments and procedures as in the two large-scale surveys described previously. The sample of the 1984

Shandong survey comprised 29,492 households, with a total of 118,998 persons (88,822 over the age of 15 years). For the 1994 survey, the sample contained 26,460 households with 84,767 persons (67,901 over the age of 15 years). The results of the 1984 survey showed that the overall lifetime prevalence of all mental disorders in Shandong Province was 0.98%, while the point prevalence rate was 0.91%. The 1994 survey, in comparison, found overall lifetime and point prevalence of all mental disorders in Shandong Province of 1.32% and 1.22%, respectively. Thus, both lifetime and point prevalence were higher than in the 1984 survey. The prevalence of alcohol dependence increased to 0.98 per 1000 and the prevalence of neurosis increased to 0.89 per 1000. There was no statistical difference in the prevalence of organic psychosis between the 1984 and 1994 surveys (Weng et al. 1998).

### 2.2.2. Epidemiological Surveys of Mental Disorders in Shenzhen City

In 1996, an epidemiological survey of mental disorders was carried out in the city of Shenzhen using the same instruments and procedures as in the two large-scale surveys that took place in 1982 and 1993. The Shenzhen survey investigated a rural and an urban sample of 500 households each, totaling 3807 persons. The overall point prevalence of all mental disorders (except neurosis) among persons aged 15 or above was estimated at 1.48%, and lifetime prevalence was estimated at 1.62%. The prevalence of schizophrenia (4.72 per 1000) was the highest among all of the mental disorders, followed by substance-related disorders (4.38 per 1000), organic psychosis (4.05 per 1000), moderate and severe mental retardation (2.36 per 1000), and mood disorders (0.34 per 1000) (Cheng et al. 1999).

### 2.2.3. Significance of Descriptive Epidemiological Data of Mental Disorders in China

Some of the results of the preceding studies, such as those involving schizophrenia, are quite similar to those in overseas studies using similar methods of assessment, whereas other results, most notably those involving the prevalence of neurotic and mood disorders, are markedly different. The consistency of results regarding psychotic disorders argues for the view that biological causes are dominant in these disorders and that this biological vulnerability is relatively stable throughout the world. The variability in the prevalence estimates of nonpsychotic disorders, in comparison, argues that cultural factors that differ across cultures play a more important role in these disorders.

These findings can be interpreted in several ways. One line of thinking is that because both the DSM and ICD diagnostic systems were developed by American and European psychiatrists and based on Western cultures, the diagnostic categories in these systems might not be valid cross-culturally. Another issue is that the evolving nature of diagnosis and classification of mental disorders makes it difficult to compare results across different surveys carried out using different methodologies and diagnostic criteria. Another possibility, of course, is that genuine differences exist in the cross-national distribution of mental disorders relating to genetic and environmental etiologic factors. Debate about these issues has aroused both interest and controversy among psychiatrists, psychologists, epidemiologists, sociologists, and anthropologists (Cooper & Sartorius 1996) as well among as governmental officers and policy makers in many countries.

## 3. METHODS

### 3.1. Instrument

The Beijing and Shanghai WMH surveys used Version 3.0 of the World Health Organization (WHO) Composite International Diagnostic Interview (CIDI) (Kessler & Üstün 2004; see also Chapter 4), a fully structured lay-administered diagnostic interview, to generate diagnoses according to the definitions and criteria of both ICD-10 (WHO 1991) and DSM-IV (American Psychiatric Association 1994) diagnostic systems. The CIDI was translated into Chinese using the standard WHO protocol in

which a team of survey experts completed the initial translation and a separate team then carried out an independent back-translation to confirm preservation of the meaning of the original English version. The translators had access to an expert panel for consultation about potentially ambiguous questions. The panel included three academic psychiatrists with epidemiological expertise, as well as a survey methodologist who was fully trained in the CIDI and was responsible for fieldwork from the Research Center for Contemporary China (RCCC) in Beijing. The expert panel evaluated the translation for content validity using information based on the results of the back-translation, as well as pilot tests with Chinese patients with mental disorders. Final revision was then carried out by the panel to ensure that lay interviewers would be able to understand the Chinese terms easily for field procedures.

Double-blinded clinical reappraisal interviews with a mixed sample of 95 inpatient and outpatient psychiatric patients and 77 normal controls, using the Structured Clinical Interview for DSM-IV (SCID) (First et al. 2002) as a standard criteria to generate diagnoses, found generally good validity and reliability with Version 2.1 of CIDI (Huang et al. 2005). As a result, no separate clinical reappraisal study was carried out of CIDI 3.0 in the Chinese WMH surveys. In the CIDI 2.1 validation, test-retest consistency was 0.74 to 1.0 among mood disorder, anxiety disorder, substance abuse, alcohol abuse, somatic disorder, schizophrenia, and other psychotic disorders. Regarding validity of CIDI 2.1, sensitivity and specificity were 88.1% and 89.6% for mood disorders, 66.7% and 94.8% for anxiety disorders, 85.7% and 98.7% for substance disorders, and 57.9% and 100% for schizophrenia and other psychotic disorders. Both hospital- and community-based clinical reappraisal studies are currently underway for CIDI 3.0 and their results will be soon available.

### 3.2. Subjects

Subjects in the Beijing and Shanghai WMH surveys were urban dwellers who met the following criteria: adults aged 18 to 70 years, living in a family household, formally registered in a nonagricultural household, and residing within the urban districts of Beijing and Shanghai. A stratified two-stage systematic selection scheme was used to select the sample with equal probability for every eligible individual in the target population. Because this sampling procedure avoids the within-household clustering that is typical of community surveys, no within-household probability of selection weight was applied to the data, increasing the efficiency of sampling. Internal subsampling reduced respondent burden by dividing the interview into two parts: Part 1 included the core diagnostic assessment; Part 2 included information about the correlates and the disorders of secondary interest. All respondents completed Part 1. All Part 1 respondents who met criteria for any disorder plus a subsample of approximately 25% of those who did not meet the criteria were administered Part 2.

Neighborhood committees (NCs) are established community organizations in urban China that were used as RCCC's preselected primary sampling units (PSUs). The sampling team first approached 50 NCs in each city to check their actual conditions against the obtained demographic data of the PSUs. A total of 47 of these NCs in Beijing and 44 in Shanghai were chosen as final PSUs for the survey. According to the predetermined sampling interval and random starting points, the desired number of households was sampled from the household registration list in each NC. The sampler then checked the address and demographic information of all the eligible members of every selected household against the RCCC's standard household sampling form (HSF). After editing the HSF, the field managers used the data to randomly select eligible persons as respondents. Of the 47 PSUs selected in Beijing, there were 4024 eligible individuals that comprised the final master sample of respondents, and 3856 respondents of the 44 selected PSUs were chosen in Shanghai. After the subjects were given a complete description of the study, written informed consent was obtained and interviews were conducted with as many of these designated respondents as possible.

The target sample size was 2500 completed interviews in each of the two cities. The actual sample size was 2633 in Beijing and 2568 in Shanghai. The response rates were 74.8% and 74.6%, respectively. Weights were applied to the data to adjust for discrepancies between the sample and population census data on the cross-classification of key sociodemographic variables. A second weight was applied to the Part 2 subsample to adjust for the oversampling of Part 1 respondents who met criteria for a core disorder.

### 3.3. Training and Field Procedures

The RCCC field managers conducted a one-day training session for field samplers in the two cities following their standard on-site training procedure. The trainers introduced the project, sampling procedures, principles, methods, and specific requirements for implementing the sampling design. The training included briefings on the field conditions and potential difficulties at different sampling stages, a demonstration interview, and practice exercises. The RCCC field managers then conducted seven days of training for the interviewers in each city following their standard on-site training procedures. This included seven main sessions: introduction, sampling design and procedures, review of the questionnaire, methods and techniques of field interviewing, briefing on field conditions, potential difficulties in different neighborhoods, and in- and out-of-classroom exercises for interviewers.

### 3.4. Measures

#### 3.4.1. Diagnostic Assessment

DSM-IV criteria were used to define the disorders included in the current chapter. The disorders included anxiety disorders (panic disorder, agoraphobia without panic disorder, specific phobia, social phobia, generalized anxiety disorder, posttraumatic stress disorder, separation anxiety disorder), mood disorders (major depressive disorder, dysthymic disorder), impulse-control disorders (conduct disorder, intermittent explosive disorder), and substance use disorders (alcohol abuse with or without dependence, drug abuse with or without dependence). Diagnostic hierarchy and organic exclusion rules were applied in making all diagnoses. Because of concerns that the recall of conduct disorder (CD), a child-adolescent onset disorder, would be low among older respondents, CD was assessed only for Part 2 respondents in the age range of 18–44 years.

On the basis of evidence that retrospective age of onset reports in structured diagnostic interviews are often erroneous (Simon et al. 1995), a special question sequence was designed to improve the accuracy of reporting. This began with questions designed to emphasize the importance of accurate response: "Can you remember your exact age of the very first time when you (had the symptom / the syndrome)?" Respondents who answered no were probed for a bound of uncertainty by moving up the age range incrementally (e.g., "Was it before you went to school?"; "Was it before age 13?"). Age of onset was set at the upper end of the bound of uncertainty (e.g., age of 12 years for respondents who reported that onset was before the beginning of their teens). Experimental research has shown that this question sequence yields more plausible responses than standard age of onset questions (Knauper et al. 1999).

### 3.4.2. Severity of 12-month Cases

A severity gradient was created that defined 12-month disorders as serious, moderate, or mild. Details of this classification and its external validation can be found elsewhere (Demyttenaere et al. 2004). Briefly put, a serious disorder included such conditions as bipolar disorder, substance dependence with a physiological dependence syndrome, and other disorders associated with a suicide plan, a suicide attempt, hospitalization, treatment with an antipsychotic medication, or severe role impairment. Respondents whose 12-month disorder did not meet criteria for serious were classified as either moderate or mild on the basis of their responses to the disorder-specific Sheehan Disability Scales (Leon et al. 1997).

### 3.4.3. Initial Lifetime Treatment Contact

Near the end of each CIDI diagnostic section, respondents were asked whether they ever had "talked to a medical doctor or other professional" about the disorder under investigation. When asking this question, the interviewer clarified that the term "other professional" was meant to apply broadly to include "psychologists, counselors, spiritual advisers, herbalists, acupuncturists, and any other healing professionals." Respondents who reported ever talking to any of these professionals about the disorder in question were then asked how old they were the first time they did so. The response to this question was used to define age of first treatment contact.

### 3.4.4. 12-month Use of Mental Health Services

All Part 2 respondents were asked whether they had ever received treatment for "problems with your emotions or nerves or your use of alcohol or drugs." Separate assessments were made for different types of professionals, support groups, self-help groups, mental health crisis hotlines (assumed to be visits with nonpsychiatrist mental health specialists), complementary alternative medical (CAM) therapies including traditional Chinese medicine, and use of other treatment settings including admissions to hospitals and other facilities (each day of admission was assumed to include a visit with a psychiatrist). Follow-up questions asked about age at first and most recent contacts, as well as the number and duration of visits in the past 12 months.

Reports of 12-month service use were classified into the following categories: psychiatrist; nonpsychiatrist mental health specialist (e.g., psychologist or other nonpsychiatrist mental health professional in any setting, social worker or counselor in a mental health specialty setting, use of a mental health hotline); general medical provider (primary-care doctor, other general medical doctor, nurse, any other health professional not previously mentioned); human services professional (religious or spiritual adviser, social worker, or counselor in any setting other than a specialty mental health setting); and CAM professional (any other type of healer such as chiropractors, participation in an Internet support group, participation in a self-help group). Psychiatrist and nonpsychiatrist specialist categories were combined into a broader mental health specialty (MHS) category; MHS was also combined with general medical (GM) into an even broader health-care (HC) category. Human services (HS) and CAM were also combined into a non–health-care (NHC) category.

### 3.4.5. Minimally Adequate 12-month Treatment

Minimally adequate treatment was defined on the basis of available evidence-based guidelines (Agency for Health Care Policy and Research 1993; Lehman & Steinwachs 1998; American Psychiatric Association 1998, 2000, 2002, 2004). Treatment was considered at least minimally adequate if the patient received either pharmacotherapy (more than 2 months of an appropriate medication for the focal disorder plus more than four visits to any type of medical doctor) or psychotherapy (more than eight visits with any health-care or human services professional lasting an average of more than 30 minutes). The decision to require more than four physician visits for pharmacotherapy was based on the fact that more than four visits for medication evaluation, initiation, and monitoring are generally recommended during the acute and continuation phases of treatment in available guidelines (Agency for Health Care Policy and Research 1993; Lehman & Steinwachs 1998; American Psychiatric Association 1998, 2000, 2002, 2004).

Appropriate medications for disorders included antidepressants for depressive disorders, mood stabilizers or antipsychotics for bipolar disorders, antidepressants or anxiolytics for anxiety disorders, antagonists or agonists (e.g., disulfiram, naltrexone, methodone) for alcohol and substance disorders, and any psychiatric drugs for impulse control disorders (Schatzberg & Nemeroff 2004). At least eight sessions were required for minimally adequate psychotherapy based on the fact that clinical trials

demonstrating effectiveness have generally included more than eight psychotherapy visits (Agency for Health Care Policy and Research 1993; Lehman & Steinwachs 1998; American Psychiatric Association 1998, 2000, 2002, 2004). For alcohol and substance disorders, self-help visits of any duration counted as psychotherapy visits. Treatment adequacy was defined separately for each 12-month disorder (i.e., a respondent with comorbid disorders could be classified as receiving minimally adequate treatment for one disorder but not for another).

### 3.5. Predictor Variables

Predictor variables in analyses of lifetime data included age of onset (AOO) of the focal disorder (coded into the categories early, middle, and late), cohort (defined by age at interview in the categories 18–34, 35–49, 50–64, 65–70), sex, and education (categorized as either current students or nonstudents with 0–6, 7–9, 10–12, or more than 13 years of education). Information on years of education was also coded as a time-varying predictor by assuming an orderly educational history for each respondent in which eight years of education corresponds to being a student up to age 14, and other lengths of education are associated with ages consistent with this benchmark (e.g., 12 years of education is assumed to correspond to being a student up to age 18).

Variables in analyses of 12-month data included sex, cohort, education (categorized as 0–6 [none and primary], 7–9 [junior high school], 10–12 [senior high school], or more than 13 [college and beyond]), and marital status (married/cohabiting, separated/widowed/divorced, never married).

### 3.6. Analysis Procedures

Survival analysis was used to make estimated projections of cumulative lifetime probability of disorders and treatment contact from year of onset. The actuarial method (Halli & Rao 1992) implemented in SAS V8.2 (SAS Institute 2001) was used for this purpose. The typical duration of delay in initial treatment contact was defined as the median number of years from disorder onset to first treatment contact among cases that eventually made treatment contact on the basis of these curves. Discrete-time survival analysis (Efron 1988) with person-year as the unit of analysis was used to examine correlates of disorders and treatment contact. Models of treatment contact were estimated twice for a given disorder: once among all respondents with a history of the disorder to study the predictors of ever making a treatment contact and a second time among the subsample who eventually made a treatment contact, to study the predictors of delay in initial contact. Basic patterns of 12-month disorders and service use were examined by computing proportions, means, and medians. Logistic regression (Hosmer & Lemeshow 1989) analysis was used to study sociodemographic predictors of having 12-month disorders, receiving any 12-month treatment in the total sample, treatment in particular sectors among those receiving any treatment, and treatment meeting criteria for minimal adequacy. Standard errors were estimated using the Taylor series method as implemented in SUDAAN (Research Triangle Institute 2002). Multivariate significance tests were made using Wald $\chi^2$ tests based on coefficient variance-covariance matrices that were adjusted for design effects using the Taylor series method. Statistical significance was evaluated using two-sided design-based tests and the 0.05 level of significance.

## 4. RESULTS

### 4.1. Lifetime Prevalence

The estimated lifetime prevalence of any DSM-IV/CIDI disorder in the Beijing and Shanghai surveys was 13.2%, 3.7% of which met criteria for two or more disorders and 1.2% for three or more disorders (Table 21.1). The most common disorders were alcohol abuse (4.7%), major depressive disorder (3.5%), and specific phobias (2.6%). Prevalence of several different disorders (social phobia, intermittent explosive disorder, alcohol abuse and/or dependence, drug abuse, any disorder, three or more disorders) was

significantly associated with age, with prevalence lowest among respondents aged 65 and older and generally highest among respondents in the age range of 18–34.

### 4.2. Projected Lifetime Risk

As not all respondents were old enough at the time of interview to have passed through the period of risk for the disorders, the proportion of respondents who will eventually develop a mental disorder is higher than the proportion with lifetime prevalence to date. We generated AOO distributions to estimate projected lifetime risk (Table 21.2), which was 18.0% for any disorder. The difference between lifetime prevalence to date and projected lifetime risk as of age 75 varied depending on the AOO distribution. For anxiety disorders, where AOO was relatively early, the difference between the two estimates was small (4.8% lifetime prevalence versus 6.0% projected lifetime risk). For intermittent explosive disorder, the only impulse-control disorder assessed for the full age range of the sample, the difference was even smaller (1.9% lifetime prevalence versus 2.1% projected lifetime risk). Differences were greater for substance use disorders (4.9% lifetime prevalence versus 6.1% projected lifetime risk), and considerably greater for mood disorders. More than half of all lifetime cases of mood disorders estimated in the sample had not yet occurred at the time of interview (3.6% lifetime prevalence versus 7.3% projected lifetime risk). At the level of individual disorders, the largest discrepancies between prevalence and projected risk were for generalized anxiety disorder and major depressive disorder, for which each of the projected lifetime risk was more than twice the lifetime prevalence to date.

For the majority of disorders, most cases had onset in the 25-year interval between the early teens (age 13) and middle age (age 44), although this varied across disorders. Median AOO (the 50th percentile of the AOO distribution in Table 21.2) was earliest for anxiety disorders (age 17), somewhat later for substance use disorders (age 25), and latest for mood disorders (age 43). The

**Table 21.1.** Lifetime prevalence for Part 1 and Part 2 samples of DSM-IV/CIDI disorders

| Diagnosis | Total % | (se) | 18–34 % | (se) | 35–49 % | (se) | 50–64 % | (se) | 65+ % | (se) | $\chi^2$ |
|---|---|---|---|---|---|---|---|---|---|---|---|
| **I. Anxiety disorders** | | | | | | | | | | | |
| Panic disorder | 0.4 | (0.1) | 0.5 | (0.3) | 0.3 | (0.1) | 0.4 | (0.2) | 1.0 | (0.6) | 3.2 |
| Generalized anxiety disorder with hierarchy | 0.8 | (0.1) | 0.4 | (0.2) | 0.8 | (0.2) | 1.1 | (0.4) | 1.4 | (0.7) | 3.4 |
| Social phobia | 0.5 | (0.1) | 0.8 | (0.2) | 0.4 | (0.1) | 0.4 | (0.3) | 0.1 | (0.1) | 10.7* |
| Specific phobia | 2.6 | (0.3) | 2.7 | (0.5) | 2.2 | (0.4) | 3.1 | (0.7) | 3.4 | (0.8) | 2.2 |
| Agoraphobia without panic | 0.0 | (0.0) | 0.1 | (0.1) | 0.0 | (0.0) | 0.0 | (0.0) | 0.1 | (0.1) | 2.1 |
| Posttraumatic stress disorder[a] | 0.3 | (0.1) | 0.3 | (0.2) | 0.2 | (0.1) | 0.4 | (0.2) | 0.0 | (0.0) | 7.7 |
| Separation anxiety disorder/ adult separation anxiety[a] | 0.7 | (0.2) | 1.7 | (0.6) | 0.2 | (0.1) | 0.0 | (0.0) | 0.0 | (0.0) | 8.9 |
| Any anxiety disorder[a] | 4.8 | (0.7) | 4.7 | (1.2) | 3.9 | (0.8) | 6.7 | (1.8) | 4.5 | (1.5) | 2.5 |
| **II. Mood disorders** | | | | | | | | | | | |
| Major depressive disorder with hierarchy | 3.5 | (0.4) | 4.1 | (0.8) | 2.9 | (0.4) | 3.9 | (0.7) | 2.6 | (0.7) | 3.5 |
| Dysthymia with hierarchy | 0.1 | (0.0) | 0.0 | (0.0) | 0.2 | (0.1) | 0.3 | (0.2) | 0.0 | (0.0) | 8.4 |
| Bipolar I–II disorders | 0.1 | (0.0) | 0.1 | (0.1) | 0.1 | (0.1) | 0.0 | (0.0) | 0.0 | (0.0) | 3.8 |
| Any mood disorder | 3.6 | (0.4) | 4.2 | (0.8) | 3.1 | (0.4) | 4.0 | (0.7) | 2.6 | (0.7) | 3.7 |
| **III. Impulse-control disorders** | | | | | | | | | | | |
| Oppositional-defiant disorder with hierarchy[b] | – | – | – | – | – | – | – | – | – | – | |
| Conduct disorder[b] | 0.5 | (0.2) | 0.5 | (0.2) | 0.7 | (0.7) | – | – | – | – | 0.1[d] |
| Attention-deficit/hyperactivity disorder[b] | – | – | – | – | – | – | – | – | – | – | |
| Intermittent explosive disorder with hierarchy | 1.9 | (0.3) | 3.1 | (0.7) | 1.6 | (0.3) | 0.7 | (0.3) | 0.0 | (0.0) | 37.9** |
| Any impulse-control disorder[b] | 4.3 | (0.9) | 3.3 | (1.1) | 7.3 | (1.8) | – | – | – | – | 3.6[d] |
| **IV. Substance disorders** | | | | | | | | | | | |
| Alcohol abuse with/without dependence | 4.7 | (0.4) | 5.4 | (0.8) | 5.7 | (0.7) | 2.2 | (0.5) | 0.9 | (0.5) | 36.4** |
| Alcohol dependence with abuse | 1.0 | (0.2) | 1.0 | (0.3) | 1.5 | (0.4) | 0.3 | (0.2) | 0.0 | (0.0) | 25.3** |
| Drug abuse with/without dependence[a] | 0.5 | (0.2) | 0.6 | (0.5) | 0.4 | (0.2) | 0.5 | (0.5) | 0.0 | (0.0) | 9.6* |
| Drug dependence with abuse[a] | 0.0 | (0.0) | 0.0 | (0.0) | 0.0 | (0.0) | 0.0 | (0.0) | 0.0 | (0.0) | 1.1 |
| Any substance disorder[a] | 4.9 | (0.7) | 6.0 | (1.2) | 5.9 | (1.0) | 2.4 | (0.7) | 1.8 | (1.6) | 15.8** |
| **V. Any disorder** | | | | | | | | | | | |
| Any[a] | 13.2 | (1.3) | 14.2 | (2.7) | 13.7 | (1.4) | 13.2 | (2.2) | 8.2 | (2.2) | 4.5 |
| Two or more disorders[a] | 3.7 | (0.5) | 4.5 | (1.1) | 4.1 | (0.8) | 3.0 | (1.3) | 1.4 | (0.4) | 16.7** |
| Three or more disorders[a] | 1.2 | (0.3) | 1.3 | (0.5) | 0.9 | (0.2) | 2.0 | (1.3) | 0.4 | (0.4) | 3.1 |

[a] Denotes Part 2 sample ($n = 1628$).

[b] Denotes disorders in Part 2 respondents and aged $\leq 39$ years ($n = 570$).

[c] ODD and ADHD was not assessed in China.

[d] The $\chi^2$ test evaluates statistical significance of age-related differences in estimated prevalence; $\chi^2$ is evaluated with one degree of freedom for conduct disorder and any impulse-control disorder.

* Significant age difference at the 0.05 level.

**Table 21.2.** Ages at selected percentiles on the standardized age of onset distributions of CIDI disorders with projected lifetime risk at age 75

| Diagnosis | Projected lifetime risk at age 75 | | Ages at selected age of onset percentiles | | | | | | | |
|---|---|---|---|---|---|---|---|---|---|---|
| | % | (se) | 5 | 10 | 25 | 50 | 75 | 90 | 95 | 99 |
| **I. Anxiety disorders** | | | | | | | | | | |
| Panic disorder[a] | – | – | – | – | – | – | – | – | – | – |
| Generalized anxiety disorder with hierarchy | 1.7 | (0.3) | 18 | 23 | 34 | 44 | 54 | 57 | 58 | 61 |
| Social phobia[a] | – | – | – | – | – | – | – | – | – | – |
| Specific phobia | 2.8 | (0.3) | 5 | 5 | 5 | 13 | 17 | 36 | 41 | 59 |
| Agoraphobia without panic[a,b] | – | – | – | – | – | – | – | – | – | – |
| Posttraumatic stress disorder[a] | – | – | – | – | – | – | – | – | – | – |
| Separation anxiety disorder/adult separation anxiety[a] | – | – | – | – | – | – | – | – | – | – |
| Any anxiety disorder | 6.0 | (0.8) | 5 | 5 | 10 | 17 | 36 | 55 | 57 | 60 |
| **II. Mood disorders** | | | | | | | | | | |
| Major depressive disorder with hierarchy | 7.2 | (0.9) | 18 | 21 | 28 | 43 | 54 | 67 | 68 | 68 |
| Dysthymia with hierarchy[a] | – | – | – | – | – | – | – | – | – | – |
| Bipolar I–II disorders[a] | – | – | – | – | – | – | – | – | – | – |
| Any mood disorder | 7.3 | (0.9) | 18 | 21 | 28 | 43 | 53 | 67 | 68 | 68 |
| **III. Impulse-control disorders** | | | | | | | | | | |
| Conduct disorder[a] | – | – | – | – | – | – | – | – | – | – |
| Intermittent explosive disorder with hierarchy | 2.1 | (0.4) | 8 | 9 | 13 | 15 | 23 | 29 | 40 | 44 |
| Any impulse-control disorder | 4.9 | (0.9) | 8 | 10 | 13 | 18 | 23 | 29 | 29 | 29 |
| **IV. Substance disorders** | | | | | | | | | | |
| Alcohol abuse with/without dependence | 5.9 | (0.5) | 18 | 19 | 21 | 26 | 33 | 41 | 46 | 49 |
| Alcohol dependence with abuse | 1.3 | (0.3) | 20 | 21 | 22 | 29 | 33 | 36 | 43 | 49 |
| Drug abuse with/without dependence[a] | – | – | – | – | – | – | – | – | – | – |
| Drug dependence with abuse[a] | – | – | – | – | – | – | – | – | – | – |
| Any substance use disorder | 6.1 | (0.8) | 18 | 19 | 21 | 25 | 31 | 39 | 51 | 53 |
| **V. Any disorder** | | | | | | | | | | |
| Any[c] | 18.0 | (1.5) | 5 | 10 | 17 | 25 | 43 | 56 | 64 | 68 |

[a] Cell size ≤30 cases; too small to estimate.

[b] Posttraumatic stress disorder and substance disorders were assessed only in the Part 2 sample ($n = 1628$).

[c] These summary measures were analyzed in the full Part 2 sample ($n = 1628$).

median AOO of any disorder was 25. Some of the disorders had onsets in a very narrow age range, with interquartile ranges (IQRs) (i.e., the number of years between the 25th and 75th percentiles of the AOO distributions) of only ten years for impulse-control disorders (ages 13–23) and for substance use disorders (ages 21–31), compared to 25 years (ages 28–53) for mood disorders and 26 years (ages 10–36) for anxiety disorders. It was found that no impulse-control disorders started after age 30.

## 4.3. Cohort Effects

The findings in Table 21.1 that lifetime prevalence was higher among younger than older respondents suggests the existence of an increase in reported risk in more recent cohorts. The implications of provisionally assuming that this pattern is genuine rather than due to methodological artifacts (e.g., age-related reporting bias or sample selection bias) can be seen by using dummy variables that define cohorts (ages 18–34,

**Table 21.3.** Cohort as a predictor of lifetime risk of DSM-IV disorders[a]

| Diagnosis | 18–34 | | 35–49 | | 50–64 | | $\chi^2$ |
|---|---|---|---|---|---|---|---|
| | OR | (95% CI) | OR | (95% CI) | OR | (95% CI) | |
| **I. Anxiety disorders** | | | | | | | |
| Panic disorder[b] | – | – | – | – | – | – | – |
| Generalized anxiety disorder with hierarchy | 3.4 | (0.8–15.0) | 1.5 | (0.3–6.5) | 1.0 | (0.3–3.6) | 5.5 |
| Social phobia[b] | – | – | – | – | – | – | – |
| Specific phobia | 0.9 | (0.5–1.8) | 0.7 | (0.4–1.3) | 0.9 | (0.5–1.6) | 2.7 |
| Agoraphobia without panic[b] | – | – | – | – | – | – | – |
| Posttraumatic stress disorder[b,c] | – | – | – | – | – | – | – |
| Separation anxiety disorder/adult separation anxiiety[b] | – | – | – | – | – | – | – |
| Any anxiety disorder[c] | 1.7 | (0.6–4.4) | 1.1 | (0.5–2.5) | 1.6 | (0.7–3.9) | 3.3 |
| **II. Mood disorders** | | | | | | | |
| Major depressive disorder with hierarchy | 22.4* | (9.8–51.0) | 4.4* | (2.3–8.6) | 2.5* | (1.4–4.5) | 76.4** |
| Dysthymia with hierarchy[b] | – | – | – | – | – | – | – |
| Bipolar I–II disorders[b] | – | – | – | – | – | – | – |
| Any mood disorder | 20.8* | (9.4–45.8) | 4.4* | (2.3–8.4) | 2.5* | (1.4–4.4) | 76.5** |
| **III. Impulse-control disorders** | | | | | | | |
| Conduct disorder[b] | – | – | – | – | – | – | – |
| Intermittent explosive disorder with hierarchy | 5.9* | (2.3–15.3) | 2.5* | (1.0–6.2) | 1.0 | (1.0–1.0) | 20.3** |
| Any impulse-control disorder | 0.5 | (0.2–1.3)[b] | 1.0 – | (1.0–1.0)– | 1.0– | (1.0–1.0)– | 1.9[e] |
| **IV. Substance use disorders** | | | | | | | |
| Alcohol abuse with/without dependence | 17.0* | (4.5–63.8) | 8.4* | (2.2–31.9) | 2.9 | (0.7–11.2) | 47.5** |
| Alcohol dependence with abuse | 10.4* | (2.8–38.8) | 5.8* | (1.6–20.8) | 1.0 | (1.0–1.0) | 12.8** |
| Drug abuse with/without dependence[b] | – | – | – | – | – | – | – |
| Drug dependence with abuse[b] | – | – | – | – | – | – | – |
| Any substance disorder | 8.2* | (1.0–67.2) | 4.0 | (0.6–28.2) | 1.5 | (0.2–11.2) | 31.9** |
| **V. Any disorder** | | | | | | | |
| Any[d] | 4.7* | (2.0–10.9) | 2.7* | (1.2–5.8) | 2.0 | (1.0–4.2) | 15.2** |

[a] Based on discrete-time survival models with person-year as the unit of analysis.

[b] Cell size ≤30 cases; too small to estimate.

[c] Estimated in the Part 2 sample ($n = 1628$).

[d] Estimated in the full Part 2 sample.

[e] $\chi^2$ is evaluated with one degree of freedom for any impulse-control disorder comparing respondents aged 18–34 to the omitted control group of respondents aged 35–49.

* Significant difference compared to the 65+-year-olds at the 0.05 level, two-sided test.

** Significant intercohort differences in global test.

35–49, 50–64, and older than 65, corresponding to cohorts born in the years 1967 or later, 1952–1966, 1937–1951, and earlier than 1937, respectively) to predict lifetime disorders using discrete-time survival analysis. Intercohort differences are significant in these models for major depressive disorder, any mood disorder, intermittent explosive disorder, and alcohol-drug use disorders (Table 21.3). In each of these cases, the odds ratios (ORs) are highest in the

**Table 21.4.** Variations in the effects of cohort (age at interview) in predicting lifetime risk of DSM-IV disorders[a]

| Age at interview | Early | | Middle | | Late | |
|---|---|---|---|---|---|---|
| | OR | (95% CI) | OR | (95% CI) | OR | (95% CI) |
| I. Anxiety disorders | | | | | | |
| 18–34 | 1.1 | (0.5–2.9) | 1.9 | (0.7–5.5) | 2.8 | (0.7–11.9) |
| 35–49 | 1.0 | (0.5–2.0) | 0.6 | (0.2–1.9) | 1.7 | (0.5–5.2) |
| 50–64 | 1.3 | (0.5–3.8) | 0.7 | (0.2–2.4) | 1.3 | (0.4–4.1) |
| 65+ | 1.0 | | 1.0 | | 1.0 | |
| | $\chi^2_{11} = 29.6^{***}$ | | $\chi^2_3 = 0.8$ | | $\chi^2_3 = 11.3^{**}$ | | $\chi^2_3 = 3.3$ |
| II. Mood disorders | | | | | | |
| 18–34 | 9.9* | (1.7–58.0) | 5.3* | (2.3–11.3) | 1.0 | (1.0–1.0) |
| 35–49 | 1.3 | (0.2–7.7) | 1.2 | (0.6–2.3) | 5.0* | (1.5–16.1) |
| 50–64 | 1.0 | (0.1–8.4) | 1.0 | | 2.3* | (1.0–5.3) |
| 65+ | 1.0 | | | | 1.0 | |
| | $\chi^2_{12} = 2.7$ | | $\chi^2_3 = 26.8^{**}$ | | $\chi^2_3 = 24.9^{**}$ | | $\chi^2_3 = 7.6^{**}$ |
| III. Substance disorders | | | | | | |
| 18–34 | 3.2 | (1.0–10.9) | 1.9 | (0.2–15.8) | 52.7* | (5.2–534.6) |
| 35–49 | 2.1 | (0.7–6.2) | 0.6 | (0.1–5.2) | 20.1* | (3.0–135.6) |
| 50–64 | 1.0 | | 0.1 | (0.0–1.6) | 6.8 | (0.8–56.4) |
| 65+ | – | | 1.0 | | 1.0 | |
| | $\chi^2_{11} = 12.6^{***}$ | | $\chi^2_3 = 3.8$ | | $\chi^2_3 = 12.7^{**}$ | | $\chi^2_3 = 30.0^{**}$ |

*Age of onset* header spans Early, Middle, Late columns.

[a] Based on discrete-time survival models with person-year as the unit of analysis. Total-sample models evaluated the significance of interactions between cohort and age of onset. This was not done for impulse-control disorders because the vast majority of such disorders have onsets in a very narrow time window. Cohort by age of onset interactions were significant in predicting each of the three outcomes. On the basis of these results, subsample models were estimated for the effects of cohort in each of the first three stages of life. All analyses were carried out in the full Part 2 sample. In the analysis of anxiety disorders was coded as absent among respondents who were not assessed for that disorder.

* Significant difference compared with the before-1936 cohorts (age $\geq$65 years) at the 0.05 level, two-sided test in the subsample of person-years defined by the column headings.

** Significant intercohort differences in the global test in the subsample of person-years.

*** Significant interaction between cohort and age of onset in the lives of respondents in the total sample.

youngest cohorts and monotonically decrease in later cohorts. The most dramatic of these effects is an OR of 20.8 in the youngest cohort for mood disorder, which means that the relative odds of having a lifetime history of mood disorder adjusting for years at risk is estimated to be 20.8 times as great among respondents in the age range 18–34 as among those in the age range of 65 and older. The OR of the youngest cohorts in predicting any disorder is considerably lower (4.7), though still substantial, owing to risk not changing for most anxiety disorders and changing less dramatically for impulse-control disorders and substance use disorders than for mood disorders.

The cohort model was elaborated to evaluate whether intercohort differences decreased significantly with increasing age, a pattern that might be expected either if lifetime risk was actually constant across cohorts, but it appeared to vary with cohort because onsets occurred earlier in more recent cohorts than in earlier cohorts (due to either secular changes in environmental triggers or age-related differences in AOO recall accuracy) or if differential mortality had an increasingly severe effect on sample selection bias with increasing age. Differences were examined separately for first onsets in the age ranges early, middle, and late on the basis of the AOO distribution summarized in Table 21.2. No evidence of decreasing cohort effects with increasing age was found for anxiety, mood disorder, or substance disorders (Table 21.4).

## 4.4. Sociodemographic Predictors

Controlling for cohort, survival analysis showed that female respondents had significantly higher lifetime risk of anxiety disorders than did their male counterparts among the 35–49 and 65 and older age groups, that male respondents had significantly higher lifetime risk of impulse-control disorders than did female respondents among the 18–34 age group, that male respondents had a significantly higher lifetime risk of substance use disorders among 18–34 and 35–49 age groups (in the same definition), and that the female–male difference was insignificant in predicting mood disorders (Table 21.5). Education was found to be significantly and inversely related to risk of anxiety disorders, but not for any of the other classes of disorders. Analysis of interactions showed that the trend of increased prevalence of substance use disorders in recent cohorts was significantly more pronounced among men than women [$\chi^2(3) = 29.6$, $p < 0.001$], but was more pronounced among women than men for prevalence of anxiety disorders [$\chi^2(3) = 12.8$, $p = 0.005$], whereas cohort effects were the same among men and women for other disorders. None of the cohort effects differed consistently across subgroups defined by level of education except for impulse-control disorders (Table 21.5).

## 4.5. 12-month Prevalence and Severity

The disorders with highest estimated 12-month prevalence are major depressive disorder (1.8%), specific phobia (1.6%), and intermittent explosive disorder (1.2%). Regarding class of disorder, impulse-control disorders are estimated to be the most prevalent (3.1%), followed by anxiety disorders (2.9%), mood disorders (1.9%), and substance use disorders (1.6%). The 12-month prevalence estimate of any disorder is 6.8% in the total sample (Table 21.6).

Among all the respondents with 12-month disorders, 14.2% are classified as serious, 33.3% as moderate, and 52.3% as mild. The distribution of severity across classes of disorder is different from the distribution of prevalence, with mood disorders having the highest percentage of cases classified as serious (21.4%) and impulse-control disorders the lowest (5.6%). Individual disorders within each class with the highest percentage of seriousness are bipolar I and II disorders (93.2%) among the mood disorders, alcohol dependence (54.6%) among the substance disorders, social phobia (24%) among the anxiety disorders, and intermittent explosive disorder (4.9%) among the impulse-control disorders (Table 21.6).

## 4.6. Association of Severity with Treatment Types

The CIDI assessed 12-month treatment by asking respondents from a long list of professionals if they ever had seen any of them either on an outpatient basis or as an in-patient for problems with their emotions, nerves, mental health, or use of substances. The present analysis grouped these professionals into four major groups: general medical (e.g., general practitioners), mental health (e.g., psychiatrists), health care (e.g., general practitioners and psychiatrists combined), and non–health care (e.g., spiritualists). Respondents with different levels of severity were compared on their treatment-seeking behavior from the four major groups of professionals. As results were very similar in the two cites, only summary results for both cities combined are reported here.

Among all respondents with at least one 12-month disorder, only 3.4% sought treatment within 12 months of the interview. Cases classified as severe or moderate had a higher proportion in seeking treatment (19.8%) than did those with no disorder (2.9%) or mild disorder (1.7%). The most common type of treatment for severe/moderate cases and noncases was general medical treatment. Among the mild cases, general medical and mental health treatment were equally common (Table 21.7).

**Table 21.5.** Variation across cohorts in the association of sex and education with first age of onset of DSM-IV disorders

| Predictors | 18–34 OR | (95% CI) | 35–49 OR | (95% CI) | 50–64 OR | (95% CI) | 65+ OR | (95% CI) | Total OR | (95% CI) | Interaction between age group and education/sex |
|---|---|---|---|---|---|---|---|---|---|---|---|
| **I. Anxiety disorder** | | | | | | | | | | | |
| i. Education[d] | | | | | | | | | | | |
| Student | 4.1 | (1.0–16.6) | 21.3 | (2.9–155.5) | 10.7* | (1.1–108.8) | 0.5 | (1.1–108.8) | 6.1* | (1.8–20.2) | |
| Low | 17.5* | (1.5–210.8) | 21.8 | (1.3–376.0*) | 35.8* | (2.8–464.9) | 1.0 | (1.0–1.0) | 16.6* | (4.3–64.1) | |
| Low/middle | 1.9 | (0.3–11.2) | 5.7 | (0.7–49.4) | 9.1 | (0.7–127.5) | | | 3.1 | (0.8–11.5) | $\chi^2_8 = 12.6$ |
| Middle | 3.8 | (0.8–17.4) | 9.763 | (0.9–105.9) | 1.0 | (1.0–1.0) | | | 4.6* | (1.2–17.5) | |
| High | 1.0 | (1.0–1.0) | 1.0 | (1.0–1.0) | – | | | | 1.0 | – | |
| $\chi^2$ | | 6.93 | | 21.2* | | 8.2* | | 1.1 | | 18.7* | |
| ii. Sex | | | | | | | | | | | |
| Female | 0.8 | (0.3–1.9) | 3.4* | (1.4–8.1) | 0.9 | (0.2–3.2) | 8.9 | (1.9–41.1) | 1.3 | (0.7–2.6) | |
| Male | 1.0 | (1.0–1.0) | 1.0 | (1.0–1.0) | 1.0 | (1.0–1.0) | 1.0 | (1.0–1.0) | 1.0 | (1.0–1.0) | $\chi^2_3 = 12.8**$ |
| $\chi^2$ | | 0.3 | | 8.1 | | 0.6 | | 8.2* | | 0.7 | |
| **II. Mood disorder** | | | | | | | | | | | |
| i. Education[d] | | | | | | | | | | | |
| Student | 1.5 | (0.5–4.3) | 0.2 | (0.0–1.1) | 1.8 | (0.1–51.6) | | | 1.1 | (0.4–3.0) | |
| Low | | | 1.2 | (0.1–11.6) | | | 0.7 | (0.0–14.6) | 0.5 | (0.1–2.7) | |
| Low/middle | 1.5 | (0.5–4.1) | 0.5 | (0.1–2.2) | 0.7 | (0.1–7.9) | 1.0 | (1.0–1.0) | 1.1 | (0.5–2.5) | $\chi^2_7 = 3.7$ |
| Middle | 1.2 | (0.5–3.1) | 0.5 | (0.1–1.7) | 1.8 | (0.3–10.0) | | | 1.1 | (0.5–2.3) | |
| High | 1.0 | (1.0–1.0) | 1.0 | (1.0–1.0) | 1.0 | (1.0–1.0) | 1.0 | (1.0–1.0) | 1.0 | (1.0–1.0) | |
| $\chi^2$ | | 0.9 | | 4.3 | | 1.5 | | 0.04 | | 1.2 | |
| ii. Sex | | | | | | | | | | | |
| Female | 0.9 | (0.4–2.1) | 0.6 | (0.2–1.6) | 2.3 | (0.3–17.7) | 1.0 | (1.0–1.0) | 0.9 | (0.5–1.8) | |
| Male | 1.0 | (1.0–1.0) | 1.0 | (1.0–1.0) | 1.0 | (1.0–1.0) | 1.0 | (1.0–1.0) | 1.0 | – | $\chi^2_2 = 1.4$ |
| $\chi^2$ | | 0.02 | | | | | | | | 0.9 | |
| **III. Impulse-control disorders** | | | | | | | | | | | |
| i. Education[d] | | | | | | | | | | | |
| Student | 4.5 | (0.7–30.8) | 1.0* | (0.0–0.6) | | | | | 1.7 | (0.3–9.3) | |
| Low | | | 14.8* | (1.4–154.0) | | | | | 1.0 | (0.0–29.7) | |
| Low/middle | 2.5 | (0.4–17.3) | 0.4 | (0.0–3.2) | | | | | 0.9 | (0.1–5.5) | $\chi^2_3 = 21.9**$ |
| Middle | 1.0 | (1.2–5.6) | 1.0 | (0.0–28.1) | | | | | 1.2 | (0.1–17.8) | |
| High | 1.0 | (1.0–1.0) | 1.0 | (1.0–1.0) | | | | | 1.0 | (1.0–1.0) | |
| $\chi^2$ | | 4.8 | | 31.7* | | | | | | 1.2 | |
| ii. Sex | | | | | | | | | | | |
| Female | 0.2* | (0.1–0.9) | 0.3 | (0.0–6.2) | | | | | 0.3 | (0.0–1.5) | |
| Male | 1.0 | (1.0–1.0) | 1.0 | (1.0–1.0) | | | – | | 1.0 | (1.0–1.0) | $\chi^2_1 = 0.03$ |
| $\chi^2$ | | 4.9* | | 0.6 | | | | | | 2.4 | |
| **IV. Substance disorders** | | | | | | | | | | | |
| i. Education[d] | | | | | | | | | | | |
| Student | 3.7 | (0.9–15.6) | 0.2* | (0.0–0.9) | | | | | 1.2 | (0.4–4.4) | |
| Low | | | 0.7 | (0.1–5.3) | 0.8 | (0.0–33.2) | | | 2.2 | (0.7–7.4) | |
| Low/middle | 2.9 | (0.7–11.8) | 0.5 | (0.1–1.9) | 2.0 | (0.2–23.4) | | | 1.5 | (0.5–4.9) | $\chi^2_5 = 9.8$ |
| Middle | 2.6 | (0.6–11.3) | 0.8 | (0.2–2.7) | 1.0 | (1.0–1.0) | | | 1.6 | (0.6–4.5) | |
| High | 1.0 | (1.0–1.0) | 1.0 | (1.0–1.0) | | | | | 1.0 | (1.0–1.0) | |
| $\chi^2$ | | 4.8 | | 10.2* | | 4.0* | | | | 2.1 | |
| ii. Sex | | | | | | | | | | | |
| Female | 0.0* | (0.0–0.1) | 0.1* | (0.0–0.4) | 0.5 | (0.1–2.1) | | | 0.1* | (0.0–0.2) | |
| Male | 1.0 | (1.0–1.0) | 1.0 | (1.0–1.0) | 1.0 | (1.0–1.0) | 1.0 | (1.0–1.0) | 1.0 | (1.0–1.0) | $\chi^2_3 = 29.6**$ |
| $\chi^2$ | | 21.0* | | 11.6* | | 1.0 | | | | 37.3* | |

**Table 21.6.** 12-month prevalence and severity of DSM-IV disorders

| Diagnosis | 12-month % | (se) | Serious % | (se) | Moderate % | (se) | Mild % | (se) |
|---|---|---|---|---|---|---|---|---|
| **Anxiety disorder** | | | | | | | | |
| Panic disorder[a] | 0.2 | (0.1) | 7.2 | (7.3) | 73.9 | (14.8) | 18.9 | (13.1) |
| Generalized anxiety disorder[a] | 0.5 | (0.1) | 3.7 | (2.6) | 60.7 | (13.7) | 35.5 | (12.9) |
| Specific phobia[a] | 1.6 | (0.2) | 17.7 | (10.4) | 42.2 | (13.9) | 40.0 | (12.3) |
| Social phobia[a] | 0.3 | (0.1) | 24.0 | (14.4) | 44.4 | (20.7) | 31.7 | (16.2) |
| Agoraphobia without panic[a] | 0.0 | (0.0) | – | – | – | – | – | – |
| Posttraumatic stress disorder[b] | 0.2 | (0.1) | 0.0 | (0.0) | 90.5 | (7.8) | 9.5 | (7.8) |
| Adult sparation anxiety[b] | 0.1 | (0.1) | 25.2 | (19.2) | 68.1 | (20.2) | 6.7 | (7.0) |
| Any anxiety disorder[c] | 2.9 | (0.5) | 14.5 | (7.0) | 46.1 | (10.1) | 39.4 | (9.2) |
| **Mood disorder** | | | | | | | | |
| Major depressive disorder[a] | 1.8 | (0.3) | 16.5 | (5.6) | 51.1 | (7.7) | 32.4 | (7.8) |
| Dysthymia[a] | 0.1 | (0.0) | 46.4 | (18.9) | 53.6 | (18.9) | 0.0 | (0.0) |
| Bipolar I–II/subthreshold[a] | 0.1 | (0.0) | 93.2 | (7.7) | 0.0 | (0.0) | 0.0 | (0.0) |
| Any mood disorder[a] | 1.9 | (0.3) | 21.4 | (6.4) | 48.4 | (7.6) | 29.8 | (7.2) |
| **Impulse disorder** | | | | | | | | |
| Oppositional-defiant disorder[c] | – | – | – | – | – | – | – | – |
| Conduct disorder[c] | 0.1 | (0.1) | 0.0 | (0.0) | 0.0 | (0.0) | 100.0 | (0.0) |
| Attention deficit disorder[c] | – | – | – | – | – | – | – | – |
| Intermittent explosive disorder[a] | 1.2 | (0.2) | 4.9 | (2.7) | 25.7 | (15.6) | 69.4 | (16.5) |
| Any impulse-control disorder[c] | 3.1 | (0.7) | 5.6 | (3.0) | 24.3 | (16.9) | 70.2 | (18.0) |
| **Substance disorder** | | | | | | | | |
| Alcohol abuse[a] | 1.3 | (0.2) | 18.7 | (8.4) | 15.4 | (5.8) | 65.9 | (9.3) |
| Alcohol dependence[a] | 0.6 | (0.2) | 54.6 | (13.7) | 45.4 | (13.7) | 0.0 | (0.0) |
| Drug abuse[b] | 0.1 | (0.0) | 10.6 | (12.0) | 15.9 | (17.2) | 73.4 | (22.5) |
| Drug dependence[b] | 0.0 | (0.0) | – | – | – | – | – | – |
| Any substance use disorder[b] | 1.6 | (0.4) | 21.3 | (7.6) | 18.1 | (5.6) | 60.6 | (9.0) |
| **Any disorder** | | | | | | | | |
| Any[b] | 6.8 | (0.9) | 14.2 | (3.8) | 33.3 | (4.9) | 52.3 | (4.4) |
| **Total sample** | | | | | | | | |
| Total sample[b] | – | – | 1.0 | (0.2) | 2.3 | (0.5) | 3.7 | (0.6) |

*Note:* Severity calculated using Part 2 weights.
[a] Using Part 1 respondents ($n = 5201$); prevalence calculated using Part 1 weights.
[b] Using Part 2 respondents ($n = 1628$); prevalence calculated using Part 2 weights.
[c] Part 2 sample (age $\leq 39$); prevalence and severity calculated using Part 2 weights for ages $\leq 39$.

## 4.7. Sociodemographic Predictors of Disorders

Analysis documented that the OR of any 12-month CIDI disorder is significantly related to age, sex, and marital status. Young age is a risk factor and being female is a protective factor. The OR of severity is significantly related to sex and marital status. Being female and never married are risk factors of severity (Table 21.8). Regarding different classes of disorders, low average income and being separated, widowed, or divorced are risk factors for mood disorders. Being never married and having completed junior high school are protective factors for impulse-control disorders. Although young age is a risk factor, female, average income, and never having been married are protective factors for substance use disorders.

**Table 21.7.** Severity by treatment

| Treatment | Severe or moderate | | Mild | | Any | | None | |
|---|---|---|---|---|---|---|---|---|
| | % | (se) | % | (se) | % | (se) | % | (se) |
| General medical | 15.2 | (7.6) | 0.0 | (0.0) | 2.3 | (0.5) | 2.0 | (0.5) |
| Mental health | 4.6 | (2.4) | 1.7 | (1.1) | 0.6 | (0.2) | 0.4 | (0.2) |
| Health care | 18.6 | (7.9) | 1.7 | (1.1) | 2.9 | (0.6) | 2.4 | (0.5) |
| Non–health care[a] | 9.1 | (7.0) | 0.0 | (0.0) | 1.0 | (0.3) | 0.7 | (0.2) |
| Any treatment | 19.8 | (8.0) | 1.7 | (1.1) | 3.4 | (0.6) | 2.9 | (0.6) |
| No treatment | 80.2 | (8.0) | 98.3 | (1.1) | 96.6 | (0.6) | 97.1 | (0.6) |
| $\chi^{2b}$ | 246.9* | | 1.2 | | 0.2 | | – | |

[a] Non–health care includes human services and CAM.
[b] Versus no-disorder group.
* $p < 0.01$.

## 4.8. Sociodemographic Predictors of Treatment

Respondents with severe and moderate disorders were significantly more likely to receive treatment than were those with mild disorders in both cities. Analysis documented that the OR of receiving treatment is significantly related to age, family income, and severity of disorders, with lower income, higher age, and severe or moderate severity being associated with higher treatment rates (Table 21.9). Sex, education, and marital status were not significantly related to treatment.

## 4.9. Lifetime Treatment: Duration of Delays in Initial Treatment Contact

Survival curves were used to project the proportion of cases that would eventually make treatment contact for each disorder. The survival curves were also used to estimate the proportion of cases that made treatment contact in the year of first onset of the disorder and the median delay among people who eventually made treatment contact after the year of first onset (Table 21.10). The proportion of cases that made treatment contact in the year of disorder onset ranges from 2.8% for substance disorders to 6.0% for mood disorders, and the proportion of cases that made treatment contact by 50 years ranges from 25.7% for substance disorders to 44.7% for anxiety disorders. Median years of delay also differ greatly

across disorders, from 1 year for mood disorders to 21 years for anxiety disorders.

## 4.10. Predictors of Failure and Delay in Initial Treatment Contact

Table 21.11 shows the predictors of failure to ever make a treatment contact among respondents with a given lifetime disorder. The most consistent predictors of failure to make a treatment contact are cohort and AOO. Cohort is significantly related to lifetime treatment contact in any anxiety disorders, alcohol abuse and alcohol abuse with dependence (0.05 level, two-sided tests), with an increasing number of treatment contacts in recent cohorts. AOO is significantly related to treatment contact in any anxiety disorders, with the number of treatment contacts collinearly relating to age at onset. There is no statistical difference between women and men in predicting initial treatment contact.

## 4.11. 12-month Treatment: Probability of 12-month Service Use

Some 3.4% of survey respondents used services to treat emotional problems in the year before the interview, including 13.2% of those with one or more 12-month DSM-IV/CIDI disorders and 2.9% of those without any such disorder (Table 21.12). The proportion of cases in health-care treatment was highest for those with any

**Table 21.8.** Sociodemographic predictors of CIDI/DSM-IV 12-month prevalence, diagnosis, and severity of diagnosis[a]

| Sociodemographic predictors | Any disorder | | Severity/disorder | | Mood | | Anxiety | | Impulse control | | Substance | |
|---|---|---|---|---|---|---|---|---|---|---|---|---|
| | OR | (95% CI) | OR | (95% CI) | OR | (95% CI) | OR | (95% CI) | OR | (95% CI) | OR | (95% CI) |
| **I. Sex** | | | | | | | | | | | | |
| Male | 1.0 | – | 1.0 | – | 1.0 | – | 1.0 | – | 1.0 | – | 1.0 | – |
| Female | 0.5 | (0.3–0.8) | 3.0 | (1.2–7.6) | 0.8 | (0.4–1.5) | 1.3 | (0.6–2.9) | 0.2 | (0.0–1.6) | 0.1 | (0.0–0.2) |
| $\chi^2_1$ | 6.9* | | 5.8* | | 0.6 | | 0.6 | | 2.4 | | 21.5* | |
| **II. Age** | | | | | | | | | | | | |
| 18–34 | 3.1 | (1.4–7.1) | 0.8 | (0.3–2.3) | 1.9 | (0.8–4.2) | 0.7 | (0.2–2.3) | 0.9 | (0.3–2.8) | 17.1 | (3.0–97.5) |
| 35–49 | 1.7 | (0.9–3.2) | 1.8 | (0.3–9.4) | 0.9 | (0.4–1.8) | 0.7 | (0.3–1.7) | 1.0 | | 6.5 | (1.6–25.7) |
| 50–64 | | | | | | | | | | | | |
| 65+ | 1.0 | – | 1.0 | – | 1.0 | – | 1.0 | – | 1.0 | – | 1.0 | – |
| $\chi^2_3$ | 7.7* | | 1.2 | | 3.7 | | 0.5 | | 0.0 | | 11.1 | |
| **III. Family income[b]** | | | | | | | | | | | | |
| Low | 1.4 | (0.6–3.2) | 0.5 | (0.1–2.4) | 1.8 | (0.8–4.2) | 3.3 | (1.3–8.7) | 1.4 | (0.2–10.8) | 0.5 | (0.2–1.6) |
| Low average | 1.3 | (0.7–2.5) | 1.9 | (0.6–5.9) | 2.7 | (1.2–6.1) | 2.2 | (0.9–5.4) | 5.8 | (1.1–29.7) | 0.1 | (0.0–1.5) |
| High average | 0.8 | (0.4–1.7) | 1.4 | (0.4–4.1) | 1.0 | (0.4–2.2) | 1.8 | (0.8–4.1) | 1.4 | (0.2–8.8) | 0.2 | (0.1–0.6) |
| High | 1.0 | – | 1.0 | – | 1.0 | – | 1.0 | – | 1.0 | – | 1.0 | – |
| $\chi^2_3$ | 5.6 | | 1.8 | | 8.7* | | 7.3 | | 5.6 | | 17.3* | |
| **IV. Marital status** | | | | | | | | | | | | |
| Married/cohabiting | 1.0 | – | 1.0 | – | 1.0 | – | 1.0 | – | 1.0 | – | 1.0 | – |
| Separate/widowed/divorced | 1.2 | (0.6–2.4) | 2.3 | (0.6–8.9) | 2.9 | (1.1–7.7) | 0.8 | (0.3–2.2) | 1.2 | (0.2–8.8) | 0.6 | (0.1–3.6) |
| Never married | 0.3 | (0.2–0.8) | 6.0 | (1.2–30.5) | 0.4 | (0.1–1.3) | 1.5 | (0.5–4.6) | 0.1 | (0.0–0.4) | 0.2 | (0.1–0.5) |
| $\chi^2_2$ | 7.3* | | 6.2* | | 8.3* | | 0.8 | | 10.3* | | 11.4* | |
| **IV. Education** | | | | | | | | | | | | |
| None and primary | 2.1 | (0.7–6.5) | 1.1 | (0.3–4.9) | 1.7 | (0.5–6.1) | 3.2 | (0.8–13.8) | 3.1 | (0.1–124.1) | 0.6 | (0.1–5.4) |
| Junior high school | 1.0 | (0.5–2.0) | 1.6 | (0.5–5.5) | 1.5 | (0.6–3.3) | 1.5 | (0.5–4.5) | 0.1 | (0.0–0.7) | 1.6 | (0.5–5.3) |
| Senior high school | 1.3 | (0.6–2.8) | 0.8 | (0.3–1.9) | 1.5 | (0.8–3.1) | 1.4 | (0.5–4.4) | 1.2 | (0.3–5.3) | 1.0 | (0.3–3.2) |
| College and beyond | 1.0 | – | 1.0 | – | 1.0 | – | 1.0 | – | 1.0 | – | 1.0 | – |
| $\chi^2_3$ | 2.6 | | 2.1 | | 1.9 | | 2.8 | | 8.5* | | 2.0 | |

[a] Using Part 2 respondents ($n = 1628$).

[b] Family income is defined in relation to the official federal poverty line for families of the size and composition of the respondent's family (Proctor and Dalaker 2002). Low income is defined as less than or equal to 1.5 times the poverty line, low-average as 1.5+ to 3 times the poverty line, high-average as 3+ to 6 times the poverty line, and high as greater than 6 times the poverty line.

* Significant at the 0.05 level, two-sided test.

**Table 21.9.** Sociodemographic predictors of 12-month treatment[a]

| Sociodemographic predictors | Treatment[b] | |
|---|---|---|
| | OR | (95% CI) |
| **I. Sex** | | |
| Male | 1.0 | – |
| Female | 1.3 | (0.5–3.0) |
| $\chi_1^2$ | 0.3 | |
| **II. Age** | | |
| 18–34 | 0.1 | (0.0–0.3) |
| 35–49 | 0.5 | (0.2–1.1) |
| 50–64 | | |
| 65+ | 1.0 | – |
| $\chi_3^2$ | 20.4* | |
| **III. Family income[b]** | | |
| Low | 9.3 | (2.3–38.0) |
| Low-average | 2.7 | (0.7–9.9) |
| High-average | 1.6 | (0.6–4.2) |
| High | 1.0 | – |
| $\chi_3^2$ | 14.1* | |
| **IV. Marital status** | | |
| Married/cohabiting | 1.0 | – |
| Separate/widowed/divorced | 0.7 | (0.1–3.0) |
| Never married | 1.2 | (0.4–4.0) |
| $\chi_2^2$ | 0.5 | |
| **IV. Education** | | |
| None and primary | 0.8 | (0.2–3.5) |
| Junior high school | 0.6 | (0.2–2.1) |
| Senior high school | 0.9 | (0.2–3.5) |
| College and beyond | 1.0 | – |
| $\chi_3^2$ | 0.8 | |

[a] Using Part 2 respondents ($n = 1628$).
[b] Controlling for disorder severity.
* Significant at the 0.05 level, two-sided test.

anxiety disorder (17.2%) and lowest for those with any substance disorder (8.6%). The proportion of cases with any mood disorder that were in treatment was not calculated because the unweighted number of cases with mood disorders was less than 30. Among all the types of treatment, most treatments occurred in the HC sectors (2.9% of respondents, representing 77.0% of those in treatments); within the HC sectors, the GM sector (2.3% of respondents, representing 55.4% of those in treatments) was the greatest.

### 4.12. Number of Visits

The median number of 12-month visits (Table 21.13) among those receiving any treatment for emotional problems was 2.3. Among all types of treatment, the median number among those receiving HC treatment (2.2) was the highest. Within the HC sectors, the median number for GM was 2.1. The mean numbers of visits were slightly higher than the median. For example, the median among patients receiving any treatment was 2.3, compared to the mean of 5.7. The means of visit for HC and GM sectors were 5.4 and 4.4, respectively, both of which were lower than the median. The greater magnitude of means than medians implies that comparatively few patients receive a disproportionately high share of all visits. The patients who used fewer services account for the majority of the respondents, whereas the patients who used more services account for the minority of the respondents. The median and the mean numbers of visits during the previous year for each disorder were not calculated because the unweighted number of cases with each disorder was less than 30.

### 4.13. Minimally Adequate Treatment

Of the treated patients with disorders, only 43.3% were classified as receiving at least minimally adequate treatment. Probabilities of treatment being at least minimally adequate for the HC and GM sectors were 40.3% and 32.9%, respectively. The percentage of patients receiving adequate treatment among people seeing professionals was 24.1%, which included 25.4% for the HC sector and 19.3% for the GM sector. The percentages of treatment that were at least minimally adequate or adequate for each disorder were not calculated because the unweighted number of cases with each disorder was less than 30.

### 4.14. Sociodemographic Predictors of Treatment

After controlling for the presence of different 12-month mental disorders, the OR of receiving any 12-month mental health treatment is significantly related to being female (Table 21.14). The

**Table 21.10.** Proportional treatment contact in the year of disorder onset and median duration of delay among cases that subsequently made treatment contact

| Diagnosis | % making treatment contact in year of onset | % making treatment contact by 50 years | Median duration of delay (years) | n |
|---|---|---|---|---|
| **I. Anxiety disorders** | | | | |
| Panic disorder | _[a] | _[a] | _[a] | _[a] |
| Generalized anxiety disorder | 7.9 | 28.5 | 20 | 59 |
| Specific phobia | 3.0 | 45.1 | 21 | 149 |
| Social phobia | _[a] | _[a] | _[a] | _[a] |
| Any anxiety disorders | 4.2 | 44.7 | 21 | 221 |
| **II. Mood disorders** | | | | |
| Major depressive episode | 5.6 | 6.9 | 1 | 180 |
| Dysthymia | _[a] | _[a] | _[a] | _[a] |
| Bipolar disorder (broad) | _[a] | _[a] | _[a] | _[a] |
| Any mood disorders | 6.0 | 7.9 | 1 | 184 |
| **III. Substance disorders** | | | | |
| Alcohol abuse | 1.9 | 20.4 | 17 | 221 |
| Alcohol abuse with dependence | 9.5 | 42.2 | 17 | 41 |
| Drug abuse[b] | _[a] | _[a] | _[a] | _[a] |
| Drug abuse with dependence[b] | _[a] | _[a] | _[a] | _[a] |
| Any substance disorders[b] | 2.8 | 25.7 | 17 | 128 |

[a] Disorder was omitted as a result of insufficient $n < 30$, but it will be included as one of the disorders in "Any" category.

[b] Assessed in the Part 2 sample ($n = 1628$).

difference between age groups, educational levels, income, and marital status, in comparison, are insignificant in predicting treatment.

## 5. DISCUSSION

Psychiatric epidemiological surveys in China have routinely used psychiatric doctors as interviewers during the past 25 years (12 collaborating units of epidemiological survey on mental disorders 1986a; Zhang et al. 1998). Although clinicians may make more valid diagnoses, there is a potential drawback of such an approach to community-based epidemiological surveys. This is because Chinese psychiatrists are accustomed to dealing almost entirely with a clinical population with severe mental disorders. As such, they may be inclined to discount less severe depressive and anxiety disorders during diagnostic assessments.

The present study is the first Chinese community survey to use laypeople to make fully structured psychiatric diagnoses. Results show that, when compared to similar Western surveys that use basically the same methodology, quite low prevalence estimates are obtained. One of the possible explanations is that people with a history of mental illness might have been less willing than others to participate in the survey, leading to reduced estimated prevalence. Another possibility is that stigma might have led survey respondents with disorders to deny symptoms of a mental disorder to interviewers whom they did not know to a far greater extent than did patients in the clinical reappraisal study who knew that the clinical interviewers were aware of their mental disorders. Yet another possibility is that the CIDI failed because it is insensitive to the symptom manifestations of people with mental disorders in the Chinese population. Only when we have

**Table 21.11.** Sociodemographic predictors of lifetime treatment contact for specific DSM-IV/CIDI disorders

| Diagnosis | Sex | | | Cohort (age at interview) | | | | | | | Age of onset | | | | | | |
|---|---|---|---|---|---|---|---|---|---|---|---|---|---|---|---|---|---|
| | Female | | | Age 18-34 | | Age 35-49 | | Age 50-64 | | | Early | | Early-average | | Late-average | | |
| | OR | (95% CI) | $\chi^2_1$ | OR | (95% CI) | OR | (95% CI) | OR | (95% CI) | $\chi^2_{1-3}$ | OR | (95% CI) | OR | (95% CI) | OR | (95% CI) | $\chi^2_{1-3}$ |
| **I. Anxiety disorders** | | | | | | | | | | | | | | | | | |
| Panic disorder | —[a] | —[a] | —[a] | —[a] | —[a] | —[a] | —[a] | —[a] | —[a] | —[a] | —[a] | —[a] | —[a] | —[a] | —[a] | —[a] | —[a] |
| Generalized anxiety disorder | 9.0 | (0.7–117.4) | 3.0 | 0.6 | (0.0–27.3) | 1.9 | (0.1–47.6) | 1.1 | (0.0–32.5) | 0.8 | 0.1* | (0.0–0.8) | 0.9 | (0.1–11.4) | 0.1 | (0.0–1.6) | 9.1* |
| Specific phobia | 0.9 | (0.4–2.4) | 0.0 | 4.8* | (1.1–21.7) | 3.0 | (0.8–11.7) | 1.3 | (0.4–4.1) | 6.2 | 0.2* | (0.0–0.5) | 0.2* | (0.0–0.6) | 0.1* | (0.0–0.6) | 14.0* |
| Social phobia | —[a] | —[a] | —[a] | —[a] | —[a] | —[a] | —[a] | —[a] | —[a] | —[a] | —[a] | —[a] | —[a] | —[a] | —[a] | —[a] | —[a] |
| Any anxiety disorders | 1.0 | (0.4–2.3) | 0.0 | 4.6* | (1.4–15.6) | 2.1 | (0.9–5.0) | 1.0 | — | 6.7* | 0.3* | (0.1–0.9) | 0.2* | (0.0–1.0) | 0.7 | (0.2–2.4) | 8.3* |
| **II. Mood disorders** | | | | | | | | | | | | | | | | | |
| Major depressive episode | 0.6 | (0.1–3.1) | 0.5 | 0.3 | (0.1–1.1) | 0.3 | (0.1–1.1) | 1.0 | — | 3.5 | 0.9 | (0.1–6.2) | 0.1* | (0.0–1.0) | 0.6 | (0.2–2.4) | 4.8 |
| Dysthymia | —[a] | —[a] | —[a] | —[a] | —[a] | —[a] | —[a] | —[a] | —[a] | —[a] | —[a] | —[a] | —[a] | —[a] | —[a] | —[a] | —[a] |
| Bipolar disorder (broad) | —[a] | —[a] | —[a] | —[a] | —[a] | —[a] | —[a] | —[a] | —[a] | —[a] | —[a] | —[a] | —[a] | —[a] | —[a] | —[a] | —[a] |
| Any mood disorders | 0.8 | (0.2–3.6) | 0.1 | 0.7 | (0.2–2.9) | 0.4 | (0.1–1.3) | 1.0 | — | 2.4 | 0.5 | (0.1–3.3) | 0.4 | (0.1–1.7) | 0.5 | (0.1–1.9) | 2.3 |
| **III. Substance disorders** | | | | | | | | | | | | | | | | | |
| Alcohol abuse | —[b] | —[b] | —[b] | 5.5* | (1.1–26.5) | 1.0 | — | 1.0 | — | 4.7* | 0.6 | (0.2–1.8) | 0.6 | (0.2–1.8) | 0.6 | (0.2–1.8) | 0.9 |
| Alcohol abuse with dependence | —[b] | —[b] | —[b] | 21.4* | (2.0–233.5) | 1.0 | — | 1.0 | — | 6.6* | 0.2 | (0.0–4.7) | 0.2 | (0.0–4.7) | 1.1 | (0.2–7.8) | 1.7 |
| Drug abuse[c] | —[a] | —[a] | —[a] | —[a] | —[a] | —[a] | —[a] | —[a] | —[a] | —[a] | —[a] | —[a] | —[a] | —[a] | —[a] | —[a] | —[a] |
| Drug abuse with dependence[c] | —[a] | —[a] | —[a] | —[a] | —[a] | —[a] | —[a] | —[a] | —[a] | —[a] | —[a] | —[a] | —[a] | —[a] | —[a] | —[a] | —[a] |
| Any substance disorders[c] | 0.4 | (0.0–6.4) | 0.5 | 1.8 | (0.2–20.1) | 0.5 | (0.1–2.0) | 1.0 | — | 3.0 | 0.5 | (0.1–3.1) | 0.5 | (0.1–3.1) | 0.8 | (0.1–5.9) | 0.6 |

[a] Disorder was omitted as a result of insufficient lifetime cases ($n < 30$), but it will be included as one of the disorders in "Any" category.

[b] Sex was used as a control variable in the model except for alcohol abuse and alcohol abuse with dependence (because of insufficient cases for female).

[c] Assessed in the Part 2 sample ($n = 1628$).

* Significant at the 0.05 level, two-sided test.

**Table 21.12.** Prevalence of 12-month mental health service use in separate service sectors by 12-month DSM-IV/CIDI disorder

| | Health care | | | | | | | Non–health care | | | | | | Any service use | | n[a] |
|---|---|---|---|---|---|---|---|---|---|---|---|---|---|---|---|---|
| | Mental health specialty | | | General medical[c] | Any | | Human services[d] | | CAM[e] | | Any | | | | | |
| | Psychiatrist | | Nonpsychiatrist[b] | Any | | | | | | | | | | | | | |
| Diagnosis | % | (se) | % | % | (se) | % | (se) | % | (se) | % | (se) | % | (se) | % | (se) | % | (se) | n[a] |
| **I. Anxiety disorders** | | | | | | | | | | | | | | | | | | |
| Generalized anxiety disorder[f] | 0 | (0) | 0 | 0 | (0) | 9.3 | (6.2) | 9.3 | (6.2) | 0 | (0) | 7.5 | (5.8) | 7.5 | (5.8) | 10.8 | (6.3) | 33 |
| Panic disorder[f] | – | | – | – | | – | | – | | – | | – | | – | | – | | 11 |
| Agoraphobia without panic[f] | – | | – | – | | – | | – | | – | | – | | – | | – | | 0 |
| Social phobia[f] | – | | – | – | | – | | – | | – | | – | | – | | – | | 18 |
| Specific phobia[f] | 0 | (0) | 0.9 | 0.9 | (1.0) | 10.2 | (4.6) | 10.2 | (4.6) | 0 | (0) | 3.0 | (2.5) | 3.0 | (2.5) | 10.7 | (4.6) | 81 |
| Separation anxiety disorder[g] | – | | – | – | | – | | – | | – | | – | | – | | – | | 2 |
| Posttraumatic stress disorder[g] | – | | – | – | | – | | – | | – | | – | | – | | – | | 4 |
| Any anxiety disorder[g] | 0.4 | (0.5) | 0.9 | 1.3 | (1.0) | 15.7 | (8.3) | 16.2 | (8.4) | 0 | (0) | 9.1 | (7.5) | 9.1 | (7.5) | 17.2 | (8.5) | 49 |
| **II. Mood disorders** | | | | | | | | | | | | | | | | | | |
| Major depressive disorder[f] | – | | – | – | | – | | – | | – | | – | | – | | – | | 0 |
| Dysthymia[f] | – | | – | – | | – | | – | | – | | – | | – | | – | | 14 |
| Bipolar disorders (broad)[f] | – | | – | – | | – | | – | | – | | – | | – | | – | | 4 |
| Any mood disorder[f] | – | | – | – | | – | | – | | – | | – | | – | | – | | 17 |
| **III. Substance disorders** | | | | | | | | | | | | | | | | | | |
| Alcohol abuse[f] | 1.2 | (1.2) | 0 | 1.2 | (1.2) | 5.3 | (5.0) | 6.5 | (5.0) | 0 | (0) | 0 | (0) | 0 | (0) | 6.5 | (5.0) | 68 |
| Alcohol abuse with dependence[f] | – | | – | – | | – | | – | | – | | – | | – | | – | | 32 |
| Drug abuse[g] | – | | – | – | | – | | – | | – | | – | | – | | – | | 1 |
| Drug abuse with dependence[g] | – | | – | – | | – | | – | | – | | – | | – | | – | | 0 |
| Any substance disorder[g] | 4.3 | (2.6) | 1.0 | 4.3 | (2.6) | 5.2 | (4.0) | 8.6 | (4.4) | 1.0 | (1.0) | 0 | (0) | 1.0 | (1.0) | 8.6 | (4.4) | 27 |
| **IV. Composite** | | | | | | | | | | | | | | | | | | |
| Any disorder[g] | 2.4 | (1.3) | 0.9 | 2.9 | (1.4) | 10.3 | (5.4) | 12.4 | (5.5) | 0.3 | (0.3) | 6.0 | (4.9) | 6.3 | (4.9) | 13.2 | (5.5) | 77 |
| No disorder[g] | 0.4 | (0.2) | 0.1 | 0.5 | (0.2) | 1.9 | (0.5) | 2.4 | (0.5) | 0.2 | (0.1) | 0.5 | (0.1) | 0.7 | (0.2) | 2.9 | (0.6) | 1551 |
| Total sample[g] | 0.5 | (0.2) | 0.1 | 0.6 | (0.2) | 2.3 | (0.5) | 2.9 | (0.6) | 0.3 | (0.1) | 0.7 | (0.3) | 1.0 | (0.3) | 3.4 | (0.6) | 1628 |

[a] Weighted number of respondents meeting criteria for each 12-month DSM-IV/CIDI disorder.
[b] Nonpsychiatrist defined as psychologists or other nonpsychiatrist mental health professional in any setting, social worker or counselor in a mental health specialty setting, use of a mental health hotline.
[c] General medical defined as primary care doctor, other general medical doctor, nurse, any other health professional not previously mentioned.
[d] Human services professional defined as religious or spiritual advisor, social worker, or counselor in any setting other than a specialty mental health setting.
[e] Complementary alternative medicine defined as any other type of healer, participation in an Internet support group, or participation in a self-help group.
[f] Using Part 1 respondents ($n = 5201$).
[g] Using Part 2 respondents ($n = 1628$).

**Table 21.13.** 12-month treatment use by service sector[a]

| | Mean number of visits | | | | Median number of visits | | | | Minimally adequate treatment | | | | Adequate treatment | | | |
|---|---|---|---|---|---|---|---|---|---|---|---|---|---|---|---|---|
| | No disorder | | Total | | No disorder | | Total | | No disorder | | Total | | No disorder | | Total | |
| | m | (se) | m | (se) | Md | (se) | Md | (se) | % | (se) | % | (se) | % | (se) | % | (se) |
| General medical[b] | 3.2 | (0.6) | 4.4 | (1.3) | 2.0 | (0.4) | 2.1 | (0.4) | 27.1 | (7.6) | 32.9 | (9.8) | 10.8 | (4.0) | 19.3 | (9.5) |
| Any health care[c] | 4.6 | (1.1) | 5.4 | (1.3) | – | – | 2.2 | (0.4) | 36.6 | (8.5) | 40.3 | (8.4) | 18.5 | (7.2) | 25.4 | (8.5) |
| Any service use[d] | 4.9 | (0.9) | 5.7 | (1.2) | 2.2 | (0.4) | 2.3 | (0.4) | 41.0 | (8.0) | 43.3 | (7.7) | 18.4 | (5.9) | 24.1 | (7.1) |

[a] The column "Any disorder" is not shown on this table as $n \leq 30$.

[b] General medical defined as primary care doctor, other general medical doctor, nurse, any other health professional not previously mentioned.

[c] The category "Any health care" includes mental health specialty, both psychiatrist and nonpsychiatrist (defined as psychologists or other nonpsychiatrist mental health professional in any setting, social worker or counselor in a mental health specialty setting, use of a mental health hotline) as well as general medical.

[d] The category "Any service use" includes those from the "Any health care" category as well as human services professionals (defined as religious or spiritual advisor, social worker, or counselor in any setting other than a specialty mental health setting) and complementary alternative medicine (defined as any other type of healer, participation in an Internet support group, or participation in a self-help group).

completed clinical reappraisal studies of CIDI 3.0 in community samples will we be able to evaluate these possibilities. On the basis of these uncertainties, the prevalence estimates reported here should be considered provisional. It is likely that these estimates are lower bounds on the true prevalence of these disorders in the metropolitan areas in which the survey was carried out.

Notwithstanding the possibility of underestimation, the prevalence estimates are nonetheless greater than those reported in the two previous major surveys of mental disorders carried out in China (Twelve collaborating units of epidemiological survey on mental disorders 1986a, 1986b; Zhang et al. 1998). In contrast to the two previous surveys, which indicated that the prevalence of mental disorders hardly changed between 1980 and the 1990s, the findings of the current study suggest that mental disorders have become more common in urban China in recent birth cohorts. There are two possible explanations for the higher prevalence estimates from this survey. First, the methodology might have been more sensitive to case finding in the Chinese context than were the methods used in the earlier surveys. In particular, the survey used rigorously trained lay interviewers to administer fully structured psychiatric diagnostic interviews that guaranteed coverage of a wide range of both serious and mild conditions. It should be emphasized again that the earlier surveys relied on clinical interviews carried out by psychiatric doctors who were accustomed to their clinical work of detecting severe mental disorders. That most of the disorders detected in the present survey were mild may lend credence to this possibility.

A second possibility is that methodological factors, such as stigma-induced concealment of symptoms, could have diminished among young Chinese respondents following societal "psychologization," resulting in greater willingness to admit such symptoms to interviewers in the WMH survey than in previous surveys. A third possibility is that AOO might be recalled incorrectly, thereby creating the false appearance of cohort effects. Although the probing strategy used in the CIDI helped to reduce this problem, it is possible that the problem was not corrected

**Table 21.14.** Demographic predictors of 12-month service use

| Demographic predictors | Any treatment | |
|---|---|---|
| | OR | (95% CI) |
| **I. Age** | | |
| 18–34 | 0.6 | (0.0–23.2) |
| 35–49 | 4.8 | (0.1–369.4) |
| 50–64 | 6.2 | (0.3–145.8) |
| 65+ | 1.0 | – |
| $\chi_3^2$ | 7.0 | |
| **II. Sex** | | |
| Male | 0.1* | (0.0–0.6) |
| Female | 1.0 | – |
| $\chi_1^2$ | 6.2* | |
| **III. Education** | | |
| 0–6 years | 13.1 | (0.5–341.3) |
| 7–9 years | 1.8 | (0.1–26.6) |
| 10–12 years | 4.3 | (0.6–32.8) |
| 13+ years | 1.0 | – |
| $\chi_3^2$ | 3.2 | |
| **IV. Marital status** | | |
| Never married | 4.9 | (0.9–28.1) |
| Separated/widowed/ divorced | 1.8 | (0.1–28.4) |
| Married/cohabiting | 1.0 | – |
| $\chi_2^2$ | 4.0 | |
| **V. Family income** | | |
| Low | 1.0 | (0.0–73.8) |
| Low-average | 14.8 | (0.6–365.7) |
| High-average | 3.3 | (0.1–106.8) |
| High | 1.0 | – |
| $\chi_1^2$ | 9.4* | |
| **VI. Any anxiety** | | |
| Yes | 4.4 | (0.2–87.9) |
| No | 1.0 | – |
| $\chi_1^2$ | 1.0 | |
| **VII. Any mood** | | |
| Yes | 10.9 | (0.2–482.7) |
| No | 1.0 | – |
| $\chi_1^2$ | 1.6 | |
| **VIII. Any substance** | | |
| Yes | 22.8 | (1.8–286.4) |
| No | 1.0 | – |
| $\chi_1^2$ | 6.2* | |

* Significant at the 0.05 level, two-sided test.

completely. Finally, the assumption of constant conditional risk of first onset in a given year of life among people of different ages, which was used to estimate lifetime risk, is implausible in the context of higher prevalence in more recent cohorts.

The general pattern of the findings in China resembles those of other WMH participating countries in several ways. Although some differences in the prevalence of certain disorders between Beijing and Shanghai exist, a similar pattern of findings is found in the two cities. These include the usual gradient of severity of disorders, higher prevalence of anxiety than mood disorders, sociodemographic risk factors, and much higher use of general medical over psychiatric help-seeking. Unlike the situation in most other countries, no significant sex difference was found in lifetime risk of any anxiety, mood, or impulse-control disorders. The reasons for this pattern are unclear. If replicated, this pattern will question the cross-national validity of the well-documented sex differences in these mental disorders.

According to the Global Burden of Disease study, mental disorders account for almost 20% of the total disease burden in China. Notwithstanding the remarkable progress in physical health (e.g., infant mortality, life expectancy) and general standard of living in the country, the central government has only recently begun to give limited attention to mental health. At the level of local governments, policy and programs on mental health receive scanty support from influential supporters and remain fragmented across multiple administrative levels. Furthermore, organized advocacy that fights for patients' right to treatment barely exists.

Although the demonstrable lifetime prevalence of mental disorders (13.2%) remains low by Western standards, it translates into an enormous number of individuals when China's population of more than 1.3 billion is considered. Moreover, estimates of lifetime rates suggest that common mental disorders such as depression and substance disorders are rising especially among the younger generation of Chinese people. As mental disorders bring about substantial productivity loss, the inadequate attention paid by the Chinese government to mental health is ironic in view of its quest for continued economic growth. In this regard, the need for multisector efforts to devise innovative policy and to implement programs that can enhance early interventions can hardly be overemphasized. Such interventions, to be effective, must take into account local political and economical circumstances unique to different regions in China.

## 5.1. Unmet Treatment Need

Previous Chinese surveys seldom measured severity of disorder or unmet treatment need. The authors conducted the first survey in China that encompassed a spectrum of DSM-IV disorders classified by severity and examined treatment. From a public health perspective, it is striking that unmet treatment is almost routine even in the two most developed cities in contemporary China. Given that China has a population of 1.3 billion, the low prevalence of mental disorders still translates into an enormous number of people with untreated disorders. The finding is indeed disturbing that 96.6% of the subjects with any disorder and 80.2% of those with moderate and severe disorders received no 12-month treatment even in Beijing and Shanghai, which have a higher than average concentrations of health-care resources including trained psychiatrists.

Even though some people did seek help from general medical practitioners, who are not adequately trained in treating mental health problems, the outcome of treatment has not been evaluated by evidence-based review. Psychiatric stigma has routinely been blamed for the undertreatment of mental disorders, especially in non-Western societies such as China. It has been a cultural tradition for Chinese people to keep their problems within the family. For example, more than 90% of people with schizophrenia in China live with and are cared for by family members only. However, the main reason for the high level of unmet treatment need is that the great majority of people with disorders do not receive any form of treatment, including from general medical practitioners who do not manifestly stigmatize. Therefore, stigma, low mental health literacy, and low perceived need cannot adequately explain the gross undertreatment. Although it may be speculated that robust family values can buffer Chinese people against mental disorders and reduce the need for professional treatment, this explanation is unlikely to account for the low level of treatment among those individuals with severe disorders.

A second possible explanation is a low level of public awareness of mental disorder in China. For decades, mental disorder has been equated with psychosis, which is thought to bring about social disruption and/or danger to others. Consequently, the idea that common symptoms such as insomnia, pains, low energy, and the like are due to mental disorders and are treatable is unpopular in the general public. A third explanation is stigma, to be emphasized again. Although the stigmatization of mental disorder is universal, it is likely to be more marked in Chinese communities. Mental disorder is commonly associated with danger, moral defect, treatment pessimism, shame to the family, rejection in the workplace, and a burden on society.

Health economists have admonished that one of the most significant casualties during China's transition to a market economy is the health-care system. Medical insurance coverage is now nonexistent in rural China and only available to about 40% of the urban population, some of whom have depleted their accounts. The consequences of such an economic reality are a waste of already-limited health-care resources and structural barriers to care. Such disparity may be reflected by the unique finding among WMH participating countries that China had a higher percentage of people with no disorder than with a mild disorder who received 12-month treatment. This is also supported by the finding that high income is associated with high treatment rates. Thus, the need for multilevel and multisector efforts to address unmet treatment should definitely be a focus of attention.

## 5.2. Limitations and Future Research

It is important to recognize several limitations of the Chinese WMH surveys that we hope to overcome in future expansion of these surveys in China. First, because of limited funding, the study sample was drawn from only two metropolitan cities, even though China is about two-thirds rural. Therefore, epidemiological studies are needed in the vast areas of rural China. Second, the survey was not conducted in a way that a meaningful number of clinical reappraisals could be used to validate or recalibrate the CIDI DSM-IV diagnoses or the assessments of severity. Third, because of the low prevalence and treatment rates, the small number of cases in specific diagnostic categories, even when data from the two cities are combined, limits the power of statistical analysis.

Theoretically speaking, to overcome these limitations, a large representative sample should be selected. However, the cost of doing so is prohibitive in China, where funding for mental health research is grossly inadequate. Consequently, it is important to devise methodological improvements that can lead to more accurate prevalence estimates with limited sample sizes. To control for information bias, it would be worthwhile for future Chinese surveys to evaluate the validity of alternative approaches to diagnostic assessment. For example, we are currently experimenting with modifications of the CIDI in which respondents are probed initially about somatic symptoms that often occur as part of mental disorders in an effort to elicit positive reports that can then be probed for related emotional, cognitive, and behavioral symptoms that would indicate the presence of mental disorders. Strategies, such as this one, that facilitate the discovery of emotional disorders need to be developed and evaluated to improve assessment of psychopathology in China. On the basis of the promising results of the Chinese WMH surveys and our subsequent ongoing substantive and methodological work with the CIDI in other Chinese metropolitan areas, we believe that the CIDI is an appropriate core instrument that can serve as the foundation for such modifications, aimed at enriching our understanding of the epidemiology of mental disorders in China.

## REFERENCES

Agency for Health Care Policy and Research (1993). *Depression Guideline Panel, Vol. 2: Treatment of major depression, Clinical Practice Guideline, No. 5.* Rockville, MD: U.S. Department of Health and Human Services, Public Health Service, Agency for Health Care Policy and Research.

American Psychiatric Association (1994). *Diagnostic and statistical manual of mental disorders (DSM-IV)*, 4th ed. Washington, DC: American Psychiatric Association.

American Psychiatric Association (1998). *Practice guideline for treatment of patients with panic disorder.* Washington, DC: American Psychiatric Association.

American Psychiatric Association (2000). *Practice guideline for treatment of patients with major depressive disorder*, 2d ed. Washington, DC: American Psychiatric Association.

American Psychiatric Association (2002). *Practice guideline for treatment of patients with bipolar disorder*, 2d ed. Washington, DC: American Psychiatric Association.

American Psychiatric Association (2004). *Practice guideline for treatment of patients with schizophrenia*, 2d ed. Washington, DC: American Psychiatric Association.

Cheng, Z. R., Gao, H., Zhang, X., Tang, Z. R., Lu, Y. W., Yang, W. Q., Cai, T., Hu, C. Y., Li, H., Li, Y. P., Zhang, Y. P. & Huang, X. Z. (1999). The epidemiological survey of mental disorders in Shenzhen. *Medical Journal of Chinese Civil Administration*, 11, 32–5 (in Chinese).

Cooper, J. E. & Sartorius, N. (1996). *Mental disorders in China: Result of the National Epidemiological Survey in 12 areas.* London: Gaskell.

Demyttenaere, K., Bruffaerts, R., Posada-Villa, J., Gasquet, I., Kovess, V., Lepine, J. P., Angermeyer, M. C., Bernert, S., Girolamo, G., Morosini, P., Polidori, G., Kikkawa, T., Kawakami, N., Ono, Y., Takeshima, T., Uda, H., Karam, E. G., Fayyad, J. A., Karam, A. N., Mneimneh, Z. N., Medina-Mora, M. E., Borges, G., Lara, G., de Graaf, R., Ormel, J., Gureje, O., Shen, Y., Huang, Y., Zhang, M., Alonso, J., Haro, J. M., Vilagut, G., Bromet, E. J., Gluzman, S., Webb, C., Kessler, R. C., Merikangas, K. R., Anthony, J. C., Korff, M. R. V., Wang, P. S., Alonso, J., Brugha, T. S., Aguilar-Gaxiola, S., Lee, S., Heeringa, S., Pennell, B. E., Zaslavsky, A. M., Üstün, T. B. & Chatterji, S. (2004). Prevalence, severity and unmet need for treatment of mental disorders in the World Health Organization World Mental Health Surveys. *Journal of the American Medical Association*, 291, 2581–90.

Efron, B. (1988). Logistic regression, survival analysis, and the Kaplan-Meier curve. *Journal of the American Statistical Association*, 83, 414–25.

First, M. B., Gibon, M., Spitzer, R. & Williams, J. B. W. (2002). *The Structured Clinical Interview for DSM-IV.* Washington, DC: American Psychiatric Press.

Halli, S. S. & Rao, K. V. (1992). *Advanced techniques of population analysis.* New York: Plenum Press.

Hosmer, D. W. & Lemeshow, S. (1989). *Applied logistic regression.* New York: John Wiley & Sons.

Huang, Y. Q., Li, S. R., Dang, W. M., Yuan, Y. B. & Liu, Z. R. (2005). Reliability and validity of the Chinese version of Composite International Diagnostic Interview, core version 2.1. Paper presented at the Sixth Annual Meeting of the Chinese Society of Psychiatry, Wuhan, China (in Chinese).

Kessler, R. C., Haro, J. M., Heeringa, S. G., Pennell, B. E. & Üstün, T. B. (2006). The World Health Organization World Mental Health Survey Initiative. *Epidemiologia e Psichiatria Sociale*, 15, 161–6.

Kessler, R. C. & Üstün, T. B. (2004). The World Mental Health (WMH) Survey Initiative version of the World Health Organization (WHO) Composite International Diagnostic Interview (CIDI). *International Journal of Methods in Psychiatric Research*, 13, 93–121.

Knauper, B., Cannell, C. F., Schwarz, N., Bruce, M. L. & Kessler, R. C. (1999). Improving the accuracy of major depression age of onset reports in the U.S. National Comorbidity Survey. *International Journal of Methods in Psychiatric Research*, 8, 39–48.

Lee, S., Fung, S. C., Tsang, A., Zhang, M. Y., Huang, Y. Q., He, Y. L., Liu, Z. R., Shen, Y. C. & Kessler, R. C. (2007). Delay in initial treatment contact after first onset of mental disorders in metropolitan China. *Acta Psychiatrica Scandinavica*, 116, 10–16.

Lee, S. & Kleinman, A. (2000). Grave new world: Is reform disease or cure for China's mentally ill? *Harvard China Review*, 2, 72–75.

Lehman, A. F. & Steinwachs, D. M. (1998). Translating research into practice: Schizophrenia patient outcomes research team (PORT) treatment recommendations. *Schizophrenia Bulletin*, 24, 1–10.

Leon, A. C., Olfson, M., Portera, L., Farber, L. & Sheehan, D. V. (1997). Assessing psychiatric impairment in primary care with the Sheehan Disability Scale. *International Journal of Psychiatry in Medicine*, 27, 93–105.

Research Triangle Institute (2002). *SUDAAN: Professional software for survey data analysis 8.01.*

Research Triangle Park, NC: Research Triangle Institute.

SAS Institute (2001). *SAS/STAT Software: Changes and enhancements, Release 8.2*. Cary, NC: SAS Publishing.

Schatzberg, A. F. & Nemeroff, C. B. (2004). *Textbook of psychopharmacology*. Washington, DC: American Psychiatric Publishing.

Shen, Y. C., Zhang, M. Y., Huang, Y. Q., He, Y. L., Liu, Z. R., Cheng, H., Tsang, A., Lee, S. & Kessler, R. C. (2006). Twelve-month prevalence, severity, and unmet need for treatment of mental disorders in metropolitan China. *Psychological Medicine*, 36, 257–68.

Simon, G. E. & Von Korff, M. (1995). Recall of psychiatric history in cross-sectional surveys: Implications for epidemiologic research. *Epidemiology Review*, 17, 221–27.

Twelve Collaborating Units of Epidemiological Survey on Mental Disorders (1986a). The methodology and data analysis of epidemiological survey on mental disorders in 12 regions in China. *Chinese Journal of Neurology and Psychiatry*, 19, 66–7 (in Chinese).

Twelve Collaborating Units of Epidemiological Survey on Mental Disorders (1986b). The prevalence of mental disorders, drug dependence and personality disorder. *Chinese Journal of Neurology and Psychiatry*, 19, 70–2 (in Chinese).

Weng, Z., Zhang, J. X., Ma, D. D., Ma, S. P., Li, X. F., Jiang, K. Q., Xu, L. Y., Chen, C. D., Cao, X. Y., Meng, G. Y., He, J. Y., Sun, L. M., Zhang, S. J., Zhu, B. J., Cui, W. C., Gong, P. J., Hu, B. W., Liu, Z. X., Mu, Z. P. & Li, X. Q. (1998). An epidemiological investigation of mental disorders in Shandong province in 1984 and 1994. *Chinese Journal of Psychiatry*, 31, 222–4 (in Chinese).

World Health Organization (WHO) (1991). *International classification of diseases (ICD-10)*. Geneva: World Health Organization.

Zhang, W. X., Shen, Y. C., Li, S. R., Chen, C. H., Huang, Y. Q., Wang, J. R., Wang, D. P., Tu, J., Ning, Z. X., Fu, L. M., Ji, L. P., Liu, Z. G., Wu, H. M., Luo, K. L., Zhai, S. T., Yan, H. J. & Meng, G. R. (1998). Epidemiological investigation on mental disorders in 7 areas of China. *Chinese Journal of Psychiatry*, 31, 69–71 (in Chinese).

# 22 Twelve-month Prevalence, Severity, and Treatment of Common Mental Disorders in Communities in Japan: The World Mental Health Japan 2002–2004 Survey

NORITO KAWAKAMI, TADASHI TAKESHIMA, YUTAKA ONO, HIDENORI UDA, YOSHIBUMI NAKANE, YOSIKAZU NAKAMURA, HISATERU TACHIMORI, NOBORU IWATA, HIDEYUKI NAKANE, MAKOTO WATANABE, YOICHI NAGANUMA, TOSHIAKI A. FURUKAWA, YUKIHIRO HATA, MASAYO KOBAYASHI, YUKO MIYAKE, AND TAKEHIKO KIKKAWA

## ACKNOWLEDGMENTS

The World Mental Health Japan (WMH-Japan) is supported by the Grant for Research on Psychiatric and Neurological Diseases and Mental Health (H13-SHOGAI-023, H14-TOKUBETSU-026, H16-KOKORO-013) from the Japan Ministry of Health, Labour, and Welfare. We would like to thank staff members, field coordinators, and interviewers of the WMH-Japan 2002–2004 Survey. The WMH-Japan 2002–2004 Survey was carried out in conjunction with the World Health Organization World Mental Health (WMH) Survey Initiative. We also thank the WMH staff for assistance with instrumentation, fieldwork, and data analysis. These activities were supported by the U.S. National Institute of Mental Health (R01MH070884), the John D. and Catherine T. MacArthur Foundation, the Pfizer Foundation, the U.S. Public Health Service (R13-MH066849, R01-MH069864, and R01 DA016558), the Fogarty International Center (FIRCA R03-TW006481), the Pan American Health Organization, Eli Lilly and Company Foundation, Ortho-McNeil Pharmaceutical, GlaxoSmithKline, and Bristol-Myers Squibb. A complete list of WMH publications can be found at http://www.hcp.med.harvard.edu/wmh/.

## I. INTRODUCTION

### 1.1. History of Psychiatric Epidemiology in Japan

A number of large-scale community-based psychiatric epidemiological surveys have been conducted in Western countries and increasingly in other parts of the world. Their findings have been used as a basis for developing policies for mental health in an entire nation and for the world as well as for understanding the etiology of and improving the classification system for mental disorders. However, psychiatric epidemiological studies have been less frequently conducted in Japan until recently (Kitamura et al. 1999; Kawakami et al. 2004; Kawakami et al. 2005).

In 1954, long before psychiatric epidemiological community surveys were carried out in their current form, a large-scale community-based survey on mental disorders of a nationally representative sample of Japan was conducted to estimate the prevalence of mental disorders and the need for mental health service (Kikkawa & Takeuchi 1980). Psychiatrists visited 23,993 residents of 4895 households at 100 survey sites that were selected by a two-stage random sampling from the whole of Japan to make clinical diagnoses of mental disorders. The survey found that 1.5% of the Japanese population currently suffered from some type of mental disorder (including psychosis, mental retardation, and epilepsy). This landmark survey in psychiatric epidemiology in Japan was conducted more than two decades before pioneering surveys by Weissman and colleagues (1978) and the ECA survey (Regier et al. 1984) in the United States, with a large number of subjects by today's standards. Similar surveys were repeated in 1963 and 1973, following the first survey, to replicate the findings. Unfortunately, at the time the surveys were conducted, no operational diagnoses of mental disorders or standardized interview instruments existed. The reliability and validity of the diagnosis depended exclusively on the clinical experience of psychiatrists. In addition, there was a serious problem in case-finding methodology, as landowners and other influential persons in each study community were used as key informants to identify possible cases of mental disorders. This approach to case-finding almost certainly led to detection bias. Strong concerns about privacy of those who suffered mental disorders prevented the government from continuing such surveys. The last survey in the series, which started in 1973, was discontinued at the midway point and permanently abandoned.

## 1.2. Low Prevalence of Mental Disorders in Asia

Cross-national psychiatric epidemiology has consistently revealed a lower prevalence of mood and anxiety disorders among East Asian countries than among Western countries. Lifetime prevalence estimates in major psychiatric epidemiological surveys of major depression ranged from 0.9% to 3.4% in South Korea (Lee et al. 1990), Taiwan (Hwu, Yeh & Chang 1989), and China (Hong Kong) (Chen et al. 1993), while a much higher prevalence (4%–15%) was reported in the United States (Kessler et al. 1994) and other Western countries (Cross-National Collaborative Group 1992; Andrade et al. 2003). The lifetime prevalence estimates of alcohol abuse and dependence were lower in surveys conducted in Taiwan and Hong Kong (less than 3%) (Hwu

et al. 1989; Chen et al. 1993; Kawakami et al. 2004) than in the United States and Europe (14%–24%) (Canino et al. 1987; Helzer et al. 1990; Kessler et al. 1994) and South Korea (11%–13%) (Lee et al. 1990). Findings from community-based psychiatric epidemiological surveys in Japan have been mixed in this regard, with one reporting comparable levels of major depression to those found in other countries (Kitamura et al. 1999) and another reporting low prevalence for mood, anxiety, and alcohol use disorders (Kawakami et al. 2004). The difference might be attributable to a difference in methodology, such as interview methods and diagnostic criteria. There is also evidence that the percentage of people with mental disorders who receive treatment is quite low in Japan (Kitamura et al. 1999), though this, too, could be a biased estimate. In light of these uncertainties, we considered it important for Japan to be included in the World Health Organization (WHO) World Mental Health (WMH) Survey Initiative.

## 2. SUBJECTS AND METHODS

### 2.1. Subjects

The World Mental Health Japan (WMH-Japan) Survey is an epidemiological survey of Japanese-speaking household residents aged 20 and older. Seven community populations in Japan were selected as study sites in 2002–2004. These sites included two urban cities (Okayama city [population: 660,000] and Nagasaki city [population: 450,000]) and five rural municipalities (Kushikino city [population: 25,000], Fukiage town [population: 8500], Ichiki town [population: 7000], Higashiichiki town [population: 14,000] in Kagoshima prefecture, and Tamano city [population: 70,000] in Okayama prefecture). These sites were selected in consideration of geographic variation, the availability of site investigators, and cooperation of the local government. Mainly as a result of the latter two factors, all survey sites were located in the western part of Japan for the 2002–2004 WMH-Japan surveys. The total response rate was 58.4% (Table 22.1). From a total of 2437

**Table 22.1.** The number of total initial sample, completed interviews and response rate by survey site in the WMH-Japan 2002–2004 survey

| | Survey site/year of survey | | | | | | | |
|---|---|---|---|---|---|---|---|---|
| | Okayama prefecture | | Nagasaki prefecture | | Kagoshima prefecture | | | |
| | Okayama | Tamano | Nagasaki | Kushikino | Fukiage | Ichiki | Higashiichiki | |
| | 2002–2003 | 2003–2004 | 2002–2003 | 2002–2003 | 2002–2003 | 2003–2004 | 2003–2004 | Total |
| Total initial sample | 1607 | 701 | 800 | 587 | 230 | 227 | 429 | 4581 |
| Completed interview | 925 | 349 | 208 | 354 | 177 | 153 | 271 | 2437 |
| Incomplete interview | 6 | | 3 | – | – | 1 | 1 | 11 |
| No contact | 80 | 28 | 296 | – | – | | | 404 |
| Refused | 397 | 242 | 280 | 185 | 40 | 61 | 116 | 1321 |
| Ineligible[a] | 199 | 82 | 13 | 48 | 13 | 12 | 41 | 408 |
| Response rate[b] | 65.7% | 56.4% | 26.4% | 65.7% | 81.6% | 71.2% | 69.8% | 58.4% |

[a] Ineligible subjects include those who were deceased, had moved, or had been institutionalized. Ineligible subjects were a small number ($n = 15$) of those who had impaired cognitive functions in the Okayama city site.

[b] Response rate = ($n$ of completed interviews)/($n$ of total initial sample – $n$ of the ineligible).

respondents, we dropped 1 respondent from Okayama city because of lack of information on marital status.

An internal sampling strategy was used in all surveys to reduce respondent burden by dividing the interview into two parts. Part 1 included a core diagnostic assessment of all respondents ($n = 2,436$) that took an average of about one hour to administer. Part 2 included questions about risk factors, consequences, other correlates, and additional disorders. In an effort to reduce respondent burden and control study costs, Part 2 was administered only to 887 of the 2436 Part 1 respondents, including all Part 1 respondents with one or more lifetime disorders plus a probability subsample of approximately 25% of other respondents. The interviews for the respondents who were not selected into Part 2 were terminated after Part 1.

Written consent was obtained from each respondent at each site. The Human Subjects Committees of Okayama University (for Okayama and Tamano), the Japan National Institute of Mental Health (for the four sites in Kagoshima prefectures), and Nagasaki University (for Nagasaki) approved the recruitment, consent, and field procedures.

## 2.2. Training and Field Procedures

The fieldwork for the WMH-Japan was carried out by a survey center at each survey site. The funding, negotiation with local government at each study site, and ethical/legal considerations were provided by headquarters at the National Institute of Mental Health (NIMH), Japan. The development of the instrument, training of the interviewers, and preparation of data analysis were supported by the technical support center at Okayama University Graduate School of Medicine and Dentistry.

Before the survey, interviewers received a five-day standardized instrument-specific training. The training included didactic sessions of general interview skills and reviews of the instrument sections, mock interviews, and role-playing exercises. Two official trainers and other assistants who were previously trained in the instrument provided the interviewers the five-day training at each survey site.

In the Okayama site, an invitation letter was sent to each subject and then an interviewer visited the subjects' homes to seek permission to participate in the survey. If the subject agreed, the interviewer conducted a face-to-face interview in the home or at the university if the participant preferred. For the four sites in Kagoshima prefecture and Tamano in Okayama prefecture, community volunteers first contacted the subjects in their homes to recruit them into the survey. When agreement was obtained, an interviewer conducted the face-to-face interview in the home or at a local community center. At the Nagasaki site, an invitation letter was sent to each subject, and an interviewer conducted the face-to-face interview with those who replied positively. When an invitation letter was mailed twice and no response was received within a month, no further effort was made to contact the individuals. Written consent was obtained from each respondent at each site.

## 2.3. Survey Instrument

The survey used the Japanese computer-assisted personal interview (CAPI) version of the WHO Composite International Diagnostic Interview (CIDI) Version 3.0 (Kessler & Üstün 2004; see also Chapter 4 of this volume), a fully structured diagnostic interview. The original English version of the instrument was translated into Japanese by a team under the supervision of the investigators. The Japanese CAPI program was tested in a preliminary survey of about 100 community residents to further modify the wordings and programs (Sakai, Ito & Takeuchi 2003). Key questions of the final draft of the Japanese version were translated back into English and sent to the WMH Data Collection Coordination Centre at the Harvard Medical School for a review to check for cross-national consistency. The reliability and validity of the Japanese version have not been fully examined. However, a pilot study using the Japanese version of CIDI with a small number of clinical psychiatric patients showed good concordance between clinical diagnosis and CIDI diagnosis of major depression and alcohol abuse/dependence (Sakai et al. 2003).

## 2.4. Measures

Disorders assessed by CIDI in the survey were (a) anxiety disorders [agoraphobia, generalized anxiety disorder, panic disorder, posttraumatic stress disorder (PTSD), social phobia, specific phobia], (b) mood disorders (bipolar I and II disorders, dysthymia, major depressive disorder), (c) disorders that share a feature of problems with impulse control (intermittent explosive disorder), and (d) substance disorders (alcohol and drug abuse and dependence). Disorders were assessed using the definitions and criteria of the American Psychiatric Association's Diagnostic and Statistical Manual of Mental Disorders, 4th ed. (DSM-IV) (American Psychiatric Association 1994). CIDI organic exclusion rules were imposed in making all diagnoses.

Twelve-month DSM-IV/CIDI disorders were classified as serious, moderate, or mild (Demyttenaere et al. 2004). Serious disorders were defined as those meeting the criteria for bipolar I disorder or substance dependence with a physiological dependence syndrome; a suicide attempt in conjunction with any other CIDI/DSM-IV disorder; reporting of at least two areas of role functioning with severe role impairment due to a mental disorder in the disorder-specific Sheehan Disability Scales (SDS) (Leon et al. 1997); or reporting of overall functional impairment at a level consistent with a Global Assessment of Functioning (GAF) (Endicott et al. 1976) of 50 or less in conjunction with any other CIDI/DSM-IV disorder. Respondents not classified as having a serious disorder were classified as moderate if interference was rated at least moderate in any SDS domain or if the respondent had substance dependence without a physiological dependence syndrome. All other disorders were classified as mild.

The 12-month treatment rate was assessed by asking respondents if they had ever seen any of a list of professionals as either an outpatient or an inpatient for problems with emotions, nerves, mental health, or use of alcohol or drugs. Professionals were classified into the following categories: (a) psychiatrist or mental health specialist (hospital visit, psychologist, other mental health providers, social worker or counselor in a mental health setting or hotline), (b) general medical (other doctor or nurse), (c) human services (religious provider, social worker or counselor in a non–mental health setting), and

(d) complementary and alternative medicine (CAM) (Internet group, self-help group, or alternative provider). Further, health-care service was defined as psychiatrist, mental health specialist, or general medical. The subjects who had used any of these services in the previous 12 months were placed in a category labeled "any treatment," and those who did not seek treatment were categorized as "no treatment."

The sociodemographic characteristics used in the analysis were age, sex, education, marital status, and income. Income was trichotomized on the basis of the median income per family member. These variables were examined as correlates of both disorder prevalence and treatment.

## 2.5. Statistical Analysis

Data are reported on prevalence, severity, and associations of severity with treatment. Simple cross-tabulations were used to calculate prevalence and severity. Logistic regression analysis was used to study sociodemographic correlates. Standard errors of descriptive statistics were estimated using the Taylor series method implemented in the SUDAAN software system (Research Triangle Institute 2002) to adjust for the weighting of cases. The logistic regression coefficients were transformed to odds ratios (ORs) and are reported below with design-adjusted 95% confidence intervals (CIs). Multivariate tests were based on Wald $\chi^2$ tests computed from design-adjusted coefficient variance-covariance matrices. Statistical significance was based on two-sided design-based tests evaluated at the 0.05 level of significance.

## 3. RESULTS

### 3.1. 12-month Prevalence and Disorder Severity

About 7% of community residents were estimated in the survey to have experienced any DSM-IV/CIDI disorder in the previous 12 months (Table 22.2), whereas about 4% of respondents experienced any anxiety disorder in

the previous 12 months and lower proportions experienced any mood disorder (1 out of every 40 respondents), any impulse-control disorder (1 out of 167 respondents), and any substance disorder (1 out of every 83 respondents). Among the specific disorders assessed in the survey, the 12-month prevalence was greater for major depressive disorder (2.1%) and specific phobia (2.4%).

Among those who had experienced a disorder in the previous 12 months, one of seven had experienced a severe disorder and about one-half had experienced a moderate disorder. In other words, 1% of the total population in Japan was estimated to have experienced a severe disorder and 3% a moderate disorder in the previous 12 months. More severe cases were likely to be among those with PTSD, dysthymia, alcohol dependence, drug abuse, and drug dependence.

### 3.2. Sociodemographic Correlates of 12-month Prevalence

Respondents who were not married at the time of the survey were three times more likely than those who were married to have any 12-month disorder and any mood disorder (Table 22.3, $p < 0.05$). The 12-month prevalence of substance use disorders was greater among men than women and among respondents aged 49 years old or younger than among older respondents ($p < 0.05$). None of the sociodemographic predictors was significantly associated with 12-month prevalence of any category of mental disorders. However, the prevalence of any disorder and any mood disorder tended to be higher among respondents aged 50–64 and among those with higher education.

### 3.3. Association of 12-month Disorder Severity with Treatment

Among respondents who had a severe or moderate disorder in the past 12 months, 24.3% had received some type of treatment, including 19.1% who obtained treatment from a mental health professional (including visits to psychiatrists and clinical psychologists) and 8.5%

**Table 22.2.** 12-month prevalence and severity of DSM-IV disorders: The WMH Japan 2002–2004 surveys

| Diagnosis | | $n$ | 12-month % | (se) | Serious[b] % | (se) | Moderate[b] % | (se) | Mild[b] % | (se) |
|---|---|---|---|---|---|---|---|---|---|---|
| Anxiety disorder | Panic disorder[a] | 8 | 0.3 | (0.1) | 17.2 | (12.0) | 48.0 | (19.9) | 34.8 | (18.6) |
| | Generalized anxiety disorder[a] | 23 | 0.8 | (0.2) | 21.3 | (8.6) | 50.5 | (10.4) | 28.2 | (10.1) |
| | Specific phobia[a] | 60 | 2.4 | (0.3) | 9.0 | (4.8) | 49.3 | (7.6) | 41.7 | (6.5) |
| | Social phobia[a] | 10 | 0.5 | (0.2) | 31.8 | (15.5) | 68.2 | (15.5) | 0.0 | (0.0) |
| | Agoraphobia without panic[a] | 5 | 0.2 | (0.1) | 24.8 | (20.1) | 75.2 | (20.1) | 0.0 | (0.0) |
| | Posttraumatic stress disorder[b] | 9 | 0.4 | (0.2) | 49.4 | (16.7) | 3.3 | (3.1) | 47.3 | (17.7) |
| | Any anxiety disorder[b] | 91 | 4.1 | (0.6) | 12.0 | (3.9) | 51.1 | (5.7) | 36.9 | (5.5) |
| Mood disorder | Major depressive disorder[a] | 52 | 2.1 | (0.3) | 16.3 | (4.4) | 59.1 | (8.0) | 24.5 | (7.4) |
| | Dysthymia[a] | 10 | 0.4 | (0.1) | 41.2 | (21.5) | 43.7 | (25.2) | 15.1 | (9.0) |
| | Bipolar I/II/subthreshold[a] | 6 | 0.3 | (0.1) | 23.3 | (18.5) | 59.1 | (26.0) | 17.6 | (17.4) |
| | Any mood disorder[a] | 60 | 2.5 | (0.4) | 18.0 | (5.6) | 58.2 | (9.3) | 23.9 | (7.4) |
| Impulse disorder | Intermittent explosive disorder[a] | 14 | 0.6 | (0.1) | 14.1 | (11.8) | 30.3 | (18.1) | 55.6 | (14.7) |
| Substance disorder | Alcohol abuse[b] | 13 | 1.0 | (0.4) | 11.3 | (6.7) | 9.5 | (6.3) | 79.3 | (11.0) |
| | Alcohol dependence[b] | 4 | 0.2 | (0.1) | 85.3 | (15.0) | 14.7 | (15.0) | 0.0 | (0.0) |
| | Drug abuse[b] | 2 | 0.1 | (0.1) | 100.0 | (0.0) | 0.0 | (0.0) | 0.0 | (0.0) |
| | Drug dependence[b] | 1 | 0.0 | (0.0) | 100.0 | (0.0) | 0.0 | (0.0) | 0.0 | (0.0) |
| | Any substance use disorder[b] | 16 | 1.2 | (0.4) | 26.8 | (9.9) | 7.8 | (5.3) | 65.4 | (11.9) |
| Any disorder | Any[b] | 142 | 7.0 | (0.8) | 13.7 | (3.3) | 46.1 | (5.5) | 40.2 | (4.6) |
| Total sample | Total sample[b] | 887 | – | – | 1.0 | (0.2) | 3.3 | (0.6) | 3.0 | (0.5) |

*Note:* Severity calculated using Part 2 weights.
[a] Part 1 sample; prevalence calculated using Part 1 weights.
[b] Part 2 sample; prevalence calculated using Part 2 weights.

from a general medical (nonpsychiatrist) physician (Table 22.4). A much smaller proportion (12.8%) of mild cases received treatment.

### 3.4. Sociodemographic Correlates of 12-month Health-care Treatment

Severity of the mental disorders was strongly and positively associated with seeking health-care treatment (Table 22.5, $p < 0.05$). Respondents who were young, who had low income, and who had low education were less likely than others with comparable disorders to seek treatment, although these associations were not strong enough to reach the conventional 0.05 level of significance.

## 4. DISCUSSION

### 4.1. Prevalence of Mental Disorders in Japan

The results in the WMH-Japan survey regarding disorder prevalence are very similar to those in other recent Japanese surveys of mental disorders (Kawakami et al. 2005; Naganuma et al. 2006). Seven percent of community residents in Japan were estimated in the WMH-Japan survey to have experienced any DSM-IV/CIDI disorder in the previous 12 months. Among specific mental disorders assessed in the survey, major depressive disorder (2.1%) and specific phobia (2.4%) were the most common. The 12-month

**Table 22.3.** Demographic correlates of 12-month DSM-IV disorders: The WMH Japan 2002–2004 surveys

| | | Any disorder | | Mood | | Anxiety | | Substance use | |
|---|---|---|---|---|---|---|---|---|---|
| | | OR | (95% CI) | OR | (95% CI) | OR | (95% CI) | OR | (95% CI) |
| Sex | Male | 1.0 | – | 1.0 | – | 1.0 | – | 1.0 | – |
| | Female | 1.6 | (0.5–4.9) | 1.6 | (0.7–3.9) | 1.9 | (0.9–4.0) | 0.1 | (0.0–0.5) |
| | $\chi^2$ | 0.6 | | 1.3 | | 3.3 | | 8.1* | |
| Age, years | 18–34 | 1.3 | (0.2–6.9) | 0.9 | (0.2–4.6) | 1.9 | (0.5–7.5) | 4.7 | (0.9–24.9) |
| | 35–49 | 1.2 | (0.2–6.1) | 0.8 | (0.1–4.3) | 1.8 | (0.5–6.2) | 4.5 | (1.1–17.9) |
| | 50–64 | 1.6 | (0.4–6.9) | 1.6 | (0.4–7.1) | 1.8 | (0.5–6.4) | 0.8 | (0.1–8.9) |
| | 65≤ | 1.0 | – | 1.0 | – | 1.0 | – | 1.0 | – |
| | $\chi^2$ | 0.7 | | 1.8 | | 1.1 | | 13.9* | |
| Income | Low | 2.0 | (0.6–6.8) | 1.0 | (0.4–2.5) | 0.9 | (0.4–2.2) | 0.3 | (0.1–1.7) |
| | Average | 1.1 | (0.3–4.1) | 0.6 | (0.2–2.4) | 0.7 | (0.3–1.9) | 3.2 | (0.4–24.1) |
| | High | 1.0 | – | 1.0 | – | 1.0 | – | 1.0 | –. |
| | $\chi^2$ | 1.5 | | 0.9 | | 0.5 | | 4.0 | |
| Marital Status | Married/cohabiting | 1.0 | – | 1.0 | – | 1.0 | – | 1.0 | – |
| | Not married | 2.8 | (1.1–7.4) | 3.1 | (1.4–7.2) | 1.2 | (0.6–2.2) | 2.2 | (0.3–14.7) |
| | $\chi^2$ | 4.8* | | 8.0* | | 0.3 | | 0.7 | |
| Education | Less than secondary | 0.4 | (0.1–2.2) | 0.1 | (0.0–0.6) | 0.6 | (0.2–2.3) | 7.5 | (0.7–82.2) |
| | Completed secondary | 0.5 | (0.1–2.2) | 0.4 | (0.1–1.4) | 0.9 | (0.4–1.9) | 2.2 | (0.2–28.7) |
| | Some college | 0.5 | (0.1–3.0) | 0.3 | (0.1–1.1) | 1.2 | (0.5–2.9) | 3.8 | (0.2–71.0) |
| | Completed college | 1.0 | – | 1.0 | – | 1.0 | – | 1.0 | – |
| | $\chi^2$ | 1.3 | | 7.7 | | 1.6 | | 5.6 | |

*Note:* Based on the Part 2 sample ($n = 887$); calculated using Part 2 weights.
* $p < 0.05$.

prevalence estimate of any DSM-IV disorder in Japan is similar to the prevalence estimates in the WMH surveys in China (Shen et al. 2006) and some European Union countries (Spain, Italy, and Germany) (ESEMeD/MHEDEA 2000 Investigators 2004), but 2–3.5 times lower than in the United States (Kessler et al. 2005), the six countries in ESEMeD (ESEMeD/MHEDEA 2000 Investigators 2004), and Mexico (Medina-Mora et al. 2005). The estimated prevalence of major depression in Japan is equal to that in China (Shen et al. 2006), but considerably lower

**Table 22.4.** Proportion of 12-month mental health treatment by the severity of mental disorders

| Treatment[a] | Severe or moderate | | Mild | | None | | Total | |
|---|---|---|---|---|---|---|---|---|
| | % | (se) | % | (se) | % | (se) | % | (se) |
| Health care | 21.6 | (4.1) | 12.3 | (4.4) | 3.5 | (0.6) | 4.6 | (0.6) |
| Mental health | 19.1 | (4.4) | 9.4 | (4.1) | 1.4 | (0.4) | 2.4 | (0.5) |
| General medical | 8.5 | (3.4) | 7.4 | (3.7) | 2.4 | (0.5) | 2.8 | (0.5) |
| Non–health care | 7.2 | (3.1) | 0.5 | (0.5) | 1.2 | (0.4) | 1.5 | (0.4) |
| Any treatment | 24.3 | (5.1) | 12.8 | (4.4) | 4.5 | (0.9) | 5.6 | (0.9) |
| No treatment | 75.7 | (5.1) | 87.2 | (4.4) | 95.5 | (0.9) | 94.4 | (0.9) |

*Note:* Non–health care includes human services and complementary and alternative medicine.
[a] Health care = general medical (nonpsychiatrist physicians) and mental health (psychiatrists and clinical psychologists).

**Table 22.5.** Demographic correlates of 12-month health-care treatment among subjects who experienced any mental disorder in the past 12 months: The WMH Japan 2002–2004 Surveys

| | | OR | (95% CI) |
|---|---|---|---|
| Sex | Male | 1.0 | – |
| | Female | 1.3 | (0.6–2.6) |
| | $\chi^2$ | 0.4 | |
| Age, years | 18–34 | 0.4 | (0.1–1.3) |
| | 35–49 | 0.5 | (0.1–1.7) |
| | 50–64 | 0.6 | (0.2–2.0) |
| | 65$\leq$ | 1.0 | – |
| | $\chi^2$ | 3.2 | |
| Income | Low | 0.6 | (0.2–2.1) |
| | Average | 0.5 | (0.3–1.1) |
| | High | 1.0 | – |
| | $\chi^2$ | 3.7 | |
| Marital status | Married/cohabiting | 1.0 | – |
| | Not married | 1.0 | (0.5–2.0) |
| | $\chi^2$ | 0.0 | |
| Education | Less than secondary | 0.4 | (0.1–1.7) |
| | Completed secondary | 1.3 | (0.5–3.6) |
| | Some college | 1.1 | (0.4–3.1) |
| | Completed college | 1.0 | – |
| | $\chi^2$ | 3.6 | |
| Severity | Severe | 12.9 | (4.3–39.1) |
| | Moderate | 5.7 | (2.4–13.8) |
| | Mild | 3.8 | (1.5–9.8) |
| | None | 1.0 | – |
| | $\chi^2$ | 48.1* | |

Note: Based on the Part 2 sample ($n = 887$); calculated using Part 2 weights.
* $p < 0.05$.

than in the United States (Kessler et al. 2003) or Europe (ESEMeD/MHEDEA 2000 Investigators 2004). The estimated prevalence of any anxiety disorder in Japan is greater than in the WMH surveys in China (Shen et al. 2006), but lower than in Western countries (Demyttenaere et al. 2004). The 12-month estimated prevalence of PTSD in the present study is greater than in the WMH surveys in China (Shen et al. 2006), similar to Mexico (Medina-Mora et al. 2005) but lower than in the United States (Kessler et al. 2005) or Europe (ESEMeD/MHEDEA 2000 Investigators 2004).

Although the preceding results are consistent with previous surveys in finding that the prevalence of mental disorders is lower in Japan than in Western countries, the 12-month prevalence estimate of alcohol abuse (1.2%) and dependence (0.2%) in Japan was similar to those in the ESEMeD surveys (0.7% and 0.3%, respectively), although lower than in the United States (Kessler et al. 2005) or Mexico (Medina-Mora et al. 2005). Cross-national variations in the prevalence of alcohol abuse/dependence should be reexamined in future research. The estimated 12-month prevalence of drug abuse/dependence was much lower than previously reported in the United States and other Western countries (ESEMeD/MHEDEA 2000 Investigators 2004; Kessler et al. 2005), a finding that is consistent with the fact that the Japanese government has a strong policy of controlling the use of illicit and other psychotropic drugs (Wada et al. 2004).

It remains unclear why mood and anxiety disorders should be less prevalent in Japan than in the United States or Europe. On the basis of data from primary care patients in 14 countries, Simon and colleagues (2002) have suggested that a cross-national difference in the prevalence of major depression is not due to a fallacy in measurement associated with a differential nature of the expression of the disorder or differential validity of assessment, but possibly to a difference in diagnostic threshold across countries. However, our study found that the prevalence of severe major depression (as well as other disorders assessed here) was also lower in Japan than in the United States (Kessler et al. 2003) and Europe (ESEMeD/MHEDEA 2000 Investigators 2004). On the basis of this result, the differential threshold explanation seems implausible. The possibilities still exist that differential validity of the CIDI or differential willingness of Japanese survey respondents to admit emotional problems to interviewers might be involved in explaining at least part of the pattern, but final evaluation of this possibility awaits the implementation of a rigorous CIDI clinical reappraisal study in Japan.

The 12-month prevalence of major depression (2.1%) in the study was almost double the six-month prevalence (1.2%) in a previous community-based survey conducted in 1997–1998 in Japan (Kawakami et al. 2004). It is noteworthy that, consistent with this finding, the Japan Ministry of Health, Labour, and Welfare reported a marked increase in treated mood disorders between the 1999 and 2002 Patient Statistics (Japan Ministry of Health Labour and Welfare 2001 and 2004). The suicide rate in Japan dramatically increased in 1998 (Lamar 2000). Although the prevalence of major depression may vary among diagnostic criteria and target communities, there is a remaining possibility that the prevalence of major depression recently increased in Japan.

## 4.2. Correlates of Mental Disorders in Japan

Mood disorders, as well as any disorder, were more prevalent among respondents who were not currently married, which is consistent with previous studies in other countries (WHO International Consortium in Psychiatric Epidemiology 2000). Although the association was not statistically significant, the higher prevalence of mood disorder among the middle-aged may reflect social distress among this generation. It is noteworthy that the suicide rate is also high in this age group in Japan (Lamar 2000). The higher prevalence of mood disorders among those with higher education observed in this study also agrees with a previous observation of a cross-national difference in the effect of education on the prevalence of mood disorder (Andrade et al. 2003), where prevalence was positively related to education in Japan but inversely related to education in the United States and the Netherlands. This replication across studies argues that this finding is reliable, and it raises questions about the special circumstances in Japan that might lead to a high prevalence of mental disorders in the socially advantaged segments of society that are typically found to have low prevalence in other countries. More detailed investigation of this interesting specification is currently underway.

## 4.3. Medical Treatment Rates for Mental Disorders in Japan

More than three-fourths of the respondents with a serious-moderate 12-month mental disorder in the WMH-Japan survey failed to receive any treatment in the months before interview. Treatment was even less common among respondents with mild 12-month disorders. These low treatment rates are roughly equal to those found in the WMH surveys in Mexico and Colombia and higher than those in China, but considerably lower than those found in the United States or Europe (Demyttenaere et al. 2004). This low treatment rate, unlike the situation in Mexico and Colombia, where the main barriers may involve access, probably more strongly involves stigma and psychological barriers to seek treatment in Japan (Jorm et al. 2005). A major objective of a mental health policy in Japan should be to provide medical treatment for those suffering from a severe or moderate mental disorder, but the results reported here suggest that the success of this agenda might hinge as much on public education and antistigma media campaigns than on the provision of treatment resources.

## 4.4. Correlates of Medical Treatments for Mental Disorders in Japan

Although the difference was not significant, it is noteworthy that those who had completed high school or attended some college were significantly more likely to seek medical treatment than were those who had graduated from college. This finding raises the possibility that individuals on each end of the educational spectrum may be reluctant to seek medical treatment for mental disorders. Those with the least education may lack knowledge of mental disorders and their treatments, and the more educated may face psychological barriers, such as fear of losing social status, a threat to job security, or humiliation, which might prevent them from seeking care. Given that this result was not statistically significant, though, replication is needed in additional waves of the WMH-Japan survey before it is considered reliable.

## 4.5. Implications for Mental Health Policy in Japan

Among 102 million adults aged 20 years or over in Japan, 7 million (7%) were estimated in the WMH-Japan survey to have experienced a DSM-IV mental disorder in the past 12 months. The present study also indicated that the majority of these people did not seek medical treatment. A primary objective of a future mental health policy in Japan should be to increase medical treatment rates for those experiencing clinically significant mental disorders. Providing education, training, and dissemination of information to communities could be a useful approach to achieve this aim. The estimated number of individuals who have experienced mental disorders could not be managed by the current psychiatrists in Japan, who numbered only 11,790 in 2002 (Japan Ministry of Health, Labour and Welfare 2003). To meet this unmet need for treatment, psychiatrists should treat cases with severe or comorbid mental disorders, whereas nonpsychiatrists should be trained to treat moderate or mild mental disorders with a liaison between nonpsychiatrists and psychiatrists. A future effort should also be made for the primary prevention of mental disorders, although the existence of so many currently untreated cases with existing mental disorders makes it important for the needs of these current cases to be addressed first. The WMH-Japan survey has obtained more data from additional communities in Japan and just finished in 2006. The final results will be coming soon.

## 4.6. The WMH-Japan Survey 2002–2004

The first reports from the WMH-Japan survey provided the prevalence estimates and treatment rates for mental disorders in Japan (Kawakami et al. 2005; Naganuma et al. 2006) using the internationally standardized method of assessment of mental disorders and help seeking, the WMH Survey Initiative Version of the WHO CIDI (Kessler & Üstün 2004). However, the sample size of the study ($n = 1663$) was still small, particularly for Part 2 interviews ($n = 477$), and limited to only three areas in Japan. In this chapter, we expanded our data to include a total of 2437 respondents living in seven areas in Japan, by adding data collected in the study years 2003–2004 (from the WMH-Japan Survey 2002–2004) to reanalyze and confirm these marked cross-national differences in the prevalences and medical treatment rates for mental disorders, and to examine their sociodemographic correlates.

## REFERENCES

American Psychiatric Association (1994). *Diagnostic and statistical manual of mental disorders (DSM-IV)*, 4th ed. Washington, DC: American Psychiatric Association.

Andrade, L., Caraveo-Anduaga, J. J., Berglund, P., Bijl, R. V., De Graaf, R., Vollebergh, W., Dragomirecka, E., Kohn, R., Keller, M., Kessler, R. C., Kawakami, N., Kilic, C., Offord, D., Üstün, T. B. & Wittchen, H.-U. (2003). The epidemiology of major depressive episodes: Results from the International Consortium of Psychiatric Epidemiology (ICPE) Surveys. *International Journal of Methods in Psychiatric Research*, 12, 3–21.

Canino, G. J., Bird, H. R., Shrout, P. E., Rubio-Stipec, M., Bravo, M., Martinez, R., Sesman, M. & Guevara, L. M. (1987). The prevalence of specific psychiatric disorders in Puerto Rico. *Archives of General Psychiatry*, 44, 727–35.

Chen, C. N., Wong, J., Lee, N., Chan-Ho, M. W., Lau, J. T. & Fung, M. (1993). The Shatin community mental health survey in Hong Kong: II. Major findings. *Archives of General Psychiatry*, 50, 125–33.

Cross-National Collaborative Group (1992). The changing rate of major depression: Cross-national comparisons. *Journal of the American Medical Association*, 268, 3098–105.

Demyttenaere, K., Bruffaerts, R., Posada-Villa, J., Gasquet, I., Kovess, V., Lepine, J. P., Angermeyer, M. C., Bernert, S., de Girolamo, G., Morosini, P., Polidori, G., Kikkawa, T., Kawakami, N., Ono, Y., Takeshima, T., Uda, H., Karam, E. G., Fayyad, J. A., Karam, A. N., Mneimneh, Z. N., Medina-Mora, M. E., Borges, G., Lara, C., de Graaf, R., Ormel, J., Gureje, O., Shen, Y., Huang, Y., Zhang, M., Alonso, J., Haro, J. M., Vilagut, G., Bromet, E. J., Gluzman, S., Webb, C., Kessler, R. C., Merikangas, K. R., Anthony, J. C., Von Korff, M. R., Wang, P. S., Brugha, T. S., Aguilar-Gaxiola, S., Lee, S., Heeringa, S., Pennell, B.-E., Zaslavsky, A. M., Üstün, T. B. & Chatterji, S. (2004).

Prevalence, severity and unmet need for treatment of mental disorders in the World Health Organization World Mental Health surveys. *Journal of the American Medical Association*, 291, 2581–90.

Endicott, J., Spitzer, R. L., Fleiss, J. L. & Cohen, J. (1976). The global assessment scale: A procedure for measuring overall severity of psychiatric disturbance. *Archives of General Psychiatry*, 33, 766–71.

ESEMeD/MHEDEA 2000 Investigators (2004). Prevalence of mental disorders in Europe: Results from the European Study of the Epidemiology of Mental Disorders (ESEMeD) project. *Acta Psychiatrica Scandinavica Supplement*, 21–7.

Helzer, J. E., Canino, G. J., Yeh, E. K., Bland, R. C., Lee, C. K., Hwu, H. G. & Newman, S. (1990). Alcoholism – North America and Asia: A comparison of population surveys with the Diagnostic Interview Schedule. *Archives of General Psychiatry*, 47, 313–9.

Hwu, H. G., Yeh, E. K. & Chang, L. Y. (1989). Prevalence of psychiatric disorders in Taiwan defined by the Chinese Diagnostic Interview Schedule. *Acta Psychiatrica Scandinavica*, 79, 136–47.

Japan Ministry of Health, Labour and Welfare (2001–2004). *Patient survey 1999 and 2002*. Tokyo: Health and Welfare Statistics Association.

Japan Ministry of Health, Labour and Welfare (2003). *Doctors, dentists and pharmacologists survey 2002*. Tokyo: Health and Welfare Statistics Association.

Jorm, A. F., Nakane, Y., Christensen, H., Yoshioka, K., Griffiths, K. M. & Wata, Y. (2005). Public beliefs about treatment and outcome of mental disorders: A comparison of Australia and Japan. *BioMed Central Medicine*, 3, 12.

Kawakami, N., Shimizu, H., Haratani, T., Iwata, N. & Kitamura, T. (2004). Lifetime and 6-month prevalence of DSM-III-R psychiatric disorders in an urban community in Japan. *Psychiatry Research*, 121, 293–301.

Kawakami, N., Takeshima, T., Ono, Y., Uda, H., Hata, Y., Nakane, Y., Nakane, H., Iwata, N., Furukawa, T. A. & Kikkawa, T. (2005). Twelve-month prevalence, severity, and treatment of common mental disorders in communities in Japan: Preliminary finding from the World Health Organization Japan Survey 2002–2003. *Psychiatry and Clinical Neurosciences*, 59, 441–52.

Kessler, R. C., Berglund, P., Demler, O., Jin, R., Koretz, D., Merikangas, K. R., Rush, A. J., Walters, E. E. & Wang, P. S. (2003). The epidemiology of major depressive disorder: Results from the National Comorbidity Survey Replication (NCS-R). *Journal of the American Medical Association*, 289, 3095–105.

Kessler, R. C., Chiu, W. T., Demler, O., Merikangas, K. R. & Walters, E. E. (2005). Prevalence, severity, and comorbidity of 12-month DSM-IV disorders in the National Comorbidity Survey Replication. *Archives of General Psychiatry*, 62, 617–27.

Kessler, R. C., McGonagle, K. A., Zhao, S., Nelson, C. B., Hughes, M., Eshleman, S., Wittchen, H.-U. & Kendler, K. S. (1994). Lifetime and 12-month prevalence of DSM-III-R psychiatric disorders in the United States: Results from the National Comorbidity Survey. *Archives of General Psychiatry*, 51, 8–19.

Kessler, R. C. & Üstün, T. B. (2004). The World Mental Health (WMH) Survey Initiative Version of the World Health Organization (WHO) Composite International Diagnostic Interview (CIDI). *International Journal of Methods in Psychiatric Research*, 13, 93–121.

Kikkawa, T. & Takeuchi, T. (1980). Mental health surveys. In *Social psychiatry and mental health part III*, ed. I. Sato & T. Miyamoto, pp. 156–88. Tokyo: Nakayama-shoten.

Kitamura, T., Fujihara, S., Iwata, N., Tomoda, A. & Kawakami, N. (1999). Epidemiology of psychiatric disorders in Japan. In *Images in psychiatry: Japan*, ed. Y. Nakane & M. Radford, pp. 37–46. Paris: World Psychiatric Association.

Lamar, J. (2000). Suicides in Japan reach a record high. *British Medical Journal*, 321, 528.

Lee, C. K., Kwak, Y. S., Yamamoto, J., Rhee, H., Kim, Y. S., Han, J. H., Choi, J. O. & Lee, Y. H. (1990). Psychiatric epidemiology in Korea – Part I: Gender and age differences in Seoul. *Journal of Nervous and Mental Disease*, 178, 242–6.

Leon, A. C., Olfson, M., Portera, L., Farber, L. & Sheehan, D. V. (1997). Assessing psychiatric impairment in primary care with the Sheehan Disability Scale. *International Journal of Psychiatry in Medicine*, 27, 93–105.

Medina-Mora, M. E., Borges, G., Lara, C., Benjet, C., Blanco, J., Fleiz, C., Villatoro, J., Rojas, E. & Zambrano, J. (2005). Prevalence, service use, and demographic correlates of 12-month DSM-IV psychiatric disorders in Mexico: Results from the Mexican National Comorbidity Survey. *Psychological Medicine*, 35, 1773–83.

Naganuma, Y., Tachimori, H., Kawakami, N., Takeshima, T., Ono, Y., Uda, H., Hata, Y., Nakane, Y., Nakane, H., Iwata, N., Furukawa, T. A. & Kikkawa, T. (2006). Twelve-month use of mental health services in four areas in Japan: Findings from the World Mental Health Japan Survey 2002–2003. *Psychiatry and Clinical Neurosciences*, 60, 240–8.

Regier, D. A., Myers, J. K., Kramer, M., Robins, L. N., Blazer, D. G., Hough, R. L., Eaton, W. W. & Locke, B. Z. (1984). The NIMH Epidemiologic Catchment

Area program: Historical context, major objectives, and study population characteristics. *Archives of General Psychiatry*, 41, 934–41.

Research Triangle Institute (2002). *SUDAAN: Professional software for survey data analysis.* Research Triangle Park, NC: Research Triangle Institute.

Sakai, A., Ito, K. & Takeuchi, K. (2003). Reliability and validity. In *A study on methods used in epidemiologic studies on mental health: 2002 research report*, ed. T. Kikkawa, pp. 107–8. Kodaira, Japan: National Institute of Mental Health, National Center of Neurology and Psychiatry.

Shen, Y. C., Zhang, M. Y., Huang, Y. Q., He, Y. L., Liu, Z. R., Cheng, H., Tsang, A., Lee, S. & Kessler, R. C. (2006). Twelve-month prevalence, severity, and unmet need for treatment of mental disorders in metropolitan China. *Psychological Medicine*, 36, 257–67.

Simon, G. E., Goldberg, D. P., Von Korff, M. & Üstün, T. B. (2002). Understanding cross-national differences in depression prevalence. *Psychological Medicine*, 32, 585–94.

Wada, K., Kikuchi, A., Nakano, R. & Ozaki, S. (2004). Current situation on drug abuse in Japan: Using a general population survey and a junior high school students survey. *Nihon Arukoru Yakubutsu Igakkai Zasshi*, 39, 28–34.

Weissman, M. M., Myers, J. K. & Harding, P. S. (1978). Psychiatric disorders in a U.S. urban community: 1975–1976. *American Journal of Psychiatry*, 135, 459–62.

WHO International Consortium in Psychiatric Epidemiology (2000). Cross-national comparisons of the prevalences and correlates of mental disorders. *Bulletin of the World Health Organization*, 78, 413–26.

# 23 Te Rau Hinengaro: The New Zealand Mental Health Survey

MARK A. OAKLEY-BROWNE, J. ELISABETH WELLS, AND KATE M. SCOTT

## ACKNOWLEDGMENTS

Te Rau Hinengaro: The New Zealand Mental Health Survey (NZMHS) was funded by the New Zealand Ministry of Health, the Alcohol Advisory Council of New Zealand, and the Health Research Council of New Zealand. Research team members are affiliated with the University of Auckland, Massey University, University of Otago (New Zealand), Monash University (Australia), the New Zealand Ministry of Health, and the World Health Organization. Members of the NZMHS Research Team are J. Baxter, M. H. Durie, S. Foliaki, C. Gale, J. Kokaua, T. K. Kingi, M. A. McGee, M. A. Oakley-Browne, K. M. Scott, R. Tapsell, C. Tukuitonga, D. Schaaf, and J. E. Wells.

We thank the WMH staff for assistance with instrumentation, fieldwork, and data analysis. These activities were supported by the U.S. National Institute of Mental Health (R01MH070884), the John D. and Catherine T. MacArthur Foundation, the Pfizer Foundation, the U.S. Public Health Service (R13-MH066849, R01-MH069864, and R01 DA016558), the Fogarty International Center (FIRCA R03-TW006481), the Pan American Health Organization, Eli Lilly and Company Foundation, Ortho-McNeil Pharmaceutical, GlaxoSmithKline, and Bristol-Myers Squibb. A complete list of WMH publications is available at http://www.hcp.med.harvard.edu/wmh/.

We thank the Kaitiaki group and the Pacific Advisory group for their input and support for this survey and we thank all the participants.

## I. INTRODUCTION

New Zealand is an island country in the southwestern Pacific. It has a population of 4.1 million and is of similar size (270,500 square kilometers) to Great Britain. More than 85% of the population lives in urban areas with the major centers being Auckland and Wellington (the capital). Twenty-two percent of the population is younger than 15 years and 16% is older than 60 years. The life expectancy at birth is 77.0 years for males and 81.3 years for females (Statistics New Zealand 2006b). The largest ethnic groups are European (80.0%), Māori (14.7%), persons of Asian descent (6.6%) and persons of Pacific descent (6.5%) (Statistics New Zealand 2002). Both Māori and English are official languages, but education is nearly all in English. The literacy rate is 99% for men and women. In 2004, the standardized unemployment rate was 3.9%. New Zealand is a high-income-group country with an annual gross domestic product (GDP) of US$80 billion and a GDP per capita of US$19,800.00 (Statistics New Zealand 2006a).

In New Zealand, the proportion of health budget to GDP is 8.3%. About 11% of the total health budget is spent on mental health (Ministry of Health 2003; World Health Organization 2005). Hospital and community-based mental health services are funded by the government. The cost of attendance at primary care is partially subsidized by the government, but patients are usually required to pay an additional fee for service. Patients are also required to pay a proportion of the costs of medications and pathology and other investigations. Private health insurance provides very limited mental health coverage. Specialist mental health services are required to target delivery of services to persons with severe mental disorder, estimated to be about 3% of the population at any time. Deinstitutionalization of specialist mental health services was completed about 15 years ago. Current provision of care is largely based within the community. Community-based mental health services form about 68% of all specialist mental health services. Persons with mild to moderate disorder are mostly cared for within primary care. Since the release of a primary care strategy in 2001 (Ministry of Health 2001), there has been increased emphasis on the integration of primary care and specialist mental health services (World Health Organization 2005).

In New Zealand, there has been no previous national survey of mental disorders in the community. Two regional surveys were conducted in the 1980s: a survey of rural and urban women living in the province of Otago (Romans-Clarkson et al. 1988; 1990) and a survey of adults aged 18–64 years living in the Christchurch urban region (Oakley-Browne et al. 1989; Wells et al. 1989). Birth cohort studies in Dunedin (University of Otago n.d.) and Christchurch (Christchurch School of Medicine & Health Sciences n.d.) have measured mental disorders, but because of the young age of these cohorts, now in their twenties and early thirties, these studies have not been able to present a comprehensive picture spanning adult age groups.

In 1997, the Australian National Mental Health Survey was carried out (Henderson, Andrews & Hall 2000; Andrews, Henderson & Hall 2001) using a version of the CIDI that focused on the past 12 months. This survey was at that time the largest such survey, the first to make DSM-IV diagnoses, and also a survey that attempted to measure disability in addition to disorder. The New Zealand Ministry of Health decided that a national study was required in New Zealand to inform policy. A tender for a pilot study was let in 1999 and was won by the present research team, which carried out consultation, a literature review, and trial interviews. To meet the New Zealand need for national data, the research team joined the WMH Survey Consortium (Kessler et al. 2006), becoming one of the countries in this international survey program. This enabled access to the revised CIDI and considerable support and advice on quality control and survey design. Because of concerns about mental health in Māori, and in Pacific peo-

ple, the Ministry of Health wanted estimates for these ethnic groups as well as national estimates. Māori are the indigenous people of New Zealand. Within New Zealand, the term "Pacific" is used to refer to people whose ethnicity is that of the indigenous inhabitants of Pacific islands such as Samoa, Tonga, the Cook Islands, and Fiji.

The objectives for the New Zealand survey as specified by the Ministry of Health were, for the total New Zealand, Māori, and Pacific populations living in New Zealand, the following:

- Describe the 1-month, 12-month, and lifetime prevalence rates of major mental disorders among people aged 16 years and over living in private dwellings, by sociodemographic variables.
- Describe patterns of and barriers to health service use for people with mental disorders.
- Describe the level of disability associated with mental disorders.
- Provide baseline data and calibrate brief instruments measuring mental disorders and psychological distress to inform the use of these instruments in future national health surveys.

All of these objectives were met within Te Rau Hinengaro ("the many minds"): The New Zealand Mental Health Survey (NZMHS).

Te Rau Hinengaro provides important information not previously available about the prevalence of mental disorders, their patterns of onset, and their impact for adults in New Zealand. Of particular note is that the survey design and sampling frame enabled the participation of sufficient numbers of Māori and Pacific people to allow estimates of acceptable precision for these ethnic groups. In the main reports for Te Rau Hinengaro, ethnicity-specific results are presented (Baxter et al. 2006a, 2006b; Foliaki et al. 2006a, 2006b; Oakley-Browne, Wells & Scott 2006; Wells et al. 2006a). However, this is not done in this chapter because, in this volume, analyses have been standardized across countries and ethnicity breakdowns differ across countries. Similarly, for comparability across countries only participants aged 18 years and older are included in the analyses presented in this chapter.

## 2. METHODS

### 2.1. Sample

The NZMHS is a nationally representative survey of the population aged 16 years and older living in private dwellings in New Zealand (Oakley-Browne et al. 2006). Results reported in this chapter are for respondents aged 18 years and older. The distinctive features of the New Zealand survey were extensive oversampling (Māori and Pacific people) and the small size of the primary sampling units (PSUs). These were census blocks (called meshblocks) originally set up to contain 40 to 70 households. The PSUs in each stratum were systematically selected from within district health boards throughout the whole country, and there was no clustering above the PSU level. Oversampling was carried out through targeting and screening. Targeting involved preferentially selecting meshblocks in one stratum. Meshblocks in which 55% or more of the population reported Pacific ethnicity in the 2001 Census of Population and Dwellings were placed in the high Pacific stratum and sampled with a much higher probability than meshblocks in the general stratum. Everyone was eligible in the high Pacific stratum. Screening occurred in the general stratum meshblocks; in about 11 households, everyone was eligible; in about 16 households, only Māori and Pacific people were eligible; and in the remaining households, only Pacific people were eligible.

Interviews were obtained from 12,992 respondents between November 2003 and December 2004. Part 1 included a core diagnostic assessment plus sections on suicidal behaviors, service use, and demographics, and it was administered to all respondents. Part 2 assessed additional disorder, measures of psychological distress and disability, and chronic physical conditions. Part 2 was administered to all Part 1 respondents who met certain criteria such as Part 1 lifetime disorders plus a probability sample of other respondents. The overall response rate was 73.3%. The NZMHS recruitment, consent, and field procedures were approved by all 14 regional ethics committees with the Auckland Y Ethics Committee serving as the lead committee.

A fuller presentation of the NZMHS sample design is presented elsewhere (Wells, McGee & Oakley-Browne 2006).

### 2.2. Measures

#### 2.2.1. Diagnostic Assessment of Lifetime and 12-month DSM-IV Disorders

DSM-IV diagnoses were made using Version 3.0 of the World Health Organization (WHO) Composite International Diagnostic Interview (CIDI) (Kessler & Üstün 2004; see also Chapter 4). This fully structured lay-administered diagnostic interview generates diagnoses according to the definitions and criteria of both the ICD-10 (World Health Organization 1991, 1993) and DSM-IV (American Psychiatric Association 1994) diagnostic systems. DSM-IV criteria are used in analyses for this chapter. A detailed discussion of the instrument is presented in Chapter 4 of this volume and is not repeated here. The disorders considered in this chapter include mood disorders (major depressive episode [MDE], dysthymia [DYS], and bipolar disorder), anxiety disorders (panic disorder [PD], agoraphobia without panic [AG], specific phobia [SP], social phobia [SoP], generalized anxiety disorder [GAD], and posttraumatic stress disorder [PTSD]), and substance disorders (alcohol and drug abuse and dependence [AA, DA, AD, DD, respectively]). Abuse is reported with or without dependence. Dependence was assessed only in those who reported abuse at any time. Lifetime diagnosis, age of onset, and the occurrence of episodes or symptoms in the past 12 months were assessed for each disorder (Oakley-Browne 2006; Oakley-Browne et al. 2006b; Wells 2006; Wells et al. 2006a). All diagnoses are considered with organic exclusions and without diagnostic hierarchy rules unless specified. As described in Chapter 6 in this volume, a blinded clinical reappraisal study using the Structured Clinical Interview for DSM-IV (SCID) (First et al. 2002) showed generally good concordance between DSM-IV diagnoses based on the CIDI and on the SCID for anxiety, mood, and substance disorders.

## 2.2.2. Severity of 12-month Cases

For this chapter, 12-month cases were classified by severity using the same algorithm as for other WMH surveys in this volume. Note that this algorithm differs slightly from that used for the New Zealand data in non-WMH publications (Wells, McGee & Oakley-Browne 2006; Wells et al. 2006a, 2006b). In those publications, the more stringent NCS-R definition was used for substance dependence (Kessler & Merikangas 2004; Kessler et al. 2005b): dependence was classified as serious only if there was serious role impairment, as defined by disorder-specific impairment questions, not just physiological impairment.

## 2.2.3. Initial Lifetime Treatment Contact

Near the end of each CIDI diagnostic section, respondents were asked whether they had ever in their life "talked to a medical doctor or other professional" about the disorder under investigation. In asking this question, the interviewer clarified that the term "other professional" was meant to apply broadly to include "psychologists, counselors, spiritual advisors, herbalists, naturopaths, homeopaths, acupuncturists, and any other healing professionals." Respondents who reported having ever talked to any of these professionals about the disorder in question were then asked how old they were the first time they did so. The response to this question was used to define age of first treatment contact (Oakley-Browne & Wells 2006; Oakley-Browne et al. 2006a).

## 2.2.4. 12-month Use of Mental Health Services

All respondents were asked whether they had ever received treatment for "problems with your emotions or nerves or your use of alcohol or drugs." Separate assessments were made for different types of professionals, support groups, self-help groups, mental health crisis hotlines (assumed to be visits with nonpsychiatrist mental health specialists), complementary and alternative medicine (CAM) therapies, and use of other treatment settings including admissions to hos-

pitals and other facilities (each day of admission was assumed to include a visit with a psychiatrist). Follow-up questions asked about age at first and most recent contacts as well as number and duration of visits in the past 12 months.

Reports of 12-month service use were classified into the following categories: psychiatrist; nonpsychiatrist mental health specialist (psychologist or other nonpsychiatrist mental health professional in any setting, social worker or counselor in a mental health specialty setting, use of a mental health hotline); general medical provider (primary care doctor, other general medical doctor, nurse, any other health professional not previously mentioned); human services professional (religious or spiritual advisor, social worker or counselor in any setting other than a specialty mental health setting); and CAM professional (any other type of healer such as chiropractors, participation in an Internet support group, participation in a self-help group). Psychiatrist and nonpsychiatrist specialist categories were combined into a broader mental health specialty (MHS) category; MHS was also combined with general medical (GM) into an even broader health care (HC) category. Human services (HS) and CAM were also combined into a non–healthcare (NHC) category.

Because the pharmacology section was omitted in New Zealand, it was not possible to calculate the percentage receiving minimally adequate treatment, using the standard WMH definitions (Wang et al. 2007a).

## 2.2.5. Predictor Variables

Predictor variables in analyses of lifetime data include age of onset (AOO) of the focal disorder (coded into the categories early, middle, and late with approximately one third in each category, cohort (defined by age at interview in the categories 18–34, 35–49, 50–64, 65+), sex, education (categorized as no educational qualifications, 10 years or less of education; some secondary school qualifications, 11 or 12 years; completed secondary school or gained trade certificate postsecondary school, 13 years; postsecondary school diploma or degree, 14 or more years), and marital status (categorized as currently married/cohabiting, previously married, or never married). The last two of these predictors vary within a given individual over time. Information on years of education was coded as a time-varying predictor by assuming an orderly educational history for each respondent in which eight years of education corresponds to being a student up to age 14, and other lengths of education are associated with ages consistent with this benchmark (e.g., 12 years of education is assumed to correspond to being a student up to age 18). However, the only temporal information about marital history was the age of first marriage.

Variables in analyses of 12-month data included sex, cohort, education, and marital status (all categorized as described previously). In addition, family income was equivalized by dividing the total income by the number in the household. The low category was up to half the median of equivalized income, low-medium was from above low up to the median, medium was from above low-medium up to two times the median, and high was above two times the median.

## 2.3. Analysis Procedures

The data were weighted to account for different probabilities of selection resulting from oversampling and the selection of one person per household, differential nonresponse, and adjustment for residual differences between the sample and the New Zealand population at the 2001 census, cross-classified by age, sex, and ethnicity (Māori, Pacific people, and the composite "other" group). An additional weight was used in the Part 2 sample to adjust for differences in probability of selection into that sample. These procedures are described in more detail elsewhere (Wells, McGee & Oakley-Browne 2006; Wells et al. 2006b). Survival analysis was used to make estimated projections of cumulative lifetime probability of disorders and treatment contact from year of onset. The actuarial method implemented in SAS V8.2 (SAS Institute 2001) was used rather than the more familiar Kaplan-

Meier method (Kaplan & Meier 1958) of generating survival curves because the former has an advantage over the latter in estimating onsets within a year. The typical duration of delay in initial treatment contact was defined on the basis of these curves as the median number of years from disorder onset to first treatment contact among cases that eventually made treatment contact.

Discrete-time survival analysis (Efron 1988) with person-year as the unit of analysis was used to examine correlates of disorders and treatment contact. Basic patterns of 12-month disorders and service use were examined by computing proportions, means, and medians. Logistic regression analysis was used to study sociodemographic predictors of having 12-month disorders, receiving any 12-month treatment in the total sample, treatment in particular sectors among those receiving any treatment, and treatment meeting criteria for minimal adequacy.

For these WMH analyses the 1318 PSUs were aggregated into pairs of adjacent sampling-error correction units (SECUs) within 166 pseudo-strata. Each SECU was formed by combining PSUs in an area to result in 25–50 interviews per SECU (50–100 interviews per stratum). Standard errors were estimated using the Taylor series method as implemented in SUDAAN (Research Triangle Institute 2002). This procedure has resulted in standard errors identical or nearly identical to those calculated using the actual survey design (comparisons available on request). Multivariable significance tests were made using Wald $\chi^2$ tests based on coefficient variance-covariance matrices that were adjusted for design effects using the Taylor series method. Statistical significance was evaluated using two-sided design-based tests and the 0.05 level of significance.

## 3. RESULTS

### 3.1. The Sample

The sociodemographic distributions of the Part 1 and Part 2 samples are shown relative to the New Zealand population in Table 23.1. The unweighted data show the effects of oversampling,

**Table 23.1.** Sociodemographic distribution of the New Zealand sample (aged 18+) compared to the population

| | Part 1 unweighted | Part 2 unweighted | Part 1 weighted[a] | Part 2 weighted[a] | Census[b] |
|---|---|---|---|---|---|
| **Sex** | | | | | |
| Male | 43.3 | 40.5 | 48.0 | 47.9 | 47.9 |
| Female | 56.7 | 59.6 | 52.0 | 52.2 | 52.1 |
| **Age** | | | | | |
| 18–24 | 10.4 | 12.4 | 14.0 | 14.0 | 12.7 |
| 25–34 | 18.9 | 20.4 | 19.1 | 19.1 | 19.4 |
| 35–44 | 22.6 | 23.6 | 21.4 | 21.7 | 21.7 |
| 45–54 | 17.6 | 18.6 | 18.0 | 18.0 | 18.2 |
| 55–64 | 13.0 | 12.4 | 12.2 | 12.3 | 12.4 |
| 65+ | 17.5 | 12.7 | 15.4 | 15.4 | 15.6 |
| **Ethnicity** | | | | | |
| Māori | 19.8 | 22.0 | 10.9 | 10.9 | 10.9 |
| Pacific | 17.0 | 17.8 | 4.5 | 4.5 | 4.5 |
| Other[c] | 63.1 | 60.2 | 84.6 | 84.6 | 84.6 |

[a] Part 1 and Part 2 samples were each poststratified to the joint distribution of sex, age, and ethnicity using the full age range of 16 years or more. For this chapter only those aged 18 or more were included for which Part 1 sample size = 12,790, Part 2 sample size = 7315.

[b] 2001 Census of Population and Dwellings. The age group 18–24 was assumed to be seven-ninths of the population aged 16–24.

[c] "Other" is a composite group consisting mainly of New Zealanders of European descent.

with Māori comprising 19.8% of the sample and Pacific comprising 17.0% of the sample. After weighting, these proportions reduced to 10.9% and 4.5%, respectively.

## 3.2. Lifetime Prevalence

The estimated lifetime prevalence of any DSM-IV/CIDI mental disorder in the New Zealand population is 39.3%, with 24.6% experiencing any anxiety disorder, 20.4% any mood disorder, and 12.4% any substance use disorder (Table 23.2). The experience of comorbidity is common, with two or more disorders occurring among 19.9% of the population, and three or more disorders occurring among 10.7% of the population. The individual disorder with the highest lifetime prevalence, by a considerable margin, is major depressive disorder (16.2%).

Age is significantly related to lifetime prevalence of disorder. For all disorder groups, the oldest age group (65+) has the lowest estimated prevalence. For anxiety and mood disorder groups, prevalences are fairly similar across the younger three age groups, but then drop off sharply in the oldest age group. For substance use disorders, there is a decrease in prevalence of disorder with increasing age.

## 3.3. Lifetime Risk

Table 23.3 shows the ages at selected percentiles on the AOO distributions of disorders and projected lifetime risk at age 75. The picture emerging from this table is that mental disorders generally begin in the earlier part of people's lives, with the median (50th percentile) AOO for any disorder being age 18. There is considerable variability in AOO both between and within disorder groups. Anxiety disorders have the earliest onset, with the median age of onset for any anxiety disorder of 14, though this ranges from 8 for SP, to 32 for GAD. Mood disorders generally occur later in life, with a median AOO of 31.

The lifetime risk of disorder for the population is 48.6% (Table 23.3). The difference

**Table 23.2.** Lifetime prevalence for Part 1 and Part 2 samples of DSM-IV/CIDI disorders

| DX group | DX | n | Total | | 18–34 | | 35–49 | | 50–64 | | 65+ | | χ² | DF | p |
|---|---|---|---|---|---|---|---|---|---|---|---|---|---|---|---|
| | | | % | (se) | % | (se) | % | (se) | % | (se) | % | (se) | | | |
| Anxiety | Panic DX | 411 | 2.8 | (0.2) | 3.1 | (0.3) | 3.4 | (0.3) | 2.2 | (0.3) | 1.4 | (0.3) | 26.6 | 3 | <0.001 |
| | GAD with hierarchy | 810 | 6.1 | (0.3) | 5.2 | (0.6) | 7.4 | (0.5) | 6.8 | (0.6) | 4.6 | (0.5) | 17.9 | 3 | 0.001 |
| | Social phobia | 1283 | 9.5 | (0.3) | 10.9 | (0.6) | 10.7 | (0.6) | 9.6 | (0.8) | 3.8 | (0.4) | 115.8 | 3 | <0.001 |
| | Specific phobia | 1548 | 10.9 | (0.4) | 12.9 | (0.7) | 11.1 | (0.6) | 11.5 | (0.8) | 5.3 | (0.6) | 89.4 | 3 | <0.001 |
| | Agoraphobia without panic | 191 | 1.2 | (0.1) | 1.3 | (0.2) | 1.8 | (0.2) | 0.8 | (0.2) | 0.5 | (0.1) | 25.7 | 3 | <0.001 |
| | PTSD[a] | 826 | 6.1 | (0.3) | 5.9 | (0.5) | 6.3 | (0.5) | 7.3 | (0.8) | 4.1 | (0.9) | 8.6 | 3 | 0.038 |
| | Any anxiety[a] | 3171 | 24.6 | (0.7) | 27.5 | (1.3) | 26.3 | (1.1) | 25.4 | (1.4) | 14.2 | (1.2) | 53.4 | 3 | <0.001 |
| Mood | MDD with hierarchy | 2084 | 16.2 | (0.4) | 16.2 | (0.8) | 18.4 | (0.8) | 17.7 | (0.9) | 9.8 | (0.8) | 69.7 | 3 | <0.001 |
| | Dysthymia with hierarchy | 303 | 2.2 | (0.2) | 2.2 | (0.3) | 2.1 | (0.3) | 2.7 | (0.4) | 1.3 | (0.3) | 11.3 | 3 | 0.012 |
| | Bipolar (broad) | 617 | 3.9 | (0.2) | 5.8 | (0.5) | 4.3 | (0.4) | 2.6 | (0.4) | 0.6 | (0.2) | 155.7 | 3 | <0.001 |
| | Any mood | 2755 | 20.4 | (0.5) | 22.1 | (0.9) | 23.1 | (0.9) | 20.8 | (1.0) | 10.6 | (0.8) | 125.7 | 3 | <0.001 |
| Substance | Alcohol abuse w/without dependence | 1649 | 11.5 | (0.4) | 17.0 | (0.9) | 11.1 | (0.6) | 9.0 | (0.7) | 4.0 | (0.5) | 176.0 | 3 | <0.001 |
| | Alcohol dependence with abuse | 663 | 4.1 | (0.2) | 6.1 | (0.5) | 4.5 | (0.4) | 2.6 | (0.4) | 0.7 | (0.2) | 153.8 | 3 | <0.001 |
| | Drug abuse w/without dependence | 749 | 5.3 | (0.3) | 10.5 | (0.7) | 4.8 | (0.4) | 1.6 | (0.3) | 0.0 | (0.0) | 376.5 | 3 | <0.001 |
| | Drug dependence with abuse | 330 | 2.2 | (0.2) | 4.4 | (0.4) | 2.2 | (0.3) | 0.3 | (0.1) | 0.0 | (0.0) | 193.4 | 3 | <0.001 |
| | Any substance | 1767 | 12.4 | (0.4) | 19.0 | (0.9) | 11.8 | (0.6) | 9.2 | (0.7) | 4.0 | (0.5) | 204.2 | 3 | <0.001 |
| All disorders | Any DX[a] | 4815 | 39.3 | (0.9) | 46.1 | (1.9) | 41.4 | (1.6) | 38.0 | (1.8) | 22.4 | (1.7) | 73.9 | 3 | <0.001 |
| | 2+ DX[a] | 2712 | 19.9 | (0.5) | 24.3 | (1.1) | 21.9 | (1.0) | 19.1 | (1.1) | 7.4 | (0.6) | 138.1 | 3 | <0.001 |
| | 3+ DX[a] | 1543 | 10.7 | (0.4) | 14.6 | (0.9) | 11.9 | (0.7) | 8.7 | (0.7) | 2.4 | (0.4) | 169.3 | 3 | <0.001 |

Age group

*Notes:* Part 1 sample size = 12,790. Part 2 sample size = 7312. Intermittent explosive disorder, oppositional-defiant disorder, attention-deficit/hyperactivity disorder, conduct disorder, and separation anxiety disorder/adult separation anxiety were not assessed in New Zealand.

[a] Part 2 sample.

**Table 23.3.** Age at selected percentiles on the standardized age of onset distributions of CIDI disorders with projected lifetime risk at age 75

| DX group | Disorder | AOO percentile 5 | AOO percentile 10 | AOO percentile 25 | AOO percentile 50 | AOO percentile 75 | AOO percentile 90 | AOO percentile 95 | AOO percentile 99 | Projected risk age 75, % | Projected risk age 75, se |
|---|---|---|---|---|---|---|---|---|---|---|---|
| Anxiety | Panic DX | 7 | 11 | 17 | 27 | 43 | 59 | 66 | 69 | 4.1 | 0.3 |
| | GAD with hierarchy | 11 | 14 | 21 | 32 | 46 | 57 | 67 | 74 | 9.1 | 0.5 |
| | Social phobia | 5 | 6 | 8 | 13 | 17 | 27 | 38 | 57 | 10.4 | 0.4 |
| | Specific phobia | 5 | 5 | 5 | 8 | 13 | 26 | 39 | 56 | 11.9 | 0.4 |
| | Agoraphobia without panic | 5 | 6 | 13 | 17 | 26 | 38 | 46 | 51 | 1.4 | 0.1 |
| | PTSD[a] | 6 | 9 | 17 | 29 | 49 | 70 | 71 | 72 | 9.9 | 1.5 |
| | Any anxiety[a] | 5 | 5 | 7 | 14 | 29 | 48 | 57 | 71 | 30.3 | 1.5 |
| Mood | MDD with hierarchy | 13 | 16 | 21 | 33 | 48 | 59 | 67 | 75 | 25.1 | 0.7 |
| | DYS with hierarchy | 8 | 11 | 15 | 26 | 41 | 54 | 59 | 68 | 2.8 | 0.2 |
| | Bipolar (broad) | 12 | 14 | 17 | 23 | 36 | 47 | 53 | 63 | 5.1 | 0.3 |
| | Any mood | 12 | 15 | 19 | 31 | 45 | 58 | 65 | 74 | 29.8 | 0.7 |
| Substance | Alcohol abuse w/without dependence | 15 | 16 | 17 | 20 | 26 | 40 | 46 | 62 | 13.8 | 0.5 |
| | Alcohol dependence with abuse | 15 | 16 | 17 | 20 | 26 | 36 | 40 | 47 | 4.8 | 0.3 |
| | Drug abuse w/without dependence | 15 | 16 | 17 | 19 | 22 | 26 | 30 | 39 | 5.9 | 0.3 |
| | Drug dependence with abuse | 14 | 15 | 17 | 19 | 23 | 28 | 31 | 39 | 2.5 | 0.2 |
| | Any substance | 14 | 15 | 17 | 19 | 25 | 38 | 46 | 62 | 14.6 | 0.5 |
| All DX | Any DX[a] | 5 | 6 | 11 | 18 | 33 | 51 | 61 | 71 | 48.6 | 1.5 |

*Notes:* Part 1 sample size = 12,790. Part 2 sample size = 7312. Intermittent explosive disorder, oppositional-defiant disorder, attention-deficit/hyperactivity disorder, conduct disorder, and separation anxiety disorder/adult separation anxiety not assessed in New Zealand.

[a] Denotes Part 2 disorder.

**Table 23.4.** Cohort as a predictor of lifetime risk of DSM-IV disorders

| Disorder | Age group | | | | | | | | | | | | $\chi^2$ | DF | p |
|---|---|---|---|---|---|---|---|---|---|---|---|---|---|---|---|
| | 18–34 | | | 35–49 | | | 50–64 | | | 65+ | | | | | |
| | OR | LCL | UCL | OR | LCL | UCL | OR | LCL | UCL | OR | LCL | UCL | | | |
| Panic DX | 7.2* | 4.4 | 11.8 | 4.6* | 2.7 | 7.8 | 2.2* | 1.3 | 3.8 | 1.0 | 1.0 | 1.0 | 82.5 | 3 | <0.001 |
| GAD with hierarchy | 3.7* | 2.6 | 5.3 | 2.8* | 2.1 | 3.7 | 1.8* | 1.3 | 2.4 | 1.0 | 1.0 | 1.0 | 72.5 | 3 | <0.001 |
| Social phobia | 3.4* | 2.6 | 4.5 | 3.1* | 2.4 | 3.9 | 2.7* | 1.9 | 3.6 | 1.0 | 1.0 | 1.0 | 89.1 | 3 | <0.001 |
| Specific phobia | 2.9* | 2.2 | 3.8 | 2.3* | 1.8 | 2.9 | 2.3* | 1.7 | 3.0 | 1.0 | 1.0 | 1.0 | 65.9 | 3 | <0.001 |
| Agoraphobia without panic | 3.9* | 1.9 | 7.8 | 4.2* | 2.1 | 8.5 | 1.8 | 0.9 | 3.9 | 1.0 | 1.0 | 1.0 | 25.7 | 3 | <0.001 |
| PTSD | 4.1* | 2.5 | 6.9 | 2.8* | 1.7 | 4.6 | 2.5* | 1.5 | 4.0 | 1.0 | 1.0 | 1.0 | 33.0 | 3 | <0.001 |
| Any anxiety | 3.4* | 2.7 | 4.2 | 2.6* | 2.1 | 3.1 | 2.1* | 1.7 | 2.7 | 1.0 | 1.0 | 1.0 | 126.3 | 3 | <0.001 |
| MDD with hierarchy | 8.6* | 6.9 | 10.6 | 4.4* | 3.5 | 5.4 | 2.7* | 2.2 | 3.3 | 1.0 | 1.0 | 1.0 | 484.0 | 3 | <0.001 |
| DYS with hierarchy | 3.9* | 2.4 | 6.1 | 2.4* | 1.5 | 3.8 | 2.4* | 1.5 | 3.9 | 1.0 | 1.0 | 1.0 | 34.3 | 3 | <0.001 |
| Bipolar (broad) | 36.5* | 18.5 | 71.7 | 15.3* | 7.6 | 30.8 | 6.8* | 3.3 | 14.0 | 1.0 | 1.0 | 1.0 | 193.4 | 3 | <0.001 |
| Any mood | 10.0* | 8.2 | 12.2 | 5.0* | 4.1 | 6.0 | 2.9* | 2.4 | 3.6 | 1.0 | 1.0 | 1.0 | 653.9 | 3 | <0.001 |
| Alcohol abuse w/without dependence | 7.6* | 5.7 | 10.0 | 3.3* | 2.5 | 4.4 | 2.4* | 1.8 | 3.3 | 1.0 | 1.0 | 1.0 | 261.6 | 3 | <0.001 |
| Alcohol dependence with abuse | 14.3* | 7.8 | 26.1 | 7.2* | 3.8 | 13.7 | 4.0* | 2.0 | 7.8 | 1.0 | 1.0 | 1.0 | 141.0 | 3 | <0.001 |
| Drug abuse w/without dependence | 873.7* | 512.0 | 1490.0 | 322.7* | 193.0 | 540.0 | 101.7* | 54.3 | 191.0 | 1.0 | 1.0 | 1.0 | 715.2 | 3 | <0.001 |
| Drug dependence with abuse | 21.2* | 9.8 | 45.7 | 8.8* | 4.0 | 19.3 | 1.0 | 1.0 | 1.0 | – | – | – | 84.3 | 2 | <0.001 |
| Any substance | 8.1* | 6.1 | 10.7 | 3.5* | 2.7 | 4.7 | 2.5* | 1.9 | 3.3 | 1.0 | 1.0 | 1.0 | 283.7 | 3 | <0.001 |
| Any DX | 5.1* | 4.2 | 6.3 | 3.1* | 2.6 | 3.8 | 2.3* | 1.9 | 2.8 | 1.0 | 1.0 | 1.0 | 295.5 | 3 | <0.001 |

*Notes:* Based on discrete-time survival models with person-year as the unit of analysis. Controls are time intervals.

* Significant at the 0.05 level.

between lifetime prevalence and lifetime risk estimates varies by disorder as a function of variability in AOO: the difference is greater for those disorders with later AOO (as survey participants of younger ages are less likely to have experienced such disorders and so less likely to have been captured by lifetime prevalence estimates).

### 3.4. Lifetime Risk by Cohort

Lifetime risk of mental disorders was estimated for the four birth cohorts corresponding to current age groups of 18–34, 35–49, 50–64, and 65+. Relative to the oldest cohort, the younger cohorts had higher risk of all disorders, with the highest odds occurring in the youngest age group (Table 23.4). As Table 23.4 indicates, there were marked differences between disorders in the extent of this cohort effect, with drug disorders showing the strongest effects, though bipolar disorder also occurred with much higher odds in the youngest cohort.

There are a number of possible explanations for this apparent cohort effect. One is that lifetime risk appears to vary across cohort because disorder onsets occur earlier in more recent cohorts. Another possibility is that disorder onsets are simply reported as occurring earlier in recent cohorts than in older cohorts because the "telescoping of recall" in older survey participants can lead them to report later onsets. In addition, older cohorts are more likely to forget onset.

Intercohort differences in the odds of disorder were examined separately for those with early, middle, and late first onsets of disorder (Tables 23.5a–c). Cohort effects were consistent across the three onset groups for anxiety disorders. For substance use disorders, however, cohort effects were significantly more pronounced among those reporting early onset of disorder ($p < 0.001$), and somewhat more pronounced among those reporting early onset of disorder for mood disorders ($p = 0.075$).

Sociodemographic predictors of lifetime risk of disorders were examined in analyses that adjusted for cohort (results not shown but available on request). Women have significantly higher risk of anxiety and mood disorders; men

have significantly higher risk of substance use disorders. People with less education are more at risk of mood and, in particular, substance use disorders.

### 3.5. Lifetime Treatment

The proportion of cases that made treatment contact in the year of disorder onset is shown in Table 23.6. The proportion making early treatment contact was highest for those with mood disorders, at 41.4%, and substantially lower for anxiety disorders (12.5%) and substance use disorders (6.6%). However, there was much variability between anxiety disorders in this regard, with greater proportions of those with PD (34.1%) and GAD (37.5%) making contact in the year of disorder onset. Table 23.6 also shows the proportion eventually making treatment contact and the median duration of delay (among those eventually making contact). It is clear from this that although the majority of those with disorder eventually seek treatment if their disorder continues, substantial minorities of those with SP and SOP do not seek treatment, and one in seven of those with bipolar disorder or AA do not seek treatment. It is also clear that delays in seeking treatment among those eventually making treatment contact are often lengthy, particularly for the phobias (23–30 years), but also for those with alcohol use disorders (12–17 years).

Women are more likely to eventually make treatment contact; this holds for all disorder groups, though not necessarily for all individual disorders (Table 23.7). Younger cohorts are generally more likely to make lifetime treatment contact. As a general rule, those with earlier-onset disorders are less likely to make treatment contact than are those with late-onset disorders, but the exception to this rule is drug use disorders, for which the differences across AOO groups in likelihood of making treatment contact are not significant.

### 3.6. 12-month Prevalence and Severity

Anxiety disorders are the most prevalent class of 12-month disorders (14.6%), followed by mood disorders (8.0%), and then substance use

**Table 23.5a.** Variation across life course in the association of cohort in predicting lifetime risk of DSM-IV disorders

| | | Age of onset | | | | | | | | |
|---|---|---|---|---|---|---|---|---|---|---|
| | | Early | | | Middle | | | Late | | |
| DX | Age group | OR | LCL | UCL | OR | LCL | UCL | OR | LCL | UCL |
| Anxiety | 18–34 | 3.8* | 2.8 | 5.3 | 3.2* | 2.3 | 4.5 | 3.4* | 2.4 | 4.9 |
| | 35–49 | 2.9* | 2.2 | 3.9 | 2.3* | 1.7 | 3.1 | 2.6* | 1.9 | 3.6 |
| | 50–64 | 2.4* | 1.7 | 3.3 | 2.3* | 1.6 | 3.3 | 2.0* | 1.4 | 2.8 |
| | 65+ | 1.0 | 1.0 | 1.0 | 1.0 | 1.0 | 1.0 | 1.0 | 1.0 | 1.0 |
| | $\chi^2$, df, $p$ | 74.7 | 3 | <0.001 | 51.1 | 3 | <0.001 | 46.1 | 3 | <0.001 |

Global $\chi^2 = 3.5$; df $= 6$; $p = 0.74$.

*Note:* Model includes time intervals and sex as controls.
* Significant at the 0.05 level.

**Table 23.5b.** Variation across life course in the association of cohort in predicting lifetime risk of DSM-IV disorders

| | | Age of onset | | | | | | | | |
|---|---|---|---|---|---|---|---|---|---|---|
| | | Early | | | Middle | | | Late | | |
| DX | Age group | OR | LCL | UCL | OR | LCL | UCL | OR | LCL | UCL |
| Mood | 18–34 | 16.2* | 9.6 | 27.2 | 9.8* | 6.7 | 14.2 | 3.9* | 1.9 | 8.2 |
| | 35–49 | 7.6* | 4.4 | 12.9 | 4.8* | 3.3 | 6.9 | 5.0* | 3.8 | 6.5 |
| | 50–64 | 4.5* | 2.5 | 8.1 | 3.3* | 2.1 | 5.1 | 2.8* | 2.2 | 3.6 |
| | 65+ | 1.0 | 1.0 | 1.0 | 1.0 | 1.0 | 1.0 | 1.0 | 1.0 | 1.0 |
| | $\chi^2$, df, $p$ | 224.7 | 3 | <0.001 | 243.1 | 3 | <0.001 | 142.6 | 3 | <0.001 |

Global $\chi^2 = 11.5$; df $= 6$; $p = 0.08$.

*Note:* Model includes time intervals and sex as controls.
* Significant at the 0.05 level.

**Table 23.5c.** Variation across life course in the association of cohort in predicting lifetime risk of DSM-IV disorders

| | | Age of onset | | | | | | | | |
|---|---|---|---|---|---|---|---|---|---|---|
| | | Early | | | Middle | | | Late | | |
| DX | Age group | OR | LCL | UCL | OR | LCL | UCL | OR | LCL | UCL |
| Substance | 18–34 | 52.3* | 20.5 | 133.3 | 13.8* | 6.6 | 29.2 | 3.3* | 2.2 | 4.8 |
| | 35–49 | 19.4* | 7.5 | 50.2 | 6.4* | 2.9 | 13.8 | 1.9* | 1.4 | 2.7 |
| | 50–64 | 6.0* | 2.1 | 16.8 | 4.5* | 2.1 | 9.7 | 1.8* | 1.3 | 2.4 |
| | 65+ | 1.0 | 1.0 | 1.0 | 1.0 | 1.0 | 1.0 | 1.0 | 1.0 | 1.0 |
| | $\chi^2$, df, $p$ | 180.4 | 3 | <0.001 | 84.5 | 3 | <0.001 | 38.9 | 3 | <0.001 |

Global $\chi^2 = 38.6$; df $= 6$; $p = <0.001$.

*Note:* Model includes time intervals and sex as controls.
* Significant at the 0.05 level.

**Table 23.6.** Proportional treatment contact at the age of disorder onset and median duration of delay among cases that subsequently made treatment contact

| | % making treatment contact at age of onset | % making treatment contact after 50 years | Median duration of delay (years) |
|---|---|---|---|
| **I. Anxiety disorders** | | | |
| Panic disorder | 34.1 | 96.4 | 5 |
| Generalized anxiety disorder | 37.5 | 90.6 | 4 |
| Specific phobia | 2.4 | 58.4 | 30 |
| Social phobia | 4.8 | 62.7 | 23 |
| Any anxiety disorders | 12.5 | 84.2 | 21 |
| **II. Mood disorders** | | | |
| Major depressive episode | 45.2 | 97.5 | 2 |
| Dysthymia | 33.5 | 98.5 | 5 |
| Bipolar disorder (broad) | 36.6 | 86.2 | 3 |
| Any mood disorders | 41.4 | 97.5 | 3 |
| **III. Substance disorders** | | | |
| Alcohol abuse with/without dependence | 8.5 | 85.7 | 17 |
| Alcohol dependence with abuse | 12.0 | 92.1 | 12 |
| Drug abuse with/without dependence | 12.7 | 94.9 | 9 |
| Drug dependence with abuse | 15.9 | 92.2 | 6 |
| Any substance disorders | 6.6 | 71.9 | 13 |

disorders (3.5%) (Table 23.8). The 12-month prevalence of any mental disorder is 20.4%, with 12.6% experiencing one disorder, 4.3% two disorders, and 3.5% three or more disorders. The severity distribution of 12-month cases is also shown in Table 23.8. Substance use disorders were the class of disorders with the highest proportion of serious cases, which is not surprising given the criteria for serious disorders. Comorbidity was strongly related to case severity, with 12.5% of those with one disorder being classified as serious cases, compared to 66.4% of those with three or more disorders being classified as serious cases.

The sociodemographic correlates of 12-month disorders are shown in Table 23.9. The same patterns for sex and age occur with 12-month disorder as occur for lifetime disorder: higher risk of mood and anxiety disorder among women, higher risk of any disorder among young people. Lower income predicted disorder as did being previously married or having never married. Education (less) predicted anxiety disorders and substance use disorders.

### 3.7. 12-month Treatment

In the previous 12 months, only 35.7% of those with a 12-month disorder sought treatment from a health-care provider for a mental health reason (Table 23.10). Slightly more than half of those with mood disorder sought treatment from a health-care provider (52.0%), with smaller proportions of those with anxiety disorders (36.0%) and substance use disorders (27.2%) making treatment contact with the health sector. Treatment was more likely to have been provided for these disorders by general medical services (e.g., family practitioners) than by mental health services. Among individual disorders, those with panic disorder were most likely to have sought help. Around 10 percent of those with any mental disorder consulted non–health-care providers for mental health problems. It is also notable

Table 23.7. Sociodemographic predictors of lifetime treatment contact for specific DSM-IV/CIDI disorders

| | Sex | | Cohort (age at interview) | | | | | Age of onset | | | | | |
| --- | --- | --- | --- | --- | --- | --- | --- | --- | --- | --- | --- | --- | --- |
| | Female | | Age 18-34 | Age 35-49 | Age 50-64 | | | Early | Early-average | Late-average | | |
| | OR (95% CI) | $\chi_1^2$ | OR (95% CI) | OR (95% CI) | OR (95% CI) | $\chi_3^2$ | | OR (95% CI) | OR (95% CI) | OR (95% CI) | $\chi_3^2$ | |
| **I. Anxiety disorders** | | | | | | | | | | | | |
| Panic disorder | 1.6* (1.1–2.3) | 5.6* | 4.4* (2.0–9.6) | 3.3* (1.6–6.7) | 1.3 (0.6–2.7) | 24.6* | | 0.1* (0.0–0.1) | 0.2* (0.1–0.3) | 0.3* (0.2–0.6) | 109.7* | |
| Generalized anxiety disorder | 1.2 (0.9–1.5) | 2.3 | 10.9* (6.2–19.2) | 6.2* (3.8–10.0) | 3.1* (2.0–4.7) | 76.0* | | 0.1* (0.1–0.1) | 0.2* (0.1–0.3) | 0.5* (0.3–0.7) | 182.4* | |
| Specific phobia | 1.2 (0.9–1.6) | 1.7 | 1.4 (0.8–2.5) | 1.0 (0.6–1.6) | 0.8 (0.5–1.4) | 7.8* | | 0.5* (0.3–0.7) | 0.5* (0.3–0.7) | 0.5* (0.4–0.7) | 26.1* | |
| Social phobia | 1.2 (0.9–1.7) | 1.7 | 2.4* (1.4–4.2) | 1.2 (0.7–2.1) | 0.7 (0.4–1.2) | 36.7* | | 0.3* (0.2–0.3) | 0.3* (0.2–0.4) | 0.4* (0.3–0.6) | 83.0* | |
| Any anxiety disorders | 1.3* (1.1–1.5) | 8.6* | 4.3* (2.9–6.3) | 2.4* (1.7–3.4) | 1.7* (1.3–2.4) | 68.8* | | 0.1* (0.1–0.1) | 0.1* (0.1–0.2) | 0.2* (0.2–0.2) | 461.0* | |
| **II. Mood disorders** | | | | | | | | | | | | |
| Major depressive episode | 1.3* (1.1–1.5) | 8.7* | 3.8* (2.6–5.4) | 2.3* (1.7–3.2) | 1.5* (1.0–2.1) | 87.8* | | 0.2* (0.2–0.3) | 0.4* (0.3–0.5) | 0.7 (0.5–0.9) | 167.8* | |
| Dysthymia | 0.9 (0.6–1.2) | 0.7 | 3.8* (1.9–7.5) | 3.1* (1.7–5.4) | 1.8* (1.0–3.2) | 21.4* | | 0.3* (0.2–0.4) | 0.6* (0.3–0.9) | 0.8 (0.5–1.3) | 43.1* | |
| Bipolar disorder (broad) | 1.7* (1.2–2.5) | 9.0* | 4.7* (1.0–21.6) | 3.1 (0.7–13.1) | 4.1 (0.9–18.2) | 6.7 | | 0.2* (0.1–0.3) | 0.3* (0.2–0.6) | 0.3* (0.2–0.5) | 43.3* | |
| Any mood disorders | 1.4* (1.2–1.6) | 16.9* | 3.7* (2.7–5.2) | 2.3* (1.7–3.1) | 1.6* (1.2–2.2) | 84.1* | | 0.2* (0.2–0.3) | 0.3* (0.3–0.4) | 0.6* (0.5–0.8) | 205.6* | |
| **III. Substance disorders** | | | | | | | | | | | | |
| Alcohol abuse with/without dependence | 1.4* (1.1–1.9) | 7.6* | 6.0* (3.0–12.1) | 3.2* (1.7–6.2) | 1.9 (1.0–3.6) | 47.2* | | 0.4* (0.3–0.6) | 0.4* (0.3–0.5) | 0.4* (0.3–0.5) | 54.1* | |
| Alcohol dependence with abuse | 1.3 (0.9–1.9) | 2.1 | 3.5 (1.0–12.9) | 2.5 (0.7–8.5) | 1.6 (0.5–5.6) | 10.6* | | 0.5* (0.3–0.7) | 0.5* (0.3–0.8) | 0.4* (0.2–0.6) | 21.6* | |
| Drug abuse with/without dependence | 1.3 (0.9–1.8) | 1.9 | 2.0 (0.9–4.5) | 1.1 (0.5–2.4) | 1.0 — | 13.1* | | 0.9 (0.5–1.5) | 1.2 (0.6–2.3) | 0.9 (0.5–1.4) | 1.3 | |
| Drug dependence with abuse | 0.9 (0.6–1.5) | 0.1 | 0.8 (0.2–2.7) | 0.5 (0.2–1.8) | 1.0 — | 3.5 | | 0.7 (0.4–1.2) | 0.6 (0.4–1.1) | 0.5 (0.2–1.1) | 4.4 | |
| Any substance disorders | 1.3* (1.0–1.7) | 4.6* | 5.6* (2.8–11.0) | 3.1* (1.6–5.9) | 1.8 (0.9–3.5) | 47.1* | | 0.4* (0.3–0.6) | 0.3* (0.2–0.4) | 0.4* (0.3–0.5) | 63.2* | |

* Significant at the 0.05 level, two-sided test.

498

**Table 23.8.** 12-month prevalence and severity of DSM-IV/CIDI disorders

| Disorder Group | Disorder | n | 12-month prevalence | | Severity[a] | | | | | |
| | | | | | Mild | | Moderate | | Serious | |
| | | | % | (se) | % | (se) | % | (se) | % | (se) |
|---|---|---|---|---|---|---|---|---|---|---|
| Anxiety disorder | Panic disorder | 252 | 1.7 | (0.1) | 20.2 | (3.8) | 32.6 | (3.9) | 47.2 | (4.3) |
| | Generalized anxiety disorder | 288 | 2.1 | (0.2) | 7.5 | (1.9) | 56.5 | (3.8) | 36.0 | (4.0) |
| | Social phobia | 690 | 5.1 | (0.2) | 21.2 | (2.0) | 46.1 | (2.5) | 32.7 | (2.1) |
| | Specific phobia | 1045 | 7.3 | (0.3) | 40.8 | (2.3) | 36.9 | (2.1) | 22.4 | (1.9) |
| | Agoraphobia without panic | 110 | 0.6 | (0.1) | 20.3 | (4.8) | 33.3 | (6.6) | 46.5 | (6.0) |
| | Posttraumatic stress disorder* | 414 | 3.0 | (0.2) | 28.3 | (3.5) | 36.2 | (3.9) | 35.5 | (3.3) |
| | Any anxiety disorder* | 1981 | 14.6 | (0.5) | 34.1 | (1.6) | 40.9 | (1.6) | 25.0 | (1.3) |
| Mood disorder | Dysthymia | 154 | 1.1 | (0.1) | 15.5 | (3.7) | 34.4 | (4.8) | 50.1 | (5.5) |
| | Major depressive disorder | 738 | 5.7 | (0.3) | 8.9 | (1.4) | 55.0 | (2.2) | 36.1 | (2.1) |
| | Bipolar disorder (broad) | 351 | 2.2 | (0.2) | 9.5 | (2.4) | 33.3 | (3.3) | 57.3 | (3.8) |
| | Any mood disorder | 1109 | 8.0 | (0.4) | 9.4 | (1.1) | 48.9 | (1.9) | 41.7 | (1.9) |
| Substance disorder | Alcohol abuse | 362 | 2.6 | (0.2) | 39.0 | (4.3) | 15.6 | (2.6) | 45.4 | (3.8) |
| | Alcohol dependence | 216 | 1.3 | (0.1) | 0.0 | (0.0) | 11.7 | (3.6) | 88.3 | (3.6) |
| | Drug abuse | 147 | 1.1 | (0.1) | 24.6 | (4.9) | 10.6 | (3.4) | 64.8 | (5.3) |
| | Drug dependence | 96 | 0.7 | (0.1) | 0.0 | (0.0) | 0.0 | (0.0) | 100.0 | (0.0) |
| | Any substance use disorder | 501 | 3.5 | (0.2) | 34.9 | (3.2) | 14.4 | (2.3) | 50.7 | (3.0) |
| Any disorder | Any* | 2690 | 20.4 | (0.6) | 32.4 | (1.2) | 41.5 | (1.4) | 26.2 | (1.0) |
| | 0 Disorders* | 4622 | 79.6 | (0.6) | 0.6 | (0.1) | 0.0 | (0.0) | 0.0 | (0.0) |
| | 1 Disorder* | 1566 | 12.6 | (0.5) | 45.4 | (1.7) | 42.2 | (1.8) | 12.5 | (1.0) |
| | 2 Disorders* | 611 | 4.3 | (0.2) | 17.0 | (1.9) | 49.1 | (2.6) | 33.9 | (2.5) |
| | 3+ Disorders* | 513 | 3.5 | (0.2) | 4.0 | (1.1) | 29.6 | (2.6) | 66.4 | (2.8) |

*Notes:* Percentages in the three severity columns are repeated as proportions of all cases and sum to 100% across each row. Sample size for Part 1 = 12,790. Sample size for Part 2 = 7312.

[a] Severity calculated using Part 2 weights.

* Part 2 sample.

Table 23.9. Demographic correlates of 12-month DSM-IV psychiatric disorders

| Variable | Label | Any mood disorder | | | Any anxiety disorder | | | Any substance disorder | | |
|---|---|---|---|---|---|---|---|---|---|---|
| | | OR | Lower 95% limit OR | Upper 95% limit OR | OR | Lower 95% limit OR | Upper 95% limit OR | OR | Lower 95% limit OR | Upper 95% limit OR |
| Sex | Male | 1.0 | – | – | 1.0 | – | – | 1.0 | – | – |
| | Female | 1.4 | 1.2 | 1.7 | 1.9 | 1.6 | 2.3 | 0.4 | 0.3 | 0.5 |
| | $\chi^2$, df, $p$ | 11.5 | 1 | 0.001 | 63.4 | 1 | <0.001 | 43.2 | 1 | <0.001 |
| Age | 18–34 | 8.5 | 5.8 | 12.6 | 4.2 | 3.0 | 5.8 | 621.0 | 112.2 | 3436.8 |
| | 35–49 | 6.7 | 4.6 | 9.7 | 3.6 | 2.6 | 4.9 | 224.3 | 41.3 | 1217.1 |
| | 50–64 | 4.4 | 2.9 | 6.7 | 3.0 | 2.2 | 4.2 | 62.7 | 10.9 | 360.3 |
| | 65≤ | 1.0 | – | – | 1.0 | – | – | 1.0 | – | – |
| | $\chi^2$, df, $p$ | 127.2 | 3 | <0.001 | 76.9 | 3 | <0.001 | 107.8 | 3 | <0.001 |
| Income | Low | 1.8 | 1.3 | 2.5 | 1.6 | 1.2 | 2.1 | 1.7 | 1.0 | 2.8 |
| | Low-average | 1.5 | 1.1 | 2.0 | 1.2 | 0.9 | 1.5 | 1.4 | 0.8 | 2.4 |
| | High-average | 1.4 | 1.1 | 1.9 | 1.1 | 0.8 | 1.4 | 1.2 | 0.7 | 2.1 |
| | High | 1.0 | – | – | 1.0 | – | – | 1.0 | – | – |
| | $\chi^2$, df, $p$ | 11.9 | 3 | 0.008 | 17.9 | 3 | <0.001 | 5.6 | 3 | 0.13 |
| Marital Status | Married/cohabiting | 1.0 | – | – | 1.0 | – | – | 1.0 | – | – |
| | Separated/widowed/divorced | 3.0 | 2.4 | 3.8 | 1.6 | 1.3 | 1.9 | 3.1 | 1.9 | 4.8 |
| | Never married | 1.6 | 1.2 | 2.0 | 1.3 | 1.0 | 1.5 | 1.8 | 1.3 | 2.6 |
| | $\chi^2$, df, $p$ | 86.2 | 2 | <0.001 | 17.8 | 2 | <0.001 | 30.6 | 2 | <0.001 |
| Education | ≤10 years | 1.0 | 0.7 | 1.3 | 1.4 | 1.1 | 1.7 | 3.9 | 2.5 | 6.0 |
| | 11–12 years | 1.0 | 0.8 | 1.3 | 1.1 | 0.9 | 1.3 | 2.1 | 1.3 | 3.2 |
| | 13 years | 0.9 | 0.7 | 1.2 | 1.1 | 0.9 | 1.4 | 2.3 | 1.4 | 3.7 |
| | 14+ years | 1.0 | – | – | 1.0 | – | – | 1.0 | – | – |
| | $\chi^2$, df, $p$ | 0.5 | 3 | 0.92 | 7.1 | 3 | 0.07 | 38.7 | 3 | <0.001 |
| Overall | $\chi^2$, df, $p$ | 2710.1 | 13 | <0.001 | 2496.4 | 13 | <0.001 | 2215.0 | 13 | <0.001 |

*Notes:* Evaluated only on Part 2 sample. Sample size for Part 2 = 7312.

**Table 23.10.** 12-month service usage in New Zealand: Percentage treated by health-care professionals among people with mental disorders

| Disorder group | Mental disorder | Measure | Type of Professional | | | | | | | | | Unweighted n with mental disorder | Weighted n with mental disorder |
|---|---|---|---|---|---|---|---|---|---|---|---|---|---|
| | | | Psychiatrist % (se) | Other mental health care % (se) | Any mental health care % (se) | General medical % (se) | Any health care % (se) | Human services % (se) | CAM % (se) | Any non-health care % (se) | Any treatment % (se) | | |
| Anxiety | GAD | % in treatment | 15.2 (2.5) | 27.9 (3.2) | 32.4 (3.2) | 46.6 (2.8) | 56.8 (2.9) | 8.7 (1.7) | 12.6 (2.2) | 18.4 (2.4) | 62.2 (3.1) | 441 | 389 |
| | Panic disorder | % in treatment | 15.8 (3.4) | 24.7 (3.9) | 29.7 (3.9) | 56.8 (3.9) | 63.3 (4.0) | 5.3 (1.6) | 12.8 (3.0) | 17.4 (3.2) | 66.1 (4.0) | 252 | 212 |
| | Agoraphobia w/o panic | % in treatment | 14.4 (4.6) | 22.0 (5.2) | 28.3 (5.7) | 43.4 (6.8) | 54.2 (6.5) | 13.7 (4.3) | 11.7 (4.3) | 22.8 (5.5) | 61.8 (6.3) | 110 | 78 |
| | Social phobia | % in treatment | 8.8 (1.4) | 14.8 (1.9) | 18.8 (2.0) | 30.0 (2.0) | 36.0 (2.3) | 6.9 (1.3) | 9.3 (1.5) | 13.0 (1.6) | 39.0 (2.3) | 690 | 646 |
| | Specific phobia | % in treatment | 5.9 (0.9) | 9.7 (1.4) | 12.0 (1.4) | 25.8 (1.5) | 29.4 (1.7) | 4.5 (0.8) | 5.5 (1.0) | 8.7 (1.3) | 32.6 (1.8) | 1045 | 928 |
| | Posttraumatic stress disorder[a] | % in treatment | 9.2 (2.6) | 23.0 (2.9) | 27.5 (3.3) | 35.0 (3.5) | 50.0 (3.9) | 8.8 (2.0) | 11.3 (2.2) | 17.7 (2.9) | 56.5 (3.8) | 414 | 220 |
| | Any anxiety disorder[a] | % in treatment | 7.0 (0.8) | 13.7 (1.1) | 16.7 (1.2) | 29.0 (1.2) | 36.0 (1.4) | 5.1 (0.6) | 7.3 (0.9) | 10.7 (1.0) | 39.5 (1.4) | 2011 | 1074 |
| Mood | Major depressive episode | % in treatment | 11.7 (1.4) | 23.1 (1.9) | 27.5 (2.1) | 45.5 (1.9) | 56.1 (2.1) | 7.3 (1.1) | 10.3 (1.5) | 15.2 (1.7) | 59.8 (2.2) | 901 | 842 |
| | Dysthymia | % in treatment | 12.0 (2.7) | 21.8 (3.2) | 25.7 (3.4) | 47.1 (3.9) | 57.4 (3.8) | 10.0 (2.1) | 8.8 (2.4) | 16.7 (3.1) | 61.6 (3.9) | 288 | 235 |
| | Bipolar disorder (broad) | % in treatment | 11.9 (2.6) | 20.9 (3.1) | 25.4 (3.3) | 35.8 (3.7) | 44.5 (3.7) | 7.3 (1.7) | 7.6 (2.0) | 12.4 (2.5) | 46.3 (3.7) | 351 | 279 |
| | Any mood disorder | % in treatment | 10.8 (1.2) | 21.7 (1.7) | 25.7 (1.8) | 42.3 (1.8) | 52.0 (2.0) | 6.8 (1.0) | 9.4 (1.3) | 14.0 (1.5) | 55.2 (2.1) | 1110 | 1018 |
| Substance | Alcohol abuse | % in treatment | 5.7 (1.7) | 10.6 (2.1) | 13.1 (2.3) | 17.2 (2.5) | 24.6 (3.0) | 2.7 (1.0) | 3.5 (1.1) | 5.9 (1.5) | 25.6 (3.0) | 362 | 330 |
| | Alcohol dependence | % in treatment | 6.7 (2.1) | 17.8 (3.5) | 20.5 (3.7) | 25.0 (4.1) | 34.5 (4.9) | 2.3 (0.9) | 7.1 (2.3) | 8.9 (2.4) | 36.2 (4.8) | 216 | 162 |
| | Drug abuse | % in treatment | 12.1 (3.6) | 19.0 (3.8) | 21.4 (4.0) | 23.9 (4.5) | 33.6 (4.9) | 4.8 (2.4) | 8.9 (2.8) | 13.0 (3.5) | 38.4 (4.9) | 147 | 140 |
| | Drug dependence | % in treatment | 14.8 (5.4) | 24.7 (5.9) | 25.7 (6.0) | 25.6 (5.6) | 35.8 (6.4) | 3.5 (1.7) | 9.2 (3.4) | 10.6 (3.6) | 40.8 (6.5) | 96 | 89 |
| | Any substance | % in treatment | 6.9 (1.6) | 12.0 (1.8) | 14.3 (2.0) | 20.2 (2.4) | 27.2 (2.7) | 2.7 (0.8) | 5.3 (1.2) | 7.2 (1.4) | 29.8 (2.8) | 501 | 447 |
| Composite | Any disorder[a] | % in treatment | 6.2 (0.6) | 13.4 (0.9) | 16.3 (1.0) | 28.7 (1.0) | 35.7 (1.1) | 4.9 (0.5) | 6.6 (0.7) | 10.0 (0.8) | 38.9 (1.2) | 2691 | 1483 |
| | No disorder[a] | % in treatment | 0.7 (0.1) | 1.9 (0.3) | 2.3 (0.3) | 4.2 (0.3) | 5.9 (0.5) | 0.7 (0.1) | 1.6 (0.3) | 2.2 (0.3) | 7.4 (0.5) | 4621 | 5800 |
| | Total Part 2 sample[a] | % in treatment | 1.8 (0.2) | 4.2 (0.3) | 5.2 (0.3) | 9.2 (0.4) | 12.0 (0.5) | 1.6 (0.2) | 2.6 (0.8) | 3.8 (0.3) | 13.8 (0.5) | 7312 | 7283 |

*Notes*: Values are percentages with standard errors in parentheses.

[a] Part 2 sample.

501

that 5.9% of the population without diagnosed 12-month disorder made a mental health visit to a health-care provider in the past 12 months.

### 3.8. Number of Visits in the Past Year

Table 23.11 shows that the median number of visits to any health-care professional for a mental health problem among those with any mental disorder was 2.3, with the highest median being for those with substance use disorders (3.9 visits vs. 2.3 for anxiety disorders and 2.9 for mood disorders). Those who were treated by mental health professionals made more visits, with a median of 5.3 visits to any mental health care professional among those with any mental disorder. The mean number of visits in the past year was much higher than the median number of visits (data not shown but available on request). For example, the mean number of visits to any health-care professional by those with any mental disorder was 9.1, and to any mental health care professional the mean was 13.2. These differences between means and medians indicate that a small number of individuals made a very large number of visits.

### 3.9. 12-month Treatment by Severity

Table 23.12 shows that case severity was associated with treatment, with slightly more than half (53.6%) of severe cases making a mental health visit to a health-care professional, compared with 37.5% of those with moderate disorder and 19.0% of those with mild disorder making a mental health visit to a health-care professional. The level of unmet need appears significant, ranging from 43.3% among serious cases to 77.6% among mild cases.

### 3.10. Sociodemographic Predictors of 12-month Treatment

Analysis of sociodemographic predictors of any treatment, controlling for the presence of any mental disorder, found that males were less likely to seek treatment for mental health problems. There was an overall age effect, with higher odds

ratios in the middle age groups and lowest in the youngest age group relative to the 65+ age group, but these differences were small. There were no other significant effects for sociodemographic variables (data not shown but available on request).

## 4. DISCUSSION

Mental disorder is common in New Zealand with 39.3% of the population aged 18 years or older having experienced a disorder at some time prior to the interview, and 48.6% projected to experience a disorder by the age of 75 years. In the past 12 months, 20.4% of the population had experienced at least one of the disorders assessed. The disorders tend to have early onset with 50% of persons developing the disorder doing so by age 18 years. Younger cohorts have higher risks of all disorders compared to older cohorts. Females have higher risk for lifetime disorder for anxiety and mood disorders; men had higher risk of substance use disorders. People with less education are more at risk of mood and substance use disorders.

These findings from the NZMHS may be compared with findings from other high-income countries (Belgium, France, Germany, Italy, Israel, Japan, the Netherlands, and the United States) in the WMH Survey Initiative. However, as not all disorders were assessed in every country (the New Zealand survey, for example, did not include impulse-control disorders), disorder-specific prevalence estimates are more comparable than are those for the prevalence of any disorder. New Zealand has high 12-month prevalence estimates of anxiety, mood, and substance use disorders relative to other high-income countries, with the exception of the United States, and relative to the 15 sites reported in 2004 (Demyttenaere et al. 2004), again with the exception of the United States.

Comparing 12-month prevalence for individual disorders with the six European sites in the European Study of the Epidemiology of Mental Disorders (ESEMeD) combined (ESEMeD 2004) shows that New Zealand has higher prevalence estimates for major depressive disorder,

**Table 23.11.** 12-month service usage in New Zealand: Median number of visits in the past year

| Disorder group | Mental disorder | Type of professional | | | | | | | | |
|---|---|---|---|---|---|---|---|---|---|---|
| | | Psychiatrist % (se) | Other mental health care % (se) | Any mental health care % (se) | General medical % (se) | Any health care % (se) | Human services % (se) | CAM % (se) | Any non–health care % (se) | Any treatment % (se) |
| Anxiety | GAD | 4.6 (1.8) | 4.6 (1.1) | 6.1 (1.1) | 1.8 (0.1) | 3.4 (0.8) | 4.0 (0.7) | 4.2 (2.2) | 4.7 (1.3) | 2.9 (0.7) |
| | Panic disorder | 5.0 (1.5) | 5.8 (1.8) | 6.5 (2.0) | 1.8 (0.1) | 2.9 (1.0) | – | – | 2.5 (0.7) | 2.6 (0.8) |
| | Agoraphobia w/o panic | – | – | – | 1.6 (0.4) | 2.6 (2.0) | – | – | – | 2.2 (1.0) |
| | Social phobia | 3.6 (1.9) | 5.9 (1.0) | 6.6 (1.5) | 1.7 (0.1) | 3.0 (0.7) | 4.3 (0.9) | 6.7 (9.3) | 5.1 (3.4) | 2.3 (0.8) |
| | Specific phobia | 5.8 (2.4) | 7.6 (2.2) | 9.2 (2.1) | 1.7 (0.1) | 2.1 (0.5) | 4.2 (1.4) | 6.1 (7.4) | 5.6 (2.6) | 1.9 (0.3) |
| | Posttraumatic stress disorder[a] | 1.9 (1.4) | 7.1 (1.6) | 6.3 (2.1) | 1.8 (0.2) | 3.3 (1.0) | 5.1 (1.1) | 7.5 (5.9) | 5.7 (1.9) | 2.0 (0.8) |
| | Any anxiety disorder[a] | 4.3 (1.2) | 5.7 (0.8) | 6.3 (0.9) | 1.6 (0.0) | 2.3 (0.4) | 3.8 (0.6) | 4.9 (1.6) | 4.9 (1.1) | 2.0 (0.3) |
| Mood | Major depressive episode | 5.6 (1.2) | 4.6 (0.7) | 5.5 (0.9) | 1.7 (0.1) | 2.9 (0.7) | 3.7 (0.9) | 4.1 (2.3) | 3.7 (1.3) | 2.5 (0.6) |
| | Dysthymia | 4.1 (1.8) | 6.3 (2.9) | 5.8 (3.7) | 1.8 (0.1) | 2.4 (0.7) | – | – | 5.1 (2.2) | 2.0 (0.7) |
| | Bipolar disorder (broad) | – | 5.4 (1.7) | 4.3 (1.2) | 1.8 (0.2) | 3.3 (0.9) | – | – | 3.6 (1.5) | 3.3 (0.9) |
| | Any mood disorder | 5.2 (0.9) | 4.7 (0.5) | 5.4 (0.9) | 1.7 (0.1) | 2.9 (0.3) | 3.5 (0.8) | 3.9 (1.8) | 3.4 (0.9) | 2.5 (0.6) |
| Substance | Alcohol abuse | – | 8.9 (2.3) | 7.7 (3.3) | 2.6 (0.5) | 5.1 (1.0) | – | – | – | 5.0 (1.0) |
| | Alcohol dependence | – | 6.0 (2.9) | 5.9 (3.3) | 2.5 (0.5) | 5.5 (1.4) | – | – | – | 5.5 (1.4) |
| | Drug abuse | – | 6.6 (1.8) | 7.0 (4.6) | – | 4.0 (2.1) | – | – | – | 3.7 (1.8) |
| | Drug dependence | – | – | – | 2.4 (1.5) | 12.1 (5.1) | – | – | – | 9.6 (5.6) |
| | Any substance | 4.7 (1.4) | 6.4 (2.3) | 7.0 (3.0) | 2.1 (0.4) | 3.9 (1.1) | – | 3.5 (1.5) | 3.3 (1.4) | 3.6 (0.9) |
| Composite | Any disorder[a] | 4.4 (0.9) | 5.0 (0.5) | 5.3 (0.7) | 1.6 (0.0) | 2.3 (0.3) | 3.3 (0.6) | 4.5 (1.2) | 4.0 (1.0) | 2.0 (0.3) |
| | No disorder[a] | – | 2.8 (1.0) | 2.5 (0.7) | 1.6 (0.1) | 1.8 (0.0) | 4.0 (0.9) | 3.3 (1.6) | 3.6 (1.2) | 1.5 (0.0) |
| | Total Part 2 Sample[a] | 3.0 (0.4) | 3.7 (0.6) | 3.9 (0.5) | 1.6 (0.0) | 1.9 (0.3) | 3.5 (0.8) | 3.7 (0.9) | 3.8 (0.7) | 1.8 (0.0) |

*Notes:* Values are medians with standard errors in parentheses. Cells with unweighted *n* less than 30 or where the standard error could not be calculated do not have medians.
[a] Part 2 sample.

**Table 23.12.** Severity by treatment

| Treatment | Severe % | (se) | Moderate % | (se) | Mild % | (se) | None % | (se) | Total % | (se) |
|---|---|---|---|---|---|---|---|---|---|---|
| General medical | 42.5 | (2.2) | 30.8 | (1.8) | 15.2 | (1.6) | 4.1 | (0.3) | 9.2 | (0.4) |
| Mental health | 32.5 | (2.2) | 14.1 | (1.6) | 5.9 | (1.1) | 2.3 | (0.3) | 5.2 | (0.3) |
| Health care | 53.6 | (2.3) | 37.5 | (1.9) | 19.0 | (1.9) | 5.8 | (0.5) | 12.0 | (0.5) |
| Non–health care[a] | 16.3 | (1.9) | 9.7 | (1.2) | 5.6 | (1.0) | 2.2 | (0.3) | 3.8 | (0.3) |
| Any treatment | 56.7 | (2.2) | 40.7 | (1.9) | 22.4 | (1.9) | 7.3 | (0.5) | 13.8 | (0.5) |
| No treatment | 43.3 | (2.2) | 59.3 | (1.9) | 77.6 | (1.9) | 92.7 | (0.5) | 86.2 | (0.5) |

[a] Non–health care includes human services and CAM.

GAD, SOP, SP, PD, AA, and AD. However, given the variation in prevalence for disorder groups across the ESEMeD countries (Demyttenaere et al. 2004), it is not straightforward to interpret the prevalences for individual disorders that have been combined across sites.

For estimates of lifetime prevalence and risk also, New Zealand is generally higher than other high-income countries (with the exception of a similar estimate for mood disorders to that of France) but lower than the United States (Kessler et al. 2007).

The NZMHS, as with most other WMH surveys, has shown an apparent cohort effect: younger age groups have higher estimates of disorder than do older age groups, or older age groups have lower than expected (on the basis of projections from incidence studies) estimates of disorder. Inspection of the standardized AOO distribution curves for GAD, PD, PTSD, and mood disorders in the WMH surveys suggests a trend toward earlier AOO in the NZMHS than in the European sites, but later AOO compared to the United States. For substance use disorders, the standardized AOO curves suggest an earlier AOO in the NZMHS compared to all the European sites and the United States.

The NZMHS shows that not quite 40% of people with a mental disorder in the past 12 months made a mental health visit within that period. Of participants with any serious disorder, 56.5% had a mental health visit to the health-care sector in the past 12 months, which compares with 62.1% in Belgium, 48.0% in France, 53.9% in Israel, 40.6% in Germany, 51.6% in Italy, 24.2%

in Japan, 49.2% in the Netherlands, 58.7% in Spain, and 59.7% in the United States (Wang et al. 2007a). Comparisons between New Zealand and other WMH sites for moderate and mild disorders are also broadly similar.

Within the NZMHS, the 12-month service use in the mental health specialty sector is 5.2%, with the range in the high-income countries in the WMH series from 2.0% in Italy to 8.8% in Germany (Wang et al. 2007a). For the general medical sector, in the NZMHS, 9.2% of participants have had contact within the previous 12 months, with the range in the WMH survey high-income countries from 2.8% in Japan to 9.3% in the United States. Among those participants using services in the NZMHS, 37.6% used mental health specialty services (the range of other high-income countries in the WMH surveys is from 37.6% in New Zealand to 52.2% in Spain), and 66.5% used general medical services (the range is from 40.4% in Israel to 71.2% in the Netherlands).

These findings suggest that although the overall rate of service use for mental health problems in New Zealand is comparable to other high-income countries in the WMH series, there is a pattern suggestive of higher general medical service use and lower mental health specialty use in New Zealand than in the other high-income countries.

New Zealand data on the proportion of persons with a disorder making treatment contact in the year of onset of the disorder is in the low to middle range as compared to other high-income countries, and the median duration of delay among cases that subsequently made treatment contact is in the middle to high range (Wang et al. 2007b). The pattern of health service use for mental disorders in New Zealand is consistent with the structure of the healthcare service system and the available resources in specialist mental health services and primary mental health. The percentage of GDP spent on health in New Zealand (8.3%) is the second lowest of the WMH high-income countries, ranging from 8.0% (Japan) to 13.9% (United States). The per capita total expenditure on health in New Zealand is the lowest of the WMH high-income countries (ranging from $1724 in New Zealand to $4887 in the United States). However, the New Zealand government spends 11.0% of the health budget on mental health services, which is the highest percentage of the WMH high-income countries (ranging from 5.0% in Japan to 11.0% in New Zealand). New Zealand has completed the deinstitutionalization of mental health services and has a well-developed community-oriented mental health service. This is reflected in the lowest number of total psychiatric beds (3.8 per 10,000 of population) of the high-income countries (ranging from 3.8 in New Zealand to 22.1 in Belgium).

New Zealand does have difficulties maintaining the mental health medical workforce and has the lowest number of psychiatrists per 100,000 of population of the WMH survey high-income countries, though it has a comparable number of psychiatric nurses and psychologists to other high-income countries (World Health Organization 2005). Within the New Zealand health system, primary care and general practitioners act as gatekeepers to specialist services and many persons with mental disorders are cared for within the primary care sector.

The NZMHS shows New Zealand to have high lifetime and 12-month prevalences compared to many other WMH survey high-income countries. The reason for this is unclear. Given the early AOO of many of the common mental disorders, one possibility is that high rates of disorder in the adult population may be associated with more exposure to adversity in the child and adolescent populations. The UNICEF report "An overview of child well-being in rich countries" (United Nations Children's Fund 2007) contains information on eight of the nine WMH survey high-income countries (information for Israel was not included in the report). The report provides an assessment of the lives and well-being of children in industrialized nations on six dimensions: material well-being, health and safety, educational well-being, family and peer relationships, behavior and risks, and subjective well-being. As a result of incomplete data, for New Zealand only three of these dimensions could be completely assessed. For the dimension of material well-being, New Zealand ranked sixth of eight WMH survey high-income countries. For the health and safety dimension, New Zealand ranked seventh out of eight WMH survey high-income countries. For educational well-being, New Zealand ranked fifth out of seven WMH survey high-income countries (Japan was not assessed on this dimension). On the dimension of family and peer relationships, New Zealand had incomplete data and could not be assessed. However, on one item (the percentage of 15-year-olds who eat the main meal of the day with their parents "several times per week") that contributed to this dimension, New Zealand ranked eighth of the eight WMH survey high-income countries. On one item (teenage fertility) that contributed to the dimension of behaviors and risks, New Zealand ranked seventh of the eight WMH survey high-income countries. Thus, New Zealand consistently tended to rank lower than other WMH survey high-income countries for the available measures of childhood well-being. In so much as the antecedents of adult disorder lie in part in adversities and experience in childhood and adolescence (Rutter 2002), the higher rates of mental disorder found in the NZMHS may be associated with less-than-optimal well-being of children in New Zealand compared to other WMH survey high-income countries.

These findings suggest a significant unmet need for treatment for people with mental disorders in the New Zealand community and emphasize the importance of mental disorders as contributors to the burden of disease in New Zealand. Future NZMHS analyses will examine barriers to obtaining treatment of mental disorders to provide information to policy makers about modifiable barriers that could be the target of future intervention efforts.

## REFERENCES

American Psychiatric Association (1994). *Diagnostic and statistical manual of mental disorders (DSM-IV)*, 4th ed. Washington, DC: American Psychiatric Association.

Andrews, G., Henderson, S. & Hall, W. (2001). Prevalence, comorbidity, disability and service utilisation: Overview of the Australian National Mental Health Survey. *British Journal of Psychiatry*, 178, 145–53.

Baxter, J., Kingi, T. K., Tapsell, R. & Durie, M. (2006a). Māori. In *Te Rau Hinengaro: The New Zealand Mental Health Survey*, ed. M. A. Oakley-Browne, J. E. Wells & K. M. Scott, pp. 139–78. Wellington: Ministry of Health.

Baxter, J., Kingi, T. K., Tapsell, R., Durie, M., McGee, M. A. & New Zealand Mental Health Survey Research Team (2006b). Prevalence of mental disorders among Māori in Te Rau Hinengaro: The New Zealand Mental Health Survey. *Australian and New Zealand Journal of Psychiatry*, 40, 914–23.

Christchurch School of Medicine & Health Sciences (n.d.). *Christchurch Health and Development Study*. Available at http://www.chmeds.ac.nz/research/chds/.

Demyttenaere, K., Bruffaerts, R., Posada-Villa, J., Gasquet, I., Kovess, V., Lepine, J. P., Angermeyer, M. C., Bernert, S., Girolamo, G., Morosini, P., Polidori, G., Kikkawa, T., Kawakami, N., Ono, Y., Takeshima, T., Uda, H., Karam, E. G., Fayyad, J. A., Karam, A. N., Mneimneh, Z. N., Medina-Mora, M. E., Borges, G., Lara, G., de Graaf, R., Ormel, J., Gureje, O., Shen, Y., Huang, Y., Zhang, M., Alonso, J., Haro, J. M., Vilagut, G., Bromet, E. J., Gluzman, S., Webb, C., Kessler, R. C., Merikangas, K. R., Anthony, J. C., Korff, M. R. V., Wang, P. S., Alonso, J., Brugha, T. S., Aguilar-Gaxiola, S., Lee, S., Heeringa, S., Pennell, B.-E., Zaslavsky, A. M., Üstün, T. B. & Chatterji, S. (2004). Prevalence, severity and unmet need for treatment of mental disorders in the World Health Organization World Mental Health Surveys. *Journal of the American Medical Association*, 291, 2581–90.

Efron, B. (1988). Logistic regression, survival analysis, and the Kaplan-Meier curve. *Journal of the American Statistical Association*, 83, 414–25.

ESEMeD/MHEDEA 2000 Investigators (2004). Prevalence of mental disorders in Europe: Results from the European Study of the Epidemiology of Mental Disorders (ESEMeD) project. *Acta Psychiatrica Scandinavica*, 420, 21–7.

First, M. B., Spitzer, R. L., Gibbon, M. & Williams, J. B. W. (2002). *Structured Clinical Interview for DSM-IV axis I disorders, research version, non-patient edition (SCID-I/NP)*. New York: Biometrics Research, New York State Psychiatric Institute.

Foliaki, S., Kokaua, J., Schaaf, D. & Tukuitonga, C. (2006a). Pacific people. In *Te Rau Hinengaro: The New Zealand Mental Health Survey*, ed. M. A. Oakley-Browne, J. E. Wells & K. M. Scott, pp. 179–208. Wellington: Ministry of Health.

Foliaki, S., Kokaua, J., Schaaf, D., Tukuitonga, C. & New Zealand Mental Health Survey Research Team (2006b). Twelve-month and lifetime prevalences of mental disorders and treatment contact among Pacific people in Te Rau Hinengaro: The New Zealand Mental Health Survey. *Australian and New Zealand Journal of Psychiatry*, 40, 924–34.

Henderson, S., Andrews, G. & Hall, W. (2000). Australia's mental health: An overview of the general population survey. *Australian and New Zealand Journal of Psychiatry*, 34, 197–205.

Kaplan, E. L. & Meier, P. (1958). Nonparametric estimation for incomplete observations. *Journal of the American Statistics Association*, 53, 457–81.

Kessler, R. C., Angermeyer, M., Anthony, J. C., de Graff, R., Demyttenaere, K., Gasquet, I., de Girolamo, G., Gluzman, S., Gureje, O., Haro, J. M., Kawakami, N., Karam, A., Levinson, D., Medina Mora, M. E., Oakley-Browne, M. A., Posada-Villa, J., Stein, D. J., Tsang, C. H. A., Aguilar-Gaxiola, S., Alonso, J., Lee, S., Heeringa, S., Pennell, B.-E., Berglund, P. A., Gruber, M., Petukhova, M., Chatterji, S. & Üstün, T. B. (2007). Lifetime prevalence and age-of-onset distributions of mental disorders in the World Health Organization's World Mental Health Surveys. *World Psychiatry*, 6, 168–76.

Kessler, R. C., Chui, W. T., Demler, O. & Walters, E. E. (2005b). Prevalence, severity and comorbidity of 12-month DSM-IV disorders in the National Comorbidity Survey Replication. *Archives of General Psychiatry*, 62, 617–27.

Kessler, R. C., Haro, J. M., Heeringa, S. G., Pennell, B.-E. & Üstün, T. B. (2006). The World Health Organization World Mental Health Survey Initiative. *Epidemiologia e Psichiatria Sociale*, 15, 161–6.

Kessler, R. C. & Merikangas, K. R. (2004). The National Comorbidity Survey Replication (NCS-R): Background and aims. *International Journal of Methods in Psychiatric Research*, 13, 60–8.

Kessler, R. C. & Üstün, T. B. (2004). The World Mental Health (WMH) Survey Initiative Version of the World Health Organization (WHO) Composite International Diagnostic Interview (CIDI). *International Journal of Methods in Psychiatric Research*, 13, 93–121.

Ministery of Health (2001). *The primary health care strategy*. Wellington: Ministry of Health.

Ministry of Health (2003). *New Zealand health and disability sector overview*. Wellington: Ministry of Health.

Oakley-Browne, M. A. (2006). Lifetime prevalence and lifetime risk of DSM-IV disorders. In *Te Rau Hinengaro: The New Zealand Mental Health Survey*, ed. M. A. Oakley-Browne, J. E. Wells & K. M. Scott, pp. 57–71. Wellington: Ministry of Health.

Oakley-Browne, M. A., Joyce, P. R., Wells, J. E., Bushnell, J. A. & Hornblow, A. R. (1989). Christchurch Psychiatric Epidemiology Study Part II: Six month and other period prevalences of specific psychiatric disorders. *Australian and New Zealand Journal of Psychiatry*, 23, 327–40.

Oakley-Browne, M. A. & Wells, J. E. (2006). Health services. In *Te Rau Hinengaro: The New Zealand Mental Health Survey*, ed. M. A. Oakley-Browne, J. E. Wells & K. M. Scott, pp. 115–38. Wellington: Ministry of Health.

Oakley-Browne, M. A., Wells, J. E., McGee, M. A. & New Zealand Mental Health Survey Research Team (2006a). Twelve-month and lifetime health service use in Te Rau Hinengaro: The New Zealand Mental Health Survey. *Australian and New Zealand Journal of Psychiatry*, 40, 855–64.

Oakley-Browne, M. A., Wells, J. E. & Scott, K. M. (2006). *Te Rau Hinengaro: The New Zealand Mental Health Survey*. Wellington: Ministry of Health.

Oakley-Browne, M. A., Wells, J. E. & Scott, K. M., McGee, M. A. & New Zealand Mental Health Survey Research Team (2006b). Lifetime prevalence and projected lifetime risk of DSM-IV disorders in Te Rau Hinengaro: The New Zealand Mental Health Survey. *Australian and New Zealand Journal of Psychiatry*, 40, 865–74.

Research Triangle Institute (2002). *SUDAAN: Professional software for survey data analysis 8.01*. Research Triangle Park, NC: Research Triangle Institute.

Romans-Clarkson, S. E., Walton, V. A., Herbison, G. P. & Mullen, P. E. (1988). Marriage, motherhood and psychiatric morbidity in New Zealand. *Psychological Medicine*, 18, 983–90.

Romans-Clarkson, S. E., Walton, V. A., Herbison, G. P. & Mullen, P. E. (1990). Psychiatric morbidity among women in urban and rural New Zealand: Psychosocial correlates. *British Journal of Psychiatry*, 156, 84–91.

Rutter, M. (2002). The interplay of nature, nurture, and developmental influences: The challenge ahead for mental health. *Archives of General Psychiatry*, 59, 996–1000.

SAS Institute (2001). *SAS/STAT software: Changes and enhancements, Release 8.2*. Cary, NC: SAS Publishing.

Statistics New Zealand (2002). *Ethnic groups: 2001 Census of Population and Dwellings*. Wellington: Statistics New Zealand.

Statistics New Zealand (2006a). *New Zealand in profile*. Wellington: Statistics New Zealand.

Statistics New Zealand (2006b). *Demographic trends 2005*. Wellington: Statistics New Zealand.

United Nations Children's Fund (UNICEF) (2007). Child poverty in perspective: An overview of child well-being in rich countries. *Innocenti Report Card 7: Innocenti Report Cards*. Florence, Italy: UNICEF Innocenti Research Centre.

University of Otago (n.d.). Dunedin Multidisciplinary Health and Development Research Unit. Available at: http://dunedinstudy.otago.ac.nz/.

Wang, P. S., Aguilar-Gaxiola, S., Alonso, J., Angermeyer, M. C., Borges, G., Bromet, E. J., Bruffaerts, R., de Girolamo, G., de Graaf, R., Gureje, O., Haro, J. M., Karam, E. J., Kessler, R. C., Kovess, V., Lane, M. C., Lee, S., Levinson, D., Ono, Y., Petukhova, M., Posada-Villa, J., Seedat, S. & Wells, J. E. (2007a). Twelve month use of mental health services in the World Health Organization World Mental Health (WMH) Surveys. *Lancet*, 370, 841–50.

Wang, P. S., Angermeyer, M., Borges, G., Bruffaerts, R., Chiu, W. T., de Girolamo, G., Fayyad, J., Gureje, O., Haro, J. M., Huang, Y.-Q., Kessler, R. C., Kovess, V., Levinson, D., Nakane, Y., Oakley-Browne, M. A., Ormel, J., Posada-Villa, J., Aguilar-Gaxiola, S., Alonso, J., Lee, S., Heeringa, S., Pennell, B.-E., Chatterji, S. & Üstün, T. B. (2007b). Delay and failure in treatment seeking after first onset of mental disorders in the World Health Organization's World Mental Health Survey Initiative. *World Psychiatry*, 6, 177–85.

Wells, J. E. (2006). Twelve-month prevalence. In *Te Rau Hinengaro: The New Zealand Mental Health Survey*, ed. M. A. Oakley-Browne, J. E. Wells & K. M. Scott, pp. 37–56. Wellington: Ministry of Health.

Wells, J. E., Joyce, P. R., Bushnell, J. A., Hornblow, A. R. & Oakley-Browne, M. A. (1989). Christchurch Psychiatric Epidemiology Study Part I: Methodology and lifetime prevalence for specific psychiatric disorders. *Australian and New Zealand Journal of Psychiatry*, 23, 315–26.

Wells, J. E., McGee, M. A. & Oakley-Browne, M. A. (2006). Methods. In *Te Rau Hinengaro: The New Zealand Mental Health Survey*, ed. M. A. Oakley-Browne, J. E. Wells & K. M. Scott, pp. 218–51. Wellington: Ministry of Health.

Wells, J. E., Oakley-Browne, M. A., Scott, K. M., McGee, M. A., Baxter, J., Kokaua, J. & New Zealand Mental Health Survey Research Team (2006a). Prevalence, interference with life and severity of 12-month DSM-IV disorders in Te Rau Hinengaro:

The New Zealand Mental Health Survey. *Australian and New Zealand Journal of Psychiatry*, 40, 845–54.

Wells, J. E., Oakley-Browne, M. A., Scott, K. M., McGee, M. A., Baxter, J., Kokaua, J. & New Zealand Mental Health Survey Research Team (2006b). Te Rau Hinengaro: The New Zealand Mental Health Survey: Overview of methods and findings. *Australian and New Zealand Journal of Psychiatry*, 40, 835–44.

World Health Organization (WHO) (1991). *International classification of diseases (ICD-10)*. Geneva: World Health Organization.

World Health Organization (WHO) (1993). *The ICD-10 classification of mental and behavioural disorders: Diagnostic criteria for research*. Geneva: World Health Organization.

World Health Organization (WHO) (2005). *Mental health atlas 2005*. Geneva: World Health Organization.

# PART THREE

# Cross-National Comparisons

# 24 Lifetime Prevalence and Age of Onset Distributions of Mental Disorders in the World Mental Health Survey Initiative

RONALD C. KESSLER, SERGIO AGUILAR-GAXIOLA, JORDI ALONSO, MATTHIAS C. ANGERMEYER, JAMES C. ANTHONY, PATRICIA A. BERGLUND, SOMNATH CHATTERJI, GIOVANNI DE GIROLAMO, RON DE GRAAF, KOEN DEMYTTENAERE, ISABELLE GASQUET, SEMYON F. GLUZMAN, MICHAEL J. GRUBER, OYE GUREJE, JOSEP MARIA HARO, STEVEN G. HEERINGA, AIMEE N. KARAM, NORITO KAWAKAMI, SING LEE, DAPHNA LEVINSON, MARIA ELENA MEDINA-MORA, MARK A. OAKLEY-BROWNE, BETH-ELLEN PENNELL, MARIA PETUKHOVA, JOSÉ POSADA-VILLA, AYELET RUSCIO, DAN J. STEIN, CHEUK HIM ADLEY TSANG, AND T. BEDIRHAN ÜSTÜN

## ACKNOWLEDGMENTS

Centralized data cleaning, coding, and analyses of the WMH data are supported by the U.S. National Institute of Mental Health (R01 MH070884), the John D. and Catherine T. MacArthur Foundation, the Fogarty International Center (FIRCA R03-TW006481), the Pan American Health Organization, the U.S. Public Health Service (R13-MH066849, R01-MH069864, and R01 DA016558), the Pfizer Foundation, Eli Lilly and Company Foundation, Ortho-McNeil Pharmaceutical, GlaxoSmith-Kline, and Bristol-Myers Squibb.

Portions of this chapter are based on: Kessler, R. C., Angermeyer, M., Anthony, J. C., de Graaf, R., Demyttenaere, K., Gasquet, I., de Girolamo, G., Gluzman, S., Gureje, O., Haro, J. M., Kawakami, N., Karam, A., Levinson, D., Medina-Mora, M. E., Oakley-Browne, M. A., Posada-Villa, J., Stein, D. J., Tsang, C. H., Aguilar-Gaxiola, S., Alonso, J., Lee, S., Heeringa, S., Pennell, B.-E., Berglund, P., Gruber, M. J., Petukhova, M., Chatterji, S., Üstun, T. B., for The WHO World Mental Health Survey Consortium (2007). Lifetime prevalence and age of onset distributions of mental disorders in the World Health Organization's World Mental Health Survey Initiative. World Psychiatry, 6(3), 168–76. Copyright

## I. INTRODUCTION

There is wide variation in the estimated lifetime prevalence of DSM-IV/CIDI disorders in the WMH surveys. Previous cross-national research found the same sort of wide variation (Kessler et al. 1994; Andrade et al. 2002; Bijl et al. 1998; Caraveo, Martinez & Rivera 1998; Kylyc 1998; Vega et al. 1998; Wittchen et al. 1998; WHO International Consortium in Psychiatric Epidemiology 2000). The highest lifetime prevalence estimate of having any disorder is 47.4% in the United States. The lowest is 12.0% in Nigeria. Although it would be interesting to speculate about possible substantive reasons for this variation, methodological explanations are also plausible (Simon et al. 2002; Cooke, Hart & Michie 2004; Chang et al. 2007) and our follow-up studies of the WMH data aimed at addressing these methodological explanations are as yet so preliminary that we will not offer any comments on substantive interpretations of cross-national differences in this first volume of WMH results. A brief overview of methodological explanations is presented at the end of this chapter. Preliminary results of the WMH methodological studies are presented in Chapter 26. On the basis of these results, we believe that it is most useful to focus readers' attention in this chapter on the important similarities in results across the WMH surveys rather than on the differences. A number of important similarities exist. These similarities, emerging as they do despite the wide variation in survey conditions, form a firm foundation for future more fine-grained analyses of the WMH data.

## 2. PREVALENCE

The first noteworthy similarity is that the DSM-IV/CIDI disorders assessed in the WMH surveys are quite common in all the countries studied. The interquartile range (IQR) (25th–75th percentiles across countries) of lifetime prevalence of any disorder across these surveys is 18.1%–36.1%. A lifetime DSM/CIDI diagnosis was found among more than one-third of respondents in five countries (Colombia, France, New Zealand, Ukraine, United States), more than one-fourth in six countries (Belgium, Germany, Lebanon, Mexico, Netherlands, South Africa), and more than one-sixth in four countries (Israel, Italy, Japan, Spain) (Table 24.1). The remaining two countries, China (13.2%) and Nigeria (12.0%), had considerably lower prevalence estimates that are likely to be downwardly biased (Gureje et al. 2006; Shen et al. 2006). Prevalence estimates for other developing countries were all above the lower bound of the IQR. This, when coupled with the fact that our clinical reappraisal studies showed prevalence estimates in developed countries to be accurate and with the possibility that prevalence estimates in less developed countries are underestimated (discussed in more detail in Chapter 26), argues persuasively that mental disorders have great public health importance throughout the world.

It is also noteworthy that all four classes of disorder considered here were important components of overall prevalence in most countries. Anxiety disorders were the most prevalent in ten countries (4.8%–31.0%, IQR: 9.9%–16.7%) and mood disorders in all but one other country (3.3%–21.4%, IQR: 9.8%–15.8%).

Impulse-control disorders were least prevalent in most countries that included a relatively full assessment of these disorders (0.3%–25.0%, IQR: 3.1%–5.7%). Substance use disorders were generally least prevalent elsewhere (1.3%–15.0%, IQR: 4.8%–9.6%). The Western European countries did not assess illicit drug abuse/dependence, though, leading to artificially low prevalence estimates (1.3%–8.9%) compared to other countries (2.2%–15.0%). Substance dependence was also assessed only in the presence of abuse, which possibly further reduces estimated prevalence (Hasin & Grant 2004). Lifetime disorder co-occurrence was also quite common in most countries, as seen by noting that the sum of prevalence across the four disorder types was generally between 30% and 50% higher than the prevalence of any disorder. Within-class co-occurrence cannot be seen in the results reported in Table 24.1, although it can be seen in the country-specific chapters reported in Part 2 of this volume by comparing the sum of disorder-specific prevalence estimates within a class of disorders to the prevalence estimate for any disorders within the class. This exercise is even stronger than between-class co-occurrence (results available on request).

## 3. AGE OF ONSET DISTRIBUTIONS

Considerable cross-national consistency exists in standardized age of onset (AOO) distributions. Impulse-control disorders have the earliest AOO distributions in most countries. This is true both in terms of early median AOOs and in terms of the narrowness of the age range of onset risk. The median AOOs of impulse-control disorders across the WMH surveys considered in this volume are 7–9 years of age for attention-deficit/hyperactivity disorder, 7–15 for oppositional-defiant disorder, 9–14 for conduct disorder, and 13–21 for intermittent explosive disorder. There is an extremely narrow age range of onset risk for impulse-control disorders in most surveys, with 80% of all lifetime attention-deficit/hyperactivity disorder beginning in the age range 4–11 and the vast majority of oppositional-defiant disorder and conduct disorder beginning between the ages of 5 and 15.

**Table 24.1.** Lifetime prevalence and projected lifetime risk as of age 75 of DSM-IV/ CIDI disorders[a]

| | Any anxiety disorder | | | | | Any mood disorder | | | | | Any impulse-control disorder | | | | | Any substance disorder | | | | | Any disorder | | | | |
|---|---|---|---|---|---|---|---|---|---|---|---|---|---|---|---|---|---|---|---|---|---|---|---|---|---|
| | Previous | | | Proj. LT risk | | Previous | | | Proj. LT risk | | Previous | | | Proj. LT risk | | Previous | | | Proj. LT risk | | Previous | | | Proj. LT risk | |
| | % | n[b] | (se) | % | (se) | % | n[b] | (se) | % | (se) | % | n[b] | (se) | % | (se) | % | n[b] | (se) | % | (se) | % | n[b] | (se) | % | (se) |
| **WHO: Regional Office for the Americas (AMRO)** | | | | | | | | | | | | | | | | | | | | | | | | | |
| Colombia | 25.3 | 948 | (1.4) | 30.9 | (2.5) | 14.6 | 666 | (0.7) | 27.2 | (2.0) | 9.6 | 273 | (0.8) | 10.3 | (0.9) | 9.6 | 345 | (0.6) | 12.8 | (1.0) | 39.1 | 1432 | (1.3) | 55.2[c] | (6.0) |
| Mexico | 14.3 | 684 | (0.9) | 17.8 | (1.6) | 9.2 | 598 | (0.5) | 20.4 | (1.7) | 5.7 | 152 | (0.6) | 5.7 | (0.6) | 7.8 | 378 | (0.5) | 11.9 | (1.0) | 26.1 | 1148 | (1.4) | 36.4[c] | (2.1) |
| United States[d] | 31.0 | 2692 | (1.0) | 36.0 | (1.4) | 21.4 | 2024 | (0.6) | 31.4 | (0.9) | 25.0 | 1051 | (1.1) | 25.6 | (1.1) | 14.6 | 1144 | (0.6) | 17.4 | (0.6) | 47.4 | 3929 | (1.1) | 55.3 | (1.2) |
| **WHO: Regional Office for Africa (AFRO)** | | | | | | | | | | | | | | | | | | | | | | | | | |
| Nigeria | 6.5 | 169 | (0.9) | 7.1 | (0.9) | 3.3 | 236 | (0.3) | 8.9 | (1.2) | 0.3 | 9 | (0.1) | –[e,h] | – | 3.7 | 119 | (0.4) | 6.4 | (1.0) | 12.0 | 440 | (1.0) | 19.5 | (1.9) |
| South Africa | 15.8 | 695 | (0.8) | 30.1 | (4.4) | 9.8 | 439 | (0.7) | 20.0 | (2.4) | –[e,h] | – | – | – | – | 13.3 | 505 | (0.9) | 17.5 | (1.2) | 30.3 | 1290 | (1.1) | 47.5 | (3.7) |
| **WHO: Regional Office for the Eastern Mediterranean (EMRO)** | | | | | | | | | | | | | | | | | | | | | | | | | |
| Lebanon | 16.7 | 282 | (1.6) | 20.2 | (1.8) | 12.6 | 352 | (0.9) | 20.1 | (1.2) | 4.4 | 53 | (0.9) | 4.6 | (1.0) | 2.2 | 27 | (0.8) | –[e] | | 25.8 | 491 | (1.9) | 32.9 | (2.1) |
| **WHO: Regional Office for Europe (EURO)** | | | | | | | | | | | | | | | | | | | | | | | | | |
| Belgium | 13.1 | 219 | (1.9) | 15.7 | (2.5) | 14.1 | 367 | (1.0) | 22.8 | (1.7) | 5.2 | 31 | (1.4) | 5.2 | (1.4) | 8.3 | 195 | (0.9) | 10.5 | (1.1) | 29.1 | 519 | (2.3) | 37.1 | (3.0) |
| France | 22.3 | 445 | (1.4) | 26.0 | (1.6) | 21.0 | 648 | (1.1) | 30.5 | (1.4) | 7.6 | 71 | (1.3) | 7.6 | (1.3) | 7.1 | 202 | (0.5) | 8.8 | (0.6) | 37.9 | 847 | (1.7) | 47.2 | (1.6) |
| Germany | 14.6 | 314 | (1.5) | 16.9 | (1.7) | 9.9 | 372 | (0.6) | 16.2 | (1.3) | 3.1 | 31 | (0.8) | 3.1 | (0.8) | 6.5 | 228 | (0.6) | 8.7 | (0.9) | 25.2 | 573 | (1.9) | 33.0 | (2.5) |
| Israel | 5.2 | 252 | (0.3) | 10.1 | (0.9) | 10.7 | 524 | (0.5) | 21.2 | (1.6) | –[f] | – | – | – | | 5.3 | 261 | (0.3) | 6.3 | (0.4) | 17.6 | 860 | (0.6) | 29.7 | (1.5) |
| Italy | 11.0 | 328 | (0.9) | 13.7 | (1.2) | 9.9 | 452 | (0.5) | 17.3 | (1.2) | 1.7 | 27 | (0.4) | –[e] | | 1.3 | 56 | (0.2) | 1.6 | (0.3) | 18.1 | 612 | (1.1) | 26.0 | (1.9) |
| Netherlands | 15.9 | 320 | (1.1) | 21.4 | (1.8) | 17.9 | 476 | (1.0) | 28.9 | (1.9) | 4.7 | 37 | (1.1) | 4.8 | (1.1) | 8.9 | 210 | (0.9) | 11.4 | (1.2) | 31.7 | 633 | (2.0) | 42.9 | (2.5) |
| Spain[g] | 9.9 | 375 | (1.1) | 13.3 | (1.4) | 10.6 | 672 | (0.5) | 20.8 | (1.2) | 2.3 | 40 | (0.8) | 2.3 | (0.8) | 3.6 | 180 | (0.4) | 4.6 | (0.5) | 19.4 | 842 | (1.4) | 29.0 | (1.8) |
| Ukraine | 10.9 | 371 | (0.8) | 17.3 | (2.0) | 15.8 | 814 | (0.8) | 25.9 | (1.5) | 8.7 | 91 | (1.1) | 9.7 | (1.3) | 15.0 | 293 | (1.3) | 18.8 | (1.7) | 36.1 | 1074 | (1.5) | 48.9 | (2.5) |
| **WHO: Regional Office for the Western Pacific (WPRO)** | | | | | | | | | | | | | | | | | | | | | | | | | |
| People's Republic of China | 4.8 | 159 | (0.7) | 6.0 | (0.8) | 3.6 | 185 | (0.4) | 7.3 | (0.9) | 4.3 | 37 | (0.9) | 4.9 | (0.9) | 4.9 | 128 | (0.7) | 6.1 | (0.8) | 13.2 | 419 | (1.3) | 18.0 | (1.5) |
| Japan | 6.9 | 155 | (0.6) | 9.2 | (1.2) | 7.6 | 183 | (0.5) | 14.1 | (1.7) | 2.8[h] | 11 | (1.0) | –[e] | | 4.8 | 69 | (0.5) | 6.2 | (0.7) | 18.0 | 343 | (1.1) | 24.4 | (1.8) |
| New Zealand | 24.6 | 3171 | (0.7) | 30.3 | (1.5) | 20.4 | 2755 | (0.5) | 29.8 | (0.7) | –[f] | – | – | – | | 12.4 | 1767 | (0.4) | 14.6 | (0.5) | 39.3 | 4815 | (0.9) | 48.6 | (1.5) |

[a] See the text for a discussion of between-county differences in the disorders included in each of the diagnostic groups.

[b] The numbers reported here are the numbers of respondents with the disorders indicated in the column heading. The denominators used to calculate prevalence estimates based on these numbers of cases are reported in Chapter 1, Table 1.1. In the case of anxiety disorders and substance disorders, the denominators are the numbers of respondents in the Part 1 sample. In the case of impulse-control disorders and any disorders, the denominators are the numbers of respondents in the Part 2 sample. In the case of mood disorders, the denominators are the numbers of respondents age ≤ 44 in the Part 2 sample.

[c] Projected lifetime risk to age 65 due to the sample including only respondents up to age 65.

[d] The results reported here for the United States differ somewhat from those in Chapter 9 as a result of updates in the coding scheme implemented in the analyses reported here compared to the analyses reported in Chapter 9.

[e] Cell size was too small to be included in analysis.

[f] Impulse disorders not assessed.

[g] The results for Spain differ somewhat from those reported in Chapter 19, as the latter used country-specific algorithms to estimate coefficients.

[h] Only IED assessed.

Although the AOO distribution is less concentrated for intermittent explosive disorder, fully half of all lifetime cases have onsets in childhood and adolescence.

The situation is more complex with anxiety disorders, as the AOO distributions fall into two distinct sets. The phobias and separation anxiety disorder all have very early AOO (medians in the age range 7–14, IQR: 8–11). Generalized anxiety disorder, panic disorder, and posttraumatic stress disorder, in comparison, have much later AOO (median 24–50, IQR: 31–41), with much wider cross-national variation than for the impulse control disorders or the phobias or separation anxiety disorder. The AOO distributions for mood disorders are similar to those for generalized anxiety disorder, panic disorder, and posttraumatic stress disorder. Specifically, lifetime prevalence of mood disorders is consistently low until the early teens, at which time a roughly linear increase begins that continues through late middle age, with a more gradual increase thereafter. The median AOO of mood disorders ranges between the late twenties and the early forties in the WMH surveys (29–43, IQR: 35–40).

The AOO distribution of substance use disorders is consistent across countries, in that few onsets occur prior to the midteens and cumulative increase in onset is rapid in adolescence and early adulthood. Considerable cross-national variation exists, though, in the sharpness of the change in the slope as well as in the age range of this change. This cross-national variation leads to wider cross-national variation in both the median and the IQR of the AOO distributions than for impulse-control disorders or phobias or separation anxiety disorder, but lower variation than for mood disorders or other anxiety disorders.

## 4. PROJECTED LIFETIME RISK

Projected lifetime risk of any disorder as of age 75 is between 17% higher (United States) and 69% higher (Israel) than estimated lifetime prevalence (IQR: 28%–44%). The highest risk-to-prevalence ratios (57%–69%) are in countries exposed to sectarian violence (Israel, Nigeria, and

South Africa). Excluding these three, there is no strong difference in ratios of developing (28%–41%) versus developed (17%–49%) countries. The highest class-specific proportional increase in projected risk is for mood disorders (45%–170%, IQR: 61%–98%) and the lowest is for impulse-control disorders (0%–14%, IQR: 0%–2%), consistent with the former having the latest and the latter having the earliest AOO distribution. The projected lifetime risk estimates suggest that approximately half the population (47%–55%) will eventually have a mental disorder in six countries (Colombia, France, New Zealand, South Africa, Ukraine, United States), approximately one-third (30%–43%) in six other countries (Belgium, Germany, Israel, Lebanon, Mexico, the Netherlands), approximately one-fourth (24%–29%) in three others (Italy, Japan, Spain), and approximately one-fifth (18%–19%) in the remaining countries (China, Nigeria).

It is noteworthy that the projected increases in lifetime prevalence of any disorder in most WMH surveys are considerably lower than the projected increases in lifetime prevalence of particular disorders, especially the disorders with the later AOO distributions. For example, the results reported in Chapter 19 for Spain show that while the proportion of the sample that is estimated eventually to have a lifetime depressive episode is roughly twice as high as the percentage who reported ever having such an episode as of their age at interview, the projected increase in the proportion of respondents having any disorder is only about one-third. The reason for this discrepancy is that many of the people who are projected to have first onsets of later-onset disorders already have a history of one or more lifetime mental disorders. New onsets, then, are likely to be onsets of secondary comorbid conditions. This is an important for two reasons. First, comorbidity is found to be associated with severity in the vast majority of WMH surveys. This means that the prevention of comorbidity might be effective in reducing the prevalence of seriously impairing mental disorders. Second, the results regarding lifetime treatment, which are discussed in the next chapter, show that delays in initial efforts to seek professional help are much greater for early-onset disorders. The latter disorders are much more likely to be temporally primary than are later-onset disorders. This raises the possibility that delays in seeking treatment for early-onset disorders might result in higher risk of the onset of secondary comorbid disorder, which, in turn, leads to an increase in the severity of mental disorders. The public health implications of these patterns are discussed in the next chapter but need to be pointed out here in our review of important similarities in the patterns of basic results across the WMH surveys.

## 5. COHORT EFFECTS

Previous research has suggested that projected lifetime risk might be increasing in recent cohorts (WHO International Consortium in Psychiatric Epidemiology 2000). Prospective tracking studies are required to monitor cohort effects directly. However, indirect approximations can be obtained in cross-sectional data using retrospective AOO reports. This was done in the WMH data using discrete-time survival analysis to predict onset of disorders across age groups 18–34, 35–49, 50–64, and 65+. As these surveys were completed between 2002 and 2005, the most recent cohorts (aged 18–34 at interview) roughly correspond to those born in the years from 1968 onward. Respondents aged 35–49 at interview correspond roughly to cohorts born in 1953–70, while those aged 50–64 were born in 1938–55, and those ages 65+ were born before 1938. The results of the survival analyses reported in Part 2 of this volume show clearly that the odds ratios for anxiety, mood, and substance use disorders are generally higher in recent cohorts than in older cohorts, while not for impulse control disorders (Tables 24.2–24.5). No meaningful difference exists between less developed and developed countries, although cross-national variation exceeds chance expectations.

## 6. DISCUSSION

It is likely that the lifetime prevalence estimates reported here are downwardly biased. Four sources of bias could have led to underestimating

prevalence in the WMH surveys. First, people with mental illness have been found to be less likely than others to participate in surveys, because of sample frame exclusions (e.g., excluding homeless people), differential mortality, and greater reluctance to participate (Allgulander 1989). Variation in the magnitude of such underrepresentation across countries could help account for the wide between-country variations in prevalence-risk estimates. Second, previous research suggests that lifetime prevalence is sometimes underreported because of respondent reluctance to admit mental illness (Cannell, Marquis & Laurent 1977). This bias might be especially strong in developing countries with no strong tradition of independent public opinion research, which could help account for the especially low prevalence-risk estimates in Nigeria and China. Third, interviewer error might have led to underreporting, especially in countries where there was an indirect incentive to rush through interviews, because interviewers were paid by the interview rather than by the hour. Fourth, the interview thresholds for defining disorders might have been too strict in some countries. As noted in Chapter 6, clinical reappraisal studies carried out in some of the countries with the highest prevalence estimates found no evidence of such bias (Haro et al. 2006). This means that the high prevalence estimates of DSM-IV/CIDI disorders found in these countries are accurate. However, it is possible, even likely in light of evidence presented in Chapter 26, that prevalence was underestimated in some of the countries that had low prevalence estimates.

A possible bias is also noteworthy with regard to the results reported here regarding projected lifetime risk: that the method used to estimate lifetime risk was based on the assumption of constant conditional risk of first onset in a given year of life across cohorts. The existence of an apparent cohort effect means that this assumption is incorrect, probably causing an underestimation of lifetime risk in younger cohorts. At the same time, AOO might have been recalled with error related to age at interview. Older people, for example, might have had a higher rate

**Table 24.2.** Intercohort differences in lifetime risk of any DSM-IV/CIDI anxiety disorder[a]

| | 18–34 | | | 35–49 | | | 50–64 | | | 65+[b] | | | χ² | df | n |
|---|---|---|---|---|---|---|---|---|---|---|---|---|---|---|---|
| | OR | (95% CI) | n | OR | (95% CI) | n | OR | (95% CI) | n | OR | (95% CI) | n | | | |
| **WHO: Regional Office for the Americas (AMRO)** | | | | | | | | | | | | | | | |
| Colombia | 1.6* | (1.2–2.1) | 825 | 1.3 | (0.9–1.8) | 906 | 1.0 | – | 379 | – | – | – | 10.0* | 2 | 2381 |
| Mexico | 2.4* | (1.6–3.4) | 896 | 1.6* | (1.1–2.4) | 840 | 1.0 | – | 359 | – | – | – | 25.3* | 2 | 2362 |
| United States[c] | 3.5* | (2.8–4.4) | 1939 | 3.4* | (2.7–4.1) | 1831 | 2.5* | (2.0–3.0) | 1213 | 1.0 | – | 709 | 159.2* | 3 | 5692 |
| **WHO: Regional Office for Africa (AFRO)** | | | | | | | | | | | | | | | |
| Nigeria | 3.1* | (1.4–6.9) | 971 | 2.3* | (1.1–4.9) | 549 | 2.8* | (1.5–5.4) | 369 | 1.0 | – | 254 | 11.1* | 3 | 2143 |
| South Africa | 2.3* | (1.3–4.0) | 2172 | 1.8* | (1.1–3.1) | 1264 | 1.3 | (0.8–2.1) | 638 | 1.0 | – | 241 | 16.5* | 3 | 4315 |
| **WHO: Regional Office for the Eastern Mediterranean (EMRO)** | | | | | | | | | | | | | | | |
| Lebanon | 3.2* | (1.6–6.2) | 349 | 2.5* | (1.2–5.1) | 348 | 1.0 | (0.5–2.1) | 199 | 1.0 | – | 135 | 24.1* | 3 | 1031 |
| **WHO: Regional Office for Europe (EURO)** | | | | | | | | | | | | | | | |
| Belgium | 2.6* | (1.3–5.0) | 254 | 1.6 | (0.8–3.2) | 331 | 1.3 | (0.6–2.6) | 278 | 1.0 | – | 180 | 14.2* | 3 | 1043 |
| France | 3.1* | (1.5–6.4) | 388 | 3.2* | (1.5–6.7) | 472 | 1.6 | (0.8–3.3) | 362 | 1.0 | – | 214 | 21.3* | 3 | 1436 |
| Germany | 3.1* | (1.9–5.1) | 316 | 2.3* | (1.4–3.9) | 436 | 2.3* | (1.3–4.1) | 345 | 1.0 | – | 226 | 21.8* | 3 | 1323 |
| Israel | 4.7* | (2.6–8.3) | 1627 | 2.7* | (1.6–4.4) | 1302 | 2.1* | (1.4–3.3) | 1069 | 1.0 | – | 861 | 27.3* | 3 | 4859 |
| Italy | 1.5 | (0.7–3.0) | 496 | 1.6 | (0.9–2.8) | 516 | 1.3 | (0.8–2.2) | 454 | 1.0 | – | 313 | 3.3 | 3 | 1779 |
| Netherlands | 3.6* | (2.1–6.1) | 264 | 4.5* | (3.0–6.8) | 358 | 3.0* | (2.0–4.6) | 302 | 1.0 | – | 170 | 60.6* | 3 | 1094 |
| Spain[d] | 3.8* | (2.2–6.5) | 545 | 2.8* | (1.5–5.2) | 556 | 1.3 | (0.8–2.2) | 456 | 1.0 | – | 564 | 28.7* | 3 | 2121 |
| Ukraine | 1.7 | (1.1–2.6) | 420 | 1.0 | (0.6–1.6) | 434 | 1.0 | (0.7–1.6) | 412 | 1.0 | – | 454 | 6.5 | 3 | 1720 |
| **WHO: Regional Office for the Western Pacific (WPRO)** | | | | | | | | | | | | | | | |
| People's Republic of China | 1.7 | (0.6–4.4) | 379 | 1.1 | (0.5–2.5) | 726 | 1.6 | (0.7–3.9) | 357 | 1.0 | – | 166 | 3.3 | 3 | 1628 |
| Japan | 5.6* | (2.2–13.8) | 155 | 2.8* | (1.3–6.1) | 219 | 2.6* | (1.2–5.6) | 295 | 1.0 | – | 218 | 14.9* | 3 | 887 |
| New Zealand | 3.4* | (2.7–4.2) | 2517 | 2.6* | (2.1–3.1) | 2474 | 2.1* | (1.7–2.7) | 1517 | 1.0 | – | 927 | 126.3* | 3 | 7435 |

[a] Based on discrete-time survival models with person-year as the unit of analysis; controls are time intervals.

[b] Referent category unless otherwise noted.

[c] The results reported here for the United States differ somewhat from those in Chapter 9 as a result of updates in the coding scheme implemented in the analyses reported here compared to the analyses reported in Chapter 9.

[d] The results for Spain differ somewhat from those reported in Chapter 19, as the latter used country-specific algorithms to estimate coefficients.

* Significant at the 0.05 level, two-sided test.

**Table 24.3.** Intercohort differences in lifetime risk of any DSM-IV/CIDI mood disorder[a]

| | 18–34 | | | 35–49 | | | 50–64 | | | 65+[b] | | | | | |
|---|---|---|---|---|---|---|---|---|---|---|---|---|---|---|---|
| | OR | (95% CI) | n | OR | (95% CI) | n | OR | (95% CI) | n | OR | (95% CI) | n | χ² | df | n |
| **WHO: Regional Office for the Americas (AMRO)** | | | | | | | | | | | | | | | |
| Colombia | 6.3* | (4.2–9.3) | 1431 | 2.3* | (1.6–3.1) | 1735 | 1.0 | – | 730 | – | – | 530 | 92.7* | 2 | 4426 |
| Mexico | 4.0* | (2.6–6.1) | 2060 | 1.6* | (1.1–2.3) | 2236 | 1.0 | – | 840 | – | – | 646 | 65.0* | 2 | 5782 |
| United States[c] | 9.5* | (7.3–12.4) | 3034 | 5.0* | (3.7–6.6) | 2865 | 3.0* | (2.3–3.9) | 1922 | 1.0 | – | 1461 | 383.6* | 3 | 9282 |
| **WHO: Regional Office for Africa (AFRO)** | | | | | | | | | | | | | | | |
| Nigeria | 3.7* | (1.8–7.6) | 3175 | 1.8 | (0.9–3.6) | 1631 | 1.2 | (0.7–2.1) | 1104 | 1.0 | – | 842 | 19.4* | 3 | 6752 |
| South Africa | 9.6* | (5.5–16.7) | 2172 | 5.5* | (3.1–9.9) | 1264 | 2.5* | (1.4–4.4) | 638 | 1.0 | – | 241 | 95.6 | 3 | 4315 |
| **WHO: Regional Office for the Eastern Mediterranean (EMRO)** | | | | | | | | | | | | | | | |
| Lebanon | 6.2* | (3.0–12.8) | 965 | 3.1* | (1.4–6.7) | 931 | 1.7 | (0.8–3.2) | 553 | 1.0 | – | 408 | 60.5* | 3 | 2857 |
| **WHO: Regional Office for Europe (EURO)** | | | | | | | | | | | | | | | |
| Belgium | 11.3* | (6.1–20.9) | 573 | 4.9* | (3.2–7.5) | 775 | 3.6* | (2.0–6.4) | 570 | 1.0 | – | 501 | 87.3* | 3 | 2419 |
| France | 9.0* | (6.0–13.5) | 743 | 3.0* | (2.2–4.2) | 942 | 1.8* | (1.2–2.6) | 719 | 1.0 | – | 490 | 146.4* | 3 | 2894 |
| Germany | 12.2* | (7.1–21.0) | 815 | 5.2* | (3.5–7.7) | 1180 | 2.4* | (1.6–3.4) | 893 | 1.0 | – | 667 | 94.4* | 3 | 3555 |
| Israel | 6.5* | (4.5–9.4) | 1627 | 2.8* | (2.0–4.0) | 1302 | 1.8* | (1.3–2.5) | 1069 | 1.0 | – | 861 | 118.4* | 3 | 4859 |
| Italy | 5.7* | (3.8–8.4) | 1326 | 3.6* | (2.6–5.0) | 1393 | 2.3* | (1.6–3.3) | 1153 | 1.0 | – | 840 | 91.3* | 3 | 4712 |
| Netherlands | 11.7* | (6.6–20.8) | 564 | 6.4* | (4.0–10.2) | 729 | 2.9* | (1.7–4.8) | 627 | 1.0 | – | 452 | 115.7* | 3 | 2372 |
| Spain[d] | 9.6* | (6.6–13.9) | 1567 | 4.2* | (3.0–5.9) | 1431 | 2.2* | (1.6–3.0) | 1024 | 1.0 | – | 1451 | 176.3* | 3 | 5473 |
| Ukraine | 1.9* | (1.4–2.4) | 1194 | 1.0 | (0.8–1.3) | 1225 | 0.9 | (0.8–1.1) | 1180 | 1.0 | – | 1126 | 38.2* | 3 | 4725 |
| **WHO: Regional Office for the Western Pacific (WPRO)** | | | | | | | | | | | | | | | |
| People's Republic of China | 20.8* | (9.4–45.8) | 1209 | 4.4* | (2.3–8.4) | 2261 | 2.5* | (1.4–4.4) | 1184 | 1.0 | – | 547 | 76.5* | 3 | 5201 |
| Japan | 23.7* | (13.4–42.0) | 410 | 7.7* | (4.5–13.2) | 571 | 3.8* | (2.4–5.8) | 764 | 1.0 | – | 691 | 146.2* | 3 | 2436 |
| New Zealand | 10.0* | (8.2–12.2) | 3949 | 5.0* | (4.1–6.0) | 4102 | 2.9* | (2.4–3.6) | 2697 | 1.0 | – | 2244 | 653.9* | 3 | 12992 |

[a] Based on discrete-time survival models with person-year as the unit of analysis; controls are time intervals.

[b] Referent category unless otherwise noted.

[c] The results reported here for the United States differ somewhat from those in Chapter 9 as a result of updates in the coding scheme implemented in the analyses reported here compared to the analyses reported in Chapter 9.

[d] The results for Spain differ somewhat from those reported in Chapter 19, as the latter used country-specific algorithms to estimate coefficients.

* Significant at the 0.05 level, two-sided test.

**Table 24.4.** Intercohort differences in lifetime risk of any DSM-IV/CIDI impulse disorders[a]

| | 18–34 | | 35–49[b] | | 50–64[c] | | 65+[c] | | $\chi^2$ | df |
|---|---|---|---|---|---|---|---|---|---|---|
| | OR | (95% CI) | OR | (95% CI) | OR | (95% CI) | OR | (95% CI) | | |
| **WHO: Regional Office for the Americas (AMRO)** | | | | | | | | | | |
| Colombia | 1.4 | (0.9–2.0) | 1.0 | – | – | – | – | – | 2.4 | 1 |
| Mexico | 1.8* | (1.2–2.9) | 1.0 | – | – | – | – | – | 7.8* | 1 |
| United States[d] | 1.2 | (1.0–1.4) | 1.0 | – | – | – | – | – | 4.0* | 1 |
| **WHO: Regional Office for Africa (AFRO)** | | | | | | | | | | |
| Nigeria[e] | – | – | – | – | – | – | – | – | – | – |
| South Africa[f] | – | – | – | – | – | – | – | – | – | – |
| **WHO: Regional Office for the Eastern Mediterranean (EMRO)** | | | | | | | | | | |
| Lebanon | 1.4 | (0.6–3.3) | 1.0 | – | – | – | – | – | 0.8 | 1 |
| **WHO: Regional Office for Europe (EURO)** | | | | | | | | | | |
| Belgium | 1.4 | (0.6–3.4) | 1.0 | – | – | – | – | – | 0.6 | 1 |
| France | 1.5 | (0.7–3.2) | 1.0 | – | – | – | – | – | 1.3 | 1 |
| Germany | 1.1 | (0.3–4.1) | 1.0 | – | – | – | – | – | 0.0 | 1 |
| Israel[f] | – | – | – | – | – | – | – | – | – | – |
| Italy[e] | – | – | – | – | – | – | – | – | – | – |
| Netherlands | 1.3 | (0.4–4.1) | 1.0 | – | – | – | – | – | 0.2 | 1 |
| Spain[g] | 1.5 | (0.5–5.3) | 1.0 | – | – | – | – | – | 0.5 | 1 |
| Ukraine | 1.4 | (0.6–3.2) | 1.0 | – | – | – | – | – | 0.8 | 1 |
| **WHO: Regional Office for the Western Pacific (WPRO)** | | | | | | | | | | |
| People's Republic of China | 0.5 | (0.2–1.3) | 1.0 | – | – | – | – | – | 1.9 | 1 |
| Japan[e] | – | – | – | – | – | – | – | – | – | – |
| New Zealand[f] | – | – | – | – | – | – | – | – | – | – |

[a] Based on discrete-time survival models with person-year as the unit of analysis; controls are time intervals.

[b] Referent category unless otherwise noted.

[c] There was no data for these age ranges as impulse disorders were estimated among Part 2 respondents in the age range 18–39/44. All countries, with the exception of Nigeria, People's Republic of China, and Ukraine (which were age restricted to ≤ 39) were age restricted to ≤ 44.

[d] The results reported here for the United States differ somewhat from those in Chapter 9 as a result of updates in the coding scheme implemented in the analyses reported here compared to the analyses reported in Chapter 9.

[e] Cell size was too small to be included in analysis.

[f] Impulse disorder was not assessed.

[g] The results for Spain differ somewhat from those reported in Chapter 19, as the latter used country-specific algorithms to estimate coefficients.

* Significant at the 0.05 level, two-sided test.

of forgetting episodes of mental illness than did younger people as a simple function of age. Simulation research has shown that a process of this sort could produce the data pattern found here as indirect evidence for a cohort effect (Giuffra & Risch 1994). Evidence for age-related bias has been documented in previous epidemiological research (Simon & Von Korff 1995), although the novel probing strategy used in the WMH surveys has been shown to minimize this problem (Knäuper et al. 1999).

As a result of these methodological considerations, the wide cross-national variation in WMH prevalence and risk estimates should be interpreted with caution. It is likely that the true between-country differences are more modest than those found in the surveys. The overall prevalence-risk estimates, in comparison, are

**Table 24.5.** Intercohort differences in lifetime risk of any DSM-IV/CIDI substance disorders[a]

| | 18–34 | | | 35–49 | | | 50–64 | | | 65+[b] | | | $\chi^2$ | df | n |
|---|---|---|---|---|---|---|---|---|---|---|---|---|---|---|---|
| | OR | (95% CI) | n | OR | (95% CI) | n | OR | (95% CI) | n | OR | (95% CI) | n | | | |
| WHO: Regional Office for the Americas (AMRO) | | | | | | | | | | | | | | | |
| Colombia | 2.3 | (1.6–3.3) | 1431 | 1.1 | (0.7–1.6) | 1735 | 1.0 | – | 730 | – | – | 530 | 39.3* | 2 | 4426 |
| Mexico | 1.7 | (1.3–2.4) | 2060 | 1.2 | (0.9–1.7) | 2236 | 1.0 | – | 840 | – | – | 646 | 12.8* | 2 | 5782 |
| United States[c] | 6.7 | (4.6–10.0) | 1939 | 4.9* | (3.5–7.0) | 1831 | 3.5* | (2.4–5.3) | 1213 | 1.0 | – | 709 | 111.0* | 3 | 5692 |
| WHO: Regional Office for Africa (AFRO) | | | | | | | | | | | | | | | |
| Nigeria | 3.4* | (1.1–10.1) | 971 | 4.9* | (1.8–13.3) | 549 | 2.9 | (1.0–8.7) | 369 | 1.0 | – | 254 | 11.8* | 3 | 2143 |
| South Africa | 2.6* | (1.3–5.4) | 2172 | 1.5 | (0.8–2.9) | 1264 | 1.0 | (0.6–1.9) | 638 | 1.0 | – | 241 | 29.1 | 3 | 4315 |
| WHO: Regional Office for the Eastern Mediterranean (EMRO) | | | | | | | | | | | | | | | |
| Lebanon[d] | – | – | – | – | – | – | – | – | – | – | – | – | – | – | – |
| WHO: Regional Office for Europe (EURO) | | | | | | | | | | | | | | | |
| Belgium | 5.0* | (2.6–9.8) | 254 | 3.6* | (1.7–7.3) | 331 | 2.6* | (1.2–5.4) | 278 | 1.0 | – | 180 | 26.7* | 3 | 1043 |
| France | 5.8* | (3.3–10.0) | 388 | 3.3* | (2.0–5.7) | 472 | 2.5* | (1.4–4.2) | 362 | 1.0 | – | 214 | 44.1* | 3 | 1436 |
| Germany | 5.6* | (2.9–10.7) | 316 | 3.7* | (2.0–6.8) | 436 | 3.9* | (2.1–7.1) | 345 | 1.0 | – | 226 | 35.0* | 3 | 1323 |
| Israel | 11.3* | (5.9–21.6) | 1627 | 4.6* | (2.4–9.0) | 1302 | 2.5* | (1.2–5.1) | 1069 | 1.0 | – | 861 | 119.9* | 3 | 4859 |
| Italy | 2.6* | (1.0–6.7) | 496 | 1.8 | (0.8–4.1) | 516 | 1.6 | (0.6–3.9) | 454 | 1.0 | – | 313 | 5.5 | 3 | 1779 |
| Netherlands | 12.4* | (7.0–21.8) | 264 | 7.0* | (3.8–13.1) | 358 | 6.8* | (3.4–13.9) | 302 | 1.0 | – | 170 | 85.3* | 3 | 1094 |
| Spain[e] | 9.3* | (3.6–24.2) | 545 | 5.0* | (1.8–13.7) | 556 | 1.5 | (0.6–4.2) | 456 | 1.0 | – | 564 | 38.1* | 3 | 2121 |
| Ukraine | 10.8* | (5.8–20.1) | 420 | 5.0* | (2.4–10.4) | 434 | 2.8* | (1.3–5.8) | 412 | 1.0 | – | 454 | 116.4* | 3 | 1720 |
| WHO: Regional Office for the Western Pacific (WPRO) | | | | | | | | | | | | | | | |
| People's Republic of China | 8.2* | (1.0–67.2) | 379 | 4.0 | (0.6–28.2) | 726 | 1.5 | (0.2–11.2) | 357 | 1.0 | – | 166 | 31.9* | 3 | 1628 |
| Japan | 1.9 | (0.6–6.0) | 155 | 2.3* | (1.1–4.9) | 219 | 2.5* | (1.1–5.7) | 295 | 1.0 | – | 218 | 6.7 | 3 | 887 |
| New Zealand | 8.1* | (6.1–10.7) | 3949 | 3.5* | (2.7–4.7) | 4102 | 2.5* | (1.9–3.3) | 2697 | 1.0 | – | 2244 | 283.7* | 3 | 12992 |

[a] Based on discrete-time survival models with person-year as the unit of analysis; controls are time intervals.

[b] Referent category unless otherwise noted.

[c] The results reported here for the United States differ somewhat from those in Chapter 9 due to updates in the coding scheme implemented in the analyses reported here compared to the analyses reported in Chapter 9.

[d] Cell size too small to be included in analysis

[e] The results for Spain differ somewhat from those reported in Chapter 19, as the latter used country-specific algorithms to estimate coefficients.

* Significant at the 0.05 level, two-sided test.

likely to be conservative, as the most plausible biases lead to underestimation. The evidence for cohort effects is more difficult to judge, as both substantive and methodological interpretations are plausible. The options are either that the prevalence of mental disorders is on the rise or that prevalence is stable but underestimated, as a result of biased estimation among older respondents.

Given the high prevalence-risk estimates even with the possibility of conservative bias, a question can be raised about the meaningfulness of these estimates. Our clinical reappraisal studies, consistent with comparable studies carried out in conjunction with previous community psychiatric epidemiological surveys (Kessler et al. 1998), show that the high prevalence estimates in the countries where prevalence is estimated to be highest are genuine (i.e., consistent with expert clinician judgments) rather than due to measurement errors in the CIDI. It is important to recognize, though, that not all mental disorders are severe. WMH measures of disorder severity were applied only to 12-month cases, so we have no way to estimate severity of lifetime cases. Analysis of 12-month cases, though, finds the majority rated mild on a clinical rating scale with categories mild, moderate, and severe (Demyttenaere et al. 2004). These cases are nonetheless meaningful, because even mild cases can be impairing and often evolve into more serious disorders over time (Kessler et al. 2003).

The AOO distributions reported here are consistent with those in previous epidemiological surveys (Christie et al. 1988; WHO International Consortium in Psychiatric Epidemiology 2000). Given the enormous personal and societal burdens of mental disorders, the finding that many cases have early AOOs suggests that public health interventions might profitably begin in childhood. Importantly, our studies of initial contact with the treatment system, which we turn to in the next chapter, show that people with these early-onset disorders often wait more than a decade before seeking treatment, and they present with seriously impairing disorders that might have been easier to treat if they had sought treatment earlier in the course of illness. Previous

studies of speed of seeking treatment have reported similar results (Olfson et al. 1998; Christiana et al. 2000; Wang et al. 2007). Interventions aimed at early detection and treatment might help reduce the persistence or severity of these largely primary anxiety and impulse-control disorders and prevent the onset of secondary disorders, a topic that we discuss in more detail in the next chapter.

## REFERENCES

Allgulander, C. (1989). Psychoactive drug use in a general population sample, Sweden: Correlates with perceived health, psychiatric diagnoses, and mortality in an automated record-linkage study. *American Journal of Public Health*, 79, 1006–10.

Andrade, L., Walters, E. E., Gentil, V., Laurenti, R. (2002). Prevalence of ICD-10 mental disorders in a catchment area in the city of São Paulo Brazil. *Social Psychiatry and Psychiatric Epidemiology*, 37, 316–25.

Bijl, R. V., van Zessen, G., Ravelli, A., de Rijk, C. & Langendoen, Y. (1998). The Netherlands Mental Health Survey and Incidence Study (NEMESIS): Objectives and design. *Social Psychiatry and Psychiatric Epidemiology*, 33, 581–6.

Cannell, C. F., Marquis, K. H. & Laurent, A. (1977). A summary of studies of interviewing methodology: 1959–1970. *Vital and Health Statistics Series* 2, 69, 77–1343.

Caraveo, J., Martinez, J. & Rivera, B. (1998). A model for epidemiological studies on mental health and psychiatric morbidity. *Salud Mental*, 21, 48–57.

Chang, S. M., Hahm, B. J., Lee, J. Y., Shin, M. S., Jeon, H. J., Hong, J. P., Lee, H. B., Lee, D. W. & Cho, M. J. (2007). Cross-national difference in the prevalence of depression caused by the diagnostic threshold. *Journal of Affective Disorders*, 106, 159–67.

Christiana, J. M., Gilman, S. E., Guardino, M., Kessler, R. C., Mickelson, K., Morselli, P. L. & Olfson, M. (2000). Duration between onset and time of obtaining initial treatment among people with anxiety and mood disorders: An international survey of members of mental health patient advocate groups. *Psychological Medicine*, 30, 693–703.

Christie, K. A., Burke, J. D. J., Regier, D. A., Rae, D. S., Boyd, J. H. & Locke, B. Z. (1988). Epidemiologic evidence for early onset of mental disorders and higher risk of drug-abuse in young-adults. *American Journal of Psychiatry*, 145, 971–5.

Cooke, D. J., Hart, S. D. & Michie, C. (2004). Cross-national differences in the assessment of psychopathy: Do they reflect variations in raters' perceptions of symptoms? *Psychological Assessment*, 16, 335–9.

Demyttenaere, K., Bruffaerts, R., Posada-Villa, J., Gasquet, I., Kovess, V., Lepine, J. P., Angermeyer, M. C., Bernert, S., de Girolamo, G., Morosini, P., Polidori, G., Kikkawa, T., Kawakami, N., Ono, Y., Takeshima, T., Uda, H., Karam, E. G., Fayyad, J. A., Karam, A. N., Mneimneh, Z. N., Medina-Mora, M. E., Borges, G., Lara, C., de Graaf, R., Ormel, J., Gureje, O., Shen, Y., Huang, Y., Zhang, M., Alonso, J., Haro, J. M., Vilagut, G., Bromet, E. J., Gluzman, S., Webb, C., Kessler, R. C., Merikangas, K. R., Anthony, J. C., Von Korff, M. R., Wang, P. S., Brugha, T. S., Aguilar-Gaxiola, S., Lee, S., Heeringa, S., Pennell, B.-E., Zaslavsky, A. M., Üstün, T. B. & Chatterji, S. (2004). Prevalence, severity, and unmet need for treatment of mental disorders in the World Health Organization World Mental Health Surveys. *Journal of the American Medical Association*, 291, 2581–90.

Giuffra, L. A. & Risch, N. (1994). Diminished recall and the cohort effect of major depression: A simulation study. *Psychological Medicine*, 24, 375–83.

Gureje, O., Lasebikan, V. O., Kola, L. & Makanjuola, V. A. (2006). Lifetime and 12-month prevalence of mental disorders in the Nigerian Survey of Mental Health and Well-Being. *British Journal of Psychiatry*, 188, 465–71.

Haro, J. M., Arbabzadeh-Bouchez, S., Brugha, T. S., de Girolamo, G., Guyer, M. E., Jin, R., Lepine, J. P., Mazzi, F., Reneses, B., Vilagut, G., Sampson, N. A. & Kessler, R. C. (2006). Concordance of the Composite International Diagnostic Interview Version 3.0 (CIDI 3.0) with standardized clinical assessments in the WHO World Mental Health surveys. *International Journal of Methods in Psychiatric Research*, 15, 167–80.

Hasin, D. S. & Grant, B. F. (2004). The co-occurrence of DSM-IV alcohol abuse in DSM-IV alcohol dependence: Results of the National Epidemiologic Survey on Alcohol and Related Conditions on heterogeneity that differ by population subgroup. *Archives of General Psychiatry*, 61, 891–6.

Kessler, R. C., McGonagle, K. A., Zhao, S., Nelson, C. B., Hughes, M., Eshleman, S., Wittchen, H.-U. & Kendler, K. S. (1994). Lifetime and 12-month prevalence of DSM-III-R psychiatric disorders in the United States: Results from the National Comorbidity Survey. *Archives of General Psychiatry*, 51, 8–19.

Kessler, R. C., Merikangas, K. R., Berglund, P., Eaton, W. W., Koretz, D. & Walters, E. E. (2003). Mild disorders should not be eliminated from the DSM-V. *Archives of General Psychiatry*, 60, 1117–22.

Kessler, R. C., Wittchen, H.-U., Abelson, J. M., McGonagle, K. A., Schwarz, N., Kendler, K. S., Knäuper, B. & Zhao, S. (1998). Methodological studies of the Composite International Diagnostic Interview (CIDI) in the U.S. National Comorbidity Survey. *International Journal of Methods in Psychiatric Research*, 7, 33–55.

Knäuper, B., Cannell, C. F., Schwarz, N., Bruce, M. L. & Kessler, R. C. (1999). Improving the accuracy of major depression age of onset reports in the U.S. National Comorbidity Survey. *International Journal of Methods in Psychiatric Research*, 8, 39–48.

Kylyc, C. (1998). *Mental health profile of Turkey: Main report*. Ankara: Ministry of Health Publications.

Olfson, M., Kessler, R. C., Berglund, P. A. & Lin, E. (1998). Psychiatric disorder onset and first treatment contact in the United States and Ontario. *American Journal of Psychiatry*, 155, 1415–22.

Shen, Y. C., Zhang, M. Y., Huang, Y. Q., He, Y. L., Liu, Z. R., Cheng, H., Tsang, A., Lee, S. & Kessler, R. C. (2006). Twelve-month prevalence, severity, and unmet need for treatment of mental disorders in metropolitan China. *Psychological Medicine*, 36, 257–67.

Simon, G. E., Goldberg, D. P., Von Korff, M. & Üstün, T. B. (2002). Understanding cross-national differences in depression prevalence. *Psychological Medicine*, 32, 585–94.

Simon, G. E. & Von Korff, M. (1995). Recall of psychiatric history in cross-sectional surveys: Implications for epidemiologic research. *Epidemiologic Reviews*, 17, 221–7.

Vega, W. A., Kolody, B., Aguilar-Gaxiola, S., Alderete, E., Catalano, R. & Caraveo-Anduaga, J. (1998). Lifetime prevalence of DSM-III-R psychiatric disorders among urban and rural Mexican Americans in California. *Archives of General Psychiatry*, 55, 771–8.

Wang, P. S., Angermeyer, M., Borges, G., Bruffaerts, R., Chiu, W. T., de Girolamo, G., Fayyad, J., Gureje, O., Haro, J. M., Huang, Y.-Q., Kessler, R. C., Kovess, V., Levinson, D., Nakane, Y., Oakley-Browne, M. A., Ormel, J., Posada-Villa, J., Aguilar-Gaxiola, S., Alonso, J., Lee, S., Heeringa, S., Pennell, B.-E., Chatterji, S. & Üstün, T. B. (2007). Delay and failure in treatment seeking after first onset of mental disorders in the WHO World Mental Health (WMH) Survey Initiative. *World Psychiatry*, 6, 177–85.

WHO International Consortium in Psychiatric Epidemiology (2000). Cross-national comparisons of the prevalences and correlates of mental disorders. WHO International Consortium in Psychiatric Epidemiology. *Bulletin of the World Health Organization*, 78, 413–26.

Wittchen, H.-U., Perkonigg, A., Lachner, G. & Nelson, C. B. (1998). Early developmental stages of psychopathology study (EDSP): Objectives and design. *European Addiction Research*, 4, 18–27.

# 25 Delay and Failure in Treatment Seeking after First Onset of Mental Disorders in the World Mental Health Survey Initiative

PHILIP S. WANG, SERGIO AGUILAR-GAXIOLA, JORDI ALONSO, MATTHIAS C. ANGERMEYER, GUILHERME BORGES, RONNY BRUFFAERTS, SOMNATH CHATTERJI, WAI-TAT CHIU, GIOVANNI DE GIROLAMO, JOHN A. FAYYAD, OYE GUREJE, JOSEP MARIA HARO, STEVEN G. HEERINGA, YUEQIN HUANG, RONALD C. KESSLER, VIVIANNE KOVESS-MASFETY, SING LEE, DAPHNA LEVINSON, YOSHIBUMI NAKANE, MARK A. OAKLEY-BROWNE, JOHAN ORMEL, BETH-ELLEN PENNELL, JOSÉ POSADA-VILLA, AND T. BEDIRHAN ÜSTÜN

## ACKNOWLEDGMENTS

Centralized data cleaning, coding, and analyses of the WMH data are supported by the U.S. National Institute of Mental Health (R01 MH070884), the John D. and Catherine T. MacArthur Foundation, the Fogarty International Center (FIRCA R03-TW006481), the Pan American Health Organization, the U.S. Public Health Service (R13-MH066849, R01-MH069864, and R01 DA016558), the Pfizer Foundation, Eli Lilly and Company Foundation, Ortho-McNeil Pharmaceutical, GlaxoSmithKline, and Bristol-Myers Squibb.

Portions of this chapter are based on Wang, P. S., Angermeyer, M., Borges, G., Bruffaerts, R., Chiu, W. T., de Girolamo, G., Fayyad, J., Gureje, O., Haro, J. M., Huang, Y., Kessler, R. C., Kovess, V., Levinson, D., Nakane, Y., Oakley-Browne, M. A., Ormel, J. H., Posada-Villa, J., Aguilar-Gaxiola, S., Alonso, J., Lee, S., Heeringa, S., Pennell, B.-E., Chatterji, S., Üstun, T. B., for The WHO World Mental Health Survey Consortium (2007). Delay and failure in treatment seeking after first onset of mental disorders in the World Health Organization's World Mental Health Survey Initiative. World Psychiatry, 6(3), 177–85.

## I. INTRODUCTION

Although the armamentarium of effective treatments for mental disorders keeps growing, few nations seem either willing or able to pay for their widespread use (Saxena, Sharan & Saraceno 2003). Indeed, the majority of people with recent episodes of mental illnesses continue to go untreated, even in economically advantaged societies (Wang et al. 2007). This reality has left many nations searching for strategies to use what limited resources they have as efficiently as possible in an effort to alleviate burden given current constraints (World Health Organization 2001).

One promising strategy is to emphasize use of treatment resources earlier in the disease courses of affected individuals, before many negative sequelae from mental illnesses develop (Kohn et al. 2004). Such an approach is supported by several lines of research. Data from preclinical studies suggest that neural "kindling" can cause untreated disorders to become more frequent, spontaneous, severe, and treatment refractory (Post & Weiss 1998). Epidemiological studies suggest that school and job failure, teenage childbearing, and early, violent, or unstable marriages are associated with early-onset untreated mental disorders (Kessler et al. 1995; Kessler et al. 1997; Kessler, Walters & Forthofer 1998). Single disorders often progress to complex comorbid disorders that are more difficult to treat and more likely to recur than less complex conditions (Kessler & Price 1993). In addition, clinical trials have shown that timely intervention can prevent suicidality (Meltzer et al. 2003).

A crucial first step in reducing delays in seeking treatment after first onset of a mental disorder is to document the current state of affairs with regard to the delays that currently exist in the population and the predictors of those delays. Very little is known about initial treatment contact, as mental health services research has focused on recent treatment of current episodes rather than initial treatment of incident cases (Leaf et al. 1985). However, the few existing studies that have examined initial treatment seeking have found that many lifetime cases eventually make contact, but usually after delaying years from when the disorders began (Olfson et al. 1998; Christiana et al. 2000; Wang et al. 2004).

A second critical step is to identify what nations can concretely do to shorten periods of untreated mental illness. Although countries employ a wide variety of national policies, delivery system designs, and means of financing mental health services, the impacts of these on delays in initial treatment seeking are unknown. Perhaps the only way to shed light on these impacts is to compare delays across countries with different policy, delivery system, and financing features (Mezzich 2003; Saxena et al. 2003). Very few such cross-national studies of delays have been conducted (Olfson et al. 1998; Christiana et al. 2000).

The current report begins to address these issues by comparing the results reported in Part 2 of this volume regarding cumulative lifetime probability of treatment contact in the WMH surveys. Two of the surveys, Ukraine and South Africa, are not included in the chapter because they did not ask about lifetime treatment contact. In the case of Ukraine, this line of investigation was considered uninformative because, as noted by Bromet and colleagues in Chapter 20, the main form of psychiatric treatment

in Ukraine is hospitalization for psychosis and organic disorders. Although Herman and colleagues reported much higher rates of outpatient treatment in South Africa in Chapter 11, there have been such massive changes in the delivery system in South Africa in recent years that information about delays in initial treatment seeking was considered uninformative. As noted in the remaining chapters in Part 2, the other WMH surveys asked respondents who met criteria for each DSM-IV/CIDI disorder whether they had ever in their lives talked to a medical doctor or other professional about the disorder under investigation and, if so, the age of first treatment contact. Survival analysis was used to compare age of onset of the disorder with age of first treatment contact as well as with probability of eventual treatment contact.

## 2. CUMULATIVE PROBABILITIES AND MEDIAN DELAYS IN TREATMENT CONTACT

The first column of Table 25.1 presents the proportions of lifetime cases with anxiety disorders making treatment contact in the year of disorder onset. The proportion ranges from a low of 0.8% in Nigeria to a high of 36.4% in Israel, with an interquartile range (IQR) (25th–75th percentiles) of 3.6%–19.8%. The proportions of lifetime cases with anxiety disorders making treatment contact by 50 years after onset are shown in the second column of Table 25.2 and range from 15.2% in Nigeria to 95.0% in Germany (IQR: 44.7%–90.7%). The median duration of delay among cases with anxiety disorders that eventually made treatment contact is shown in the third column of Table 25.1. Among the fraction of cases making treatment contacts, delays were shortest in Israel (median delay of 3.0 years) and longest in Mexico (median delay of 30.0 years). Between-country differences are statistically significant differences ($F_{15,726} = 95,259.7$; $p < 0.001$). Delays are generally longer in developing countries than in developed countries.

As shown in Table 25.2, the proportions of lifetime cases with mood disorders making treatment contact in the year of disorder onset range

**Table 25.1.** Proportional treatment contact in the year of onset of any anxiety disorder and median duration of delay among cases that subsequently made treatment contact

| | Making treatment contact in year of onset % (se) | Making treatment contact by 50 years % (se) | Median duration of delay in years % (se) |
|---|---|---|---|
| WHO: Regional Office for the Americas (AMRO) | | | |
| Colombia | 2.9 (0.6) | 41.6 (3.9) | 26.0 (1.5) |
| Mexico | 3.6 (1.1) | 53.2 (18.2) | 30.0 (5.1) |
| United States | 11.3 (0.7) | 87.0 (2.4) | 23.0 (0.6) |
| WHO: Regional Office for Africa (AFRO) | | | |
| Nigeria | 0.8 (0.5) | 15.2 (2.6) | 16.0 (4.2) |
| WHO: Regional Office for the Eastern Mediterranean (EMRO) | | | |
| Lebanon | 3.2 (1.1) | 37.3 (11.5) | 28.0 (3.9) |
| WHO: Regional Office for Europe (EURO) | | | |
| Belgium | 19.8 (2.8) | 84.5 (4.9) | 16.0 (3.5) |
| France | 16.1 (1.8) | 93.3 (1.9) | 18.0 (1.8) |
| Germany | 13.7 (1.8) | 95.0 (2.3) | 23.0 (2.3) |
| Israel | 36.4 (0.9) | 90.7 (1.3) | 3.0 (0.1) |
| Italy | 17.1 (2.1) | 87.3 (8.5) | 28.0 (2.2) |
| Netherlands | 28.0 (3.7) | 91.1 (2.8) | 10.0 (1.6) |
| Spain | 23.2 (2.0) | 86.6 (5.2) | 17.0 (3.2) |
| WHO: Regional Office for the Western Pacific (WPRO) | | | |
| People's Republic of China | 4.2 (2.0) | 44.7 (7.2) | 21.0 (3.1) |
| Japan | 11.2 (2.4) | 63.1 (6.2) | 20.0 (2.4) |
| New Zealand[a] | 12.5 (0.8) | 84.2 (2.5) | 21.0 (0.8) |

[a] The results for New Zealand differ somewhat from those reported in Chapter 23, as the latter used country-specific algorithms to estimate coefficients.

from lows of 6.0% in Nigeria and China to a high of 52.1% in Netherlands (IQR: 16.0%–42.7%). The proportions of cases with mood disorders making treatment contact by 50 years ranges from 7.9% in China to 98.6% in France (IQR: 56.8%–96.4%). Among cases with mood disorders eventually making treatment contact, the median duration of delay was shortest in three Western European (Belgium, the Netherlands, and Spain) and two Asian (China and Japan) countries (median delay of 1.0 years in each) and longest in Mexico (median delay of 14.0 years). The delays among cases with mood disorders differ significantly across countries ($F_{15,726} = 47,368.1$; $p < 0.001$). Comparison of Tables 25.1 and 25.2 reveals that delays were generally shorter for mood disorders than for anxiety disorders.

The proportions of lifetime cases with substance use disorders making treatment contact in the year of disorder onset range from a low of 0.9% in Mexico to a high of 18.6% in Spain (IQR: 2.8%–13.2%) (Table 25.3). By 50 years, the proportions of cases with substance use disorders making treatment contact range from 19.8% in Nigeria to 86.1% in Germany (IQR: 25.7%–66.6%). Cases with substance use disorders eventually making treatment contact had the shortest delays in Spain (median delay of 6.0 years) and the longest in Belgium (median delay of 18.0 years). The delays among cases with substance use disorders differ significantly across countries ($F_{15,726} = 21,505.3$; $p < 0.001$). These delays appear to be generally intermediate between those for mood and anxiety disorders.

**Table 25.2.** Proportional treatment contact in the year of onset of any mood disorder and median duration of delay among cases that subsequently made treatment contact

| | Making treatment contact in year of onset % (se) | Making treatment contact by 50 years % (se) | Median duration of delay in years % (se) |
|---|---|---|---|
| **WHO: Regional Office for the Americas (AMRO)** | | | |
| Colombia | 18.7 (2.7) | 66.6 (3.7) | 9.0 (1.6) |
| Mexico | 16.0 (2.2) | 69.9 (8.5) | 14.0 (3.1) |
| United States | 35.4 (1.2) | 94.8 (2.5) | 4.0 (0.2) |
| **WHO: Regional Office for Africa (AFRO)** | | | |
| Nigeria | 6.0 (1.7) | 33.3 (7.2) | 6.0 (3.3) |
| **WHO: Regional Office for the Eastern Mediterranean (EMRO)** | | | |
| Lebanon | 12.3 (2.0) | 49.2 (5.2) | 6.0 (2.1) |
| **WHO: Regional Office for Europe (EURO)** | | | |
| Belgium[a] | 47.8 (2.7) | 93.7 (2.5) | 1.0 (0.3) |
| France[a] | 42.7 (2.1) | 98.6 (1.4) | 3.0 (0.3) |
| Germany[a] | 40.4 (3.8) | 89.1 (5.0) | 2.0 (0.4) |
| Israel | 31.9 (0.8) | 92.7 (0.5) | 6.0 (0.3) |
| Italy[a] | 28.8 (3.0) | 63.5 (5.9) | 2.0 (0.5) |
| Netherlands[a] | 52.1 (2.9) | 96.9 (1.7) | 1.0 (0.3) |
| Spain[a] | 48.5 (2.3) | 96.4 (3.1) | 1.0 (0.3) |
| **WHO: Regional Office for the Western Pacific (WPRO)** | | | |
| People's Republic of China | 6.0 (2.2) | 7.9 (2.6) | 1.0 (2.0) |
| Japan | 29.6 (4.0) | 56.8 (7.3) | 1.0 (0.7) |
| New Zealand[b] | 41.4 (1.3) | 97.5 (1.0) | 3.0 (0.2) |

[a] Used major depressive episode instead of any mood disorder.

[b] The results for New Zealand differ somewhat from those reported in Chapter 23, as the latter used country-specific algorithms to estimate coefficients.

## 3. CORRELATES OF LIFETIME TREATMENT CONTACT

Results from the discrete-time survival models of lifetime treatment contact for anxiety disorders are shown in Table 25.4. Female sex is significantly associated with a higher likelihood of making initial treatment contact in four countries. Significant, monotonic relationships between being in younger cohorts and higher probabilities of treatment contact exist in 13 countries. Cases with earlier ages of onset of their anxiety disorders were significantly less likely to make treatment contact in 14 countries.

Correlates of lifetime treatment contact for mood disorders are shown in Table 25.5. Female sex is significantly associated with higher likelihoods of treatment contact in three countries.

Significant, generally monotonic relationships between being in younger cohorts and higher probabilities of treatment contact exist in ten countries. Earlier ages of onset are significantly associated with lower likelihoods of making treatment contact for mood disorders in 13 countries.

For substance use disorders, female sex is significantly associated with greater initial treatment contact in one country (see Table 25.6). There are significant, generally monotonic relationships between being in younger cohorts and higher probabilities of initial treatment contact in eight countries. Having an earlier age of onset is significantly associated with a lower likelihood of initial treatment contact for substance disorders in eight countries.

**Table 25.3.** Proportional treatment contact in the year of onset of any substance use disorder and median duration of delay among cases that subsequently made treatment contact

| | Making treatment contact in year of onset % (se) | Making treatment contact by 50 years % (se) | Median duration of delay in years % (se) |
|---|---|---|---|
| **WHO: Regional Office for the Americas (AMRO)** | | | |
| Colombia | 3.6 (0.8) | 23.1 (7.1) | 11.0 (5.0) |
| Mexico | 0.9 (0.5) | 22.1 (4.8) | 10.0 (3.3) |
| United States[a] | 10.0 (0.8) | 75.5 (3.8) | 13.0 (1.2) |
| **WHO: Regional Office for Africa (AFRO)** | | | |
| Nigeria[a] | 2.8 (1.7) | 19.8 (7.2) | 8.0 (1.8) |
| **WHO: Regional Office for the Eastern Mediterranean (EMRO)** | | | |
| Lebanon[a] | _[b] | _[b] | _[b] |
| **WHO: Regional Office for Europe (EURO)** | | | |
| Belgium | 12.8 (4.8) | 61.2 (17.7) | 18.0 (5.8) |
| France | 15.7 (5.4) | 66.5 (14.1) | 13.0 (3.7) |
| Germany | 13.2 (5.7) | 86.1 (8.6) | 9.0 (3.9) |
| Israel | 2.0 (0.5) | 48.0 (2.4) | 12.0 (0.5) |
| Italy | _[b] | _[b] | _[b] |
| Netherlands | 15.5 (5.4) | 66.6 (7.9) | 9.0 (3.1) |
| Spain | 18.6 (7.6) | 40.1 (14.1) | 6.0 (4.9) |
| **WHO: Regional Office for the Western Pacific (WPRO)** | | | |
| People's Republic of China[a] | 2.8 (1.8) | 25.7 (9.0) | 17.0 (3.7) |
| Japan[a] | 9.2 (5.1) | 31.0 (7.8) | 8.0 (4.6) |
| New Zealand[c] | 6.3 (0.8) | 84.8 (15.4) | 17.0 (1.3) |

[a] Assessed in the Part 2 sample.

[b] Disorder was omitted as a result of insufficient cases ($n < 30$).

[c] The results for New Zealand differ somewhat from those reported in Chapter 23, as the latter used country-specific algorithms to estimate coefficients.

## 4. DISCUSSION

Several potential limitations should be kept in mind when interpreting these results. Most important is the possibility that respondents might have failed to recall events occurring over their lifetimes. For example, those not seeking treatment may have been more likely to forget or normalize symptoms than those who sought treatment. Unfortunately, we cannot evaluate this possibility or whether it occurred differentially across countries. However, it is worth noting that, to the extent this kind of differential recall failure occurred, we underestimated failures and delays in initial treatment seeking.

Even when events were recalled, they may have been dated inaccurately. Studies of memory processes show that the most common form of dating error is telescoping, in which past experiences are recalled as having occurred more recently than they actually did. Questions that focus memory search and bound recall uncertainty were embedded in WMH surveys to help respondents recall ages of onset and age of initial treatment contact (Kessler et al. 2000; Kessler & Üstün 2004). However, to the extent these efforts were not successful, it is again likely that delays in initial treatment seeking were underestimated in the WMH surveys.

Our examinations of contacts with providers in the prior year, which are discussed in Chapter 27, revealed that many patients fail to receive adequate treatment (Wang et al. 2007). To the extent that initial contacts with providers also

Table 25.4. Sociodemographic predictors of lifetime treatment contact of any anxiety disorder

| | Sex | | | Cohort (age at interview) | | | | | | | Age of onset | | | | | | |
| | Female | | | Age 18–34 | | Age 35–49 | | Age 50–64 | | | Early | | Early-average | | Late-average | | |
| | OR | (95% CI) | $\chi^2$ | OR | (95% CI) | OR | (95% CI) | OR | (95% CI) | $\chi^2$ | OR | (95% CI) | OR | (95% CI) | OR | (95% CI) | $\chi^2$ |
|---|---|---|---|---|---|---|---|---|---|---|---|---|---|---|---|---|---|
| **WHO: Regional Office for the Americas (AMRO)** | | | | | | | | | | | | | | | | | |
| Colombia | 1.1 | (0.7–1.8) | 0.1 | 3.4* | (1.4–8.2) | 1.6 | (0.8–3.3) | 1.0 | – | 9.6* | 0.2* | (0.1–0.3) | 0.3* | (0.2–0.6) | 0.3* | (0.1–0.5) | 33.4* |
| Mexico | 1.1 | (0.6–1.8) | 0.1 | 2.3 | (0.8–6.4) | 2.3 | (0.8–6.4) | 1.0 | – | 2.6 | 0.2* | (0.1–0.3) | 0.2* | (0.1–0.3) | 0.2* | (0.1–0.3) | 59.1* |
| United States | 1.3* | (1.0–1.6) | 5.4* | 2.5* | (1.9–3.3) | 1.4* | (1.1–1.8) | 1.2 | (0.9–1.6) | 62.6* | 0.2* | (0.2–0.2) | 0.2* | (0.2–0.3) | 0.2* | (0.2–0.3) | 326.4* |
| **WHO: Regional Office for Africa (AFRO)** | | | | | | | | | | | | | | | | | |
| Nigeria | 1.1 | (0.4–3.3) | 0.0 | 0.6 | (0.1–3.0) | 0.1* | (0.0–0.7) | 0.3 | (0.1–1.9) | 7.9* | 0.3* | (0.2–0.7) | 0.6 | (0.2–2.0) | 0.5 | (0.2–1.5) | 10.1* |
| **WHO: Regional Office for the Eastern Mediterranean (EMRO)** | | | | | | | | | | | | | | | | | |
| Lebanon | 0.5 | (0.2–1.2) | 2.5 | 1.9 | (0.2–20.0) | 1.3 | (0.1–11.3) | 0.8 | (0.1–6.9) | 2.6 | 0.1* | (0.0–0.3) | 0.2* | (0.1–0.4) | 0.7 | (0.3–1.5) | 28.7* |
| **WHO: Regional Office for Europe (EURO)** | | | | | | | | | | | | | | | | | |
| Belgium | 1.2 | (0.7–2.1) | 0.4 | 4.7* | (1.6–13.6) | 3.0* | (1.2–7.5) | 1.3 | (0.6–2.8) | 14.8* | 0.1* | (0.1–0.3) | 0.1* | (0.0–0.3) | 0.2* | (0.1–0.5) | 63.5* |
| France | 1.5* | (1.1–2.1) | 8.8* | 4.5* | (2.5–8.1) | 2.3* | (1.3–4.2) | 1.3 | (0.7–2.5) | 52.2* | 0.2* | (0.1–0.3) | 0.2* | (0.1–0.3) | 0.3* | (0.2–0.5) | 82.4* |
| Germany | 1.5* | (1.1–2.1) | 6.6* | 4.5* | (2.7–7.5) | 2.3* | (1.5–3.7) | 1.5 | (0.8–2.9) | 59.8* | 0.2* | (0.1–0.3) | 0.2* | (0.1–0.3) | 0.2* | (0.1–0.5) | 43.5* |
| Israel | 1.0 | (0.6–1.5) | 0.0 | 5.0* | (1.8–13.9) | 3.2* | (1.4–7.4) | 1.9 | (0.9–4.0) | 10.0* | 0.4 | (0.2–1.0) | 0.5 | (0.3–1.1) | 0.6 | (0.3–1.2) | 3.7 |
| Italy | 1.1 | (0.7–1.5) | 0.1 | 2.6* | (1.3–5.2) | 2.1* | (1.2–3.7) | 1.4 | (0.7–2.9) | 16.0* | 0.1* | (0.1–0.2) | 0.1* | (0.1–0.2) | 0.3* | (0.2–0.5) | 101.8* |
| Netherlands | 1.1 | (0.7–1.6) | 0.2 | 3.0* | (1.8–5.1) | 2.5* | (1.6–3.7) | 1.0 | – | 26.8* | 0.1* | (0.0–0.2) | 0.1* | (0.1–0.3) | 0.4* | (0.2–0.7) | 52.0* |
| Spain | 1.0 | (0.7–1.6) | 0.0 | 3.3* | (1.9–5.7) | 2.0* | (1.1–3.7) | 0.8 | (0.5–1.3) | 38.5* | 0.1* | (0.0–0.1) | 0.1* | (0.0–0.2) | 0.2* | (0.1–0.4) | 96.2* |
| **WHO: Regional Office for the Western Pacific (WPRO)** | | | | | | | | | | | | | | | | | |
| People's Republic of China | 1.0 | (0.4–2.3) | 0.0 | 4.6* | (1.4–15.6) | 2.1 | (0.9–5.0) | 1.0 | – | 6.7 | 0.3* | (0.1–0.9) | 0.2* | (0.0–1.0) | 0.7 | (0.2–2.4) | 8.3* |
| Japan | 0.9 | (0.5–1.6) | 0.3 | 5.6* | (1.8–17.2) | 1.7 | (0.8–3.7) | 1.3 | (0.5–3.3) | 14.1* | 0.1* | (0.0–0.1) | 0.1* | (0.1–0.2) | 0.4 | (0.2–1.0) | 63.5* |
| New Zealand[a] | 1.3* | (1.1–1.5) | 8.6* | 4.3* | (2.9–6.3) | 2.4* | (1.7–3.4) | 1.7* | (1.3–2.4) | 68.8* | 0.1* | (0.1–0.1) | 0.1* | (0.1–0.2) | 0.2* | (0.1–0.2) | 461.0* |

[a] The results for New Zealand differ somewhat from those reported in Chapter 23, as the latter used country-specific algorithms to estimate coefficients.

* Significant at the 0.05 level, two-sided test.

**Table 25.5.** Sociodemographic predictors of lifetime treatment contact of any mood disorder

| | Sex | | | Cohort (age at interview) | | | | | | | Age of onset | | | | | |
| | Female | | | Age 18–34 | | Age 35–49 | | Age 50–64 | | | Early | | Early-average | | Late-average | | |
| | OR | (95% CI) | χ² | OR | (95% CI) | OR | (95% CI) | OR | (95% CI) | χ² | OR | (95% CI) | OR | (95% CI) | OR | (95% CI) | χ² |
|---|---|---|---|---|---|---|---|---|---|---|---|---|---|---|---|---|---|
| **WHO: Regional Office for the Americas (AMRO)** | | | | | | | | | | | | | | | | | |
| Colombia | 1.5 | (0.9–2.3) | 2.7 | 3.2* | (1.3–7.7) | 1.7 | (1.0–3.2) | 1.0 | – | 6.7 | 0.2* | (0.1–0.4) | 0.3* | (0.2–0.7) | 0.8 | (0.5–1.3) | 33.6* |
| Mexico | 1.6* | (1.0–2.4) | 4.6* | 2.1 | (0.9–4.9) | 1.7 | (0.8–3.3) | 1.0 | – | 3.1 | 0.3* | (0.2–0.6) | 0.5* | (0.2–0.9) | 0.8 | (0.4–1.6) | 25.1* |
| United States | 1.3* | (1.1–1.5) | 10.2* | 4.4* | (3.2–6.1) | 3.1* | (2.3–4.1) | 1.9* | (1.4–2.6) | 115.5* | 0.2* | (0.1–0.3) | 0.3* | (0.2–0.3) | 0.4* | (0.3–0.6) | 176.7* |
| **WHO: Regional Office for Africa (AFRO)** | | | | | | | | | | | | | | | | | |
| Nigeria | 1.4 | (0.5–3.6) | 0.5 | 2.7 | (0.3–22.4) | 0.5 | (0.1–3.7) | 1.0 | – | 6.8* | 2.6 | (0.2–33.6) | 1.2 | (0.0–31.2) | 3.3 | (0.3–41.1) | 3.0 |
| **WHO: Regional Office for the Eastern Mediterranean (EMRO)** | | | | | | | | | | | | | | | | | |
| Lebanon | 1.1 | (0.7–1.8) | 0.2 | 13.8* | (2.3–83.0) | 8.8* | (1.5–51.1) | 5.0 | (0.8–30.8) | 13.4* | 0.4* | (0.2–0.8) | 0.2* | (0.1–0.7) | 0.7 | (0.3–1.4) | 10.6* |
| **WHO: Regional Office for Europe (EURO)** | | | | | | | | | | | | | | | | | |
| Belgium[a] | 1.4 | (0.9–2.1) | 2.5 | 3.9* | (1.2–12.5) | 3.9 | (1.5–10.5) | 1.7 | (0.7–4.0) | 14.5* | 0.2* | (0.1–0.6) | 0.4* | (0.2–0.9) | 0.6* | (0.4–0.9) | 14.2* |
| France[a] | 1.3 | (0.9–1.8) | 2.9 | 5.7* | (3.1–10.5) | 4.4* | (2.4–8.0) | 2.0* | (1.1–3.5) | 44.3* | 0.2* | (0.1–0.4) | 0.4* | (0.2–0.8) | 0.6 | (0.3–1.2) | 54.9* |
| Germany[a] | 1.2 | (0.8–2.0) | 0.9 | 1.9 | (0.7–5.1) | 1.2 | (0.6–2.8) | 1.2 | (0.5–2.5) | 6.3 | 0.3* | (0.1–0.6) | 0.5 | (0.2–1.0) | 1.1 | (0.5–2.1) | 22.5* |
| Israel | 1.1 | (0.9–1.5) | 0.7 | 5.4* | (2.9–10.0) | 4.0* | (2.3–6.8) | 2.3* | (1.4–3.7) | 30.9* | 0.3* | (0.2–0.6) | 0.4* | (0.2–0.6) | 0.6 | (0.4–1.0) | 20.8* |
| Italy[a] | 1.4 | (0.9–2.0) | 2.6 | 1.4 | (0.7–2.8) | 1.6 | (0.8–2.9) | 1.1 | (0.6–2.1) | 2.8 | 0.4 | (0.2–0.8) | 0.8 | (0.4–1.6) | 0.8 | (0.4–1.4) | 15.7* |
| Netherlands[a] | 0.9 | (0.7–1.3) | 0.1 | 3.9* | (1.7–8.9) | 2.7* | (1.6–4.4) | 1.0 | – | 18.5* | 0.1* | (0.0–0.3) | 0.3* | (0.1–0.6) | 0.5* | (0.3–0.8) | 27.1* |
| Spain[a] | 1.2 | (0.8–1.8) | 1.1 | 1.9 | (0.9–3.8) | 2.7* | (1.4–5.1) | 1.3 | (0.8–2.1) | 11.3* | 0.4* | (0.2–0.8) | 0.4* | (0.2–0.9) | 0.7 | (0.4–1.2) | 8.3* |
| **WHO: Regional Office for the Western Pacific (WPRO)** | | | | | | | | | | | | | | | | | |
| People's Republic of China | 0.8 | (0.2–3.6) | 0.1 | 0.7 | (0.2–2.9) | 0.4 | (0.1–1.3) | 1.0 | – | 2.4 | 0.5 | (0.1–3.3) | 0.4 | (0.1–1.7) | 0.5 | (0.1–1.9) | 2.3 |
| Japan | 1.6 | (0.8–3.5) | 1.7 | 3.9* | (1.1–13.4) | 2.0 | (0.7–6.2) | 1.5 | (0.6–4.2) | 5.0 | 0.2* | (0.0–0.6) | 0.5 | (0.2–1.3) | 0.8 | (0.4–1.9) | 9.8* |
| New Zealand[b] | 1.4* | (1.2–1.6) | 16.9* | 3.7* | (2.7–5.2) | 2.3* | (1.7–3.1) | 1.6* | (1.2–2.2) | 84.1* | 0.2* | (0.2–0.3) | 0.3* | (0.3–0.4) | 0.6* | (0.5–0.8) | 205.6* |

[a] Used major depressive episode instead of any mood disorder.

[b] The results for New Zealand differ somewhat from those reported in Chapter 23, as the latter used country-specific algorithms to estimate coefficients.

* Significant at the 0.05 level, two-sided test.

**Table 25.6.** Sociodemographic predictors of lifetime treatment contact of any substance use disorder

| | Sex | | | Cohort (age at interview) | | | | | | | Age of onset | | | | | | |
|---|---|---|---|---|---|---|---|---|---|---|---|---|---|---|---|---|---|
| | Female | | | Age 18–34 | | Age 35–49 | | Age 50–64 | | | Early | | Early-average | | Late-average | | |
| | OR | (95% CI) | χ² | OR | (95% CI) | OR | (95% CI) | OR | (95% CI) | χ² | OR | (95% CI) | OR | (95% CI) | OR | (95% CI) | χ² |
| **WHO: Regional Office for the Americas (AMRO)** | | | | | | | | | | | | | | | | | |
| Colombia | 0.8 | (0.3–2.5) | 0.1 | 9.1* | (1.6–51.0) | 5.3* | (1.0–28.2) | 1.0 | – | 6.7* | 0.2* | (0.0–0.9) | 0.4 | (0.1–2.1) | 0.2 | (0.0–0.9) | 7.9* |
| Mexico | 2.8 | (0.8–9.5) | 2.9 | 3.6 | (0.7–18.1) | 0.8 | (0.2–2.9) | 1.0 | – | 8.0* | 0.8 | (0.2–3.6) | 1.3 | (0.3–5.7) | 1.7 | (0.5–5.5) | 2.0 |
| United States[a] | 1.2 | (0.8–1.6) | 1.0 | 3.4* | (1.7–6.8) | 1.7 | (0.9–3.1) | 1.3 | (0.7–2.3) | 18.2* | 0.6* | (0.4–0.8) | 0.6* | (0.4–0.8) | 0.6* | (0.4–0.8) | 14.4* |
| **WHO: Regional Office for Africa (AFRO)** | | | | | | | | | | | | | | | | | |
| Nigeria[a] | —[b] | | | 4.7 | (0.6–34.6) | 2.3 | (0.7–7.9) | 1.0 | – | 3.5 | 0.1 | (0.0–1.7) | 0.5 | (0.1–3.0) | 0.2 | (0.0–2.8) | 3.1 |
| **WHO: Regional Office for the Eastern Mediterranean (EMRO)** | | | | | | | | | | | | | | | | | |
| Lebanon[a] | —[b] | —[b] | —[b] | —[b] | | —[b] | | —[b] | | —[b] | —[b] | | —[b] | | —[b] | | —[b] |
| **WHO: Regional Office for Europe (EURO)** | | | | | | | | | | | | | | | | | |
| Belgium | 0.7 | (0.1–8.3) | 0.1 | 35.9* | (1.1–1163.4) | 35.9* | (1.1–1163.4) | 35.9* | (1.1–1163.4) | 4.5* | 0.1* | (0.0–0.2) | 0.1 | (0.0–0.2) | 0.1 | (0.0–0.2) | 25.7* |
| France | 0.8 | (0.2–3.2) | 0.2 | 0.2 | (0.0–3.2) | 0.7 | (0.1–4.8) | 1.0 | – | 2.1 | 0.4 | (0.1–2.6) | 0.4 | (0.1–2.6) | 0.4 | (0.1–2.6) | 1.0 |
| Germany | 1.4 | (0.4–5.3) | 0.2 | 4.3 | (0.5–37.5) | 4.3 | (0.5–37.5) | 1.0 | – | 1.9 | 0.2 | (0.0–1.2) | 0.1* | (0.0–0.3) | 1.0 | (0.3–3.1) | 12.6* |
| Israel | 0.2 | (0.0–1.3) | 2.8 | 9.5* | (1.8–49.7) | 3.8* | (1.0–14.7) | 1.0 | – | 7.3* | 0.7 | (0.2–2.8) | 0.3 | (0.1–1.5) | 2.2 | (0.7–7.6) | 8.5* |
| Italy | —[b] | | | —[b] | | —[b] | | —[b] | | —[b] | —[b] | | —[b] | | —[b] | | —[b] |
| Netherlands | 0.6 | (0.1–2.9) | 0.4 | 1.4 | (0.1–24.1) | 1.7 | (0.1–19.6) | 0.4 | (0.0–5.1) | 2.1 | 0.0* | (0.0–0.7) | 0.2* | (0.0–1.1) | 0.1* | (0.0–0.3) | 18.3* |
| Spain | 1.5 | (0.1–41.2) | 0.1 | 8.1* | (1.4–46.8) | 1.0 | – | 1.0 | – | 5.8* | 0.0* | (0.0–0.1) | 0.0* | (0.0–0.7) | 0.2 | (0.0–1.7) | 16.0* |
| **WHO: Regional Office for the Western Pacific (WPRO)** | | | | | | | | | | | | | | | | | |
| People's Republic of China[a] | 0.4 | (0.0–6.4) | 0.5 | 1.8 | (0.2–20.1) | 0.5 | (0.1–2.0) | 1.0 | – | 3.0 | 0.5 | (0.1–3.1) | 0.5 | (0.1–3.1) | 0.8 | (0.1–5.9) | 0.6 |
| Japan[a] | 0.4 | (0.1–3.3) | 0.7 | 3.6 | (0.1–203.0) | 0.3* | (0.1–0.7) | 0.3* | (0.1–0.7) | 9.5* | 0.2 | (0.0–5.3) | 0.4 | (0.0–3.1) | 1.3 | (0.3–5.2) | 2.5 |
| New Zealand[c] | 1.3* | (1.0–1.7) | 4.6* | 5.6* | (2.8–11.0) | 3.1* | (1.6–5.9) | 1.8 | (0.9–3.5) | 47.1* | 0.4* | (0.3–0.6) | 0.3* | (0.2–0.4) | 0.4* | (0.3–0.5) | 63.2* |

[a] Assessed in the Part 2 sample.

[b] Disorder was omitted as a result of insufficient lifetime cases ($n < 30$).

[c] The results for New Zealand differ somewhat from those reported in Chapter 23, as the latter used country-specific algorithms to estimate coefficients.

* Significant at the 0.05 level, two-sided test.

fail to result in any treatment or in adequate regimens, we have underestimated failure and delays in receipt of effective treatment. Furthermore, we were only able to study predictors of failure to make treatment contact that could be retrospectively dated. We also limited potential predictors to variables for which a priori hypotheses have been raised regarding treatment delay or failure, to reduce the possibility of chance findings (Olfson et al. 1998; Christiana et al. 2000; Wang et al. 2004).

Finally, we cannot be certain that the failures and delays in initial treatment seeking observed here are of clinical or public health significance. Alternatively, those who failed to make prompt initial contacts may have largely had self-limiting or less serious disorders (Narrow et al. 2002). However, more detailed analyses of some data on treatment delays show that even people with severe and impairing disorders often have substantial delays in initial treatment contact (Wang et al. 2004). Furthermore, the preclinical, epidemiological, and trial data reviewed previously suggest that even milder disorders, if left untreated, lead to greater severity, additional psychiatric comorbidity, and negative social and occupational functioning (Kessler et al. 1995; Kessler et al. 1997; Kessler et al. 1998).

Keeping these limitations in mind, our results reveal two major problems in the initial treatment-seeking process for mental disorders that are pervasive across the WMH countries. The first problem is that many lifetime cases never make any treatment contacts for their disorders. This problem is particularly common in developing countries, where the financial and structural barriers to accessing mental health services are most formidable (Saxena et al. 2003). Failure to seek help also appears to be greatest for conditions with low perceived needs for treatment, such as substance use disorders, where more than half of all lifetime cases failed to make any treatment contact in the majority of countries (Leaf et al. 1985; Mojtabai, Olfson & Mechanic 2002).

The second problem is that even among cases that do eventually seek help, there are perva-sive delays before treatment contacts are made. The typical delays observed here last for years or even decades after disorder onset. Initial treatment contacts appear to be fastest for mood disorders, perhaps because these disorders have been targeted in some countries by educational campaigns, primary care quality-improvement programs, and treatment advances (Jacobs 1995; Hirschfeld et al. 1997; Olfson et al. 2002). On the other hand, the longer delays for anxiety disorders may be due to the earlier age of onset of some conditions (e.g., phobias), fewer associated impairments, and even fear of providers or treatments involving social interactions (e.g., talking therapies, group settings, waiting rooms) (Leaf et al. 1985; Solomon & Gordon 1988; Wang et al. 2007).

Women have been shown in prior research to be more likely than men to translate nonspecific feelings of distress into conscious recognition that they have emotional problems, perhaps explaining the significantly higher rates of initial treatment contact by women in some countries (Kessler, Brown & Broman 1981). More recent cohorts were also significantly more likely to make eventual treatment contact, which perhaps suggests a positive outcome of programs recently attempted in some countries to destigmatize and increase awareness of mental illness, of screening and outreach initiatives, of the introduction and direct-to-consumer promotion of new treatments, and of the expansion of insurance programs (Regier et al. 1988; Ridgely & Goldman 1989; Jacobs 1995; Hirschfeld et al. 1997; Spitzer et al. 1999; Sturm 1999; Olfson et al. 2002; Rosenthal et al. 2002; Demyttenaere et al. 2004). Consistent with prior research (Olfson et al. 1998; Christiana et al. 2000; Wang et al. 2004), early-onset disorders were associated with lower probabilities of initial treatment contact in most countries. One explanation for this finding may be that minors need the help of parents or other adults to seek treatment, and recognition is often low among these adults unless symptoms are severe (Morrissey-Kane & Prinz 1999; Janicke, Finney & Riley 2001). In addition, child- and adolescent-onset mental disorders may be associated with normalization of symptoms or development of coping strategies (e.g., social withdrawal in social phobias) that interfere with help seeking later in life. Finally, lack of accessible child mental health services may also be an important issue in many countries.

Although these results document the failure and delay in initial treatment seeking for mental disorders that are occurring worldwide, additional research will be needed to clarify what policy makers can concretely do to address them at the local and national levels. At the local level, it is critical to identify whether and through what specific programs long periods of untreated mental illness can be reduced. Cost-efficient interventions that can be applied in schools, clinics, or health-care systems, consisting of aggressive outreach and prompt treatment of new cases, are just emerging. Long-term intervention trials currently in the field will shed light on the extent to which these model programs prevent subsequent negative clinical, social, educational, and occupational outcomes (MTA Cooperative Group 1999; Beidel, Turner & Morris 2000). Programs of public education, school or primary care–based screening, disease management, or coordination and referral between non–health-care and health-care professions, may also prove helpful in this regard (Regier et al. 1988; Connors 1994; Jacobs 1995; Velicer et al. 1995; Weaver 1995; Carleton et al. 1996; Morrissey-Kane & Prinz 1999; Aseltine & DeMartino 2004).

Furthermore, it will be critical to clarify what can be done at the national level to minimize failure and delay in initial treatment contact. General and mental health care policies, delivery system designs, and levels or mechanisms of financing mental health services may have enormous impacts on the timeliness of treatment seeking. Policy makers currently lack rigorous data on these impacts, including whether impacts are positive, negative, as intended, or inadvertent. Linking data such as those of the WHO Project ATLAS on existing policies, delivery systems, and financing of mental health care, to WMH survey data on failure and delay in initial treatment may offer a novel way to shed light on these impacts and help guide future policy decisions (Mezzich 2003; Saxena et al. 2003).

## REFERENCES

Aseltine, R. H., Jr. & DeMartino, R. (2004). An outcome evaluation of the SOS Suicide Prevention Program. *American Journal of Public Health*, 94, 446–51.

Beidel, D. C., Turner, S. M. & Morris, T. L. (2000). Behavioral treatment of childhood social phobia. *Journal of Consulting and Clinical Psychology*, 68, 1072–80.

Carleton, R. A., Bazzarre, T., Drake, J., Dunn, A., Fisher, E. B., Jr., Grundy, S. M., Hayman, L., Hill, M. N., Maibach, E. W., Prochaska, J., Schmid, T., Smith, S. C., Jr., Susser, M. W. & Worden, J. W. (1996). Report of the Expert Panel on Awareness and Behavior Change to the Board of Directors, American Heart Association. *Circulation*, 93, 1768–72.

Christiana, J. M., Gilman, S. E., Guardino, M., Kessler, R. C., Mickelson, K., Morselli, P. L. & Olfson, M. (2000). Duration between onset and time of obtaining initial treatment among people with anxiety and mood disorders: An international survey of members of mental health patient advocate groups. *Psychological Medicine*, 30, 693–703.

Connors, C. K. (1994). The Connors Rating Scales: Use in clinical assessment, treatment planning and research. In *Use of psychological testing for treatment planning and outcome assessment*, ed. M. Maruish, pp. 550–78. Hillsdale, NJ: Lawrence Erlbaum Associates.

Demyttenaere, K., Bruffaerts, R., Posada-Villa, J., Gasquet, I., Kovess, V., Lepine, J. P., Angermeyer, M. C., Bernert, S., de Girolamo, G., Morosini, P., Polidori, G., Kikkawa, T., Kawakami, N., Ono, Y., Takeshima, T., Uda, H., Karam, E. G., Fayyad, J. A., Karam, A. N., Mneimneh, Z. N., Medina-Mora, M. E., Borges, G., Lara, C., de Graaf, R., Ormel, J., Gureje, O., Shen, Y., Huang, Y., Zhang, M., Alonso, J., Haro, J. M., Vilagut, G., Bromet, E. J., Gluzman, S., Webb, C., Kessler, R. C., Merikangas, K. R., Anthony, J. C., Von Korff, M. R., Wang, P. S., Brugha, T. S., Aguilar-Gaxiola, S., Lee, S., Heeringa, S., Pennell, B.-E., Zaslavsky, A. M., Üstün, T. B. & Chatterji, S. (2004). Prevalence, severity, and unmet need for treatment of mental disorders in the World Health Organization World Mental Health Surveys. *Journal of the American Medical Association*, 291, 2581–90.

Hirschfeld, R. M. A., Keller, M. B., Panico, S., Arons, B. S., Barlow, D., Davidoff, F., Endicott, J., Froom, J., Goldstein, M., Gorman, J. M., Marek, R. G., Maurer,

T. A., Meyer, R., Phillips, K., Ross, J., Schwenk, T. L., Sharfstein, S. S., Thase, M. E. & Wyatt, R. J. (1997). The national depressive and manic-depressive association consensus statement on the undertreatment of depression. *Journal of the American Medical Association*, 277, 333–40.

Jacobs, D. G. (1995). National depression screening day: Educating the public, reaching those in need of treatment and broadening professional understanding. *Harvard Review of Psychiatry*, 3, 156–9.

Janicke, D. M., Finney, J. W. & Riley, A. W. (2001). Children's health care use: A prospective investigation of factors related to care-seeking. *Medical Care*, 39, 990–1001.

Kessler, R. C., Berglund, P. A., Foster, C. L., Saunders, W. B., Stang, P. E. & Walters, E. E. (1997). Social consequences of psychiatric disorders, II: Teenage parenthood. *American Journal of Psychiatry*, 154, 1405–11.

Kessler, R. C., Brown, R. L. & Broman, C. L. (1981). Sex differences in psychiatric help-seeking: Evidence from four large-scale surveys. *Journal of Health and Social Behavior*, 22, 49–64.

Kessler, R. C., Foster, C. L., Saunders, W. B. & Stang, P. E. (1995). Social consequences of psychiatric disorders, I: Educational attainment. *American Journal of Psychiatry*, 152, 1026–32.

Kessler, R. C. & Price, R. H. (1993). Primary prevention of secondary disorders: A proposal and agenda. *American Journal of Community Psychology*, 21, 607–33.

Kessler, R. C. & Üstün, T. B. (2004). The World Mental Health (WMH) survey initiative version of the World Health Organization (WHO) Composite International Diagnostic Interview (CIDI). *International Journal of Methods in Psychiatric Research*, 13, 93–121.

Kessler, R. C., Walters, E. E. & Forthofer, M. S. (1998). The social consequences of psychiatric disorders, III: Probability of marital stability. *American Journal of Psychiatry*, 155, 1092–6.

Kessler, R. C., Wittchen, H.-U., Abelson, J. M. & Zhao, S. (2000). Methodological issues in assessing psychiatric disorder with self-reports. In *The science of self-report: Implications for research and practice*, ed. A. A. Stone, J. S. Turrkan, C. A. Bachrach, J. B. Jobe, H. S. Kurtzman & V. S. Cain, pp. 229–35. Mahwah, NJ: Lawrence Erlbaum Associates.

Kohn, R., Saxena, S., Levav, I. & Saraceno, B. (2004). The treatment gap in mental health care. *Bulletin of the World Health Organization*, 82, 858–66.

Leaf, P. J., Livingston, M. M., Tischler, G. L., Weissman, M. M., Holzer, C. E. & Myers, J. K. (1985). Contact with health professionals for the treatment of psychiatric and emotional problems. *Medical Care*, 23, 1322–37.

Meltzer, H. Y., Alphs, L., Green, A. I., Altamura, A. C., Anand, R., Bertoldi, A., Bourgeois, M., Chouinard, G., Islam, M. Z., Kane, J., Krishnan, R., Lindenmayer, J. P. & Potkin, S. (2003). Clozapine treatment for suicidality in schizophrenia: International Suicide Prevention Trial (InterSePT). *Archives of General Psychiatry*, 60, 82–91.

Mezzich, J. E. (2003). From financial analysis to policy development in mental health care: The need for broader conceptual models and partnerships. *Journal of Mental Health Policy and Economics*, 6, 149–50.

Mojtabai, R., Olfson, M. & Mechanic, D. (2002). Perceived need and help-seeking in adults with mood, anxiety, or substance use disorders. *Archives of General Psychiatry*, 59, 77–84.

Morrissey-Kane, E. & Prinz, R. J. (1999). Engagement in child and adolescent treatment: The role of parental cognitions and attributions. *Clinical Child and Family Psychology Review*, 2, 183–98.

MTA Cooperative Group (1999). A 14-month randomized clinical trial of treatment strategies for attention-deficit/hyperactivity disorder: The MTA Cooperative Group, Multimodal Treatment Study of Children with ADHD. *Archives of General Psychiatry*, 56, 1073–86.

Narrow, W. E., Rae, D. S., Robins, L. N. & Regier, D. A. (2002). Revised prevalence estimates of mental disorders in the United States: Using a clinical significance criterion to reconcile 2 surveys' estimates. *Archives of General Psychiatry*, 59, 115–23.

Olfson, M., Kessler, R. C., Berglund, P. A. & Lin, E. (1998). Psychiatric disorder onset and first treatment contact in the United States and Ontario. *American Journal of Psychiatry*, 155, 1415–22.

Olfson, M., Marcus, S. C., Druss, B., Elinson, L., Tanielian, T. & Pincus, H. A. (2002). National trends in the outpatient treatment of depression. *Journal of the American Medical Association*, 287, 203–9.

Post, R. M. & Weiss, S. R. (1998). Sensitization and kindling phenomena in mood, anxiety, and obsessive-compulsive disorders: The role of serotonergic mechanisms in illness progression. *Biological Psychiatry*, 44, 193–206.

Regier, D. A., Hirschfeld, R. M., Goodwin, F. K., Burke, J. D., Jr., Lazar, J. B. & Judd, L. L. (1988). The NIMH Depression, Awareness, Recognition, and Treatment program: Structure, aim, and scientific basis. *American Journal of Psychiatry*, 145, 1351–7.

Ridgely, M. S. & Goldman, H. H. (1989). Mental health insurance. In *Handbook on mental health policy in the United States*, ed. D. A. Rochefort, pp. 341–61. Westport, CT: Greenwood Press.

Rosenthal, M. B., Berndt, E. R., Donohue, J. M., Frank, R. G. & Epstein, A. M. (2002). Promotion of prescription drugs to consumers. *New England Journal of Medicine*, 346, 498–505.

Saxena, S., Sharan, P. & Saraceno, B. (2003). Budget and financing of mental health services: Baseline information on 89 countries from WHO's project atlas. *Journal of Mental Health Policy and Economics*, 6, 135–43.

Solomon, P. & Gordon, B. (1988). Outpatient compliance of psychiatric emergency room patients by presenting problems. *Psychiatric Quarterly*, 59, 271–83.

Spitzer, R. L., Kroenke, K., Williams, J. B. W. & The Patient Health Questionnaire Study Group (1999). Validation and utility of a self-report version of the PRIME-MD: The PHQ Primary Care Study. *Journal of the American Medical Association*, 282, 1737–44.

Sturm, R. (1999). Tracking changes in behavioral health services: How have carve-outs changed care? *Journal of Behavioural Health Services Research*, 26, 360–71.

Velicer, W. F., Hughes, S. L., Fava, J. L., Prochaska, J. O. & DiClemente, C. C. (1995). An empirical typology of subjects within stage of change. *Addictive Behaviors*, 20, 299–320.

Wang, P. S., Aguilar-Gaxiola, S., Alonso, J., Angermeyer, M. A., Borges, G., Bromet, E. J., Bruffaerts, R., de Girolamo, G., de Graaf, R., Gureje, O., Haro, J. M., Karam, E. G., Kessler, R. C., Kovess, V., Lane, M. C., Lee, S., Levinson, D., Ono, Y., Petukhova, M., Posada-Villa, J., Seedat, S. & Wells, J. (2007). Worldwide use of mental health services for anxiety, mood, and substance disorders: Results from 17 countries in the WHO World Mental Health (WMH) Surveys. *Lancet*, 370, 841–50.

Wang, P. S., Berglund, P. A., Olfson, M. & Kessler, R. C. (2004). Delays in initial treatment contact after first onset of a mental disorder. *Health Services Research*, 39, 393–415.

Weaver, A. J. (1995). Has there been a failure to prepare and support parish-based clergy in their role as frontline community mental health workers: A review. *Journal of Pastoral Care*, 49, 129–47.

World Health Organization (WHO) (2001). The World Health Report 2001: Mental health: New understanding, new hope. Available at http://www.who.int/whr2001/.

# 26 Prevalence and Severity of Mental Disorders in the World Mental Health Survey Initiative

RONALD C. KESSLER, SERGIO AGUILAR-GAXIOLA, JORDI ALONSO,
MATTHIAS C. ANGERMEYER, JAMES C. ANTHONY, TRAOLACH S. BRUGHA,
SOMNATH CHATTERJI, GIOVANNI DE GIROLAMO, KOEN DEMYTTENAERE,
SEMYON F. GLUZMAN, OYE GUREJE, JOSEP MARIA HARO, STEVEN G.
HEERINGA, IRVING HWANG, ELIE G. KARAM, TAKEHIKO KIKKAWA,
SING LEE, JEAN-PIERRE LÉPINE, MARIA ELENA MEDINA-MORA,
KATHLEEN RIES MERIKANGAS, JOHAN ORMEL, BETH-ELLEN PENNELL,
JOSÉ POSADA-VILLA, T. BEDIRHAN ÜSTÜN, MICHAEL R. VON KORFF,
PHILIP S. WANG, ALAN M. ZASLAVSKY, AND MINGYUAN ZHANG

## ACKNOWLEDGMENTS

Centralized data cleaning, coding, and analyses of the WMH data are supported by the U.S. National Institute of Mental Health (R01 MH070884), the John D. and Catherine T. MacArthur Foundation, the Fogarty International Center (FIRCA R03-TW006481), the Pan American Health Organization, the U.S. Public Health Service (R13-MH066849, R01-MH069864, and R01 DA016558), the Pfizer Foundation, Eli Lilly and Company Foundation, Ortho-McNeil Pharmaceutical, GlaxoSmith-Kline, and Bristol-Myers Squibb.

## I. INTRODUCTION

Readers who have examined the many chapters in Part 2 and compared results across these chapters or who have read Chapter 24 know that prevalence estimates vary widely across the WMH surveys considered in this volume. As noted in Chapter 24, where we discussed lifetime prevalence estimates, methodological explanations for cross-national variations in prevalence estimates are so plausible that we do not offer substantive interpretations of these differences in this volume. Instead, we focus on important similarities in results across the WMH surveys. In the case of 12-month prevalence, the vast majority of WMH surveys show 12-month mental disorders to be commonly occurring and often seriously impairing. This chapter discusses these similarities.

## 2. PREVALENCE

The highest 12-month prevalence estimate among these surveys is 27.0% in the United States and the lowest is 6.0% in Nigeria. It should be noted that these estimates differ slightly from those reported in Part 2 for all countries due to several updates to the diagnostic algorithms implemented subsequent to the time those reports were prepared. The interquartile range (IQR) (the range after excluding the highest and lowest four surveys) of the prevalence estimates is 9.8%–19.1% (Table 26.1). Between one-fourth and one-fifth of the population in five of the countries considered here is estimated to meet criteria for one of the DSM-IV disorders assessed in the surveys at some time in the 12 months before interview (Colombia, France, New Zealand, Ukraine, United States). Between one-sixth and one-eighth of the population is estimated to have one or more of these 12-month disorders in five other WMH countries (Belgium, Lebanon, Mexico, Netherlands, South Africa). Twelve-month prevalence estimates are between 6.0% (Nigeria) and 11.2% (Germany) in the other WMH surveys.

**Table 26.1.** 12-month prevalence of DSM-IV/CIDI disorders

| | Anxiety | | Mood | | Impulse[a] | | Substance | | Any | |
|---|---|---|---|---|---|---|---|---|---|---|
| | % | (se) | % | (se) | % | (se) | % | (se) | % | (se) |
| **WHO: Regional Office for the Americas (AMRO)** | | | | | | | | | | |
| Colombia | 14.4 | (1.0) | 7.0 | (0.5) | 4.4 | (0.4) | 2.8 | (0.4) | 21.0 | (1.0) |
| Mexico | 8.4 | (0.6) | 4.7 | (0.3) | 1.6 | (0.3)[e] | 2.3 | (0.3) | 13.4 | (0.9) |
| United States | 19.0 | (0.7) | 9.7 | (0.4) | 10.5 | (0.7) | 3.8 | (0.4) | 27.0 | (0.9) |
| **WHO: Regional Office for Africa (AFRO)** | | | | | | | | | | |
| Nigeria | 4.2 | (0.5) | 1.1 | (0.2) | 0.1 | (0.0)[f,h] | 0.9 | (0.2) | 6.0 | (0.6) |
| South Africa | 8.2 | (0.6)[b,c] | 4.9 | (0.4)[d] | 1.9 | (0.3)[f,g,h] | 5.8 | (0.5) | 16.7 | (1.0) |
| **WHO: Regional Office for the Eastern Mediterranean (EMRO)** | | | | | | | | | | |
| Lebanon | 12.2 | (1.2) | 6.8 | (0.7) | 2.6 | (0.7)[h] | 1.3 | (0.8) | 17.9 | (1.7) |
| **WHO: Regional Office for Europe (EURO)** | | | | | | | | | | |
| Belgium | 8.4 | (1.4) | 5.4 | (0.5)[d] | 1.7 | (1.0)[e] | 1.8 | (0.4)[i] | 13.2 | (1.5) |
| France | 13.7 | (1.1) | 6.5 | (0.6)[d] | 2.4 | (0.6)[e] | 1.3 | (0.3)[i] | 18.9 | (1.4) |
| Germany | 8.3 | (1.1) | 3.3 | (0.3)[d] | 0.6 | (0.3)[e] | 1.2 | (0.2)[i] | 11.0 | (1.3) |
| Israel | 3.6 | (0.3)[b,c] | 6.4 | (0.4) | – | –[e,f,g,h] | 1.3 | (0.2) | 10.0 | (0.5) |
| Italy | 6.5 | (0.6) | 3.4 | (0.3)[d] | 0.4 | (0.2)[e] | 0.2 | (0.1)[i] | 8.8 | (0.7) |
| Netherlands | 8.9 | (1.0) | 5.1 | (0.5)[d] | 1.9 | (0.7)[e] | 1.9 | (0.3)[i] | 13.6 | (1.0) |
| Spain | 6.6 | (0.9) | 4.4 | (0.3)[d] | 0.5 | (0.2)[e] | 0.7 | (0.2)[i] | 9.7 | (0.8) |
| Ukraine | 6.8 | (0.7)[b,c] | 9.0 | (0.6)[d] | 5.7 | (1.0)[f,h] | 6.4 | (0.8) | 21.4 | (1.3) |
| **WHO: Regional Office for the Western Pacific (WPRO)** | | | | | | | | | | |
| People's Republic of China | 3.0 | (0.5) | 1.9 | (0.3) | 3.1 | (0.7)[f,h] | 1.6 | (0.4) | 7.1 | (0.9) |
| Japan | 4.2 | (0.6)[b] | 2.5 | (0.4) | 0.2 | (0.1)[f,g,h] | 1.2 | (0.4) | 7.4 | (0.9) |
| New Zealand | 15.0 | (0.5)[b] | 8.0 | (0.4) | – | –[e,f,g,h] | 3.5 | (0.2) | 20.7 | (0.6) |

*Notes:* Anxiety disorders include agoraphobia, adult separation anxiety disorder, generalized anxiety disorder, panic disorder, posttraumatic stress disorder, social phobia, and specific phobia. Mood disorders include bipolar disorders, dysthymia, and major depressive disorder. Impulse-control disorders include intermittent explosive disorder, and reported persistence in the past 12 months of symptoms of three child-adolescent disorders (attention-deficit/hyperactivity disorder, conduct disorder, and oppositional-defiant disorder). Substance disorders include alcohol or drug abuse with or without dependence. In the case of substance dependence, respondents who met full criteria at some time in their life and who continue to have any symptoms are considered to have 12-month dependence even if they currently do not meet full criteria for the disorder. Organic exclusions were made as specified in the DSM-IV.

[a] Impulse disorders restricted to age ≤39 (China, Ukraine, Nigeria) or to age ≤44 (all other countries).

[b] Adult separation anxiety disorder was not assessed.

[c] Specific phobia was not assessed.

[d] Bipolar disorders were not assessed.

[e] Intermittent explosive disorder was not assessed.

[f] Attention-deficit/hyperactivity disorder was not assessed.

[g] Conduct disorder was not assessed.

[h] Oppositional-defiant disorder was not assessed.

[i] Only alcohol abuse with or without dependence were assessed. No assessment was made of other drug abuse with or without dependence.

Relative prevalence estimates are quite consistent across surveys. Anxiety disorders are the most common disorders in all but three countries (higher prevalence of mood disorders in Israel and Ukraine; higher prevalence of impulse-control disorders in China), with prevalence in the range 3.0%–19.0% (IQR: 6.5%–12.2%). Mood disorders are next most common in all but three countries (higher prevalence of substance disorders in South Africa and of

**Table 26.2.** Prevalence of 12-month DSM-IV/CIDI disorders by severity across countries[a]

|  | Serious | | Moderate | | Mild | |
|---|---|---|---|---|---|---|
|  | % | (se) | % | (se) | % | (se) |
| **WHO: Regional Office for the Americas (AMRO)** | | | | | | |
| Colombia | 23.1 | (2.1) | 41.0 | (2.6) | 35.9 | (2.1) |
| Mexico | 25.7 | (2.4) | 33.9 | (2.2) | 40.5 | (2.6) |
| United States | 25.2 | (1.4) | 39.2 | (1.2) | 35.7 | (1.4) |
| **WHO: Regional Office for Africa (AFRO)** | | | | | | |
| Nigeria | 12.8 | (3.8) | 12.5 | (2.6) | 74.7 | (4.2) |
| South Africa | 25.7 | (1.8) | 31.5 | (2.2) | 42.8 | (2.2) |
| **WHO: Regional Office for the Eastern Mediterranean (EMRO)** | | | | | | |
| Lebanon | 22.4 | (3.1) | 42.6 | (4.7) | 35.0 | (5.5) |
| **WHO: Regional Office for Europe (EURO)** | | | | | | |
| Belgium | 31.8 | (4.2) | 37.8 | (3.3) | 30.4 | (4.8) |
| France | 18.5 | (2.5) | 42.7 | (3.0) | 38.8 | (3.6) |
| Germany | 21.3 | (2.5) | 42.6 | (4.6) | 36.1 | (4.3) |
| Israel | 36.8 | (2.4) | 35.2 | (2.3) | 28.0 | (2.1) |
| Italy | 15.9 | (2.7) | 47.6 | (3.8) | 36.5 | (3.9) |
| Netherlands | 30.7 | (3.4) | 31.0 | (3.7) | 38.3 | (4.6) |
| Spain | 19.3 | (2.4) | 42.3 | (4.0) | 38.4 | (4.7) |
| Ukraine | 22.9 | (1.8) | 39.4 | (2.9) | 37.7 | (3.5) |
| **WHO: Regional Office for the Western Pacific (WPRO)** | | | | | | |
| People's Republic of China | 13.8 | (3.7) | 32.2 | (4.9) | 54.0 | (4.6) |
| Japan | 13.2 | (3.1) | 45.5 | (5.3) | 41.3 | (4.6) |
| New Zealand | 25.3 | (1.0) | 40.8 | (1.4) | 33.9 | (1.2) |

[a] See the text for a description of the coding rules used to define the severity levels.

impulse-control disorders in the United States and China), with prevalence in the range 1.1%–9.7% (IQR: 3.4%–6.8%). Substance disorders (lifetime prevalence: 0.2%–6.4%; IQR: 1.2%–2.8%) and impulse-control disorders (lifetime prevalence: 0.1%–10.5%; IQR: 0.6%–2.6%) are consistently less prevalent across the surveys. If we use the terms "high" and "low" to refer to the five highest and five lowest prevalence estimates in each column of the table, the United States and Colombia have consistently high prevalence estimates across all classes of disorder, Netherlands and Ukraine are high on three of four, Nigeria and Shanghai are consistently low, and Italy is low on three of four.

## 3. SEVERITY

The proportions of disorders (Table 26.2) classified as serious (12.8%–36.8%; IQR: 18.5%–

25.7%) or moderate (12.5%–47.6%; IQR: 33.9%–42.6%), using the definitions of those terms described in the chapters of Part 2, are generally smaller than the proportions with a mild disorder. As with the results in Table 26.1, it should be noted that these estimates differ slightly from those reported in Part 2 for all countries, as a result of several updates to the diagnostic algorithms implemented subsequent to the time those reports were prepared. The proportion of disorders classified mild is substantial: from 28.0% in Israel to 74.7% in Nigeria (IQR: 35.7%–40.5%). The severity distribution among cases varies significantly across countries ($\chi^2_{32} = 153.5$, $p < 0.001$), with severity not strongly related either to region or to development status. There are substantial positive associations, though, between overall prevalence of any disorder and both the proportion of cases classified as serious (Pearson $r = 0.46$, $p < 0.001$) and the proportion of cases classified as either serious or moderate (Pearson $r = 0.77$, $p < 0.001$).

The finding of a positive association between estimated prevalence and severity across countries is potentially important because it speaks to an issue that has been raised in the methodological literature regarding the possibility of biased prevalence estimates. Two separate research groups found an opposite sort of effect. A report comparing results from the Korean Epidemiologic Catchment Area (KECA) Study (Chang et al. 2007) with results from a parallel survey in the United States, argued that the lower estimated prevalence of major depression in the KECA than the U.S. survey was due, at least in part, to a higher threshold for reporting depression among people in the Korean population than in the United States. In support of this assertion, the investigators showed that Koreans diagnosed as depressed with an earlier version of the CIDI, which was the diagnostic instrument used in the KECA survey, had considerably higher levels of role impairment than did respondents diagnosed as depressed using the same instrument in the United States.

A similar finding was reported in a methodological study carried out as part of the WHO Collaborative Study on Psychological Problems in General Health Care (PPG) (Üstün & Sartorius 1995). In that study, nearly 26,000 primary care patients in 14 countries were assessed using an earlier version of the CIDI that included an evaluation of current symptoms of depression. As in the WMH surveys, substantial cross-national variation was found in the prevalence of major depression. However, the investigators found that the average amount of impairment associated with depression across countries was inversely proportional to the estimated prevalence of depression in those countries (Simon et al. 2002; Chang et al. 2007). This result is consistent with the possibility that the substantial differences in estimated prevalence of depression in the PPG study might be due, at least in part, to cross-national differences in diagnostic thresholds. However, as shown in Table 26.2, we do not replicate this result in the WMH surveys. The countries with the lowest prevalence estimates of the DSM-IV disorders assessed in the WMH

surveys also have the lowest reported levels of impairment associated with those disorders.

## 4. SEVERITY AND IMPAIRMENT

It is important to note that the severity classification used in the WMH surveys was validated by documenting a consistently monotonic association between reported disorder severity and mean number of days out of role associated with the disorders (Table 26.3). This association is statistically significant in all but four surveys. Respondents with serious disorders in most surveys reported at least 40 days in the past year when they were totally unable to carry out usual activities because of these disorders (IQR: 56.7–135.9 days). The mean days out of role for mild disorders, in comparison, is in the range of 11.7–68.9 days, whereas the mean for moderate disorders is intermediate between these extremes (21.1–109.4 days; IQR: 39.3–65.3 days). When we compare between-country differences in these means with between-country differences in prevalence, using the same logic as in the previous section, we once again find a positive association between prevalence and this indicator of role impairment. For example, in the three countries with the highest estimated overall 12-month prevalence (United States, Ukraine, New Zealand), the mean number of days out of role associated with disorders classified as severe is in the range of 98.1–142.5, compared to means in the range of 48.7–56.7 in the three countries with the lowest 12-month prevalence estimates (Nigeria, China, Japan).

## 5. DISCUSSION

The WMH results regarding 12-month prevalence are consistent with those of earlier surveys in showing that mental disorders are highly prevalent (Cross National Collaborative Group 1994; Weissman et al. 1996a; Weissman et al. 1996b; Weissman et al. 1997) and often associated with serious role impairment (Wells et al. 1989; Ormel et al. 1994; Kessler & Frank 1997). We found substantial cross-national variation in these results. One broad pattern consistent with previous research is that prevalence

**Table 26.3.** Association between severity of 12-month DSM-IV/CIDI disorders and days out of role

| | Serious | | Moderate | | Mild | | Wald F[a] | (p-value) |
|---|---|---|---|---|---|---|---|---|
| | Mean | (se) | Mean | (se) | Mean | (se) | | |
| **WHO: Regional Office for the Americas (AMRO)** | | | | | | | | |
| Colombia | 53.0 | (8.9) | 33.7 | (6.7) | 15.6 | (3.0) | 10.8* | (<0.001) |
| Mexico | 42.8 | (6.9) | 26.3 | (5.3) | 11.7 | (2.7) | 11.7* | (<0.001) |
| United States | 135.9 | (6.9) | 65.3 | (4.6) | 35.7 | (2.7) | 126.1* | (<0.001) |
| **WHO: Regional Office for Africa (AFRO)** | | | | | | | | |
| Nigeria | 56.7 | (22.3) | 51.5 | (18.8) | 25.9 | (7.4) | 1.6 | (0.20) |
| South Africa | 73.1 | (9.7) | 49.3 | (6.5) | 32.5 | (4.8) | 9.1* | (<0.001) |
| **WHO: Regional Office for the Eastern Mediterranean (EMRO)** | | | | | | | | |
| Lebanon | 81.4 | (10.6) | 42.0 | (9.5) | 13.6 | (5.4) | 14.4* | (<0.001) |
| **WHO: Regional Office for Europe (EURO)** | | | | | | | | |
| Belgium | 96.1 | (26.0) | 59.9 | (11.6) | 42.5 | (9.6) | 3.7* | (0.025) |
| France | 105.7 | (14.3) | 71.8 | (16.5) | 67.6 | (17.3) | 2.7 | (0.07) |
| Germany | 77.8 | (18.1) | 33.2 | (8.2) | 45.7 | (12.1) | 2.2 | (0.12) |
| Israel | 184.6 | (12.5) | 109.4 | (10.1) | 44.6 | (9.1) | 41.8* | (<0.001) |
| Italy | 178.5 | (25.6) | 55.6 | (10.9) | 41.7 | (11.2) | 11.7* | (<0.001) |
| Netherlands | 140.7 | (19.9) | 87.1 | (17.1) | 68.9 | (22.7) | 4.0* | (0.018) |
| Spain | 131.5 | (15.8) | 56.6 | (10.0) | 57.4 | (22.0) | 8.1* | (<0.001) |
| Ukraine | 142.5 | (14.5) | 103.2 | (9.2) | 51.6 | (9.9) | 13.9* | (<0.001) |
| **WHO: Regional Office for the Western Pacific (WPRO)** | | | | | | | | |
| People's Republic of China | 48.7 | (18.4) | 21.1 | (5.2) | 21.3 | (7.2) | 1.5 | (0.23) |
| Japan | 51.0 | (17.3) | 39.3 | (10.6) | 22.5 | (6.4) | 3.7* | (0.024) |
| New Zealand | 98.1 | (5.9) | 54.6 | (3.4) | 36.4 | (3.6) | 40.7* | (<0.001) |

[a] No demographic controls were used.

* Significant association between severity and days out of role at the 0.05 level.

is low in Asian countries (Cross National Collaborative Group 1994; Weissman et al. 1996a; Weissman et al. 1996b; Weissman et al. 1997; Simon et al. 2002). It is noteworthy that prevalence and severity estimates are likely to be conservative because of the sample selection bias documented in previous methodological studies, whereby survey nonrespondents tend to have significantly higher rates and severity of mental illness than do respondents (Allgulander 1989; Eaton et al. 1992; Kessler et al. 1994; Kessler & Merikangas 2004). In addition, we would expect reporting bias among respondents to be conservative. Although good concordance was observed between diagnoses based on the CIDI and those based on blinded clinical reinterviews in the countries that participated in the coordinated WMH clinical reappraisal studies reported in Chapter 6, these studies were all conducted in developed Western countries. It remains possible that the accuracy of CIDI diagnoses could be lower odds ratios in other countries because of greater reluctance on the part of respondents in those countries to admit emotional problems to a stranger who comes to their home to carry out a survey, lower relevance of DSM-IV diagnoses to symptom experiences in less developed countries, or higher thresholds for reporting symptoms in less developed countries.

We addressed the last of these possibilities in this chapter with data on the cross-national association between estimated prevalence and reported severity of disorders. Contrary to the findings of two previous studies on this issue (Simon et al. 2002; Chang et al. 2007), we found that cross-national variation in estimated prevalence is positively associated with variation in the reported level of impairment associated with mental disorders. This argues against the possibility that higher symptom thresholds explain the lower prevalence estimates in some WMH countries, as we would expect such a process to result in especially high levels of impairment associated with the disorders found in those countries.

Another possibility, though, is that we underestimated prevalence in some countries because the DSM categories are less relevant to symptom expression in some countries than in others. We

did not investigate this possibility in the WMH surveys, but rather assumed that DSM categories apply equally well to all countries. A sophisticated analysis of the possibility that DSM categories might not apply equally to all countries was carried out as part of the WHO Collaborative Study on Psychological Problems in General Health Care (Üstün & Sartorius 1995). In that study, an analysis of cross-national variation in the structure of depressive symptom was carried out using item response theory methods (Simon et al. 2002). The results showed clearly that both the latent structure of depressive symptoms and the associations between specific depressive symptoms and this latent structure, were very similar across the countries studied. These results argue strongly against the suggestion that the large cross-national variation in estimated prevalence of depression is due to cross-national differences in the nature of depression. Comparable psychometric analyses have not yet been completed for other disorders, though, so it remains possible that cross-national differences exist in latent structure that might play a part in explaining the substantial differences in 12-month prevalence documented in the WMH surveys. New methodological studies are being carried out by WMH collaborators to investigate this possibility.

Although results are still preliminary, an intriguing early finding reported in the next chapter is that the countries with the lowest disorder prevalence estimates also have the highest proportions of treated cases classified as subthreshold, that is, as not meeting criteria for any of the DSM-IV/CIDI disorders assessed in the WMH interview. This finding at least indirectly raises the possibility that the assessments in the CIDI are less adequate in capturing the psychopathological syndromes that are common in all the WMH countries. In particular, the syndromes associated with treatment in low-prevalence countries are not well characterized by the CIDI. Additional WMH clinical reappraisal studies using flexible and culturally sensitive assessments of psychopathology to explore this finding empirically are currently under way in both developed and developing countries.

## REFERENCES

Allgulander, C. (1989). Psychoactive drug use in a general population sample, Sweden: Correlates with perceived health, psychiatric diagnoses, and mortality in an automated record-linkage study. *American Journal of Public Health*, 79, 1006–10.

Chang, S. M., Hahm, B. J., Lee, J. Y., Shin, M. S., Jeon, H. J., Hong, J. P., Lee, H. B., Lee, D. W. & Cho, M. J. (2007). Cross-national difference in the prevalence of depression caused by the diagnostic threshold. *Journal of Affective Disorders*, 106, 159–67.

Cross National Collaborative Group (1994). The cross national epidemiology of obsessive compulsive disorder. *Journal of Clinical Psychiatry*, 55 (suppl.), 5–10.

Eaton, W. W., Anthony, J. C., Tepper, S. & Dryman, A. (1992). Psychopathology and attrition in the Epidemiologic Catchment Area Study. *American Journal of Epidemiology*, 135, 1051–9.

Kessler, R. C. & Frank, R. G. (1997). The impact of psychiatric disorders on work loss days. *Psychological Medicine*, 27, 861–73.

Kessler, R. C., McGonagle, K. A., Zhao, S., Nelson, C. B., Hughes, M., Eshleman, S., Wittchen, H.-U. & Kendler, K. S. (1994). Lifetime and 12-month prevalence of DSM-III-R psychiatric disorders in the United States: Results from the National Comorbidity Survey. *Archives of General Psychiatry*, 51, 8–19.

Kessler, R. C. & Merikangas, K. R. (2004). The National Comorbidity Survey Replication (NCS-R): Background and aims. *International Journal of Methods in Psychiatric Research*, 13, 60–8.

Ormel, J., Von Korff, M., Üstün, T. B., Pini, S., Korten, A. & Oldehinkel, T. (1994). Common mental disorders and disability across cultures: Results from the WHO Collaborative Study on Psychological Problems in General Health Care. *Journal of the American Medical Association*, 272, 1741–8.

Simon, G. E., Goldberg, D. P., Von Korff, M. & Üstün, T. B. (2002). Understanding cross-national differences in depression prevalence. *Psychological Medicine*, 32, 585–94.

Üstün, T. B. & Sartorius, N. (1995). *Mental health in general health care: An international study*. New York: John Wiley & Sons.

Weissman, M. M., Bland, R. C., Canino, G. J., Faravelli, C., Greenwald, S., Hwu, H. G., Joyce, P. R., Karam, E. G., Lee, C. K., Lellouch, J., Lépine, J.-P., Newman, S. C., Rubio-Stipec, M., Wells, J. E., Wickramaratne, P. J., Wittchen, H. & Yeh, E. K. (1996a). Cross-national epidemiology of major depression and bipolar disorder. *Journal of the American Medical Association*, 276, 293–9.

Weissman, M. M., Bland, R. C., Canino, G. J., Faravelli, C., Greenwald, S., Hwu, H. G., Joyce, P. R., Karam, E. G., Lee, C. K., Lellouch, J., Lépine, J.-P., Newman, S. C., Oakley-Browne, M. A., Rubio-Stipec, M., Wells, J. E., Wickramaratne, P. J., Wittchen, H.-U. & Yeh, E. K. (1997). The cross-national epidemiology of panic disorder. *Archives of General Psychiatry*, 54, 305–9.

Weissman, M. M., Bland, R. C., Canino, G. J., Greenwald, S., Lee, C. K., Newman, S. C., Rubio-Stipec, M. & Wickramaratne, P. J. (1996b). The cross-national epidemiology of social phobia: A preliminary report. *International Clinical Psychopharmacology*, 11 (suppl. 3), 9–14.

Wells, K. B., Stewart, A., Hays, R. D., Burnam, M., Rogers, W., Daniels, M., Berry, S., Greenfield, S. & Ware, J. (1989). The functioning and well-being of depressed patients: Results from the Medical Outcomes Study. *Journal of the American Medical Association*, 262, 914–19.

# 27 Recent Treatment of Mental Disorders in the World Mental Health Survey Initiative

PHILIP S. WANG, SERGIO AGUILAR-GAXIOLA, JORDI ALONSO, MATTHIAS
C. ANGERMEYER, GUILHERME BORGES, EVELYN J. BROMET, RONNY
BRUFFAERTS, SOMNATH CHATTERJI, GIOVANNI DE GIROLAMO, RON DE
GRAAF, OYE GUREJE, JOSEP MARIA HARO, STEVEN G. HEERINGA, ELIE G.
KARAM, RONALD C. KESSLER, VIVIANNE KOVESS-MASFETY, MICHAEL C.
LANE, SING LEE, DAPHNA LEVINSON, YUTAKA ONO, BETH-ELLEN
PENNELL, MARIA PETUKHOVA, JOSÉ POSADA-VILLA, KATHLEEN
SAUNDERS, SORAYA SEEDAT, YUCUN SHEN, T. BEDIRHAN ÜSTÜN, AND
J. ELISABETH WELLS

## ACKNOWLEDGMENTS

Centralized data cleaning, coding, and analyses of the WMH data are supported by the U.S. National Institute of Mental Health (R01 MH070884), the John D. and Catherine T. MacArthur Foundation, the Fogarty International Center (FIRCA R03-TW006481), the Pan American Health Organization, the U.S. Public Health Service (R13-MH066849, R01-MH069864, and R01 DA016558), the Pfizer Foundation, Eli Lilly and Company Foundation, Ortho-McNeil Pharmaceutical, GlaxoSmithKline, and Bristol-Myers Squibb.

Portions of this chapter are based on Wang, P. S., Aguilar-Gaxiola, S., Alonso, J., Angermeyer, M. C., Borges, G., Bromet, E. J., Bruffaerts, R., de Girlolamo, G., de Graaf, R., Gureje, O., Haro, J. M., Karam, E. G., Kessler, R. C., Kovess, V., Lane, M. C., Lee, S., Levinson, D., Ono, Y., Petukhova, M., Posada-Villa, J., Seedat, S., Wells, J. E. (2007). Use of mental health services for anxiety, mood, and substance disorders in 17 countries in the WHO World Mental Health Surveys. Lancet, 370(9590), 841–50. Copyright © 2007, Elsevier. All rights reserved. Reproduced with permission.

## I. INTRODUCTION

The WHO Global Burden of Disease (GBD) study concluded that neuropsychiatric conditions are the leading causes of disability worldwide, accounting for 37% of all healthy life years lost from disease (Lopez et al. 2006). This high burden of neuropsychiatric conditions exists, according to the GBD investigators, even in low- and middle-income countries, which may be least able to bear such burdens. Although efficacious and tolerable treatments are increasingly available, even economically advantaged societies experience competing priorities and budgetary constraints (Tasman, Kay & Lieberman 2003). As a result, knowing how to provide effective mental health care has become imperative worldwide (Hu 2003). Unfortunately, most countries suffer from a lack of data to guide decisions, absent or competing visions for resources, and near-constant pressures to cut insurance and entitlements (Mechanic 1994).

A first step in helping countries redesign their mental health care systems and optimally allocate resources is to document the services currently being used as well as the extent and nature of unmet needs for treatment. This can be

**Table 27.1.** 12-month service use by sectors in the WMH surveys

| | Among respondents[a] | | | | | | | | | | | | | | | Among respondents using services[b] | | | | | | | | | | | |
|---|---|---|---|---|---|---|---|---|---|---|---|---|---|---|---|---|---|---|---|---|---|---|---|---|---|---|---|
| | Any treatment | | | Mental health specialty | | | General medical | | | Human services | | | CAM[c] | | | Mental health specialty | | | General medical | | | Human services | | | CAM[c] | | |
| Country | n | % | (se) | n | % | (se) | n | % | (se) | n | % | (se) | N | % | (se) | n | % | (se) | n | % | (se) | n | % | (se) | n | % | (se) |
| WHO: Regional Office for the Americas (AMRO) | | | | | | | | | | | | | | | | | | | | | | | | | | | |
| Colombia | 217 | 5.5 | (0.6) | 126 | 3.0 | (0.4) | 82 | 2.3 | (0.4) | 19 | 0.5 | (0.2) | 10 | 0.2 | (0.1) | 126 | 53.4 | (4.8) | 82 | 41.7 | (5.1) | 19 | 9.2 | (2.8) | 10 | 3.7 | (1.4) |
| Mexico | 240 | 5.1 | (0.5) | 121 | 2.8 | (0.3) | 92 | 1.7 | (0.3) | 15 | 0.3 | (0.1) | 45 | 1.0 | (0.2) | 121 | 53.6 | (4.2) | 92 | 33.1 | (4.0) | 15 | 6.2 | (2.0) | 45 | 20.0 | (3.4) |
| United States | 1477 | 17.9 | (0.7) | 738 | 8.8 | (0.5) | 773 | 9.3 | (0.4) | 266 | 3.4 | (0.3) | 247 | 2.8 | (0.2) | 738 | 48.8 | (1.7) | 773 | 51.8 | (1.3) | 266 | 18.8 | (1.1) | 247 | 15.6 | (1.0) |
| WHO: Regional Office for Africa (AFRO) | | | | | | | | | | | | | | | | | | | | | | | | | | | |
| Nigeria | 57 | 1.6 | (0.3) | 5 | 0.1 | (0.1) | 42 | 1.1 | (0.2) | 14 | 0.5 | (0.2) | 1 | 0.0 | (0.0) | 5 | 8.3 | (3.7) | 42 | 66.6 | (10.1) | 14 | 30.9 | (10.2) | 1 | 1.1 | (1.1) |
| South Africa | 675 | 15.4 | (1.0) | 108 | 2.5 | (0.8) | 440 | 10.2 | (0.8) | 169 | 3.7 | (0.4) | 161 | 3.7 | (0.3) | 108 | 16.3 | (2.2) | 440 | 66.4 | (2.5) | 169 | 24.0 | (1.9) | 161 | 23.8 | (2.1) |
| WHO: Regional Office for the Eastern Mediterranean (EMRO) | | | | | | | | | | | | | | | | | | | | | | | | | | | |
| Lebanon | 77 | 4.4 | (0.6) | 18 | 1.0 | (0.3) | 53 | 2.9 | (0.5) | 11 | 0.8 | (0.3) | 0 | 0.0 | (0.0) | 18 | 22.3 | (5.7) | 53 | 66.6 | (7.4) | 11 | 17.5 | (6.1) | 0 | 0.0 | (0.0) |
| WHO: Regional Office for Europe (EURO) | | | | | | | | | | | | | | | | | | | | | | | | | | | |
| Belgium | 187 | 10.9 | (1.4) | 96 | 5.2 | (0.7) | 147 | 8.2 | (1.3) | 6 | 0.4 | (0.2) | 12 | 0.7 | (0.3) | 96 | 47.9 | (4.4) | 147 | 75.5 | (3.8) | 6 | 3.7 | (1.8) | 12 | 6.5 | (2.9) |
| France | 272 | 11.3 | (1.0) | 111 | 4.4 | (0.5) | 214 | 8.8 | (0.9) | 10 | 0.4 | (0.2) | 9 | 0.5 | (0.3) | 111 | 39.4 | (3.6) | 214 | 78.4 | (3.3) | 10 | 3.4 | (1.2) | 9 | 4.3 | (2.1) |
| Germany | 183 | 8.1 | (0.8) | 100 | 3.9 | (0.6) | 102 | 4.2 | (0.6) | 16 | 1.0 | (0.4) | 15 | 0.6 | (0.2) | 100 | 48.5 | (4.8) | 102 | 51.7 | (5.1) | 16 | 12.2 | (4.5) | 15 | 7.4 | (2.5) |
| Israel | 421 | 8.8 | (0.4) | 215 | 4.4 | (0.3) | 169 | 3.6 | (0.3) | 71 | 1.6 | (0.2) | 42 | 0.8 | (0.1) | 215 | 50.5 | (2.6) | 169 | 40.4 | (2.6) | 71 | 18.0 | (2.0) | 42 | 9.6 | (1.5) |
| Italy | 141 | 4.3 | (0.4) | 55 | 2.0 | (0.3) | 107 | 3.0 | (0.3) | 15 | 0.4 | (0.1) | 4 | 0.1 | (0.0) | 55 | 47.1 | (5.1) | 107 | 70.9 | (4.8) | 15 | 9.1 | (2.4) | 4 | 1.5 | (0.7) |
| Netherlands | 202 | 10.9 | (1.2) | 105 | 5.5 | (1.0) | 141 | 7.7 | (1.1) | 14 | 0.6 | (0.2) | 27 | 1.5 | (0.4) | 105 | 51.0 | (6.0) | 141 | 71.2 | (6.1) | 14 | 5.4 | (1.6) | 27 | 13.5 | (3.8) |
| Spain | 375 | 6.8 | (0.5) | 200 | 3.6 | (0.4) | 249 | 4.4 | (0.4) | 11 | 0.1 | (0.1) | 20 | 0.2 | (0.1) | 200 | 52.2 | (3.6) | 249 | 64.9 | (3.4) | 11 | 2.1 | (0.8) | 20 | 3.5 | (1.0) |
| Ukraine | 212 | 7.2 | (0.8) | 39 | 1.2 | (0.3) | 135 | 4.0 | (0.7) | 47 | 1.7 | (0.4) | 29 | 1.0 | (0.3) | 39 | 17.2 | (3.8) | 135 | 55.4 | (7.1) | 47 | 24.1 | (5.1) | 29 | 14.4 | (4.0) |
| WHO: Regional Office for the Western Pacific (WPRO) | | | | | | | | | | | | | | | | | | | | | | | | | | | |
| People's Republic of China | 74 | 3.4 | (0.6) | 19 | 0.6 | (0.2) | 41 | 2.3 | (0.5) | 6 | 0.3 | (0.1) | 18 | 0.7 | (0.3) | 19 | 18.0 | (5.9) | 41 | 68.5 | (6.8) | 6 | 7.4 | (3.8) | 18 | 21.2 | (7.3) |
| Japan | 92 | 5.6 | (0.9) | 43 | 2.4 | (0.5) | 47 | 2.8 | (0.5) | 8 | 0.8 | (0.5) | 13 | 0.6 | (0.2) | 43 | 42.5 | (5.5) | 47 | 50.2 | (8.2) | 8 | 15.0 | (6.7) | 13 | 11.1 | (4.7) |
| New Zealand | 1592 | 13.8 | (0.5) | 585 | 5.2 | (0.3) | 1122 | 9.2 | (0.4) | 203 | 1.6 | (0.2) | 265 | 2.6 | (0.3) | 585 | 37.6 | (1.8) | 1122 | 66.5 | (1.8) | 203 | 11.5 | (1.1) | 265 | 19.0 | (1.7) |
| $\chi^2_{16}$ | 764.6[a] | | (<0.001) | 679.6[a] | | (<0.001) | 732.2[a] | | (<0.001) | 262.9[a] | | (<0.001) | 388.0[a] | | (<0.001) | 232.4[a] | | (<0.001) | 207.3[a] | | (<0.001) | 201.8[a] | | (<0.001) | 223.1[a] | | (<0.001) |

[a] Percentages among respondents are based on entire Part 2 samples.
[b] Percentages are based on respondents using any 12-month services.
[c] CAM: Complementary and alternative medicine.

especially helpful when such data are presented in a cross-national perspective that allows policy makers to make comparisons of service use and unmet needs in countries with different mental health care systems. Such comparisons can help uncover optimal financing, national policies, and delivery systems for mental health care. Unfortunately, few cross-national studies are available (Kessler et al. 1997; Bijl et al. 2003). The results reported in Part 2 of this volume take a first step in the direction of presenting data of this sort. It is useful, though, to compare the country-specific results in those papers regarding levels, types, and adequacy of mental health service use in an explicit cross-national perspective. We do this in the current chapter.

## 2. 12-MONTH USE OF MENTAL HEALTH SERVICES

Respondents using any mental health services in the prior 12 months varied significantly across the 17 WMH countries considered here, from a low of 1.6% in Nigeria to a high of 17.9% in the United States ($\chi^2_{16} = 764.6$, $p < 0.0001$), with generally smaller proportions in treatment in low- or middle-income versus high-income countries (Table 27.1 and Table 27.2). As with the results in Chapter 24, it should be noted that these estimates differ slightly from those reported in Part 2 for all countries as a result of several updates to the diagnostic algorithms implemented subsequent to the time those reports were prepared. The proportions receiving services also tended to correspond with countries' overall spending on health care (World Health Organization n.d.) (Table 27.2). The largest proportions used general medical (GM), followed by mental health specialty (MHS) sectors, with the exceptions of Mexico, Colombia, and Israel, where this was reversed. Smaller proportions used human services (HS) and complementary-alternative medical (CAM) sectors. The right-hand columns of Table 27.1 present proportions using specific sectors among respondents receiving any 12-month services. With the exception of the two Latin American countries and Israel, the sectors used most frequently by treated respondents were GM followed by MHS; again, smaller proportions used HS and CAM.

**Table 27.2.** Health-care spending and level of economic development of each WMH country

| Country | National health-care budget as a percentage of total GDP* | Level of economic development |
|---|---|---|
| Nigeria | 3.4 | Low |
| PRC[†] Beijing | 5.5 | Low-middle |
| PRC[†] Shanghai | 5.5 | Low-middle |
| Colombia | 5.5 | Low-middle |
| South Africa | 8.6 | Low-middle |
| Ukraine | 4.3 | Low-middle |
| Lebanon | 12.2 | High-middle |
| Mexico | 6.1 | High-middle |
| Belgium | 8.9 | High |
| France | 9.6 | High |
| Germany | 10.8 | High |
| Italy | 8.4 | High |
| Israel | 8.7 | High |
| Japan | 8.0 | High |
| Netherlands | 8.9 | High |
| New Zealand | 8.3 | High |
| Spain | 7.5 | High |
| United States | 13.9 | High |

* World Health Organization. Project Atlas: Resources for Mental Health and Neurological Disorders. Available at http://www.who.int/globalatlas/dataQuery/default. asp.
[†] People's Republic of China.

## 3. SERVICE USE BY SEVERITY OF MENTAL DISORDERS

Significant, generally monotonic, relationships exist between disorder severity and probability of service use in every country except China (Table 27.3). This pattern makes it clear that there is some rationality in the allocation of mental health care resources in the vast majority of countries. In spite of these dose-response relationships, though, only between 11.0% (China) and 62.1% (Belgium) of serious cases received any service in the prior year. Lower proportions of moderate and mild cases generally received services in the prior year. Numerically small but still meaningful numbers of those apparently without disorders used treatments (ranging from 1.0% in Nigeria to 9.7% in the United States). Cross-national differences were significant in all severity categories, with generally

**Table 27.3.** Percentages using 12-month services by severity of mental disorders in the WMH surveys[a]

| Country | Severe | | | Moderate | | | Mild | | | None | | | Test of difference in probability of treatment by severity | |
|---|---|---|---|---|---|---|---|---|---|---|---|---|---|---|
| | n | %[b] | (se) | n | %[b] | (se) | n | %[b] | (se) | n | %[b] | (se) | $\chi^2_3$ | (p-value) |
| **WHO: Regional Office for the Americas (AMRO)** | | | | | | | | | | | | | | |
| Colombia | 54 | 27.8 | (4.8) | 47 | 10.3 | (2.0) | 30 | 7.8 | (1.6) | 86 | 3.4 | (0.6) | 96.1* | (<0.001) |
| Mexico | 52 | 25.8 | (4.3) | 53 | 17.9 | (2.9) | 33 | 11.9 | (2.3) | 102 | 3.2 | (0.4) | 132.9* | (<0.001) |
| United States | 385 | 59.7 | (2.4) | 394 | 39.9 | (1.3) | 219 | 26.2 | (1.7) | 479 | 9.7 | (0.6) | 668.5* | (<0.001) |
| **WHO: Regional Office for Africa (AFRO)** | | | | | | | | | | | | | | |
| Nigeria | 8 | 21.3 | (11.9) | 6 | 13.8 | (7.4) | 14 | 10.0 | (3.0) | 29 | 1.0 | (0.3) | 27.7* | (<0.001) |
| South Africa | 45 | 26.2 | (3.6) | 66 | 26.6 | (3.9) | 67 | 23.1 | (3.2) | 497 | 13.4 | (0.9) | 41.0* | (<0.001) |
| **WHO: Regional Office for the Eastern Mediterranean (EMRO)** | | | | | | | | | | | | | | |
| Lebanon | 22 | 20.1 | (5.2) | 19 | 11.6 | (3.1) | 7 | 4.0 | (1.6) | 29 | 3.0 | (0.7) | 34.9* | (<0.001) |
| **WHO: Regional Office for Europe (EURO)** | | | | | | | | | | | | | | |
| Belgium | 46 | 62.1 | (9.2) | 30 | 38.4 | (8.3) | 13 | 12.7 | (4.6) | 98 | 6.8 | (1.1) | 227.1* | (<0.001) |
| France | 56 | 48.0 | (6.4) | 70 | 29.4 | (4.0) | 43 | 22.4 | (3.4) | 103 | 7.0 | (1.1) | 82.6* | (<0.001) |
| Germany | 30 | 40.6 | (8.9) | 39 | 23.9 | (4.7) | 27 | 20.5 | (5.2) | 87 | 5.9 | (0.9) | 54.5* | (<0.001) |
| Israel | 81 | 53.9 | (4.0) | 54 | 32.6 | (3.7) | 19 | 14.4 | (3.2) | 267 | 6.0 | (0.4) | 368.1* | (<0.001) |
| Italy | 29 | 51.6 | (6.5) | 38 | 25.9 | (4.2) | 21 | 17.8 | (4.5) | 53 | 2.2 | (0.4) | 192.7* | (<0.001) |
| Netherlands | 57 | 49.2 | (6.6) | 36 | 31.3 | (7.2) | 15 | 16.1 | (6.0) | 94 | 7.7 | (1.3) | 66.8* | (<0.001) |
| Spain | 79 | 58.7 | (4.9) | 93 | 37.4 | (5.0) | 35 | 17.3 | (4.3) | 168 | 3.9 | (0.5) | 446.1* | (<0.001) |
| Ukraine | 49 | 25.7 | (3.2) | 68 | 21.2 | (3.6) | 19 | 7.6 | (2.6) | 76 | 4.4 | (0.8) | 81.2* | (<0.001) |
| **WHO: Regional Office for the Western Pacific (WPRO)** | | | | | | | | | | | | | | |
| People's Republic of China | 5 | 11.0 | (5.4) | 11 | 23.5 | (10.9) | 3 | 1.7 | (1.2) | 55 | 2.9 | (0.6) | 16.1* | (0.001) |
| Japan[c] | 10 | 24.2 | (5.0) | 16 | 24.2 | (5.0) | 9 | 12.8 | (4.4) | 57 | 4.5 | (0.9) | 44.5*[c] | (<0.001) |
| New Zealand | 458 | 56.6 | (2.2) | 421 | 39.8 | (1.9) | 184 | 22.2 | (1.9) | 529 | 7.3 | (0.5) | 644.8* | (<0.001) |
| $\chi^2_{16}$[d] | 186.9* | (<0.001) | | 145.6* | (<0.001) | | 104.1* | (<0.001) | | 330.0* | (<0.001) | | | |

[a] Percentages are based on entire Part 2 samples.

[b] Percentages are based on respondents using any services within each level of severity.

[c] Severe and moderate cases were combined into one category for Japan and the percentage using services was displayed in both columns. The $\chi^2$ test was two degrees of freedom for this country.

[d] $\chi^2_{16}$ is from a model predicting any 12-month service use among respondents within each level of severity.

* Significant at the 0.05 level, two-sided test.

less service use in low- and middle-income than in high-income countries.

It is noteworthy that further analysis of the respondents who received treatment for emotional problems despite not meeting criteria for a DSM-IV/CIDI disorder showed that the vast majority of them either had a lifetime disorder that was in partial remission or a subthreshold syndrome that was associated with meaningful role impairment (Druss et al. 2007). These findings indicate that there is little evidence of inappropriate mental health treatment among people with no need.

## 4. MENTAL HEALTH SPECIALTY USE BY SEVERITY OF DISORDERS

Table 27.4 presents associations between disorder severity and use of the MHS sector among respondents receiving services. Statistical power was low in these analyses because of the small numbers of treated respondents. Nevertheless, significant relationships between severity and use of MHS sectors were found in only 6 of 17 countries. Even in those countries where such a relationship exists, meaningful proportions of mild and noncases consumed MHS services.

## 5. CONTINUITY AND ADEQUACY OF TREATMENTS

Among respondents initiating treatments, those receiving any follow-up care varied significantly between 70.2% in Germany and 94.5% in Italy (Table 27.5). Although the proportions were generally smaller in low- and middle-income countries than in high-income countries, there were notable exceptions to this pattern. Significant relationships between disorder severity and the probability of receiving follow-up care existed in only seven countries. As a result, receiving at least some follow-up care among treatment initiators was by no means universal among severe cases and was quite common among apparent noncases.

Among respondents using services, those who received treatments that were potentially minimally adequate varied significantly between 10.4% in Nigeria and 42.3% in France (Table 27.6). Proportions were generally smaller in lower-income countries, with the low rate in the United States (18.1%) being a notable exception. There were significant relationships between severity and receiving minimally adequate treatment in only five countries; as a result, substantial fractions of severe cases using services failed to receive minimally adequate treatment, whereas many noncases received substantial treatment resources.

## 6. DISCUSSION

We found that disorder severity is strongly related to treatment in all countries. This finding is consistent with two previous large-scale survey investigations of the relationship between severity and treatment (Kessler et al. 1997; Bijl et al. 2003). Correction for response bias would likely strengthen this relationship. The most reasonable interpretation is that demand for treatment is related to severity, presumably mediated by distress and impairment. A question could be raised as to whether this is merely a matter of demand or whether the treatment system is also more responsive to severe cases. Some indirect indication of system responsiveness can be gleaned from the findings that treatment intensity, as indicated by proportional treatment in the specialty sector and number of visits, is greater for serious than other treated cases in most WMH countries.

Despite this evidence of rationality in treatment resource allocation, we found disturbingly high levels of unmet need for mental health treatment worldwide, even among respondents with the most serious disorders. The situation appears to be direst in developing nations, with only small fractions of severe cases receiving any form of care in the prior year; however, even in developed Western nations, roughly half of severe cases receive no services. Most plausible study limitations (e.g., sample bias, response bias) would lead to underestimation of unmet need for treatment, which means that these estimates are almost certainly conservative.

Among the minority of cases receiving some services, even fewer are likely to have been effectively treated. Some received non–health-care

**Table 27.4.** Percentages using mental health specialty sectors among respondents using any services in the WMH surveys[a]

| Country | Severe | | | Moderate | | | Mild | | | None | | | Test of difference in probability of treatment by severity (1 or 3 df)[d] | |
|---|---|---|---|---|---|---|---|---|---|---|---|---|---|---|
| | n | %[b] | (se) | n | %[b] | (se) | n | %[b] | (se) | n | %[b] | (se) | χ² | (p-value) |
| **WHO: Regional Office for the Americas (AMRO)** | | | | | | | | | | | | | | |
| Colombia | 30 | 62.9 | (8.3) | 28 | 47.1 | (8.0) | 19 | 62.2 | (10.3) | 49 | 48.8 | (8.3) | 1.9 | (0.60) |
| Mexico | 26 | 60.3 | (8.0) | 30 | 59.1 | (6.8) | 15 | 51.0 | (11.2) | 50 | 50.4 | (7.0) | 1.1 | (0.78) |
| United States | 250 | 66.0 | (2.4) | 182 | 45.0 | (3.3) | 91 | 41.5 | (3.1) | 215 | 43.8 | (2.6) | 59.6* | (<0.001) |
| **WHO: Regional Office for Africa (AFRO)** | | | | | | | | | | | | | | |
| Nigeria | 1 | –[c] | –[c] | 0 | –[c] | –[c] | 3 | 9.5 | (4.5) | 1 | 9.5 | (4.5) | 1.4 | (0.24) |
| South Africa | 14 | 35.9 | (7.6) | 13 | 19.7 | (5.9) | 12 | 15.5 | (5.6) | 69 | 14.1 | (2.0) | 15.4* | (0.002) |
| **WHO: Regional Office for the Eastern Mediterranean (EMRO)** | | | | | | | | | | | | | | |
| Lebanon | 7 | 35.6 | (9.2) | 5 | 35.6 | (9.2) | 1 | 14.0 | (7.3) | 5 | 14.0 | (7.3) | 3.1 | (0.08) |
| **WHO: Regional Office for Europe (EURO)** | | | | | | | | | | | | | | |
| Belgium | 25 | 58.6 | (9.8) | 17 | 48.6 | (10.9) | 6 | –[c] | –[c] | 48 | 43.4 | (7.0) | 1.5 | (0.68) |
| France | 27 | 49.7 | (8.6) | 26 | 33.8 | (8.3) | 13 | 34.1 | (7.0) | 45 | 40.1 | (6.9) | 2.4 | (0.50) |
| Germany | 17 | 46.4 | (12.1) | 27 | 68.9 | (8.9) | 12 | –[c] | –[c] | 44 | 47.4 | (6.2) | 9.8* | (0.020) |
| Israel | 39 | 47.4 | (5.7) | 31 | 55.7 | (7.1) | 10 | –[c] | –[c] | 135 | 50.0 | (3.3) | 1.1 | (0.76) |
| Italy | 10 | –[c] | –[c] | 11 | 33.8 | (10.6) | 7 | –[c] | –[c] | 27 | 63.6 | (7.5) | 7.0 | (0.07) |
| Netherlands | 34 | 66.9 | (7.3) | 22 | 45.2 | (15.5) | 7 | –[c] | –[c] | 42 | 47.5 | (9.2) | 2.5 | (0.48) |
| Spain | 52 | 65.4 | (7.3) | 55 | 61.3 | (5.5) | 19 | 41.2 | (10.4) | 74 | 45.8 | (6.5) | 5.6 | (0.13) |
| Ukraine | 15 | 34.8 | (6.8) | 9 | 16.2 | (8.2) | 3 | –[c] | –[c] | 12 | 12.5 | (5.3) | 8.6* | (0.035) |
| **WHO: Regional Office for the Western Pacific (WPRO)** | | | | | | | | | | | | | | |
| People's Republic of China | 3 | –[c] | –[c] | 2 | –[c] | –[c] | 3 | 16.7 | (6.8) | 11 | 16.7 | (6.8) | 0.2 | (0.64) |
| Japan | 7 | –[c] | –[c] | 13 | –[c] | –[c] | 5 | 34.2 | (6.0) | 18 | 34.2 | (6.0) | 12.0* | (<0.001) |
| New Zealand | 232 | 57.4 | (2.9) | 140 | 34.7 | (3.4) | 49 | 26.3 | (4.3) | 164 | 32.0 | (2.9) | 63.1* | (<0.001) |

[a] Percentages are based on entire Part 2 samples.

[b] Percentages are those in any mental health treatment among respondents using any services within each level of severity.

[c] Percentages not reported if the number of respondents using any services in a level of severity <30.

[d] One degree of freedom $\chi^2$ tests were performed for Nigeria, Lebanon, Japan and People's Republic of China, where combined severe and moderate was compared against combined mild and none category. Three degree of freedom tests were performed for all other countries.

* Significant at the 0.05 level, two-sided test.

**Table 27.5.** Percentages receiving follow-up treatment[a] among respondents using services in the WMH surveys

| Country | Any severity | | | Severe | | | Moderate | | | Mild | | | None | | | Test of difference in probability of follow-up treatment by severity (1 or 3 df)[e] | |
|---|---|---|---|---|---|---|---|---|---|---|---|---|---|---|---|---|---|
| | n | %[b] | (se) | n | %[c] | (se) | n | %[c] | (se) | n | %[c] | (se) | n | %[c] | (se) | $\chi^2$ | (p-value) |
| **WHO: Regional Office for the Americas (AMRO)** | | | | | | | | | | | | | | | | | |
| Colombia | 158 | 72.0 | (4.3) | 49 | 92.6 | (3.5) | 31 | 73.1 | (7.9) | 20 | 61.7 | (11.3) | 58 | 63.6 | (7.9) | 12.3* | (0.006) |
| Mexico | 180 | 74.5 | (4.4) | 40 | 85.5 | (4.2) | 41 | 76.6 | (6.7) | 25 | 84.3 | (6.9) | 74 | 67.8 | (7.7) | 6.0 | (0.11) |
| United States | 1313 | 86.8 | (1.4) | 362 | 93.2 | (1.7) | 354 | 88.4 | (2.0) | 187 | 83.0 | (2.9) | 410 | 83.3 | (2.6) | 17.2* | (0.001) |
| **WHO: Regional Office for Africa (AFRO)** | | | | | | | | | | | | | | | | | |
| Nigeria | 47 | 76.3 | (8.7) | 6 | _[d] | _[d] | 6 | _[d] | _[d] | 13 | 74.6 | (9.2) | 22 | 74.6 | (9.2) | 0.4 | (0.51) |
| South Africa | 601 | 89.1 | (1.7) | 42 | 93.9 | (3.9) | 63 | 95.7 | (3.0) | 58 | 87.4 | (3.7) | 438 | 88.0 | (2.2) | 3.0 | (0.39) |
| **WHO: Regional Office for the Eastern Mediterranean (EMRO)** | | | | | | | | | | | | | | | | | |
| Lebanon | 62 | 78.9 | (6.9) | 17 | 84.1 | (4.4) | 15 | 84.1 | (4.4) | 7 | 75.7 | (10.2) | 23 | 75.7 | (10.2) | 0.8 | (0.37) |
| **WHO: Regional Office for Europe (EURO)** | | | | | | | | | | | | | | | | | |
| Belgium | 165 | 84.3 | (3.9) | 42 | 84.4 | (9.5) | 27 | 84.3 | (10.4) | 12 | _[d] | _[d] | 84 | 83.1 | (5.1) | 3.1 | (0.38) |
| France | 235 | 86.0 | (3.9) | 49 | 87.5 | (4.7) | 65 | 97.3 | (1.6) | 35 | 89.7 | (4.4) | 86 | 80.0 | (6.9) | 7.8 | (0.05) |
| Germany | 152 | 70.2 | (5.1) | 28 | 89.2 | (8.5) | 37 | 97.1 | (0.7) | 23 | _[d] | _[d] | 64 | 61.1 | (7.4) | 66.4* | (<0.001) |
| Israel | 364 | 86.1 | (1.8) | 73 | 90.7 | (3.2) | 48 | 89.2 | (4.2) | 17 | _[d] | _[d] | 226 | 83.6 | (2.4) | 3.3 | (0.34) |
| Italy | 129 | 94.5 | (1.5) | 28 | _[d] | _[d] | 34 | 93.1 | (3.7) | 19 | _[d] | _[d] | 48 | 94.4 | (2.4) | 1.3 | (0.73) |
| Netherlands | 183 | 85.9 | (4.3) | 53 | 96.4 | (2.1) | 35 | 98.9 | (1.2) | 15 | _[d] | _[d] | 80 | 78.5 | (7.2) | 10.0* | (0.007) |
| Spain | 341 | 88.8 | (2.6) | 73 | 95.3 | (1.9) | 86 | 92.6 | (3.0) | 33 | 90.8 | (6.2) | 149 | 84.7 | (4.7) | 5.8 | (0.12) |
| Ukraine | 167 | 79.1 | (3.8) | 44 | 92.3 | (3.6) | 51 | 82.3 | (4.5) | 14 | _[d] | _[d] | 58 | 71.8 | (7.0) | 12.5* | (0.006) |
| **WHO: Regional Office for the Western Pacific (WPRO)** | | | | | | | | | | | | | | | | | |
| People's Republic of China | 56 | 77.6 | (6.0) | 4 | _[d] | _[d] | 6 | _[d] | _[d] | 3 | 80.8 | (6.8) | 43 | 80.8 | (6.8) | 1.0 | (0.33) |
| Japan | 83 | 89.8 | (2.6) | 9 | _[d] | _[d] | 13 | _[d] | _[d] | 9 | 91.2 | (3.3) | 52 | 91.2 | (3.3) | 0.9 | (0.33) |
| New Zealand | 1394 | 85.7 | (1.3) | 421 | 92.5 | (1.4) | 368 | 88.7 | (1.8) | 151 | 83.5 | (3.2) | 454 | 81.0 | (2.8) | 15.1* | (0.002) |
| $\chi^2_{16}$[f] | | 67.1* (<0.001) | | | 25.4 (0.06) | | | 71.5* (<0.001) | | | 21.3 (0.13) | | | 47.9* (<0.001) | | | |

[a] Follow-up treatment was defined as receiving 2 or more visits to any service sector, or being in ongoing treatment at interview.

[b] Percentages are based on entire Part 2 samples.

[c] Percentages are those receiving follow-up treatment among those in treatment within each level of severity.

[d] Percentages not reported if the number of cases with any treatment in a level of severity <30.

[e] One degree of freedom chi-square tests were performed for Nigeria, Lebanon, Japan, and People's Republic of China, where combined severe and moderate was compared against combined mild and none category. Three degree of freedom tests were performed for all other countries.

[f] $\chi^2_{13}$ is from a model predicting follow-up treatment among respondents in each level of severity that used any 12-month services.

* Significant at the 0.05 level, two-sided test.

**Table 27.6.** Percentages receiving minimally adequate treatment[a] among respondents using services in the WMH surveys

| Country | Any severity | | | Severe | | | Moderate | | | Mild | | | None | | | Test of difference in probability of minimally adequate treatment by severity (1, 2, or 3 df)[e] | |
|---|---|---|---|---|---|---|---|---|---|---|---|---|---|---|---|---|---|
| | n | %[b] | (se) | n | %[c] | (se) | n | %[c] | (se) | n | %[c] | (se) | n | %[c] | (se) | $\chi^2$ | (p-value) |
| **WHO: Regional Office for the Americas (AMRO)** | | | | | | | | | | | | | | | | | |
| Colombia | 33 | 14.7 | (3.4) | 11 | 23.1 | (8.5) | 7 | 21.7 | (10.5) | 3 | 6.3 | (4.6) | 12 | 10.1 | (3.5) | 4.7 | (0.20) |
| Mexico | 42 | 15.2 | (2.7) | 8 | 11.3 | (4.5) | 13 | 28.6 | (6.3) | 6 | 19.8 | (5.8) | 15 | 11.3 | (4.0) | 10.5* | (0.014) |
| United States | 302 | 18.1 | (1.1) | 160 | 41.8 | (3.2) | 101 | 24.8 | (2.1) | 41 | 4.9 | (0.8) | – | – | – | 114.0* | (<0.001) |
| **WHO: Regional Office for Africa (AFRO)** | | | | | | | | | | | | | | | | | |
| Nigeria | 1 | 10.4 | (9.8) | 0 | –[d] | | 0 | –[d] | | 0 | 12.4 | (11.8) | 1 | 12.4 | (11.8) | | |
| South Africa | 0 | –[g] | | 0 | –[g] | | 0 | –[g] | | 0 | –[g] | | 0 | –[g] | | | |
| **WHO: Regional Office for the Eastern Mediterranean (EMRO)** | | | | | | | | | | | | | | | | | |
| Lebanon | 18 | 24.5 | (7.1) | 5 | 24.0 | (6.2) | 3 | 24.0 | (6.2) | 3 | 24.8 | (10.7) | 7 | 24.8 | (10.7) | 0.0 | (0.95) |
| **WHO: Regional Office for Europe (EURO)** | | | | | | | | | | | | | | | | | |
| Belgium | 78 | 33.6 | (5.2) | 23 | 42.5 | (8.5) | 12 | 35.5 | (12.6) | 5 | –[d] | | 38 | 29.4 | (6.2) | 1.7 | (0.63) |
| France | 113 | 42.3 | (5.4) | 29 | 57.9 | (8.5) | 28 | 36.5 | (6.6) | 15 | 41.5 | (9.7) | 41 | 40.2 | (8.3) | 3.4 | (0.34) |
| Germany | 91 | 42.0 | (6.1) | 21 | 67.3 | (10.7) | 21 | 53.3 | (8.4) | 14 | –[d] | | 35 | 35.4 | (8.8) | 6.1 | (0.11) |
| Israel | 148 | 35.1 | (2.5) | 28 | 34.4 | (5.4) | 21 | 40.3 | (6.8) | 6 | –[d] | | 93 | 34.3 | (3.1) | 0.7 | (0.87) |
| Italy | 45 | 33.0 | (5.1) | 12 | –[d] | | 11 | 35.7 | (9.4) | 6 | –[d] | | 16 | 29.9 | (7.4) | 3.5 | (0.32) |
| Netherlands | 98 | 34.4 | (5.0) | 37 | 65.7 | (9.2) | 19 | 34.1 | (10.2) | 10 | –[d] | | 32 | 21.9 | (5.2) | 23.2* | (<0.001) |
| Spain | 152 | 37.3 | (3.3) | 41 | 47.5 | (7.5) | 37 | 43.6 | (5.6) | 20 | 44.8 | (9.9) | 54 | 30.1 | (4.4) | 8.5* | (0.037) |
| Ukraine | 0 | –[g] | | 0 | –[g] | | 0 | –[g] | | 0 | –[g] | | 0 | –[g] | | | |
| **WHO: Regional Office for the Western Pacific (WPRO)** | | | | | | | | | | | | | | | | | |
| People's Republic of China | 19 | 24.1 | (7.0) | 0 | –[d] | | 3 | –[d] | | 2 | 20.1 | (5.9) | 14 | 20.1 | (5.9) | 0.8 | (0.36) |
| Japan | 35 | 31.8 | (6.8) | 6 | –[d] | | 6 | –[d] | | 5 | 27.9 | (7.0) | 18 | 27.9 | (7.0) | 4.4* | (0.037) |
| New Zealand | 0 | –[g] | | 0 | –[g] | | 0 | –[g] | | 0 | –[g] | | 0 | –[g] | | | |
| $\chi^2_{12}$[f] | 117.0* (<0.001) | | | 41.0* (<0.001) | | | 31.2* (0.002) | | | 25.9* (0.011) | | | 96.7* (<0.001) | | | | |

[a] Minimally adequate treatment was defined as receiving eight or more visits to any service sector, or four or more visits and at least one month of medication, or being in ongoing treatment at interview.

[b] Percentages based on entire Part 2 samples.

[c] Percentages are those receiving minimally adequate treatment among those in treatment within each level of severity.

[d] Percentages not reported if the number of cases with any treatment in a level of severity <30.

[e] The test was not performed for Nigeria because there was only one (unweighted) case with adequate treatment. One degree of freedom chi-square tests were performed for Lebanon, Japan, and People's Republic of China, where combined severe and moderate was compared against combined mild and none category. Two degree of freedom test was performed for the United States, where the mild and none categories were collapsed. Three degree of freedom tests were performed for all other countries.

[f] $\chi^2_{13}$ is from a model predicting minimally adequate treatment among respondents in each level of severity that used any 12-month services.

[g] The questions on pharmacoepidemiology were not asked in Ukraine, South Africa, or New Zealand.

* Significant at the 0.05 level, two-sided test.

services from CAM and human services sectors despite growing questions over the efficacy and safety of such treatments (Niggemann & Gruber 2003). In many countries, nearly one-quarter of those initiating treatments failed to receive any follow-up care. Consistent with prior studies, only a minority of treatments were observed to meet minimal standards for adequacy (Agency for Health Care Policy and Research 1993; Lehman & Steinwachs 1998; Wang et al. 2005; American Psychiatric Association 2006).

High levels of unmet need worldwide are not surprising, given the findings from the WHO Project Atlas that much lower mental health expenditure exists in virtually all countries around the world than is indicated by the estimated magnitude of the societal burden of mental illnesses (Saxena, Sharan & Saraceno 2003; Lopez et al. 2006). The generally greater unmet needs found in low- and middle-income countries are due to these nations spending often less than 1% of their already-low health-care budgets on mental health care, and relying heavily on out-of-pocket spending by a citizenry ill equipped to pay for the treatment of emotional problems (Saxena et al. 2003). Notable exceptions to this general rule of greater unmet need in developing than developed countries may be explained by variation in levels of investment in health care. For example, South Africa's high rates of treatment might reflect its greater spending (8.6% of gross domestic product [GDP]) on health care than any low- or middle-income country studied, and even some high-income countries; on the other hand, Japan's and Italy's smaller rates of treatment may reflect less spending (8.0% and 8.4% of GDP, respectively) than other high- and even some low- and middle-income countries (World Health Organization n.d.).

Additional research is needed to understand how the limited mental health resources available in most countries can be optimally allocated. The fact that the majority of people in treatment in most countries were subthreshold cases is striking in light of the fact that so many serious cases are untreated. This finding raises the possibility that the problem of unmet need for treatment among serious cases not merely is a matter of limited treatment resources but

also might be a matter of the misallocation of treatment resources. Another possibility, of course, is that the CIDI is less able to characterize the psychopathological syndromes in some countries than in others.

Assuming for the moment that misallocation is a problem, a major practical difficulty in revising allocation of treatment resources is that system barriers often constrain reallocation options. This is especially true in a decentralized system as in the United States. For example, there is no obvious mechanism by which constraining access to psychotherapy among middle-class women with mild mental disorders in the United States would result in an increase in treatment of low-income people with serious mental illness.

Another complexity in reorganizing allocation of treatment resources is that misallocation is partly due to differences in perceived need for treatment that are unrelated to objective severity, and to differences in access associated either with insurance coverage or with financial resources (Katz et al. 1997; Kessler et al. 1997; Bijl et al. 2003). A good illustration of this problem is found in a report comparing the mental health care delivery systems in the United States and Ontario, which showed that these two systems differ along exactly these lines. A higher proportion of people with serious mental illness were treated in Ontario than the United States because of lower constraints on access among people unable to pay in Ontario than in the United States, while a higher proportion of mild cases were treated in the United States than Ontario because of significantly higher perceived need for treatment among insured middle-class people with mild disorders in the United States. Although a number of structural possibilities exist to modify constraints on access, it is unclear how one would modify perceived need to align demand with true need for treatment.

A final complexity in reallocating treatment resources is that optimal allocation rules are not obvious. The simplistic strategy of not treating any mild disorders is almost certainly suboptimal (Narrow et al. 2002), as we know that many people with mild disorders, especially young people, go on to develop serious mental disorders (Kessler et al. 2003). To the extent that early intervention can prevent progression, early treatment of mild cases might be quite cost effective (Kessler & Price 1993). It is difficult to act on this insight, though, as we lack good information either about the characteristics of mild cases that predict risk of progression to more serious disorders or about the effectiveness of interventions for mild cases in preventing this progression. A new focus on the development and evaluation of secondary prevention programs for the early treatment of mild cases is needed to guide rationalization of treatment resource allocation.

Turning from the complexities or resource allocation to other issues raised by the WMH results, a clear observation is that the GM sector is for most countries the largest source of mental health services. This may reflect conscious attempts by policy makers to broaden access to services rather than concentrate resources on the relatively fewer patients with access to specialty sectors (Rosenheck et al. 1998). It may also reflect gatekeeping by primary care physicians employed in some countries to reserve specialty treatment for severe cases (Forrest 2003). Whatever the rationale, future research is need to ensure that mental health care received in the GM sector is not of low intensity and adequacy, as has been observed both in the WMH data and in other studies (Wang et al. 2005). In particular, the proportion of patients receiving at least minimally adequate treatment is generally lower among patients treated in the GM sector than in the MHS sector. This pattern suggests that efforts are needed to focus on mental health treatment quality improvement in primary care. Although the literature in this area is scant, especially in low-income countries, promising models exist that need to be evaluated more broadly (den Boer et al. 2005; Araya et al. 2006; Bass et al. 2006).

The results reported in the chapters of Part 2 concerning predictors of service use are generally consistent with prior research. The young may be more dependent on others than are the middle-aged, and therefore reluctant to access services (Morrissey-Kane & Prinz 1999); on the other hand, the elderly may avoid seeking mental health care because of the greater perceived stigma of mental disorders and treatments

among people in this age range (Leaf et al. 1985). Higher rates of treatment among women than among men may be explained by women's diminished perceptions of stigma and their greater abilities to translate nonspecific feelings of distress into conscious recognition of having a mental health problem (Kessler, Brown & Broman 1981).

Effects of greater income in predicting treatment were variable across the WMH surveys. In countries where positive associations exist, this may reflect the formidable influences of financial barriers on seeking treatment (Wells et al. 1986). On the other hand, the negative associations found in other countries may be explained by the fact that only the poor qualify for entitlements in some countries (Wells et al. 1986). More educated respondents may also have greater resources; alternatively, the higher treatment rates of well-educated respondents may reflect the fact that some modalities (e.g., psychotherapies) place an emphasis on knowledge and cognitive processes. The generally greater use of mental health services among those not married may indicate the power of relationship loss, strife, or social impairments as motivators for seeking treatment (Leaf et al. 1985).

These results have implications in several areas. First, alleviating the problem of widespread undertreatment will almost certainly require expansion of treatment resources and governmental as well as private means of financing mental health services. Second, there is also a pressing need to devise rational, transparent, and ethical allocation rules. In many countries it is not clear whether to focus resources on those with the greatest needs or on larger numbers with milder disorders (e.g., to prevent negative sequelae), whether to deliver services through primary versus specialty sectors or through inpatient versus community settings, and whether to provide mental health services on parity with those for general medical disorders (Callahan 1994). Ideally these questions would be answered through formal analyses of the burdens from illnesses and the cost-effectiveness of treatments (Gold et al. 1996). Unfortunately, rigorous data to compare disease burdens and weigh the costs and benefits of different regimens are largely lacking (Rosenheck et al. 1998). In the absence of such rational schemata, decisions regarding resource allocation are often made on the basis of simple cost-minimization and even attitudinal factors such as stigma and desire to punish persons perceived as being personally responsible for their problems (Corrigan & Watson 2003).

Finally, when rational, transparent, and ethical priorities have been set, policy makers need specific designs that they can implement to achieve their goals. Some techniques employed in managed care systems (e.g., gatekeeping, increased cost sharing, usage review, prior approval) could presumably be brought to bear on unnecessary use but not on underuse – in fact, they may worsen unmet needs for treatment. Furthermore, these elements from largely developed nations, such as the United States, may not be translatable to other countries and circumstances. The impacts of other policies, delivery system features, and means of financing that policy makers could implement are essentially unknown. For these reasons, collection of detailed data on the mental health policies, delivery system features, and means of financing mental health care in different countries is a promising area for future research (Saxena et al. 2003). When merged with WMH surveys on the use and adequacy of treatments, such combined data could shed light on the impacts of policies, delivery system, and financing features and help policy makers choose ones that achieve their desired goals (Mezzich 2003).

## REFERENCES

Agency for Health Care Policy and Research (1993). *Depression guideline panel, Volume 2: Treatment of major depression, clinical practice guideline, No 5.* Rockville, MD: U.S. Department of Health and Human Services, Public Health Service, Agency for Health Care Policy and Research.

American Psychiatric Association (2006). *Practice guidelines for treatment of psychiatric disorders: Compendium 2006.* Arlington, VA: American Psychiatric Association Press.

Araya, R., Flynn, T., Rojas, G., Fritsch, R. & Simon, G. (2006). Cost-effectiveness of a primary care treatment program for depression in low-income women in Santiago, Chile. *American Journal of Psychiatry*, 163, 1379–87.

Bass, J., Neugebauer, R., Clougherty, K. F., Verdeli, H., Wickramaratne, P., Ndogoni, L., Speelman, L., Weissman, M. & Bolton, P. (2006). Group interpersonal psychotherapy for depression in rural Uganda: 6-month outcomes: Randomised controlled trial. *British Journal of Psychiatry*, 188, 567–73.

Bijl, R. V., de Graaf, R., Hiripi, E., Kessler, R. C., Kohn, R., Offord, D. R., Üstün, T. B., Vicente, B., Vollebergh, W. A., Walters, E. E. & Wittchen, H.-U. (2003). The prevalence of treated and untreated mental disorders in five countries. *Health Affairs (Millwood)*, 22, 122–33.

Callahan, D. (1994). Setting mental health priorities: Problems and possibilities. *Milbank Quarterly*, 72, 451–70.

Corrigan, P. W. & Watson, A. C. (2003). Factors that explain how policy makers distribute resources to mental health services. *Psychiatric Services*, 54, 501–7.

den Boer, P. C., Wiersma, D., Russo, S. & van den Bosch, R. J. (2005). Paraprofessionals for anxiety and depressive disorders. *Cochrane Database of Systematic Reviews*, 2, CD004688.

Druss, B. G., Wang, P. S., Sampson, N. A., Olfson, M., Pincus, H. A., Wells, K. B. & Kessler, R. C. (2007). Understanding mental health treatment in persons without mental diagnoses: Results from the National Comorbidity Survey Replication. *Archives of General Psychiatry*, 64, 1196–203.

Forrest, C. B. (2003). Primary care in the United States: Primary care gatekeeping and referrals: Effective filter or failed experiment? *British Medical Journal*, 326, 692–5.

Gold, M. R., Siegel, J. E., Russell, L. B. & Weinstein, M. C., eds. (1996). *Cost-effectiveness in health and medicine.* New York: Oxford University Press.

Hu, T. W. (2003). Financing global mental health services and the role of WHO. *Journal of Mental Health Policy and Economics*, 6, 135–43.

Katz, S. J., Kessler, R. C., Frank, R. G., Leaf, P. & Lin, E. (1997). Mental health care use, morbidity, and socioeconomic status in the United States and Ontario. *Inquiry*, 34, 38–49.

Kessler, R. C., Brown, R. L. & Broman, C. L. (1981). Sex differences in psychiatric help-seeking: Evidence from four large-scale surveys. *Journal of Health and Social Behavior*, 22, 49–64.

Kessler, R. C., Frank, R. G., Edlund, M., Katz, S. J., Lin, E. & Leaf, P. (1997). Differences in the use of psychiatric outpatient services between the United States and Ontario. *New England Journal of Medicine*, 336, 551–7.

Kessler, R. C., Merikangas, K. R., Berglund, P., Eaton, W. W., Koretz, D. S. & Walters, E. E. (2003). Mild disorders should not be eliminated from the

DSM-V. *Archives of General Psychiatry*, 60, 1117–22.

Kessler, R. C. & Price, R. H. (1993). Primary prevention of secondary disorders: A proposal and agenda. *American Journal of Community Psychology*, 21, 607–33.

Leaf, P. J., Livingston, M. M., Tischler, G. L., Weissman, M. M., Holzer, C. E., III & Myers, J. K. (1985). Contact with health professionals for the treatment of psychiatric and emotional problems. *Medical Care*, 23, 1322–37.

Lehman, A. F. & Steinwachs, D. M. (1998). Translating research into practice: Schizophrenia patient outcomes research team (PORT) treatment recommendations. *Schizophrenia Bulletin*, 24, 1–10.

Lopez, A. D., Mathers, C. D., Ezzati, M., Jamison, D. T. & Murray, C. J. L., eds. (2006). *Global burden of disease and risk factors*. New York: Oxford University Press/World Bank.

Mechanic, D. (1994). Establishing mental health priorities. *Milbank Quarterly*, 72, 501–14.

Mezzich, J. E. (2003). From financial analysis to policy development in mental health care: The need for broader conceptual models and partnerships. *Journal of Mental Health Policy and Economics*, 6, 149–50.

Morrissey-Kane, E. & Prinz, R. J. (1999). Engagement in child and adolescent treatment: The role of parental cognitions and attributions. *Clinical Child and Family Psychology Review*, 2, 183–98.

Narrow, W. E., Rae, D. S., Robins, L. N. & Regier, D. A. (2002). Revised prevalence estimates of mental disorders in the United States: Using a clinical significance criterion to reconcile 2 surveys' estimates. *Archives of General Psychiatry*, 59, 115–23.

Niggemann, B. & Gruber, C. (2003). Side-effects of complementary and alternative medicine. *Allergy*, 58, 707–16.

Rosenheck, R., Armstrong, M., Callahan, D., Dea, R., Del Vecchio, P., Flynn, L., Fox, R. C., Goldman, H. H., Horvath, T. & Munoz, R. (1998). Obligation to the least well off in setting mental health service priorities: A consensus statement. *Psychiatric Services*, 49, 1273–4, 1290.

Saxena, S., Sharan, P. & Saraceno, B. (2003). Budget and financing of mental health services: Baseline information on 89 countries from WHO's Project Atlas. *Journal of Mental Health Policy and Economics*, 6, 135–43.

Tasman, A., Kay, J. & Lieberman, J. A., eds. (2003). *Psychiatry*, 2d ed. Chichester, UK: John Wiley & Sons.

Wang, P. S., Lane, M., Olfson, M., Pincus, H. A., Wells, K. B. & Kessler, R. C. (2005). Twelve-month use of mental health services in the United States: Results from the National Comorbidity Survey Replication. *Archives of General Psychiatry*, 62, 629–40.

Wells, K. B., Manning, W. G., Duan, N., Newhouse, J. P. & Ware, J. E., Jr. (1986). Sociodemographic factors and the use of outpatient mental health services. *Medical Care*, 24, 75–85.

World Health Organization (n.d.). Project Atlas: Resources for mental health and neurological disorders. Available at http://www.who.int/globalatlas/dataQuery/default.asp (accessed July 6, 2006).

# PART FOUR

# Conclusions

# 28 Overview and Future Directions for the World Mental Health Survey Initiative

RONALD C. KESSLER AND T. BEDIRHAN ÜSTÜN

## I. INTRODUCTION

As noted in the introduction to this volume, although surveys of mental disorders have been carried out since the end of World War II (Leighton 1959; Langner & Michael 1963; Hagnell 1966), cross-national comparisons were hampered by inconsistencies in diagnostic methods. This situation changed in the 1980s with the development of the Diagnostic Interview Schedule (DIS), the first psychiatric diagnostic interview designed for use by lay interviewers (Bland, Orn & Newman 1988). The DIS was a landmark development in psychiatric epidemiology, as it led to a series of parallel surveys being carried out in a number of countries (Bland et al. 1988; Hwu, Yeh & Cheng 1989; Lépine et al. 1989; Robins & Regier 1991), the comparative analysis of these surveys by a cross-national group of collaborators who were precursors to the collaborators in the WMH Survey Initiative (Weissman et al. 1994; Weissman et al. 1996; Weissman et al. 1996; Weissman et al. 1997), and the subsequent development of the CIDI from the DIS along with the implementation of many CIDI surveys throughout the world (Kessler et al. 1994; Andrade et al. 2002; Bijl et al. 1998; Caraveo, Martinez & Rivera 1998; Kylyc 1998; Vega et al. 1998; Wittchen et al. 1998; Andrade et al. 2002).

The DIS and CIDI surveys that came before the WMH surveys generated results similar to those in the WMH in finding that even though prevalence varied widely across countries, more than one-third of respondents typically met criteria for a lifetime CIDI disorder (WHO International Consortium in Psychiatric Epidemiology 2000) and that most mental disorders were untreated (Alegria et al. 2000; Bijl et al. 2003). Before concluding, though, that unmet need for treatment of mental disorders is a major problem, it is important to recognize that many mental disorders are mild and transitory. This was not a focus of the initial DIS or CIDI surveys, which were designed to estimate prevalence rather than severity. However, the high prevalence estimates in these surveys raised concerns that even the richest of countries could not afford to treat all people with a mental disorder (Regier et al. 1998; Regier et al. 2000). Motivated by this concern, secondary analyses of some of these early surveys developed post hoc measures of severity and carried out analyses using these measures that concluded that up to half of 12-month mental disorders were mild and that treatment was consistently correlated with severity and disability (Narrow et al. 2002; Bijl et al. 2003). These analyses also found that between one-third and two-thirds of even the most serious cases in these surveys received no treatment, which raised concerns about unmet need for treatment.

These results were limited because they were based on superficial and arbitrary measures of disorder severity, with no distinction made between the true severity of the disorder and its other daily life consequences (i.e., disability). In addition, the analyses of treatment were hampered by the fact that they did not include measures of treatment adequacy. Furthermore, as there was no coordination across the different surveys and as the DIS and CIDI did not include a standard set of questions about treatment, valid cross-national comparisons of treatment could not be made. Finally, these surveys were carried out mostly in developed countries, which made it impossible to examine the extent to which results were similar in all parts of the world and in countries that differ in level of development. The WMH surveys were designed, in part, to address these limitations (Kessler 1999) by expanding the CIDI in ways described in Chapter 4 to include detailed questions about disorder severity, disability, and treatment (Kessler & Üstün 2004) and by carrying out surveys that made use of this expanded instrument in a wider range of countries than in the past.

In many cases, the WMH surveys produced the first general population data on the descriptive epidemiology of mental disorders ever available to the policy makers in participating countries. In other cases, the WMH surveys produced updates on data that was available from previous surveys. Even in the latter cases, though, the WMH surveys went well beyond earlier surveys in a number of respects. The most notable of these advances for purposes of the current volume involve the two areas noted in the previous paragraph, the assessment of disorder severity and the assessment treatment adequacy, although there are many other advances that will be highlighted in future WMH volumes. We found that mental (and substance) disorders are commonly occurring, that similar forms of symptomatology exist in different cultures, and that the correlates of mental disorders (e.g., the high female-to-male ratio for anxiety and mood disorders and the high male-to-female ratio for impulse-control and substance disorders) are remarkably similar across countries. We also found that, despite the fact that mental disorders are often quite disabling, they are undertreated in all the countries studied.

Because of the importance of the advances of the WMH surveys in studying disorder severity and treatment adequacy for the results reported in this volume, a few words are in order about these topics before discussing other issues.

## 2. DISORDER SEVERITY

Disorder severity is important to assess in light of the consistent evidence in previous epidemiological surveys that mental disorders are highly prevalent and often untreated. Before concluding from these results that unmet need for treatment of mental disorders is a major problem, we have to recognize that many mental disorders are mild, self-limiting, and possibly not in need of treatment. As noted in Chapter 26, disorder severity was not a primary focus of attention in previous DIS or CIDI surveys. Prevalence was the main focus in these surveys. However, the high prevalence estimates in these surveys raised concerns that even the richest of countries could not afford to treat all the people with a mental disorder (Regier et al. 1998; Regier et al. 2000). This question, in turn, led to more focused questions regarding the extent to which probability of treatment is related to severity and the extent to which seriously disabling disorders are treated.

The WMH surveys are distinct from earlier DIS-CIDI surveys in that they include explicit measures of disorder severity, which we examined in this volume, and separate measures of disability. The latter include both a global measure of functioning, the WHO Disability Assessment Schedule (WHO-DAS) (World Health Organization 1998), and a disorder-specific measure of disability, the Sheehan Disability Scales (SDS) (Leon et al. 1997). Only the SDS was used in the current volume, but the WHO-DAS will be the focus of considerable attention in the next volume in the WMH series. As we have seen in this volume, only a minority of the mental disorders assessed in the WMH surveys were seriously disabling. This finding speaks to the widespread skepticism of critics regarding the high prevalence estimates found in previous DIS-CIDI surveys, which have variously been criticized as due to errors in the interview schedules used in these surveys (Regier et al. 1998) or to the over inclusiveness of the DSM or ICD diagnostic systems (Narrow et al. 2002). The clinically validated WMH results make it quite clear that ICD and DSM disorders assessed in the WMH surveys are, in fact, highly prevalent in the general population of many countries and that the high overall prevalence estimates are not due to errors in the CIDI classification rules. The fact that only a minority of these cases are seriously disabling means that the proportion of the general population that has a seriously disabling mental disorder is much smaller than the proportion that meets criteria for any ICD or DSM disorder. This comparatively low prevalence of seriously disabling ICD or DSM disorders will presumably be seen by critics as more plausible than the very high undifferentiated (with respect to severity) prevalence estimates reported in previous DIS-CIDI surveys.

The question still remains, of course, whether the ICD or DSM systems are overinclusive; that is, whether the many people who are classified as having a mildly or moderately disabling ICD or DSM mental disorder should be classified as meeting ICD or DSM criteria rather than as being subthreshold cases. An argument has been made that the ICD or DSM criteria should be tightened to exclude mild cases based on the fact that the number of people with mild disorders is so large that it is impossible to treat all of them even in resource-rich countries (Narrow et al. 2002). The results reported in this volume provide no information that evaluates this recommendation. However, an earlier report from a ten-year follow-up of an earlier CIDI survey carried out by the WMH collaborators in the United States shed some light on this matter by showing that the mild cases in the baseline survey had significantly elevated risk (compared to baseline noncases) of becoming serious cases at follow-up, as indicated by high risk of such outcomes as suicide attempt, hospitalization for a mental illness, and psychiatric disability (Kessler et al. 2003).

It is interesting to note that the recommendation to narrow the ICD and DSM criteria is coming at a time when various professional associations in other branches of medicine are calling for a lowering of the thresholds for a number of common disease definitions. Examples include new proposed definitions of hypercholesterolemia (Downs et al. 1998), diabetes (Expert Committee on the Diagnosis and Classification of Diabetes Mellitus 1997), and hypertension (Joint National Committee on Prevention, Detection, Evaluation, and Treatment of High Blood Pressure 1997). These recommendations are based not only on prospective

epidemiological findings, which show that people who are borderline subthreshold cases of these disorders have significantly elevated odds of severe adverse outcomes, but more important on long-term treatment effectiveness trials that document a positive cost–benefit ratio in providing early treatment to these subthreshold cases (Medical Research Council Working Party 1985; Downs et al. 1998).

It is noteworthy that the 2.0–4.0 elevated odds ratios (ORs) of subsequent serious adverse mental health outcomes associated with mild baseline ICD or DSM mental disorders are compare in magnitude to the ORs found in prospective studies of the subthreshold cases that are now being proposed for inclusion in expanded definitions of the physical disorders mentioned previously. The missing element in the case of the mild mental disorders is evidence about the benefit of early treatment. We do not know about the effectiveness of early intervention with mild mental disorders in preventing progression to more severe disorders. We do know from the WMH survey results reported in this volume that some mental disorders (most notably the phobias, separation anxiety disorder, and a number of impulse-control disorders) typically start at much earlier ages than other disorders. We also know from epidemiological surveys including the WMH series that these early-onset disorders are often highly comorbid with later-onset mental disorders and that seriously disabling disorders are concentrated within these comorbid disorder clusters (Kessler et al. 1994; Kessler et al. 2005). We have also seen in this volume, though, that delays in obtaining initial treatment for early-onset disorders are typically substantial. As a result, little is known about the long-term effects of early intervention with early-onset mild cases, which makes it impossible to appeal to evidence regarding the cost–benefit ratio of such treatment to make a decision about whether to retain mild disorders in the DSM and ICD systems.

As a response to the question of whether mild disorders should be excluded from the classification systems, our preference is that mild disorders be retained, at least provisionally, in the revised DSM and ICD systems, both of which are currently under review for revision within the next five years (Kupfer, First & Regier 2002; Üstün 2002). We say this for two reasons. First, rather than reify our ignorance about the effectiveness of treating mild disorders by ruling such disorders out of consideration in the revised DSM and ICD diagnostic schemes, we believe that we should highlight the importance of this knowledge gap by retaining mild cases in the definition of disorders and by encouraging research aimed at developing and evaluating the effectiveness of the early treatment of mild cases.

The reader might wonder why this same kind of research could not be carried out while defining currently classified mild cases as subthreshold in the revised DSM and ICD systems. It could. Indeed, as noted earlier, this is exactly what was done in research on subthreshold diabetes, hypertension, and hypercholesterolemia. However, we have a second reason for preferring to retain mild cases in the revised systems that addresses this issue: that the WMH data show clearly that mild DSM disorders are as clinically significant as the vast majority of the cases of chronic physical disorders that are currently included in the ICD system. The evidence on this point is one focus of the second WMH volume in this series, so we will only briefly sketch out the evidence here. As noted in Chapter 4, the WMH surveys included assessments of the prevalence and disabilities associated with commonly occurring chronic physical conditions such as asthma, cancer, diabetes, and heart disease. The WHO-DAS and SDS, the same scales used to assess the disability associated with mental disorders, were also used to assess the disability associated with these physical disorders. Systematic comparisons showed that the disability associated with the mental disorders was consistently higher, on average, than the disability associated with the physical disorders (Ormel et al. 2008). This was true despite the fact that a high proportion of the mental disorders were rated mild according to the WMH classification scheme. Even these ostensibly mild disorders, as it turned out, were more disabling than many chronic physical disorders. In light of this fact, in conjunction with the considerations

raised in the preceding few paragraphs, we can see no rationale for excluding mild mental disorders from the revised DSM and ICD systems.

## 3. TREATMENT ADEQUACY

The treatment of mental disorders is much more variable than the treatment of most physical disorders. This is true because many different kinds of professionals purport to provide help with emotional problems, including physician mental health professionals (psychiatrists, behavioral neurologists), other medical doctors (who largely prescribe medications but in some cases also offer brief psychotherapies), a wide range of nonphysician mental health professionals (psychologists, marriage and family counselors, psychiatric social workers), a similarly wide range of human services professionals (most notably, human services caseworkers and religious/spiritual advisors), and complementary-alternative medical (CAM) providers (e.g., traditional medicine providers, acupuncturists, self-help group moderators, and other CAM providers). Previous psychiatric epidemiological research, while attempting to capture the variety of such treatment modalities, did not collect the depth of information captured in the WMH surveys.

We collected this detailed information to assess not only the presence of treatment but also the adequacy of treatment in relation to published treatment guidelines. We were in the fortunate position of having well-developed practice guidelines for the treatment of mental disorders that have been developed over more than a decade. Our analyses of these data in conjunction with the larger analysis of treatment in the WMH data documented a disturbing fact: that unmet need for treatment of mental disorders has three components, each of which is of substantial importance. The first is that only a minority of people with mental disorders in the countries we studied were receiving treatment for these disorders. The second is that even though a high proportion of chronic cases eventually obtain treatment, substantial delays in obtaining treatment are pervasive. The third is that the quality of treatment, once it is provided, is often inadequate in relation to published treatment guidelines.

The third of these components is a critical one that, with a few notable exceptions (Wells et al. 1999; Wang, Berglund & Kessler 2000), has not been the subject of sustained attention in previous psychiatric epidemiological studies. It is critical because the other components are to some extent irrelevant unless available treatment meets at least minimum standards of adequacy. Indeed, a recent analysis of the cost-effectiveness of screening for depression in primary care concluded that repeated screening of this sort would not currently be cost-effective because of the generally low quality of depression treatment in primary care (Valenstein et al. 2001). The recommendation was that treatment quality-improvement initiatives needed to be developed and implemented before it would be cost-effective to launch interventions aimed at increasing depression detection and treatment. Although this cost-effectiveness analysis was carried out with a focus on depression treatment in the United States, the WMH results show clearly that a similar problem of low treatment quality exists in all the countries considered for all other commonly occurring mental disorders.

What can be done to correct this problem of low treatment quality? This is a question that goes beyond the scope of the current volume to address. However, it is important to note that the WMH surveys include some information that can be used to address at least one part of this question: the part that concerns patient compliance with treatment regimens. This will be a focus of a future WMH volume on mental health service use. A further analysis of the WMH data shows that one part of the problem of inadequate treatment is due to the fact that many patients receive too few visits (Wang et al. 2007). The problem of too few visits, in turn, is due in part to a high proportion of patients dropping out of treatment before a full course of treatment is completed (Edlund et al. 2002). Little is known about patterns and determinants of treatment dropout because virtually all studies of dropout have been carried out in single treatment settings, which makes it impossible to study

structural determinants that are, for the most part, constants within single settings (Baekeland & Lundwall 1975; Bischoff & Sprenkle 1993; Ogrodniczuk, Joyce & Piper 2005). However, this problem can be addressed in the WMH surveys, as information is available about treatment dropout from representative samples of patients across all treatment settings. This makes it possible to study structural determinants of treatment dropout. In addition, the WMH surveys collected information about reasons for dropout from patients who quit treatment for emotional problems, which can be used to expand on the small literature on this topic (e.g., Todd, Deane & Bragdon 2003; Roe et al. 2006). Data analysis of these WMH data on reasons for treatment termination is currently underway.

## 4. LIMITATIONS OF THE INITIAL WMH WORK

It is to be expected that an undertaking as large and ambitious as the WMH Survey Initiative has limitations. Although a number of criticisms that point to these limitations have been raised in print by commentators (Weich & Araya 2004; Jorm 2006; Henderson & Andrews in press), it might be useful to consider all the major criticisms and limitations and discuss our approach to handling them in future WMH work. On the basis of the published criticisms and our own reflections, we believe that three sets of issues warrant discussion. The first concerns a question of whether descriptive surveys like the WMH surveys are needed in light of the existence of many previous surveys of a similar sort. The second concerns a series of issues concerning WMH survey design limitations. The third concerns the possibility of measurement error in the assessment of mental disorders in the WMH surveys.

### 4.1. Do We Need More Descriptive Surveys?

A criticism raised by some commentators is that the descriptive epidemiology of mental disorders is by now so well known in its broad fundamentals (i.e., that the prevalence of mental disorders is high and the proportion of cases in treatment is low) that we do not need to carry out any more expensive, large-scale epidemiological surveys to document yet again these same predictable results (Weich & Araya 2004). We agree that many of the basic patterns documented in this volume would be considered predictable by experts in the field. However, we want to point out that the WMH surveys collected much more than basic descriptive data, even though the results reported in this first volume of WMH results focus on basic descriptive data.

Furthermore, we disagree with the view that the WMH surveys would be unnecessary even if they did nothing more than collect basic descriptive data. As noted earlier, the WMH surveys in many of the participating countries are the first representative general population surveys ever carried out to assess the prevalence and correlates of mental disorders. Predictable though the results of these surveys might have been considered prior to the time the surveys were launched, there is great political value in obtaining data on the societal burden of mental disorders in countries where such data did not previously exist, even when the results of the survey are similar to the results found in previous surveys in other countries. In addition, the WMH design allows us to carry out a number of additional analyses that have never before been undertaken. For example, the separate assessments of diagnosis, severity, and disability in the WMH surveys allows us to compare the severity and disability of mental disorders with those of commonly occurring physical illnesses and to document the relative share of global disease burden due to mental disorders. This work on global disease burden, which is currently under way, will be the first-ever empirical research to implement broad-based, comparative general population–based studies of comparative disease-related disability.

An additional value of the WMH surveys is that they are helping to build a new generation of psychiatric epidemiologists who are capable of carrying out future community epidemiological studies that can be used to monitor trends in the prevalence and correlates of mental disorders over time and evaluate the effects of various policy interventions. There is an old adage that says,

"You can't manage what you can't measure." The WMH surveys have made it possible to measure mental illness, disability (i.e., role functioning) related to mental illness, treatment, quality of treatment, and barriers to treatment. The WMH data allow policy makers in each participating country empirically to confirm or disconfirm prior conceptions about the magnitude of the problem of mental illness in their populations. The data can be used to help target future interventions along the lines described in the previous section of this chapter. The WMH data represent a baseline against which the effects of future policy interventions can be evaluated in trend studies. These are also very valuable uses that exist irrespective of whether the basic descriptive findings in the surveys are the same or different from those in previous surveys.

## 4.2. Design Considerations

The WMH surveys are cross-sectional rather than longitudinal. They are naturalistic rather than experimental. As a result, the surveys are in a much better position to study point-in-time descriptive patterns than to study change over time or to make inferences about cause and effect. Yet policymakers often pose questions that require inferences to be made about change over time or about cause and effect relationships. We are aware of these limitations of the WMH design.

The cross-sectional design feature can, of course, be expanded over time to include either trend surveys (i.e., repeat surveys with new samples designed to monitor aggregate population changes), panel surveys (i.e., repeat surveys with the same respondents designed to study within-person change), or mixed panel-trend surveys. Several of the WMH surveys are being expanded in one or more of these ways. The longitudinal data collected in these new surveys will be of great value in allowing inferences to be made about change based on prospective data rather than based on the retrospective data collected in the baseline WMH surveys.

Even in the absence of these prospective data, we have not hesitated to make inferences about some aspects of change from the retrospective reports collected in the baseline WMH surveys, although we tried to be clear in presenting these results that they were provisional because they were based on retrospective reports. This was most notable in our analyses of retrospective reports about lifetime prevalence, age of onset, and delays in initial attempts to seek treatment for incident mental disorders. As we described when presenting those results, special question-wording sequences and memory-priming probes were developed in an effort to facilitate complete recall and accurate dating. We are aware, of course, that errors in reporting inevitably remained despite our use of these strategies, but we felt that it was preferable to have access to provisional information based on these retrospective reports than no data at all about temporal patterns.

We should note that quite different decisions have been made by some other psychiatric epidemiologists who have carried out surveys of mental disorders that focused exclusively on current disorders to avoid retrospective recall bias (Jenkins et al. 1997). Our view is that this approach is unnecessarily restrictive in light of the fact that this design does not actually remove retrospective recall. Methodological studies of memory failure show that recall bias of some sort exists in reports that ask about recall periods as short as a single day (Stone & Broderick 2007; Shiffman in press). The recall period typically used in psychiatric epidemiological studies that focus on "current" disorders, in comparison, is the past 30 days, which is long enough that some recall failure certainly exists in these reports. This recall failure will, of course, be lower over a 30-day recall period than over a one-year recall period or a lifetime recall period for the same kind of question, but as the ability to recall generally decreases with the length of the recall interval, it is important to recognize that the kinds of questions one can reasonably ask vary as a function of length of recall.

We would not ask a respondent to tell us, for example, how many days he was sad in his entire life, although we might ask this question about the past 30 days. However, we could reasonably ask about lifetime hospitalization for depression or about lifetime suicide attempts on the basis of the assumption that these events would be sufficiently vividly recalled that we could collect accurate information about them even over a very long recall period. In light of this fact, it strikes us as needlessly restrictive to limit all questions in psychiatric epidemiological surveys to experiences that occurred in the recent past. Our approach has consequently been to include rather detailed recall questions in the WMH surveys that ask about experiences that happened in the past 30 days, less detailed questions about experiences that occurred in the past 12 months, and even less detailed questions about experiences that occurred over the entire lifetime. All the while, we have been alert to the fact that recall bias can exist in all these reports and that prospective data collection could be used to assess the magnitude of this bias. This strikes us as a more intelligent approach than merely declaring all information about experiences that occurred more than 30 days ago beyond the realm of accurate reporting.

The issue of how to deal with the fact that policy makers often ask questions about cause-effect relationships in a naturalistic study is a separate matter. It is clear that causal inferences cannot be made legitimately from naturalistic data. As a result, we are careful in interpreting WMH data to be clear that the associations we examine are descriptive rather than causal. There were few, if any, statements in the current volume that interpreted associations in causal terms. At the same time, provisional causal interpretations of naturalistic data can sometimes be useful in promoting thought experiments that subsequently lead to more definitive intervention studies. We speculated previously, for example, about the possibility that early intervention to treat mild disorders might lead to the prevention of secondary disorders or to a reduction in the lifetime persistence and/or severity of primary disorders. We did this with an explicit recognition that the WMH data provide no basis for making causal inferences about the associations found between temporally primary and secondary comorbid conditions.

This is a legitimate use of descriptive epidemiological data, as such provisional analyses can lead to targeted experimental interventions. For example, an earlier wave of the WMH survey in the United States observed that major depression is associated with an enormous amount of disability in work performance among employed people with versus without depression (Kessler & Frank 1997), which raised the question of whether expanded efforts to detect and treat workers with depression would have a positive return on investment from the employer's perspective (Kessler et al. 1999). Based on the results of simulations that made use of epidemiological data to generate estimates of prevalence and impact on work performance and treatment trial data to generate estimates of the likely impact of expanded treatment on work performance (Wang et al. 2006), the decision was made to launch a major experimental workplace treatment effectiveness trial, the results of which showed that expanded outreach-treatment of depressed workers can, in fact, have a positive return on investment from the employer's perspective (Wang et al. 2007).

It is also important to mention for the sake of completeness that descriptive epidemiological data can sometimes be used to make provisional causal inferences by making use of information about quasi-experimental variation in exposure to some presumed causal factor (e.g., Lu 1999; Brookhart et al. 2007). For example, if information available outside of the survey makes researchers aware of geographic variation in access to a particular medication, possibly as a result of a formulary rule that is imposed in one area or another, this information can sometimes be used to help make provisional estimates of the causal effect of the medication on outcomes measured in the survey (Schneeweiss et al. 2007). However, this approach goes well beyond the types of analysis presented in the current volume and will only seldom be used in future WMH analyses.

## 4.3. The Accuracy of Disorder Assessments

An important potential limitation is that the reliability and validity of the diagnoses made in the WMH surveys might vary considerably across countries. Although, as shown in Chapter 6, good

concordance was observed between diagnoses made with the CIDI and those from blind clinical reinterviews in the countries that participated in the coordinated WMH CIDI clinical reappraisal studies, these studies were all conducted in developed Western countries. It is possible that the accuracy of CIDI diagnoses is worse in other countries because the concepts and phrases used to describe mental syndromes are less consonant with cultural concepts in those countries than in developed Western countries, because absence of a tradition of free speech and anonymous public-opinion surveying leads to greater reluctance to admit emotional problems than in developed Western countries, or because survey implementation (e.g., translation, field quality-control monitoring, data cleaning, and coding) was carried out with less care than in other countries. The fact that the countries with the lowest disorder prevalence estimates had the highest proportions of treated respondents classified as subthreshold cases is indirectly consistent with this possibility that prevalence was underestimated in these countries. Clinical reappraisal studies are currently under way in both developed and less developed WMH countries in all major regions of the world to evaluate the issue of cross-national differences in CIDI diagnostic validity and to make revisions to the WMH study protocol in ways appropriate to address the problems found in these methodological studies.

A deeper version of the same concern is that the DSM and ICD diagnostic systems might not make sense is some countries; that the structure of psychopathology might be fundamentally different in some parts of the world, so that some disorders, such as depression or panic disorder, might not exist or that culture-bound syndromes are in common occurrence and are not adequately characterized by the diagnoses included in the CIDI. We want to be clear in noting, though, that the first part of this deep concern, involving the absence of various ICD or DSM anxiety or mood or impulse-control disorders in one or more of the WMH countries, has not been voiced by any of the culturally competent mental health professionals who are either collaborating in the WMH Survey Initiative or who are consulting with WMH collaborators in their countries. Interesting questions have been raised, in comparison, about cross-national differences in the expression of various disorders, such as variation in social anxiety disorder in Asian countries, where a high value is placed on not offending others (Choy et al. 2007). Variations of this sort are captured in the CIDI. Questions have also been raised, furthermore, about some variants on the disorders assessed in the CIDI that might constitute culture-related specific syndromes (Tseng 2006) that are not captured in the core version of the CIDI. Efforts are under way to expand the CIDI to capture these syndromes in future expansions of the WMH surveys.

## 5. FUTURE DIRECTIONS

The WMH collaborative is continuing to grow both in breadth and depth. In terms of breadth, the past year saw the addition of national surveys in Bulgaria, India, Iraq, and Romania and a regional survey in Brazil to the WMH series, and several additional countries are discussing the possibility of launching WMH surveys in the coming year. In terms of depth, the WMH collaborators in the past year have expanded their joint studies beyond the basic descriptive domain considered in the current volume to a wide range of other areas of investigation. The WMH work groups are currently studying a number of important sociodemographic correlates of mental disorders from a cross-national perspective, most notably gender differences and social class differences.

Other work groups are studying substantive risk factors for mental disorders, including, most notably, childhood adversities and traumatic life experiences. Another WMH work group is studying barriers to treatment, including patterns and determinants of treatment dropout. A large work group is considering the many societal costs of mental disorders, including the effects of early-onset disorders on life-course trajectories (e.g., reduced educational attainment, early marriage, marital instability, low earnings) and the effects of recent disorders on current role functioning.

A related line of analysis is examining health preferences and utilities associated with mental and physical disorders in terms of standard measures of visual analogue, time trade-off, and willingness to pay (Gyrd-Hansen 2005; Torrance 2006). It is expected that this body of evidence, together with the findings about the descriptive epidemiology of mental disorders, will contribute importantly to the comprehensive empirical update of global burden of disease estimates currently being undertaken by the WHO and IHME (Murray et al. 2007).

An area of special interest to many WMH collaborators is comorbidity between mental disorders and physical disorders (Demyttenaere et al. 2007; Ormel et al. 2007; Scott et al. 2007; Gureje et al. 2008; Scott et al. 2008). This will be the focus of the second volume in this series. Another area of special interest is the information collected in the WMH surveys on the epidemiology of suicidal ideation, plans, gestures, and attempts (Borges et al. 2006; Nock & Kessler 2006; Nock et al. 2008). This will be the focus of the third volume in this series. The results of these and other WMH studies published in journal articles can be found on the WMH Web site at http://www.hcp.med.harvard.edu, while expanded presentations of the results will be presented in the annual volumes in this series.

## REFERENCES

Alegria, M., Bijl, R. V., Lin, E., Walters, E. E. & Kessler, R. C. (2000). Income differences in persons seeking outpatient treatment for mental disorders: A comparison of the U.S. with Ontario and The Netherlands. *Archives of General Psychiatry*, 57, 383–91.

Andrade, L., Walters, E. E., Gentil, V. & Laurenti, R. (2002). Prevalence of ICD-10 mental disorders in a catchment area in the city of São Paulo, Brazil. *Social Psychiatry and Psychiatric Epidemiology*, 37, 316–25.

Baekeland, F. & Lundwall, L. (1975). Dropping out of treatment: A critical review. *Psychological Bulletin*, 82, 738–83.

Bijl, R. V., de Graaf, R., Hiripi, E., Kessler, R. C., Kohn, R., Offord, D. R., Üstün, T. B., Vicente, B., Vollebergh, W. A., Walters, E. E. & Wittchen, H.-U. (2003). The prevalence of treated and untreated mental disorders in five countries. *Health Affairs (Millwood)*, 22, 122–33.

Bijl, R. V., van Zessen, G., Ravelli, A., de Rijk, C. & Langendoen, Y. (1998). The Netherlands Mental Health Survey and Incidence Study (NEMESIS): Objectives and design. *Social Psychiatry and Psychiatric Epidemiology*, 33, 581–6.

Bischoff, R. J. & Sprenkle, D. H. (1993). Dropping out of marriage and family therapy: A critical review of research. *Family Process*, 32, 353–75.

Bland, R. C., Orn, H. & Newman, S. C. (1988). Lifetime prevalence of psychiatric disorders in Edmonton. *Acta Psychiatrica Scandinavica*, 77 (suppl. 338), 24–32.

Borges, G., Angst, J., Nock, M. K., Ruscio, A. M., Walters, E. E. & Kessler, R. C. (2006). A risk index for 12-month suicide attempts in the National Comorbidity Survey Replication (NCS-R). *Psychological Medicine*, 36, 1747–57.

Brookhart, M. A., Rassen, J. A., Wang, P. S., Dormuth, C., Mogun, H. & Schneeweiss, S. (2007). Evaluating the validity of an instrumental variable study of neuroleptics: Can between-physician differences in prescribing patterns be used to estimate treatment effects? *Medical Care*, 45, S116–22.

Caraveo, J., Martinez, J. & Rivera, B. (1998). A model for epidemiological studies on mental health and psychiatric morbidity. *Salud Mental*, 21, 48–57.

Choy, Y., Schneier, F. R., Heimberg, R. G., Oh, K. S. & Liebowitz, M. R. (in press). Features of the offensive subtype of Taijin-Kyofu-Sho in U.S. and Korean patients with DSM-IV social anxiety disorder. *Depression Anxiety*.

Demyttenaere, K., Bruffaerts, R., Lee, S., Posada-Villa, J., Kovess, V., Angermeyer, M. C., Levinson, D., de Girolamo, G., Nakane, H., Mneimneh, Z., Lara, C., de Graaf, R., Scott, K. M., Gureje, O., Stein, D. J., Haro, J. M., Bromet, E. J., Kessler, R. C., Alonso, J. & Von Korff, M. (2007). Mental disorders among persons with chronic back or neck pain: Results from the World Mental Health Surveys. *Pain*, 129, 332–42.

Downs, J. R., Clearfield, M., Weis, S., Whitney, E., Shapiro, D. R., Beere, P. A., Langendorfer, A., Stein, E. A., Kruyer, W. & Gotto, A. M., Jr. (1998). Primary prevention of acute coronary events with lovastatin in men and women with average cholesterol levels: Results of AFCAPS/TexCAPS, Air Force/Texas Coronary Atherosclerosis Prevention Study. *Journal of the American Medical Association*, 279, 1615–22.

Edlund, M. J., Wang, P. S., Berglund, P. A., Katz, S. J., Lin, E. & Kessler, R. C. (2002). Dropping out of mental health treatment: Patterns and predictors among epidemiological survey respondents in the United States and Ontario. *American Journal of Psychiatry*, 159, 845–51.

Expert Committee on the Diagnosis and Classification of Diabetes Mellitus (1997). Report of the Expert Committee on the Diagnosis and Classification of Diabetes Mellitus. *Diabetes Care*, 20, 1183–97.

Gureje, O., Von Korff, M., Kola, L., Demyttenaere, K., He, Y., Posada-Villa, J., Lepine, J. P., Angermeyer, M. C., Levinson, D., de Girolamo, G., Iwata, N., Karam, A., Luiz Guimaraes Borges, G., de Graaf, R., Browne, M. O., Stein, D. J., Haro, J. M., Bromet, E. J., Kessler, R. C. & Alonso, J. (2008). The relation between multiple pains and mental disorders: Results from the World Mental Health Surveys. *Pain*, 135, 82–91.

Gyrd-Hansen, D. (2005). Willingness to pay for a QALY: Theoretical and methodological issues. *Pharmacoeconomics*, 23, 423–32.

Hagnell, O. (1966). *A prospective study of the incidence of mental disorder: A study based on 24,000 person years of the incidence of mental disorders in a Swedish population together with an evaluation of the aetiological significance of medical, social, and personality factors.* Lund, Sweden: Svenska Bokforlaget.

Henderson, S. & Andrews, G. (in press). The yield from national surveys of mental health. *International Psychiatry*.

Hwu, H. G., Yeh, E. K. & Cheng, L. Y. (1989). Prevalence of psychiatric disorders in Taiwan defined by the Chinese diagnostic interview schedule. *Acta Psychiatrica Scandinavica*, 79, 136–47.

Jenkins, R., Bebbington, P., Brugha, T., Farrell, M., Gill, B., Lewis, G., Meltzer, H. & Petticrew, M. (1997). The National Psychiatric Morbidity surveys of Great Britain: Strategy and methods. *Psychological Medicine*, 27, 765–74.

Joint National Committee on Prevention, Detection, Evaluation, and Treatment of High Blood Pressure, (1997). The sixth report of the Joint National Committee on Prevention, Detection, Evaluation, and Treatment of High Blood Pressure. *Archives of Internal Medicine*, 157, 2413–46.

Jorm, A. F. (2006). National surveys of mental disorders: Are they researching scientific facts or constructing useful myths? *Australian and New Zealand Journal of Psychiatry*, 40, 830–4.

Kessler, R. C. (1999). The World Health Organization International Consortium in Psychiatric Epidemiology (ICPE): Initial work and future directions – the NAPE lecture 1998. *Acta Psychiatrica Scandinavica*, 99, 2–9.

Kessler, R. C., Barber, C., Birnbaum, H. G., Frank, R. G., Greenberg, P. E., Rose, R. M., Simon, G. E. & Wang, P. (1999). Depression in the workplace: Effects on short-term disability. *Health Affairs (Millwood)*, 18, 163–71.

Kessler, R. C., Chiu, W. T., Demler, O., Merikangas, K. R. & Walters, E. E. (2005). Prevalence, severity, and comorbidity of 12-month DSM-IV disorders in the National Comorbidity Survey Replication. *Archives of General Psychiatry*, 62, 617–27.

Kessler, R. C. & Frank, R. G. (1997). The impact of psychiatric disorders on work loss days. *Psychological Medicine*, 27, 861–73.

Kessler, R. C., McGonagle, K. A., Zhao, S., Nelson, C. B., Hughes, M., Eshleman, S., Wittchen, H.-U. & Kendler, K. S. (1994). Lifetime and 12-month prevalence of DSM-III-R psychiatric disorders in the United States: Results from the National Comorbidity Survey. *Archives of General Psychiatry*, 51, 8–19.

Kessler, R. C., Merikangas, K. R., Berglund, P., Eaton, W. W., Koretz, D. S. & Walters, E. E. (2003). Mild disorders should not be eliminated from the DSM-V. *Archives of General Psychiatry*, 60, 1117–22.

Kessler, R. C. & Üstün, T. B. (2004). The World Mental Health (WMH) Survey Initiative Version of the World Health Organization (WHO) Composite International Diagnostic Interview (CIDI). *International Journal of Methods in Psychiatric Research*, 13, 93–121.

Kupfer, D. J., First, M. B. & Regier, D. A. (2002). *A research agenda for DSM-IV*. Washington, DC: American Psychiatric Press.

Kylyc, C. (1998). *Mental health profile of Turkey: Main report*. Ankara, Turkey: Ministry of Health Publications.

Langner, T. S. & Michael, S. T. (1963). *Life stress and mental health: The Midtown Manhattan Study*. London: Collier-Macmillan.

Leighton, A. H. (1959). *My name is Legion.* The Stirling County Study, Vol. 1. New York: Basic Books.

Leon, A. C., Olfson, M., Portera, L., Farber, L. & Sheehan, D. V. (1997). Assessing psychiatric impairment in primary care with the Sheehan Disability Scale. *International Journal of Psychiatry in Medicine*, 27, 93–105.

Lépine, J.-P., Lellouch, J., Lovell, A., Teherani, M., Ha, C., Verdier-Taillefer, M. G. & Rambourg, N. (1989). Anxiety and depressive disorders in a French population: Methodology and preliminary results. *Psychiatry and Psychobiology*, 4, 267–74.

Lu, M. (1999). The productivity of mental health care: An instrumental variable approach. *Journal of Mental Health Policy and Economics*, 2, 59–71.

Medical Research Council Working Party (1985). MRC trial of treatment of mild hypertension: Principal results. *British Medical Journal*, 291, 97–104.

Murray, C. J., Lopez, A. D., Black, R., Mathers, C. D., Shibuya, K., Ezzati, M., Salomon, J. A., Michaud, C. M., Walker, N. & Vos, T. (2007). Global burden of disease 2005: Call for collaborators. *Lancet*, 370, 109–10.

Narrow, W. E., Rae, D. S., Robins, L. N. & Regier, D. A. (2002). Revised prevalence estimates of mental disorders in the United States: Using a clinical significance criterion to reconcile 2 surveys' estimates. *Archives of General Psychiatry*, 59, 115–23.

Nock, M. K., Borges, G., Bromet, E. J., Alonso, J., Angermeyer, M., Beautrais, A., Bruffaerts, R., Chiu, W. T., de Girolamo, G., Gluzman, S., de Graaf, R., Gureje, O., Haro, J. M., Huang, Y., Karam, E., Kessler, R. C., Lépine, J.-P., Levinson, D., Medina-Mora, M. E., Ono, Y., Posada-Villa, J. & Williams, D. (2008). Cross-national prevalence and risk factors for suicide ideation, plans, and attempts. *British Journal of Psychiatry*, 192, 98–105.

Nock, M. K. & Kessler, R. C. (2006). Prevalence of and risk factors for suicide attempts versus suicide gestures: Analysis of the National Comorbidity Survey. *Journal of Abnormal Psychology*, 115, 616–23.

Ogrodniczuk, J. S., Joyce, A. S. & Piper, W. E. (2005). Strategies for reducing patient-initiated premature termination of psychotherapy. *Harvard Review of Psychiatry*, 13, 57–70.

Ormel, J., Petukhova, M., Chatterji, S., Aguilar-Gaxiola, S., Alonso, J., Angermeyer, M. C., Bromet, E. J., Burger, H., Demyttenaere, K., de Girolamo, G., Haro, J. M., Karam, E., Kawakami, N., Lepine, J. P., Medina-Mora, M. E., Posada-Villa, J., Scott, K., Üstün, T. B., Von Korff, M., Williams, D., Zhang, M. & Kessler, R. C. (2008). Disability and treatment of specific mental and physical disorders across the world: Results from the WHO World Mental Health Surveys. *British Journal of Psychiatry*, 192, 368–75.

Ormel, J., Von Korff, M., Burger, H., Scott, K., Demyttenaere, K., Huang, Y. Q., Posada-Villa, J., Lépine, J.-P., Angermeyer, M. C., Levinson, D., de Girolamo, G., Kawakami, N., Karam, E., Medina-Mora, M. E., Gureje, O., Williams, D., Haro, J. M., Bromet, E. J., Alonso, J. & Kessler, R. (2007). Mental disorders among persons with heart disease: Results from World Mental Health surveys. *General Hospital Psychiatry*, 29, 325–34.

Regier, D. A., Kaelber, C. T., Rae, D. S., Farmer, M. E., Knauper, B., Kessler, R. C. & Norquist, G. S. (1998). Limitations of diagnostic criteria and assessment instruments for mental disorders: Implications for research and policy. *Archives of General Psychiatry*, 55, 109–15.

Regier, D. A., Narrow, W. E., Rupp, A., Rae, D. S. & Kaelber, C. T. (2000). The epidemiology of mental disorder treatment need: Community estimates of medical necessity. In *Unmet need in psychiatry*, ed. G. Andrews & S. Henderson, pp. 41–58. Cambridge, UK: Cambridge University Press.

Robins, L. N. & Regier, D. A. (1991). *Psychiatric disorders in America: The Epidemiologic Catchment Area Study.* New York: Free Press.

Roe, D., Dekel, R., Harel, G. & Fennig, S. (2006). Clients' reasons for terminating psychotherapy: A quantitative and qualitative inquiry. *Psychology and Psychotherapy*, 79, 529–38.

Schneeweiss, S., Setoguchi, S., Brookhart, A., Dormuth, C. & Wang, P. S. (2007). Risk of death associated with the use of conventional versus atypical antipsychotic drugs among elderly patients. *Canadian Medical Association Journal*, 176, 627–32.

Scott, K. M., Bruffaerts, R., Simon, G. E., Alonso, J., Angermeyer, M., de Girolamo, G., Demyttenaere, K., Gasquet, I., Haro, J. M., Karam, E., Kessler, R. C., Levinson, D., Medina Mora, M. E., Oakley-Browne, M. A., Ormel, J., Villa, J. P., Uda, H. & Von Korff, M. (2008). Obesity and mental disorders in the general population: Results from the world mental health surveys. *International Journal of Obesity*, 32, 192–200.

Scott, K. M., Von Korff, M., Ormel, J., Zhang, M. Y., Bruffaerts, R., Alonso, J., Kessler, R. C., Tachimori, H., Karam, E., Levinson, D., Bromet, E. J., Posada-Villa, J., Gasquet, I., Angermeyer, M. C., Borges, G., de Girolamo, G., Herman, A. & Haro, J. M. (2007). Mental disorders among adults with asthma: Results from the World Mental Health Survey. *General Hospital Psychiatry*, 29, 123–33.

Shiffman, S. (2008). Ecological momentary assessment. *Annual Review of Clinical Psychology*, 4, 1–32.

Stone, A. A. & Broderick, J. E. (2007). Real-time data collection for pain: Appraisal and current status. *Pain Medicine*, 8 (suppl. 3), S85–93.

Todd, D. M., Deane, F. P. & Bragdon, R. A. (2003). Client and therapist reasons for termination: A conceptualization and preliminary validation. *Journal of Clinical Psychology*, 59, 133–47.

Torrance, G. W. (2006). Utility measurement in healthcare: The things I never got to. *Pharmacoeconomics*, 24, 1069–78.

Tseng, W. S. (2006). From peculiar psychiatric disorders through culture-bound syndromes to culture-related specific syndromes. *Transcultural Psychiatry*, 43, 554–76.

Üstün, T. B. (2002). WHO perspectives on international classification. *Psychopathology*, 35, 62–6.

Valenstein, M., Vijan, S., Zeber, J. E., Boehm, K. & Buttar, A. (2001). The cost-utility of screening for depression in primary care. *Annals of Internal Medicine*, 134, 345–60.

Vega, W. A., Kolody, B., Aguilar-Gaxiola, S., Alderete, E., Catalano, R. & Caraveo-Anduaga, J. (1998). Lifetime prevalence of DSM-III-R psychiatric disorders among urban and rural Mexican Americans in California. *Archives of General Psychiatry*, 55, 771–8.

Wang, P. S., Aguilar-Gaxiola, S., Alonso, J., Angermeyer, M. C., Borges, G., Bromet, E. J., Bruffaerts, R., de Girolamo, G., de Graaf, R., Gureje, O., Haro, J. M., Karam, E. G., Kessler, R. C., Kovess, V., Lane, M. C., Lee, S., Levinson, D., Ono, Y., Petukhova, M., Posada-Villa, J., Seedat, S. & Wells, J. E. (2007). Use of mental health services for anxiety, mood, and substance disorders in 17 countries in the WHO world mental health surveys. *Lancet*, 370, 841–50.

Wang, P. S., Berglund, P. & Kessler, R. C. (2000). Recent care of common mental disorders in the United States: Prevalence and conformance with evidence-based recommendations. *Journal of General Internal Medicine*, 15, 284–92.

Wang, P. S., Patrick, A., Avorn, J., Azocar, F., Ludman, E., McCulloch, J., Simon, G. & Kessler, R. (2006). The costs and benefits of enhanced depression care to employers. *Archives of General Psychiatry*, 63, 1345–53.

Wang, P. S., Simon, G. E., Avorn, J., Azocar, F., Ludman, E. J., McCulloch, J., Petukhova, M. Z. & Kessler, R. C. (2007). Telephone screening, outreach, and care management for depressed workers and impact on clinical and work productivity outcomes: A randomized controlled trial. *Journal of the American Medical Association*, 298, 1401–11.

Weich, S. & Araya, R. (2004). International and regional variation in the prevalence of common mental disorders: Do we need more surveys? *British Journal of Psychiatry*, 184, 289–90.

Weissman, M. M., Bland, R. C., Canino, G. J., Faravelli, C., Greenwald, S., Hwu, H. G., Joyce, P. R., Karam, E. G., Lee, C. K., Lellouch, J., Lépine, J.-P., Newman, S. C., Rubio-Stipec, M., Wells, J. E., Wickramaratne, P. J., Wittchen, H. & Yeh, E. K. (1996). Cross-national epidemiology of major depression and bipolar disorder. *Journal of the American Medical Association*, 276, 293–9.

Weissman, M. M., Bland, R. C., Canino, G. J., Faravelli, C., Greenwald, S., Hwu, H. G., Joyce, P. R., Karam, E. G., Lee, C. K., J., L., Lépine, J.-P., Newman, S. C., Oakley-Browne, M. A., Rubio-Stipec, M., Wells, J. E., Wickramaratne, P. J., Wittchen, H.-U. & Yeh, E. K. (1997). The cross-national epidemiology of panic disorder. *Archives of General Psychiatry*, 54, 305–9.

Weissman, M. M., Bland, R. C., Canino, G. J., Greenwald, S., Hwu, H. G., Lee, C. K., Newman, S. C., Oakley-Browne, M. A., Rubio-Stipec, M., Wickramaratne, P. J. et al. (1994). The cross national epidemiology of obsessive compulsive disorder: The Cross National Collaborative Group. *Journal of Clinical Psychiatry*, 55 (suppl.), 5–10.

Weissman, M. M., Bland, R. C., Canino, G. J., Greenwald, S., Lee, C. K., Newman, S. C., Rubio-Stipec, M. & Wickramaratne, P. J. (1996). The cross-national epidemiology of social phobia: a preliminary report. *International Clinical Psychopharmacology*, 11 (suppl 3), 9–14.

Wells, K. B., Schoenbaum, M., Unutzer, J., Lagomasino, I. T. & Rubenstein, L. V. (1999). Quality of care for primary care patients with depression in managed care. *Archives of Family Medicine*, 8, 529–36.

WHO International Consortium in Psychiatric Epidemiology (2000). Cross-national comparisons of the prevalences and correlates of mental disorders. *Bulletin of the World Health Organization*, 78, 413–26.

Wittchen, H.-U., Perkonigg, A., Lachner, G. & Nelson, C. B. (1998). Early developmental stages of psychopathology study (EDSP): Objectives and design. *European Addiction Research*, 4, 18–27.

World Health Organization (WHO) (1998). *The WHO Disability Assessment Schedule II (WHODAS II)*. Geneva: World Health Organization.

# Index